The Oncogene Handbook

The Oncogene Handbook

Robin Hesketh

Department of Biochemistry, University of Cambridge, UK

Academic Press

Harcourt Brace & Company, Publishers

London   San Diego   New York   Boston
Sydney   Tokyo   Toronto

ACADEMIC PRESS LIMITED
24–28 Oval Road
LONDON NW1 7DX

United States Edition published by
ACADEMIC PRESS INC.
San Diego, CA 92101

Typeset by Photo·graphics, Honiton, UK
Printed and bound in Great Britain at the Bath Press, Avon

Contents

Foreword

This book has its origin in my accumulated notes for research and undergraduate lectures over the past 15 years. The realization of the potential usefulness of this material as the basis for a book providing a comprehensive summary of what is known about the genes that cause cancer came almost coincidentally with the awareness that any further delay would probably render such a project impossible, so fast is the oncofacts mountain rising. The organization of the book is intended to make a vast amount of data readily accessible so that, for example, individual genes can be rapidly located and specific features of a gene and its product(s) and their involvement in human and animal cancers determined. It is hoped that the layout and content will make the book of use to research workers, to clinicians and to final year undergraduates with a particular interest in the molecular and cellular biology of cancer.

I started to write *The Oncogene Handbook* at the behest of Dr Susan King of Academic Press (now of Wiley Liss) to whom I am deeply grateful. Without her seemingly limitless enthusiasm this book probably never would have been started and most certainly would not have been finished. I am also indebted beyond words to many colleagues who made the time to offer detailed comments and suggestions about individual sections of the book and also to provide general encouragement. Any omissions or errors that remain are entirely my responsibility. I trust that they will accept that simply listing their names in alphabetical order in no way diminishes my gratitude.

Mariano Barbacid (Bristol-Myers Squibb Pharmaceutical Research Institute, Princeton), Jenny Barna (Department of Biochemistry, University of Cambridge), Glenn Begley (Walter and Eliza Hall Institute of Medical Research, Melbourne), Anton Berns (The Netherlands Cancer Institute, Amsterdam), Carmen Birchmeier (Max Delbruck Laboratory, Cologne), David Brown (Department of Virology, University of Cambridge), Franco Calabi (Royal Postgraduate Medical School, Hammersmith Hospital), Sara Courtneidge (European Molecular Biology Laboratory, Heidelberg), Albert Deisseroth (MD Anderson Cancer Center, Houston), Christine Dozier (Institut Pasteur, Lille), Robert Eisenman (Fred Hutchinson Cancer Research Center, Seattle), David Ellar (Department of Biochemistry, University of Cambridge), Christine Ellis (Chester Beatty, London), Jon Frampton (European Molecular Biology Laboratory, Heidelberg), Jacques Ghysdael (Institut Curie, Orsay), Thomas Gilmore (Biology Department, Boston University), Thomas Graf (European Molecular Biology Laboratory, Heidelberg), Michele Grieco (Dipartmento di Biologia e Patologia Cellulare e Moleculare, University of Naples), Gerard Grosveld (Erasmus Universiteit, Rotterdam), Hidesaburo Hanafusa (The Rockefeller University, New

York), Michael Hanley (Department of Biological Chemistry, University of California, Davis), Nick Hastie (MRC Human Genetics Unit, Edinburgh), Mike Hayman (State University of New York), Tim Hunt (Imperial Cancer Research Fund Laboratories, London), Tony Hunter (The Salk Institute), Tony Kouzarides (Department of Pathology, University of Cambridge), Jo Milner (Department of Biology, University of York), Tony Minson (Department of Virology, University of Cambridge), Kiyoshi Miyagawa (Genetics Division, National Cancer Center Research Institute, Tokyo), Jenny Morton (Department of Pharmacology, University of Cambridge), Jane Osbourn (Department of Clinical Pharmacology, Addenbrooke's Hospital, Cambridge), Richard Osborne (Department of Clinical Oncology, Addenbrooke's Hospital, Cambridge), Tony Pawson (Samuel Lunenfeld Research Institute, Mount Sinai Hospital, Toronto), Angel Pellicer (Department of Pathology, New York University Medical Center), Gordon Peters (Imperial Cancer Research Fund, London), Jo Peters (MRC Radiobiology Unit, Didcot), Alastair Reith (Ludwig Institute for Cancer Research, London), Keith Robbins (National Institutes of Health, Bethesda), Richard Roden (National Institutes of Health, Bethesda), Larry Rohrschneider (Fred Hutchinson Cancer Research Center, Seattle), Craig Sorenson (Oncogene Science, New York), Stephen Storm (National Cancer Institute, Frederick, Maryland), Pramod Sutrave (National Cancer Institute, Frederick, Maryland), Julie Turner (Department of Pathology, University of Cambridge), George Vande Woude (Frederick Cancer Research and Development Center, Frederick, Maryland), Bjorn Vennstrom (Department of Molecular Biology, Karolinska Institute, Stockholm).

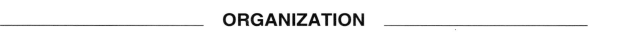

ORGANIZATION

Chapter 1 is a summary of the principal developments in our understanding of oncogenes together with a discussion of patterns of oncogene expression in human tumours and a summary of the present position with regard to gene therapy for human cancers. Chapter 2 comprises tables of the major categories of oncogenes. The properties of oncogenes that do not have individual sections in Chapter 3 are given in supplements to the tables. In Chapter 3 a constant format has been adopted for each of the sections on individual oncogenes: this includes the following headings (with minor modifications for individual genes as appropriate): Related genes, Cross-species homology, Transformation (Man, Animals, *In vitro*, Transgenic animals), Table of properties (Nucleotides, Chromosomes, Exons, mRNA size and half-life, Amino acids, Mass, Protein half-life), Cellular location, Tissue location, Protein function, Structure of the proviral genome, Gene structure, Protein structure, Protein sequences, Databank file names and accession numbers, References (divided into Reviews and Papers). In the tables of properties the nucleotide entries indicate the size of the genomic region (human unless otherwise indicated) over which the cellular gene is distributed and the size of the complete viral genome.

The Appendix contains summaries of the life-cycle of retroviruses and the genomic structure of HIV and HTLV-1.

The references quoted at the end of each section are intended to cover the major facts and to cite the most recent work, thereby enabling readers to acquaint themselves rapidly with a particular area. They are not intended to form a comprehensive list and I trust that authors of the many publications that are not specifically referenced, even though their findings have contributed to the overall picture, will appreciate the rationale upon which selection has been made.

NOMENCLATURE

The recommendations of the International Standing Committee on human gene nomenclature have been followed. Thus human genes are written in italicized capitals and their gene products in non-italicized capitals (Shows *et al.*, 1987). For genes of other species the nomenclature recommended for murine genes has been followed. Thus genes are italicized with an initial capital letter followed by lower case letters; the corresponding proteins are written in non-italicized capitals (Lyon, 1984). In the individual genes sections (Chapter 3) the official designation is given at the outset but for some genes the commonly accepted form is used thereafter to avoid confusion. These are human *ABL1* (*ABL*), the avian *Erb* genes (*ErbA* and *ErbB*), *EPHT* (*EPH*), *TP53*/TP53 (*P53*/p53) and *RB1* (*RB*) and *NME1*/*NME2* (*NM23*). The designations *TGFβ* and *TCRβ* are also used, rather than *TGFB* and *TCRB*.

Viral oncogenes are referred to by trivial names of the form v-*onc* (e.g. v-*myc*), that is, the names do not imply target cell specificity of function (Coffin *et al.*, 1981). The gene products are referred to as "p", "gp", "pp", or "P" followed by the molecular mass in kilodaltons to indicate "protein", "glycoprotein", "phosphoprotein", or "polyprotein" respectively, and an additional italicized superscript indicates the gene encoding the protein (e.g. pp60$^{v\text{-}src}$). Hyphenated superscripts denote polyproteins derived from two genes (e.g. gp180$^{gag\text{-}src}$). Suffixes -a, -b, etc. denote inserts in the same virus that can code for different proteins via distinct RNAs (e.g. *Erba*, *Erbb*).

References

Coffin, J.M., Varmus, H.E., Bishop, M.J., Essex, M., Hardy, W.D., Martin, G.S., Rosenberg, N.E., Scolnick, E.M., Weinberg, R.A. and Vogt, P.K. (1981). Proposal for naming host cell-derived inserts in retrovirus genomes. J. Virol., 40, 953–957.

Lyon, M.F. (1984). Rules for nomenclature of genes, chromosome anomalies and inbred strains. Mouse News Letter, 72, 2–27.

Shows, T.B., McAlpine, P.J., Boucheix, C., Collins, F.S., Conneally, P.M., Frezac, J., Gershowitz, H., Goodfellow, P.N., Hall, J.G., Issitt, P., Jones, C.A., Knowles, B.B., Lewis, M., McKusick, V.A., Meisler, M., Morton, N.E., Rubinstein, P., Schanfield, M.S., Schmickel, R.D., Skolnick, M.H., Spence, M.A., Sutherland, G.R., Traver, M., Van Cong, N. and Willard, H.F. (1987). Guidelines for human gene nomenclature. Cytogenet. Cell Genetics, 46, 11–28.

CHAPTER 1

Introduction

Oncogenes are genes that cause cancer and it now seems probable that the interplay between the products of oncogenes is central to the development of most, if not all, cancer cells. Cellular oncogenes may be defined as genes which, under certain conditions, are capable of inducing neoplastic transformation of cells. They arise by the modification through mutation or change in the control of expression of a normal gene, referred to as a "proto-oncogene" (Huebner and Todaro, 1969; Bishop *et al.*, 1979). In addition to oncogenes that arise within the cellular genome, some viruses carry oncogenes as part of their genome. The oncogenes of tumorigenic RNA viruses are derived from cellular proto-oncogenes; such viruses can rapidly transform cells in culture and induce tumours in appropriate host animals. Some DNA viruses are also tumorigenic but in general there is no evidence that the oncogenes they express are derived from cellular progenitors.

The notion that cancer might be caused by genetic abnormality originated in the early nineteenth century when it was noted that predisposition to cancer seemed to run in families (Norris, 1820). By the turn of the century it had been observed using light microscopy that the chromosomes from cancer cells were frequently of abnormal length or shape when compared with those from normal cells (Hansemann, 1890; Boveri, 1914). More recent discoveries suggest that there is a connection between susceptibility to cancer and an impaired ability of cells to repair damaged DNA and that the mutagenic potential of a substance is related to its carcinogenicity. This general picture was completed by the revelation implied above that cellular genes (proto-oncogenes) in another form (oncogenes) cause neoplastic growth.

The *in vitro* paradigm of the neoplastic cancer cell is the transformed cell. The derivation of transformed cells from normal cells in culture is generally thought to involve "immortalization" of the cells so that they escape the normal limitation on growth of a finite number of division cycles. Such "established cell lines" are assumed to be partially transformed and a variety of carcinogenic agents can cause them subsequently to undergo full transformation to a state of unregulated growth resembling that of cancer cells. Transformed cells may be distinguished morphologically and by their decreased dependence on exogenous growth factors and are generally, although not invariably, tumorigenic when transplanted into immunologically compatible animals. There are presently about 100 known oncogenes that, under certain conditions, can release cells from the normal controls of growth, mortality and location to cause neoplastic transformation. It is probable that the majority of genes that possess oncogenic potential have now been identified and this figure of approximately 100 proto-oncogenes from about 30 000

1

functional human genes thereby sets an upper limit to the number of points at which the bio-chemical pathways controlling normal cell growth might be subverted by oncoproteins. The actual number of distinct mechanisms is probably much smaller, however, as oncogenes fall into groups of similar activity (e.g. tyrosine kinases, guanine nucleotide binding, etc., see Table 1.1) which are presumed to act at the same point in a pathway. In the main, oncogene activation is the result of somatic events (i.e. what we do to ourselves) rather than genetic causes. It is, in other words, a consequence of evolution (mutation and selection) within the body of one animal.

TUMOUR VIRUSES AND THE IDENTIFICATION OF ONCOGENES

Oncogenes were first directly identified in viruses capable of inducing tumours in animals or of transforming cells *in vitro*. Many such viruses have RNA genomes and this family of "retro-viruses" replicate through a DNA intermediate in infected cells (e.g. avian leukosis virus (ALV) and mouse mammary tumour virus (MMTV)). The oncogenes carried by such viruses are strongly homologous in sequence to normal cellular genes (proto-oncogenes) that are themselves highly conserved in evolution. Many DNA viruses are also oncogenic (e.g. SV40, polyoma, adenovirus and papillomavirus) although, as noted above, their transforming genes have not yet been shown to have proto-oncogene homologues within the normal genome, save for the pres-ence of *BCL2* sequences in the Epstein–Barr virus *BHRF1* gene (see **DNA Tumour Viruses, EBV**).

Retroviruses are usually weakly pathogenic or apathogenic (e.g., ALV) although they are associated with a variety of chronic diseases. Productive infection has little effect on the host cell and progeny virus particles are released by budding from the plasma membrane without cell lysis. The basic genomes of retroviruses contain three genes (Fig. 1.1, see Appendix for details of the life-cycle of retroviruses).

Those retroviruses that can cause rapid neoplasia in infected organisms do so because they have acquired genes derived from normal cellular counterparts and the inappropriate expression of these transduced genes (or oncogenes) perturbs the normal regulation of cell growth. However, despite the fact that retroviruses induce cancers in a wide range of mammals and birds, no retrovirally borne gene has yet been demonstrated to be directly oncogenic in humans, including those in the genomes of the HIV and HTLV families (see Appendix).

For all retroviruses that have been studied, with the exception of some strains of Rous sarcoma virus (RSV), the acquisition of an oncogene disrupts the sequence of one or more of the *gag*, *pol* or *env* genes, rendering the virus replication-defective. A specific example of the proviral struc-ture of a naturally occurring oncogenic retrovirus, selected for illustrative purposes, is shown in Fig. 1.2 in which the *gag* sequence remains but all of *pol* and most of *env* is replaced by

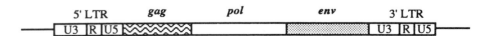

Fig. 1.1 Structure of a typical DNA provirus. U3, R and U5 within the long terminal repeat (LTR) regions refer to sequences derived from the 3' and 5' ends of the viral genome (see Appendix). *gag* (encoding the capsid protein of the virus), *pol* (reverse transcriptase) and *env* (the spike protein of the outer envelope) are the three major structural and replicative genes. The lines indicate cellular DNA.

cellular (*Fos*) sequences. Replication of such defective viruses occurs in the presence of a helper virus that expresses complete *gag*, *pol* and *env* genes.

The identification of oncogenes

The major steps in the experimental analysis of tumour viruses that led to the exposure of cancer genes began with the demonstration by Rous that cell-free filtrates of chicken sarcomas gave rise to sarcomas when inoculated into normal birds (Rous, 1911). As Rous himself observed, "The...transmission of a true neoplasm by means of a cell-free filtrate assumes exceptional importance". Similar experiments at about this time had shown that avian leukaemia could be transmitted horizontally by cell-free preparations (Ellerman and Bang, 1909), although leukosis was not at that time recognized as a cancer.

Very little further progress occurred until the late 1950s, when the development of electron microscopic techniques enabled the infectious agent in these experiments to be recognized as a virus (Bernhard, 1960). In 1965 Fried, by treating polyoma virus with nitrous acid, derived a conditional mutation that was temperature-sensitive in its ability to transform normal hamster cells to neoplastic cells *in vitro*. This was a remarkable achievement, but DNA tumour viruses have subsequently proved difficult to work with in this context because their oncogenes may be involved in the expression and replication of viral DNA and they kill the cells in which they replicate.

The crucial retroviral experiment was performed by Martin (1970) who used the chemical mutagen *N*-methyl-*N*′-nitro-*N*-nitrosoguanidine (MNNG) to obtain a temperature-sensitive mutant of RSV. With this mutant Martin was able to show that chick fibroblasts could be transformed to a fully neoplastic state by the expression of part of the viral genome alone, and

```
     Rat  ←──┬──→ U₃                              U₃ ←──┬──→ R      R ←──┬──→ U₅
(1) CGGGCTGTAT│TGAAAGACCC── (363)CCAAT── (414)TATAAA── (441)GGC│GCG ── (510)CA│TC──
                           CAT              TATA                │
                                                               Cap

            U₅ ←──┐                                    ┌──→ p75
── (575)GGGGTCTTTCATT│TGGGGGCTCGTCCGGGAT── (1079)TAT┌──→p15   p15 ←──┬──→ p12
            I.R.              P.B.S.             │GGG ── (1464)TAC│CCT
                                              Met Gly             Tyr Pro

    p12 ←──┬──→ p30      gag ←──┬──→ fos      fos ←──┬──→ fox       p75 ←──┐
── (1719)TTC│CCA ── (2007)GAA│GAC ── (2716)GCT│TTA ── (2742)TAG└──
       Phe Pro          Glu Asp            Phe

    fox ←──┬──→ env    Δp15E ←──┐              ┌──→ U₃            U₃ ←──┬──→ R
── (3166)AGT│AAA ── (3176)TAA└── (3226)│ATTGAAAGACCCC ── (3657)GGC│GCG ──
                                        I.R.

                 R ←──┬──→ U₅             U₃ ←──┬──→ Rat
── (3706)AATAAA ── (3725)GCA│TCC ── (3791)GGGGTCTTTCA│GTATGTAAT(3811)A
   (A)ₙ signal
```

Fig. 1.2 Principal structural features of a complete provirus. The FBR murine sarcoma virus encodes p75$^{gag\text{-}fos}$, the sequence for which includes eight C-terminal amino acids encoded by nucleotides derived from cellular sequences (*Fox*) distinct from *Fos*. The *gag* gene encodes p15, p12 and p30. Δp15E indicates the end of the residual *env* gene. I.R. indicates 13 nucleotide inverted repeats at the ends of the LTRs that are identical to those found in other C-type murine retroviruses: the AA and TT pairs that mark the 5′ and 3′ ends, respectively, of the LTRs of unintegrated DNA in murine retroviruses have been lost at the proviral junctions. PBS: primer binding site. The four nucleotides flanking the proviral termini are identical (open bars). Figures in parentheses indicate the number of the following base (van Beveren *et al.*, 1984).

that sustained expression was required to maintain that state – an experiment that Bishop has described as ushering in the "age of oncogenes" (Bishop, 1985). We now know that in RSV a single gene, *Src*, is responsible for rapid oncogenesis.

Perhaps the most remarkable observation of the whole story came from screening total DNA in chickens (Stehelin *et al.*, 1976) when it emerged that the *Src* gene was not viral after all but is present in the normal genome all the time. These results led the way to the conclusion that highly conserved proto-oncogenes are present in normal cellular DNA in low copy number in virtually all members of the animal kingdom. This finding implied, though did not establish, the unification of the fields of retroviral research and cancer: if a normal gene misbehaving was responsible for retrovirally transmitted cancers in animals, then perhaps the same kind of mechanism might be involved in human tumours that arose spontaneously or were chemically induced and that apparently were not in any way due to viruses. This was particularly encouraging in that neither at that time nor since has any evidence accumulated that retroviruses directly cause cancers in humans.

Further evidence that genes that had been normal at one time could become determinants of transformation came in the late 1970s from experiments in which the transfection of DNA from cell lines transformed by chemical carcinogens into normal cells gave rise to transformed phenotypes (Shih *et al.*, 1979). Shortly thereafter, oncogenes began to be identified by transfection of cells *in vitro* with DNA taken from human tumours. The transfected cells were tumorigenic when injected into syngeneic animals and the genes responsible were shown to be homologous to the transforming genes of retroviruses. This was first shown by Der and his colleagues for *RAS* (Der *et al.*, 1982) and in fact the majority of the genes subsequently detected by this method have been members of the *RAS* family. During this period, Erikson and his colleagues were able to show that the *Src* gene product, pp60^{src}, is a tyrosine kinase and that normal cells express low levels of the same protein (Collett and Erikson, 1978; Collett *et al.*, 1981). This was a striking finding because tyrosine phosphorylation is rare in cells: only 1 in 2000 of the phosphate groups linked to proteins are attached to tyrosine residues. Since then it has become clear that many other oncogenes encode kinases, several of which are tyrosine-specific (Table 1.1) and when activated increase total cellular phosphotyrosine content by up to tenfold. pp60^{src} has subsequently been shown to act on many substrates but those that are essential mediators of transformation remain to be unequivocally identified (see **SRC**).

The observation that confirmed the normal origins of oncogenes was made in 1983 by Waterfield and his colleagues who showed that the transforming gene of simian sarcoma virus (v-*sis*) encodes a protein that is identical to the N-terminal 109 residues of the B chain of platelet-derived growth factor (PDGF; Waterfield *et al.*, 1983). PDGF is a normal growth factor secreted by platelets that stimulates the proliferation of fibroblasts. This discovery indicated that the v-*sis* viral oncogene was derived from a normal growth factor gene. The simplest explanation for the evolution of v-*sis* is that cells infected with simian sarcoma virus will continuously produce an autocrine growth factor. Shortly thereafter it was shown that the v-*erbB* gene codes for part of the epidermal growth factor (EGF) receptor, that other oncogenes (v-*fms*, *Met* and v-*ros*) are similarly derived from normal transmembrane receptors and that *ErbA* encodes a high-affinity thyroid hormone receptor (see individual oncogenes).

How are proto-oncogenes activated by retroviruses?

Two general mechanisms account for the way in which transduced retroviral genes might promote cancers, even though the genes derive from normally harmless, or even necessary, cellular genes:

1 The integration of viral DNA is potentially mutagenic: it can damage cellular genes directly

or influence their expression by bringing them under the control of powerful regulatory elements in the viral genome (sometimes called "insertional mutagenesis" (Kung *et al.*, 1991)). Both types of event are examples of *cis* activation. A further version of insertional mutagenesis may occur when the inserted provirus encodes a protein (i.e. viral) that can regulate transcription of a cellular gene – a form of *trans* activation independent of the respective locations of the proviral integration site and the normal gene within the host genome.

Proviral insertion may occur anywhere in the host cell genome but, for a number of viruses, groups of preferred integration sites have been identified (Fig. 1.3). Such sites are sometimes adjacent to the loci of known proto-oncogenes but may also lie in proximity to previously unidentified genes (see Table 2.5, Chapter 2). Genes that have been detected through being targets for insertional activation or mutation by viruses include *Ahi-1*, *Evi-1*, *Evi-2*, *Mlvi-1*, *Mlvi-2*, *Mlvi-3* and *Pvt-1* and for each of these common integration sites there is a significant frequency of double viral integration.

2 Recombination between retroviral and cellular genomes can insert a cellular gene in the viral genome, the cellular gene thus becoming oncogenic. This process is called "transduction". Because the cellular gene is now regulated by viral promoters its expression is independent of the site of proviral integration within chromosomal DNA. The oncoprotein expressed may be comprised of cellular information (possibly altered) or may be a viral–cellular fusion protein.

As a consequence of insertional mutagenesis the action of viral promoters beyond the control of the cell may cause sustained overexpression of a normal host gene, leading to neoplastic growth. Most proto-oncogenes can transform established cell lines (although not primary explants of normal cells) when they are expressed at high levels. This was first observed in chicken lymphomas in which *Myc* was activated by retroviral DNA inserted upstream, within or downstream of the gene (Fig. 1.3). Proviral insertion of ALV into the chicken genome is nearly always in the same transcriptional orientation as *Myc*, giving rise to promoter insertion in which transcription of the gene is initiated from the viral promoter. Insertions in the opposite orientation or 3' of the coding sequences are presumed to activate transcription by the ALV LTR functioning as a *cis* enhancer. In mammals infected by murine leukaemia virus (MuLV) the converse situation occurs: over 90% of viral insertions are in the opposite orientation to the gene with the viral sequences acting as an enhancer.

It is evident, therefore, that genes activated by viral insertion can mediate tumorigenesis but it seems certain that additional, undefined factors are involved. Thus, MMTV insertion can activate the *Wnt-1*, *Wnt-2*, *Wnt-3*, *Wnt-4* or *Hst* genes, of which only *Wnt*-2 and *Hst* reside on the same chromosome. However, in MMTV-induced tumours that are histologically identical these genes may be activated collectively or only individually.

During transduction genes usually acquire mutations that can convert proto-oncogenes into oncogenes. Capture of cellular DNA by retroviruses generally involves trimming of either end of the gene. This may be critical in allowing enhanced expression (see **SRC** for comparison of v-*src* and *Src*). In some cases single-point mutations are sufficient to activate oncogenic potential, for example, in *Ras* and *Neu*.

Retroviral infection is often harmless (if the viral genome lacks an oncogene) but even retroviruses that do not carry oncogenes can induce disease in susceptible hosts. However, they act more slowly and do not readily transform cells *in vitro*. Such viruses work by insertional activation of cellular proto-oncogenes. Known genes can be examined by Southern blot analysis to determine whether they are rearranged by viral integration in tumours. Novel genes can be detected by searching for proviral integration sites common to independent tumours: since retroviruses integrate into a large number of sites in the host genome, the probability of two such tumours having identical proviral integrations is very low.

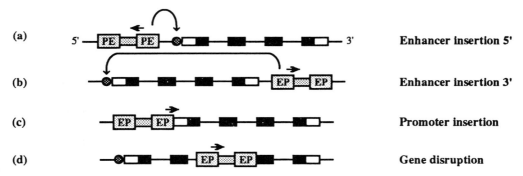

Fig. 1.3 Proviral activation of a cellular gene. E and P represent the viral enhancer and promoter elements within the LTR of the provirus. (a) Insertion 5′ to the cellular gene in the opposite orientation such that E is in close proximity to the cellular gene promoter (circle). (b) 3′ Insertion minimizing the distance between E and the cellular promoter. (c) Replacement of the cellular gene promoter by that of the virus. (d) Proviral integration within the cellular gene (Peters, 1991). Potential avian or rodent oncogenes affected by viral insertion include, in addition to *Myc* and *Wnt-1*, *ErbB*, *Hst*, *Int-2*, *Mos*, *Myb*, *Hras-1*, RMO-*Wnt-1*, *Pim-1* and *Raf* (see Table 2.5, Chapter 2). During the induction of erythroleukaemia by insertional mutagenesis of ALV, the *ErbB* gene (encoding the receptor for epidermal growth factor, EGFR) is truncated at the N-terminus, giving rise to a gene closely similar to v-*erbB* which arises from transduction. Integration sites regulating *Myb* expression occur in introns both 5′ and 3′ of the exons homologous to v-*myb* and *Wnt-2* and *Hst* expression is altered by integration in 5′ or 3′ non-coding sequences.

The long latency of most neoplasms suggests that multiple steps are involved in the development of the disease. This concept is illustrated by the finding that in a number of retroviral infections distinct transforming genes (detectable by transfection of DNA into NIH 3T3 cells) are activated. Thus ALV-induced chicken lymphomas express *Blym-1* in addition to *Myc*, and MMTV-induced mouse mammary carcinomas express *Hst-1* and combinations of the *Int* and *Wnt* families. Activated transforming genes have now been detected in a wide variety of primary tumours and derived cell lines of avian, rodent and human origin. The involvement of multiple genes in human cancers is discussed below (page 16).

Much of our understanding of the molecular biology of oncogenes has come from the study of tumour viruses and yet the variety of behaviour attributable to the oncoproteins that they express remains bewildering. Some tumour viruses are oncogenic only in animals not their host in nature whilst others are oncogenic in their natural host. Some do not transform cells in culture and yet are powerful oncogenes in animals. As will be discussed in the following sections, there is also great diversity in the oncoproteins synthesized by DNA and RNA tumour viruses: oncoproteins may attack the nucleus, cytoplasm or plasma membrane (see page 9) but, although their cellular location may be known and specific protein functions are gradually being revealed, for the most part the manner in which the expression of multiple oncogenes integrates to cause cancers is not understood. From what is known, no correlation can be drawn between how proteins act and the nature of the tumour induced.

How are proto-oncogenes activated in humans?

In normal cells proto-oncogene activation may occur by mutation, DNA rearrangement or oncogene amplification (Fig. 1.4). Point mutations may arise from the action of chemicals or radiation. For example, the transfection experiments that revealed activated *RAS* genes in human tumours led to the finding that, for *RAS*, the transformation from normal proto-oncogene to oncogene was due to substitution of a single base, resulting in the exchange of valine for glycine or glutamine for lysine at residues 12 or 61 respectively (see **RAS**).

The mechanisms of chromosome translocation and amplification can provide a novel promoter for the cellular gene. The exchange of genetic material can occur between homologous or non-homologous chromosomes and can either be a balanced, reciprocal event or can involve loss of material from one or both junctions. Alternatively, inversion of segments within a chromosome may occur without net loss, or interstitial deletions may give rise to shortened chromosomes. Burkitt's lymphoma and human chronic myeloid leukaemia are characterized by chromosome exchange between non-homologous chromatids. In some B cell leukaemias the proto-oncogene comes under the control of the immunoglobulin promoter and enhancer. In Burkitt's lymphoma the gene involved is *MYC* and this releases transcription of *MYC* from normal controls so that it may be expressed at inappropriate times as well as being overexpressed. Damage to the translocated gene may also increase mRNA stability.

Gene amplification, thought to play a role in later stages of cancer, frequently involves proto-oncogenes. The process expands the number of copies of a gene which can lead to excess production of oncogene message and protein. Amplification of *MYC* and *MYCL* has frequently been observed in small cell carcinoma of the lung. Amplified genes may also have undergone mutation and, for *KRAS2* at least, there is evidence that amplification of the normal gene may occur in parallel with mutation of that gene.

DNA tumour viruses

The double-stranded DNA viruses of the adenovirus, herpesvirus, poxvirus and papovavirus families possess oncogenic potential. Most adenoviruses are tumorigenic in newborn rodents and

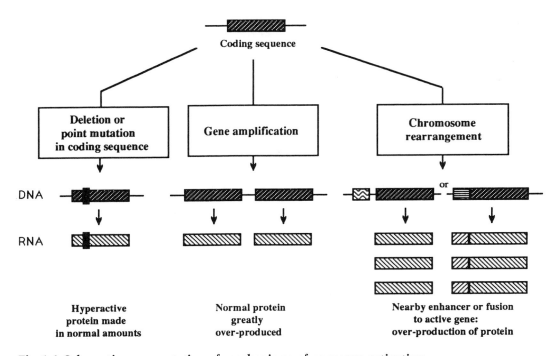

Fig. 1.4 Schematic representation of mechanisms of oncogene activation.

will transform cells from such animals *in vitro*. The papovaviruses polyoma virus and simian vacuolating virus 40 (SV40) are also highly tumorigenic in rodent cells whereas in monkey cells (permissive cells) they enter the lytic cycle that leads to lysis of the infected cells and release of progeny viruses. A major difference between DNA viruses and retroviruses is that the former replicate autonomously without being integrated into the host chromosome. DNA viral genes, including those with oncogenic potential, have therefore evolved to encode proteins that are essential for the continuation of the life-cycle of the virus. Hence the oncogenes of DNA viruses differ from those of retroviruses, possession of which confers no advantage on the virus.

In the early phase of SV40 infection the major proteins synthesized are the large T and small t antigens (see **DNA Tumour Viruses**). T Antigen is the only viral protein necessary for viral DNA replication, achieved by its binding to and unwinding DNA and then interacting with DNA polymerase α. T Antigen alone is a potent transforming agent whereas t antigen, although not necessary for either transformation or viral replication, enhances both processes. The polyoma locus encodes three early proteins, t antigen, middle t antigen and T antigen, of which middle t antigen is the strongest transforming protein. Adenoviruses encode two classes of early mRNA (E1A and E2B), from which alternative splicing patterns generate a range of proteins. Two E1A proteins of adenovirus 5 have been shown to act as transcription factors and to possess transforming activity. The E1B region does not possess transforming capacity but can promote that of E1A. The general mechanism by which these different viral proteins cause transformation is by forming complexes with host cell proteins. Thus both E1A proteins and SV40 and polyoma T antigens form specific complexes with the tumour suppressor retinoblastoma gene product (p105^{RB}) and these and other viral proteins share a sequence motif essential for interaction with p105^{RB} (see **Tumour Suppressor Genes**). SV40 T antigen also forms complexes with the product of the tumour suppressor gene *P53* at a site separate from that binding p105^{RB} and p53 also associates with E1B. These observations suggest that the transforming potential of SV40 T antigen lies in its capacity to bind to and inactivate p105^{RB} and p53, both of which are expressed in normal cells. The polyoma antigens do not bind p53 but it is probable that the increasing number of proteins being detected in complexes with these and other DNA viral antigens will include tumour suppressor gene products that are presently unknown (see **DNA Tumour Viruses**).

NORMAL CELL GROWTH AND THE FUNCTIONS OF ONCOPROTEINS

Activation of normal cell growth

The stimulation of normal cell proliferation occurs as a consequence of the activation of biochemical pathways by growth factors (or mitogens) interacting with their receptors on the plasma membrane (Fig. 1.5). There are many different growth factors (e.g. PDGF, EGF, insulin, bombesin) and a single cell often possesses a variety of types of receptor. There are, however, only four known intracellular second messengers that can be activated by the interaction of a growth factor with its receptor:

1 Cyclic AMP, produced by the action of adenylate cyclase, a membrane-bound enzyme stimulated by many different signal–receptor complexes (e.g. prostaglandin E_2). Cyclic AMP-dependent protein kinases regulate many cellular processes.

2 Cyclic GMP, produced by the action of guanylate cyclase (e.g. cyclic GMP concentrations are modulated in retinal cells in response to light). Cyclic GMP directly regulates membrane cation channels in photoreceptor cells and mediates other processes including the relaxation of smooth muscle.

3 The elevation of the free, intracellular concentration of Ca^{2+} ($[Ca^{2+}]_i$), usually caused by the action of inositol 1,4,5-trisphosphate released during the hydrolysis of phosphatidylinositol 4,5-bisphosphate ($PtdIns(4,5)P_2$). Many growth factors cause $PtdIns(4,5)P_2$ hydrolysis when they activate their specific receptors on the cell surface (e.g. PDGF, bombesin, anti-T cell receptor antibody).

4 Activated protein tyrosine kinases. These enzymes, often intrinsic to the receptor molecule, are activated by many growth factors (e.g. EGF, PDGF, bombesin).

One growth factor may recognize both receptors that activate adenylate cyclase and receptors that cause elevation of $[Ca^{2+}]_i$: such receptors are often, but not invariably, on different types of cell. Furthermore, the activation of tyrosine kinase(s) may be coupled to a mechanism for increasing $[Ca^{2+}]_i$.

The activation of second messengers causes the enhanced transcription of ~100 genes within 6 h. Of these, the "immediate early response genes" are activated within the first hour and include ornithine decarboxylase, the overexpression of which may cause transformation (see Table 1.1), and the proto-oncogene families of *Jun* and *Fos*. The proto-oncogenes *Myc* and *Myb* are also transcriptionally activated, approximately 2 h and 6 h respectively after cell stimulation.

In normal, untransformed cells the consistent pattern of a correlation between the early stages of proliferation and the expression of the proto-oncogenes *Ets*, *Fos*, *Jun* and *Myc* clearly suggests that these proto-oncogenes function as essential mediators of the biochemical pathways that regulate proliferation and that their corresponding oncogenic forms may act via sustained perturbation of normal growth control mechanisms.

It should also be noted that normal growth factors synthesized in an appropriate setting may act as "promoters" in the early stages of the development of cancers. Gastric releasing peptide (GRP or mammalian bombesin) functions as an autocrine growth factor in small cell lung cancer: these tumour cells produce large amounts of the peptide which causes $PtdIns(4,5)P_2$ hydrolysis and an increase in $[Ca^{2+}]_i$ (Minna, 1988), characteristic responses of cells entering the cell cycle. In this situation the growth factor may act selectively to promote the proliferation of a clone of tumour cells.

What do oncoproteins do?

The gene products of *Ets*, *Fos*, *Jun* and *Myc* and their oncogenic equivalents function as nuclear transcription factors. In addition to controlling mRNA synthesis, only three basic ways are known by which the products of oncogenes can interfere with normal cell function (Table 1.1, Hunter, 1991): (1) protein phosphorylation (Tyr, Ser, Thr), (2) metabolic regulation via G proteins, and (3) participation in DNA replication. The latter is established for DNA tumour viruses but there is no evidence that oncogenes derived from proto-oncogenes work in this way.

Class 1 (Table 1.1) includes the v-*sis* gene product referred to earlier, that appears to function as an autocrine growth factor providing sustained activation of proliferation via a normal plasma membrane receptor. v-*sis* encodes the B chain subunit of PDGF and in some cells a v-*sis* homodimer of PDGF is released that has a structure and activity similar to that of PDGF-BB. Hence, one possibility is that the cells proliferate indefinitely by an autocrine mechanism, although no increase in tyrosine phosphorylation corresponding to that caused by activation of the PDGF

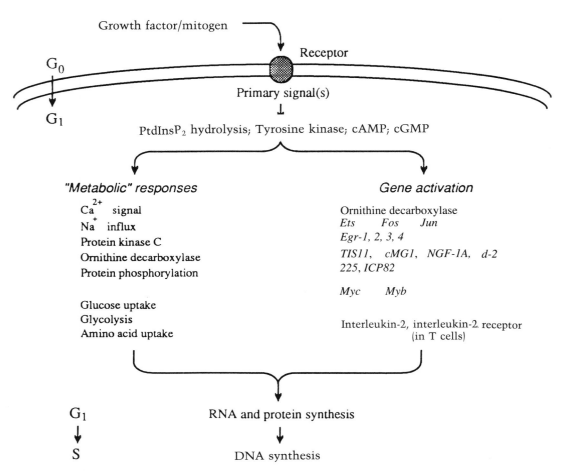

Fig. 1.5 Biochemical events during proliferation in eukaryotic cells. The interaction of growth factors with their receptors on the cell surface causes quiescent, somatic cells to leave G_0, traverse G_1 and enter S phase, whereupon cells are normally committed to at least one round of the cell cycle. Following the generation of one or more primary signals a sequence of "metabolic" events occurs that includes ionic changes, increased ornithine decarboxylase activity, protein phosphorylation and enhanced glycolytic flux. In parallel with and independent of these events the coordinated transcription of ~100 genes is activated (Almendral *et al.*, 1988; Zipfel *et al.*, 1989). The "immediate early response genes" activated within approximately 1 h include ornithine decarboxylase, *Ets-1* and *Ets-2*, the *Jun* family (*Jun, JunB* and *JunD*), the *Fos* family (*Fos, Fra1, Fra2* and *FosB*), serum response factor (SRF), the steroid hormone receptors *Nurk77, N10, NGFI-B, TIS1* and the early growth response family (*Egr-1* (also known as *Zpf-6, Zif-268, Krox24 NGFI-A* or *TIS8*; Sukhatme *et al.*, 1988), *Egr-2* (*Krox20*; Joseph *et al.*, 1988), *Egr-3* (Patwardhan *et al.*, 1991) and *Egr-4*), *TIS11* (or *TTP* or *Nup475*; Ma and Herschman, 1991) and the homologous *cMG1* (Gomperts *et al.*, 1990), *TTP, Nup475*, fibronectin, fibronectin receptor β subunit, β-actin, α-tropomyosin (Ryseck *et al.*, 1989), *NGFI-A, CEF-4* (or *9E3*, related to interleukin-8; Gonneville *et al.*, 1991), *CEF-5 d-2, c25, rIRF-1*, p27, *Mtf*, the glucose transporter, *KC, N51, JE, TIS10, Cyr61, PC4, TIS7, Snk* (serum-inducible kinase; Simmons *et al.*, 1992) and *Pip92* (see Herschman, 1991 for review).

In HTLV-1-infected T cells the TAX1 protein activates the *JUN* and *FOS* families, *EGR1* and *EGR2* and two other genes, *ICP82* and *225* (Hijikata *et al.*, 1990; Wright *et al.*, 1990).

Myc mRNA is detectable within 2 h, *Myb* within 6 h. The T-cell-specific genes for interleukin-2 and its receptor are detectable after 8 h.

Table 1.1. *Functional classification of oncogene products*

Class 1. Growth factor related proteins:
  PDGFB/Sis, INT2, HSTF1/HST1

Class 2. Tyrosine kinases:
  Receptor-like tyrosine kinases: EPH, EGFR/ERBB, FMS, KIT, MET, HER2/NEU, TRK
  Non-receptor tyrosine kinases: ABL, FPS/FES
  Membrane-associated non-receptor tyrosine kinases: SRC, FGR, FYN, HCK, LCK, YES

Class 3. Receptors lacking protein kinase activity:
  MAS

Class 4. Membrane-associated G proteins:
  HRAS, KRAS2, NRAS, GSP, GIP2

Class 5. Cytoplasmic protein serine kinases:
  BCR, MOS, PIM1, RAF/MIL

Class 6. Protein serine-, threonine- and tyrosine kinase:
  Sty

Class 7. Cytoplasmic regulators:
  CRK

Class 8. DNA binding proteins (transcription factors) or proteins located mostly in the nucleus:
  FOS, JUN, ETS, MYC, MYB, REL, ERBA, P53

Class 9. Mitochondrial membrane factor:
  BCL2

Class 10. Function unknown:
  LCO

This table is a selected list of prominent oncogenes: for a complete list see Table 2.5 in Chapter 2.

receptor has yet been detected. There are three possibilities that could account for the fact that v-SIS but not PDGF causes transformation: (1) it has abnormal activity compared to PDGF; (2) it causes the receptor to be processed abnormally; and (3) it acts at an anomalous site within the cell. There is some evidence for the latter in that the v-*sis* product may not need to leave the cell to evoke neoplastic growth but may combine with an intracellular receptor.

In addition to v-SIS and the transcription factors, oncogene products may be located in or attached to the plasma membrane or in the cytosol (Fig. 1.6). Thus, in principle, oncogenesis may occur as the result of perturbation at any point on the normal biochemical pathways that control proliferation.

Oncogenes that encode tyrosine kinase receptor-like proteins are generally considered to exert their effects through the sustained activation of their kinase domain. All tyrosine-specific protein kinases share sequence homology over ~300 amino acids although some, for example, PDGFR, contain an insert region (Fig 1.7).

The transforming activity of avian erythroblastosis virus (AEV) arises from v-*erbB* which encodes a truncated form of the EGFR that has lost the ligand binding domain and remains active as a protein tyrosine kinase, independent of EGF. v-ERBB has also lost a C-terminal region that includes an autophosphorylation site, presumed important for normal function. It is, however, difficult to show that v-ERBB has sustained tyrosine kinase activity. The major substrate for the activated EGFR is a 42 kDa protein, detected in some but not all cells transformed by oncogenes encoding a tyrosine kinase. In general, little is known about protein substrates for the EGFR or v-ERBB. Nevertheless, it would appear that the oncogenic action of v-ERBB is due to: (a) sustained tyrosine kinase activity, and (b) absence of downregulation of the receptor on account of the missing EGF binding site.

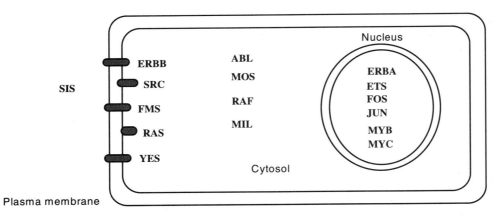

Fig. 1.6 Cellular location of some oncogene products. A selected number of oncoproteins is shown to illustrate that they may act as extracellular growth factors (SIS), as ligand-independent membrane-associated proteins (ERBB, SRC, FMS, RAS, YES), as cytosolic factors (ABL, MOS, RAF, MIL) or in the nucleus, where they are presumed to function as transcription factors (ERBA, ETS, FOS, JUN, MYB, MYC).

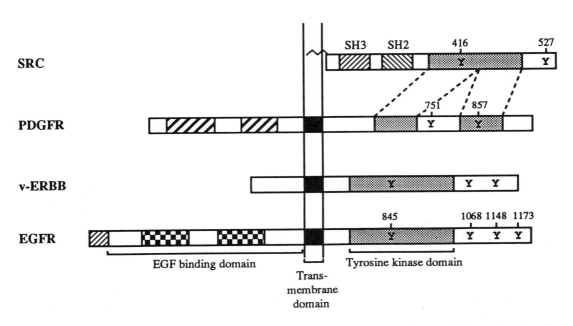

Fig. 1.7 SRC, v-ERBB and the transmembrane receptors for epidermal growth factor (EGF) and platelet-derived growth factor (PDGF). The kinase domains are homologous but that of the PDGF receptor is divided by a kinase insert region. v-ERBB is homologous to the EGF receptor but truncated at both ends, resulting in the loss of the ligand binding region and of a C-terminal regulatory tyrosine residue.

In general for the cytoplasmic and plasma membrane oncoproteins (e.g. v-*ras*, v-*src*, v-*erbB*, etc.) it appears that mutation in the cellular genes releases the translation products from the normal allosteric controls. As exemplified by v-ERBB, however, specific phosphorylation targets for the oncogenic tyrosine kinases that are involved in cell transformation remain largely undiscovered (see ***THR/ErbA, EGFR/ErbB-1, HER2/Neu, HER3*** and ***HER4, SRC*** and ***RAS***).

Nuclear oncoproteins

The early response proto-oncogenes that encode transcription factors are of particular interest in that they may regulate, either positively or negatively, genes that are directly involved in growth control. Although much is known about the interactions of these proteins with DNA *in vitro* (Table 1.2), their function *in vivo* remains largely obscure. The following is a general summary of what is currently known of the effects on transcription of the major nuclear oncoproteins FOS, JUN, ETS, MYB, MYC, REL and ERBA. The individual sections should be consulted for details and references relating to specific proteins.

The members of the *Fos* and *Jun* families are the major components of the transcription factor AP-1. Cellular expression (by transfection) of several oncogenes (*Fos, Mos, Ras, Raf, Src* or polyoma middle T) induces AP-1 activity and AP-1-binding enhancer elements occur in the *cis* control regions of a number of genes that are strongly expressed in transformed cells, including collagenase, metallothionein IIA and stromelysin. FOS cannot dimerize with itself and dimerization between FOS and JUN or between members of the JUN family is necessary for DNA binding. Eighteen different dimeric combinations can thus be formed from within the FOS and JUN families. DNA binding occurs by interaction between the leucine zipper regions (see *JUN*) of the proteins that lie next to basic, DNA binding domains. JUN proteins also bind with high affinity to the cAMP response element (CRE) and JUN, but not FOS, proteins dimerize with some members of the CREB family, the dimers formed binding preferentially to the CRE. The capacity of JUN to interact with cAMP signalling pathways by forming JUN–CREB dimers thus provides an additional group of transcription factors. The basic and leucine zipper regions are present in both the normal and oncogenic forms of FOS and JUN and mutations that prevent dimerization decrease the transforming potential of v-*fos* and v-*jun*. In fibroblasts that have been stimulated by serum all the products of the *Fos* and *Jun* gene families coexist but the extent and temporal pattern of expression varies. These genes are also differentially expressed during development. This suggests that these proteins have distinct functions that are probably mediated by the wide range of affinities for AP-1 sites of the different dimeric forms. Thus JUN dimers have a tenfold greater affinity for AP-1 than JUNB or JUND: in JUN–FOS dimers the affinity and the half-life of interaction with DNA depends on the specific FOS protein involved (FOSB>FRA1>FOS). Furthermore, single base substitutions in the regions immediately flanking the AP-1 sequence (or the CRE element) can cause a tenfold change in binding affinity. These *in vitro* determinations of relative affinities are consistent with the finding that *Jun* with *Hras-1* is a more potent transforming combination than *JunB* and *Hras-1* and that JUNB expressed at high levels inhibits the transforming potential of *Jun*.

The oncogenic form of *Jun* is derived from *Jun*, the principal change being the loss of a 27 amino acid N-terminal region (δ) that is not well conserved in JUNB and JUND. The δ region appears to facilitate or stabilize the interaction of an inhibitor protein present in some cells

Table 1.2. *Oncoproteins that act as transcription factors*

	Transcription factors	DNA target sequence
ETS	ETS1, ETS2	GC^C/$_G$GGAAGT
FOS	FOS, FOSB, FRA1, FRA2	TGA^C/$_G$TCA (AP-1)
		TGACGTCA (CRE)
JUN	JUN, JUNB, JUND	TGA^C/$_G$TCA (AP-1)
MYB	MYB	C^A/$_C$GTTA^A/$_G$
MYC	MYC/MAX	CACGTG
REL	REL/NF-κB	GGG^A/$_G$NT^T/$_C$^{T}/$_C$CC
ERBA	ERBA/T$_3$	TCAGGTCATGACCTGA

with the A1 transcription activation domain of JUN. v-JUN and JUN bind equally well to the AP-1 site but in HeLa cells that express the inhibitory protein, v-JUN is a much stronger transcriptional activator. Thus the deletion of δ in v-JUN releases the oncoprotein from regulation by the inhibitory protein. However, JUN from which δ has been deleted is still less effective at activating transcription than v-*jun*, indicating the importance of the three additional mutations that occur in v-*jun*. JUN–FOS heterodimers do not appear to bind the inhibitory protein.

In the FOS family, although the leucine zipper and basic domains are essential for DNA binding, the regulation of transcription from AP-1 sites is also dependent on net negative charge in a C-terminal region, usually conferred by phosphorylation (Hunter and Karin, 1992). In both v-FOS and the truncated form of the normal protein FOS, FOSB2, the C-terminus is deleted: such proteins form dimers with JUN that bind to AP-1 but do not activate transcription from AP-1 promoters or suppress *Fos* transcription. Thus the effect of FOSB2 is to compete with normal FOS thereby decreasing the concentration of active FOS–JUN dimers.

The ETS family of transcription factors show strong homology in their DNA binding domains across a wide range of species. Their expression is modulated by growth stimuli during differentiation and from their distribution it appears that they are tissue-specific regulators of gene expression. ETS1 and ETS2 activate transcription through the PEA3 motif (CACTTCCT) that is present in the oncogene responsive domain (ORD) of the polyoma enhancer, where it overlaps an AP-1 site (GTTAGTCA). The co-expression of p68^{ets-1} together with FOS and JUN causes a large, synergistic increase in transcription directed by the ORD (Wasylyk *et al.*, 1990).

The MYB protein contains transcriptional activation and negative regulatory domains as well as a domain that binds directly to the DNA sequence PyAAC^G/$_T$G to activate transcription. MYB DNA binding activity is negatively regulated via phosphorylation by casein kinase II. The cellular activity of this enzyme is increased by the action of some growth factors (e.g. insulin), but not by others (e.g. PDGF), suggesting that proliferation may involve the suppression of MYB-controlled genes. The changes in casein kinase II activity during proliferation remain to be fully characterized, however, and all that can be said at present is that growth factors can indirectly control the transcription-regulating capacity of MYB. The casein kinase II phosphorylation site is in the N-terminal region of MYB but in all oncogenic forms of MYB N-terminal mutations cause the deletion of this site together with most of the negative regulatory domain. These changes result in DNA binding that is independent of a normal regulatory mechanism and in an enhanced level of transcription due to the loss of the inhibitory region.

The MYC proteins (MYC, MYCN and MYCL) each contain basic, helix–loop–helix and leucine zipper domains. Each forms heterodimers with the protein MAX (which also contains all three motifs) that bind specifically to DNA. MAX expression is independent of MYC and MAX may thus regulate transcription of genes independently of *Myc*. The specificity of MYC–DNA interaction appears to be due to the fact that MAX is the only known helix–loop–helix protein that forms dimers with MYC.

The DNA binding domains of the REL oncoproteins are strongly homologous to the DNA binding subunits of the transcription factors NF-κB and KBF1. v-REL thus appears to be a transcription factor but is unique in that it transforms cells equally effectively whether it is located in the cytoplasm or the nucleus. v-REL has, however, lost the strong transcription activating element in the C-terminus of REL and appears by itself to be a weak activator of transcription. C-Terminal loss may promote movement to the nucleus (C-terminal removal does allow the protein to move to the nucleus but v-REL to which the C-terminus of REL has been attached remains cytoplasmic and yet still transforms). v-REL forms complexes with REL and with three proteins to which REL binds, two of which (p115/p124) may be precursors of NF-κB. Thus v-REL may deplete the cell of transcription factor precursors or bind directly to NF-κB or REL DNA target sequences. In any of these mechanisms v-REL would be acting as a dominant negative oncogene (see v-*erbA*).

The v-*erbB* and v-*erbA* genes are both carried by the avian erythroblastosis virus AEV-ES4. The v-*erbA* gene is the oncogenic homologue of *ErbA*, the thyroid hormone receptor (THR), and it increases the transforming potential of other oncogenes, including v-*erbB*. ERBA appears to be permanently bound to the THR response element. The physiological ligand for ERBA (triiodothyronine, T_3) stimulates transcription by over 50-fold. v-ERBA represses transcription to a level similar to that caused by ERBA but is insensitive to T_3. Thus v-ERBA causes sustained repression and is acting as a dominant negative oncogene. The N- and C-terminal truncations occurring in the conversion of *ErbA* to v-*erbA* affect only its hormone responsiveness, not its capacity to bind to DNA. An additional mutation removes a phosphorylation site from ERBA, the loss of which is essential for the effects of v-*erbA* on transformation.

Summary

The nuclear proto-oncogenes fall into two major categories: those that only interact with DNA as complexes with other proteins (FOS–JUN, MYC and probably REL) and those that, in monomeric form, possess a high affinity for specific DNA sequences (ETS, MYB and ERBA). The activity as transcription factors of proteins in both of these categories can be regulated by phosphorylation, for example FOS and MYB, and this may well be a general mechanism. The modulation of the activity of relevant kinases (e.g. casein kinase II) by growth factors provides one mechanism by which transcriptional regulation mediated by these proto-oncogene products may be coupled to proliferation.

The FOS–JUN system, thus far unique in its resolved complexity, illustrates the way in which the transcriptional control exerted by various heterodimeric combinations may undergo subtle modulation during cell development or proliferation as the extent of transcription and translation of different members of the families changes.

In each of the examples discussed above, formation of the oncogene involves the loss of the C-terminus of the normal cellular gene. This does not affect the DNA binding capacity of any these proteins but it invariably alters the effect that the bound protein can exert on transcription. Thus v-FOS and v-ERBA bind normally to promoter regions but v-FOS is unable to suppress *Fos* transcription and v-ERBA is insensitive to T_3. The effect of each is that of a dominant negative oncogene and resembles the dominant negative mutations that may occur in the tumour suppressor gene *P53* that cause the formation of complexes betweeen mutant and wild-type p53, inhibiting the function of the latter.

It should be noted that structural modifications leading to altered transcriptional regulation are not confined to the products of oncogenes but occur during normal cell development, usually by alternative splicing. This provides a mechanism by which the biological function of a single gene can be expanded and *Src*, *Hras-1*, *Abl*, *Myb* and *Fos* have been shown to generate more than one product by this means.

The alternative product of *Myb* (*Mbm-2*) is a truncated version of MYB that retains the DNA binding and nuclear localization regions but has lost the regulatory regions required for transcriptional activation. Expression of normal *Myb* blocks differentiation whereas the effect of *Mbm-2* transcription is to enhance differentiation. Similarly, FOSB2 possesses normal FOS binding functions but not *trans*-activation potential. Thus *Mbm-2* interferes with *Myb* function during mouse erythroid leukaemia cell differentiation and FOSB inhibits *trans* activation by v-FOS, FOS or FOSB, acting effectively as a *trans*-negative regulator.

The proteins encoded by the DNA tumour viruses adenovirus (E1A), polyoma (middle T antigen), SV40 (T antigen) and human papilloma virus (HPV)-16 (E7) are potent regulators of viral transcription. As occurs with the proto-oncogene transcription factors, most of these DNA tumour virus proteins can immortalize primary cells and cooperate with other oncoproteins (typically *Ras*) to transform. These proteins contain limited stretches of homologous sequence, particularly to region 2 of E1A; this is one of the three conserved sequences (18–46 amino acids long) that confer function on E1A, regions 1 and 2 being essential for transformation and region 3 for transcriptional activation. Thus E1A region 2 has been replaced by the corresponding SV40 sequence to generate a chimeric protein with full transforming activity. In E1A at least, transforming and transcription regulating activities appear separable. The expression of *RAS* itself may also be activated by several of the transcription factors mentioned earlier because the human *RASN* promoter includes binding sites for AP-1, CREB, MYC and MYB.

The *Fos* promoter and E1A and T antigen bind the retinoblastoma protein (as well as other proteins), suggesting a common mechanism based on the short homologous regions of the nuclear oncoproteins. Nevertheless, it is established that, for E1A at least, p105^{RB} binding alone is insufficient to cause transformation (see **Tumour Suppressor Genes**).

A wealth of knowledge has accumulated concerning the molecular biology of oncogenes and their normal counterparts. Furthermore, there is a strong correlation between normal growth activation and the expression of a group of nuclear proto-oncogenes that function as transcription factors. Nevertheless, almost nothing is known of the cellular role of the products of these genes or indeed whether proto-oncogenes have functions other than those relating to control of proliferation.

GENERAL CONSEQUENCES OF ONCOGENE EXPRESSION

The epidemiology of cancer strongly suggests that to drive a cell through the various stages preceding the production of a tumour *in vivo* requires the accumulation of several genetic lesions. *In vitro* cellular studies generally support the notion that transformation is at least a two-stage process, one oncogene being needed for immortalization and another for transformation. Thus, primary fibroblasts can often be transformed to a focal growth phenotype (anchorage-independent) by expression of a single oncogene (e.g. *Src*, *Ras*, *Raf*, *Mos*, *Trk*, *Fos*, *Sis*, or SV40 large T antigen). Full transformation, however, generally requires the expression of two complementing oncogenes, typically *Ras* and *Myc*. For example, mutant *RAS* from human tumours only transforms embryonic rat cells when supplemented with other oncogenes in transfected cells, e.g. the E1A adenovirus gene, large T antigen of polyoma, cellular *Myc* or v-*myc*. However, massive overexpression of a single gene can probably override this distinction, thus v-*myc* alone can transform embryonic cells.

In experimental animals the chemical induction of tumours generally requires the sequential application of two types of agent: an "initiator" and a "promoter". The initiator is usually a mutagen that has irreversible effects and must be administered before the promoter. These model systems indicate that the initiating event in tumorigenesis is mutation and that subsequent tumour progression may be mediated by either genetic or epigenetic mechanisms.

In humans the multi-step nature of neoplastic development may be readily distinguished in some forms of the disease. In cervical cancer the initiating event is probably infection with human papillomavirus. Subsequently cervical dysplasia (cervical intraepithelial neoplasia, CIN) may arise. CIN Types I, II and III represent progressively more severe forms in the development of malignant cervical carcinoma. However, the development of an abnormal cell clone (CIN Types I and II) is usually followed by its disappearance and only very infrequently does it give rise to a still more abnormal clone of fully invasive cells (Hollingworth and Barton, 1988). The fact that smoking significantly increases the probability of cervical tumour progression indicates the importance of environmental factors that may not operate through genetic mechanisms.

The detailed studies of malignant colorectal carcinomas indicate that they develop from benign adenomas in a process requiring mutation of at least four genes (Table 1.3; Fearon and Vogelstein, 1990). Prominent among the abnormalities that characterize colorectal carcinomas are the acquisition of mutations in *RAS* and deletions in chromosomes 5q, 18q and 17p. Although mutations in *RAS* and chromosome 17p usually appear at a relatively advanced stage of colorectal carcinoma development, the sequence in which they and the 5q (*APC* and *MCC*) and 18q (*DCC*) changes arise varies between different tumours. This fact has led to the suggestion that the development of malignant colorectal carcinoma requires an overall accumulation rather than a fixed sequence of somatic mutations. It may also be noted that, although the majority of colorectal carcinomas show mutations in *RAS* (50%), 17p (>75%) and 18q (>70%), this disease is typical of the vast majority of cancers in that there is no combination of genetic abnormalities that correlates absolutely with its development.

The region deleted in chromosome 17p in most colorectal neoplasms contains the tumour suppressor gene *P53*. Mutations in the single-copy *P53* gene are the most frequent genetic changes yet shown to be associated with human cancers and point mutations, deletions or insertions in *P53* occur in 70% of all tumours. The rare, autosomal dominant Li–Fraumeni syndrome arises from *P53* mutations inherited through the germ line (Srivastava *et al.*, 1990): 50% of the carriers develop diverse cancers by 30 years of age, compared with 1% in the normal population. In general, however, *P53* mutations are somatic and occur with high frequency in all types of lung cancer, in over 60% of breast tumours and in ~40% of brain tumours (astrocytomas), frequently in combination with the activation of other oncogenes (Table 1.3). Nevertheless, despite the high frequency of *P53* mutations, individual forms of cancer are not characterized by a specific combination of genetic defects. The most notable exception to the pattern of variable expression of cancer genes in histologically identical tumours is provided by the retinoblastoma (*RB*) gene, both alleles of which are defective in all retinoblastomas. However, inactivation of this tumour suppressor gene also occurs in other neoplasms (Table 1.3), for example, Wilms' kidney tumour, breast cancer and small-cell lung carcinoma (SCLC), and individuals with retinoblastoma are particularly susceptible to the development of sarcomas. The frequency of RB inactivation in tumours other than retinoblastoma varies widely. It is mutated with high frequency in SCLCs and most osteosarcomas and soft tissue sarcomas: in non-SCLCs (e.g. adenocarcinomas, squamous cell carcinomas or large cell carcinomas), however, *RB* mutations are infrequent although some tumours of this type have been shown to be defective in both *RB* and *P53*. *P53* mutations are common in some non-SCLCs (squamous cell carcinomas) but not in others (adenocarcinomas), whereas chromosomal deletions affecting *HRAS*, *RAF1* and *INT2* are relatively common (occurring in 18–50% of cases examined) in both these types of SCLC.

In breast cancer, bladder cancer and some other adenocarcinomas there is a correlation

Table 1.3. *Combinations of oncogenes frequently associated with some human cancers*

Affected loci	Tumour
APC, MCC, DCC, KRAS2, P53	Colorectal carcinoma
HRAS, MYC	Cervical carcinoma
MYB, MYC, EGFR, HER2, HRAS, P53, RB1, BRCA1, BCL1, HSTF1, INT2	Breast carcinoma
JUN, MYC, MYCN, MYCL, HRAS, RB1, P53, RAF1	Lung carcinoma
HRAS, P53, RAF1, INT2	Squamous cell carcinoma
MYC, BLYM	Burkitt's lymphoma
P53 (EGFR, MYC, MYCN, GLI, HER2, PDGFB, ROS, TGFα)	Astrocytoma
ABL	Chronic myeloid leukaemia

between the degree of *HER2* overexpression and tumour stage. In one study *HER2* expression has been shown to be inversely correlated with the expression of *MYB*. Overexpression of the EGF receptor (EGFR) has been reported to be associated with oestrogen-receptor negative breast tumours: thus *EGFR* and *MYB* expression provide indicators of a poor or good prognosis, respectively. Deletion of genes is also relatively common in human breast cancer. Inactivation of the breast cancer gene *BRCA1* on chromosome 17q, a putative tumour suppressor gene, occurs in the majority of cases (Smith *et al.*, 1992) and the *RB* gene is inactivated in ~20% of primary carcinomas. In ~65% of cases there is allelic loss of the *P53* gene on chromosome 17. The retained *P53* allele frequently contains point mutations although some tumours retain one normal allele. Between 20% and 50% of breast carcinomas contain non-random loss of heterozygosity for specific locations on chromosomes 1q, 3p or 11p at which specific genes have not been identified and virtually all chromosomes show some susceptibility to allelic imbalance either as an increase in allele copy number (~25%) or as loss of heterozygosity (Devilee *et al.*, 1991).

The *EGFR* gene is also amplified in cell lines derived from squamous carcinomas, glioblastomas and bladder carcinomas. *MYC*, *MYCL* and *MYCN* amplification is frequently associated with both breast carcinomas and lung tumours. In breast carcinomas the combination of enhanced *MYC* and *HER2* expression is indicative of a particularly poor prognosis. Amplification of *MYC* is almost invariably associated with the translocation occurring in Burkitt's lymphoma and is accompanied by the activation of the transforming gene *BLYM1*.

A variety of lymphoid neoplasms are frequently associated with chromosomal translocations where the breakpoints are adjacent to the *BCL* genes. The region containing *BCL1* is also amplified in approximately 20% of breast and squamous cell carcinomas. In breast carcinomas *BCL1* is usually co-amplified with *HSTF1* and *INT2* and, in a very small proportion of cases, *SEA* which is located on the same chromosome. The proteins encoded by these genes have not been fully characterized, however, and evidence for their involvement in tumorigenesis remains circumstantial.

The chromosome translocation involving *ABL* occurs in over 95% of cases of chronic myeloid leukaemia (CML) and in 25% of adult acute lymphocytic leukaemias. The translocation involves the loss of N-terminal ABL sequences (as happens during retroviral transduction when *Abl* is juxtaposed to viral *gag*) and the activation of the ABL protein tyrosine kinase. The *ABL* gene is also amplified tenfold in CML. There is clear evidence for the involvement of the *RAS* family (*HRAS*, *KRAS2* and *NRAS*) in a wide range of cancers. In all cancers the average incidence of *RAS* mutations is approximately 15% but in pancreatic carcinomas, for example, *KRAS2* mutations occur in 95% of tumours. In general, mutations in *RAS* reduce its GTPase activity, the oncogenic protein thus remaining in an active, GTP-bound state. The cellular role of *RAS* remains unclear. *GSP* and *GIP2* are also genes the products of which regulate GTPase activity: for *GSP* and *GIP2*, however, oncogenic mutations cause a sustained elevation of cyclic AMP that appears to promote thyroid carcinomas and ovarian tumours.

All of the oncogenes included in Table 1.4 have been shown to be activated in at least one type of human tumour. However, with the exception of *ABL* in CML, the frequency of their involvement varies widely and for a considerable number (e.g. *YES*) is confined to isolated reports.

V. GENE THERAPY FOR CANCER

The facility with which exogenous genes may be introduced into somatic cells offers the possibility of effective treatment for most if not all cancers. Thus far the main approaches have

Table 1.4. *Individual proto-oncogenes activated in human cancers*

Proto-oncogene	Method of identification
Abl, Egfr, Myc, Hras-1, Kras-2, Src	Retrovirus
ABL, BEK, EGFR, HER2, HER3, FGR, FLG, FPS, GLI, JUN, MET, MYB, MYC, MYCN, MYCL, PIM1, KRAS2, YES	Amplification
DBL, EPH, ETS-1, FOS, FPS/FES, FYN, KIT, LCK, SEA	Overexpression
ABL, BCL1, BCL2, BCL3, BCR, BTG1, CAN, DEK, ETS, ELK, ERG, ETS, HOX11, LCK, LYL1, MLL, MOS, MYC, PML, PVT1, RBTN1, RBTN2, REL, SET, SIL, TAL1, TAL2, TAN1	Translocation
BLYM, HSTF1, LCA, MAS, MCF3, MET, HER2, RAF, NRAS, RET, TRK, TLM	Transfection
GSP, GIP2	Adenylyl cyclase activity

utilized either (a) anti-sense oligodeoxynucleotides, (b) drug targeting, (c) the production of cytokines or (d) the introduction of genes the expression of which reverses the effects of dominant oncogenes or of mutated tumour suppressor genes (Gutierrez *et al.*, 1992). Virtually all applications directed towards human cancers have utilized retroviral vectors for gene transduction (Miller, 1992; see Glossary). This method uses non-infectious virions that can transfer exogenous genes with high efficiency (30–50%) and precise integration into the DNA of almost all types of eukaryotic cell. Four principal types of application employing this techniques have so far shown promise as forms of anti-cancer therapy.

1 The incorporation of specific promoters into retroviral vectors has led to the technique of virally directed enzyme prodrug therapy (VDEPT). This has been used, for example, to permit the expression of herpes simplex thymidine kinase specifically in hepatoma cells through the activation of the α-fetoprotein promoter (Huber *et al.*, 1991). The prodrug 6-methoxypurine arabinonucleoside (araM) is a good substrate for thymidine kinase and is converted to the cytotoxic metabolite araATP within the tumour cells.

2 Genetic modification of tumour infiltrating cells (TIL) has been accomplished by transduction of a retroviral vector expressing an active tumour necrosis factor (TNF) gene into cells from patients with melanoma (Rosenberg, 1992). TIL have been grown *in vitro* in the presence of interleukin-2 (IL-2) from tumour cell samples of a wide variety of human cancers, including colon, breast, bladder, melanoma, renal, lymphoma and neuroblastoma. TIL infiltrate and accumulate within developing tumours and hence high local concentrations of synthesized, diffusible cytokine encoded by the vector are delivered to the site of the tumour without requirement for high systemic doses. The administration of TNF–TIL together with IL-2 has been effective in causing tumour regression in patients with melanoma and this technique is clearly suitable for the introduction of other cytokines and agents with potential therapeutic value into TIL.

3 Antisense oligodeoxynucleotides expressed from transduced retroviral vectors have been used to modulate the tumorigenicity or metastatic potential of a number of oncogenes including *ABL, MYB, MYC, MYCN, RAF1, RAS, SCL, Src*, HPV E7, *RB1* and *P53* (see individual oncogene sections).

4 The expression of a variety of genes has been shown either to modulate the metastatic potential of transformed cells or to cause their reversion to a normal phenotype. Thus in some cells *in vivo* tumorigenicity is reduced by the expression from retroviral vectors of the *JE*/MCP-1 gene (Rollins and Sunday, 1991), *NM23* (Leone *et al.*, 1991) or $\alpha_5\beta_1$ integrin (fibronectin receptor; Giancotti and Ruoslahti, 1990). *In vitro* invasiveness is decreased when the highly metastatic cell line B16-F10 is transfected with a plasmid expressing βm-actin (Sadano *et al.*, 1990). Furthermore, the expression of antisense RNA directed against the cell adhesion molecule

E-cadherin or against tissue inhibitors of metalloproteinases (TIMP) can confer metastatic capacity (see **Tumour Suppressor Genes: Cadherins**). The expression of antisense oligodeoxynucleotide directed against human type I regulatory subunit (RI_α) of the cAMP-dependent protein kinase arrests the growth of human and rodent cancer cells *in vitro* and antisense RII_α blocks cAMP-inducible growth inhibition and differentiation. Cell growth is also inhibited by retroviral vector expression of RII_β (Cho-Chung *et al.*, 1991).

Genes the expression of which induces reversion of transformed cells to a normal morphology include in *Krev-1/Rap-1 Kras-2*-transformed cells (see **RAS**) and wild-type genes inserted to replace defective copies of the tumour suppressor genes *P53*, retinoblastoma, Wilms' kidney tumour or neurofibromatosis type 1 (see **Tumour Suppressor Genes**).

Reviews

Bishop, M.J. (1985). Viral oncogenes. Cell, 42, 23–38.

Copeland, N.G. and Jenkins, N.A. (1990). Retroviral integration in murine myeloid tumors to identify *Evi-1*, a novel locus encoding a zinc-finger protein. Adv. Cancer Res., 54, 141–157.

Cory, S. (1986). Activation of cellular oncogenes in hemopoietic cells by chromosome translocation. Adv. Cancer Res., 47, 189–234.

Fearon, E.R. and Vogelstein, B. (1990). A genetic model for colorectal tumorigenesis. Cell, 61, 759–767.

Gutierrez, A.A., Lemoine, N.R. and Sikora, K. (1992). Gene therapy for cancer. Lancet, 339, 715–721.

Herschman, H.R. (1991). Primary response genes induced by growth factors and tumor promoters. Annu. Rev. Biochem., 60, 281–319.

Hunter, T. (1991). Cooperation between oncogenes. Cell, 64, 249–270.

Hunter, T. and Karin, M. (1992). The regulation of transcription by phosphorylation. Cell, 70, 375–387.

Kung, H.J., Boerkoel, C. and Carter, T.H. (1991). Retroviral mutagenesis of cellular oncogene: a review with insights into the mechanism of insertional activation. Curr. Top. Microbiol. Immunol., 171, 1–25.

Miller, A.D. (1992). Human gene therapy comes of age. Nature, 357, 455–460.

Nusse, R. (1986). The activation of cellular oncogenes by retroviral insertion. Trends Genet., 2, 244–247.

Peters, G. (1991). Inappropriate expression of growth factor genes in tumors induced by mouse mammary tumor virus. Seminars Virol., 2, 319–328.

Rosenberg, S.A. (1992). The immunotherapy and gene therapy of cancer. J. Clin. Oncol., 10, 180–199.

Papers

Almendral, J.M., Sommer, D., MacDonald-Bravo, H., Burckhardt, J., Perera, J. and Bravo, R. (1988). Complexity of the early genetic response to growth factors in mouse fibroblasts. Mol. Cell. Biol., 8, 2140–2148.

Bernhard, W. (1960). The detection and study of tumor viruses with the electron microscope. Cancer Res., 20, 712–727.

Bishop, M.J., Courtneidge, S.A., Levinson, A.D., Oppermann, H., Quintrell, N., Sheiness, D.K., Weiss, S.R. and Varmus, H.E. (1979). Origin and function of avian retrovirus transforming genes. Cold Spring Harbor 39, 919–930.

Boveri, T. (1914). Zur Frage der Entstelung maligner Tumoren. Vol. 1., Gustav Fischer Verlag, Jena.

Cho-Chung, Y.S., Clair, T., Tortora, G., Yokozaki, H. and Pope, S. (1991). Suppression of malignancy targeting the intracellular signal transducing protein of cAMP: the use of site-selective cAMP analogs, antisense strategy, and gene transfer. Life Sci., 48, 1123–1132.

Collett, M.S. and Erikson, R.L. (1978). Protein kinase activity associated with the avian sarcoma virus *src* gene product. Proc. Natl Acad. Sci. USA, 75, 2021–2024.

Collett, M.S., Purchio, A.F. and Erikson, R.L. (1981). Avian sarcoma virus-transforming protein pp60^{src} shows protein kinase activity specific for tyrosine. Nature, 285, 167–169.

Der, C.J., Krontiris, T.G. and Cooper, G.M. (1982). Transforming genes of human bladder and lung carcinoma cell lines are homologous to the *ras* genes of Harvey and Kirsten sarcoma viruses. Proc. Natl Acad. Sci. USA, 79, 3637–3640.

Devilee, P., van Vliet, M., van Sloun, P., Kuipers Dijkshoorn, N., Hermans, J., Pearson, P.L. and Cornelisse, C.J. (1991). Allelotype of human breast carcinoma: a second major site for loss of heterozygosity is on chromosome 6q. Oncogene, 6, 1705–1711.

Ellerman, V. and Bang, O. (1909). Experimentelle Leukamie bei Huhnern. Z. Hyg. Infekt., 62, 231 & Zentralbt. Bacteriol., 46, 595.

Frieben, A. (1902). Cancroid des rechten Handruckens. Fortschritte auf dem Gebiete Rongenstrahlen, 6, 106.

Fried, M. (1965). L-Transforming ability of a temperature-sensitive mutant of polyoma virus. Proc. Natl Acad. Sci. USA, 53, 486–491.

Giancotti, F.G. and Ruoslahti, E. (1990). Elevated levels of the $\alpha_5\beta_1$ fibronectin receptor suppress the transformed phenotype of Chinese hamster ovary cells. Cell, 60, 849–859.

Gomperts, M., Pascall, J.C. and Brown, K.D. (1990). The nucleotide sequence of a cDNA encoding an EGF-inducible gene indicates the existence of a new family of mitogen-induced genes. Oncogene, 5, 1081–1083.

Gonneville, L., Martins, T.J. and Bedard, P.-A. (1991). Complex expression pattern of the CEF-4 cytokine in transformed and mitogenically stimulated cells. Oncogene, 6, 1825–1833.

Hansemann, D. (1890). Uber asymmetrische Zellteilung in Epithelkrebsen und deren biologische Bedeutung. Virchows Archiv fur pathologische Anatomie und Physiologie und fur klinische Medicin, 119, 299–326.

Hijikata, M., Kato, N., Sato, T., Kagami, Y. and Shimotohno, K. (1990). Molecular cloning and characterization of a cDNA for a novel phorbol-12-myristate-13-acetate-responsive gene that is highly expressed in an adult T-cell leukemia cell line. J. Virol., 64, 4632–4639.

Hollingworth, A. and Barton, S. (1988). The natural history of early cervical neoplasia and cervical papillomavirus infection. Cancer Surveys, 7, 519–527.

Huber, B.E., Richards, C.A. and Krenitsky, T.A. (1991). Retroviral-mediated gene therapy for the treatment of hepatocellular carcinoma: an innovative approach for cancer therapy. Proc. Natl Acad. Sci. USA, 88, 8039–8043.

Huebner, R.J. and Todaro, G.J. (1969). Oncogenes of RNA tumor viruses as determinants of cancer. Proc. Natl Acad. Sci. USA, 64, 1087–1094.

Joseph, L.J., Le Beau, M.M., Jamieson, G.A., Acharya, S., Shows, T.B., Rowley, J.D. and Sukhatme, V.P. (1988). Molecular cloning, sequencing, and mapping of EGR2, a human early growth response gene encoding a protein with "zinc-binding finger" structure. Proc. Natl Acad. Sci. USA, 85, 7164–7168.

Leone, A., Flatow, U., King, C.R., Sandeen, M.A., Margulies, I.M.K., Liotta, L.A. and Steeg, P.S. (1991). Reduced tumor incidence, metastatic potential, and cytokine responsiveness of nm23-transfected melanoma cells. Cell, 65, 25–35.

Ma, Q. and Herschman, H.R. (1991). A corrected sequence for the predicted protein from the mitogen-inducible TIS11 primary response gene. Oncogene, 6, 1277–1278.

Martin, G.S. (1970). Rous sarcoma virus: a function required for the maintenance of the transformed state. Nature, 227, 1021–1023.

Minna, J.D. (1988). Autocrine growth factor production, chromosomal deletions and oncogene activation in the pathogenesis of lung cancer. Lung Cancer, 4, P6–P10.

Norris, W. (1820). Case of fungoid disease. Edin. Med. Surg. J., 16, 562–565.

Patwardhan, S., Gashler, A., Siegel, M.G., Chang, L.C., Joseph, L.J., Shows, T.B., Le Beau, M.M. and Sukhatme, V.P. (1991). EGR3, a novel member of the Egr family of genes encoding immediate-early transcription factors. Oncogene, 6, 917–928.

Rollins, B.J. and Sunday, M.E. (1991). Suppression of tumor formation in vivo by expression of the JE gene in malignant cells. Mol. Cell. Biol., 11, 3125–3131.

Rous, P. (1911). A sarcoma of the fowl transmissible by an agent separable from the tumor cells. J. Exp. Med., 13, 397–411.

Ryseck, R.-P., MacDonald-Bravo, H. Zerial, M. and Bravo, R. (1989). Coordinate induction of fibronectin, fibronectin receptor, tropomyosin, and actin genes in serum-stimulated fibroblasts. Exp. Cell Res., 180, 537–545.

Sadano, H., Taniguchi, S. and Baba, T. (1990). Newly identified type of β actin reduces invasiveness of mouse B16 melanoma. FEBS Letts., 271, 23–27.

Shih, C., Shilo, B.-Z., Goldfarb, M.P., Dannenberg, A. and Weinberg, R.A. (1979). Passage of phenotypes of chemically transformed cells via transfection of DNA and chromatin. Proc. Natl Acad. Sci. USA, 76, 5714–5718.

Simmons, D.L., Neel, B.G., Stevens, R., Evett, G. and Erikson, R.L. (1992). Identification of an early-growth-response gene encoding a novel putative protein kinase. Mol. Cell. Biol., 12, 4164–4169.

Smith, S.A., Easton, D.F., Evans, D.G.R. and Ponder, B.A.J. (1992). Allele losses in the region 17q12-21 in familial breast and ovarian cancer involve the wild-type chromosome. Nature Genetics, 2, 128–131.

Srivastava, S., Zou, Z., Pirollo, K., Blattner, W. and Chang, E.H. (1990). Germ-line transmission of a mutated *p53* gene in a cancer-prone family with Li–Fraumeni syndrome. Nature, 348, 747–749.

Stehelin, D., Varmus, H.E., Bishop, M.J. and Vogt, P.K. (1976). DNA related to the transforming gene(s) of avian sarcoma viruses is present in normal avian DNA. Nature, 260, 170–173.

Sukhatme, V.P., Cao, X., Chang, L.C., Tsai-Morris, C.-H., Stamenkovich, D., Ferreira, P.C.P., Cohen, D.R., Edwards, S.A., Shows, T.B., Curran, T., Le Beau, M.M. and Adamson, E.D. (1988). A zinc finger-encoding gene coregulated with c-*fos* during growth and differentiation, and after cellular depolarization. Cell, 53, 37–43.

van Beveren, C., Enami, S., Curran, T. and Verma, I.M. (1984). FBR murine osteosarcoma virus. J. Virol., 135, 229–243.

Wasylyk, B., Wasylyk, C., Flores, P., Begue, A., Leprince, D. and Stehelin, D. (1990). The c-*ets* proto-oncogenes encode transcription factors that cooperate with c-fos and c-jun for transcriptional activation. Nature, 346, 191–193.

Waterfield, M.D., Scrace, G.T., Whittle, N., Stroobant, P., Johnsson, A., Wasteson, A., Westermark, B., Heldin, C.-H., Huang, J.S. and Deuel, T.F. (1983). Platelet-derived growth factor is structurally related to the putative transforming protein p28^{sis} of simian sarcoma virus. Nature, 304, 35–39.

Wright, J.J., Gunter, K.C., Mitsuya, H., Irving, S.G., Kelly, K. and Siebenlist, U. (1990). Expression of a zinc finger gene in HTLV-I and HTLV-II-transformed cells. Science, 248, 588–591.

Zipfel, P.F., Irving, S.G., Kelly, K. and Siebenlist, U. (1989). Complexity of the primary response to mitogenic activation of human T cells. Mol. Cell. Biol., 9, 1041–1048.

CHAPTER 2

Major Categories of Oncogenes

Table 2.1. *Oncogenes transduced by retroviruses*

Gene/locus	Activating virus	Associated tumours
Abl	Ab-MuLV/HZ2-FeSV	T lymphoid/sarcoma
Akt	AKT8	Thymoma
Cbl	Cas NS-1	B lymphomas
Cyl-1	MuLV	Lymphomas
Crk	ASV CT10	Sarcoma
ErbA/ErbB	AEV-ES4	Erythroid
ErbB	ALV/RPL25/RPL28	Erythroid
Ets	AEV-E26	Erythroid
Fgr	GR-FeSV	Sarcoma
Fms	SM-FeSV and HZ5-FeSV	Sarcoma
Fos	FBJ- and FBR-MuSV	Sarcoma
Fps/Fes	FSV	Sarcoma
Jun	ASV 17	T lymphomas
Kit	HZ4-FeSV	Sarcoma
Maf	AS42	Sarcoma
Mos	Mo-MuSV	B-lymphoid/sarcoma
Mpl	MyLV	Erythroid
Myb	MuLV, ALV	B-lymphoid, myeloid
Myc	ALV, MuLV, REV, FeLV	T and B cell lymphomas
Qin	ASV 31	Sarcoma
Raf/Mil/Mht	MuSV	Carcinoma/lymphoma
Hras	ALV	Nephroblastic
Kras	F-MuLV	Erythroid
Rel	REV	B lymphomas
Ros	ASV UR2	Sarcoma
Ryk	RPL30	Sarcoma
Sea	AEV-S13	Erythroid/sarcoma
Sis	SSV	Glioblastoma
Ski	SKV	Carcinoma
Src	RSV	Sarcoma
Yes	Esh and Y73	Sarcoma

AEV: avian erythroblastosis virus; AKT8: leukaemia virus isolated from lymphomatous AKR mice; ALV: avian leukosis virus; ASV: avian sarcoma virus; FeLV: feline leukaemia virus: F-MuLV: Friend murine leukaemia virus; FSV: Fujinami sarcoma virus; GaLV: gibbon ape leukaemia virus; G-MuLV: Gross murine leukaemia virus; GR-FeSV: Gardner–Rasheed feline sarcoma virus; HZ4-FeSV: Hardy–Zuckerman 4 feline sarcoma virus; Mo-MuLV: Moloney murine luekaemia virus; MMTV: mouse mammary tumour virus; MuSV: murine sarcoma virus; MyLV: myeloproliferative luekaemia virus; REV: reticuloendotheliosis virus; RPL30: acute avian retrovirus; RSV: Rous sarcoma virus; SFFV: spleen focus forming virus; SKV: Sloan Kettering virus; SM-FeSV: Susan McDonough feline sarcoma virus; SSV: simian sarcoma virus.

Genes shown in bold type are discussed in individual sections in Chapter 3. For summaries of genes in plain type see Table 2.2 Supplement.

Table 2.2. *Oncogenes activated by retroviral insertion*

Gene/locus	Chromosomal location	Activating virus/System	Associated tumours
A. Mouse mammary tumour virus			
Hst-1/kFGF	7	BR6	Mammary
Wnt-1 (*Int-1*) and *Int-2*	15	BALB/cfC3H; BR6; C3H; GR; GRf; C3Hf; *Mus cervicolor*	Mammary
Int-3	17	BR6; Czech II	Mammary
Wnt-3 (*Int-4*)	11	BALB/cfC3H; GR	Mammary
Int-5	9	BALB/c	Mammary
B. Murine leukaemia viruses			
Ahi-1	10	Mo-MuLV (Abelson)	Pre-B cell
Bla-1	?	Eμ-*Myc* transgenics	B cell
Bmi-1/*Bup*	2	Eμ-*Myc* transgenics	B cell
Pal-1	5	Eμ-*Myc* transgenics	B cell
CSF-1[1]	3	BALB/c eco	Monocytic
Dsi-1	4	Mo-MuLV (rat)	T cell
Evi-2	11	MuLV (BXH-2)	Myeloid
Fim-1	13	F-MuLV	Myeloid
Fim-2/**Fms**	18	F-MuLV	Myeloid
Fim-3 (or *Evi-1* or *CB-1*)	3	F-MuLV	Myeloid
Fis-1 (or *Cyl-1*)	7	F-MuLV	Myeloid, lymphoid
Fli-1	9	F-MuLV	Erythroid
Gin-1	19	Gross A	T cell
Lck	4	Mo-MuLV	T cell
Mlvi-1 (or *Pvt*, *Mis-1* or *RMO-int-1*)	15	AKR, AKXD, Mo-MuLV (rat)	T cell
Mlvi-2, -3, -4	15	Mo-MuLV (rat)	T cell
Myb	10	Mo-MuLV (Abelson); Cas-Br-M	Myeloid NFS-60 cell line
Myc	15	AKR; AKXD, Gross A; MCF247; MCF69L1; Mo-MuLV (rat); Soule; Eμ-Pim-1 transgenics	T cell
Nmyc-1	12	MCF247; Mo-MuLV Eμ-Pim-1 transgenics	T cell
Pim-1	17	AKR; AKXD; MCF247; MCF1233; MCF69L1	T cell
		AKXD	Non-T cell
		ΔMo-MuLV + SV	B-lymphoblastic
Pim-2	17	AKXD; Mo-MuLV; Transplanted	T cell
Hras	7	Mo-MuLV	T cell
Kras	6	F-MuLV	Myeloid
Sic-1	9	Cas-Br-E MuLV	Non-B, non-T cell
Spi-1	2	SFFV	Erythroid
P53	11	F-MuLV; SFFV	Erythroid
		Abelson MuLV	Lymphoid
Tpl-1/**Ets-1**	9	Mo-MuLV	T cell
Vin-1	6	RadLV	T cell
C. Avian retroviruses			
Bic		UR2AV + RAV-2	Lymphomas
Erbb		RAV-1	Erythroblastosis
Myb		RAV-1; EU-8; UR2AV + RAV-2	Lymphomas
Myc		ALV; REV (CSV); RPV	B-lymphomas
		RPV	Adencarcinoma
		REV	T-lymphoma
Nov		MAV1	Myeloblastosis
Hras		MAV	Nephroblastoma
Blym		ALV	B-lymphoma
Rel		ALV	B-lymphoma

Table 2.2. *Continued*

Gene/locus	Activating virus/System	Associated tumours
D. Other systems		
Erythropoietin receptor[2]	SFFV	Erythroid
Flvi-1	FeLV	T cell
His-1, His-2	Cas-Br Mo-MuLV (IL-3-dependent)	Myeloid
Hox-2.4[3]	IAP	WEHI-3B
IL2[4]	GaLV	T cell line
IL3[5]	IAP	WEHI-3B
IL2R[6]	IAP	Lymphoma cell line
Mos	IAP	Plasmacytoma
Myc	IAP	Plasmacytoma
Myc	F-MuLV	T cell
Myc	Retrotransposon	Canine
Pim-1	F-MuLV	T cell

Source: Peters, G. (1990). Oncogenes at viral integration sites. Cell Growth Differ. 1, 503–510.
For abbreviations see Table 2.1; RadLV: BL.VL3 radiation leukaemia virus; IAP: intracisternal A particle.
References for genes shown in bold type are given in the individual sections in Chapter 3. Summaries/references for genes shown in plain type are in Table 2.2 Supplement, except for those with superscript numbers, references for which are as follows:

[1]*CSF-1*: Baumbach, W.R., Colston, E.M. and Cole, M.D. (1988). Integration of the BALB/c ecotropic provirus into the colony-stimulating factor-1 growth factor locus in a *Myc* retrovirus-induced murine monocyte tumor. J. Virol., 62, 3151–3155.

[2]Erythropoietin receptor: Lacombe, C., Chretien, S., Lemarchandel, V., Mayeux, P., Romeo, P.-H., Gisselbrecht, S. and Cartron, J.-P. (1991). Spleen focus-forming virus long terminal repeat insertional activation of the murine erythropoietin receptor gene in the T3Cl-2 Friend leukemia cell line. J. Biol. Chem., 266, 6952–6956.

[3]*Hox-2.4*: Blatt, C., Aberdam, D., Schwartz, R. and Sachs, L. (1988). DNA rearrangement of a homeobox gene in myeloid leukemic cells. EMBO J., 7, 4283–4290.
Kongsuwan, K., Allen, J. and Adams, J.M. (1989). Expression of Hox-2.4 homeobox gene directed by proviral insertion in a myeloid leukemia. Nucleic Acids Res., 17, 1881–1892.

[4]*IL2*: Chen, S.J., Holbrook, N.J., Mitchell, K.F., Vallone, C.A., Greengard, J.S., Crabtree, G.R. and Lin, Y. (1985). A viral long terminal repeat in the interleukin 2 gene of a cell line that constitutively produces interleukin 2. Proc. Natl. Acad. Sci. USA., 82, 7284–7288.

[5]*IL3*: Algate, P.A. and McCubrey, J.A. (1993). Autocrine transformation of hemopoietic cells resulting from cytokine message stabilization after intracisternal A particle transposition. Oncogene, 8, 1221–1232.

[6]*IL2R*: Kono, T., Doi, T., Yamada, G., Hatakeyama, M., Minamoto, S., Tsudo, M., Miyasaka, M., Miyata, T. and Taniguchi, T. (1990). Murine interleukin 2 receptor β chain: dysregulated gene expression in lymphoma line EL-4 caused by proviral insertion. Proc. Natl. Acad. Sci. USA., 87, 1806–1810.
Peters, G. (1990). Oncogenes at viral integration sites. Cell Growth & Differentiation, 1, 503–510.

Table 2.2. Supplement. *Oncogenes activated by retroviral insertion (summaries)*

Ahi-1

Abelson *h*elper *i*ntegration site. Relatively common (16%) integration site in Abelson virus-induced murine, pre-B cell lymphomas. Transcripts from this 53 kb region have not been detected.

Poirer, Y., Kozak, C. and Jolicoeur, P. (1988). Identification of a common helper provirus integration site in Abelson murine leukemia virus-induced lymphoma DNA. J. Virol., 62, 3985–3992.

Bic

Bic is a common integration site in late lymphomas that are often metastatic. Frequent activation of *Bic* and *Myc* within one tumour.

Clurman, B.E. and Hayward, W.S. (1989). Multiple proto-oncogene activations in avian leukosis virus-induced lymphomas: evidence for stage-specific events. Mol. Cell. Biol., 9, 2657–2664.

Bla-1, Bmi-1 and Bup

Bla-1

Integration locus of Mo-MuLV in 14% of B cell lymphomas generated in Eμ-*myc* transgenic mice (van Lohuizen *et al.*, 1991a).

Bmi-1

B cell-specific *Mo-MuLV* integration site *1*. Gene encodes 324 amino acids (expressed protein: 45–47 kDa: predicted 37.5 kDa; Haupt *et al.*, 1991). Mainly nuclear: includes motifs characteristic of transcriptional regulators with an N-terminal putative zinc finger, nuclear import signal (KRRR), helix–loop–helix domain (residues 165–220), three potential *N*-linked glycosylation sites, C-terminal PEST sequences (264–299) and serine-rich domain (van Lohuizen *et al.*, 1991a). Ten exons: major transcript from exon 1a: minor from exon 1b. The sequence predicts one ORF starting in exon 2 (AUG at position 471) and terminating at UAG (position 1444). Integration locus of Mo-MuLV in up to 50% of B cell lymphomas generated in Eμ-*Myc* transgenic mice. Two proviral integration sites detected (positions 297 and 377 in exon 1). Mouse *Bmi-1* has 41% and 34% identity with the *Drosophila Psc* and *Su(z)2* genes, respectively (van Lohuizen *et al.*, 1991b). BMI1 and MEL18 are >60% identical in amino acid sequence (Goebl, 1991).

Sequence of BMI1

```
  (1)   MHRTTRIKITELNPHLMCVLCGGYFIDATTIIECLHSFCKTCIVRYLETSKYCPICDVQV
 (61)   HKTRPLLNIRSDKTLQDIVYKLVPGLFKNEMKRRRDFYAAHPSADAANGSNEDRGEVADE
(121)   EKRIITDDEIISLSIEFFDQSRLDRKVNKEKPKEEVNDKRYLRCPAAMTVMHLRKFLRSK
(181)   MDIPNTFQIDVMYEEEPLKDYYTLMDIAYIYTWRRNGPLPLKYRVRPTCKRMKMSHQRDG
(241)   LTNAGELESDSGSDKANSPAGGVPSTSSCLPSPSTPVQSPHPQFPHISSTMNGTSNSPSA
(301)   NHQSSFASRPRKSSLNGSSATSSG(324)
```

Underlined: zinc finger domain (18–56).

Bup

*Bmi-1 up*stream: gene with at least 7 exons upstream from *Bim-1*. Expression is increased in cell lines compared with normal cells but it is not known whether it contributes to lymphoma-genesis (Haupt *et al.*, 1991).

Goebl, M.G. (1991). The *bmi*-1 and *mel*-18 gene products define a new family of DNA-binding proteins involved in cell proliferation and tumorigenesis. Cell, 66, 623.

Haupt, Y., Alexander, W.S., Barri, G., Klinken, S.P. and Adams, J.M. (1991). Novel zinc finger gene implicated as myc collaborator by retrovirally accelerated lymphomagenesis in Eμ-*myc* transgenic mice. Cell, 65, 753–763.

van Lohuizen, M., Verbeek, S., Scheijen, B., Wientjens, E., van der Gulden, H. and Berns, A. (1991a). Identification of cooperating oncogene in Eμ-*myc* transgenic mice by provirus tagging. Cell, 65, 737–752.

van Lohuizen, M., Frasch, M., Wientjens, E. and Berns, A. (1991b). Sequence similarity between the mammalian *bmi-1* proto-oncogene and the Drosophila regulatory genes *Psc* and *Su(z)2*. Nature, 353, 353–355.

Blym

Originally detected by transfection of NIH 3T3 fibroblasts with DNA from chickens infected with ALV. *Blym* has no homology with known viral oncogenes. A human transforming gene homologue (chromosome 1p32; Diamond *et al.*, 1984) has been isolated from Burkitt's lymphomas (Diamond *et al.*, 1983; Goubin *et al.*, 1983).

Sequence of human BLYM

```
(1)  MTLRGLRLQWRKQLKMRARPCLLEKRKKIVSYISFLLSDLKGTLAIDSLYSLQFAGGN (58)
```

Diamond, A., Cooper, G.M., Fitz, J. and Lane, M.A. (1983). Identification and molecular cloning of the human B-*lym* transforming gene activated in Burkitt's lymphomas. Nature, 305, 112–116.

Diamond, A., Devine, J.M. and Cooper, G.A. (1984). Nucleotide sequence of a human *Blym* transforming gene activated in Burkitt's lymphoma. Science, 225, 516–519.

Goubin, G., Goldman, D.S., Luce, J., Neiman, P.E. and Cooper, G.M. (1983). Molecular cloning and nucleotide sequence of a transforming gene detected by transfection of chicken B-cell lymphoma DNA. Nature, 302, 114–119.

Dsi-1

A 13.5 kb region with proviral insertions in 10–20% of Mo-MuLV-induced thymomas in rats.

Vijaya, S., Steffen, D.L., Kozak, C. and Robinson, H.L. (1987). *dsi*-1, a region with frequent proviral insertions in Moloney murine leukemia virus-induced rat thymomas. J. Virol., 61, 1164–1170.

Evi-2

Ecotropic viral integration site 2. Evi-2 defines a cluster of viral integration sites. Within this region there is a potential 223 amino acid ORF (24 kDa): this putative proto-oncogene encodes a transmembrane glycoprotein, the hydrophobic region including a leucine zipper domain. The 5′ exon of *Evi-2B* (homologous to human *EVI2B*, 17q11.2), lies approximately 2.8 kb from the 3′ end of *Evi-2A*, in the midst of a cluster of viral integration sites identified in retrovirus-induced myeloid tumours; thus, *Evi-2B* may function as an oncogene in these tumours. The human homologue of *Evi-2* is tightly linked to the neurofibromatosis locus and may thus be involved in human disease (see **Tumour Suppressor Genes: NF1**). Altered expression of *Evi-2* may predispose cells to myeloid disease.

Some viral integrations produce premature termination of *Evi-2* mRNA but most leave the *Evi-2* coding region intact and appear to alter expression either through an enhancer mechanism or by the insertion of viral LTRs. Double viral integrations may occur in *Evi-2*, as also in other common integration sites including *P53*, *Ahi-1*, *Mlvi-1*, *Mlvi-2* and *Pvt-1*.

Ben-David, Y., Prideaux, V.R., Chow, V., Benchimol, S. and Bernstein, A. (1988). Inactivation of the p53 oncogene by internal deletion or retroviral integration in erythroleukemic cell lines induced by Friend leukemia virus. Oncogene, 3, 179–185.

Buchberg, A.M., Bedigian, H.G., Jenkins, N.A. and Copeland, N.G. (1990). *Evi-2*, a common integration site involved in murine myeloid leukemogenesis. Mol. Cell. Biol., 10, 4658–4666.

Graham, M., Adams, J.M. and Cory, S. (1985). Murine T lymphomas with retroviral inserts in the chromosomal 15 locus for plasmacytoma variant translocations. Nature, 314, 740–743.

Hicks, G.G. and Mowat, M. (1988). Integration of Friend murine leukemia virus into both alleles of the p53 oncogene in an erythroleukemia cell line. J. Virol., 62, 4752–4755.

Poirer, Y., Kozak, C. and Jolicoeur, P. (1988). Identification of a common helper provirus integration site in Abelson murine leukemia virus-induced lymphoma DNA. J. Virol., 62, 3985–3992.

Tsichlis, P.N., Strauss, P.G. and Lohse, M.A. (1985). Concerted DNA rearrangements in Moloney murine leukemia virus-induced thymomas: a potential synergistic relationship in oncogenesis. J. Virol., 56, 258–267.

Fis-1

The *Fis-1* integration site is <300 kb from the 5' end of the mouse *Cyl-1* (cyclin D1) locus and the 3' end of *Cyl-1* is ~75 kb from *Hst-1* and *Int-2*. Viral integrations in this region may be functionally equivalent to the *BCL1* translocations (see ***BCL1***) that activate cyclin D1 expression in some human B cell malignancies.

Lammie, G.A., Smith, R., Silver, J., Brookes, S., Dickson, C. and Peters, G. (1992). Proviral insertions near cyclin D1 in mouse lymphomas: a parallel for BCL1 translocations in human B-cell neoplasms. Oncogene, 7, 2381–2387.

Silver, J. and Kozak, C. (1986). Common proviral integration region on mouse chromosome 7 in lymphomas and myelogenous leukemias induced by Friend murine leukaemia virus. J. Virol., 57, 526–533.

Fim

Friend integration myeloid. Fim-1 (human homologue *FIM1*, 6p23–p22.3). No RNA product has been detected. *Fim-2* spans the 5' end of the *Fms* (colony stimulating factor 1 receptor (*CSF1R*)) gene (Buchberg *et al.*, 1989). *Fim-3* (also called *CB-1* or *Evi-1* (ecotropic viral integration site *1*) is the site of retroviral insertion in ~15% of murine myeloid leukaemias. Transcription is activated by retroviral insertion in either of two 5' non-coding exons. Alternative splicing generates 4.7 kb and 5.7 kb mRNAs encoding 718 and 1072 amino acids, respectively (Bordereaux *et al.*, 1990). The larger (120 kDa) protein contains ten zinc finger motifs in two domains 380 amino acids apart and an acidic domain located C-terminal to the zinc fingers. The 718 residue protein lacks the sixth and seventh zinc fingers of p120. EVI1 binds to the synthesized consensus sequence TGACAAGATAA (Perkins *et al.*, 1991). Expression: oocyte development: not in normal haematopoietic cells.

The human homologue (*EVI1*, chromosome 3q26, 5.3/6.0 kb mRNA) is 94% homologous in amino acid sequence (145 kDa) to mouse EVI1. High levels are expressed in human endometrial carcinoma cells. An alternatively spliced form has a 315 amino acid deletion that includes both zinc fingers. In acute myelogenous leukaemia (AML) transformation and inhibition of differentiation of myeloid cells *EVI1* can be activated by chromosomal translocation (Bartholomew and Ihle, 1991; Morishita *et al.*, 1992).

Sequence of EVI1/FIM3

```
 (1)   MKSEEDPHEPMAPDIHEERQHRCEDCDQLFESKAELADHQKFPCSTPHSAFSMVEEDLQQ
(61)   NLESESDLREIHGNQDCKECDRVFPDLQSLEKHMLSHTEEREYKCDQCPKAFNWKSNLIR
(121)  HQMSHDSGKHYECENCAKVFTDPSNLQRHIRSQHVGARAHACPECGKTFATSSGLKQHKH
```

```
 (181)   IHSSVKPFICEVCHKSYTQFSNLCRHKRMHADCRTQIKCKDCGQMFSTTSSLNKHRRFCE
 (241)   GKNHFAAGGFFGQGISLPGTPAMDKTSMVNMSHANPGLADYFGTNRHPAGLTFPTAPGFS
 (301)   FSFPGLFPSGLYHRPPLIPASPPVKGLSSTEQSNKCQSPLLTHPQILPATQDILKALSKH
 (361)   PPVGDNKPVELLPERSSEERPLEKISDQSESSDLDDVSTPSGSDLETTSGSDLESDLESD
 (421)   KEKCKENGKMFKDKVSPLQNLASITNKKEHNNHSVFSASVEEQSAVSGAVNDSIKAIASI
 (481)   AEKYFGSTGLVGLQDKKVGALPYPSMFPLPFFPAFSQSMYPFPDRDLRSLPLKMEPQSPS
 (541)   EVKKLQKGSSESPFDLTTKRKDEKPLTSGPSKPSGTPATSQDQPLDLSMGSRGRASGTKL
 (601)   TEPRKNHVFGEKKGSNMDTRPSSDGSLQHARPTPFFMDPIYRVEKRKLTDPLEALKEKYL
 (661)   RPSPGFLFHPQMSAIENMAEKLESFSALKPEASELLQSVPSMFSFRAPPNTLPENLLRKG
 (721)   KERYTCRYCGKIFPRSANLTRHLRTHTGEQPYRCKYCDRSFSISSNLQRHVRNIHNKEKP
 (781)   FKCHLCDRCFGQQTNLDRHLKKHENGNMSGTATSSPHSELESAGAILDDKEDAYFTEIRN
 (841)   FIGNSNHGSQSPRNMEERMNGSHFKDKKALATSQNSDLLDDEEVEDEVLLDEEDEDNDIP
 (901)   GKPRKELGVTRLDEEIPEDDYEEAGALEMSCKASPVRYKEEDYKSGLSALDHIRHFTDSL
 (961)   KMREMEENQYTDAELSSISSSHVPEELKQTLHRKSKSQAYAMMLSLSDKDSLHPTSHSSS
(1021)   NVWHSMARAAAESSAIQSISHV(1042)
```

Underlined: zinc finger domains (21–44, 75–97, 103–125, 131–154, 160–182, 188–210, 217–239, 724–746, 752–775, 781–803). Italics: acidic domain (877–928).

Bartholomew, C. and Ihle, J.N. (1991). Retroviral insertions 90 kilobases proximal to the *Evi-1* myeloid transforming gene activate transcription from the normal promoter. Mol. Cell. Biol., 11, 1820–1828.
Bordereaux, D., Fichelson, S., Tambourin, P. and Gisselbrecht, S. (1990). Alternative splicing of the *Evi-1* zinc finger gene generates mRNAs which differ by the number of zinc finger motifs. Oncogene, 5, 925–927.
Buchberg, A.M., Jenkins, N.A. and Copeland, N.G. (1989). Localization of the murine macrophage colony-stimulating factor gene to chromosome 3 using interspecific backcross analysis. Genomics, 5, 363–367.
Buchberg, A.M., Bedigian, H.G., Jenkins, N.A. and Copeland, N.G. (1990). *Evi-2*, a common integration site involved in murine myeloid leukemogenesis. Mol. Cell. Biol., 10, 4658–4666.
Morishita, K., Parker, D.S., Mucenski, M.L., Jenkins, N.A., Copeland, N.G. and Ihle, J.N. (1988). Retroviral activation of a novel gene encoding a zinc finger protein in IL-3-dependent myeloid leukemia cell lines. Cell, 54, 831–840.
Morishita, K., Paganas, E., Douglas, E.C. and Ihle, J.N. (1990). Unique expression of the human *Evi-1* gene in an endometrial carcinoma cell line: sequence of cDNAs and structure of alternatively spliced transcripts. Oncogene, 5, 963–971.
Morishita, K., Parganas, E., Willman, C.L., Whittaker, M.H., Drabkin, H., Oval, J., Taetle, R., Valentine, M.B. and Ihle, J.N. (1992). Activation of *EVI1* gene expression in human acute myelogenous leukemias by translocations spanning 300–400 kilobases on chromosome band 3q26. Proc. Natl Acad. Sci. USA, 89, 3937–3941.
Perkins, A.S., Fishel, R., Jenkins, N.A. and Copeland, N.G. (1991). *Evi-1*, a murine zinc finger proto-oncogene, encodes a sequence-specific DNA-binding protein. Mol. Cell. Biol., 11, 2665–2674.
Sola, B., Fichelson, S., Bordereaux, D., Tambourin, P.E. and Gisselbrecht, S. (1986). *fim-1* and *fim-2*: two new integration regions of Friend murine leukemia virus in myeloblastic leukemias. J. Virol., 60, 718–725.
Sola, B., Simon, D., Mattei, M.-G., Fichelson, S., Bordereaux, D., Tambourin, P.E., Guenet, J.-L. and Gisselbrecht, S. (1988). *fim-1*, *fim-2/c-fms*, and *fim-2*, three common integration sites of Friend murine leukemia virus in myeloblastic leukemias, map to mouse chromosomes 13, 18, and 3, respectively. J. Virol., 62, 3973–3978.

Fli-1, Fli-2

Friend *l*eukaemia *i*ntegration-*1*, -*2*. Genes flanking common integration sites for F-MuLV or SFFV. *Fli-1* encodes a member of the *Ets* family (Sels *et al.*, 1992). cDNA adjacent to *Fli-2* is homologous to human RNP A1 (RNA binding protein) involved in RNA splicing and is inactivated in an erythroleukaemia cell line. *Fli-1* is activated in 75% of erythroleukaemias induced by Friend murine leukaemia virus. Human FLI1 encodes a 452 amino acid protein that is 85% homologous to ERG2 (see ETS). The 5′ ETS homology domain of this protein is shared only by FLI1, c-ETS1, ETS2, GABPα and ERG (Ben-David *et al.*, 1991; Prasad *et al.*, 1992).

Ben-David, Y., Giddens, E.B., Letwin, K. and Bernstein, A. (1991). Erythroleukemia induction by Friend murine leukemia virus: insertional activation of a new member of the *ets* gene family, *fli-1*, closely linked to c-*ets*-1. Genes Devel., 5, 908–918.

Prasad, D.D., Rao, Y.N. and Reddy, E.S. (1992). Structure and expression of human *fli-1* gene. Cancer Res., 52, 5833–5837.

Sels, F.T., Langer, S., Schulz, A.S., Silver, J., Sitbon, M. and Friedrich, R.W. (1992). Friend murine leukemia virus is integrated at a common site in most primary spleen tumours of erythroleukemic animals. Oncogene, 7, 643–652.

Flvi-1

Flvi-1 is the only locus other than *Myc* at which FeLV proviral integration has been detected in multiple, independent tumours, integrations occurring over a 2.4 kb region of *Flvi-1*. Integration is in the same transcriptional orientation with respect to the *Flvi-1* locus but *Flvi-1* transcripts have not been isolated. The murine homologue of *Flvi-1* (chromosome 2) is adjacent to *Spi-1*.

Levesque, K.S., Bonham, L. and Levy, L.S. (1990). *flvi-1*, a common integration domain for feline leukemia virus in naturally occurring lymphomas of a particular type. J. Virol., 64, 3455–3462.

Levesque, K.S., Mattei, M.-G. and Levy, L.S. (1991). Evolutionary conservation and chromosomal localization of *flvi-1*. Oncogene, 6, 1377–1379.

Gin-1

Represents a 26 kb region that is a common integration site of Gross A MuLV in T cell lymphomas.

Villemur, R., Monzak, Y., Rassart, E., Kozak, C. and Jolicoeur, P. (1987). Identification of a new common provirus integration site in Gross passage A murine leukemia virus-induced mouse thymoma DNA. Mol. Cell. Biol., 7, 512–522.

His-1

His-1 maps near the proximal breakpoint for a deletion observed in >90% of radiation-induced leukaemias. The human *HIS1* locus maps to chromosome 2q14–q21.

Askew, D.S., Bartholomew, C., Buchberg, A.M., Valentine, M.B., Jenkins, N.A., Copeland, N.G. and Ihle, J.N. (1991). *His*-1 and *His*-2: identification and chromosomal mapping of two commonly rearranged sites of viral integration in a myeloid leukemia. Oncogene, 6, 2041–2047.

Int-3

2.4 kb mRNA, 552 amino acids, 57 kDa. Integration occurs within the transcription unit of *Int-3* whereas activation of *Wnt-1/Int-1*, *Int-2*, *Hst-1* or *Wnt-3/Int-4* by MMTV does not perturb the coding regions (Gallahan *et al.*, 1987). Murine *Int-3* contains motifs related to those in *S. cerevisiae cdc*10 that are ~50% identical to an intracellular region of *Drosophila notch* (Robbins *et al.*, 1992). *Int-3* transforms mouse mammary epithelial cells (Robbins *et al.*, 1992).

Gallahan, D. and Callahan, R. (1987). Mammary tumorigenesis in feral mice: identification of a new *int* locus in mouse mammary tumor virus (Czech II)-induced mammary tumors. J. Virol., 61, 66–74.

Gallahan, D., Kozak, C. and Callahan, R. (1987). A new common integration region (*int*-3) for mouse mammary tumor virus on mouse chromosome 17. J. Virol., 61, 218–220.

Robbins, J., Blondel, B.J., Gallahan, D. and Callahan, R. (1992). Mouse mammary tumor gene *int*-3: a member of the *notch* gene family transforms mammary epithelial cells. J. Virol., 66, 2594–2599.

Int-5

Integration site of MMTV in three chemically induced mammary hyperplasias. The region encodes 3.3 and 4.0 kb mRNAs. The sequence is highly conserved in several mammalian species including man and appears to be involved in early events in some *in vivo* models of chemical carcinogenesis.

Morris, V.L., Rao, T.R., Kozak, C.A., Gray, D.A., Lee Chan, E.C.M., Cornell, T.J., Taylor, C.B., Jones, R.F. and McGrath, C.M. (1991). Characterization of *int*-5, a locus associated with early events in mammary carcinogenesis. Oncogene Res., 6, 53–63.

Mlvi-1, Mlvi-2 and Mlvi-3

Mlvi-1 defines the region to which Ig domains are translocated in the less frequent forms of murine plasmacytoma. *Mlvi-1* (also denoted *Pvt-1* (plasmacytoma *variant translocation*), RMO-*int*-1) is a common Mo-MuLV proviral integration site in murine thymomas, equivalent to *Mis-1* (Moloney *integration site-1*) in rats and the human *Pvt-1*-like region that maps to 8q24 (Villeneuve *et al.*, 1986). t(2;8) Burkitt's lymphoma variants involve the *Pvt-1*-like region that maps 100–500 kb 3' of *MYC* (Mengle-Gaw and Rabbitts, 1987) and murine *Mlvi-1* maps 270 kb 3' of *Myc*. A tumour-specific RNA (~10 kb) is present in tumours carrying a provirus in *Mlvi-1* (Tsichlis *et al.*, 1989).

Mlvi-2 and *Mlvi-3* are additional common proviral integration domains identified in virus-induced rat thymic lymphomas (Kozak *et al.*, 1985). Present on different chromosomes in rat, *Mlvi-1* and *Mlvi-2* are both rearranged in some tumours. The murine homologues of *Mlvi-1* and *Mlvi-2* map to distinct regions of chromosome 15.

Copeland, N.G. and Jenkins, N.A. (1990). Retroviral integration in murine myeloid tumors to identify *evi-1*, a novel locus encoding a zinc-finger protein. Adv. Cancer Res., 54, 141–157.

Graham, M., Adams, J.M. and Cory, S. (1985). Murine T lymphomas with retroviral inserts in the chromosomal 15 locus for plasmacytoma variant translocations. Nature, 314, 740–743.

Kozak, C.A., Strauss, P.G. and Tsichlis, P.N. (1985). Genetic mapping of a cellular DNA region involved in induction of thymic lymphomas (*Mlvi-1*) to mouse chromosome 15. Mol. Cell. Biol., 5, 894–897.

Lemay, G. and Jolicoeur, P. (1984). Rearrangement of a DNA sequence homologous to a cell-virus junction fragment in several Moloney murine leukemia virus-induced rat thymomas. Proc. Natl Acad. Sci. USA, 81, 38–42.

Mengle-Gaw, L. and Rabbitts, T.H. (1987). A human chromosome 8 region with abnormalities in B cell, HTLV-1[+] T cell and c-*myc* amplified tumours. EMBO J., 6, 1959–1965.

Mucenski, M.L., Gilbert, D.J., Taylor, B.A., Jenkins, N.A. and Copeland, N.G. (1987). Common sites of viral integration in lymphomas arising in AKXD recombinant inbred mouse strains. Oncogene Res., 2, 33–48.

Tsichlis, P.N., Shepherd, B.M. and Bear, S.E. (1989). Activation of the *mlvi-1/mis*1/*pvt*-1 locus in Moloney murine leukemia virus-induced T-cell lymphomas. Proc. Natl Acad. Aci. USA, 86, 5487–5491.

Villeneuve, L., Rassart, E., Jolicoeur, P., Graham, M. and Adams, J.M. (1986). Proviral integration site *Mis-1* in rat thymomas corresponds to the *pvt*-1 translocation breakpoint in murine plasmacytomas. Mol. Cell. Biol., 6, 1834–1837.

Mlvi-4

Maps 30 kb 3' of *Myc* between *Myc* and *Mlvi-1*. Proviral insertion at *Mlvi-4* activates transcription of a gene transcribed in the same orientation as *Myc* giving rise to 3.0 and 10.0 kb mRNAs. Low levels of 3.0 and 5.5 kb *Mlvi-4* transcripts are present in normal thymus and spleen.

Tsichlis, P.N., Lee, J.S., Bear, S.E., Lazo, P.A., Patriotis, C., Gustafson, E., Shinton, S., Jenkins, N.A., Copeland, N.G., Huebner, K., Croce, C., Levan, G. and Hanson, C. (1990). Activation of multiple genes by provirus integration in the *mlvi-4* locus in T-cell lymphomas induced by Moloney murine leukemia virus. J. Virol., 64, 2236–2244.

Nov

Nov encodes a putative 32 kDa secreted chicken protein. *Nov* is not transcribed in adult kidney cells but is activated by proviral insertion of myeloblastosis-associated virus type 1 (MAV1). The expression of the N-terminal truncated product of *Nov* transforms chicken embryo fibroblasts *in vitro* (Joliot *et al.*, 1992). The homologous human locus maps to chromosome 8q24.1 and another homologous human gene (connective tissue growth factor, *CTGF*) is located on chromosome 6q23.1 proximal to *MYB* (Martinerie *et al.*, 1992).

Joliot, V., Martinerie, C., Dambrine, G., Plassiart, G., Brisac, M., Crochet, J. and Perbal, B. (1992). Proviral rearrangements and overexpression of a new cellular gene (*nov*) in myeloblastosis-associated virus type 1-induced nephroblastomas. Mol. Cell. Biol., 12, 10–21.

Martinerie, C., Viegas-Pequignot, E., Guenard, I., Dutrillaux, B., Nguyen, V.C., Bernheim, A. and Perbal, B. (1992). Physical mapping of human loci homologous to the chicken *nov* proto-oncogene. Oncogene, 7, 2529–2534.

Pal-1

Integration locus of Mo-MuLV in 38% of B cell lymphomas generated in Eμ-*Myc* transgenic mice.

van Lohuizen, M., Verbeek, S., Scheijen, B., Wientjens, E., van der Gulden, H. and Berns, A. (1991). Identification of cooperating oncogene in Eμ-*myc* transgenic mice by provirus tagging. Cell, 65, 737–752.

Pim-2

In primary tumours integration near *Pim-2* is rare but is common in subclones obtained by transplantation of primary tumour cells. Insertion near *Pim-2* is thus a late event in tumour progression, frequently preceded by insertion near the *Myc* and *Pim-1* loci.

Breuer, M.L., Cuypers, H.T. and Berns, A. (1989). Evidence for the involvement of *pim-2*, a new common proviral insertion site, in progression of lymphomas. EMBO J., 8, 743–747.

Spi-1

SFFV proviral integration (or *sfpi-1*). The Friend virus complex includes an acutely oncogenic, replication defective component, SFFV. In SFFV it is the recombinant *env* gene, rather than a transduced cellular gene, that is the transforming agent. Erythroid tumours frequently contain the SFFV provirus integrated within the *Spi-1* domain. *Spi-1* encodes a 1.4 kb mRNA the predicted product of which is identical to the macrophage and B cell-specific transcription factor PU.1 (Moreau-Gachelin *et al.*, 1990; Paul *et al.*, 1991).

The *ETS*-related PU.1 is involved in differentiation and binds to the PU box (5'-CCGAGGAA-3'; Goebl *et al.*, 1990). The human homologue (11p12–p11.2; mRNA 1.4 kb) is expressed in a wide range of carcinomas and sarcomas (Ray *et al.*, 1990). Human PU.1 activates transcription from the *CD11b* promoter, a gene encoding an integrin cell surface receptor that is expressed on mature monocytes, macrophages, granulocytes and natural killer cells (Pahl *et al.*, 1993). Human SPIB is 43% identical in protein sequence to SPI1 and also contains an ETS DNA binding domain. *SPIB* (and the murine homologue) is expressed in a variety of haematopoietic cell lines (Ray *et al.*, 1992).

Sequences of human and mouse SPI1

```
Human SPI1 (1)    MEGFPLVPPPSEDLVPYDTDLYQRQTHEYYPYLSSDGESHSDHYWDFHPHHVHSEFESF
Mouse SPI1 (1)    ----S-TA---D---T--SE----PM-D--SFVG------------SA----NNEFEN

          (60)    AENN FTELQSVQPPQLQQLYRHMELEQMHVLDTPMVPPHPSLG HQVSYLP RMCLQYP
          (60)    FPE-H-----------------------------------TGLS------MR---FP-Q

         (117)    SLSPA QPSSDEEEGERQSPPLEVSDGEADGLEPGPGLLPGETGSKKKIRLYQFLLDLLR
         (120)    T----HQQ---------------------------------H-----------------

         (176)    SGDMKDSIWWVDKDKGTFQFSSKHKEALAHRWGIQKGNRKKMTYQKMARALRNYGKTGEV
         (180)    -----------------------------------------------------------

         (236)    KKVKKKLTYQFSGEVLGRGGLAERRHPPH (264 amino acids; M_r 30 408)
         (240)    -----------------------L--- (266 amino acids; M_r 30 674)
```

Underlined: the human ETS domain 159–247.

Goebl, M.G., Klemsz, M.J., McKercher, S.R, Celada, A., van Beveren, C. and Maki, R.A. (1990). The PU.1 transcription factor is the product of the putative oncogene *spi-1*. Cell, 61, 1165–1166.

Moreau-Gachelin, F., Ray, D., Tambourin, P. and Tavitian, A. (1990). The putative oncogene SPI-1 encodes a transcription factor. Oncogene 5, 941.

Pahl, H.L., Scheibe, R.J., Zhang, D.-E., Chen, H.-M., Galson, D.L., Maki, R.A. and Tenen, D.G. (1993). The proto-oncogene PU.1 regulates expression of the myeloid-specific CD11b promoter. J. Biol. Chem., 268, 5014–5020.

Paul, R., Schuetze, S., Kozak, S.L., Kozak, C.A. and Kabat, D. (1991). The *Sfpi-1* proviral integration site of Friend erythroleukemia encodes the *ets*-related transcription factor Pu.1. J. Virol., 65, 464–467.

Ray, D., Culine, S., Tavitian, A. and Moreau-Gachelin, F. (1990). The human homologue of the putative proto-oncogene Spi-1: characterization and expression in tumors. Oncogene, 5, 663–668.

Ray, D., Bosselut, R., Ghysdael, J., Mattei, M.-G., Tavitian, A. and Moreau-Gachelin, F. (1992). Characterization of Spi-B, a transcription factor related to the putative oncoprotein Spi-1/PU.1. Mol. Cell. Biol., 12, 4297–4304.

Tpl-1

Tpl-1 (tumour progression locus 1) lies 1.2 cM from *Ets-1* and is activated by MoMuLV in rat thymomas. Although the genes are distinct, they are closely related.

Bear, S.E., Bellacosa, A., Lazo, P.A., Jenkins, N.A., Copeland, N.G., Hanson, C., Levan, G. and Tsichlis, P.N. (1989). Provirus insertion in *tpl-1*, an *ets*-1-related oncogene, is associated with tumor progression in Moloney murine leukemia virus-induced rat thymic lymphomas. Proc. Natl Acad. Sci. USA, 86, 7495–7499.

Vin-1

Integration region in ~5% of RadLV-induced thymomas. Proviral integration is at the 5′ end of the first coding exon and in opposite transcriptional orientation to the *Vin-1* gene. The human homologue of *Vin-1* is cyclic D2 that maps to chromosome 12.

Hanna, Z., Jankowski, M., Tremblay, P., Jiang, X., Milatovich, A., Francke, U. and Jolicoeur, P. (1993). The *Vin-1* gene, identified by proviral insertional mutagenesis, is the cyclin D2. Oncogene, 8, 1661–1666.
Tremblay, P.J., Kozak, C.A. and Jolicoeur, P. (1992). Identification of a novel gene, *vin-1*, in murine leukemia virus-induced T-cell leukemias by provirus insertional mutagenesis. J. Virol., 66, 1344–1353 and 5176.

Databank file names and accession numbers

	GENE	*EMBL*	*SWISSPROT*	*REFERENCES*
Mouse	*Bmi-1*	Mmbmi1 M64067 Mmbmi1b M64068	BMI1_MOUSE P25916	Haupt *et al.*, 1991
	Mo-MuLV integration site	Mmbmi1a M64279		van Lohuizen *et al.*, 1991b
Mouse	*Evi-1*	Mmev1 M64494 Mm2fp M21829	EVI1_MOUSE P14404	Bartholomew and Ihle, 1991 Morishita *et al.*, 1988
Mouse	*Int-3*	Mmin3mam M80456		Robbins *et al.*, 1992
Human	*BLYM1*	Hsblym1 K01884	TBLV_HUMAN P01124	Diamond *et al.*, 1984
Human	*SPI1* (PU.1)	Hsspi1 X52056	PU1_HUMAN P17947	Ray *et al.*, 1990 Moreau-Gachelin *et al.*, 1990
Mouse	*Spi-1* (PU.1)	Mmspi14 X17463 Mmpu1 M32370 Mmsfpi1 M38252	PU1_MOUSE P17433	Moreau-Gachelin *et al.*, 1989, 1990 Klemsz *et al.*, 1990 Paul *et al.*, 1991

Table 2.3. *Oncogenes at chromosomal translocations*

ABL	BCR
AML1	*ETO*
BCL1, BCL2, BCL3	Immunoglobulin heavy chain
BTG1	Deletion
CAN	*DEK/SET*
FLI1	*EWS*
HOX11	T cell receptor β/δ chain
IL2	*BCM*
IL3	Immunoglobulin heavy chain
LYL1	T cell receptor β chain
MLL (ALL1)	*AF4/AF9/ENL*
MYC	Immunoglobulin loci
PBX1 (PRL)	*E2A*
PLZF	*RARA*
PML	*RARA*
RBTN1	T cell receptor δ chain
RBTN2	T cell receptor δ chain
SIL	***TAL1***
TAL1	T cell receptor α/β chain
TAL2	T cell receptor β chain
TAN1	Deletion

Table 2.3. Supplement. *Oncogenes at chromosomal translocations*

Chimeric genes

Gene   *PBX1/PRL* (1q23)   *Translocation*   t(1;19)(q23;p13.3)   *Leukaemia*   Pre-B ALL
E2A (19p13.3)

E2A normally encodes the related helix–loop–helix transcription factors E12 and E47 (3.5 kb mRNA ubiquitously expressed). The 1;19 translocation in many pre-B acute lymphoblastic leukaemias links the 5′ coding portion of *E2A* to the homeobox gene *PBX1* (pre B-cell leukaemia transcription factor 1). The fusion protein contains 484 E2A amino acids and either 259 or 342 PBX1 amino acids. E2A–PBX1 may therefore contribute to the pathogenesis of leukaemia (Visvader *et al.*, 1991).

Sequences of PBX proteins

```
PBX1a  (1)   MDEQ    PRLMHSHAGVGM AGHP   GLSQHLQDGAGGTEGEGG     RKQDIGDILQQIMTITDQSLD
PBX2   (1)   ---RLLGP-PPGGGRG-L-LVS-E-   -GPGEPPG-GDPGG-S--VPGGRG-------------------
PBX3a  (1)   --D-    S-MLQTL---NL ---SVQG-MALPPPPHGHEGADGD-    ---------H-----------
PBX1b  (1)   ----    ----------- ----   -----------------     ---------------------
PBX3b  (1)   --D-    S-MLQTL---NL ---SVQG-MALPPPPHGHEGADGD-    ---------H-----------

PBX1a  (60)  EAQARKHALNCHRMKPALFNVLCEIKEKTVLSIRGAQEEEPTDPQLMRLDNMLLAEGVAG
PBX2   (70)  ----K-------------S---------G----SS-----V----------------
```

```
PBX3a   (63)   ----K--------------S---------G---------D-P---------------S-
PBX1b   (60)   ------------------------------------------------------------
PBX3b   (63)   ----K--------------S---------G---------D-P---------------S-

PBX1a  (120)   PEKGGGSAAAAAAAAASGGAGS DNSVEHSDYRAKLSQIRQIYHTELEKYEQACNEFTTHV
PBX2   (130)   ------------------GV-P---I------S--A---H---S--------------
PBX3a  (123)   ------------------S- ---I---------T----------------------
PBX1b  (120)   ------------------ ------------------------------------
PBX3b  (123)   ------------------S- ---I---------T----------------------

PBX1a  (180)   MNLLREQSRTRPISPKEIERMVSIIHRKFSSIQMQLKQSTCEAVMILRSRFLDARRKRRNF
PBX2   (181)   -------------VA---M-----------A------------------------------
PBX3a  (183)   --------------------G---------------------------------------
PBX1b  (180)   ------------------------------------------------------------
PBX3b  (183)   --------------------G---------------------------------------

PBX1a  (241)   NKQATEILNEYFYSHLSNPYPSEEAKEELAKKCGITVSQVSNWFGNKRIRYKKNIGKFQEE
PBX2   (242)   S-----V-----------------------------------------------------
PBX3a  (244)   S-------------------------------------S----------------------
PBX1b  (241)   ------------------------------------------------------------
PBX3b  (244)   S-------------------------------------S----------------------

PBX1a  (302)   ANIYAAKTAVTATNVSA   HGSQANSPSTPNSAGSSSSFNMSNSGDLFMSVQSLNGDSYQ
PBX2   (303)   -----V----SV-QGGH    -RTS--TP-S----GG---L-G---M-LGMPG------S
PBX3a  (305)   --L---------AHAV-AAVQNN-T---T---- ---G---LP----M--NM---------
PBX1b  (302)   ----------------    --------------GYPSPCYQPDRRIQ (347)
PBX3b  (305)   --L---------AHAV-AAVQNN-T---T---- ----PS---S-G-L- (351)

PBX1a  (360)   GAQVGANVQSQVDTLRHVISQTGGYSDGLAASQMYSPQGISANGGWQDATTPSSVTSPTEGPGSVHSDTSN (430)
PBX2   (359)   A          ---ES---SMG P---G-N-GGG-I---REMR---S--E-V-------------------- (430)
PBX3a  (365)   -S---------------------N---------GGNSL---HNLN------------------------- (434)
```

Dashes indicate identity with PBX1a except for the PBX3b sequence after residue 332 when the comparison is with PBX1b (Monica *et al.*, 1991).

Kamps, M.P., Murre, C., Sun, X.-H. and Baltimore, D. (1990). A new homeobox gene contributes the DNA binding domain of the t(1;19) translocation protein in pre-B ALL. Cell, 60, 547–555.

Monica, K., Galili, N., Nourse, J., Saltman, D. and Cleary, M.L. (1991). *PBX2* and *PBX3*, new homeobox genes with extensive homology to the human proto-oncogene *PBX1*. Mol. Cell. Biol., 11, 6149–6157.

Visvader, J., Begley, C.G. and Adams, J.M. (1991). Differential expression of the LYL, SCL and E2A helix–loop–helix genes within the hemopoietic system. Oncogene, 6, 187–194.

Gene   PML (15q21)   *Translocation*   t(15;17) (q21;q11–22)   *Leukaemia*   APL
RARA (17q21)

The reciprocal translocation results in a fusion between the retinoic acid receptor α gene (17q21) and the *PML* (*p*romyelocytic *l*eukaemia) gene on chromosome 15. The normal *PML* gene comprised of 9 exons (2.8 kb DNA) is alternatively spliced giving rise to numerous isoforms (48–98 kDa) with differing C-termini (Fagioli *et al.*, 1992). *PML* is one of a family of genes encoding putative transcription factors (containing "The Cysteine Chapel Motif", C_3HC_4) that includes *Bmi-1, Mel-18* and *Rag-1*.

Structures of RARA, RARB, RARG *and* PML *and* PML–RARA

Chimeric isoforms (797/955 amino acids, 90/106 kDa) having 394/552 amino acids from PML in place of the first 59 of the RARA N-terminus have been described (PML–RARA; Kakizuka *et al.*, 1991; de The *et al.*, 1991). However, multiple PML–RARA isoforms co-exist due to (i)

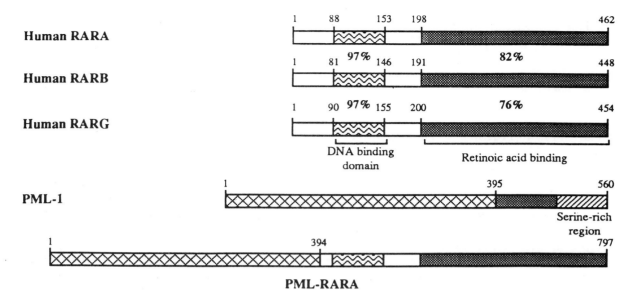

PML-RARA

variable breaking of chromosome 15 within three *PML* breakpoint cluster regions (*BCR1*, *BCRL2* and *BCRL3*), (ii) alternative splicing of *PML*, and (iii) alternative use of two *RARA* polyadenyl-ation sites (Tong *et al.*, 1992; Pandolfi *et al.*, 1992; Chen *et al.*, 1992). In HL60 cells the fusion protein (PML–RARA) is a hormone-dependent transcription factor with enhanced *transactiv*-ation capability compared with wild-type RARA that may act as a dominant negative oncogene to inhibit myeloid differentiation. In HepG2 cells, however, PML–RARA is a poor inducer. Hence the fusion protein is a cell- and sequence-specific transcription factor.

PML protein shows a punctate distribution in the nucleus: the fusion protein is distributed in a nuclear corona: co-expression of the fusion and wild-type forms restores the punctate distri-bution of PML.

The second form of hybrid mRNA transcribed from this breakpoint is *RARA–PML* comprising 503 bp of *RARA* exon II fused 5′ to 1.76 kb of *PML* (Chang *et al.*, 1992). Two types of *RARA–PML* junctions occur resulting from chromosome 15 breakage at two different points (Alcalay *et al.*, 1992). Multiple *RARA–PML* fusion transcripts arise from differing assemblies of *PML* exons. PML–RARA and RARA–PML can be co-expressed in APL.

Alcalay, M., Zangrilli, D., Fagioli, M., Pandolfi, P.P., Mencarelli, A., Lo Coco, F., Biondi, A., Grignani, F. and Pelicci, P.G. (1992). Expression pattern of the *RARα–PML* fusion gene in acute promyelocytic leuke-mia. Proc. Natl Acad. Sci. USA, 89, 4840–4844.

Chang, K.-S., Stass, S.A., Chu, D.-T., Deaven, L.L., Trujillo, J.M. and Freireich, E.J. (1992). Characterization of a fusion cDNA (RAR/*myl*) transcribed from the t(15;17) translocation breakpoint in acute promyelo-cytic leukemia. Mol. Cell. Biol., 12, 800–810.

Chen, S.-J., Chen, Z., Chen, A., Tong, J.-H., Dong, S., Wang, Z.-Y., Waxman, S. and Zelent, A. (1992). Occurrence of distinct *PML–RARα* fusion gene isoforms in patients with acute promyelocytic leukemia detected by reverse transcriptase/polymerase chain reaction. Oncogene, 7, 1223–1232.

de The, H., Lavau, C., Marchio, A., Chomienne, C., Degos, L. and Dejean, A. (1991). The PML–RARα fusion mRNA generated by the t(15;17) translocation in acute promyelocytic leukemia encodes a func-tionally altered RAR. Cell, 66, 675–684.

Fagioli, M., Alcalay, M., Pandolfi, P.P., Venturini, L., Mencarelli, A., Simeone, A., Acampora, D., Grignani, F. and Pelicci, P.G. (1992). Alternative splicing of PML transcripts predicts coexpression of several carb-oxy-terminally different protein isoforms. Oncogene, 7, 1083–1091.

Kakizuka, A., Miller, W.H., Umesono, K., Warrell, R.P., Frankel, S.R., Murty, V.V.V.S., Dmitrovsky, E. and Evans, R.M. (1991). Chromosomal translocation t(15;17) in human acute promyelocytic leukemia fuses RARα with a novel putative transcription factor, PML. Cell, 66, 663–674.

Pandolfi, P.P., Alcalay, M., Fagioli, M., Zangrilli, D., Mencarelli, A., Diverio, D., Biondi, A., Lo Coco, F., Rambaldi, A., Grignani, F., Rochette-Egly, C., Gaube, M.-P., Chambon, P. and Pelicci, P.G. (1992). Genomic variability and alternative splicing generate multiple PML/RARα transcripts that encode aberrant PML proteins and PML/RARα isoforms in acute promyeolocytic leukemia. EMBO J., 11, 1397–1407.

Tong, J.-H., Dong, S., Geng, J.-P., Huang, W., Wang, Z.-Y., Sun, G.-L., Chen, S.-J., Chen, Z., Larsen, C.-J. and Berger, R. (1992). Molecular rearrangements of the *MYL* gene in acute promyelocytic leukemia (APL, M3) define a breakpoint cluster region as well as some molecular variants. Oncogene, 7, 311–316.

Gene	*PLZF* (11q23)	*Translocation*	t(11;17) (q23–q21.1)	*Leukaemia*	APL
	RARA (17q21)				

The reciprocal translocation fuses the coding sequences of *PLZF* (promyelocytic leukaemia zinc finger) in-frame either upstream of the *RARA* B region or downstream of the A1 and A2 regions that are unique to the *RARA* isoforms (Chen *et al.*, 1993). In addition to *PLZF(A)–RARA* expressed from the *PLZF* promoter on the derivative 11q+ chromosome, both forms of the reciprocal mRNA (*RARA1–PLZF* and *RARA2–PLZF*) are expressed from the derivative 17q chromosome. PLZF (74 kDa) is a potential transcription factor containing nine zinc finger motifs. *PLZF* is transcribed in normal bone marrow and in peripheral blood mononuclear cells but not in lymphoid tissues or cell lines.

Sequence of PLZF

```
  (1)   MDLTKMGMIQLQNPSHPTGLLCKANQMRLAGTLCDVVIMVDSQEFHAHRTVLACTSKMFE
 (61)   ILFHRNSQHYTLDFLSPKTFQQILEYAYTATLQAKAEDLDDLLYAAEILEIEYLEEQCLK
(121)   MLETIQASDDNDTEATMADGGAEEEEDRKARYLKNIFISKHSSEESGYASVAGQSLPGPM
(181)   VDQSPSVSTSFGLSAMSPTKAAVDSLMTIGQSLLQGTLQPPAGPEEPTLAGGGRHPGVAE
(241)   VKTEMMQVDEVPSQDSPGAAESSISGGMGDKVEERGKEGPGTPTRSSVITSARELHYGRE
(301)   ESAEQVPPPAEAGQAPTGRPEHPAPPPEKHLGIYSVLPNHKADAVLSMPSSVTSGLHVQP
(361)   ALAVSMDFSTYGGLLPQGFIQRELFSKLGELAVGMKSESRTIGEQCSVCGVELPDNEAVE
(421)   QHRKLHSGMKTYGCELCGKRFLDSLRLRMHLLAHSAGAKAFVCDQCGAQFSKEDALETHR
                                                            Δ
(481)   QTHTGTDMAVFCLLCGKRFQAQSALQQHMEVHAGVRSYICSECNRTFPSHTALKRRLRSH
(541)   TGDHPYECEFCGSCFRDESTLKSHKRIHTGEKPYECNGCDKKFSLKHQLETHYRVHTGEK
(601)   PFECKLCHQRSRDYSAMIKHLRTHNGASPYQCTICTEYCPSLSSMQKHMKGHKPEEIPPD
(661)   WRIEKTYLYLCYV (673)
```

The full sequence represents PLZF(B). The sequence fusing to RARA (PLZF(A)) lacks the 123 underlined residues that may correspond to an alternatively spliced exon. The nine zinc finger regions are italicized. Δ Indicates the breakpoint within PLZF.

Chen, Z., Brand, N.J., Chen, A., Chen, S.-J., Tong, J.-H., Wang, Z.-Y. Waxman, S. and Zelent, A. (1993). Fusion between a novel Kruppel-like zinc finger gene and the retinoic acid receptor-α locus due to a variant t(11;17) translocation associated with acute promyelocytic leukemia. EMBO J., 12, 1161–1167.

Gene	*CAN* (6p23)	*Translocation*	t(6;9)(p23;q34)	*Leukaemia*	AML
	DEK (9q34)				
	SET (9q34)				

Breakpoints occur within 8 kb, 360 kb telomeric of *ABL* at introns (*icb*-6 and *icb*-9) in the Cain (*CAN*) gene. The normal *CAN* transcript is 7.5 kb: after the translocation a 5.5 kb *CAN* mRNA is transcribed from 6p⁻ (von Lindern *et al.*, 1990). The *SET* gene (2.0 or 2.7 kb mRNAs encoding 32 kDa) may also fuse to *CAN* to form a 155 kDa chimeric protein (von Lindern *et al.*, 1992a,b).

Sequence of CAN

```
   (1)   MGDEMDAMIPEREMKDFQFRALKKVRIFDSPEELPKERSSLLAVSNKYGLVFAGGASGL
  (60)   QIFPTKNLLIQNKPGDDPNKIVDKVQGLLVPMKFPIHHLALSCDNLTLSACMMSSEYGSI
 (120)   IAFFDVRTFSNEAKQQKRPFAYHKLLKDAAGMVIDMKWNPTVPSMVAVCLADGSIDVLQV
 (180)   TETVKVCATLPSTVAVTSVCWSPKGKQLAVGKQNGTVVQYLPTLQEKKVIPCPPFYESDH
 (240)   PVRVLDVLWIGTYVFAIVYAAADGTLETSPDVVMALLPKKEEKHPEIFVNFMEPCYGSCT
 (300)   ERQHHYYLSYIEEWDLVLAASAASTEVSILARQSDQINWESWLLEDSSRAELPVTDKSDD
 (360)   SLPMGVVVDYTNQVEITISDEKTLPPAPVLMLLSTDGVLCPFYMINQNPGVKSLIKTPER
 (420)   LSLEGERQPKSPGSTPTTPTSSQAPQKLDASAAAAPASLPPSSPAAPIATFSLLPAGGAP
 (480)   TVFSFGSSSLKSSATVTGEPPSYSSGSDSSKAAPGPGPSTFSFVPPSKASLAPTPAASPV
 (540)   APSAASFSFGSSGFKPTLESTPVPSVSAPNIAMKSSFPPSTSAVKVNLSEKFTAAATSTP
 (600)   VSSSQSAPPMSPFSSASKPAASGPLSHPTPLSAPPSSVPLKSSVLPSPSGRSAQGSSSPV
 (660)   PSMVQKSPRITPPAAKPGSPQAKSLQPAVAEKQGHQWKDSDPVMAGIGEEIAHFQKELEE
 (720)   LKARTSKACFQVGTSEEMKMLRTESDDLHTFLLEIKETTESLHGDISSLKTTLLEGFAGV
 (780)   EEAREQNERNRDSGYLHLLYKRPLDPKSEAQLQ EIRRLHQYVKFAVQDVNDVLDLEWDQH
                                              Δ
 (840)   LEQKKKQRHLLVPERETLFNTLANNREIINQQRKRLNHLVDSLQQLRLYKQTSLWSLSSA
 (900)   VPSQSSIHSFDSDLESLCNALLKTTIESHTKSLPKVPAKLSPMKQAQLRNFLAKRKTPPV
 (960)   RSTAPASLSRSAFLSQRYYEDLDEVSSTSSVSQSLESEDARTSCKDDEAVVQAPRHAPVV
(1020)   RTPSIQPSLLPHAAPFAKSHLVHGSSPGVMGTSVATSASKIIPQGADSTMLATKTVKHGA
(1080)   PSPSHPISAPQQLAAAALRRQMASQAPAVNTLTESTLKNVPQVVNVQELKNNPATPSTAM
(1140)   GSSVPYSTAKTPHPVLTPVAANQAKQGSLINSLKPSGPTPASGQLSSGDKASGTAKIETA
(1200)   VTSTPSASGQFSKPFSFSPSGTGFNFGIITPTPSSNFTAAQGATPSTKESSQPDAFSSGG
(1260)   GSKPSYEAIPESSPPSGITSASNTTPGEPAASSSRPVAPSGTALSTTSSKLETPPSKLGE
(1320)   LLFPSSLAGETLGSFSGLRVGQADDSTKPTNKASSTSLTSTQPTKTSGVPSGFNFTAPPV
(1380)   LGKHTEPPVTSSATTTSVAPPAATSTSSTAVFGSLPVTSAGSSGVISFGGTSLSAGKTSF
(1440)   SFGSQQTNSTVPPSAPPPTTAATPLPTSFPTLSFGSLLSSATTPSLPMSAGRSTEEATSS
(1500)   ALPEKPGDSEVSASAASLLEEQQSAQLPQAPPQTSDSVKKEPVLAQPAVSNSGTAASSTS
(1560)   LVALSAEATPATTGVPDARTEAVPPASSFSVPGQTAVTAAAISSAGPVAVETSSTPIASS
(1620)   TTSIVAPGPSAEAAAFGTVTSGSSVFAQPPAASSSSAFNQLTNNTATAPSATPVFGQVAA
(1680)   STAPSLFGQQTGSTASTAAATPQVSSSGFSSPAFGTTAPGVFGQTTFGQASVFGQSASSA
(1740)   ASVFSFSQPGFSSVPAFGQPASSTPTSTSGSVFGAASSTSSSSSFSFGQSSPNTGGGLFG
(1800)   QSNAPAFGQSPGFGQGGSVFGGTSAATTTAATSGFSFCQASGFGSSNTGSVFGQAASTGG
(1860)   IVFGQQSSSSSGSVFGSGNTGRGGGFFSGLGGKPSQDAANKNPFSSASGGFGSTATSNTS
(1920)   NLFGNSGAKTFGGFASSSFGEQKPTGTFSSGGGSVASQGFGFSSPNKTGGFGAAPVFGSP
(1980)   PTFGGSPGFGGVPAFGSAPAFTSPLGSTGGKVFGEGTAAASAGGFGFGSSSNTTSFGTLA
(2040)   SQNAPTFGSLSQQTSGFGTQSSGFSGFGSGTGGFSFGSNNSSVQGFGGWRS(2090)
```

Δ Indicates breakpoint in the t(6;9) translocation. Underlined: putative leucine zipper and amphipathic helices.

Sequence of DEK

```
   (1)   MSASAPAAEGEGTPTQPASEKEPEMPGPREESEEEEDEDDEEEEEEEKEKSLIVEGKRE
  (60)   KKKVERLTMQVSSLQREPFTIAQGKGQKLCEIERIHFFLSKKKTDELRNLHKLLYNRPGT
 (120)   VSSLKKNVGQFSGFPFEKGSVQYKKKEEMLKKFRNAMLKSICEVLDLERSGVNSELVKRI
 (180)   LNFLMHPKPSGKPLPKSKKTCSKGSKKERNSSGMARKAKRTKCPEILSDESSSDEDEKKN
 (240)   KEESSDDEDKESEEEPPKKTAKREKPKQKATSKSKKSVKSANVKKADSSTTKKNQNSSKK
 (300)   ESESEDSSDDEPLIKKLKKPPTDEELKETIKKLLASANLEEVTMKQICKK VYENYPTYDL
                                                              Δ
 (360)   TERKDFIKTTVKELIS (375)
```

Δ Indicates breakpoint in the t(6;9) translocation.

Sequence of SET

```
   (1)   MSAQAAKVSKKELNSNHDGADETSEKEQQEAIEHIDEVQNEIDRLNEQASEEILKVEQ
  (60)   KYNKLRQPFFQKRSELIAKIPNFWVTTFVNHPQVSALLGEEDEEALHYLTRVEVTEFEDI
```

```
(120)  KSGYRIDFYFDENPYFENKVLSKEFHLNESGDPSSKSTEIKWKSGKDLTKRSSQTQNKAS
(180)  RKRQHEEPESFFTWFTDHSDAGADELGEVIKDDIWPNPLQYYLVPDMDDEEGEGEEDDDD
(240)  DEEEEGLEDIDEEGDEDEGEEDEDDDEGEEGE EDEGEDD (277)
                                          Δ
```

Underlined: acidic C-terminus. Δ Indicates SET–CAN fusion point.

von Lindern, M., Poustka, A., Lerach, H. and Grosveld, G. (1990). The (6;9) chromosome translocation, associated with a specific subtype of acute nonlymphocytic leukemia, leads to aberrant transcription of a target gene on 9q34. Mol. Cell. Biol., 10, 4016–4026.

von Lindern, M., van Baal, S., Wiegant, J., Raap, A., Hagemeijer, A. and Grosveld, G. (1992a). can, a putative oncogene associated with myeloid leukemogenesis, may be activated by fusion of its 3' half to different genes: characterization of the set gene. Mol. Cell. Biol., 12, 3346–3355.

von Lindern, M., Fornerod, M., van Baal, S., Jaegle, M., de Wit, T., Buijs, A. and Grosveld, G. (1992b). The translocation (6;9), associated with a specific subtype of acute myeloid leukemia, results in the fusion of two genes, dek and can, and the expression of a chimeric, leukemia-specific dek-can mRNA. Mol. Cell. Biol., 12, 1687–1697.

Gene	IL2 (4q26)	Translocation	t(4;16)(q26;p13.1)	Leukemia	T cell
	BCM (16p13)				lymphoma

The BCM (B cell maturation) gene is expressed in mature B cells (1.2 kb mRNA) and encodes a putative transmembrane protein of unknown function. The translocation places the first three exons of the interleukin-2 gene before an in-frame sequence encoding the final 181 amino acids of BCM (Laabi et al., 1992). One important consequence of this rearrangement is the impairment of function of IL-2 in T cell growth and differentiation.

Sequence of BCM

```
  (1)   MLQMAGQCSQNEYFDSLLHACIPCQLRCSSNTPPLTCQRYCNASVTNSVKGTNAILWTC
 (60)   LGLSLIISLAVFVLMFLLRKISSEPLKDEFKNTGSGLLGMANIDLEKSRTGDEIILPRGL
(120)   EYTVEECTCEDCIKSKPKVDSDHCFPLPAMEEGATILVTTKTNDYCKSLPAALSATEIEK
(180)   SISAR (184)
```

Laabi, Y., Gras, M.P., Carbonnel, F., Brouet, J.C., Berger, R., Larsen, C.J. and Tsapis, A. (1992). A new gene, BCM, on chromosome 16 is fused to the interleukin 2 gene by a t(4;16)(q26;p13) translocation in a malignant T cell lymphoma. EMBO J., 11, 3897–3904.

Gene	SIL (1p33)	Translocation	t(1;14)	Leukaemia	T-ALL

SIL (SCL interrupting locus): highly conserved mammalian gene. SIL fuses with SCL/TAL1 through the action of the V(D)J recombinase system, even though neither gene encodes an antigen receptor (see TAL1). (T cell receptor (TCR) genes that normally rearrange during T cell ontogeny are common sites for chromosomal translocation in T cell leukaemias.) SIL (>70 kb, 18 exons, alternative 5' exons) encodes a normal 5.5 kb mRNA (143 kDa protein; Aplan et al., 1991). The rearrangement (which occurs in ~20% of ALL patients) is similar in effect to the t(1;14) translocation. An interstitial deletion removes most of the SIL gene, splicing SIL exon 1 to TAL1 exon 3 and the 3' TAL1 exons (4, 5 and 6).

Sequence of SIL

```
  (1)   MEPIYPFARPQMNTRFPSSRMVPFHFPPSKCALWNPTPTGDFIYLHLSYYRNPKLVVTEK
 (61)   TIRLAYRHANENKKNSSCFLLGSLTADEDEEGVTLTVDRFDPGREVPECLEITPTASLPG
```

```
(121)  DFLIPCKVHTQELCSREMIVHSVDDFSSALKALQCHICSKDSLDCGKLLSLRVHITSRES
(181)  LDSVEFDLHWAAVTLANNFKCTPVKPIPIIPTALARNLSSNLNISQVQGTYKYGYLTMDE
(241)  TRKLLLLLESDPKVYSLPLVGIWLSGITHIYSPQVWACCLRYIFNSSVQERVFSESGNFI
(301)  IVLYSMTHKEPEFYECFPCDGKIPDFRFQLLTSKETLHLFKNVEPPDKNPIRCELSAESQ
(361)  NAETEFFSKASKNFSIKRSSQKLSSGKMPIHDHDSGVEDEDEFSPRPIPSPHPVSQKISKI
(421)  QPSVPELSLVLDGNFIESNPLPTPLEMVNNENPPLINHLEHLKPLQPQLYDEKHSPEVEA
(481)  GEPSLRGIPNQLNQDKPALLRHCKVRQPPAYKKGNPHTRNSIKPSSHNGPSHDIFEKLQT
(541)  VSAGNVQNEEYPIRPSTLNSRQSSLAPQSQPHDFVFSPHNSGRPMELQIPTPPLPSYCST
(601)  NVCRCCQHHSHIQYSPLNSWQGANTVGSIQDVQSEALQKHSLFHPSGCPALYCNAFCSSS
(661)  SPIALRPQGDMGSCSPHSNIEPSPVARPPSHMDLCNPQPCTVCMHTPKTESDNGMMGLSP
(721)  DAYRFLTEQDRQLRLLQAQIQRLLEAQSLMPCSPKTTAVEDTVQAGRQMELVSVEAQSSP
(781)  GLHMRKGVSIAVSTGASLFWNAAGEDQEPDSQMKQDDTKISSEDMNFSVDINNEVTSLPG
(841)  SASSLKAVDIPSFEESNIAVEEEFNQPLSVSNSSLVVRKEPDVPVFFPSGQLAESVSMCL
(901)  QTGPTGGASNNSETSEEPKIEHVMQPLLHQPSDNQKIYQDLLGQVNHLLNSSSKETEQPS
(961)  TKAVIISHECTRTQNVYHTKKKTHHSRLVDKDCVLNATLKQLRSLGVKIDSPTKVKKNAH
(1021) NVDHASVLACISPEAVISGLNCMSFANVGMSGLSPNGVDLSMEANAIALKYLNENQLSQL
(1081) SVTRSNQNNCDPFSLLHINTDRSTVGLSLISPNNMSFATKKYMKRYGLLQSSDNSEDEEE
(1141) PPDNADSKSEYLLNQNLRSIPEQLGGQKEPSKNDHEIINCSNCESVGTNADTPVLRNITN
(1201) EVLQTKAKQQLTEKPAFLVKNLKPSPAVNLRTGKAEFTQHPEKENEGDITIFPESLQPSE
(1261) TLKQMNSMNSVGTFLDVKRLRQLPKLF (1287)
```

The underlined sequence encoded by exon 7 is spliced out of a minority of mRNAs.

Aplan, P.D., Lombardi, D.P. and Kirsch, I.R. (1991). Structural characterization of *SIL*, a gene frequently disrupted in T-cell acute lymphoblastic leukemia. Mol. Cell. Biol., 11, 5462–5469.

Gene	*FLI1* (11q24)	*Translocation*	t(11;22)(q24;q12)	Ewing's
	EWS (22q12)			sarcoma

The C-terminal region of EWS includes a putative RNA binding domain. The translocation substitutes this region of EWS with the ETS DNA binding domain present in the C-terminus of FLI1 (Delattre *et al.*, 1992). Variant forms of the chimeric protein contain an additional 84 amino acids of EWS (Type 3) or 22 amino acids from FLI1 (Type 2).

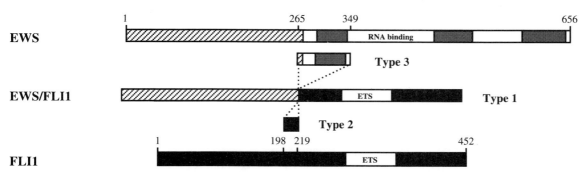

Sequence of EWS

```
EWS      (1)    MASTDYSTYSQAAAQQGYSAYTAQPTQGYAQTTQAYGQQSYGTYGQPTDVSYTQAQTTAT
EWS      (61)   YGQTAYATSYGQPPTGYTTPTAPQAYSQPVQGYGTGAYDTTTATVTTTQASYAAQSAYGT
EWS      (121)  QPAYPAYGQQPAATAPTRPQDGNKPTETSQPQSSTGGYNQPSLGYGQSNYSYPQVPGSYP
EWS      (181)  MQPVTAPPSYPPTSYSSTQPTSYDQSSYSQQNTYGQPSSYGQQSSYGQQSSYGQQPPTSY
EWS      (241)  PPQTGSYSQAPSQYSQQSSSYGQQSSFRDHPSSMGVYGQESGGFSGPGENRSMSGPDNR
EWS/FLI1                                              NPSYDSVRRGAWGNNMNSGLNKSPPLGGAQTISKNT
EWS      (301)  GRGRGGFDRGGMSRGGRGGGRGGMGSAGERGGFNKPGGPMDEGPDLDLGPPVDPDEDSDN
EWS/FLI1        EQRPQPDPYQILGPTSSRLANPGSSGQIQLWQFLLELLKDSANASCITWEGTNGE
EWS      (361)  SAIYVQGLNDSVTLDDLADFFKQCGVVKMNKRTGQPMIHIYLDKETGKPKGDATVSYEDP
```

```
EWS     (421)   PTAKAAVEWFDGKDFQGSKLKVSLARKKPPMNSMRGGLPPREGRGMPPPLRGGPGGPGGP
EWS     (481)   GGPMGRMGGRGGDRGGFPPRGPRGSRGNPSGGGNVQHRAGDWQCPNPGCGNQNFAWRTEC
EWS     (541)   NQCKAPKPEGFLPPPFPPPGGDRGRGGPGGMRGGRGGLMDRGGPGGMFRGGRGGDRGGFR
EWS     (601)   GGRGMDRGGFGGGRRGGPGGPPGPLMEQMGGRRGGRGGPGKMDKGEHRQERRDRPY(656)
```

Codons 265 and 349 (underlined) are split in the two chimeric transcripts. The FLI1 sequence extending from codon 265 in the Type 1 chimeric protein is indicated.

Delattre, O., Zucman, J., Plougastel, B., Desmaze, C., Melot, T., Peter, M., Kovar, H., Joubert, I., de Jong, P., Rouleau, G., Aurias, A. and Thomas, G. (1992). Gene fusion with an *ETS* DNA-binding domain caused by chromosome translocation in human tumours. Nature, 359, 162–165.

Helix–loop–helix proteins

Gene	LYL1 (19p13.2)	Translocation	t(7;19)(q35;p13.2)	Leukaemia	T cell leukaemia line

Translocation involves a breakpoint within the first intron of *LYL1* and the juxtaposition of the gene to the TCRβ gene (7q35) in opposite transcriptional orientation and with the loss of a 5′ non-coding *LYL1* exon. The predicted mouse LYL1 helix–loop–helix protein (chromosome 8) is 78% identical to human LYL1 (Kuo *et al.*, 1991). Expressed in most B lineage cell lines (mRNAs 1.5–1.8 kb and 2.0–2.3 kb; Visvader *et al.*, 1991) but not in T cells, its deregulated expression contributes to T cell neoplasms.

Sequence of human LYL1

```
  (1)    MTEKAEMVCAPSPAPAPPPKPASPGPPQVEEVGHRGGSSPPRLPPGVPVISLGHSRPPGV
 (61)    AMPTTELGTLRPPLLQLSTLGTAPPTLALHYHPHPFLNSVYIGPAGPFSIFPSSRLKRRP
(121)    SHCELDLAEGHQPQKVARRVFTNSRERWRQQNVNGAFAELRKLLPTHPPDRKLSKNEVLR
(181)    LAMKYIGFLVRLLRDQAAALAAGPTPPGPRKRPVHRVPDDGPRRGSGRRAEAAARSQPAP
(241)    PADPDGSPGGAARPIKMEQTALSPEVR (267)
```

Underlined: DNA binding domain (136–199). Italics: amphipathic helices homologous to those contained in TAL1 and TAL2.

Kuo, S.S., Mellentin, J.D., Copeland, N.G., Gilbert, D.J., Jenkins, N.A. and Cleary, M.L. (1991). Structure, chromosome mapping, and expression of the mouse *lyl*-1 gene. Oncogene, 6, 961–968.
Mellentin, J.D., Smith, S.D. and Cleary, M.L. (1989). *lyl*-1, a novel gene altered by chromosomal translocation in T cell leukemia, codes for a protein with a helix–loop–helix DNA binding motif. Cell 58, 77–83.
Visvader, J., Begley, C.G. and Adams, J.M. (1991). Differential expression of the LYL, SCL and E2A helix–loop–helix genes within the hemopoietic system. Oncogene, 6, 187–194.

Gene	TAL1 (1p32)	Translocation	t(1;14)(p32;q11)	Leukaemia	T-ALL

The helix–loop–helix domain of *TAL1*-encoded proteins (also called *SCL* and *TCL5*) interacts with the helix–loop–helix proteins E12 and E47 and the heterodimers recognize the E box DNA enhancer motif. Thus TAL1 may normally regulate T cell differentiation (see **TAL1**). *TAL1* encodes two proteins: pp42^{TAL1} (331 amino acids) and pp22^{TAL1} (residues 176–331 of pp42). Ser122 of pp42^{TAL1} is phosphorylated *in vitro* by ERK1 protein kinase and in intact cells after stimulation by EGF (Cheng *et al.*, 1993a). *TAL1* is structurally altered in ~30% of T-ALL cases, either by a 90 kb deletion or translocation to the TCRα/δ chain gene (14q11) and there is one reported example in which the gene is not disrupted, the breakpoint occurring 25 kb downstream of *TAL1* (Xia *et al.*, 1992).

Chen, Q., Cheng, J.-T., Tsai, L.-H., Schneider, N., Buchanan, G.F., Carroll, A., Crist, W., Ozanne, B., Siciliano, M.J. and Baer, R. (1990). The *tal* gene undergoes chromosome translocation in T cell leukemia and potentially encodes a helix–loop–helix protein. EMBO J., 9, 415–424.

Cheng, J.-T., Cobb, M.H. and Baer, R. (1993a). Phosphorylation of the TAL1 oncoprotein by the extracellular-signal-regulated protein kinase ERK1. Mol. Cell. Biol., 13, 801–808.

Cheng, J.-T., Hsu, H.-L., Hwang, L.-Y. and Baer, R. (1993b). Products of the *TAL1* oncogene: basic helix–loop–helix proteins phosphorylated at serine residues. Oncogene, 8, 677–683.

Xia, Y., Brown, L., Tsan, J.T., Yang, Y.-C., Siciliano, M.J., Crist, W.M., Carroll, A.J. and Baer, R. (1992). The translocation (1;14)(p34;q11) in human T-cell leukemia: chromosome breakage 25 kilobase pairs downstream of the *TAL1* protooncogene. Genes, Chromosomes & Cancer, 4, 211–216.

Gene	TAL2 (9q34)	*Translocation*	t(7;9)(q35;q34)	*Leukaemia*	T-ALL

TAL2 is located 33 kbp from the chromosome 9 breakpoint of t(7;9)(q35;q34). The translocation juxtaposes *TAL2* with *TCRβ* sequences on chromosome 7 and *TAL2* is transcribed (3.5 and 5.0 kb mRNAs) in the SUP-T3 T cell line that carries t(7;9)(q35;q34). TAL2 is highly homologous to TAL1 and LYL1 and all contain helix–loop–helix and DNA binding domains.

Sequences of human and mouse TAL2

```
Human TAL1      (1)    GPHTKVVRRIFTNSRERWRQQNVNGAFAELRKLIPTHPPDKKLSKNEILRLAMKYINFLA
Human TAL2      (1)     NSNMTRKIFTNTRERWRQQNVNSAFAKLRKLIPTHPPDKKLSKNETLRLAMRYINFLV
Mouse TAL2             -LD-------------  ---S--N-------------------------------------

Human TAL1     (61)    KLLNDQEEEGTQRAKTGKDPVVGAGGGGGGGGGGAPPDDLLQDVLSPNSSCGSSLDGAAS
Human TAL2     (59)    KVLGEQSLQQTGVAAQGNILGLFPQGPHLPGLEDRTLLENYQVPSPGPSHHIP (111)
Mouse TAL2            -------H--------------PKTR--DED-----ND-R--------GA- (111)

Human TAL1    (121)    PDSYTEEPAPKHTARSLHPAMLPAADGAGPR (151)
```

Underlined: amphipathic helices.

Xia, Y., Brown, L., Yang, C.Y.-C., Tsan, J.T., Siciliano, M.J., Espinosa, R., Le Beau, M.M. and Baer, R.J. (1991). *TAL2*, a novel helix–loop–helix gene activated by the (7;9)(q34;q32) translocation in human T-cell leukemia. Proc. Natl Acad. Sci. USA, 88, 11416–11420.

LIM proteins

Gene	RBTN1 (11p15)	*Translocation*	t(11;14)(p15;q11)	*Leukaemia*	T-ALL
	RBTN2 (11p13)		t(11;14)(p13;q11)		

The translocation t(11;14)(p13;q11) occurs in ~20% of childhood T cell acute lymphoblastic leukaemias (T-ALL). It frequently involves the *TCRδ* gene on chromosome 14q11 that lies between the *TCRα* constant and variable genes. *RBTN1* (also called *T cell translocation gene 1* (*TTG1*) or rhombotin 1; 11p15) and *RBTNL1* (rhombotin-like 1, also called *RBTN2* or *TTG2*; 11p13) are two genes deregulated by translocations of *TCRδ* from 14q11 (Boehm *et al.*, 1988; McGuire *et al.*, 1989; Royer-Pokora *et al.*, 1991). *RBTN1* is predominantly expressed in the central nervous system whereas *RBTN2* is widely expressed and a similar pattern has been detected for the murine proteins (Foroni *et al.*, 1992). The proteins are 48% homologous and contain two copies each of the cysteine-rich LIM motif (CX_2–C–X_{17-19}––H–X_2–C–X_2–C–X_2–C–X_{7-11}–(C)–X_8–C; Boehm *et al.*, 1991; Michelson *et al.*, 1993). Mice bearing an *Rbtn-1* transgene develop T cell lymphomas in a manner that correlates with the extent of *Rbtn-1* mRNA expression (McGuire *et al.*, 1992; Fisch *et al.*, 1992).

Sequence of human rhombotin 2 (RBTNL1)

```
 (1)   MSSAIERKSLDPSEEPVDEVLQIPPSLLTCGGCQQNIGDRYFLKAIDQYWHEDCLSCDLC
(61)   GCRLGEVGRRLYYKLGRKLCRRDYLRLFGQDGLCASCDKRIRAYEMTMRVKDKVYHLECF
(121)  KCAACQKHFCVGDRYLLINSDIVCEQDIYEWTKINGMI (158)
```

Underlined: the LIM motifs (30–89 and 94–153).

Boehm, T., Baer, R., Lavenir, I., Forster, A., Waters, J.J., Nacheva, E. and Rabbitts, T.H. (1988). The mechanism of chromosomal translocation t(11;14) involving the T-cell receptor Cδ locus on human chromosome 14q11 and a transcribed region of chromosome 11p15. EMBO J., 7, 385–394.

Boehm, T., Foroni, L., Kaneko, Y., Perutz, M.F. and Rabbitts, T.H. (1991). The rhombotin family of cysteine-rich LIM-domain oncogenes: distinct members are involved in T-cell translocations to human chromosomes 11p15 and 11p13. Proc. Natl Acad. Sci. USA, 88, 4367–4371.

Fisch, P., Boehm, T., Lavenir, I., Larson, T., Arno, J., Forster, A. and Rabbitts, T.H. (1992). T-cell acute lymphoblastic lymphoma induced in transgenic mice by the *RBTN1* and *RBTN2* LIM-domain genes. Oncogene, 7, 2389–2397.

Foroni, L., Boehm, T., White, L., Forster, A., Sherrington, P., Liao, X.B., Brannan, C.I., Jenkins, N.A., Copeland, N.G. and Rabbitts, T.H. (1992). The rhombotin gene family encode related LIM-domain proteins whose differing expression suggests multiple roles in mouse development. J. Mol. Biol., 226, 747–761.

McGuire, E.A., Hockett, R.D., Pollock, K.M., Bartholdi, M.F., O'Brien, S.J. and Korsmeyer, S.J. (1989). The t(11;14)(p15;q11) in a T-cell acute lymphoblastic leukemia cell line activates multiple transcripts, including *ttg-1*, a gene encoding a potential zinc finger protein. Mol. Cell. Biol., 9, 2124–2132.

McGuire, E.A., Rintoul, C.E., Sclar, G.M. and Korsmeyer, S.J. (1992). Thymic overexpression of *ttg-1* in transgenic mice results in T-cell acute lymphoblastic leukemia/lymphoma. Mol. Cell. Biol., 12, 4186–4196.

Michelsen, J.W., Schmeichel, K.L., Beckerle, M.C. and Winge, D.R. (1993). The LIM motif defines a specific zinc-binding protein domain. Proc. Natl Acad. Sci. USA, 90, 4404–4408.

Royer-Pokora, B., Loos, U. and Ludwig, W.-D. (1991). TTG-2, a new gene encoding a cysteine-rich protein with the *LIM* motif, is overexpressed in acute T-cell leukemia with the t(11;14)(p13;q11). Oncogene, 6, 1887–1893.

Homeodomain proteins

Gene   HOX11 (10q24)   *Translocation*   t(10;14)(q24;q11)   *Leukaemia*   T-ALL
                                           t(7;10)(q35;q24)

HOX11 (also called *TCL3*) shares homology with the developmentally regulated homeobox genes of *Drosophila* and mammals (Dear *et al.*, 1993). It is transcriptionally activated by translocation to either *TCRβ* (7q35) or *TCRδ* (14q11) that occurs in up to 7% of T-ALLs (Kennedy *et al.*, 1991). The t(10;14) translocation juxtaposes *HOX11* head-to-tail with the TCR δ chain gene. *HOX11* is expressed in normal T cells and in an unaltered form in some T cell lines (Lu *et al.*, 1992).

Sequence of HOX11

```
 (1)   MEHLGPHHLHPGHAEPISFGIDQILNSPDQGGCMGPASRLQDGEYGLGCLVGGAYTYGG
(60)   GGSAAATGAGGAGAYGTGGPGGPGGPAGGGGACSMGPLTGSYNVNMALAGGPGPGGGGGS
```

```
(120)  SGGAGALSAAGVIRVPAHRPLAGAVAHPQPLATGLPTVPSVPAMPGVNNLTGLTFPWMES
(180)  NRRYTKDRFTGHPYQNRTPPKKKKPRTSFTRLQICELEKRFHRQKYLASAERAALAKALK
(240)  MTDAQVKTWFQNRRTKWRRQTAEEREAERQQANRILLQLQQEAFQKSLAQPLPADPLCVH
(300)  NSSLFALQNLQPWSDDSTKITSVTSVASACE (330)
```

Dear, T.N., Sanchez-Garcia, I. and Rabbitts, T.H. (1993). The *HOX11* gene encodes a DNA-binding nuclear transcription factor belonging to a distinct family of homeobox genes. Proc. Natl Acad. Sci. USA, 90, 4431–4435.

Lu, M., Zhang, N. and Ho, A.D. (1992). Genomic organization of the putative human homeobox proto-oncogene HOX-11 (*TCL-3*) and its endogenous expression in T cells. Oncogene, 7, 1325–1330.

Kennedy, M.A., Gonzalez-Sarmiento, R., Kees, U.R., Lampert, F., Dear, N., Boehm, T. and Rabbitts, T.H. (1991). *HOX11*, a homeobox-containing T-cell oncogene on human chromosome 10q24. Proc. Natl Acad. Sci. USA, 88, 8900–8904.

Anti-proliferative genes

Gene   BTG1 (12q22)   *Translocation*   t(8;12)(q24;q22)   *Leukaemia*   B-CLL

B-cell translocation gene *1* (*BTG1*: 1.8 kb mRNA) maps to chromosome 12q22, is maximally expressed in G_o/G_1 phases of the cell cycle and is 60% homologous to the immediate early response gene *PC3* induced in PC12 cells by NGF (Roualt *et al.*, 1992). Overexpression of *BTG1* inhibits NIH 3T3 cell proliferation. The *BTG1* locus is deleted in >40% testicular or extragonadal non-seminomatous germ cell tumours.

Sequence of BTG1

```
(1)    MHPFYTRAATMIGEIAAAVSFISKFLRTKGLTSERQLQTFSQSLQELLAEHYKHHWFPE
(60)   KPCKGSGYRCIRINHKMDPLIGQAAQRIGLSSQELFRLLPSELTLWVDPYEVSYRIGEDG
(120)  SICVLYEASPAGGSTQNSTNVQMVDSRISCKEELLLGRTSPSKNYNMMTVSG (171)
```

Roualt, J.-P., Rimokh, R., Tessa, C., Paranhos, G., Ffrench, M., Duret, L., Garoccio, M., Germain, D., Samarut, J. and Magaud, J.-P. (1992). *BTG1*, a member of a new family of antiproliferative genes. EMBO J., 11, 1663–1670.

Others

Gene   IL3 (5q31)   *Translocation*   t(5;14)(q31;q32)   *Leukaemia*   Acute pre-B cell

Translocation joins the immunoglobulin heavy chain gene (chromosome 14) to the *IL3* promoter resulting in overexpression of *IL3*. Acute pre-B cell leukaemia may thus involve an IL-3 autocrine loop, although as overexpression of *IL3* in mice is not sufficient to induce leukaemia, it is probable that other oncogenes are involved (Meeker *et al.*, 1990).

Meeker, T.C., Hardy, D., Willman, C., Hogan, T. and Abrams, J. (1990). Activation of the interleukin-3 gene by chromosome translocation in acute lymphocytic leukemia with eosinophilia. Blood, 76, 285–289.

Gene   TAN1 (9q34)   *Translocation*   t(7;9)(q34;q34.3)   *Leukaemia*   T-ALL

The 9q34.3 region is transcriptionally activated by translocation during rearrangement of the D–J segments of TCRβ (Reynolds *et al.*, 1987) and at least five translocations involving the TCRβ gene showing cytogenetic breakpoints at 7q34–35 have been detected. In t(7;9)(q34;q34.3) the second locus involved is *TAN1* on chromosome 9. *TAN1* (translocation-associated *Notch* homologue: highly homologous to *Drosophila Notch*) encodes an 8.3 kb mRNA (2555 amino acid ORF) expressed in normal fetal human tissues and the mouse homologue is expressed in many normal adult cells. Most abundant in lymphoid tissues. Breakpoints within 100 bp of a *TAN1* intron have been detected in ALL: the products of such genes would encode a TAN1 protein lacking its normal extracellular domain (Ellisen *et al.*, 1991).

Sequence of TAN1

```
  (1)  MPPLLAPLLCLALLPALAARGPRCSQPGETCLNGGKCEAANGTEACVCGGAFVGPRCQD
 (60)  PNPCLSTPCKNAGTCHVVDRRGVADYACSCALGFSGPLCLTPLDNACLTNPCRNGGTCDL
(120)  LTLTEYKCRCPPGWSGKSCQQADPCASNPCANGGQCLPFEASYICHCPPSFHGPTCRQDV
(180)  NECGQKPRLCRHGGTCHNEVGSYRCVCRATHTGPNCERPYVPCSPSPCQNGGTCRPTGDV
(240)  THECACLPGFTGQNCEENIDDCPGNNCKNGGACVDGVNTYNCPCPPEWTGQYCTEDVDEC
(300)  QLMPNACQNGGTCHNTHGGYNCVCVNGWTGEDCSENIDDCASAACFHGATCHDRVASFYC
(360)  ECPHGRTGLLCHLNDACISNPCNEGSNCDTNPVNGKAICTCPSGYTGPACSQDVDECSLG
(420)  ANPCEHAGKCINTLGSFECQCLQGYTGPRCEIDVNECVSNPCQNDATCLDQIGEFQCMCM
(480)  PGYEGVHCEVNTDECASSPCLHNGRCLDKINEFQCECPTGFTGHLCQDVDECASTPCKNG
(540)  AKCLDGPNTYTCVCTEGYTGTHCEVDIDECDPDPCHYGSCKDGVATFTCLCRPGYTGHHC
(600)  ETNINECSSQPCRLRGTCQDPDNAYLCFCLKGTTGPNCEINLDDCASSPCDSGTCLDKID
(660)  GYECACEPGYTGSMCNSNIDECAGNPCHNGGTCEDGINGFTCRCPEGYHDPTCLSEVNEC
(720)  NSNPCVHGACRDSLNGYKCDCDPGWSGTNCDINNNECESNPCVNGGTCKDMTSGIVCTCR
(780)  EGFSGPNCQTNINECASNPCLNKGTCIDDVAGYKCNCLLPYTGATCEVVLAPCAPSPCRN
(840)  GGECRQSEDYESFSCVCPTAGAKGQTCEVDINECVLSPCRHGASCQNTHGXYRCHCQAGY
(900)  SGRNCETDIDDCRPNPCHNGGSCTDGINTAFCDCLPGFRGTFCEEDINECASDPCRNGAN
(960)  CTDCVDSYTCTCPAGFSGIHCENNTPDCTESSCFNGGTCVDGINSFTCLCPPGFTGSYCQ
(1020) HVVNECDSRPCLLGGTCQDGRGLHRCTCPQGYTGPNCQNLVHWCDSSPCKNGGKCWQTHT
(1080) QYRCECPSGWTGLYCDVPSVSCEVAAQRQGVDVARLCQHGGLCVDAGNTHHCRCQAGYTG
(1140) SYCEDLVDECSPSPCQNGATCTDYLGGYSCKCVAGYHGVNCSEEIDECLSHPCQNGGTCL
(1200) DLPNTYKCSCPRGTQGVHCEINVDDCNPPVDPVSRSPKCFNNGTCVDQVGGYSCTCPPGF
(1260) VGERCEGDVNECLSNPCDARGTQNCVQRVNDFHCECRAGHTGRRCESVINGCKGKPCKNG
(1320) GTCAVASNTARGFICKCPAGFEGATCENDARTCGSLRCLNGGTCISGPRSPTCLCLGPFT
(1380) GPECQFPASSPCLGGNPCYNQGTCEPTSESPFYRCLCPAKFNGLLCHILDYSFGGGAGRD
(1440) IPPPLIEEACELPECQEDAGNKVCSLQCNNHACGWDGGDCSLNFNDPWKNCTQSLQCWKY
(1500) FSDGHCDSQCNSAGCLFDGFDCQRAEGQCNPLYDQYCKDHFSDGHCDQGCNSAECEWDGL
(1560) DCAEHVPERLAAGTLVVVVLMPPEQLRNSSFHFLRELSRVLHTNVVFKRDAHGQQMIFPY
(1620) YGREEELRKHPIKRAAEGWAAPDALLGQVKASLLPGGSEGGRRRRELDPMDVRGSIVYLE
(1680) IDNRQCVQASSQCFQSATDVAAFLGALASLGSLNIPYKIEAVQSETVEPPPPAQLHFMYV
(1740) AAAAFVLLFFVGCGVLLSRKRRXQHGQLWFPEGFKVSEASKKKRREXLGEDSVGLKPLKN
(1800) ASDGALMDDNQNEWGDEDLETKKFRFEEPVVLPDLDDQTDHRQWTQQHLDAADLRMSAMA
(1860) PTPPQGEVDADCMDVNVRGPDGFTPLMIASCSGGGLETGNSEEEEDAPAVISDFIYQGAS
(1920) LHNQTDRTGETALHLAARYSRSDAAKRLLEASADANIQDNMGRTPLHAAVSADAQGVFQI
(1980) LIRNRATDLDARMHDGTTPLILAARLAVEGMLEDLINSHADVNAVDDLGKSALHWAAAVN
(2040) NVDAAVVLLKNGANKDMQNNREETPLFLAAREGSYETAKVLLDHFANRDITDHMDRLPRD
(2100) IAQERMHHDIVRLLLDEYNLVRSPQLHGAPLGGTPTLSPPLCSPNGYLGSLKPGVQGKKVR
(2160) KPSSKGLACGSKEAKDLKARRKKSQDGKGCLLDSSGMLSPVDSLESPHGYLSDVASPPLL
```

```
(2220)  PSPFQQSPSVPLNHLPGMPDTHLGIGHLNVAAKPEMAALGGGGRLAFETGPPRLSHLPVA
(2280)  SGTSTVLGSSSGGALNFTVGGSTSLNGQCEWLSRLQSGMVPNQYNPLRGSVAPGPLSTQA
(2340)  PSLQHGMVGPLHSSLAASALSQMMSYQGLPSTRLATQPHLVQTQQVQPQNLQMQQQNLQP
(2400)  ANIQQQQSLQPPPPPPQPHLGVSSAASGHLGRSFLSGEPSQADVQPLGPSSLAVHTILPQ
(2460)  ESPALPTSLPSSLVPPVTAAQFLTPPSQHSYSSPVENTPSHQLQVPEHPFLTPSPESPDQ
(2520)  WSSSSPHSNVSDWSEGVSSPPTSMQSQIARIPEAFK  (2555)
```

Arrows indicate beginnings of the 36 tandemly repeated epidermal growth factor cysteine repeats. Underlined: beginning of the three *Notch/lin-12* cysteine repeats. Italics: six regions with homology to the *Saccharomyces pombe cdc*10 gene product.

Ellisen, L.W., Bird, J., West, D.C., Soreng, A.L., Reynolds, T.C., Smith, S.D. and Sklar, J. (1991). *TAN-1*, the human homolog of the Drosophila *Notch* gene, is broken by chromosomal translocations in T lymphoblastic neoplasms. Cell, 66, 649–661.

Reynolds, T.C., Smith, S.D. and Sklar, J. (1987). Analysis of DNA surrounding the breakpoints of chromosome translocations involving the β T cell receptor gene in human lymphoblastic neoplasms. Cell, 50, 107–117.

Gene	*MLL* (11q23)	*Translocations*	t(4;11)(q21;q23)	*Leukaemia*	AML
	AF4 (4q21)				
	AF9 (9q22)		t(9;11)(q22;q23)		
	ENL (19p13.3)		t(11;19)(q23;p13.3)		

The *MLL* (*m*yeloid/*l*ymphoid, or *m*ixed-*l*ineage, *l*eukaemia, also called *ALL1*) gene is rearranged in acute leukaemias with interstitial deletions or translocations between chromosome 11 and chromosomes 1, 4, 6, 9, 10 or 19. *MLL* spans ~100 kb and contains at least 21 exons encoding a protein of >3968 amino acids (Gu *et al.*, 1992; Tkachuk *et al.*, 1992). In normal pre-B cells 2.0, 11.5, 12.0 and 12.5 kb *MLL* mRNAs are detected (McCabe *et al.*, 1992). MLL shares regions homology with the *Drosophila trithorax* gene product, including six zinc finger domains. A 12.5 kb transcript of *MLL* spans the breakpoint junctions of the translocations (Ziemin-van der Poel *et al.*, 1992). mRNAs of 11.5, 11.25, 11.0 kb and other truncated transcripts expressed in cells with the 11q23 translocation may represent abnormal forms arising from the translocation (Yamamoto *et al.*, 1993). The t(4;11) translocation cleaves the *MLL* gene within the coding region, resulting in the fusion of the *MLL* ORF with the *AF4* gene (ALL-1 fused gene from chromosome 4) and the predicted production of two chimeric proteins. In t(11;19) *MLL* is fused to the *ENL* (*e*leven-*n*ineteen *l*eukaemia) gene (Tkachuk *et al.*, 1992) on chromosome 19 and in the t(9;11) abnormality to the *AF9* gene (Nakamura *et al.*, 1993).

Gu, Y., Nakamura, T., Alder, H., Prasad, R., Canaani, O., Cimino, G., Croce, C. and Canaani, E. (1992). The t(4;11) chromosome translocation of human acute leukemias fuses the *ALL-1* gene, related to Drosophila *trithorax*, to the *AF-4* gene, Cell, 71, 701–708.

McCabe, N.R., Burnett, R.C., Gill, H.J., Thirman, M.J., Mbangkollo, D., Kipiniak, M., van Melle, E., Ziemin-van der Poel, S., Rowley, J.D. and Diaz, M.O. (1992). Cloning of cDNAs of the *MLL* gene that detect DNA rearrangements and altered RNA transcripts in human leukemic cells with 11q23 translocations. Proc. Natl Acad. Sci. USA, 89, 11794–11798.

Nakumura, T., Alder, H., Gu, Y., Prasad, R., Canaani, O., Kamada, N., Gale, R.P., Lange, B., Crist, W.M., Nowell, P.C., Croce, C.M. and Canaani, E. (1993). Genes on chromosomes 4, 9, and 19 involved in 11q23 abnormalities in acute leukemia share sequence homology and/or common motifs. Proc Natl Acad. Sci. USA, 90, 4631–4635.

Tkachuk, D.C., Kohler, S and Cleary, M.L. (1992). Involvement of a homolog of Drosophila trithorax by11q23 chromosomal translocations in acute leukemias. Cell, 71, 691–700.

Yamamoto, K., Seto, M., Akao, Y., Iida, S., Nakazawa, S., Oshimura, M., Takahashi, T. and Ueda, R. (1993). Gene rearrangement and truncated mRNA in cell lines with 11q23 translocation. Oncogene, 8, 479–485.

Ziemin-van der Poel, S., McCabe, N.R., Gill, H.J., Espinosa, R., Patel, Y., Harden, A., Rubinelli, P., Smith, S.D., LeBeau, M.M., Rowley, J.D. and Diaz, M.O. (1992). Identification of a gene, *MLL*, that spans the breakpoint in 11q23 translocations associated with human leukemias. Proc. Natl Acad. Sci. USA, 88, 10735–10739.

Gene	*AML1* (8q22)	*Translocation*	t(8;21)(q22;q22)	*Leukaemia*	AML
	ETO (21q22)				

Breakpoints of the t(8;21) translocation occur within the *AML1* gene on chromosome 21 (Miyoshi *et al.*, 1991). Four species of mRNA (2.1, 4.3, 5.4 and 8.2 kb) occur in normal cells. The AML1 protein has homology with the *Drosophila* segmentation gene product *runt* and the α subunit of the polyoma virus enhancer binding protein 2 (PEBP2α). The murine homologue of *AML1*, *PEBP2αB* is highly expressed in both B cell and T cell lines (Bae *et al.*, 1993). The fusion product AML1–ETO is transcribed from the t(8;21) translocation breakpoint but *ETO* is not normally expressed in myeloid cells although a 5.5 kb transcript occurs in the lung (Chang *et al.*, 1993).

Sequence of AML1

```
  (1)   MRIPVDASTSRRFTPPSTALSPGKMSEALPLGAPDAGAALAGKLRSGDRSMVEVLADHP
 (60)   GELVRTDSPNFLCSVLPTHWRCNKTLPIAFKVVALGDVPDGTLVTVMAGNDENYSAELRN
(120)   ATAAMKNQVARFNDLRFVGRSGRGKSFTLTITVFTNPP QVATYHRAIKITVDGPREPRRH
                         ───────    Δ
(180)   RQKLDDQTKPGSLSFSERLSELEQLRRTAMRVSPHHPAPTPNPRASLNHSTAFNPQPQSQ
(240)   MQEEDTAPWRC(250)
```

Underlined: putative ATP or GTP binding site. Δ Indicates site of breakpoints occurring in t(8;21) translocations.

Bae, S.C., Yamaguchi-Iwai, Y., Ogawa, E., Maruyama, M., Inuzuka, M., Kagoshima, H., Shigesaada, K., Satake, M. and Ito, Y. (1993). Isolation of *PEBP2αB* cDNA representing the mouse homolog of human acute myeloid leukemia gene, *AML1*. Oncogene, 8, 809–814.

Chang, K.-S., Fan, Y.-H., Stass, S.A., Estey, E.H., Wang, G., Trujillo, J.M., Erickson, P. and Drabkin, H. (1993). Expression of *AML1–ETO* fusion transcripts and detection of minimal residual disease in t(8;21)-positive acute myeloid leukemia. Oncogene, 8, 983–988.

Miyoshi, H., Shimiizu, K., Maseki, N., Kaneko, Y. and Ohki, M. (1991). t(8;21) breakpoints on chromosome 21 in acute myeloid leukemia are clustered within a limited region of a single gene, *AML1*. Proc. Natl Acad. Sci. USA, 88, 10431–10434.

ALL: acute lymphoblastic leukaemia; AML: acute myeloid leukaemia; APL: acute promyelocytic leukaemia (a subtype of AML); ANLL: acute nonlymphocytic leukaemia; B-CLL: chronic B cell lymphocytic leukaemia; CML: chronic myelogenous leukaemia; T-ALL: acute T cell leukaemia.

Reviews

Rabbitts, T.H. (1991). Translocations, master genes and differences between the origins of acute and chronic leukemias. Cell, 67, 641–644.

Sawyers, C.L., Denny, C.T. and Witte, O.N. (1991). Leukemia and the disruption of normal hematopoiesis. Cell, 64, 337–350.

Databank file names and accession numbers

	GENE	EMBL	SWISSPROT	REFERENCES
Human	AF-4	L13773		Nakamura et al., 1993
	AF-9	L13743		Nakamura et al., 1993
Human	ALL/AF-9	L13744		Nakamura et al., 1993
	ALL/MLL/HRX	Hshrx L04284		Tkachuk et al., 1992
Human	AML1	Hsaml1 D10570, D90525		Miyoshi et al., 1991
		Hsaml1bd M83215		
Human	BCM	Hsbcm Z14954		Laabi et al., 1992
	BCM-IL2	Hsil2bcm Z14955		
	Breakpoint regions	(Hsc16ba Z14317;		
		(Hsc16bb Z14318;		
		(Hsc16bc Z14319;		
		(Hsc16bd Z14320		
Human	BTG1	Hsbtg1 X61123		Roualt et al., 1992
Human	CAN	Hscan X64228		von Lindern et al., 1992b
Human	DEK	Hsdek9 X64229		von Lindern et al., 1992b
Human	ENL	Hsen1 L04285		Tkachuk et al., 1992
Human	EWS	Hsews X66899		Delattre et al., 1992
Human	HOX11	Hshox M75952		Kennedy et al., 1991
				Lu et al., 1992
Human	LYL1	Hslyl1a M22637	LYL1_HUMAN P12980	Mellentin et al., 1989
		Hslyl1b M22638		
Mouse	Lyl-1	Mmlyl1 X55055		Kuo et al., 1991
		Mmlyl122 X57686		Visvader et al., 1991
		Mmlyl16 X57687		
Human	PBX1a, PBX1b	Hspbx1ab M864546		Monica et al., 1991
	PBX2	Hspbx2 X59842		
	PBX3	Hspbx3 X59841		
Human	PML	Hspmlex23 X63631		Pandolfi et al., 1992
	PML–RARA	Hspmlrark X63647		Fagioli et al., 1992
Human	PLZF	Z19002		Chen et al., 1993
Human	PRL/E2A	Hstraa1 M31522		Kamps et al., 1990
Human	RBTN1	Hsrhom2A M64357		Boehm et al., 1991
		Hsrhom3A M64358		
		Hstcrdrho M64361		
	RBTN2, RBTN3			Foroni et al., 1992
Mouse	Rbtn-1			Foroni et al., 1992
	Rbtn-2	Mmrhom2a M64359		Boehm et al., 1991
		Mmrhom2b M64360		
	Rbtn-3			Foroni et al., 1992
Human	RBTN2	Hsttg2 X61118	RHM2_HUMAN P25791	Royer-Pokora et al., 1991
Human	SET	Hsset M93651		von Lindern et al., 1992a
Human	SIL	Hssil M74558		Aplan et al., 1991
Human	TAL1	Hstal1aa X51990		Chen et al., 1990
				Cheng et al., 1993b

	GENE	EMBL	SWISSPROT	REFERENCES
Human	*TAL2*	Hstal M81078		Xia *et al.*, 1991
Mouse	*Tal-2*	Mmtal M81077		Xia *et al.*, 1991
Human	*TAN1*	Hstan1 M73980		Ellisen *et al.*, 1991

Table 2.4. *Tumour suppressor genes detected in human tumours*

Gene	Chromosomal locus	Neoplasms
APC	5q21–22	Familial adenomatosis polyposis (FAP)
BRCA1	17q12–21	Breast and ovarian cancer
CMAR/CAR	16q	Breast, prostate cancers
DCC	18q21	Colon carcinoma
α-inhibin (*INHA*)	2q33–qter	Gonadal tumours?
MEN1	11q13	Parathyroid, pancreatic and pituitary and adrenal cortex tumours
NF1	17q11.2	Neurofibromatosis type 1
NF2	22q12	Neurofibromatosis type 2
NM23	17q21.3	Neuroblastoma, colon carcinoma
PHB	17q21	Breast carcinoma
P53	17p13.1	Breast, colon and lung carcinoma, osteosarcoma, astrocytoma
RB	13q14	Retinoblastoma, breast, bladder and lung carcinoma, osteosarcoma
VHL	3p25–p26	von Hippel–Lindau disease
WT1	11p12	Wilms' tumour
	11p15.5	Wilms' tumour
	16q22.1–23.2	Liver carcinoma
	3p21	Lung carcinoma
	3p12–14	Kidney carcinoma
	1p36.1	Neuroblastoma

Table 2.5. *Functions of oncoproteins*

Class 1. Growth factors:
PDGFB/SIS, INT2, HSTF1/HST1, WNT1/WNT3

Class 2. Tyrosine kinases:
Receptor-like tyrosine kinases:
EPH (ECK, EEK, ELK, ERK, CEK, HEK, MEK, NUK, SEK), **EGFR/ERBB, FMS, KIT**, TYK1/LTK, **MET, HER2/NEU, RET, ROS**, RYk, **SEA**, TIE, **TRK**, UFO
Non-receptor tyrosine kinases:
ABL1 (ARG), CSK/CYL, **FPS/FES**, (FER/TYK3), TKF
Membrane-associated non-receptor tyrosine kinases:
SRC, SRC-related kinases: Blk, **FGR, FYN, HCK, LCK**, LYN/SYN, TKL, **YES**

Class 3. Receptors lacking protein kinase activity:
MAS, MPL

Class 4a. Membrane-associated G proteins:
HRAS, KRAS, NRAS, GSP, GIP2

Table 2.5. *Continued*

Class 4b. Guanine nucleotide exchange proteins:
SDC25

Class 4c. RHO/RAC binding proteins:
BCR, DBL, ECT2

Class 5. Cytoplasmic protein serine kinases:
BCR, Clk (& Nek), EST/COT, **MOS, PIM1, RAF/MIL**

Class 6. Protein serine-, threonine- and tyrosine kinase:
STY

Class 7. Cytoplasmic regulators:
BCL1, CRK, NCK, ornithine decarboxylase, PEM

Class 8. Transcription factors:
BCL3, CBL, ERBA, ETS (ELK), EVI1*, **FOS (FOSB, ΔFOSB, FRA1, FRA2)**, GLI, HOX2.4, HOX7.1, HOX11†, **JUN, (JUNB, JUND)**, LYL1, **MYB (MBM2), MYC, MYCL, MYCN**, Qin, RBTN1†, RBTN2†, **REL, TAL1, SKI**, TRE, VAV

Class 9. Mitochondrial membrane factor:
BCL2

Class 10. Function unknown:
AKT, DLK, LCO/LCA, NRL (MAF), MEL, MELF, SCC, TLM

This table lists gene products that have been shown to be tumorigenic or that are specifically expressed in at least one type of tumour cell. Those in bold type are described in individual sections in Chapter 3. Entries in brackets are discussed in the preceding bold type entry. Oncoproteins in plain text, selected on the arbitrary basis of having not more than eight references cited, are summarized in Table 2.5 Supplement. *Summarized in Table 2.2 Supplement. †Summarized in Table 2.3 Supplement.

Table 2.5 supplement. *Functions of oncogenes (summaries)*

Akt

Akt is the oncogene of the transforming retrovirus AKT8 isolated from a spontaneous mouse thymoma (Staal, 1987). The mouse gene (chromosome 12) has two known human homologues, *AKT1* (chromosome 14q32; amplified in a primary gastric adenocarcinoma) and *AKT2* (Staal *et al.*, 1988). AKT1 is 98% homologous to the mouse AKT protein (Bellacosa *et al.*, 1993). v-*akt* encodes a tripartite *gag* (p12, p15, Δp30)–X–*Akt* product that is a protein kinase C-related serine/threonine kinase highly expressed in the thymus (Bellacosa *et al.*, 1991). *AKT* contains an SH2 domain in its regulatory region.

Sequence of v-AKT

```
  (1)  MGQTVTTPLSLTLEHWGDVQRIASNQSVDVKKRRWVTFCSAEWPTFGVGWPQDGTFNLD
 (60)  IILQVKSKVFSPGPHGHPDQVPYIVTWEAIAYEPPPWVKPFVSPKLSLSPTAPILPSGPS
(120)  TQPPPRSALYPALTPSIKPRPSKPQVLSDNGGPLIDLLTEDPPPYGEQGPSSSDGDGDRE
(180)  EATSTPEIPAPSPMVSRLRGKRDPPAAVSTTSRAFPLRLGGNGQLQYWPFSSSDLYNWKN
(240)  NNPSFSEDPGKLTALIESVLTTHAREETLIIIPGLPLSLGATDTMNDVAIVKEGWLHKRG
(300)  EYIKTWRPRYFLLKNDGTFIGYKERPQDVDQRESPLNNFSVAQCQLMKTERPRPNTFIIR
(360)  CLQWTTVIERTFHVETPEEREEWATAIQTVADGLKRQEEETMDFRSGSPSDNSGAEEMEV
(420)  SLAKPKHRVTMNEFEYLKLLGKGTFGKVILVKEKATGRYYAMKILKKEVIVAKDEVAHTL
(480)  TENRVLQNSRHPFLTALKYSFQTHDRLCFVMEYANGGELFFHLSRERVFSEDRARFYGAE
(540)  IVSALDYLHSEKNVVYRDLKLENLMLDKDGHIKITDFGLCKEGIKDGATMKTFCGTPEYL
(600)  APEVLEDNDYGRAVDWWGLGVVMYEMMCGRLPFYNQDHEKLFELILMEEIRFPRTLGPEA
(660)  KSLLSGLLKKDPTQRLGGGSEDAKEIMQHRFFANIVWQDVYEKKLSPPFKPQVTSETDTR
(720)  YFDEEFTAQMITITPPDQDDSMECVDSERRPHFPQFSYSASGTA (763)
```

Bellacosa, A., Testa, J.R., Staal, S.P. and Tsichlis, P.N. (1991). A retroviral oncogene, *akt*, encoding a serine–threonine kinase containing an SH-2-like region. Science, 254, 274–277.

Bellacosa, A., Franke, T.F., Gonzalez-Portal, E., Datta, K., Taguuchi, T., Gardner, J., Cheng, J.Q., Testa, J.R. and Tsichlis, P.N. (1993). Structure, expression and chromosomal mapping of c-*akt*: relationship to v-*akt* and its implications. Oncogene, 8, 745–754.

Staal, S.P. (1987). Molecular cloning of the *akt* oncogene and its human homologues *AKT1* and *AKT2*: amplification of *AKT1* in a primary human gastric adenocarcinoma. Proc. Natl Acad. Sci. USA, 84, 5034–5037.

Staal, S.P., Huebner, K., Croce, C.M., Parsa, N.Z. and Testa, J.R. (1988). The *AKT1* proto-oncogene maps to human chromosome 14, band q32. Genomics, 2, 96–98.

Blk

Blk is a member of the *Src* tyrosine kinase family (*Blk, Fgr, Fyn, Hck, Lck/Tkl, Lyn, Src, Yes*). In the mouse and in cell lines *Blk* is specifically expressed in the B cell lineage (Dymecki *et al.*, 1990).

Sequence of mouse BLK

```
  (1)   MGLLSSKRQVSEKGKGWSPVKIRTQDKAPPPLPPLVVFNHLAPPSPNQDPDEEERFVVALFDYAAVNDR
 (70)   DLQVLKGEKLQVLRSTGDWWLARSLVTGREGYVPSNFVAPVETLEVEKWFFRTISRKDAERQLLAPMNKA
(140)   GSFLIRESESNKGAFSLSVKDITTQGEVVKHYKIRSLDNGGYYISPRITFPTLQALVQHYSKKGDGLCQK
(210)   LTLPCVNLAPKNLWAQDEWEIPRQSLKLVRKLGSGQFGEVVMGYYKNNMKVAIKTLKEGTMSPEAFLGEA
(280)   NVMKTLQHERLVRLYAVVTREPIYIVTEYMARGCLLDFLKTDEGSRLSLPRLIDMSAQVAEGMAYIERMN
(350)   SIHRDLRAANILVSETLCCKIADFGLARIIDSEYTAQEGAKFPIKWTAPEAIHFGVFTIKADVWSFGVLL
(420)   MVIVTYGRVPYPGMSNPEVIRSLEHGYRMPCPETCPPELYNDIITECWRGRPEERPTFEFLQSVLEDFYT
(490)   ATEGQYELQP (499)
```

Dymecki, S.M., Niederhuber, J.E. and Desiderio, S.V. (1990). Specific expression of a tyrosine kinase gene, *blk*, in B lymphoid cells. Science, 247, 332–336.

Clk

Clk (CDC28/cdc2⁺-*like* kinase) was detected in mouse erythroleukaemia cells. CLK has intrinsic serine/threonine and tyrosine kinase activity and a C-terminal *cdc*2 kinase domain. It is closely related to *nek* (nimA-related kinase), a putative serine/threonine kinase (2.2 kb mRNA; 774 amino acids) related to nimA that is expressed in the central nervous system and reproductive system and regulates the G_2–M phase transition in *Aspergillus nidulans* (Ben-David *et al.*, 1991).

Sequence of mouse CLK

```
  (1)   MRHSKRTYCPDWDERDWDYGTWRSSSSHKRKKRSHSSAREQKRCRYDHSKTTDSYYLES
 (60)   RSINEKAYHSRRYVDEYRNDYMGYEPGHPYGEPGSRYQMHSSKSSGRSGRSSYKSKHRSR
(120)   HHTSQHHSHGKSHRRKRSRSVEDDEEGHLICQSGDVLSARYEIVDTLGEGAFGKVVECID
(180)   HKVGGRRVAVKIVKNVDRYCEAAQSEIQVLEHLNTTDPHSTFRCVQMLEWFEHRGHICIV
(240)   FELLGLSTYDFIKENSFLPFRMDHIRKMAYQICKSVNFLHSNKLTHTDLKPENILFVKSD
(300)   YTEAYNPKMKRDERTIVNPDIKVVDFGSATYDDEHHSTLVSTRHYRAPEVILALGWSQPC
(360)   DVWSIGCILIEYYLGFTVFPTHDSREHLAMMERILGPLPKHMIQKTRKRRYFHHDRLDWD
(420)   EHSSAGRYVSRRCKPLKEFMLSQDAEHEFLFDLVGKILEYDPAKRITLKEALKHPFFYPL
(480)   KKHT (483)
```

Ben-David, Y., Letwin, K., Tannock, L., Bernstein, A. and Pawson, T. (1991). A mammalian protein kinase with potential for serine/threonine and tyrosine-phosphorylation is related to cell cycle regulators. EMBO J., 10, 317–325.

CSK

CSK (*C*onsensus tyrosine-*l*acking *k*inase) cDNA was isolated from the K562 human leukaemia cell line, chromosome 15 (Partanen *et al.*, 1991). *CYL* is probably identical to *CSK* (*c-src k*inase; Nada *et al.*, 1991). The 12 exons of *CSK* (Brauninger *et al.*, 1993) give rise to 2.6 and 3.4 kb mRNAs expressed ubiquitously. The deduced 450 amino acid sequence lacks signal and transmembrane regions but contains tyrosine kinase, SH2 and SH3 domains. CSK lacks the highly conserved tyrosine autophosphorylation site (Tyr416) and also Tyr527 of SRC. It has no myristylation signal. It specifically phosphorylates Tyr527 of p60^{src} from neonatal rat brain (see **SRC**). CSK specifically phosphorylates p56^{lck} in human T cells (see **LCK**). *CYL/CSK* is distinct from murine *Cyl-1*, *Cyl-2* and *Cyl-3* that are homologous to human cyclins D1, D2 and D3 (see Tables 2.1 and 2.2 and **BCL1**).

Sequence of CSK

```
  (1)  MSAIQASWPSGTECIAKYNFHGTAEQDLPFCKGDVLTIVAVTKDPNWYKAKNKVGREGII
 (61)  PANYVQKREGVKAGTKLSLMPWFHGKITREQAERLLYPPETGLFLVRESTNYPGDYTLCV
(121)  SCEGKVEHYRIMYHASKLSIDEEVYFENLMQLVEHYTTDADGLCTRLIKPKVMEGTVAAQ
(181)  DEFYRSGWALNMKELKLLQTIGKGEFGDVMLGDYRGNKVAVKCIKNDATAQAFLAEASVM
(241)  TQLRHSNLVQLLGVIVEEKGGLYIVTEYMAKGSLVDYLRSRGRSVLGGDCLLKFSLDVCE
(301)  AMEYLEGNNFVHRDLAARNVLVSEDNVAKVSDFGLTKEASSTQDTGKLPVKWTAPEALRE
(361)  KKFSTKSDVWSFGILLWEIYSFGRVPYPRIPLKDVVPRVEKGYKMDAPDGCPPAVYDVMK
(421)  NCWHLDAATRPTFLQLREQLEHIRTHELHL (450)
```

Italics: SH3 domain. Underlined: SH2 domain.

Brauninger, A., Karn, T., Strebhardt, K. and Rubsamen-Waigmann, H. (1993). Characterization of the human CSK locus. Oncogene, 8, 1365–1369.

Nada, S., Okada, M., MacAuley, A., Cooper, J.A. and Nakagawa, H. (1991). Cloning of a complementary DNA for a protein tyrosine kinase that specifically phosphorylates a negative regulatory site of p60^{src}. Nature, 351, 69–72.

Partanen, J., Armstrong, E., Bergman, M., Makela, T.P., Hirvonen, H., Huebner, K. and Alitalo, K. (1991). cyl encodes a putative cytoplasmic tyrosine kinase lacking the conserved tyrosine autophosphorylation site (Y416^{src}). Oncogene, 6, 2013–2018.

DLK

DLK (*D*elta-*l*ike) is a putative transmembrane protein (42 kDa, human and mouse, 86.2% identical), highly homologous to invertebrate homeotic proteins including *delta* and *notch* and is a member of the EGF-like superfamily (Laborda *et al.*, 1993). *DLK* is expressed in normal adrenal gland and placenta and in some neuroendocrine tumour cell lines, including a subset of small-cell lung carcinoma cell lines.

Sequence of mouse and human DLK

```
Mouse DLK   (1)   MIATGALLRVLLLLLAFGHSTYGAECDPPCDPQYGFCEADNVCRCHVGWEGPLCDKCVTA
Human DLK   (1)   -T--E-----------------F-A-N--N----D---------------Q---S

Mouse DLK  (61)   PGCVNGVCKEPWQCICKDGWDGKFCEIDVRACTSTPCANNGTCVDLEKGQYECSCTPGFS
Human DLK  (61)   ---LH-L-G--G----T-----EL-DR-----S----------S-DG-L-----A--Y-

Mouse DLK (121)   GKDCQHKAGPCVINGSPCQHGGACVDDEGQASHASCLCPPGFSGNFCEIVAATNSCTPNP
Human DLK (121)   -----K-D-------------T------R-------------------  ------
```

```
Mouse DLK  (181)  CENDGVCTDIGGDFRCRCPAGFVDKTCSRPVSNCASGPCQNGGTCLQHTQVSFECLCKPP
Human DLK  (179)  ---------------------I--------T----S--------------Y------E

Mouse DLK  (241)  FMGPTCAKKRGASPVQVTHLPSGYGLTYRLTPGVHELPVQQPEQHILKVSMKELNKSTPL
Human DLK  (239)  -T-L--V---AL--Q---R-------A----------------HR----------K---

Mouse DLK  (301)  LTEGQAICFTILGVLTSLVVLGTVAIVFLNKCETWVSNLRYNHTFRKKKNLLLQYNSGEE
Human DLK  (299)  ----------------------G-----------------ML-------------D

Mouse DLK  (361)  LAVNIIFPEKIDMTTFNKEAGDEEI (385)
Human DLK  (359)  ---------------S-------- (383)
```

Underlined: signal sequence. Italics: transmembrane domain.

Laborda, J., Sausville, E.A., Hoffman, T. and Notario, V. (1993). *dlk*, a putative mammalian homeotic gene differentially expressed in small cell lung carcinoma and neuroendocrine tumor cell line. J. Biol. Chem., 268, 3817–3820.

Ect-2

Ect-2 was detected by transfection of NIH 3T3 cells with mouse keratinocyte cDNA (Miki *et al.*, 1993). The oncogenic potential of ECT2 is activated by N-terminal truncation. The central 255 amino acid sequence of ECT2 is similar to that of BCR, DBL and CDC24, all of which regulate RHO-like GTP-binding proteins.

Sequence of ECT2

```
  (1)    MLNLVLCFTGFRKKEELVKLVTLVHHMGGVIRKECNSKVTHLVANCTQGEKFRVAVSLG
 (60)    TPIMKPEWIYKAWERRNEQCFCAAVDDFRNEFKVPPFQDCILSFLGFSDEEKHSMEEMTE
(120)    MQGGSYLPVGDERCTHLIVEENTVKDLPFEPSKKLFVVKQEWFWGSIQMDARAGETMYLY
(180)    EKANTPELKKSVSLLSLSTPNSNRKRRRLKETLAQLSRETDLSPFPPRKRPSAEHSLSIG
(240)    SLLDISNTPESSIHYGETPKSCAKSSRSSTPVPPKQSARWQVAKELYQTESNYVNILATI
(300)    IQLFQVPLEEEGQRGGPILAPEEIKTIFGSIPDIFDVHMKIKDDLEDLIANWDESRSIGD
(360)    IFLKYAKDLVKTYPPFVNFFEMSKEMIIKCEKQKPRFHAFLKINQAKPECGRQSLVELLI
(420)    RPVQRLPSVALLLNDLKKHTADENPDKSTLEKAIGSLKEVMTHINEDKRKTEAQKQIFDV
(480)    VYEVDGCPANLLSSHRSLVQRVETVSLGEHPCDRGEQVTLFLFNDCLEIARKRHKVIGTF
(540)    RSPHDRTRPPASLKHIHLMPLSQIKKVLDIRETEDCHNAFALLVRPPTEQANVLLSFQMT
(600)    SEELPKESWLKMLCRHVANTICKADAENLMYVADPESFEVNTKDMDSTLSRASRAIKKTS
(660)    KKVTRAFSFSKTPKRALRMALSSSHSSEGRSPPSSGKLAVSRLSSTSSLAGIPSPSLVSL
(720)    PSFFERRSHTLSRSTTHLI (738)
```

Underlined: region of sequence homology with BCR, DBL and CDC24.

Miki, T., Smith, C.L., Long, J.E., Eva, A. and Fleming, T.P. (1993). Oncogene *ect2* is related to regulators of small GTP-binding proteins. Nature, 362, 462–465.

EST/COT

EST was identified by transfection of NIH 3T3 cells with DNA from a Ewing sarcoma cell line (Chan *et al.*, 1993). It is the cellular proto-oncogene of *COT* (cancer Osaka thyroid), a cytoplasmic serine kinase identified by transfection of the hamster-derived cell line SHOK with DNA from a cell line derived from human anaplastic thyroid cancer. *COT* encodes 46 kDa and 52 kDa proteins, probably by utilizing alternative AUG initiation codons (Aoki *et al.*, 1991). Over-expression of *COT* transforms NIH 3T3 cells or SHOK cells (Miyoshi *et al.*, 1991). *EST* mRNA (3.2 kb) is expressed at low level in human fibroblasts and epithelial cells and is oncogenically activated either by overexpression or by gene rearrangement. In COT the 69 C-terminal amino acids of EST are replaced by an unrelated sequence of 18 residues.

Sequence of EST/COT

```
  (1)   MEYMSTGSDNKEEIDLLIKHLNVSDVIDIMENLYASEEPAVYEPSLMTMCQDSNQNDERS
 (61)   KSLLLSGQEVPWLSSVRYGTVEDLLAFANHISNTAKHFYGQRPQESGILLNMVITPQNGR
(121)   YQIDSDVLLIISNTAKHFYGQRPQESGILLKVYLAQDIKTKKRMACKLIPVDQFKPSDVE
(181)   IQACFRHENIAELYGAVLWGETVHLFMEAGEGGSVLEKLESCGPMREFEIIWVTKHVLKG
(241)   LDFLHSKKVIHHDIKPSNIVFMSTKAVLVDFGLSVQMTEDVYFPKDLRGTEIYMSPEVIL
(301)   CRGHSTKADIYSLGATLIHMQTGTPPWVKRYPRSAYPSYLYIIHKQAPPLEDIADDCSPG
(361)   MRELIEASLERNPNHRPRAADLLKHEALNPPREDQPRCQSLDSALLERKRLLSRKELELP
```
COT   `GHQVIHEGSSTNDPNNSC` (415)
EST (421)   `ENIADSSCTGSTEESESEMLKRQRSLYIDLGALAGYFNLVRGPPTLEYG` (467)

Aoki, M., Akiyama, T., Miyoshi, J. and Toyoshima, K. (1991). Identification and characterization of protein products of the *cot* oncogene with serine kinase activity. Oncogene, 6, 1515–1519.

Chan, A.M.-L., Chedid, M., McGovern, E.S., Popescu, N.C., Miki, T. and Aaronson, S.A. (1993). Expression cDNA cloning of a serine kinase transforming gene. Oncogene, 8, 1329–1333.

Miyoshi, J., Higashi, T., Mukai, H., Ohuchi, T. and Kakunaga, T. (1991). Structure and transforming potential of the human *cot* oncogene encoding a putative protein kinase. Mol. Cell. Biol., 11, 4088–4096.

GSP and GIP2

GSP is an oncogene arising from mutation of the α_s subunit of the G_s stimulatory regulator of adenylate cyclase (Landis *et al.*, 1989). Detected in growth hormone-secreting human pituitary tumours in which the activity of adenylate cyclase is constitutively elevated and responds weakly to growth hormone-releasing hormone (GHRH). Mutation sites: Arg201 and Gln227. Mutations inhibit GTPase activity and cause sustained activation of adenylate cyclase and elevation of cAMP (Clementi *et al.*, 1990). They have been detected in three from 39 differentiated thyroid tumour samples (Suarez *et al.*, 1991). In thyrocytes cAMP elevation stimulates proliferation and *GSP* mutations may therefore promote thyroid carcinomas. Gln227 in α_s is equivalent to Gln61 of $p21^{ras}$.

GIP2 is a mutant α_{i2} gene detected in ~30% of adrenal cortex and endocrine ovarian tumours (Lyons *et al.*, 1990) in which Arg179 is replaced with either His or Cys. G_i proteins inhibit adenylate cyclase (Wong *et al.*, 1991) and the inference from these findings is that mitogens active in these tissues act via α_{i2}, although as yet there is no evidence for this. The expression of GTPase-deficient α_{i2} transforms rat-1 fibroblasts (Gupta *et al.*, 1992).

Clementi, E., Malgaretti, N., Meldolesi, J. and Taramelli, R. (1990). A new constitutively activating mutation of the Gs protein α subunit-*gsp* oncogene is found in human pituitary tumours. Oncogene, 5, 1059–1061.

Gupta, S.K., Gallego, C., Lowndes, J.M., Pleiman, C.M., Sable, C., Eisfelder, B.J. and Johnson, G.L. (1992). Analysis of the fibroblast transformation potential of GTPase-deficient *gip2* oncogenes. Mol. Cell. Biol., 12, 190–197.

Landis, C.A., Masters, S.B., Spada, A., Pace, A.M., Bourne, H.R. and Vallar, L. (1989). GTPase inhibiting mutations activate the α chain of G_s and stimulate adenylyl cyclase in human pituitary tumours. Nature, 340, 692–696.

Lyons, J., Landis, C.A., Harsh, G., Vallar, L., Grunewald, K., Feichtinger, H., Duh, Q.-Y., Clark, O.H., Kawasaki, E., Bourne, H.R. and McCormick, F. (1990). Two G protein oncogenes in human endocrine tumors. Science, 249, 655–659.

Suarez, H.G., du Villard, J.A., Caillou, B., Schlumberger, Parmentier, C. and Monier, R. (1991). *gsp* mutations in human thyroid tumours. Oncogene, 6, 677–679.

Wong, Y.H., Federman, A., Pace, A.M., Zachary, I., Evans, T., Pouyssegur, J. and Bourne, H.R. (1991). Mutant alpha subunits of G_{i2} inhibit cyclic AMP accumulation. Nature, 351, 63–65.

GLI

GLI1 encodes a 118 kDa protein related to *Drosophila cid* with five repeats of the zinc finger motif. It is expressed in embryonal carcinoma cells (human chromosome 12q13–q14.3, murine 10) but not in adult tissues (Kinzler *et al.*, 1988). Enhanced expression of *GLI* has been detected in some (~7%) astrocytomas of relatively high malignant potential (Salgaller *et al.*, 1991). When co-expressed with E1A, GLI has a functional activity analogous to that of RAS and transforms primary cells (Ruppert *et al.*, 1991). GLI2 is 89% identical to GLI1, and GLI2 and GLI3 (1596 amino acids) are 96% identical (Ruppert *et al.*, 1990).

Sequence of human GLI1

```
  (1)    MFNSMTPPPISSYGEPCCLRPLPSQGAPSVGTEGLSGPPFCHQANLMSGPHSYGPARET
 (60)    NSCTEGPLFSSPRSAVKLTKKRALSISPLSDASLDLQTVIRTSPSSLVAFINSRCTSPGG
(120)    SYGHLSIGTMSPSLGFPAQMNHQKGPSPSFGVQPCGPHDSARGGMIPHPQSRGPFPTCQL
(180)    KSELDMLVGKCREEPLEGDMSSPNSTGIQDPLLGMLDGREDLEREEKREPESVYETDCRW
(240)    DGCSQEFDSQEQLVHHINSEHIHGERKEFVCHWGGCSRELRPFKAQYMLVVHMRRHTGEK
(300)    PHKCTFEGCRKSYSRLENLKTHLRSHTGEKPYMCEHEGCSKAFSNASDRAKHQNRTHSNE
(360)    KPYVCKLPGCTKRYTDPSSLRKHVKTVHGPDAHVTKRHRGDGPLPRAPSISTVEPKRERE
(420)    GGPIREESRLTVPEGAMKPQPSPGAQSSCSSDHSPAGSAANTDSGVEMTGNAGGSTEDLS
(480)    SLDEGPCIAGTGLSTLRRLENLRLDQLHQLRPIGTRGLKLPSLSHTGTTVSRRVGPPVSL
(540)    ERRSSSSSSISSAYTVSRRSSLASPFPPGSPPENGASSLPGLMPAQHYLLRARYASARGG
(600)    GTSPTAASSLDRIGGLPMPPWRSRAEYPGYNPNAGVTRRASDPAQAADRPAPARVQRFKS
(660)    LGCVHTPPTVAGGGQNFDPYLPTSVYSPQPPSITENAAMDARGLQEEPEVGTSMVGSGLN
(720)    PYMDFPPTDTLGYGGPEGAAAEPYGARGPGSLPLGPGPPTNYGPNPCPQQASYPDPTQET
(780)    WGEFPSHSGLYPGPKALGGTYSQCPRLEHYGQVQVKPEQGCPVGSDSTGLAPCLNAHPSE
(840)    GPPHPQPLFSHYPQPSPPQYLQSGPYTQPPPDYLPSEPRPCLDFDSPTHSTGQLKAQLVC
(900)    NYVQSQQELLWEGGGREDAPAQEPSYQSPKFLGGSQVSPSRAKAPVNTYGPGFGPNLPNH
(960)    KSGSYPTPSPCHENFVVGANRASHRAAAPPRLLPPLPTCYGPLKVGGTNPSCGHPEVGRL
(1020)   GGGPALYPPPEGQVCNPLDSLDLDNTQLDFVAILDEPQGLSPPPSHDQRGSSGHTPPP
(1080)   SGP1PNMAVGNMSVLLRSLPGETEFLNSSA  (1106)
```

Underlined: zinc finger domains.

Kinzler, K.W., Ruppert, J.M., Bigner, S.H. and Vogelstein, B. (1988). The *GLI* gene is a member of the *Kruppel* family of zinc finger proteins. Nature, 332, 371–374.

Ruppert, J.M., Kinzler, K.W., Wong, A.J., Bigner, S.H., Kao, F.T., Law, M.L., Seuanez, H.N., O'Brien, S.J. and Vogelstein, B. (1988). The GLI–Kruppel family of human genes. Mol. Cell. Biol., 8, 3104–3113.

Ruppert, J.M., Vogelstein, B., Arheden, K. and Kinzler, K.W. (1990). *GLI3* encodes a 190-kilodalton protein with multiple regions of GLI similarity. Mol. Cell. Biol., 10, 5408–5415.

Ruppert, J.M., Vogelstein, B. and Kinzler, K.W. (1991). The zinc finger protein GLI transforms primary cells in cooperation with adenovirus E1A. Mol. Cell. Biol., 11, 1724–1728.

Salgaller, M., Pearl, D. and Stephens, R. (1991). *In situ* hybridization with single-stranded RNA probes to demonstrate infrequently elevated *gli* mRNA and no increased *ras* mRNA levels in meningiomas and astrocytomas. Cancer Lett., 57, 243–253.

HOX2.4

HOX2.4 is a homeobox-containing gene transcriptionally activated in WEHI-3B mouse myeloid leukaemia cells. NIH 3T3 fibroblasts expressing activated *Hox-2.4* are tumorigenic in nude mice (Aberdam *et al.*, 1991).

Partial sequence of human HOX2.4

```
(1)   AAAGRRRGRQTYSRYQTLELEKEFLFNPYLTRKRRIEVSHALGLTERQVKIWFQNRRMK
(60)  WKKENNKDKFP (70)
```

Underlined: DNA binding region.

Aberdam, D., Negreanu, V., Sachs, L. and Blatt, C. (1991). The oncogenic potential of an activated hox-2.4 homeobox gene in mouse fibroblasts. Mol. Cell. Biol., 11, 554–557.

Giampaolo, A., Acampora, D., Zappavigna, V., Pannese, M., D'Esposito, M., Care, A., Faiella, A., Stornaiuolo, A., Russo, G., Simeone, A., Boncinelli, E. and Peschle, C. (1989). Differential expression of human *HOX-2* genes along the anterior–posterior axis in embryonic central nervous system. Differentiation, 40, 191–197.

HOX7.1

HOX7.1 is a homeobox-containing gene expressed throughout the limb bud in proliferating, undifferentiated cells. Expression of *HOX7.1* transforms myogenic cells and renders them tumorigenic in nude mice (Song *et al.*, 1992).

Song, K., Wang, Y. and Sassoon, D. (1992). Expression of *Hox-7.1* in myoblasts inhibits terminal differentiation and induces cell transformation. Nature, 360, 477–481.

LCO

LCO (liver cancer oncogene; (also *LCA*) is a human transforming gene (chromosome 2q14–q21). It has homology with known viral oncogenes (Tokino *et al.*, 1988). *LCO* was detected by NIH 3T3 fibroblast transfection with DNA from a primary liver carcinoma (Ochiya *et al.*, 1986).

Tokino, T., Satoh, H., Yoshida, M.C., Ochiya, T. and Matsubara, K. (1988). Regional localisation of the LCA oncogene to human chromosome region 2q14–q21. Cytogenet. Cell Genet., 48, 63–64.

Ochiya, T., Fujiyama, A., Fukushige, S., Hatada, I. and Matsubara, K. (1986). Molecular cloning of an oncogene from a human hepatocellular carcinoma. Proc. Natl Acad. Sci. USA, 83, 4993–4997.

Ltk

Murine *Ltk* (human homologue *TYK1*) is a putative transmembrane tyrosine kinase. It is a member of the *Ros*/insulin family. Human chromosome 15q13–21: 14 exons occupying 7.5 kb of genomic DNA: mouse forms 90% homologous. mRNA 2.4/2.8/3.2 kb. *Ltk* is expressed in murine B lymphocyte precursors and forebrain neurons. The lymphoid form (69 kDa) uses a CUG translational start codon and has a 110 amino acid extracellular domain. The brain form (75 kDa) derives from an alternatively spliced mRNA and has 61 additional amino acids in the extracellular domain (Haase *et al.*, 1991). C1300 neuroblastoma cells express 3.2 kb mRNAs that differ by the same 183 kb alternatively spliced exon that distinguishes brain from lymphoid mRNAs (Snijers *et al.*, 1993). The lymphoid protein and at least one of the C1300 LTK receptors are located in the endoplasmic reticulum. *LTK* mRNA is expressed with high frequency in human leukaemias (Ben-Neriah and Bauskin, 1988; Maru *et al.*, 1990).

Sequence of human LTK/TYK1

```
  (1)  MGCWGQLLVWFGAAGAILCSSPGSQETFLRSSPLPLASPSPRDPKVSAPPSILEPASPLN
 (61)  SPGTEGSWLFSTCGASGRHGPTQTQCDGAYAGTSVVVTVGAAGQLRGVQLWRVPGPGQYL
(121)  ISAYGAAGGKGAKNHLSRAHGVFVSAIFSLGLGESLYILVGQQGEDACPGGSPESQLVCL
(181)  GESRAVEEHAAMDGSEGVPGSRRWAGGGGGGGGGATYVFRLRAGELEPLLVAAGGGGRAYL
(241)  RPRDRGRTQASPEKLENRSEAPGSSGGRGGAAGGDASETDNLWADGEDGVSFIHPSSELFL
(301)  QPLAVTENHGEVEIRRHLNCSHCPLRDCQWQAELQLAECLCPEGMELAVDNVTCMDLHKP
(361)  PGPLVLMVAVVATSTLSLLMVCGVLILVKQKKWQGLQEMRLPSPELELSKLRTSAIRTAP
(421)  NPYYCQVGLGPAQSWPLPPGVTEVSPANVTLLRALGHGAFGEVYEGLVIGLPGDSSPLQV
(481)  AIKTLPELCSPQDELDFLMEALIISKFRHQNIVRCVGLSLRATPRLILLELMSGGDMKSF
(541)  LRHSRPHLGQPSPLVMRDLLQLAQDIAQGCHYLEENHFIHRDIAARNCLLSCAGPSRVAK
(601)  IGDFGMARDIYRASYYRRGDRALLPVKWMPPEAFLEGIFTSKTDSWSFGVLLWEIFSLGY
(661)  MPYPGRTNQEVLDFVVGGGRMDPPRGCPGPVYRIMTQCCWQHEPELRPSFASILERLQYCT
(721)  QDPDVLNSLLPMELGPTPEEEGTSGLGNRSLECLRPPQPQELSPEKLKSWGGSPLGPWLS
(781)  SGLKPLKSRGLQPQNLWNPTYRS (802)
```

Underlined: signal sequence. Italics: transmembrane domain.

Ben-Neriah, Y. and Bauskin, A.R. (1988). Leucocytes express a novel gene encoding a putative transmembrane protein-kinase devoid of an extracellular domain. Nature, 333, 672–676.

Bernards, A. and de la Monte, S. (1990). The *ltk* receptor tyrosine kinase is expressed in pre-B lymphocytes and cerebral neurons and uses a non-AUG translational initiator. EMBO J., 9, 2279–2287.

Haase, V.H., Snijders, A.J., Cooke, S.M., Teng, M.N., Kaul, D., LeBeau, M.M., Bruns, G.A.P. and Bernards, A. (1991). Alternatively spliced *ltk* mRNA in neurons predicts a receptor with a larger putative extracellular domain. Oncogene, 6, 2319–2325.

Krolewski, J.J. and Dalla-Favera, R. (1991). The *ltk* gene encodes a novel receptor-type protein tyrosine kinase. EMBO J., 10, 2911–2919.

Maru, Y., Hirai, H. and Takaku, F. (1990). Human *ltk*: gene structure and preferential expression in human leukemic cells. Oncogene Res., 5, 199–204.

Snijers, A.J., Haase, V.H. and Bernards, A. (1993). Four tissue-specific mouse *ltk* mRNAs predict tyrosine kinases that differ upstream of their transmembrane segment. Oncogene, 8, 27–35.

LYN

LYN is a member of the *SRC* tyrosine kinase family (formerly *SYN*). It is highly homologous to the kinase domain of *LCK* and v-*yes* but has a different mRNA transcript size (3.2 kb), tissue expression and chromosome location (8q13–qter). The *LYN* promoter lacks TATA or CAAT boxes but contains four GC-rich regions, a cAMP-responsive element, an octamer-binding motif, PEA3-like motifs and an NF-κB-binding sequence. In T cells transcription is induced by the HTLV-1: encoded p40^{TAX} protein (Uchiumi *et al.*, 1992). Common splicing patterns indicate that *Src*, *Fgr*, *Fyn*, *Lyn* and *Yes* are derived from a common gene but each differs in C-terminus and tissue-specific expression and thus, presumably, in function. Two LYN proteins (53 kDa, 56 kDa) detected in human and murine cell lines and tissues derive from alternative splicing that deletes 21 amino acids from a region 24 amino acids C-terminal of the translation initiation codon (Stanley *et al.*, 1991; Yi *et al.*, 1991). p53^{LYN} and p56^{LYN} are physically associated with IgM on B cells and cross-linking IgM increases the kinase activity of LYN kinase and of LYN-associated phosphatidylinositol 3-kinase (Yamanashi *et al.*, 1992). In the rat basophilic leukaemia cell line RBL-2H3 the kinase activity of both p56^{lyn} and pp60^{src} is increased after cellular stimulation via the high-affinity IgE receptor (Eiseman and Bolen, 1992). p56^{lyn} immunoprecipitates with both the activated IgE and Thy-1 receptors (Draberova and Draber, 1993) and may therefore be responsible for the tyrosine phosphorylation of the β and γ subunits of the activated receptor. Association of p54^{lyn} and p58^{lyn}, together with pp62^{yes} and pp60^{fyn}, with a major signalling receptor also occurs in human platelets and in some cell lines (see **YES**). Related forms of *LYN* have been detected in the spleen (Brunati *et al.*, 1991).

Sequence of human LYN

```
  (1)   MGCIKSKGKDSLSDDGVDLKTQPVRNTERTIYVRDPTSNKQQRPVPESQLLPGQRFQTK
 (60)   DPEEQGDIVVALYPYDGIHPDDLSFKKGEKMKVLEEHGEWWKAKSLLTKKEGFIPSNYVA
(120)   KLNTLETEEWFFKDITRKDAERQLLAPGNSAGAFLIRESETLKGSFSLSVRDFDPVHGDV
(180)   IKHYKIRSLDNGGYYISPRITFPCISDMIKHYQKQADGLCRRLEKACISPKPQKPWDKDA
(240)   WEIPRESIKLVKRLGAGQFGEVWMGYYNNSTKVAVKTLKPGTMSVQAFLEEANLMKTLQH
(300)   DKLVRLYAVVTREEPIYIITEYMAKGSLLDFLKSDEGGKVLLPKLIDFSAQIAEGMAYIE
(360)   RKNYIHRDLRAANVLVSESLMCKIADFGLARVIEDNEYTAREGAKFPIKWTAPEAINFGC
(420)   FTIKSDVWSFGILLYEIVTYGKIPYPGRTNA451DVMTALSQGYRMPRVENCPDELYDIM
(480)   KMCWKEKAEERPTFDYLQSVLDDFYTATEGQYQQQP (512).
```

Domains: two myristate attachment sites; 253–261 and 275 ATP binding; 397, 508 autophosphorylation; 68–119 SH3.

Brunati, A.M., Donella-Deana, A., Ralph, S., Marchiori, F., Borin, G., Fischer, S. and Pinna, L.A. (1991). Stimulation by NaCl, polylysine and heparin of two forms of spleen tyrosine protein kinase immunologically related with the protein expressed by *lyn* oncogene. Biochim. Biophys. Acta, 1091, 123–126.

Draberova, L. and Draber, P. (1993). Thy-l glycoprotein and src-like protein-tyrosine kinase p53/p56*lyn* are associated in large detergent-resistant complexes in rat basophilic leukemic cells. Proc. Natl Acad. Sci. USA, 90, 3611–3615.

Eiseman, E. and Bolen, J.B. (1992). Engagement of the high-affinity IgE receptor activates *src* protein-related tyrosine kinases. Nature, 355, 78–80.

Semba, K., Nishizawa, M., Miyajima, N., Yoshida, M.C., Sukegawa, J., Yamanashi, Y., Sasaki, M., Yamamoto, T. and Toyoshima, K. (1986). *Yes*-related protooncogene, *syn*, belongs to the protein-tyrosine kinase family. Proc. Natl Acad. Sci. USA, 83, 5459–5463.

Stanley, E., Ralph, S., McEwen, S., Boulet, I., Holtzman, D.A., Lock, P. and Dunn, A.R. (1991). Alternatively spliced murine *lyn* mRNAs encode distinct proteins. Mol. Cell. Biol., 11, 3399–3406.

Uchiumi, F., Semba, K., Yamanashi, Y., Fujisawa, J.-I., Yoshida, M., Inoue, K., Toyoshima, K. and Yamamoto, T. (1992). Characterization of the promoter region of the *src* family gene *lyn* and its *trans* activation by human T-cell leukemia virus type I-encoded p40*tax*. Mol. Cell. Biol., 12, 3784–3795.

Yamanashi, Y., Fukushige, S., Semba, K., Sukegawa, J., Miyajima, N., Matsubara, K., Yamamoto, T. and Toyoshima, K. (1987). The *yes*-related cellular gene *lyn* encodes a possible tyrosine kinase similar to p56*lck*. Mol. Cell. Biol., 7, 237–243.

Yamanashi, Y., Fukui, Y., Wongsasant, B., Kinoshita, Y., Ichimori, Y., Toyoshima, K. and Yamamoto, T. (1992). Activation of src-like protein-tyrosine kinase lyn and its association with phosphatidylinositol 3-kinase upon B-cell antigen receptor-mediated signaling. Proc. Natl Acad. Sci USA, 89, 1118–1122.

Yi, T., Bolen, J.B. and Ihle, J.N. (1991). Hematopoietic cells express two forms of *lyn* kinase differing by 21 amino acids in the amino terminus. Mol. Cell. Biol., 11, 2391–2398.

Maf/NRL

Maf is an oncogene of the avian transforming retrovirus AS42 isolated from a chicken musculoaponeurotic fibrosarcoma (Kawai *et al.*, 1992). The predicted *gag–maf* fusion protein contains 864 amino acids (95 kDa) and is a putative nuclear protein with a leucine zipper motif. The human homologue of *Maf* may therefore be associated with the development of desmoid tumours. The v-*maf* product (Nishizawa *et al.*, 1989) is strongly homologous to the NRL protein (*n*eural *r*etina *l*eucine zipper) that is expressed in retina and retinoblastoma cells (Swaroop *et al.*, 1992).

Sequence of human NRL

```
  (1)   MALPPSPLAMEYVNDFDLMKFEVKREPSEGRPGPPTASLGSTPYSSVPPSPTFSEPGMVG
 (61)   ATEGTRPGLEELYWLATLQQQLGAGEALGLSPEEAMELLQGQGPVPVDGPHGYYPGSPEE
```

```
(121)    TGAQHVQLAERFSDAALVSMSVRELNRQLRGCGRDEALRLKQRRRTLKNRGYAQACRSKR
(181)    LQQRRGLEAERARLAAQLDALRAEVARLARERDLYKARCDRLTSSGPGSGDPSHLFL (237)
```

The basic motif (italics) and the leucine zipper regions (leucines underlined) are similar to those of the FOS/JUN family. NRL is 75% similar to v-MAF over the 97 amino acids of the basic and leucine zipper regions.

Kawai, S., Goto, N., Kataoka, K., Saegusa, T., Shinno-Kohno, H. and Nishizawa, M. (1992). Isolation of the avian transforming retrovirus, AS42, carrying the v-*maf* oncogene and initial characterization of its gene product. Virology, 188, 778–784.

Nishizawa, M., Kataoka, K., Goto, N., Fujiwara, K.T. and Kawai, S. (1989). v-*maf*, a viral oncogene that encodes a "leucine zipper" motif. Proc. Natl Acad. Sci. USA, 86, 7711–7715.

Swaroop, A., Xu, J., Pawar, H., Jackson, A., Skolnick, C. and Agarwal, N. (1992). A conserved retina-specific gene encodes a basic motif/leucine zipper domain. Proc. Natl Acad. Sci. USA, 89, 266–270.

MEL

MEL is a transforming gene from the human melanoma cell line NK14 (Padua *et al.*, 1984). It occupies 16 kbp at the chromosome locus 19cen–p13.2 (3.5 kb mRNA). The translocation breakpoints that occur in melanoma and small-cell lung carcinoma map to 19p. *LYL1* and the immunoglobulin enhancer binding protein E2A genes are involved in the t(7:19) and t(1:19) translocations that occur in acute lymphoblastic anaemia.

NIH 3T3 cells are transformed by DNA from three melanoma cell lines (NK14, MeWo, Mel Swift). In Mel Swift the transforming agent is an activated *Nras* gene.

MEL has homology with RAS (40% identity) and mouse YPT1 (51% identity, 87% homology) proteins. The human and mouse proteins are 96% homologous. Human MEL differs in only six amino acids from the sequence of dog RAB8. The effector site (residues 35–42) differs from that of RAS but is highly conserved between MEL, RAB and YPT. MEL differs from RAB/YPT in having a RAS-type C-terminal CAAX box.

Sequence of human MEL

```
  (1)    MAKTYDYLFKLLLIGDSGVGKTCVLFRFSEDAFNSTFISTIGIDFKIRTIELDGKRIKLQ
 (61)    IWDTAGQERFRTITTAYYRGAMGIMLVYDITNEKSFDNIRNWIRNIEEHASADVEKMILG
(121)    NKCDVNDKRQVSKERGEKLALDYGIKFMETSAKANINVENAFFTLARDIKAKMDKKWKAT
(181)    APGSNQGVKITPDQQKRSSFFRCVLL (206)
```

Padua, R.A., Barras, N. and Currie, G. (1984). A novel transforming gene in a human malignant melanoma cell line. Nature, 311, 671–673.

Nimmo, E.R., Sanders, P.G., Padua, R.A., Hughes, D., Williamson, R. and Johnson, K.J. (1991). The *MEL* gene: a new member of the *RAB/YPT* class of *RAS*-related genes. Oncogene, 6, 1347–1351.

MelF

Overexpressed in the murine erythroleukaemia cell line F5-5, *MelF* encodes a 395 amino acid protein that is the homologue of human CD43 (leukosialin) lymphocyte surface antigen (Misawa and Shibuya, 1992). *MelF* expression is 30- to 50-fold higher in erythroleukaemia cell lines than in spleen cells uninfected by SFFV.

Misawa, Y. and Shibuya, M. (1992). Amplification and rearrangement of *MelF*/mouse CD43 (leukosialin) gene encoding a highly glycosylated membrane protein gp120 in Friend erythroleukemia cells. Oncogene, 7, 919–926.

MPL

MPL is the human homologue of the v-*mpl* oncogene transduced by the *m*yelo*p*roliferative *l*eukemia retrovirus (Vigon *et al.*, 1992). It is detected in the human erythroleukaemia (HEL) cell line as co-expressed major (3.7 kb) and minor (2.8 kb) mRNAs (*MPLP* and *MPLK*, respectively). MPL has structural and amino acid homology with the cytokine receptor superfamily that includes the "WS motif" (WSXWS), although the WS motif is not essential for the oncogenic properties of MPLV (Benit *et al.*, 1993). The extracellular region can be divided into two subunits, as can those of the IL-3 receptor and the human granulocyte–macrophage colony stimulating factor β chain.

Sequences of human MPLP and MPLK and v-MPL

```
Human-MPL    (1)   MPSWALFMVTSCLLLAPQNLAQVSSQDVSLLASDSEPLKCFSRTFEDLTCFWDEEEAAPS
            (61)   GTYQLLYAYPREKPRACPLSSQSMPHFGTRYVCQFPDQEEVRLFFPLHLWVKNVFLNQTR
           (121)   TQRVLFVDSVGLPAPPSIIKAMGGSQPGELQISWEEPAPEISDFLRYELRYGPRDPKNST
           (181)   GPTVIQLIATETCCPALQRPHSASALDQSPCAQPTMPWQDGPKQTSPSREASALTAEGGS
           (241)   CLISGLQPGNSYWLQLRSEPDGISLGGSWGSWSLPVTVDLPGDAVALGLQCFTLDLKNVT
           (301)   CQWQQQDHASSQGFFYHSRARCCPRDRYPIWENCEEEEKTNPGLQTPQFSRCHFKSRNDS
           (361)   IIHILVEVTTAPGTVHSYLGSPFWIHQAVRLPTPNLHWREISSGHLELEWQHPSSWAAQE
           (421)   TCYQLRYTGEGHQDWKVLEPPLGARGGTLELRPRSRYRLQLRARLNGPTYQGPWSSWSDP
v-MPL        (1)                                             ------A--S----------------A--P-

Human-MPLP  (481)   TRVETATETAWISLVTALHLVLGLSAVLGLLLLRWQFPAHYRRLRHALWPSLPDLHRVLG
Human-MPLK  (481)                                                       YRPRQAGDWRWTRWSRTC
v-MPL        (33)   A--S-GS-----T-----L---S---L------K----------------------

Human-MPLP  (541)   QYLRDTAALSPPKATVSDTCEEVEPSLLEILPKSSERTPLPLCSSQAQMDYRRLQPSCLG
Human-MPLK  (541)   KQAFLVRSVT-DLRPPPVRTYGFALPARHLWDSPRLLTL (579)
v-MPL        (93)   ----------S----T-S--------------S------P--P-----G---C LR (151)

Human-MPLP  (601)   TMPLSVCPPMAESGSCCTTHIANHSYLPLSYWQQP (635)
```

Underlined: signal sequence. Italics: transmembrane sequence. MPLP and MPLK have identical N-termini up to the nine amino acids following the transmembrane domain.

Benit, L., Cocault, C.L., Wendling, F. and Gisselbrecht, S. (1993). The 'WS motif' common to v-*mpl* and members of the cytokine receptor superfamily is dispensable for myeloproliferative leukemia virus pathogenicity. Oncogene, 8, 787–790.
Vigon, I., Mornon, J.-P., Cocault, L., Mitjavila, M.-T., Tambourin, P., Gisselbrecht, S. and Souyri, M. (1992). Molecular cloning and characterization of *MPL*, the human homolog of the v-*mpl* oncogene: identification of a member of the hematopoietic growth factor receptor superfamily. Proc. Natl Acad. Sci. USA, 89, 5640–5644.

NCK

The *NCK* gene was cloned from a human melanoma expression library and encodes a highly conserved, 47 kDa protein comprised of three SH3 domains followed by one SH2 domain that is widely expressed in mammalian tissues (Lehmann *et al.*, 1990). Overexpression of *NCK* transforms 3Y1 rat fibroblasts (Chou *et al.*, 1992) and NIH 3T3 cells (Li *et al.*, 1992). However, in contrast to cells transformed by v-*crk*, these cells do not have grossly elevated levels of phospho-tyrosine. In human and murine cells NCK protein is phosphorylated on tyrosine, serine and threonine residues following stimulation by EGF or PDGF and NCK associates with the receptors for these ligands via its SH2 domain (Li *et al.*, 1992). NCK is also phosphorylated in RBL-2H3 cells in response to cross-linking of high-affinity IgE receptors, in PC12 cells by the action of NGF, in Jurkat cells by activation of the T cell receptor, in Daudi cells by IgM cross-linking, in U937 cells by activation of the low-affinity IgG receptor (Park and Rhee, 1992), and in v-*src*-transformed cells (see **SRC**) and may therefore mediate signal transduction pathways initiated by activated plasma membrane protein tyrosine kinases.

Sequence of NCK

```
  (1)    MAEEVVVVAKFDYVAQQEQELDIKKNERLWLLDDSKSWWRVRNSMNKTGFVPSNYVERK
 (60)    NSARKASIVKNLKDTLGIGKVKRKPSVPDSASPADDSFVDPGERLYDLNMPAYVKFNYMA
(120)    EREDELSLIKGTKVIVMEKCSDGWWRGSYNGQVGWFPSNYVTEEGDSPLGDHVGSLSEKL
(180)    AAVVNNLNTGQVLHVVQALYPFSSSNDEELNFEKGDVMDVIEKPENDPEWWKCRKINGMV
(240)    GLVPKNYVTVMQNNPLTSGLEPSPPQCDYIRPSLTGKFAGNPWYYGKVTRHQAEMALNER
(300)    GHEGDFLIRDSESSPNDFSVSLKAQGKNKHFKVQLKETVYCIGQRKFSTMEELVEHYKKA
(360)    PIFTSEQGEKLYLVKHLS(377)
```

SH3 domains: residues 1–61, 106–165 and 190–252; SH2 domain: residues 282–374.

Chou, M.M., Fajardo, J.E. and Hanafusa, H. (1992). The SH2- and SH3-containing nck protein transforms mammalian fibroblasts in the absence of elevated phosphotyrosine levels. Mol. Cell. Biol., 12, 5834–5842.

Lehmann, J.M., Riethmuller, G. and Johnson, J.P. (1990). Nck, A melanoma cDNA encoding a cytoplasmic protein consisting of the src homology units SH2 and SH3. Nucleic Acids Res., 18, 1048.

Li, W., Hu, P., Skolnik, E.Y., Ullrich, A. and Schlessinger, J. (1992). The SH2 and SH3 domain-containing nck protein is oncogenic and a common target for phosphorylation by different surface receptors. Mol. Cell. Biol., 12, 5824–5833.

Park, D. and Rhee, S.G. (1992). Phosphorylation of nck in response to a variety of receptors, phorbol myristate acetate, and cyclic AMP. Mol. Cell. Biol., 12, 5816–5823.

Ornithine decarboxylase (ODC1)

The human *ODC1* gene maps to chromosome 2p25 and a processed pseudogene maps to 7cen–qter (Hickok *et al.*, 1992). The gene contains 12 exons and the promoter contains a TATA box, GC boxes, a cAMP-responsive element and AP-1, AP-2 and NF-1 binding sites. The mouse and rat genes are of similar structure. ODC is a cytoplasmic enzyme (half-life ~10 min) that catalyses the formation of putrescine from ornithine and is the key regulator of polyamine synthesis. Essential for cell proliferation, its expression is rapidly activated (10- to 20-fold) by many hormones (including growth hormone, corticosteroids, testosterone or EGF) and oncogenes and the overexpression of ornithine decarboxylase can itself cause cell transformation (Auvinen *et al.*, 1992) or cooperate with activated oncogenes to do so (Chiao *et al.*, 1991; see **RAS**).

Sequence of human ODC

```
  (1)    MNNFGNEEFDCHFLDEGFTAKDILDQKINEVSSSDDKDAFYVADLGDILKKHLRWLKAL
 (60)    PRVTPFYAVKCNDSKAIVKTLAATGTGFDCASKTEIQLVQSLGVPPPERIIYANPCKQVSQ
(120)    IKYAANNGVQMMTFDSEVELMKVARAHPKAKLVLRIATDDSKAVCRLSVKFGATLRTSRL
```

```
(180)  LLERAKELNIDVVGVSFHVGSGCTDPETFVQAISDARCVFDMGAEVGFSMYLLDIGGGFP
(240)  GSEDVKLKFEEITGVINPALDKYFPSDSGVRIIAEPGRYYVASAFTLAVNIIAKKIVLKE
(300)  QTGSDDEDESSEQTFMYYVNDGVYGSFNCILYDHAHVKPLLQKRPKPDEKYYSSSIWGPT
(360)  CDGLDRIVERCDLPEMHVGDWMLFENMGAYTVAAASTFNGFQRPTIYYVMSGPAWQLMQQ
(420)  FQNPDFPPEVEEQDASTLPVSCAWESGMKRHRAACASASINV (461)
```

Serine 303 is phosphorylated by casein kinase II.

Auvinen, M., Paasinen, A., Andersson, L.C. and Holtta, E. (1992). Ornithine decarboxylase activity is critical for cell transformation. Nature, 360, 355–358.

Chiao, P.J., Kannan, P., Yim, S.O., Krizman, D.B., Wu, T.-A., Gallick, G.E. and Tainsky, M.A. (1991). Susceptibility to *ras* oncogene transformation is correlated with signal transduction through growth factor receptors. Oncogene, 6, 713–720.

Hickok, N.J., Wahlfors, J., Crozat, A., Halmekyto, M., Alhonen, L., Janne, J. and Janne, O.A. (1992). Human ornithine decarboxylase-encoding loci: nucleotide sequence of the expressed gene and characterization of a pseudogene. Gene, 93, 257–263.

Pem

Pem transcripts occur in immortalized and tumorigenic cell lines and are expressed in murine placenta and embryos in a stage-specific manner but not in adult tissues (Wilkinson *et al.*, 1991). The predicted 210 amino acid protein has serine/threonine kinase phosphorylation sites and may be a cytosolic signal regulator.

Sequence of mouse PEM

```
  (1)  MEAEGSSRKVTRLLRLGVKEDSEEQHDVKAEAFFQAGEGRDEQGAQGQPGVGAVGTEGEG
 (61)  EELNGGKGHFGPGAPGPMGDGDKDSGTRAGGVEQEQNEPVAEGTESQENGNPGGRQMPSR
(121)  ALGSPSYRLRELESILQRTNSFDVPREDLDRLMDACVSRVQNWFKIRRAAARRTRRRATP
(181)  VPEHFRGTFECPACRGVRWGERCPFATPRF (210)
```

Wilkinson, M.F., Kleeman, J., Richards, J. and MacLeod, C.L. (1991). A novel oncofetal gene is expressed in a stage-specific manner in murine embryonic development. Devel. Biol., 141, 451–455.

Qin

Oncogene of the avian sarcoma virus 31. *Qin* encodes a protein related to the transcription factor family that includes hepatocyte nuclear factor 3 (HNF-3) and the *Drosophila* homeotic regulator fork head (Li and Vogt, 1993).

Li, J and Vogt, P.K. (1993). The retroviral oncogene *qin* belongs to the transcription factor family that includes the homeotic gene fork head. Proc. Natl Acad. Sci. USA, 90, 4490–4494.

RYK

v-*ryk* is the oncogene of the RPL30 acute avian retrovirus isolated from chickens. It contains a 1.39 kb cellular sequence that encodes a tyrosine kinase domain inserted in the *env* sequence to encode a P69[gp37-ryk] fusion oncoprotein (Jia *et al.*, 1992). RPL30 transforms chick embryo fibroblasts and induce sarcomas following injection into the wing webs of chickens. Murine RYK is a receptor tyrosine kinase with unusual motifs in the kinase domain (Hovens *et al.*, 1992). Human RYK has been cloned from an IL-1-stimulated hepatoma cDNA library (Stacker *et al.*, 1993).

Sequences of human and mouse RYK

```
Human RYK   (1)   MRGAARLGRPGRSCLPGPALRAAAAPALLLARCAVAAAAGLRAAAARPRPPELQSASAGPS
Mouse RYK   (1)                                              MLPPAAPV-GPGR-P----

          (61)   VSLYLSEDEVRRLIGLDAELYYVRNDLISHYALSFNLLVPSETNFLHFTWHAKSKVEYKL
          (20)   ------------L-----------------------------------------------

         (121)   GFQVDNVLAMDMPQVNISVQGEVPRTLSVFRVELSCTGKVDSEVMILMQLNLTVNSSKNF
          (80)   ----N-FV--G-------A---G-------------------------------------

         (181)   TVLNFKRRKMCYKKLEEVKTSALDKNTSRTIYDPVHAAPTTSTR VFYISVGVCCAVIFLV
         (140)   ------------------------------------------------------------

         (241)   AIILAVLHLHNMKRIELDDSISASSSSQGLSQPSTQTTQYLRADTPNNATPITS   YPT
         (200)   ---------S----------------------------------------SSG---

         (298)   LRIEKNDLRSVTLLEAKGKVKDIAISRERITLKDVLQEGTFGRIFHGILIDEKDPNKEKQ
         (260)   ----------------A-----G--------------S---------V---R------

         (358)   AFVKTVKDQASEIQVTMMLTESCKLRGLHHRNLLPITHVCIEEGEKPMVILPYMNWGNLK
         (320)   T----------V-----------------------------------------V------

         (418)   LFLRQCKLVEANNPQAISQQDLVHMAIQIACGMSYLARREVIHKDLAARNCVIDDTLQVK
         (380)   ----------------------------------------R---------------

         (478)   ITDNALSRDLFPMDYHCLGDNENRPVRWMALESLVNNEFSSASDVWAFGVNSLWELMTLG
         (440)   ----------------------------------------------- T--------

         (538)   QTPYTLDIDPFEMAAYLKDGYRIAQPITCPDELFAVMACCWALDPEERPRFQQLVQCLTE
         (499)   ---- V-------------------N-------------------K---------

         (598)   FHAALGAYV (606)
         (558)   --------- (566)
```

Italics: transmembrane domain.

Hovens, C.M., Stacker, S.A., Andres, A.-C., Harpur, A.G., Ziemiecki, A. and Wilks, A.F. (1992). RYK, a receptor tyrosine kinase-related molecule with unusual kinase domain motifs. Proc. Natl Acad. Sci. USA, 89, 11818–11822.

Jia, R., Mayer, B.J., Hanafusa, T. and Hanafusa, H. (1992). A novel oncogene, v-*ryk*, encoding a truncated receptor tyrosine kinase is transduced into the RPL30 virus without loss of viral sequences. J. Virol., 66, 5975–5987.

Stacker, S.A., Hovens, C.M., Vitali, A., Pritchard, M.A., Baker, E., Sutherland, G.R. and Wilks, A.F. (1993). Molecular cloning and chromosomal localisation of the human homologue of a receptor related to tyrosine kinases (RYK). Oncogene, 8, 1347–1356.

Scc

Susceptibility to colon cancer genes 1–4 present on mouse chromosomes 2, 7, 11 and 10, respectively (Moen *et al.*, 1992). *Scc-1* is distinct from the homologues of genes known to be associated with colon cancer in humans (*FAP/APC*, *MCC*, *DCC*, *KRAS* and *TP53*).

Moen, C.J.A., Snoek, M., Hart, A.A.M. and Demant, P. (1992). *Scc-1*, a novel colon cancer susceptibility gene in the mouse: linkage to *CD44* (*Ly*-24, *pgp*-1) on chromosome 2. Oncogene, 7, 563–566.

SDC25

*Saccharomyces cerevisiae sdc*25 encodes a protein with C-terminal GDP/GTP exchange activity for mammalian RAS proteins *in vitro* and is tumorigenic when expressed in NIH 3T3 cells (Barlat *et al.*, 1993).

Barlat, I., Schweighoffer, F., Chevallier-Multon, M.C., Duchesne, M., Fath, I., Landais, D., Jacquet, M. and Tocque, B. (1993). The *Saccharomyces cerevisiae* gene product SDC25 C-domain functions as an oncoprotein in NIH 3T3 cells. Oncogene, 8, 215–218.

Sty

Sty is a serine-, threonine- and tyrosine-phosphorylating kinase cloned from an embryonal carcinoma cell line (Howell *et al.*, 1991). Its 1.8 kb mRNA encodes a 57 kDa protein that is highly basic and contains a nuclear localization signal.

Sequence of mouse STY

```
  (1)  MRHSKRTYCPDWDERDWDYGTWRSSSSHKRKKRSHSSAREQKRCRYDHSKTTDSYYLESR
 (61)  SINEKAYHSRRYVDEYRNDYMGYEPGHPYGEPGSRYQMHSSKSSGRSGRSSYKSKHRSRH
(121)  HTSQHHSHGKSHRRKRSRSVEDDEEGHLICQSGDVLSARYEIVDTLGEGAFGKVVECIDH
(181)  KVGGRRVAVKIVKNVDRYCEAAQSEIQVLEHLNTTDPHSTFRCVQMLEWFEHRGHICIVF
(241)  ELLGLSTYDFIKENSFLPFRMDHIRKMAYQICKSVNFLHSNKLTHTDLKPENILFVKSDY
(301)  TEAYNPKMKRDERTIVNPDIKVVDFGSATYDDEHHSTLVSTRHYRAPEVILALGWSQPCD
(361)  VWSIGCILIEYYLGFTVFPTHDSREHLAMMERILGPLPKHMIQKTRKRRYFHHDRLDWDE
(421)  HSSAGRYVSRRCKPLKEFMLSQDAEHEFLFDLVGKILEYDPAKRITLKEALKHPFFYPLK
(481)  KHT(483)
```

Howell, B.W., Afar, D.E., Lew, J., Douville, E.M., Icely, P.L., Gray, D.A. and Bell, J.C. (1991). STY, a tyrosine-phosphorylating enzyme with sequence homology to serine/threonine kinases. Mol. Cell. Biol., 11, 568–572.

TIE

TIE (tyrosine kinase with *Ig* and *EGF* homology domains) is a human receptor tyrosine kinase (chromosome 1p33–p34) highly expressed in endothelial cells lines and in some myeloid leukaemia cell lines (Partanen *et al.*, 1992). The extracellular domain of TIE contains three EGF homology motifs between two Ig-like loops with three fibronectin type III repeats adjacent to the transmembrane region. Murine *Tek* is closely related to *TIE* (Dumont *et al.*, 1993).

Sequence of TIE

```
  (1)  MVWRVPPFLLPILFLASHVGAAVDLTLLANLRLTDPQRFFLTCVSGEAGAGRGSDAWGPP
 (61)  LLLEKDDRIVRTPPGPPLRLARNGSHQVTLRGFSKPSDLVGVFSCVGGAGARRTRVIYVH
(121)  NSPGAHLLPDKVTHTVNKGDTAVLSARVHKEKQTDVIWKSNGSYFYTLDWHEAQDGRFLL
(181)  QLPNVQPPSSGIYSATYLEASPLGSAFFRLIVRGCGAGRWGPGCTKECPGCLHGGVCHDH
(241)  DGECVCPPGFTGTRCEQACREGRFGQSCQEQCPGISGCRGLTFCLPDPYGCSCGSGWRGS
(301)  QCQEACAPGHFGADCRLQCQCQNGGTCDRFSGCVCPSGWHGVHCEKSDRIPQILNMASEL
(361)  EFNLETMPRINCAAAGNPFPVRGSIELRKPDGTVLLSTKAIVEPEKTTAEFEVPRLVLAD
(421)  SGFWECRVSTSGGQDSRRFKVNVKVPPVPLAAPRLLTKQSRQLVVSPLVSFSGDGPISTV
(481)  RLHYRPQDSTMDWSTIVVDPSENVTLMNLRPKTGYSVRVQLSRPGEGGEGAWGPPTLMTT
(541)  DCPEPLLQPWLEGWHVEGTDRLRVSWSLPLVPGPLVGDGFLLRLWDGTRGQERRENVSSP
(601)  QARTALLTGLTPGTHYQLDVQLYHCTLLGPASPPAHVLLPPSGPPAPRHLHAQALSDSEI
```

```
(661)  QLTWKHPEALPGPISKYVVEVQVAGGAGDPLWIDVDRPEETSTIIRGLNASTRYLFRMRA
(721)  SIQGLGDWSNTVEESTLGNGLQAEGPVQESRAAEEGLDQQLILAVVGSVSATCLTILAAL
(781)  LTLVCIRRSCLHRRRTFTYQSGSGEETILQFSSGTLTLTRRPKLQPEPLSYPVLEWEDIT
(841)  FEDLIGEGNFGQVIRAMIKKDGLKMNAAIKMLKEYASENDHRDFAGELEVLCKLGHHPNI
(901)  INLLGACKNRGYLYIAIEYAPYGNLLDFLRKSRVLETDPAFAREHGTASTLSSRQLLRFA
(961)  SDAANGMQYLSEKQFIHRDLAARNVLVGENLASKIADFGLSRGEEVYVKKTMGRLPVRWM
(1021) AIESLNYSVYTTKSDVWSFGVLLWEIVSLGGTPYCGMTCAELYEKLPQADRMEQPRNCDD
(1081) EVYELMRQCWRDRPYERPPFAQIALQLGRMLEARKAYVNMSLFENFTYAGIDATAEEA (1138)
```

Underlined: signal sequence. Italics: transmembrane region.

Dumont, D.J., Gradwohl, G.J., Fong, G.-H., Auerbach, R. and Breitman, M.L. (1993). The endothelial-specific receptor tyrosine kinase, *tek*, is a member of a new subfamily of receptors. Oncogene, 8, 1293–1301.

Partanen, J., Armstrong, E., Makela, T.P., Korhonen, J., Sandberg, M., Renkonen, R., Knuutila, S., Huebner, K. and Alitalo, K. (1992). A novel endothelial cell surface receptor tyrosine kinase with extracellular epidermal growth factor homology domains. Mol. Cell. Biol., 12, 1698–1707.

TKF

TKF (tyrosine *k*inase related to *f*ibroblast growth factor receptor) is a cytosolic protein tyrosine kinase and the fourth member of the fibroblast growth factor receptor family (see **HSTF1/Hst-1**: Holtrich *et al.*, 1991). *TKF* is expressed in the lung and some lung-derived tumours and in malignancies not derived from lung tissues.

Sequences of human TKF *and the catalytic domains of* FLG, BEK *and* FGFR3

```
TKF     (1)    HPRPPATVQKLSRFPLARQ  FSLESGSSGKSSSSLVRGVRLSSS  GPALLAGLVSLDL
FLG     (410)  SQMAVHKLA-SIPLRRQVT  V-AD-SA-MN-GVL---PS-----  -TPM---VSEYE-
BEK     (409)  FSSQ--VHKLTK-I--R--VTV-A--S--MN-NTP---ITTRL--TADTPM---VSEYE-
FGFR3   (404)  KGLGSP--H-I-----K--  V----NA-MS-NTP---IA----G  EGPT--NVSE-E-

TKF     (57)   PLDPLWEFPRDRLVLGKPLGEGCFGQVVRAEAFGMDPARPDQASTVAVKMLKDNASDKDL
FLG     (466)  -E--R--L------------------L---I-L-KDK-NRVTK------SD-TE---
BEK     (469)  -E--K------K-T-------------M---V-I-KDK-KE-V--------D-TE---
FGFR3   (460)  -A--K--LS-A--T-------------M---I-I-KD-AAKPV--------D-T----

TKF     (117)  ADLVSEMEVMKLIGRHKNIINLLGVCTQEGPLYVIVECAAKGNLREFLRARRPPGPDLSP
FLG     (526)  S--I----M--M--K---------A---D--------Y-S------Y-Q------LEYCY
BEK     (529)  S-------M--M--K---------A---D--------Y-S------Y--------MEY-Y
FGFR3   (520)  S-------M--M--K-----N---A---G-----L--Y-A--------------L-Y-F

TKF     (177)  DGPRSSEGPLSFPVLVSCAYQVARGMQYLESRKCIHRDLAARNVLVTEDNVMKIADFGLA
FLG     (586)  NPSHNP-EQ--SKD------------E--A-K----------------------------
BEK     (589)  -IN-VP-EQMT-KD----T--L----E--A-Q---------------N----------
FGFR3   (580)  -TCKPP-EQ-T-KD-----------E--A-Q----------------------------

TKF     (237)  RGVHHIDYYKKTSNGRLPVKWMAPEALFDRVYTHQSDVWSFGILLWEIFTLGGSPYPGIP
FLG     (646)  -DI---------T----------------I-----------V-------------V-
BEK     (649)  -DINN------T-----------------------------V-M--------------
FGFR3   (640)  -D--NL------T----------------------------V---------------

TKF     (297)  VEELFSLLREGHRMDRPPHCPPELYGLMRECWHAAPSQRPTFKQLVEALDKVL LAVSEE
FLG     (706)  -----K--K------K-SN-TN---MM--D----V-----------D--RIVA-TSNQ-
BEK     (709)  -----K--K------K-AN-TN---MM--D----V-----------D--RI-T-TTN--
FGFR3   (700)  -----K--K------K-AN-THD--MI----------------D--R--TVTSTD-

TKF     (357)  YLDLRLTFGPYSPSGGDASSTCSSS  DSVFSHDPLPLGSSSFPFGSGSGVQT (404)
FLG     (766)  ----SMPLDQ----FP-TR-STC--GE------E---EEPCLPRHPAQLANGGLKRR (822)
```

```
BEK    (769)   ----SQPLEQ----YP-TR-S---G D-----P--M-YEPCLPQYPHINGSVKT (827)
FGFR3  (760)   ----SAP-EQ---GGQ-TP-SS--G DD---A--L--PAPP-SGGSRT (806)
```

Holtrich, U., Brauninger, A., Strebhardt, K. and Rubsamen-Waigmann, H. (1991). Two additional protein-tyrosine kinases expressed in human lung: fourth member of the fibroblast growth factor receptor family and an intracellular protein-tyrosine kinase. Proc. Natl Acad. Sci. USA, 88, 10411–10415.

Tlm

Tlm was detected by transfection of mouse T cell lymphoma DNA. It transforms NIH 3T3 fibroblasts with high efficiencies (Lane *et al.*, 1984). It is not homologous to *Blym-1* or to retroviral transforming genes (Lane and Tobin, 1990). The *Tlm* homologue is expressed in human neoplasms.

Sequence of mouse TLM

```
  (1)   MRTHLLLSRPQSSRGPAAGHRARHTDLLVLLESPAPVLSTVMMCLLWWPAPAKITSHSLI
 (61)   QLTNQCVCLYFAPGHMCVWVLPGQACSMALQSFFLVSLWLLPWQNPARFFLPSLINRGFF
(121)   DSMSPLQCTLVLSVVLASLVQWLAVSIHLCICKALSGPLRRQPYQAPFSMYFLVSTIVSG
(181)   FGNCIWDESPGGTVSGLSFSISSTLLSPYLLMYFVLLLRRHGSTMPNFLRNCQTDFQSGC
(241)   TSLQSHQQWRSVLLSPHPRQHLLPSEFLILAILTGVRWNLRVVLICISLMTKDVFNCFSA
(301)   IRDSSVDNPLFSSVPHF (317)
```

Lane, M.A. and Tobin, M.B. (1990). Genomic sequence of the mouse oncogene tlm. Nucleic Acids Res., 18, 3410.

Lane, M.A., Sainten, A., Doherty, K. and Cooper, G.M. (1984). Isolation and characterization of a stage-specific transforming gene, *Tlym*-I, from T cell lymphomas. Proc. Natl Acad. Sci. USA, 81, 2227–2231.

TRE

TRE is a *r*ecombinant gene isolated from NIH 3T3 fibroblasts *t*ransfected with human Ewing's sarcoma DNA (Nakamura *et al.*, 1988). It contains three major genetic elements derived from chromosomes 5, 18 and 17 (5' to 3'). The 3' region encodes an ORF (786 amino acids) with potential nucleic acid binding sites and is transcribed in a wide variety of human cancer cells (Nakamura *et al.*, 1992).

Sequence of TRE

```
  (1)   MDMVENADSLQAQERKDILMKYDKGHRAGLPEDKGPEPVGINSSIDRFGILHETELPPVT
 (61)   AREAKKIRREMTRTSKWMEMLGEWETYKHSSKLIDRVYKGIPMNIRGPVWSVLLNIQEIK
(121)   LKNPGRYQIMKERGKRSSEHIHHIDLDVRTTLRNHVFFRDRYGAKQRELFYILLAYSEYN
(181)   PEVGYCRDLSHITALFLLYLPEEDAFWALVQLLASERHSLPGFHSPNGGTVQGLQDQQEH
(241)   VVPKSQPKTMWHQDKEGLCGQCASLGCLLRNLIDGISLGLTLRLWDVYLVEGEQVLMPIT
(301)   SIALKVQQKRLMKTSRCGLWARLRNQFFDTWAMNDDTVLKHLRASTKKLTRKQGDLPPP̲M̲
(361)   P̲Q̲R̲L̲P̲H̲A̲R̲Q̲H̲T̲P̲L̲P̲L̲G̲S̲A̲D̲Y̲R̲R̲V̲V̲S̲V̲R̲P̲Q̲G̲P̲H̲R̲D̲P̲K̲D̲S̲R̲D̲A̲A̲K̲R̲E̲Q̲G̲S̲L̲A̲P̲R̲P̲V̲P̲A̲S̲R̲G̲G̲
(421)   K̲T̲L̲C̲K̲G̲Y̲R̲Q̲A̲P̲P̲G̲P̲P̲A̲Q̲F̲Q̲R̲P̲I̲C̲S̲A̲S̲P̲P̲W̲A̲S̲R̲F̲S̲T̲P̲C̲P̲G̲G̲A̲V̲R̲E̲D̲T̲Y̲P̲V̲G̲T̲Q̲G̲V̲P̲S̲L̲A̲L̲A̲
(481)   Q̲G̲G̲P̲Q̲G̲S̲W̲R̲F̲L̲E̲W̲K̲S̲M̲P̲R̲L̲P̲T̲D̲L̲D̲I̲G̲G̲P̲W̲F̲P̲H̲Y̲D̲F̲E̲R̲S̲C̲W̲V̲R̲A̲I̲S̲Q̲E̲D̲Q̲L̲A̲T̲C̲W̲Q̲A̲E̲H̲C̲G̲
(541)   E̲V̲H̲N̲K̲D̲M̲S̲W̲P̲E̲E̲M̲S̲F̲T̲A̲N̲S̲S̲K̲I̲D̲R̲Q̲K̲V̲P̲T̲E̲K̲G̲A̲T̲G̲L̲S̲N̲L̲G̲N̲T̲C̲F̲M̲N̲S̲S̲I̲Q̲C̲V̲S̲N̲T̲Q̲P̲L̲T̲Q̲
(601)   Y̲F̲I̲S̲G̲R̲H̲L̲Y̲E̲L̲N̲R̲T̲N̲P̲I̲G̲M̲K̲G̲H̲M̲A̲K̲C̲Y̲G̲D̲L̲V̲Q̲E̲L̲W̲S̲G̲T̲Q̲K̲S̲V̲A̲P̲L̲K̲L̲R̲R̲T̲I̲A̲K̲Y̲A̲P̲K̲F̲D̲G̲
(661)   F̲Q̲Q̲Q̲D̲S̲Q̲E̲L̲L̲A̲F̲L̲L̲D̲G̲L̲H̲E̲D̲L̲N̲R̲V̲H̲E̲K̲P̲Y̲V̲E̲L̲K̲D̲S̲D̲G̲R̲P̲D̲W̲E̲V̲A̲A̲E̲A̲W̲D̲N̲H̲L̲R̲R̲N̲R̲S̲I̲I̲V̲
(721)   D̲L̲F̲H̲G̲Q̲L̲R̲S̲Q̲V̲K̲C̲K̲T̲C̲G̲H̲I̲S̲V̲R̲F̲D̲P̲F̲N̲F̲L̲S̲L̲P̲L̲P̲M̲D̲S̲Y̲M̲D̲L̲E̲I̲T̲V̲I̲K̲L̲D̲G̲T̲T̲P̲V̲R̲Y̲G̲L̲R̲L̲
(781)   N̲M̲D̲E̲K̲Y̲T̲G̲L̲K̲K̲Q̲L̲R̲D̲L̲C̲G̲L̲N̲S̲E̲Q̲I̲L̲L̲A̲E̲V̲H̲D̲S̲N̲I̲K̲NFPQDNQKVQLSVSGFLCAFEIPVP
(841)   SSPISASSPTQIDFSSSPSTNGMFTLTTNGDLPKPIFIPNGMPNTVVPCGTEKNFTNGMV
              ISPLHHLQMECSP(786)
```

```
  (901)  NGHMPSLPDSPFTGYIIAVHRKMMRTELYFLSPQENRPSLFGMPLIVPCTVHTQKKDLYD
  (961)  AVWIQVSWLARPLPPQEASIHAQDRDNCMGYQYPFTLRVVQKDGISCAWCPQYRFCRGCK
 (1021)  IDCGEDRAFIGNAYIAVDWHPTALHLRYQTSQERVVDKHESVEQSRRAQAEPINLDSCLR
 (1081)  AFTSEEELGESEMYYCSKCKTHCLATKKLDLWRLPPFLIIHLKRFQFVNDQWIKSQKIVR
 (1141)  FLRESFDPSAFLVPRDPALCQHKPLTPQGDELSKPRILAREVKKVDAQSSAGKEDMLLSK
 (1201)  SPSSLSANISSSPKGSPSSSRKSGTSCPSSKNSSPNSSPRTLGRSKGRLRLPQIGSKNKP
 (1261)  SSSKKNLDASKENGAGQICELADALSRGHMRGGSQPELVTPQDHEVALANGFLYEHEACG
 (1321)  NGCGDGYSNGQLGNHSEEDSTDDQREDTHIKPIYNLYAISCHSGILSGGHYITYAKNPNC
 (1381)  KWYCYNDSSCEELHPDEIDTDSAYILFYEQQGIDYAQFLPKIDGKKMADTSSTDEDSESD
 (1441)  YEKYSMLQ (1448)
```

The sequence is for clone 210; underlined regions are unique to clone 213. An additional variant in clone 213 commences at residue 360 (GPTALGRRCVRGSPQPV) and terminates after these 17 amino acids. Non-expression of the second underlined region gives rise to a truncated protein of 786 amino acids (Nakamura *et al.*, 1992).

Nakamura, T., Hillova, J., Mariage-Samson, R. and Hill, M. (1988). Molecular cloning of a novel oncogene generated by DNA recombination during transfection. Oncogene Res., 2, 357–370.

Nakamura, T., Hillova, J., Mariage-Samson, R., Onno, M., Huebner, K., Cannizzaro, L.A., Boghosian-Sell, Croce, C. and Hill, M. (1992). A novel transcriptional unit of the tre oncogene widely expressed in human cancer cells. Oncogene, 7, 733–741.

UFO

UFO *u*nidentified *f*unction *o*f its protein (also *FGFR4*, *JTK2* or *AXL* (Greek *anexelekto*, uncontrolled)) was isolated by a DNA transfection assay from human chronic myelogenous leukaemia (Janssen *et al.*, 1991). Overexpression of *UFO* transforms NIH 3T3 cells. A 2682 bp human *UFO* ORF encodes a 140 kDa (894 amino acid) transmembrane receptor tyrosine kinase that is translated from 3.2 and 5.0 kb mRNAs in bone marrow and tumour cell lines. Different isoforms are generated by alternative splicing of exon 10 (Schulz *et al.*, 1993). UFO is 56% identical in sequence with BEK and FLG (see **HSTF1/Hst-1**). A 4 kb mRNA homologue is expressed in mice. The extracellular domain includes two Ig-like loops and two fibronectin type III domains (thus comprising another insulin receptor subclass in addition to the insulin receptor and the *EPH* class). Murine *Ufo* (chromosome 7) encodes a protein that is 87.6% identical with human UFO (Faust *et al.*, 1992).

Sequence of UFO

```
   (1)  MRLLLALLGVLLSVPGPPVLSLEASEEVELEPCLAPSLEQQEQELTVALGQPVRLCCGRA
  (61)  ERGGHWYKEGSRLAPAGRVRGWRGRLEIASFLPEDAGRYLCLARGSMIVLQNLTLITGDS
 (121)  LTSSNDDEDPKSHRDPSNRHSYPQQAPYWTHPQRMEKKLHAVPAGNTVKFRCPAAGNPTP
 (181)  TIRWLKDGQAFHGENRIGGIRLRHQHWSLVMESVVPSDRGTYTCLVENAVGSIRYNYLLD
 (241)  VLERSPHRPILQAGLPANTTAVVGSDVELLCKVYSDAQPHIQWLKHIVINGSSFGAVGFP
 (301)  YVQVLKTADINSSEVEVLYLRNVSAEDAGEYTCLAGNSIGLSYQSAWLTVLPEEDPTWTA
 (361)  AAPEARYTDIILYASGSLALAVLLLLAGLYRGQALHGRHPRPPATVQKLSRFPLARQFSL
 (421)  ESGSSGKSSSSLVRGVRLSSSGPALLAGLVSLDLPLDPLWEFPRDRLVLGKPLGEGCFGQ
 (481)  VVRAEAFGMDPARPDQASTVAVKMLKDNASDKDLADLVSEMEVMKLIGRHKNIINLLGVC
 (541)  TQEGPLYVIVECAAKGNLREFLRARRPPGPDLSPDGPRSSEGPLSFPVLVSCAYQVARGM
 (601)  QYLESRKCIHRDLAARNVLVTEDNVMKIADFGLARGVHHIDYYKKTSNGRLPVKWMAPEA
 (661)  LFDRVYTHQSDVWSFGILLWEIFTLGGSPYPGIPVEELFSLLREGHRMDRPPHCPPELYG
 (721)  LMRECWHAAPSQRPTFKQLVEALDKVLLAVSEEYLDLRLTFGPYSPSGGDASSTCSSSDS
 (781)  VFSHDPLPLGSSSFPFGSGVQT (802)
```

Underlined: Ig-like loops. Italics: transmembrane domain.

Faust, M., Ebensperger, C., Schulz, A.S., Schleithoff, L., Hameister, H., Bartram, C.R. and Janssen., J.W.G. (1992). The murine *ufo* receptor: molecular cloning, chromosomal localization and *in situ* expression analysis. Oncogene, 7, 1287–1293.

Janssen, J.W.G., Schulz, A.S., Steenvoorden, A.C.M., Schmidberger, M., Strehl, S., Ambros, P.F. and Bartram, C.R. (1991). A novel putative tyrosine kinase receptor with oncogenic potential. Oncogene, 6, 2113–2120.

Partenen, J., Makela, T.P., Alitalo, R., Lehvaslaiho, H. and Alitalo, K. (1990). Putative tyrosine kinases expressed in K-562 human leukemia cells. Proc. Natl Acad. Sci. USA, 87, 8913–8917.

Partenen, J., Makela, T.P., Eerola, E., Korhonen, J., Hirvonen, H., Claesson-Welsh, L. and Alitalo, K. (1991). FGFR-4, a novel acidic fibroblast growth factor receptor with a distinct expression pattern. EMBO J., 10, 1347–1354.

O'Bryan, J.P., Frye, R.A., Cogswell, P.C., Neubauer, A., Kitch, B., Prokop, C., Espinosa, R., Le Beau, M.M., Earp, H.S. and Liu, E.T. (1991). *axl*, a transforming gene isolated from primary human myeloid leukemia cells, encodes a novel receptor tyrosine kinase. Mol. Cell. Biol., 11, 5016–5031.

Schulz, A.S., Schleithoff, L., Faust, M., Bartram, C.R. and Janssen, J.W.G. (1993). The genomic structure of the human UFO receptor. Oncogene, 8, 509–513.

VAV

Normal human *VAV* appears to be specifically expressed in cells of haematopoietic origin (erythroid, lymphoid, myeloid) regardless of their differentiation lineage. Human *VAV* maps to chromosome region 19p13.2 (Martinerie *et al.*, 1990), a region involved in karyotypic abnormalities in a variety of malignancies including melanomas and leukaemias. The gene was first identified by *in vitro* replacement of 67 N-terminal proto-VAV amino acids by 19 Tn5 transposase residues (Katzav *et al.*, 1989). VAV is a weak NIH 3T3 cell transforming agent; transformation is greatly enhanced by truncation of the N-terminal helix–loop–helix/leucine zipper region (Katzav *et al.*, 1991). p95^{vav} undergoes rapid and transient tyrosine phosphorylation following activation of the T cell receptor or in response to EGF or PDGF in transfected NIH 3T3 cells (Bustelo *et al.*, 1992; Margolis *et al.*, 1992) and in human haematopoietic cells after stimulation of KIT by stem cell factor (see **KIT**; Alai *et al.*, 1992). The central domain (198–434) shares homology with DBL, BCR, CDC24 and CDC25 (see **ABL**).

VAV proteins also contain a cysteine-rich domain that includes two putative metal binding regions, Cys–X$_2$–Cys–X1$_3$–Cys–X$_2$–Cys and His–X$_2$–Cys–X$_6$–Cys–X$_2$–His. Mutations in these regions may completely abolish transforming activity (Coppola *et al.*, 1991).

Sequence of human VAV *(see also* DBL*)*

```
  (1)    MNVSYWAIWTRENASAKRKQFLCLKNIRTFLSTCCEKFGLKRSELFEAFDLFDVQDFGK
 (60)    VIYTLSALSWTPIAQNRGIMPFPTEEESVGDEDIYSGLSDQIDDTVEEDEDLYDCVENEE
(120)    AEGDEIYEDLMRSEPVSMPPKMTEYDKRCCCLREIQQTEEKYTDTLGSIQQHFLKPLQRF
(180)    LKPQDIEIIFINIEDLLRVHTHFLKEMKEALGTPGAPNLYQVFIKYKERFLVYGRYCSQV
(240)    ESASKHLDRVAAAREDVQMKLEECSQRANNGRFTARPADGAYAASSQISPPSPGAGETHA
(300)    GGDGARKLRLALDAMRDLAQCVNEVKRDNETLRQITNFQLSIENLDQSLAHYGRPKIDGE
(360)    LKITSVERRSKMDRYAFLLDKALLICKRRGDSYDLKDFVNLHSFQVRDDSSGDRDNKKWS
(420)    HMFLLIEDQGAQGYELFFKTRELKKKWMEQFEMAISNIYPENATANGHDFQMFSFEETTS
(480)    CKACQMLLRGTFYQGYRCHRCRASAHKECLGRVPPCGRHGQDFPGTMKKDKLHRRAQDKK
(540)    RNELGLPKMEVFQEYYGLPPPPGAIGPFLRLNPGDIVELTKAEAEQNWWEGRNTSTNEIG
(600)    WFPCNRVKPYVHGPPQDLSVHLWYAGPMERAGAESILANRSDGTFLVRQRVKDAAEFAIS
(660)    IKYNVEVKHTVKIMTAEGLYRITEKKAFRGLTELVEFYQQNSLKDCFKSLDTTLQFPFKE
(720)    PEKRTISRPAVGSTKYFGTAKARYDFCARDRSELSLKEGDIIKILNKKGQQGWWRGEIYG
(780)    RVGWFPANYVEEDYSEYC (797)
```

Underlined: two zinc finger domains. There are two putative nuclear localization signals (438–445 and 527–534). VAV contains N-terminal helix–loop–helix and leucine zipper domains. Human and mouse VAV are 95% homologous.

Adams, J.M., Houston, H., Allen, J., Lints, T. and Harvey, R. (1992). The hematopoietically expressed *vav* proto-oncogene shares homology with the *dbl* GDP-GTP exchange factor, the *bcr* gene and a yeast gene (CDC24) involved in cytoskeletal organization. Oncogene, 7, 611–618.

Alai, M., Mui, A.L.-F., Cutler, R.L., Bustelo, X.R., Barbacid, M. and Krystal, G. (1992). Steel factor stimulates the tyrosine phosphorylation of the proto-oncogene product, p95^{vav}, in human hemopoietic cells. J. Biol. Chem., 267, 18021–18025.

Bustelo, X.R., Ledbetter, J.A. and Barbacid, M. (1992). Product of *vav* proto-oncogene defines a new class of tyrosine protein kinase substrates. Nature, 356, 68–71.

Coppola, J., Bryant, S., Koda, T., Conway, D. and Barbacid, M. (1991). Mechanism of activation of the *vav* protooncogene. Cell Growth Differ., 2, 95–105.

Katzav, S., Martin-Zanca, D. and Barbacid, M. (1989). *vav*, a novel human oncogene derived from a locus ubiquitously expressed in hematopoietic cells. EMBO J., 8, 2283–2290.

katzav, S., Cleveland, J.L., Heslop, H.E. and Pulido, D. (1991). Loss of the amino-terminal helix-loop-helix domain of the *vav* proto-oncogene activates its transforming potential. Mol. Cell. Biol., 11, 1912–1920.

Martinerie, C., Cannizzaro, L.A., Croce, C.M., Huebner, K., Katzav, S. and Barbacid, M. (1990). The human VAV proto-oncogene maps to chromosome region 19p12–19p13.2. Hum. Genet., 86, 65–68.

Margolis, B., Hu, P., Katzav, S., Li, W., Oliver, J.M., Ullrich, A., Weiss, A. and Schlessinger, J. (1992). Tyrosine phosphorylation of *vav* proto-oncogene product containing SH2 domain and transcription factor motifs. Nature, 356, 71–74.

Databank file names and accession numbers

	GENE	EMBL	SWISSPROT	REFERENCES
Mouse	Akt	X65687		Bellacosa *et al.*, 1993
Mouse (AKT8)	v-*akt*	Aktakta M80675; M61767		Bellacosa *et al.*, 1991
Human	COT			Miyoshi *et al.*, 1991
Rat	Csk	Rptyk1 X58631		Nada *et al.*, 1991
Chicken	Csk	Ggsrcka M85039		
Human	CYL	Hscylctk X60114		Partanen *et al.*, 1991
Human	DLK	Z12172		Laborda *et al.*, 1993
Mouse	Dlk	Mmdlkhomm Z12171		Laborda *et al.*, 1993
Mouse	Ect2			Miki *et al.*, 1993
Human	EST	Z14138		Chan *et al.*, 1993
Human	GLI1	Hsgli X07384	GLI_HUMAN P08151	Kinzler *et al.*, 1988
Human	GLI2	Hsgli21 M20672 Hsgli22 M20673	GLI2_HUMAN P10070	Ruppert *et al.*, 1988
Human	GLI3	Hsgli3 M20674	GLI3_HUMAN P10071	Ruppert *et al.*, 1988
Human	HOX2.4	Hshox24 X16173	HM24_HUMAN P17481	Giampaolo *et al.*, 1989
Human	JTK2	Hsjtk2 M59373; M37781		Partanen *et al.*, 1990
Human	LYN	Hslyn M16038	KLYN_HUMAN P07948	Yamanashi *et al.*, 1987
Human	LTK	Hsltk X60702		Krolewski and Dalla-Favera, 1991
Human	MEL			Nimmo *et al.*, 1991
Human	NCK	Hsnck X17576	NCK_HUMAN P16333	Lehmann *et al.*, 1990

	GENE	EMBL	SWISSPROT	REFERENCES
Human	ODC1	Hssodb M33764 Hsodc M16650 Hsodcg X16277 Hsodc1 X55362 Hsodc1a M81740	DCOR_HUMAN P11926	Hickok *et al.*, 1990
Mouse	Mel			Nimmo *et al.*, 1991
Human	Mplk	Hshmplk M90102		Vigon *et al.*, 1992
Human	Mplp	Hshmplp M90103		Vigon *et al.*, 1992
ASV 31	qin	L10719		Li and Vogt, 1993
Human	TIE	Hstiemr X60957		Partanen *et al.*, 1992
Human	TKF			Holtrich *et al.*, 1991
Human	TRE	Hstre210 X63546 (clone 210)		Nakamura *et al.*, 1992
Human	TRE	Hstre213 X63547 (clone 213)		Nakamura *et al.*, 1992
Human	UFO	Hsjtk2 M59373; M37781 Hsfgr4 X57205	FGR4_HUMAN P22455	Partanen *et al.*, 1990 Janssen *et al.*, 1991 Schulz *et al.*, 1993
Human	VAV	Hsvavpo X16316 Gbo:Humvavpo M59834	VAV_HUMAN P15498	Katzav *et al.*, 1989 Katzav *et al.*, 1991
Mouse	Blk	Mmtkblk M30903	KBLK_MOUSE P16277	Dymecki *et al.*, 1990
Mouse	Clk	Mmclkmrna X57186 Mmltk X07984	KCLK_MOUSE P22518	Ben-David *et al.*, 1991
Mouse	Ltk	Mmltk2 X52621	KLTK_MOUSE P08923	Ben-Neriah *et al.*, 1990 Bernards and de la Monte, 1990
Mouse	LynA	Mmlyna M57696		Yi *et al.*, 1991
Mouse	LynB	Mmlynb M57697		Yi *et al.*, 1991
Human	NRL v-maf	Hsnrlgp; M81840 Aafvmaf; M26769	TMAF_AVIS4 P23091	Swaroop *et al.*, 1992 Nishizawa *et al.*, 1989
Mouse	Pem			Wilkinson *et al.*, 1991
Mouse	Sty	Mmstykin M38381	KCLK_MOUSE P22518	Howell *et al.*, 1991
Mouse	Tlm	Mmonctlm X52634	TLM_MOUSE P17408	Lane and Tobin, 1990
Mouse	Vav	Mmvavpo M59833		Katzav *et al.*, 1991
Chicken	Ryk	Arevryk M92847		Jia *et al.*, 1992
Mouse	Ryk	M98547		Hovens *et al.*, 1992
Chicken	Tkl	Ggtckl J03579		Strebhardt *et al.*, 1987

Table 2.6. *Chromosome locations of human proto-oncogenes*

1	ECK	10q24	HOX11
1	EEK	11p12–p11.2	SPI1
1	ERK	11p13	RBTNL1
1	TPR	11p13	WT1
1p13	NRAS	11p15	RBTN1
1p32	BLYM	11p15.5	HRAS
1p32	MYCL1	11q13	BCL1
1p32	TAL1	11q13	INT2
1p32–p31	JUN	11q13	MEN1
1p33	SIL	11q13	SEA
1p33–p34	TIE	11q13.3	HSTF1
1p34	MPL	11q23	MLL
1p35–p32	LCK	11q23	PLZF
1p36.2–p36.1	FGR	11q23–q24	ERGB
1q22–q24	SKI	11q23.3	ETS1
1q23	PBX1	11q23.3–qter	CBL
1q23–q24	TRK	11q24	FLI1
1q23–q31	TRKB	12p12.1	KRAS2
1q23–q31	TRKC	12p13	HST2
1q24–q25	ABL2 (ARG)	12q13	HER3
2p13–p12	REL	12q13	WNT1
2p24.1	MYCN	12q13–q14.3	GLI1
2p25	ODC1	12q22	BTG1
2q14–q21	HIS1	13q12	FLT1
2q14–q21	LCO	13q12	FLT3/FLK2
2q33–qter	INHA	13q14.2	RB1
3p24.1–p22	THRB	14q24.3	FOS
3p25	RAF1	14q32	AKT
3p25–p26	VHL	14q32.3	ELK2
3q22	RYK	15	CSK
3q26	EVI	15q13–q21	LTK
4q21	AF4	15q21	PML
4	FLK1/KDR	15q25–q26	FPS/FES
4q11–q21	KIT	16q	CMAR/CAR
5/17/18 (elements)	TRE	16q22.1	UVO
5q21	FER	17p13.1	TP53
5q21	MCC	17q11.2	EV12B
5q21–q22	APC	17q11.2	NF1
5q31.3–q33.2	FGFA	17q11.2–q12	THRA1
5q33.3–q34	CSF1R	17q12–q21	BRCA1
5q35	FLT4	17q21	PHB
6p21	PIM1	17q21	RARA
6p23–p22.3	FIM1	17q21–q22	HER2
6q21	FYN	17q21–q22	WNT3
6q21–q22	ROS1	17q21.3	NME1, NME2
6q22–q23	MYB	18q21	BCL2
6q23	CAN	18q21	DCC
6q24–q27	MAS	18q21.3	YES1
7p13–p12	EGFR	19p13.2	LYL1
7p15	MYCLK1	19p13.2	JUNB
7q31	MET	19p13.2	JUND
7q31	WNT2	19p13.2	VAV
7q32–q36	EPHT	19p13.3	ENL
7q33–q36	RAFB1	19cen–p13.2	MEL
8p12	FLT2	19q13.1	BCL3
8q11–q12	MOS	19q13.1	UFO
8q13–qter	LYN	20q11	HCK
8q22	MYBL1	20q13.3	SRC
8q22	AML1	21q22	ETO
8q24	MYC	21q22.3	ERG
8q24	PVT1	21q22.3	ETS2
8q24.1	NOV	22q11.2	BCR
9q22	AF9	22q12	EWS
9p34.1	ABL1	22q12	NF2
9q34	DEK	22q12.3–q13.1	PDGFB
9q34	SET	Xp11.2	ELK1
9q34	TAL2	Xp11.2	RAFA1
9q34	TAN1	Xp11.3–p11.23	TIMP
10p11.2	EST	Xq13	MYBL2
10q11.2	RET	Xq27	DBL

```
PhK   (25)  LG.G.SS.V..C(19) YAVKII.(16)E(4)E(2)I(32)GE....L (23) ALH....VH RDL KPENILL (6) K(2)DFG(12)E(2)G .  PS YLAPEII(15)D.W..G(8)G..PP(14)G(30)R(43)                            [318]
cGPK  (365) LG.G.FG.V..V(9)  FAMKIL.(10)E(4)E(2)I(31)GE....L (23) YLH... IY RDL KPENILL (6) K(2)DFG(12)T(2)G .  PE YLAPEII (9)D.W..G(8)G..PP(14)G(28)R(43)                            [644]
cAPK  (48)  LG.G.FG.V..V(9)  YAMKIL.(10)E(4)E(2)I(31)GE....L (23) YLH... IY RDL KPENLLI (6) Q(2)DFG(10)T(2)G .  PE YLAPEII (9)D.W..G(8)G..PP(14)G(26)R(43)                            [323]
v-SRC (273) LG.G.FG.V..G(7)  VAIKTLK                        (45) GS.L.L (22)GM.Y.E...YVH RDL RAANILV (6) K(2)DFG(9) Y(4)GAKF PIKWTAPE (11) D.W..G(9)G..PY(14)G(27)RP.F(5) QLLPACVLEVAE  [526]
SRC   (273) LG.G.FG.V..G(7)  VAIKTLK                        (45) GS.L.L (22)GM.Y.E...YIH RDL RAANILV (6) K(2)DFG(9) Y(4)GAKF PIKWTAPE (11) D.W..G(9)G..PY(14)G(27)RP.F(5)FLEDYFTSTEPQYQPGENL [530]
YES   (557) LG.G.FG.V..G(7)  VAIKTLK                        (45) GS.L.L (22)GM.Y.E...YIH RDL RAANILV (6) K(2)DFG(9) Y(4)GAKF PIKWTAPE (11) D.W..G(9)G..PY(14)G(27)RP.F(12) AAEPSGT      [812]
FGR   (410) LG.G.FG.V..G(7)  VAVKTLK                        (45) GS.L.L (22)GM.Y.E...YIH RDL RAANILV (6) K(2)DFG(9) Y(4)GAKF PIKWTAPE (11) D.W..G(9)G..PY(14)G(27)RP.F(13) PQQM         [663]
ABL   (370) LG.G.YG.V..G(8)  VAVKTLK                        (45) GN.L.L (22)AM.Y.E...FIH RDL AARNCLV (6) K(2)DFG(9) Y(4)GAKF PIKWTAPE (11) D.W..G(9)G..PY(14)G(27)RP.F(40)              [647]
FPS   (927) LG.G.FG.V..G(8)  VAVKTLK                        (46) GD.L.L (21)GM.Y.E...CIH RDL AARNCLV (6) K(2)DFG(9) Y(4)GMKQIPVKWTAPE (11) D.W..G(9)G..PY(14)G(27)RP.F(15)             [1182]
FES   (703) LG.G.FG.V..G(7)  VAVKTLK                        (49) GD.L.L (21)GM.Y.E...CIH RDL AARNCLV (6) K(2)DFG(9) Y(4)GLRLVPVKWTAPE (11) D.W..G(9)G..PW(14)G(27)RP.F(15)            [958]
MET  (1102) IG.G.FG.V..G(11) CAVKSLN                        (49) GD.R..I (21)AM.YLA...FVH RDL AARNCML (6) K(2)DFG(9) Y(7)GAKL PVKWMALE (11) D.W..G(9)G..PY(14)G(27)RP.F(60)           [1408]
ROS   (264) LG.G.FG.V..G(14) VAVKTLK                        (48) GD.L.L (27)GC.Y.E...FIH RDL AARNCLV (6) K(2)DFG(9) Y(4)GEGLLPVRHMAPE (11) D.W..G(9)G..PY(14)G(27)RP.F(40)            [562]
FAK   (403) LG.G.FG.V..G(11) VAIKTCK                        (47) GE.R..I (21)AL.Y.E...FVH RDI AARNVLV (6) K(2)DFG(9) Y(4)GKSKL PIKWMAPE (11) D.W..G(9)G..PF(14)G(27)RP.F(384)         [1028]
EGFR  (695) LG.G.FG.V..G(12) VAIK.L.                        (47) GC.L.V (21)GM.Y.E...LVH RDL AARNVLV (6) K(2)DFG(11)Y(3)G..KV PIKWMALE (11) D.W..G(9)G..PY(14)G(27)RP.F(128)PEY(75)DNPDY(20)ENAEY(13) [1186]
ERBB  (144)                        I                                                                                                                         QDDFLPTSCS              [604]
Ins-R(1029) LG.G.FG.V..G(13)VAVKTVN                         (48) GD.K..L (30)GM.Y.N...FVH RDL AARNCMV (6) K(2)DFG(9) Y(6)GL LPVRWMAPE (11) D.W..G(9)A..PY(14)G(27)RP.F(99)           [1382]
PDGFR (606) LG.G.FG.V..A(13)VAVRMLK                         (49) GDLV..L(119)GM.F.A...CVH RDL AARNVLI (6) K(2)DFG(10)Y(3)GSTFLPLKWMAPE (11) D.W..G(9)G..PY(15)G(27)RP.F(155)         [1106]
                                                                 K.I                                      *
```

Fig. 2.1. **Sequence homology between protein kinases.** PhK: phosphorylase kinase; cAPK: c-AMP-dependent protein kinase; cGPK: cGMP-dependent protein kinase; c-SRC. Underlined sequences represent the residue corresponding to the autophosphorylation site of c-SRC. Underlined sequences represent the three EGFR phosphorylation sites (Tyr1068, 1148 and 1173). For ERBB only the residues in the sequences shown that differ from those of the EGFR are indicated; the C-terminus does not contain the equivalent of Tyr1173 in the EGFR. The shaded box marks the ATP-binding consensus site [G.G.FG.V --- VA.K]. The solid box marks the phosphorylation consensus site [RDL(3)N.L(10)DFG..K[16–21)APE[11]D.W..G.L.E]. These consensus sequences are absolutely conserved between cAPK and a number of other kinases including the yeast p34 kinases encoded by *cdc2* and *cdc28*. K.I. indicates the kinase insert region contained in the 119 amino acid region of the PDGFR.

CHAPTER 3

Individual oncogenes

ABL/BCR

v-*abl* is the transforming gene of the replication-defective Abelson murine leukaemia virus (Ab-MuLV), originally isolated from a mouse infected with Moloney murine leukaemia virus (Mo-MuLV) after chemical thymectomy (Abelson and Rabstein, 1970). Mo-MuLV is an NB-trophic retrovirus. v-*abl* is also carried by the ABL-MYC murine retrovirus derived from Ab-MuLV (Largaespada *et al.*, 1992). The Hardy–Zuckerman 2 feline sarcoma virus (HZ2-FeSV) has also transduced the (feline) *Abl* gene to become an acute transforming virus (Besmer *et al.*, 1983).

ABL (*ABL1*) is the human homologue of *Abl*.

BCR (*b*reakpoint *c*luster *r*egion) is the first defined member of a small gene family localized on human chromosome 22 (Groffen *et al.*, 1984).

Related genes

ABL contains regions homologous to the kinase and homology regions 2 and 3 (SH2, SH3) of SRC (see **SRC**). The *Drosophila melanogaster Dash* gene is 89% homologous (77% identical) to human *ABL1* (Henkemeyer *et al.*, 1988) and *Caenorhabditis elegans* also expresses a highly conserved *Abl* homologue that is 62% homologous to the v-*abl* tyrosine kinase region (Goddard *et al.*, 1986).

Other *Abl*-related genes detected by screening genomic libraries are *ABL2/ARG*, *EPH* detected in an erythropoietin-producing human hepatocellular carcinoma cell line (ETL-1; Hirai *et al.*, 1987), NCP94, TKR11 and TKR16 (Foster *et al.*, 1986). *ABL2/ARG* (Abelson-related gene; 12 kb, human chromosome 1q24–q25) produces a 145 kDa protein containing SH2, SH3 and tyrosine kinase domains and, like *Abl*, is expressed as two proteins differing only in N-termini due to alternative splicing. Like *ABL*, *ARG* is expressed in a wide variety of tissues (Kruh *et al.*, 1990; Perego *et al.*, 1991).

There are three *BCR* related loci, *BCR2*, *BCR3* and *BCR4* (Croce *et al.*, 1987).

Cross-species homology

ABL: 85% overall; 99% and 96% in the N-terminal 500 and C-terminal 130 amino acids, respectively (human and mouse).

Transformation

MAN

Over 90% of chronic myeloid leukaemia (CML) cases involve a balanced translocation t(9;22)(q34,q11) of a fragment of the long arm of chromosome 9 to the long arm of chromosome 22, generating a shortened, hybrid chromosome (the Philadelphia chromosome, Ph[1], Nowell and Hungerford, 1960). The Ph[1] chromosome also occurs in 10–20% of patients with acute lymphoblastic leukaemias (ALL).

The proliferation *in vitro* of blast cells from CML patients is selectively suppressed by antisense oligodeoxynucleotides directed against the *BCR–ABL* junction (Szczylik *et al.*, 1991).

ANIMALS

Mo-MuLV induces lymphocytic leukaemias in mice (Reddy *et al.*, 1980). Cell-free extracts from the original lymphosarcoma induced by the combination of Mo-MuLV and prednisolone caused the rapid induction of bone marrow and lymphatic tumours following injection into mice, due to the action of the replication defective Ab-MuLV. HZ2-FeSV causes sarcomas.

Proviral integration of Mo-MuLV or Ab-MuLV into the *Myb* locus induces a subset of lymphoid neoplasms (see **MYB**).

The ABL-MYC retrovirus, in which *Myc* is expressed under the control of the herpes simplex virus thymidine kinase gene promoter, rapidly induces plasmacytomas in mice in the absence of pristane treatment, indicating that v-*abl* and *Myc* act synergistically to transform mature B cells (Largaespada *et al.*, 1992). The induction of plasmacytomas rather than the pre-B cell lymphomas induced by Ab-MuLV indicates that the constitutive overexpression of *Myc* permits maturation of infected immature B cells (Weissinger *et al.*, 1993).

IN VITRO

Ab-MuLV does not transform primary fibroblasts but does transform haematopoietic cells, NIH 3T3 fibroblasts and lymphoid cells and is thus unique among murine retroviruses (Rosenberg *et al.*, 1975; Scher and Siegler, 1975). However, although v-*abl* transforms NIH 3T3 cells, the majority of Ab-MuLV-infected cells in a population undergo growth arrest in the G_1 phase of the cell cycle (Renshaw *et al.*, 1992).

Viral mutants with defective kinase activity do not transform cells *in vitro* (Witte *et al.*, 1980).

Ab-MuLV-transformed fibroblasts are tumorigenic on injection into syngeneic mice. $P210^{bcr-abl}$, $P185^{bcr-abl}$ or v-ABL proteins induce both lymphoid and myeloid colonies in bone marrow cells, although only the lymphoid colonies are tumorigenic (Kelliher *et al.*, 1993).

In general the *BCR–ABL* gene product is non-transforming: $P210^{bcr-abl}$ stimulates the growth of immature lymphoid cells from bone marrow after retroviral gene transfer and $P185^{bcr-abl}$ is a more potent growth promoter (McLaughlin *et al.*, 1987, 1989). In rat-1 cells, however, $P210^{bcr-abl}$ is weakly transforming and its tumorigenicity is strongly enhanced by the co-expression of v-*myc* (Lugo and Witte, 1989). The *gag–bcr–abl* fusion protein is a potent fibroblast and lymphoid cell transforming agent *in vitro* (Scher and Siegel, 1975; Witte *et al.*, 1980) and induces an acute, pre-B cell leukaemia *in vivo* (Abelson and Rabstein, 1970).

Overexpression of *Myc* acts synergistically with the expression of *Abl* oncogenes in transformation, whereas dominant negative mutations in MYC that leave the dimerization motif intact (deletion of amino acids 106–143 in the transcriptional activation domain or insertion of four serine residues between positions 373 and 374 in the DNA binding domain, see **MYC**) reduce transformation by v-*abl* or by $P185^{bcr-abl}$ (Sawyers *et al.*, 1992).

TRANSGENIC MICE

Haematopoietic stem cells expressing v-*abl* initiate leukaemogenesis in mice (Chung *et al.*, 1991). Animals with a homozygous deletion of *Abl* (Abl^{m1}) have increased perinatal mortality (within the first 2 weeks after birth) and have a major decrease in the level of B cell progenitors and a lesser depression in the concentration of developing (CD4+/CD8+) T cells (Schwartzberg *et al.*, 1991; Tybulewicz *et al.*, 1991).

Mice transgenic for a *Bcr–Abl* P190 DNA construct develop aggressive leukaemias with early onset and rapid progression, consistent with there being a critical role for the *Bcr–Abl* gene product of the Ph¹ chromosome in human leukaemia (Heisterkamp *et al.*, 1990). Plasmacytoma development in *Abl* transgenic mice occurs after a translocation in *Myc* that causes overexpression of MYC protein and is accelerated by crossing with transgenic *Myc* mice (Rosenbaum *et al.*, 1992).

	ABL/Abl	*BCR*	*v-abl*
Nucleotides			
Human	225 kb	130 kb	5668 bp (Ab-MuLV, P120)
Chromosome			
Human	9q34.1	22q11.2	
Mouse	2		
Exons	12 (including two alternative first exons, 1a and 1b)	21	
mRNA (kb)			
Human	6.0/7.0 (Two specific promoters utilize exon 1a or 1b: mRNAs 1a and 1b are equivalent to mouse Type I and IV mRNAs, respectively (Fainstein *et al.*, 1989).)	4.5/6.7	6.3 (Ab-MuLV P160$^{gag\text{-}abl}$) ~5.5 (P90$^{gag\text{-}abl}$, P100$^{gag\text{-}abl}$, P120$^{gag\text{-}abl}$) 4.6 (P92$^{gag\text{-}abl}$)
Mouse	5.3/6.5 (additional 4.2 kb in testis: Meijer *et al.*, 1987). (Types I, II, III and IV: these have four alternative divergent 5′ sequences encoded by differential splicing of exons 1a and 1b to a common 3′ sequence). Types II and IV: 6.5 kb mRNA; Type I: 5.3 kb mRNA.		
mRNA half-life (h)	0.5	4 4 (*BCR–ABL*)	
Amino acids			
Human	1130 (1a) 1148(1b)	1271	918 (P120)
Mouse	1123, 1117, 1118, 1142 (Types I, II, III, IV; Ben-Neriah *et al.*, 1986)		
Mass (kDa)			
Human (predicted) (expressed)	123 pp145^{ABL} (with alternative N-termini)	143 160	P160, P120 (+P90, P100 both weakly oncogenic)
Mouse	pp150^{abl}		

Cellular location

pp145^{abl}: mainly nuclear, some cytoplasmic/plasma membrane (Renshaw *et al.*, 1988); P210$^{bcr\text{-}abl}$: cytoplasm (Dhut *et al.*, 1991).

BCR: Cytoplasm.

v-*abl*: Plasma membrane (substrate adhesion points).

Tissue location

Abl: Widespread but is particularly strongly expressed in the spleen, testis and thymus (Van Etten *et al.*, 1989). In germ cells there is a novel transcript, restricted to post-meiotic spermatogenic cells (Ponzetto and Wolgemuth, 1985).

BCR: Widely expressed in many types of human haematopoietic and non-haematopoietic cells and cell lines (Collins *et al.*, 1987).

Protein function

ABL

ABL has weak tyrosine kinase activity. It does not transform fibroblasts even when over-expressed whether or not it is N-terminally myristylated. N-Terminal deletions activate tyrosine protein kinase and transformation potential. In addition to being a tyrosine kinase, ABL has a sequence-specific DNA binding activity for the EP element present in the enhancers of several viruses (hepatitis B virus, polyomavirus) and in the *Myc* promoter (Dikstein *et al.*, 1992). DNA binding activity is lost in the mutant P210$^{bcr-abl}$ protein (see below).

ABL and v-ABL proteins do not function as receptors and specific targets for their tyrosine kinase activity have not been characterized, although transformation by Ab-MuLV causes phosphorylation of enolase, vinculin and p42 and serine phosphorylation of ribosomal protein S6. The tyrosine kinase activity of v-ABL causes erythroid bursts in fetal liver cells in the absence of erythropoietin, renders the proliferation of mast cells and other types of cell independent of IL-3 (Cook *et al.*, 1985; Mathey-Prevot *et al.*, 1986; Rovera *et al.*, 1987) and in fibroblasts reduces the number of EGFRs and stimulates secretion of an EGF-like growth factor. All myristylated, tyrosine kinase-active forms of ABL associate with phosphatidylinositol-3-kinase (Varticovski *et al.*, 1991).

The serum-responsive genes *Fos*, *Jun* and *Myc* are selectively activated by v-*abl* in NIH 3T3 cells undergoing Ab-MuLV-induced transformation (Renshaw *et al.*, 1992). Transfection of v-*abl* activates the *Fos* promoter linked to heterologous genes, independent of protein kinase C (Hori *et al.*, 1990). CAT transcription directed by the SRE or TRE is also activated by v-*abl* and by *Raf*, consistent with there being a mechanism by which v-ABL can phosphorylate and thereby activate RAF (see **RAS**). In murine myeloid FDL-P1 cells, however, although v-*abl* (and also *Fms*, *Src* or *Trk*) abrogate the requirement for IL-3 and stimulate *Myc* transcription, v-*abl* does not induce *Fos* or *Jun* transcription although these genes are expressed during IL-3 stimulation (Cleveland *et al.*, 1989).

All ABL proteins (p150^{abl}, p160^{v-abl}, P210$^{bcr-abl}$) are phosphorylated at two C-terminal sites by protein kinase C (Pendergast *et al.*, 1987), the principal target being Ser1012 (human; 1004 mouse). As the region involved is not required either for ABL kinase activity or for transformation by v-ABL, the significance of this is unclear.

When Swiss 3T3 fibroblasts are transformed with Ab-MuLV, there is no amplification or rearrangement of *Fos*, *Myc* or *P53* (Colledge *et al.*, 1989) although in NIH 3T3 cells similarly transformed 4- to 16-fold amplification of *Myc* occurs. Thus transformation of Swiss 3T3 cells by v-*abl* does not require activation of *Myc* (or *Fos* or *P53*) and this is not selected for in tumorigenesis induced by these cells. However, in rat-1 fibroblasts, primary mouse bone marrow pre-B cells and transgenic mice the expression of *Myc* is essential for transformation by *Abl* oncogenes (Rosenbaum *et al.*, 1992; Sawyers *et al.*, 1992). These observations suggest that either *Abl* and *Myc* oncogenes activate independent, synergistic pathways or that one of the effects of the expression of *Abl* oncogenes is to activate *Myc*. Activated ABL proteins may cause modulation of the normal mechanisms that regulate growth factor-stimulated proliferation (for example, by activating phosphatidylinositol metabolism or the transcription of early genes including *Fos*), an inference strengthened by the finding that ABL is phosphorylated by p34^{cdc2} (Kipreos and Wang, 1990, 1992).

BCR

p160^{BCR} has serine/threonine protein kinase activity, encoded by the first exon (Maru and Witte, 1991), contains a central domain with homology to sequences having guanine nucleotide exchange activity and has a C-terminal domain (absent in P210$^{BCR-ABL}$ and P185$^{BCR-ABL}$) that possesses *in vitro* GTPase-activating protein activity (Diekmann *et al.*, 1991).

Structure of the Ab-MuLV genome and translation products

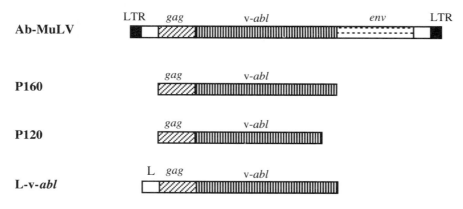

Ab-MuLV contains sequences derived from its natural helper virus, Mo-MuLV, as do other transforming viruses. Retroviral transduction deletes *pol*, *env* and some of *gag* from the viral genome and the SH3 domain from *Abl* (Wang *et al.*, 1984). The *gag–abl* hybrid proteins contain the entire sequence of p15^{gag} and p12^{gag} and the first 21 amino acids of p30^{gag} fused to *Abl* sequences (Reddy *et al.*, 1983). Upstream fusion of *gag* provides a myristylated N-terminus (Gly2 of p15^{gag}) that directs membrane localization. These two modifications to ABL activate tyrosine phosphorylation and transformation (as with SRC).

The two prototype strains of Ab-MuLV encode different v-ABL proteins (P120 and P160), and variants encoding 90 kDa and 100 kDa proteins have also been isolated (Rosenberg *et al.*, 1980). The 6.3 kb genomic RNA of P160 uses different translation start sites to yield L-v-*abl* and P160$^{gag-abl}$. P160$^{gag-abl}$ has tyrosine kinase and transforming activity. L-v-*abl* has an additional leader sequence and no tyrosine kinase activity.

The P120 and P160 forms of v-*abl* have 114 codons from the 5′ end of *Abl* replaced by 240 *gag* codons. P120 (918 amino acids, 240 *gag*, 678 v-*abl*) has an in-frame deletion of 263 codons and a point mutation (G to A) immediately downstream of the deletion (codon 832 of *Abl* (type I) cDNA). The mutation at position 832 also occurs in P160. The major deletion in P120 accounts for the difference in molecular weight between P120 and P160. In P160 the region deleted in the formation of P120 contains two frame-shift mutations that change the sequence of 23 amino acids in the centre of ABL. The variant forms (P90 and P100) have arisen from frame-shift mutations in P120 that cause premature termination of the encoded protein. In addition to the coding sequence deletions, the P120 form of v-*abl* has also lost a 765 nucleotide, non-coding, 3′ region during transduction of the cellular gene (Reddy *et al.*, 1983; Wang *et al.*, 1984).

P120 is not glycosylated: P160 has a glycosylation signal in the leader sequence of *gag*: a point mutation in this region can give rise to a non-glycosylated form. The 5′ *gag* sequences are not necessary for fibroblast transformation but their removal greatly reduces lymphoid cell transformation, possibly by decreasing the stability of the protein in these cells (Prywes *et al.*, 1983).

A viral strain carrying a further deletion in v-*abl* generates a 4.6 kb mRNA encoding P92*gag-abl* that is completely defective in transformation.

The HZ2-FeSV gene contains 439 amino acids derived from the cat *Abl* gene: 51 codons at the 5′ end have been replaced by 344 codons of *gag* and 633 codons at the 3′ end by 200 *pol* codons.

Sequences of v-ABL and human ABL (type 1a)

```
v-ABL    (1)    MGQTVTTPLSLTLGHWKDVERIAHNQSVDVKKRRWVTFCSAEWPTFNVGWPRDGTFNRDLITQVKIKVF

v-ABL    (70)   SPGPHGHPDQVPYIVTWEALAFDPPPWVKPFVHPKPPPPLPPSAPSLPLEPPLSTPPRSSLYPALTPSLG
ABL      (1)                                                                MLEICLKLVGCKSKKGLS

         (140)  AKPKPQVLSDSGGPLIDLLTEDPPPYRDPRPPPSDRDGNGGEATPAGEAPDPSPMASRLRGRREPPVADS
         (19)   SSSSCYLEEALQRPVASDFEPQGLSEAARWNSKENLLAGPSENDPNLFVALYDFVASGDNTLSITKGEKL

                               gag * abl
         (210)  TTSQAFPLRTGGNGQLQYWPFSSSDLYITPVNSLEKHSWYHGPVSRNAAEYLLSSGINGSFLVRESESSP
         (89)   RVLGYNHNGEWCEAQTKNGQGWVPSN--------------------P-----------------

         (280)  GQRSISLRYEGRVYHYRINTASDGKLYVSSESRFNTLAELVHHHSTVADGLITTLHYPAPKRNKPTIYGV
         (159)  S-----------------------------------------------------------V---

         (350)  SPNYDKWEMERTDITMKHKLGGGEYGEVYEGVWKKYSLTVAVKTLKEDTMEVEEFLKEAAVMKEIKHPNL
         (229)  --------------------Q---------------------------------------------

         (420)  VQLLGVCTREPPFYIITEFMTYGNLLDYLRECNRQEVSAVVLLYMATQISSAMEYLEKKNFIHRDLAARN
         (299)  -----------------------------------N-----------------------------

         (490)  CLVGENHLVKVADFGLSRLMTGDTYTAHAGAKFPIKWTAPESLAYNKFSIKSDVWAFGVLLWEIATYGMS
         (369)  -----------------------------------------------------------------

         (560)  PYPGIDLSQVYELLEKDYRMERPEGCPEKVYELMRACWQWNPSDRPSFAEIHQAFETMFQESSISDEVEK
         (439)  ------P------------K---------------------------------------------
                                  +                                    +
         (630)  ELGKRGTRGGAGSMLQAPELPTKTRTCRRAAEQKDAPDTPELLHTKGLGESDALDSEPAVSPLLPRKERG
         (509)  ----Q-VR-AVSTL-----------S-----HR-TT-V--MP-S--Q----P--H-----------

         (700)  PPDGSLNEDERLLPRDRKTNLFSALIKKKKKHAPTPPKRSSSFREMDGQPDRRGASEDDSRELCNGTTSS
         (579)  --E-G---------K-K-------------T----------------E----G-EEG-DIS--ALAF

         (770)  HLRRSRAYQVPKGQQWGWL PNGAFREPGNSGFRSPHMWKKSSTLTGSRLAAAEEESGMSSSKRFLRSCS
         (649)  TPLDTADPAKSPKPSN-AGV----L--S-G-------L---------S----TG---G-G-----------

         (839)  ASCMPHGARDTEWRSVTLPRDLPSAGKQFDSSTFGGHKSEKPALPRKRTSESRSEQVAKSTAMPLPGWLK
         (719)  V--V----K------------Q-T-R------------------KAG-N--D--TRG-VT-P-RLV-

         (909)  KNEEAAEEGFKDT ESSPGSSPPSLTPKLLRRQVTASPSSGLSHKKEATKGSASGMGTPATAEPAPPSNK
         (789)  ------D-V---IM---------N----P------VA-A---P--E--W----L-TPAA-EPV  T-TS-
```

ABL/BCR

```
v-ABL   (978)  VG      LSKASSEEMRVRRHKHSSESPGRDKGRLAKLKPAPPPPPACTG KA GKPAQSPSQE AGEA
ABL     (857)  A-SGAPRGT--GPA--S----------------K-S----------ASAG--G---S-R-G--A----

       (1039)  GGPTKTKCTSLAMDAVNTDPTKAGPPGEGLRKPVPPSVPKPQSTAKPPGTPTSPVSTP ST APAPSPLA
        (927)  VLGA---A--- V----S-AA-PSQ-----K---L-AT----P ---S---I--APV-L--LPS-S-A--

       (1107)  GDQQPSSAAFIPLISTRVSLRKTRQPPERIASGTITKGVVLDSTEALCLAISRNSEQMASHSAVLEAGKN
        (995)  ---PS-T -------------------P ---A-----------------G----------------

       (1177)  LYTFCVSYVDSIQQMRNKFAFREAINKLESNLRELQICPATASSGPAATQDFSKLLSSVKEISDIVRR (1245)
       (1063)  --------------------------N---------S-G----------------------Q- (1130)
```

Dashes represent identical amino acids. The v-ABL (p160) sequence to the right of * is identical with the murine ABL sequence. Underlined amino acids are common to the phosphotyrosine acceptor sites of ABL, v-ABL, v-FES, v-FPS, v-SRC and v-YES. + Indicates the serine and threonine residues phosphorylated by p34^{cdc2} (Ser588 and Thr566 in the 559–596 region of murine Type IV ABL; Kipreos and Wang, 1990). The underlined region (v-ABL 664–927) is deleted in P120 with the insertion of an additional alanine residue.

ABL protein structure and alternative N-terminal sequences

(a)

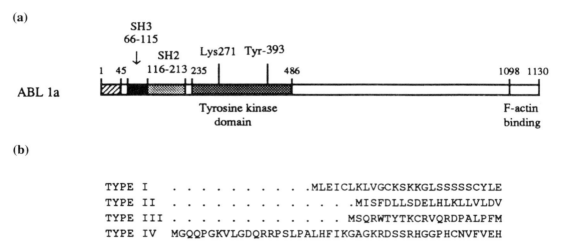

(b)

```
TYPE I    . . . . . . . . . . .MLEICLKLVGCKSKKGLSSSSSCYLE
TYPE II   . . . . . . . . . . . .MISFDLLSDELHLKLLVLDV
TYPE III  . . . . . . . . . . MSQRWTYTKCRVQRDPALPFM
TYPE IV   MGQQPGKVLGDQRRPSLPALHFIKGAGKRDSSRHGGPHCNVFVEH
```

(a) Major domains in human type 1a ABL. Cross-hatched box: exon 1a product. Black box: SH3 domain. Shaded boxes: SH2 and tyrosine kinase domains. Lys271 (Lys290 in type 1b ABL) is essential for kinase activity. The highly conserved SH2 motif FLVRES is critical for binding to tyrosine phosphorylated proteins and transforming potential (Mayer et al., 1992; Zhu et al., 1993). Amino acids 1098–1130 represent an F-actin binding domain homologous to those in ARG and Drosophila D-ABL (McWhirter and Wang, 1993). The affinity of ABL for F-actin is enhanced by the BCR sequences present in BCR–ABL.

(b) Sequences of the unique N-termini encoded by the four alternative first exons of murine Abl (Ben-Neriah et al., 1986). Type I encodes a sequence identical to that of human exon 1a. Type IV encodes a sequence that differs from human 1b only by the replacement of Arg29 and Asp30 by Lys29 and Glu30, respectively (Shtivelman et al., 1986). Types I and IV are ubiquitously expressed.

The structure of the SH2 domain of ABL in solution has been shown by multidimensional NMR spectroscopy to comprise a compact sphere with a large three-stranded antiparallel β sheet (βI, 32–38; βII, 44–51; and βIII, 54–60), a second smaller β sheet (βIV, 61–63; βV, 67–70; βVI, 74–77) and a C-terminal α helix enclosing the hydrophobic core (Overduin *et al.*, 1992). The putative phosphotyrosyl binding site is formed by conserved residues in the large β sheet and in a short amphipathic helix (αI, 17–25). The four residues at the binding site are Arg18, Arg36, His57 and Arg59.

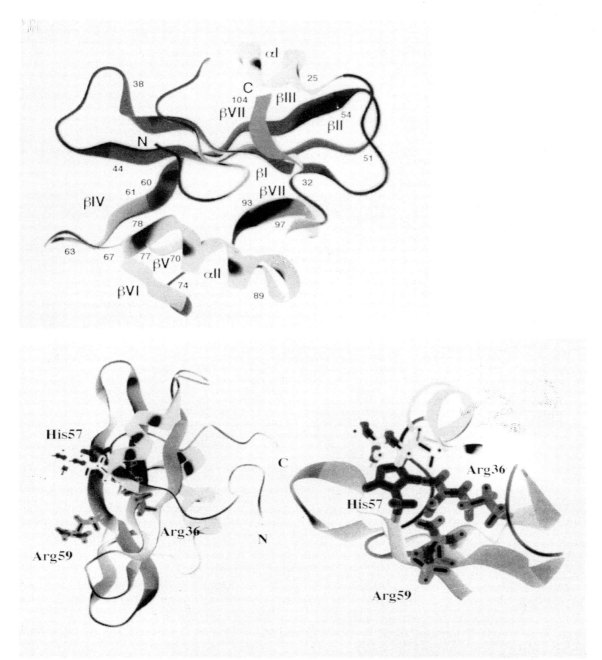

(From Overduin, M., Rios, C.B., Mayer, B.J., Baltimore, D. and Cowburn, D. (1992). Three-dimensional solution structure of the src homology 2 domain of c-*abl*. Cell, 70, 697–704.)

Sequence of human BCR

```
  (1)   MVDPVGFAEAWKAQFPDSEPPRMELRSVGDIEQELERCKASIRRLEQEVNQERFRMIYLQTLLAKEKKS
 (70)   YDRQRWGFRRAAQAPDGASEPRASASRPQPAPADGADPPPAEEPEARPDGEGSPGKARPGTARRPGAAAS
(140)   GERDDRGPPASVAALRSNFERIRKGHGQPGADAEKPFYVNVEFHHERGLVKVNDKEVSDRISSLGSQAMQ
(210)   MERKKSQHGAGSSVGDASRPPYRGRSSESSCGVDGDYEDAELNPRFLKDNLIDANGGSRPPWPPLEYQPY
(280)   QSIYVGGMMEGEGKGPLLRSQSTSEQEKRLTWPRRSYSPRSFEDCGGGYTPDCSSNENLTSSEEDFSSGQ
(350)   SSRVSPSPTTYRMFRDKSRSPSQNSQQSFDSSSPPTPQCHKRHRHCPVVVSEATIVGVRKTGQIWPNDGE
                  **
(420)   GAFHGDADGSFGTPPGYGCAADRAEEQRRHQDGLPYIDDSPSSSPHLSSKGRGSRDALVSGALESTKASE
(490)   LDLEKGLEMRKWVLSGILASEETYLSHLEALLLPMKPLKAAATTSQPVLTSQQIETIFFKVPELYEIHKE
(560)   FYDGLFPRVQQWSHQQRVGDLFQKLASQLGVYRAFVDNYGVAMEMAEKCCQANAQFAEISENLRARSNKD
(630)   AKDPTTKNSLETLLYKPVDRVTRSTLVLHDLLKHTPASHPDHPLLQDALRISQNFLSSINEEITPRRQSM
(700)   TVKKGEHRQLLKDSFMVELVEGARKLRHVFLFTELLLCTKLKKQSGGKTQQYDCKWYIPLTDLSFQMVDE
(770)   LEAVPNIPLVPDEELDALKIKISQIKSDIQREKRANKGSKATERLKKKLSEQESLLLLMSPSMAFRVHSR
(840)   NGKSYTFLISSDYERAEWRENIREQQKKCFRSFSLTSVELQMLTNSCVKLQTVHSIPLTINKEDDESPGL
                  ++
(910)   YGFLNVIVIHSATGFKQSSNLYCTLEVDSFGYFVNKAKTRVYRDTAEPNWNEEFEIELEGSQTLRILCYEK
(980)   CYNKTKIPKEDGESTDRLMGKGQVQLDPQALQDRDWQRTVIAMNGIEVKLSVKFNSREFSLKRMPSRKQT
(1050)  GVFGVKIAVVTKRERSKVPYIVRQCVEEIERRGMEEVGIYRVSGVATDIQALKAAFDVNNKDVSVMMSEM
(1120)  DVNAIAGTLKLYFRELPEPLFTDEFYPNFAEGIALSDPVAKESCMLNLLLSLPEANLLTFLFLLDHLKRV
(1190)  AEKEAVNKMSLHNLATVFGPTLLRPSEKESKLPANPSQPITMTDSWSLEVMSQVQVLLYFLQLEAIPAPD
(1260)  SKRQSILFSTEV(1271)
```

Underlined: region of homology with DBL, VAV, CDC24 and CDC25. Italics: p21^{rac}–GAP activity region. ** Indicates the breakpoint in P185$^{BCR-ABL}$(426). ++ Indicates breakpoint in P210$^{BCR-ABL}$ (927).

Structural features of p160^{BCR}

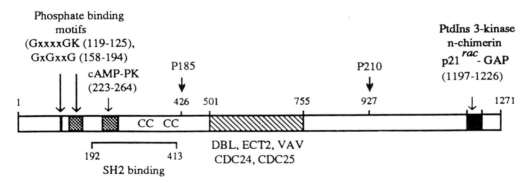

Thick line and shaded boxes: phosphate binding motifs and region of weak homology with cAMP-dependent protein kinases (223–264: VxxxxRxPxxxxSSxxxxxVxxxxxxxxLxxRFLKDxxxDxN). Cross-hatched box: homology with amino acid region 498–735 of DBL (function unknown), 198–434 of VAV, 166–420 of ECT2 (Miki *et al.*, 1993) and residues 163–400 of *Saccharomyces cerevisiae* CDC24 (regulates cytokinesis in yeast) and CDC25 (Cen *et al.*, 1992). Black box: GAP activity for p21^{rac}, homology with a p21^{rho} GAP, phosphatidylinositol 3-kinase 85 kDa subunit and *n*-chimaerin (which also has GAP activity for p21^{rac}, Diekmann *et al.*, 1991). The C-termini of the portions incorporated into P185$^{BCR-ABL}$ and P210$^{BCR-ABL}$ are indicated (P185, P210). The N-terminal 63 amino acids mediate binding to actin (McWhirter and Wang, 1991).

Serine/threonine-rich regions of BCR (192–242 and 298–413) bind to the SH2 domain of ABL in a high-affinity, phosphotyrosine-independent interaction (Pendergast *et al.*, 1991a; Muller *et al.*, 1992). This interaction is essential for BCR–ABL-mediated transformation: for the chimeric

BCR–ABL proteins the interaction may be inter- or intramolecular. The effect of the interaction may arise via interference with the binding of a cellular inhibitor to ABL regulatory domains (see below). *In vitro* p160*BCR* possesses autophosphorylating activity and phosphorylates histones and casein on serine residues. The kinase domain lies within exon 1 (426 amino acids, 10% serine) and has a novel nucleotide binding region containing two pairs of cysteine residues (324 & 332, 388 & 395) that is essential for the phosphotransferase activity of BCR (Maru and Witte, 1991; Liu *et al.*, 1993). The kinase, SH2-binding and GAP activities of BCR indicate its possible importance in cell signalling pathways.

ABL tyrosine kinase activation

ABL tyrosine kinase activity may be activated by:

1 The formation of the fusion BCR–ABL protein in which BCR sequences replace the ABL first exon (see below).
2 Deletion of the non-catalytic SH3 homology region. Evidence from mutational studies of ABL is consistent with the SH3 region being a negative regulatory element, as it is for SRC. Thus deletion of 114 codons from the 5′ end of *Abl* (including SH3) confers high oncogenic activity, as assayed by NIH 3T3 fibroblast transformation (Jackson and Baltimore, 1989; Shore *et al.*, 1990). Deletion of 53 codons from the 5′ end that includes the deletions in HZ2-FeSV and *Bcr–Abl* but retention of the SH3 region gives only low transforming activity. The G to A mutation in codon 823 that occurs in v-*abl* strongly increases tyrosine kinase activity and transforming potential. The retention of an N-terminal myristylation site (for which the first 14 amino acids of type IV ABL suffices) is essential for transforming activity. ABL differs from members of the SRC family of protein tyrosine kinases in that it does not contain a C-terminal regulatory tyrosine (Tyr527 in SRC).
3 Hyperexpression of ABL (>500-fold more than the normal endogenous concentration). The activation of ABL kinases in cells hyperexpressing the protein may reflect the presence of cellular factors that normally inhibit the kinase by non-covalent interaction. Tyrosine kinase activity is not detectable in the normal human ABL proteins (types 1a and 1b) until they have been immunoprecipitated and the lysate components removed, indicating that intracellular inhibitor(s) are normally present (Pendergast *et al.*, 1991b).

Chromosomal translocations in the formation of Philadelphia chromosome

(a) The standard 9:22 reciprocal translocation occurs in about 92% of CML cases with a Ph¹ chromosome, resulting in a *BCR–ABL* chimeric gene on that chromosome. This translocation places *ABL* within the *BCR* gene on chromosome 22: the fused *BCR–ABL* gene encodes an 8.5 kb mRNA containing the *BCR* exons 5′ of the breakpoint and all *ABL* exons except the first alternative exon. The product of the gene is P210*BCR-ABL*. Ph¹ chromosome breakpoints occur between exons 1a and 2 and also between exons 1a and 1b. Thus in some CML patients the *ABL* gene located on the Ph¹ chromosome retains an intact exon 1a. In the other cases the translocated portion of chromosome 22 moves to some chromosome other than 9 (Rowley, 1982).

(b) *ABL* and *BCR* gene structures. Black boxes: *ABL* exons (10) homologous to those expressed in v-*abl* and occupying ~32 kb. Cross-hatched boxes: *ABL* exons 1a and 1b (48 kb and 225 kb from the 3′ end of the gene, respectively). Exon 1a encodes 26 amino acids (identical in murine exon I), exon 1b encodes 45 amino acids (42 of which are identical to the murine

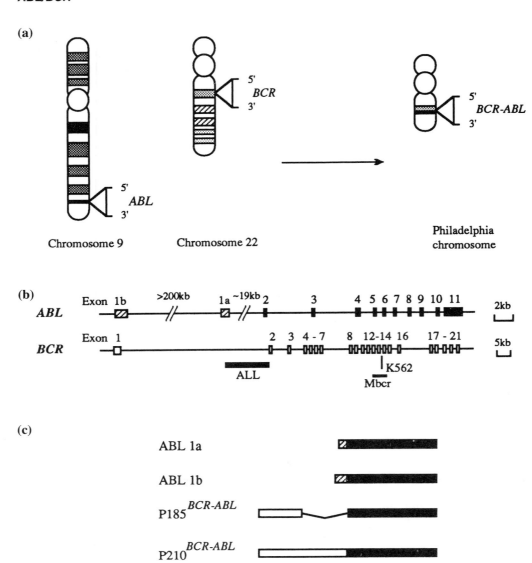

(a)

Chromosome 9   Chromosome 22   Philadelphia chromosome

(b)

(c)

ABL 1a

ABL 1b

P185^{BCR-ABL}

P210^{BCR-ABL}

exon IV sequence, see above). The chromosome 9 breakpoint can be 5' of exon 1b, i.e. over 200 kb from exon 2, the most 5' exon of *ABL* that is homologous to v-*abl* sequences.

Open boxes: *BCR* exons: intron 1 spans 68 kb. Mbcr: major breakpoint cluster region (5.8 kb) in which breakpoints in CML are located. Breakpoints occur in the introns between *BCR* exons 12, 13 and 14 (Sowerby *et al.*, 1993). Twenty-six codons from the 5' end of *ABL* are replaced by 927 codons from the *BCR* gene and fused to 1104 amino acids from ABL. P210^{BCR-ABL} is encoded by an 8.5 kb mRNA. Two minor breakpoint cluster regions (mbcr2 and mbcr3) are located within the 3' half of the first *BCR* intron. The breakpoint in the *ABL* sequence is in close proximity to that occurring in the generation of v-*abl*: thus the mechanism of activation of *ABL* in CML and by Ab-MuLV is similar, although the N-terminal deletion in v-*abl* is much larger and internal/frame-shift mutations do not occur in the *BCR–ABL* gene.

ALL: the 3′ region of intron 1 in which Mbcr negative, Ph¹–positive ALL breakpoints occur giving rise to a 7 kb *BCR–ABL* mRNA (1.8 kb from *BCR* exon 1 and 5.2 kb from the same *ABL* exons as in CML) that is translated into P185$^{BCR-ABL}$ (426 *BCR*-encoded amino acids fused to 1104 from *ABL*; Clark *et al.*, 1988). In ALL the breakpoints may also occur within Mbcr (Hermans *et al.*, 1987).

K562: indicates the breakpoint in the K562 CML-derived cell line (Heisterkamp *et al.*, 1988). An additional breakpoint within the first *BCR* intron occurs in one of the copies of *BCR–ABL* in this cell line but K562 cells produce only P210$^{BCR-ABL}$, not P185. In K562 cells the *BCR–ABL* region of the Ph¹ chromosome is amplified by 4- to 8-fold but the cells also possess un-amplified copies of normal chromosome 22.

P210$^{BCR-ABL}$ associates in tight complexes in K562 cells with p160^{BCR} and with a 53 kDa protein (ph-P53) that is distinct from the *P53* tumour suppressor gene product (Campbell *et al.*, 1990). ph-P53 also binds to BCR proteins in Ph¹-negative cells. Three related 41 kDa proteins have been identified as potential substrates of P210$^{BCR-ABL}$ (Freed and Hunter, 1992).

In the KBM-5 CML-derived cell line alternative mRNAs are formed by splicing at least two exons distinct from *BCR* exon 1 to *BCR* exon 2 to encode 7.7 kb mRNA and a p190 protein (Romero *et al.*, 1989).

(c) Structures of types 1a and 1b ABL and the chimeric proteins P185$^{BCR-ABL}$ and P210$^{BCR-ABL}$, indicating the coding regions of the genes from which they are derived. The variation in gene sizes arising from the range of breakpoints within the two major regions is removed by splicing to generate similar sized (7.7 kb and 8.7 kb) mRNAs encoding the fusion proteins. Both forms of BCR–ABL retain the SH3 domain and lack a myristylation signal, but tyrosine kinase activity is conferred by the additional N-terminal domain, specifically by sequences encoded by the first *BCR* exon (Muller *et al.*, 1991). P210$^{BCR-ABL}$ has a tyrosine kinase activity similar to that of v-ABL. P185$^{BCR-ABL}$ has a fivefold greater tyrosine kinase activity, is a more potent transforming agent and is more often associated with acute than with chronic leukaemia. Bone marrow reconstitution experiments in mice indicate that P185 and P210 induce similar patterns of haematological diseases (granulocytic, myelomonocytic and lymphocytic leukaemias) but P185-infected marrow causes more aggressive forms that have shorter latency periods than those resulting from P210 infection (Kelliher *et al.*, 1991), consistent with the transgenic data summarized above (see page 77).

The human 1a and 1b *ABL* promoter sequences show high homology (Zhu *et al.*, 1990). The 1b promoter contains at least 12 protein binding elements, including seven Sp-1 motifs and four CCAAT boxes but no TATA box. The 1a promoter contains seven Sp-1 sites and a TTAA sequence that may function as a TATA box. However, the 1a promoter Sp-1 sites do not bind protein, as indicated by DNAase protection assays. This may be significant in that in CML an intact copy of all *ABL* exons including 1a and its promoter sequence is often present on the Ph¹ chromosome (see below). The mouse 1a promoter does bind protein at several sites but it shares little sequence homology with the corresponding human region.

The *BCR* promoter occupies ~1 kb 5′ to exon 1 and contains six Sp-1 consensus sequences, two CCAAT boxes and no TATA-like boxes (Shah *et al.*, 1991). The 5′ non-coding region augments transformation by both P210 and P185$^{BCR-ABL}$ *in vitro* and includes an open reading frame encoding a putative 18 amino acid peptide (Gishizky *et al.*, 1991).

Data bank file names and accession numbers

	GENE	EMBL	SWISSPROT	REFERENCES
Ab-MuLV	v-abl	Reamlv V01541	KABL_MLVAB P00521	Reddy et al., 1983
		Reabl K00010		Groffen et al., 1983
Ab-MLV	v-abl	Reabmlva X02963		Lee et al., 1985
HZ2-FeSV	v-abl	Refcshz2 M15805	KABL_FSVHY P10447	Bergold et al., 1987
Human	ABL1	Hsabla M14752		Fainstein et al., 1989
Human	ABL1	Hsabl X16416	KABL_HUMAN P00519	Groffen et al., 1983 Shtivelman et al., 1986
Human	ARG	Hsargcaa M35296		Kruh et al., 1990
Human	BCR	Hsbcrr X02596	BCR_HUMAN P11274	Shah et al., 1991
		Hsbcr Y00661		Hariharan and Adams, 1987
		Hsbcrabl M15025		Heisterkamp et al., 1985
		M24603; M15025		Lifshitz et al., 1988 Mes-Masson et al., 1986, 1987
Mouse	Abl (5' end)	Mmabl1 K02290	KABL_MOUSE P00520	Wang et al., 1984
		Mmablts J02995		
Feline	Abl	sequence unknown		

Reviews

Konopka, J.B. and Witte, O.N. (1985). Activation of the abl oncogene in murine and human leukemias. Biochim. Biophys. Acta, 823, 1–17.
Ramakrishnan, L. and Rosenberg, N. (1989). abl genes. Biochim. Biophys. Acta, 989, 209–224.
Rosenberg, N. and Witte, O. (1988). The viral and cellular forms of the Abelson (abl) oncogene. Adv. Virus Res., 35, 39–81.

Papers

Abelson, H.T. and Rabstein, L.S. (1970). Lymphosarcoma: Virus-induced thymic-independent disease in mice. Cancer Res., 30, 2213–2222.
Ben-Neriah, Y., Bernards, A., Paskind, M., Daley, G.Q. and Baltimore, D. (1986). Alternative 5' exons in c-abl mRNA. Cell, 44, 577–586.
Bergold, P.J., Blumenthal, J.A., D'Andrea, E., Snyder, H.W., Lederman, L., Silverstone, A., Nguyen, H. and Besmer, P. (1987). Nucleic acid sequence and oncogenic properties of the HZ2 feline sarcoma virus v-abl insert. J. Virol., 61, 1193–1202.
Besmer, P., Hardy, W.S., Zuckerman, E.E., Bergold, P., Lederman, L. and Snyder, H.W. (1983). The Hardy–Zuckerman 2-FeSV, a new feline retrovirus with oncogene homology to Abelson MuLV. Nature, 303, 825–828.
Campbell, M.L., Li, W. and Arlinghaus, R.B. (1990). P210BCR–ABL is complexed to P160 BCR and ph-P53 proteins in K562 cells. Oncogene, 5, 773–776.

Cen, H., Papageorge, A.G., Zippel, R., Lowy, D.R. and Zhang, K. (1992). Isolation of multiple mouse cDNAs with coding homology to *Saccharomyces cerevisiae CDC25*: identification of a region related to bcr, vav, dbl and CDC24. EMBO J., 11, 4007–4015.

Chung, S.-W., Wong, P.M.C., Durkin, H., Wu, Y.-S. and Petersen, J. (1991). Leukemia initiated by hemopoietic stem cells expressing the v-*abl* oncogene. Proc. Natl Acad. Sci. USA, 88, 1585–1589.

Clark, S.S., McLaughlin, J., Timmons, M., Pendergast, A.M., Ben-Neriah, Y., Dow, L.W., Crist, W., Rovera, G., Smith, S.D. and Witte, O.N. (1988). Expression of a distinctive *BCR–ABL* oncogene in Ph[1]-positive acute lymphoblastic leukemia (ALL). Science, 239, 775–777.

Cleveland, J.L., Dean, M., Rosenberg, N., Wang, J.Y.J. and Rapp, U.R. (1989). Tyrosine kinase oncogenes abrogate interleukin-3 dependence of murine myeloid cells through signaling pathways involving c-*myc*: conditional regulation of c-*myc* transcription by temperature-sensitive v-*abl*. Mol. Cell. Biol., 9, 5685–5695.

Colledge, W.H., Gebhardt, A., Edge, M.D. and Bell, J.C. (1989). Analysis of A-MuLV transformed fibroblast lines for amplification of the c-*myc*, p53 and c-*fos* nuclear proto-oncogenes. Oncogene, 4, 753–757.

Collins, S., Coleman, H. and Groudine, M. (1987). Expression of bcr and bcr–abl transcripts in normal and leukemic cells. Mol. Cell. Biol., 7, 2870–2876.

Cook, W.D., Metcalf, D., Nicola, N.A., Burgess, A.W. and Walker, F. (1985). Malignant transformation of a growth factor-dependent myeloid cell line by Abelson virus without evidence of an autocrine mechanism. Cell, 41, 677–683.

Croce, C.M., Huebner, K., Isobe, M., Fainstain, E., Lifshitz, B., Shtivelman, E. and Canaani, E. (1987). Mapping of four distinct *BCR*-related loci to chromosome region 22q11: order of *BCR* loci relative to chronic myelogenous leukemia and acute lymphoblastic leukemia breakpoints. Proc. Natl Acad. Sci. USA, 84, 7174–7178.

Dhut, S., Chaplin, T. and Young, B.D. (1991). Normal c-*abl* gene protein – a nuclear component. Oncogene, 6, 1459–1464.

Diekmann, D., Brill, S., Garrett, M.D., Totty, N., Hsuan, J., Monfried, C., Hall, C., Lim, L. and Hall, A. (1991). *Bcr* encodes a GTPase-activating protein for $p21^{rac}$. Nature, 351, 400–402.

Dikstein, R., Heffetz, D., Ben-Neriah, Y. and Shaul, Y. (1992). c-abl has a sequence-specific enhancer binding activity. Cell, 69, 751–757.

Fainstein, E., Einat, M., Gokkel, E., Marcelle, C., Croce, C.M., Gale, R.P. and Canaani, E. (1989). Nucleotide sequence analysis of human *abl* and *bcr–abl* cDNAs. Oncogene 4, 1477–1481.

Foster, D.A., Levy, J.B., Daley, G.Q., Simon, M.C. and Hanafusa, H. (1986). Isolation of chicken cellular DNA sequences with homology to the region of viral oncogenes that encodes the tyrosine kinase domain. Mol. Cell. Biol., 6, 325–331.

Freed, E. and Hunter, T. (1992). A 41-kilodalton protein is a potential substrate for the $p210^{bcr-abl}$ protein-tyrosine kinase in chronic myelogenous leukemia cells. Mol. Cell. Biol., 12, 1312–1323.

Gishizky, M.L., McLaughlin, J., Prendergast, A.M. and Witte, O.N. (1991). The 5′ non-coding region of the BCR/ABL oncogene augments its ability to stimulate the growth of immature lymphoid cells. Oncogene, 6, 1299–1306.

Goddard, J.M., Weiland, J.J. and Capecchi, M.R. (1986). Isolation and characterization of *Caenorhabditis elegans* DNA sequences homologous to the v-*abl* oncogene. Proc. Natl Acad. Sci. USA, 83, 2172–2176.

Groffen, J., Heisterkamp, N., Reynolds, F.H. and Stephenson, J.R. (1983). Homology between phosphotyrosine acceptor site of human c-*abl* and viral oncogene products. Nature, 304, 167–169.

Groffen, J., Stephenson, J.R., Heisterkamp, N., de Klein, A., Bartram, C.R. and Grosveld, G. (1984). Philadelphia chromosomal breakpoints are clustered within a limited region, bcr, on chromosome 22. Cell, 36, 93–99.

Hariharan, I.K. and Adams, J.M. (1987). cDNA sequence for human bcr, the gene that translocates to the *abl* oncogene in chronic myeloid leukaemia. EMBO J., 6, 115–119.

Heisterkamp, N., Stam, K., Groffen, J., De Klein, A. and Grosveld, G. (1985). Structural organization of the bcr gene and its role in the Ph′ translocation. Nature, 315, 758–761.

Heisterkamp, N., Knopper, E. and Groffen, J. (1988). The first BCR gene intron contains breakpoints in Philadelphia chromosome positive leukemia. Nucleic Acids Res., 16, 10069–10081.

Heisterkamp, N., Jenster, G., ten Hoeve, J., Zovich, D., Pattengale, P.K. and Groffen, J. (1990). Acute leukemia in bcr/abl transgenic mice. Nature, 344, 251–253.

Henkemeyer, M.J., Bennett, R.L., Gertler, F.B. and Hoffmann, F.M. (1988). DNA sequence, structure, and tyrosine kinase activity of the *Drosophila melanogaster* Abelson proto-oncogene homolog. Mol. Cell. Biol., 8, 843–853.

Hermans, A., Heisterkamp, N., von Lindern, M., van Baal, S., Meijer, D., van der Plas, D., Wiedemann, L.M., Groffen, J., Bootsma, D. and Grosveld, G. (1987). Unique fusion of bcr and c-*abl* genes in Philadelphia chromosome positive acute lymphoblastic leukemia. Cell, 51, 33–40.

Hirai, H., Maru, Y., Hagiwara, K., Nishida, J. and Takaku, F. (1987). A novel putative tyrosine kinase receptor encoded by the *eph* gene. Science, 238, 1717–1720.

Hori, Y., Kaibuchi, K., Fukumoto, Y., Oku, N. and Takai, Y. (1990). Activation of the serum-response and TPA-response elements by expression of the v-*abl* protein: comparison of the mode of action of the v-*abl* protein with those of protein kinase C, cyclic AMP-dependent protein kinase, and the activated c-*raf* protein. Oncogene, 5, 1201–1206.

Jackson, P. and Baltimore, D. (1989). N-terminal mutations activate the leukemogenic potential of the myristoylated form of c-*abl*. EMBO J., 8, 449–456.

Kelliher, M., Knott, A., McLaughlin, J., Witte, O.N. and Rosenberg, N. (1991). Differences in oncogenic potency but not target cell specificity distinguish the two forms of the *BCR/ABL* oncogene. Mol. Cell. Biol., 11, 4710–4716.

Kelliher, M.A., Weckstein, D.J., Knott, A.G., Wortis, H.H. and Rosenberg, N. (1993). ABL oncogenes directly stimulate two distinct target cells in bone marrow from 5-fluorouracil-treated mice. Oncogene, 8, 1249–1256.

Kipreos, E.T. and Wang, J.Y.J. (1990). Differential phosphorylation of c-*abl* in cell cycle determined by *cdc-2* kinase and phosphatase activity. Science, 248, 217–220.

Kipreos,E.T. and Wang, J.Y.J. (1992). Cell cycle-regulated binding of c-Abl tyrosine kinase to DNA. Science, 256, 382–385.

Kruh, G.D., Perego, R., Miki, T. and Aaronson, S.A. (1990). The complete coding sequence of *arg* defines the Abelson subfamily of cytoplasmic tyrosine kinases. Proc. Natl Acad. Sci. USA, 87, 5802–5806.

Largaespada, D.A., Kaehler, D.A., Mishak, H., Weissinger, E., Potter, M., Mushinski, J.F. and Risser, R. (1992). A retrovirus that expresses v-*abl* and c-*myc* oncogenes rapidly induces plasmacytomas. Oncogene, 7, 811–819.

Lee, R., Paskind, M., Wang, J.Y.J. and Baltimore D. (1985). Abelson (P160) murine leukemia virus (Ab-MLV) *abl* gene. In Weiss, R., Teich, N., Varmus, H. and Coffin J. (eds) RNA Tumor Viruses: 861–868. Cold Spring Harbor Laboratory.

Lifshitz, B., Fainstein, E., Marcelle, C., Shtivelman, E., Amson, R., Gale, R.P. and Canaani, E. (1988). *bcr* genes and transcripts. Oncogene, 2, 113–117.

Liu, J., Campbell, M., Guo, J.Q., Lu, D., Xian, Y.M., Andersson, B.S. and Arlinghaus, R.B. (1993). BCR–ABL tyrosine kinase is autophosphorylated or transphosphorylates P160 BCR on tyrosine predominantly within the first BCR exon. Oncogene, 8, 101–109.

Lugo, T.G. and Witte, O.N. (1989). The BCR–ABL oncogene transforms rat-1 cells and cooperates with v-*myc*. Mol. Cell. Biol., 9, 1263–1270.

McLaughlin, J., Chianese, E. and Witte, O.N. (1987). *In vitro* transformation of immature hematopoietic cells by the P210$^{bcr/abl}$ oncogene product of the Philadelphia chromosome. Proc. Natl Acad. Sci. USA, 84, 6558–6562.

McLaughlin, J., Chianese, E. and Witte, O.N. (1989). Alternative forms of the *BCR–ABL* oncogene have quantitatively different potencies for stimulation of immature lymphoid cells. Mol. Cell. Biol., 9, 1866–1874.

McWhirter, J.R. and Wang, J.Y.J. (1991). Activation of tyrosine kinase and microfilament-binding functions of c-*abl* by bcr sequences in *bcr/abl* fusion proteins. Mol. Cell. Biol., 11, 1553–1565.

McWhirter, J.R. and Wang, J.Y.J. (1993). An actin-binding function contributes to transformation by the Bcr–Abl oncoprotein of Philadelphia chromosome-positive human leukemias. EMBO J., 12, 1533–1546.

Maru, Y. and Witte, O.N. (1991). The *BCR* gene encodes a novel serine/threonine kinase activity within a single exon. Cell, 67, 459–468.

Mathey-Prevot, B., Nabel, G., Palacios, R. and Baltimore, D. (1986). Abelson virus abrogation of interleukin-3 dependence in a lymphoid cell line. Mol. Cell. Biol., 6, 4133–4135.

Mayer, B.J., Jackson, P.K., van Etten, R. and Baltimore, D. (1992). Point mutations in the *abl* SH2 domain coordinately impair phosphotyrosine binding in vitro and transforming activity in vivo. Mol. Cell. Biol., 12, 609–618.

Meijer, D., Hermans, A., von Lindern, M., van Agthoven, T., de Klein, A., Mackenbach, P., Grootegoed, A., Talarico, D., Della Valle, G. and Grosveld, G. (1987). Molecular characterization of the testes specific c-*abl* mRNA in mouse. EMBO J., 6, 4041–4048.

Mes-Masson, A.M., McLaughlin, J., Daley, G.Q., Paskind, M. and Witte, O.N. (1986). Overlapping cDNA clones define the complete coding region for the P210-c-*abl* gene product associated with chronic myelogenous leukemia cells containing the Philadelphia chromosome. Proc. Natl Acad. Sci. USA, 83, 9768–9772.

Mes-Masson, A.M., McLaughlin, J., Daley, G.Q., Paskind, M. and Witte, O.N. (1987). Overlapping cDNA clones define the complete coding region for the P210-c-*abl* gene product associated with chronic myelogenous leukemia cells containing the Philadelphia chromosome: Correction. Proc. Natl Acad. Sci. USA, 84, 2507.

Miki, T., Smith, C.L., Long, J.E., Eva, A. and Fleming, T.P. (1993). Oncogene *ect2* is related to regulators of small GTP-binding proteins. Nature, 362, 462–465.

Muller, A.J., Young, J.C., Pendergast, A.-M., Pondel, M., Landau, N.R., Littman, D.R. and Witte, O.N. (1991). *BCR* first exon sequences specifically activate the *BCR/ABL* tyrosine kinase oncogene of Philadelphia chromosome-positive human leukemias. Mol. Cell. Biol., 11, 1785–1792.

Muller, A.J., Pendergast, A.-M., Havlik, M.H., Puil, L., Pawson, T. and Witte, O.N. (1992). A limited set of SH2 domains binds BCR through a high-affinity phosphotyrosine-independent interaction. Mol. Cell. Biol., 12, 5087–5093.

Nowell, P.C. and Hungerford, D.A. (1960). A minute chromosome in human granulocytic leukemia. Science, 132, 1497–1499.

Overduin, M., Rios, C.B., Mayer, B.J., Baltimore, D. and Cowburn, D. (1992). Three-dimensional solution structure of the src homology 2 domain of c-abl. Cell, 70, 697–704.

Pendergast, A.M., Traugh, J.A. and Witte, O.N. (1987). Normal cellular and transformation-associated abl proteins share common sites for protein kinase C phosphorylation. Mol. Cell. Biol., 7, 4280–4289.

Pendergast, A.M., Muller, A.J., Havlik, M.M., Maru, Y. and Witte, O.N. (1991a). BCR sequences essential for transformation by the *BCR–ABL* oncogene bind to the ABL SH2 regulatory domain in a non-phosphotyrosine-dependent manner. Cell, 66, 161–171.

Pendergast, A.M., Muller, A.J., Havlik, M.H., Clark, R., McCormick, F. and Witte, O.N. (1991b). Evidence for regulation of the human ABL tyrosine kinase by a cellular inhibitor. Proc. Natl Acad. Sci. USA, 88, 5927–5931.

Perego, R., Ron, D. and Kruh, G.D. (1991). *Arg* encodes a widely expressed 145 kDa protein-tyrosine kinase. Oncogene, 6, 1899–1902.

Ponzetto, C. and Wolgemuth, D.J. (1985). Haploid expression of a unique c-*abl* transcript in the mouse male germ line. Mol. Cell. Biol., 5, 1791–1794.

Prywes, R., Foulkes, J.G., Rosenberg, N. and Baltimore, D. (1983). Sequences of A-MuLV protein needed for fibroblast and lymphoid cell transformation. Cell, 34, 569–579.

Reddy, E.P., Dunn, C.Y. and Aaronson, S.A. (1980). Different lymphoid cell targets for transformation by replication-competent Moloney and Rauscher mouse leukemia viruses. Cell, 19, 663–669.

Reddy, E.P., Smith, M.J. and Srinivasan, A. (1983). Nucleotide sequence of Abelson murine leukemia virus genome: Structural similarity of its transforming gene product to other *onc* gene products with tyrosine-specific kinase activity. Proc. Natl Acad. Sci. USA, 80, 3623–3627 and 7372–7373.

Renshaw, M.W., Capozza, A. and Wang, J.Y.J. (1988). Differential expression of type-specific c-abl mRNAs in mouse tissues and cell lines. Mol. Cell. Biol., 8, 4547–4551.

Renshaw, M.W., Kipreos, E.T., Albrecht, M.R. and Wang, J.Y.J. (1992). Oncogenic v-abl tyrosine kinase can inhibit or stimulate growth, depending on the cell context. EMBO J., 11, 3941–3951.

Romero, P., Beran, M., Shtalrid, M., Andersson, B., Talpaz, M. and Blick, M. (1989). Alternative 5′ end of the *bcr–abl* transcript in chronic myelogenous leukemia. Oncogene, 4, 93–98.

Ron, D., Zannini, M., Lewis, M., Wickner, R.B., Hunt, L.T., Graziani, G., Tronick, S.R., Aaronson, S.A. and Eva, A. (1991). A region of proto-*dbl* essential for its transforming activity shows sequence similarity to a yeast cell cycle gene, CDC24, and the human breakpoint cluster gene, *bcr*. New Biologist, 3, 372–379.

Rosenbaum, H., Harris, A.W., Bath, M.L., McNeall, J., Webb, E., Adams, J.M. and Cory, S. (1992). An Eμ-v-*abl* transgene elicits plasmacytomas in concert with an activated *myc* gene. EMBO J., 9, 897–905.

Rosenberg, N. and Witte, O. (1980). Abelson murine leukemia virus mutants with alterations in the Ab-MuLV-specific p120 molecule. J. Virol., 33, 340–348.

Rosenberg, N., Baltimore, D. and Scher, C.D. (1975). *In vitro* transformation of lymphoid cells by Abelson murine leukemia virus. Proc. Natl Acad. Sci. USA, 72, 1932–1936.

Rosenberg, N., Clark, D.R. and Witte, O. (1980). Abelson murine leukemia virus mutants deficient in kinase activity and lymphoid cell transformation. J. Virol., 36, 766–774.

Rovera, G., Valtieri, M., Mavilio, F. and Reddy, E.P. (1987). Effect of Abelson murine leukemia virus on granulocyte differentiation and IL3 dependence of a murine progenitor cell line. Oncogene, 1, 29–35.

Rowley, J.D. (1982). Identification of the constant chromosome regions involved in human hematologic malignant disease. Science, 216, 749–751.

Sawyers, C.L., Callahan, W. and Witte, O.N. (1992). Dominant negative MYC blocks transformation by *ABL* oncogenes. Cell, 70, 901–910.

Scher, C.D. and Siegler, R. (1975). Direct transformation of 3T3 cells by Abelson murine leukemia virus. Nature, 253, 729–731.

Schwartzberg, P.L., Stall, A.M., Hardin, J.D., Bowdish, K.S., Humaran, T., Boast, S., Harbison, M.L., Robertson, E.J. and Goff, S.P. (1991). Mice homozygous for the *abl*[m1] mutation show poor viability and depletion of selected B and T cell populations. Cell, 65, 1165–1175.

Shah, N.P., Witte, O.N. and Denny, C.T. (1991). Characterization of the *BCR* promoter in Philadelphia chromosome-positive and -negative cell lines. Mol. Cell. Biol., 11, 1854–1860.

Shore, S.K., Bogart, S.L. and Reddy, E.P. (1990). Activation of murine c-*abl* protooncogene: effect of a point mutation on oncogene activation. Proc. Natl Acad. Sci. USA, 87, 6502–6506.

Shtivelman, E., Lifshitz, B., Gale, R.P., Roe, B.A. and Canaani, E. (1986). Alternative splicing of RNAs transcribed from the human *abl* gene and from the *bcr–abl* fused gene. Cell, 47, 277–284.

Sowerby, S.J., Kennedy, M.A., Fitzgerald, P.H. and Morris, C.M. (1993). DNA sequence analysis of the major breakpoint cluster region of the BCR gene rearranged in Philadelphia-positive human leukemias. Oncogene, 8, 1679–1683.

Szczylik, C., Skorski, T., Nicolaides, N.C., Manzella, L., Malaguarnera, L., Venturelli, D., Gewirtz, A.M. and Calabretta, B. (1991). Selective inhibition of leukemia cell proliferation by BCR–ABL antisense oligodeoxynucleotides. Science, 253, 562–565.

Tybulewicz, V.L.J., Crawford, C.E., Jackson, P.K., Bronson, R.T. and Mulligan, R.C. (1991). Neonatal lethality and lymphopenia in mice with a homozygous disruption of the c-*abl* proto-oncogene. Cell, 65, 1153–1163.

Van Etten, R.A., Jackson, P. and Baltimore, D. (1989). The mouse type IV c-*abl* gene product is a nuclear protein, and activation of transforming ability is associated with cytoplasmic localization. Cell, 58, 669–678.

Varticovski, L., Daley, G.Q., Jackson, P., Baltimore, D. and Cantley, L.C. (1991). Activation of phosphatidylinositol 3-kinase in cells expressing *abl* oncogene variants. Mol. Cell. Biol., 11, 1107–1113.

Wang, J.Y.J., Ledley, F., Goff, S., Lee, R., Groner, Y. and Baltimore D. (1984). The mouse c-*abl* locus: Molecular cloning and characterization. Cell 36, 349–356.

Weissinger, E.M., Mischak, H., Goodnight, J., Davidson, W.F. and Mushinski, J.F. (1993). Addition of constitutive c-*myc* expression to Abelson murine leukemia virus changes the phenotype of the cells transformed by the virus from pre-B-cell lymphomas to plasmacytomas. Mol. Cell. Biol., 13, 2578–2585.

Witte, O.N., Goff, S., Rosenberg, N. and Baltimore, D. (1980). A transformation defective mutant of Abelson murine leukemia lacks protein kinase activity. Proc. Natl Acad. Sci. USA, 77, 4993–4997.

Zhu, Q.S., Heisterkamp. N. and Groffen, J. (1990). Characterization of the human ABL promoter regions. Oncogene, 5, 885–891.

Zhu, G., Decker, S.J., Mayer, B.J. and Saltiel, A.R. (1993). Direct analysis of the binding of the *abl* Src homology 2 domain to the activated epidermal growth factor receptor. J. Biol. Chem., 268, 1775–1779.

BCL1, BCL2 and BCL3

BCL1 (*B cell leukaemia/lymphoma-1*) was detected with a probe specific for chromosome 11 in DNA isolated from a chronic lymphocytic leukaemia (CLL) cell line (Tsujimoto *et al.*, 1984). *BCL2* was detected with a probe specific for chromosome 18 in DNA isolated from an acute lymphocytic leukaemia cell line of the pre-B cell type (Tsujimoto *et al.*, 1984). *BCL3* was detected by molecular cloning of the breakpoint junction of the 14;19 translocation (Ohno *et al.*, 1990).

Related genes

BCL1

Identical to human cyclin D1 (Xiong *et al.*, 1991) and related to other cyclins. The murine homologue is *Cyl-1* (see Tables 2.5 and Supplement; Matsushime *et al.*, 1991).

BCL2

Weak homology to Epstein–Barr virus protein BHRF1 (Cleary *et al.*, 1986; Lee and Yates, 1992, see **DNA Tumour Viruses: EBV**) and *Caenorhabditis elegans ced-9* (Hengartner *et al.*, 1992).

BCL3

The seven ankyrin repeat regions (Lux *et al.*, 1990) are homologous to those in the human immediate early response gene *MAD3* (Haskill *et al.*, 1991), the β subunit of the heteromeric DNA binding protein GABP (Thompson *et al.*, 1991), *TAN1* (Ellisen *et al.*, 1991), *LYT10* (Neri *et al.*, 1991), *notch* (*D. melanogaster*), *Xotch* (*Xenopus laevis*), *Lin-12* and *Glp-1* (*Caenorhabditis elegans*), SW14/SW16 (*Saccharomyces cerevisiae*), *cdc*10 (*S. pombe*). *BCL3* is related to human I-κBα (37 kDa) and is a member of the I-κB family (Kerr *et al.*, 1992).

Cross-species homology

BCL1: Highly conserved in humans, mice, rats, pigs, cows. BCL2: Domain II (human residues 34–85) 64% identical (mouse and human); 26% identical (human and chicken). Other regions of the protein between 77% and 100% identical (human, mouse and chicken). BCL3: Protein and nucleic acid sequences 80% homologous (humans and mice).

Transformation

BCL1

The t(11;14)(q13;q32) translocation, in which *BCL1* on chromosome 11 translocates to become juxtaposed to J_H on chromosome 14, occurs in several B cell malignancies (diffuse, small and large cell lymphomas), B cell chronic lymphocytic leukaemia (CLL) and multiple myeloma.

points map ~110 kb 5' (centromeric) to the BCL1 gene. BCL1 is also overexpressed
nes carrying the t(11;14)(q13;q32) translocation (Seto et al., 1992).
part of an 11q13 region that includes CYCD1 (PRAD1, ~150 kb telomeric to BCL1)
2 and HSTF1 that is amplified in 15–20% of human breast and squamous cell carci-
Theillet et al., 1990) and in bladder tumours (Proctor et al., 1991). In breast tumours,
howe, r, BCL1 expression is not invariably associated with that of INT2 and HSTF1 (Faust and
Meeker, 1992). BCL1 is overexpressed in a rare form of benign parathyroid tumour (Motokura
et al., 1991).

In some human breast cancer cell lines there is evidence that BCL1 (cyclin D1) and other
cyclin genes are either overexpressed or encode transcripts with enhanced stability relative to
that observed in normal cells (Keyomarsi and Pardee, 1993) and differential expression of cyclins
D1 and D2 has been detected in B lymphoid cell lines (Palmero et al., 1993).

BCL2

The chromosomal translocation t(14;18)(q32;q21) is a specific abnormality of human lymphoid
neoplasms that occurs in >85% of follicular small cleaved B cell lymphomas and ~20% of
diffuse lymphomas (Tanaka et al., 1992). The major breakpoint region (mbr) on chromosome
18, involved in 60% of these cases, is within the 3' untranslated part of BCL2 -exon 3 (Limpens
et al., 1991). The minor cluster region (mcr) [40%] is ~20 kb downstream of BCL2. Additional
breakpoints occur at the 5' and 3' ends of BCL2 (Weiss et al., 1987). These translocations place
the BCL2 gene in the Ig heavy chain locus (chromosome 14) and create a BCL2–Ig fusion gene.
However, although the neoplastic germinal centres in most follicular lymphomas express high
levels of BCL2 protein whereas normal germinal centres do not, BCL2 is also present in normal
T and B cells and in hairy cell leukaemias and Ki-1 lymphomas that do not involve the 14;18
translocation (Pezzella et al., 1990, 1992).

In ~10% of chronic lymphocytic leukaemia (CLL) cases BCL2 is translocated to the Igκ or Igλ
light chain gene. Translocations may juxtapose the genes head-to-head (t(18;22)(q21;q11)) or
head-to-tail (t(2;18)(p11;q21); Tashiro et al., 1992).

High expression of BCL2 occurs in some human neuroblastoma cell lines and lower levels of
the protein occur in a variety of other neural crest-derived tumours and tumour cell lines,
including some neuroepitheliomas, Ewing's sarcomas, neurofibromas and melanomas (Reed et
al., 1991).

BCL2 expressed from a retroviral vector does not morphologically transform NIH 3T3 cells,
render FDCP-1 cells tumorigenic or immortalize normal bone marrow cells, but does immortalize pre-B cells from Eμ-Myc transgenic mice, some of which become tumorigenic. In addition,
whilst not abolishing the growth factor requirements of some established haematopoietic cell
lines, it promotes their extended survival in G_o in the absence of growth factors (Vaux et al.,
1988). BCL2 also blocks MYC-induced apoptosis (Fanidi et al., 1992). Mice transgenic for a
BCL2–Ig fusion gene show an expansion of the lymphoid compartment predominantly caused
by an increase in B220+, IgM/IgD+ B cells. Mature B cells from these mice show a survival
advantage in vitro (McDonnell et al., 1989). Mice doubly transgenic for BCL2 and Myc under
the control of the Ig_H enhancer show hyperproliferation of pre-B and B cells and develop tumours
which appear at earlier times than in Eμ-Myc mice and display the phenotype of primitive
haematopoietic cells (Strasser et al., 1990). Thus, by extending cell survival, BCL2 may increase
the chance of secondary genetic changes responsible for tumorigenicity.

BCL3

The (14;19)(q32;q13.1) translocation occurs in some cases of B cell chronic lymphocytic leukaemia (B-CLL): BCL3 is adjacent to the breakpoints involved. Rearrangement of a gene desig-

nated *BCL3* and *BCL5* (17q22) has been reported in prolymphocytic leukaemia (Gauwerky *et al.*, 1989) but this gene is unrelated to the chromosome 19 B-CLL-associated gene.

	BCL1/Bcl-1	*BCL2/Bcl-2*	*BCL3/Bcl-3*
Nucleotides (kb)		>370	~10–11
Chromosome			
Human	11q13	18q21	19q13.1
Mouse		1	7
Exons			
Human		3	>7
Mouse		2	
mRNA (kb)			
Human	4.4/1.5 (major) (4.2 minor) (differential polyadenylation)	3.5, 5.5 and 8.5 (3.5 alternatively spliced) Half-life short (~2.5 h) when transcribed from the normal or translocated gene (Seto *et al.*, 1988)	2.1–2.3
Mouse	3.8/4.5 (major) 6.0 (minor)	2.4/7.5	1.8
Amino acids			
Human	295	239 (BCL2α)/205 (BCL2β) (overlapping reading frames: only C-termini differ)	446
Mouse	295	236 (mBCL2α)/199 (mBCL2β)	
Chicken		233	
Mass (kDa)			
(predicted)	33.4	26 (BCL2α)/22 (BCL2β)	46.8
(expressed)	34	28/30	
pI	4.9	(BCL2α, alternative AUGs)	9.4 (predicted)

Cellular location

BCL1: Cytoplasmic.
BCL2α: Inner mitochondrial membrane.
BCL2β: Cytoplasmic (Tanaka *et al.*, 1993).
BCL3: Nuclear.

Tissue location

Bcl-1: This is expressed in many cells, including proliferating macrophages, but not in cells of other lymphoid or myeloid lineages. In mouse macrophages expression is induced by CSF1. Transcription varies during the cell cycle, being maximal in G_1 (Matsushime *et al.*, 1991).

Bcl-2: This is generally expressed in tissues characterized by apoptotic cell turnover and restricted to long-lived progenitor cells and select post-mitotic cells that have an extended lifespan (Villuendas *et al.*, 1991). It is restricted within germinal centres to the follicular mantle and to portions of the light zone implicated in the selection and maintenance of plasma cells and memory B cells. *Bcl-2* is expressed in surviving T cells in the thymic medulla and in proliferating precursors, but not in post-mitotic maturation stages, of all haematopoietic lineages. It is also expressed in glandular epithelium under hormonal or growth factor control, in complex differentiating epithelium characterized by long-lived stem cells and in some neurons (Hockenbery *et al.*, 1991). It is expressed in normal and malignant plasma cells from myeloma patients (Hamilton *et al.*, 1991; Pettersson *et al.*, 1992) and in a number of human lymphoid and myeloid cell lines and tissues (Delia *et al.*, 1992; Haury *et al.*, 1993). The human *BCL2* 5′ untranslated region contains a unique negative regulatory element (NRE), the activity of which may vary during B cell development (Young and Korsmeyer, 1993).

Mouse *Bcl-2* is expressed in all newborn tissues but in the adult is detectable at high levels only in the thymus and spleen (Negrini *et al.*, 1987).

Chicken *Bcl-2* is highly expressed in the thymus and widely expressed in other tissues in both the embryo and adult (Eguchi *et al.*, 1992).

Bcl-3: B lymphocytes. In mouse tumours it is present in follicular centre mature B cells and large pre-B cells but not in small pre-B cells (Bhatia *et al.*, 1991).

Protein function

BCL1

Unknown. Binds to and activates p34^{cdc2} kinase. It is phosphorylated in G_1. In human lung fibroblasts D type cyclins associate with many other proteins, including the proliferating cell nuclear antigen (PCNA; Xiong *et al.*, 1992).

BCL2

Overexpression of BCL2 inhibits apoptosis induced by deprivation of growth factors (Korsmeyer, 1992; Garcia *et al.*, 1992). Thus, overexpression of BCL2 blocks the apoptotic death of IL-3- or IL-7-dependent, pre-B lymphocyte cell lines (Hockenbery *et al.*, 1990; Borzillo *et al.*, 1992) and of sympathetic neurons deprived of nerve growth factor (Garcia *et al.*, 1992). The expression of high levels of BCL2 also blocks glucocorticoid-induced apoptosis of pre-B lymphocytes by a mechanism that requires the concurrent repression of *MYC* (Alnemri *et al.*, 1992a; see **MYC**). In fibroblasts in which the overexpression of MYC is induced, the apoptotic cell death that would normally occur is prevented by the co-expression of BCL2 (Bissonnette *et al.*, 1992; Fanidi *et al.*, 1992). Thus the proto-oncogenes *Myc* and *Bcl-2* can cooperate to prevent apoptosis and cause continuous cell proliferation in the absence of mitogens, although the cells do not appear to be transformed. However, although stable expression of BCL2 renders WEHI-231 B cells more resistant to cell death induced by heat shock, it does not prevent IgM receptor-mediated cell death, indicating that other proteins may be involved in apoptosis (Cuende *et al.*, 1993).

In transgenic mice that overexpress *Bcl-2*, the lifetime of immunoglobulin-secreting cells and memory B cells is extended and the proportion of CD4⁻8⁺ thymocytes is increased (Nunez *et al.*, 1990; Sentman *et al.*, 1991). The response to immunization is enhanced, consistent with reduced death of activated T cells (Strasser *et al.*, 1991), and the overproduction of BCL2 substantially alters the V_H gene repertoire in B cells (Yeh *et al.*, 1991). *Bcl-2* transgenic mice have also been derived in which T cell survival is prolonged (Katsumata *et al.*, 1992). Thus *Bcl-2* sustains immune responsiveness.

Expression of full-length human BCL2 in baculovirus-infected insect cells prevents cell death by inhibiting virally induced DNA damage (Alnemri *et al.*, 1992b) and prevents lytic infection by Sindbis virus giving rise to persistent productive infection (Levine *et al.*, 1993).

BCL2 may be functionally equivalent to the product of the Epstein–Barr virus early gene BHRF1 (see **DNA Tumour Viruses, EBV**).

BCL3

Probable transcription factor. Phosphorylated BCL3 (Nolan *et al.*, 1993) functions as a form of I-κB specific for the p50 subunit of NF-κB (see **REL**), inhibiting its translocation to the nucleus and binding to DNA (Hatada *et al.*, 1992; Naumann *et al.*, 1993) and increasing κB-dependent *trans* activation in intact cells by acting as an anti-repressor of inhibitory p50–NF-κB homodimers (Franzoso *et al.*, 1992). BCL3 does not inhibit the DNA binding activity of REL protein or its ability to *trans*-activate genes linked to a κB motif (Kerr *et al.*, 1992). However, BCL3 also associates tightly with homodimers of p50B, a protein closely related to p50 (Bours *et al.*, 1993). Formation of the BCL3–p50 ternary complex permits BCL3 directly to *trans*-activate transcription via κB sites.

mRNA expression increases sevenfold in normal human T cells between 15 min and 8 h after stimulation by PHA (Ohno *et al.*, 1990). Mouse *Bcl-3* is abundantly expressed in B cell lines just prior to the Ig switch, which event may promote the recombination that occurs between *Bcl-3* and Ig$_H$ in B-CLL-associated chromosomal translocations.

Protein structure

BCL1: Cyclin D1. ~33% identical to human cyclin A.

BCL2: Lacks a signal sequence but has a C-terminal hydrophobic region (19 amino acids in human BCL2) (Chen-Levy *et al.*, 1989).

BCL3: The N-terminal region is proline-rich and the C-terminal region serine- and proline-rich. The central domain (120–359) contains seven tandem ankyrin repeats (33–37 amino acids each) (see **Related genes**, above).

Sequence of human BCL1

```
  (1)  MEHQLLCCEVETIRRAYPDANLLNDRVLRAMLKAEETCAPSVSYFKCVQKEVLPSMRKI
 (60)  VATWMLEVCEEQKCEEEVFPLAMNYLDRFLSLEPVKKSRLQLLGATCMFVASKMKETIP
(119)  LTAEKLCIYTDNSIRPEELLQMELLLVNKLKWNLAAMTPHDFIEHFLSKMPEAEENKQI
(178)  IRKHAQTFVALCATDVKFISNPPSMVAAGSVVAAVQGLNLRSPNNFLSYYRLTRFLSRV
(237)  IKCDPDCLRACQEQIEALLESSLRQAQQNMDPKAAEEEEEEEEEVDLACTPTDVRDVDI(295)
```

Sequence comparison of BCL1 with four A-type cyclins

```
1.  [55]   MRKIVATWMLEVCEEQKCEEEVFPLAMNYLDRFLSLEPVKKSRLQLLGATCMFVA
2.  [209]  --A-LVD-LV--G--Y-LQN-TLH--V--I-----SMS-LRGK---V-TAA-LL-
3.  [195]  --T-LVD-LV--G--Y-LHT-TLY----------CMS-LRGK---V-TAAILL-
4.  [194]  --C-LVD-LV--S--D-LHR-TLF-GV--I-----KIS-LRGK---V--AS--L-
5.  [234]  --S-LID-LV--S--Y-LDT-TLY-SVF------QMA-VR-K---V-TAA-YI-
```

```
1.          SKMKETIPLTAEKLCIYTDNSIRPEELLQMELLLVNKLKWNLAAMTPHDFIEHFL  [130]
2.          --FE-IY-PEVAEFVYI--DTYTKKQV-R--H-VLKV-TFD---P-VNQ-LTQYF  [113]
3.          --YE-IY-PDVDEFVYI--DTYSKKQ--R--HV-LKV-AFD-TVP-VNQ-LLQY-  [113]
4.          A-YE-IY-PEVGEFVFL--D-YTKAQV-R--QVILKI-SFD-CTP-AYV--NTYA  [147]
5.          A-YE-IY-PEVGEFVFL--D-YTKAQV-R--QVILKI-SFD-CTP-AYV--NTYA  [147]
```

1. Human BCL1; 2. human cyclin A; 3. *Xenopus laevis* cyclin A; 4. *Spisula solidissima* cyclin A; 5. *Drosophila melanogaster* cyclin A. Dashes indicate identical residues. Numbers in brackets refer to the number of amino acids preceding and following each sequence shown.

Sequences of human, mouse and chicken BCL2α and BCL2β

```
Human BCL2α     (1)    MAHAGRTGYDNREIVMKYIHYKLSQRGYEWDAG DVGAAPPGAAPAPGIFSSQPGHTPHP
Mouse BCL2α     (1)    --Q----------------------------- -AD---L----T-----F--ESN-M-
Chicken BCL2α   (1)    ---P--R--------L------------D-A--E-RPPV--AP---AA     PAAVA

Human BCL2α    (60)    AASRDPVARTSPLQTPAAPGAAAGPALSPVPPVVHLTLRQAGDDFSRRYRRDFAEMSSQL
Mouse BCL2α    (60)    -VHREMA------RPLV-    T---------C---T--R------------------
Chicken BCL2α  (54)    --GASSHH-PE-PGSA--SEVPPAEG-R-A--GVHLA------E-----Q----Q--G--

Human BCL2α   (120)    HLTPFTARGRFATVVEELFRDGVNWGRIVAFFEFGGVMCVESVNREMSPLVDNIALWMTE
Mouse BCL2α   (117)    ---------------------------------------------------------
Chicken BCL2α (114)    -------H---VA--------------------------------------------T----

Human BCL2α   (180)    YLNRHLHTWIQDNGGWDAFVELYGPSMRPLFDFSWLSLKTLLSLALVGACITLGAYLGHK  (239)
Mouse BCL2α   (177)    ------------------------------------------PWV-------------  (236)
Chicken BCL2α (174)    -------N--------------N----------I----I---V--------------  (233)

Human BCL2β   (180)    ---------------VGASGDVSLG (205)
Mouse BCL2β   (177)    ---------------VGACLVE (199)
Chicken BCL2β (174)    -------N--------VRACASLSSTGGWLVGFAVTSVGGRKV (216)
```

Dashes indicate identity with human BCL2α. In human and mouse, BCL2α and BCL2β are identical up to amino acid 195 and BCL2β sequences are only shown from residue 180. The sequence shown is that of Tsujimoto and Croce (1986). The following positions differ in Cleary *et al.* (1986): 96 = T, 110 = R, 117 = R, 237 = G. Underlined: domain II (human residues 34–85) that is 64% conserved between mouse and human BCL2 but poorly conserved in the chicken protein.

Sequence of human BCL3

```
BCL3          (1)    MDEGPVDLRTRPKAAGLPGAALPLRKRPLRAPSPEPAAPRGAAGLVVPLDPLRGGCDLP
BCL3         (60)    AVPGPPHGLARPEALYYPGALLPLYPTRAMGSPFPLVNLPTPLYPMMCPMEHPLSADIAM
                            ⟶ 1                           1 ⟷ 2
p105        (537)    AVQ--N--SV--L-IIHLHSQL-RD-LEVTSGLISDDIINMR-D-Y----------KQE
BCL3        (120)    ATRADEDGDTPLHIAVVQGNLPAVHRLVNLFQQGGREL    DIYNNLRQTPLHLAVITTLP
MAD-3/IkB    (68)    QQLT----SF--L-IIHEEKALTMEVIRQVKGDLAF-    NFQ---Q----------NQ-
                            2 ⟶ 3                           3 ⟷ 4
p105        (596)    D--ED-LR---DLSL---L-NSVL---AKEGHDKV-SI--KHKKAAL-L    DHPNG---
BCL3        (178)    SVVRLLVTAGASPMALDRHGQTAAHLACEHRSPTCLRALLDSAAPGTLDL    EARNYDGL
MAD-3/IkB   (125)    EIAEA-LG--CD-ELR-FR-N-PL-----QGCLASVGV-TQ-CTTPH-HSILK-T--N-H
```

```
p105      (654)  N-I-L-MMSNSLPCLL--VAA---VN-QEQ----TA-HL---HDNI-LAGC--LE-DAHV
BCL3      (236)  TALHVAVNTECQETVQLLLERGADIDAVDIKSGRSPLIHAVENNSLSMVQLLLQHGANV
MAD-3/IkB (185)  -C--L-SIHGYLGI-E--VSL---VN-QEPCN--TA-HL--DLQNPDL-S---KC--D-

p105      (713)  DSTT-D-TTP-DI-A---STR-AAL-KAA---PLVE   NFEPLYDLDDSWENAGEDE
BCL3      (295)  NAQMYSGSSALHSASGRGLLPLVRTLVRSGADS
MAD-3/IkB (244)  -RVT-Q-Y-PYQLTW--PSTRIQQQ-GQLTLENLQMLPESEDEESYDTESEFTEFTEDE

p105      (766)   GVVPGT---DM-T-WQ-F---N--PYE-EF--DDLL
BCL3      (328)  SLKNCHNDTPLMVARSRRVIDILRGKATRPASTSQPDPSPDRSANTSPESSSRLSSNGLL

BCL3      (388)  SASPSSSPSQSPPRDPPGFPMAPPNFFLPSPSPPAFLPFAGVLRGPGRPVPPSPAPGGS (446)

Ankyrin          N-----GψTPLHψAA--GH---V--LL--GA--
                 D
Consensus        N--GφTPLHψA--------V--LL--GA--
                 D     SA
```

Numbered arrows indicate the seven ankyrin repeats. The alignment of these conserved regions is shown for p105 (the NF-κB precursor) and MAD3/I-κB: Dashes indicate identity with BCL3. Italics: acidic region absent in BCL3. ψ Hydrophobic residue, φ = hydrophilic residue. Consensus refers to the BCL3, p105, MAD3 consensus.

Databank file names and accession numbers

	GENE	EMBL	SWISSPROT	REFERENCES
Human	BCL1	Hsbcl1 M73554	CG1D_HUMAN P24385	Withers et al., 1991
		Hsprad1cy X59789; X59485		
Mouse	Bcl-1	Mdcyl1 M64403	CG1D_MOUSE P25322	Matsushime et al., 1991
Human	BLC2α	Hsbcl2a M13994	BCA2A_HUMAN P10415	Tsujimoto and Croce, 1986
		Hsbcl2c M14745		Cleary et al., 1986
Human	BCL2β	Hsbcl2b M13995	BC2B_HUMAN P10416	Tsujimoto and Croce, 1986
Mouse	Bcl-2α	Mmbcl2 M16506	BC2A_MOUSE P10417	Negrini et al., 1987
Mouse	Bcl-2β	Mmbcl2 M16506	BC2B_MOUSE P10418	Negrini et al., 1987
Chicken	Bcl-2	Ggbcl1 D11381, Ggbcl2 D11382		Eguchi et al., 1992
Human	BLC3	Hsbclaa M31731	BCL3_HUMAN P20749	Ohno et al., 1990
		Hsbcl3aa M31732		
Mouse	Bcl-3	MmbclIII M90397		Bhatia et al., 1991

Review

Korsmeyer, S.J. (1992). *Bcl-2* initiates a new category of oncogene: regulators of cell death. Blood, 80, 879–886.

Papers

Alnemri, E.S., Fernandes, T.F., Haldar, S., Croce, C.M. and Litwack, G. (1992a). Involvement of BCL2 in glucocorticoid-induced apoptosis of human pre-B-leukemias. Cancer Res., 52, 491–495.

Alnemri, E.S., Robertson, N.M., Fernandes, T.F., Croce, C.M. and Litwack, G. (1992b). Overexpressed full-length human BCL2 extends the survival of baculovirus-infected Sf9 insect cells. Proc. Natl Acad. Sci. USA, 89, 7295–7299.

Bhatia, K., Huppi, K., McKeithan, T., Siwarski, D., Mushinski, J.F. and Magrath, I. (1991). Mouse BCL3: cDNA structure, mapping and stage-dependent expression in B lymphocytes. Oncogene, 6, 1569–1573.

Bissonnette, R.P., Echeverri, F., Mahboubi, A. and Green, D.R. (1992). Apoptotic cell death induced by c-*myc* is inhibited by *BCL2*. Nature, 359, 552–554.

Borzillo, G.V., Endo, K. and Tsujimoto, Y. (1992). *BCL2* confers growth and survival advantage to interleukin 7-dependent early pre-B cells which become factor independent by a multistep process in culture. Oncogene, 7, 869–876.

Bours, V., Franzoso, G., Azarenko, V., Park, S., Kanno, T., Brown, K. and Siebenlist, U. (1993). The oncoprotein Bcl-3 directly transactivates through κB motifs via association with DNA-binding p50B homodimers. Cell, 72, 729–739.

Chen-Levy, Z., Nourse, J. and Cleary, M.L. (1989). The *BCL2* candidate proto-oncogene product is a 24-kilodalton integral membrane protein highly expressed in lymphoid cell lines and lymphomas carrying the t(14;18) translocation. Mol. Cell. Biol., 9, 701–710.

Cleary, M.L., Smith, S.D. and Sklar, J. (1986). Cloning and structural analysis of cDNAs for *BCL2* and a hybrid *BCL2*/immunoglobulin transcript resulting from the t(14;18) translocation. Cell, 47, 19–28.

Cuende, E., Ales-Martinez, J.E., Ding, L., Gonzales-Garcia, M., Martinez-A.C. and Nunez, G. (1993). Programmed cell death by *bcl-2*-dependent and independent mechanisms in B lymphoma cells. EMBO J., 12, 1555–1560.

Delia, D., Aiello, A., Soligo, D., Fontanella, E., Melani, C., Pezzella, F., Pierotti, M.A. and Della-Porta, G. (1992). *BCL2* proto-oncogene expression in normal and neoplastic human myeloid cells. Blood, 79, 1291–1298.

Eguchi, Y., Ewert, D.L. and Tsujimoto, Y. (1992). Isolation and characterization of the chicken *BCL2* gene: expression in a variety of tissues including lymphoid and neuronal organs in adult and embryo. Nuc. Acids Res., 20, 4187–4192.

Ellisen, L.W., Bird, J., West, D.C., Soreng, A.L., Reynolds, T.C., Smith, S.D. and Sklar, J. (1991). *TAN-1*, the human homolog of the Drosophila *Notch* gene, is broken by chromosomal translocations in T lymphoblastic neoplasms. Cell, 66, 649–661.

Fanidi, A., Harrington, E.A. and Evan, G.I. (1992). Cooperative interaction between c-*myc* and *BCL2* proto-oncogenes. Nature, 359, 554–556.

Faust, J.B. and Meeker, T.C. (1992). Amplification and expression of the *BCL1* gene in human solid tumor cell lines. Cancer Res., 52, 2460–2463.

Franzoso, G., Bours, V., Park, S., Tomita-Yamaguchi, M., Kelly, K. and Siebenlist, U. (1992). The candidate oncoprotein BCL3 is an antagonist of p50/NF-κB-mediated inhibition. Nature, 359, 339–342.

Garcia, I., Martinou, I., Tsujimoto, Y. and Martinou, J.-C. (1992). Prevention of programmed cell death of synpathetic neurons by the *BCL2* proto-oncogene. Science, 258, 302–304.

Gauwerky, C.E., Huebner, K., Isobe, M., Nowell, P.C. and Croce, C.M. (1989). Activation of MYC in a masked t(8;17) translocation results in an aggressive B-cell leukemia. Proc. Natl Acad. Sci. USA, 86, 8867–8871.

Hamilton, M.S., Barker, H.F., Ball, J., Drew, M., Abbot, S.D. and Franklin, I.M. (1991). Normal and neoplastic human plasma cells express *BCL2* antigen. Leukemia, 5, 768–771.

Haskill, S., Beg, A.A., Tompkins, S.M., Morris, J.S., Yurochko, A.D., Sampson-Johannes, A., Mondal, K., Ralph, P. and Baldwin, A.S. (1991). Characterization of an immediate-early gene induced in adherent monocytes that encodes Iκ-B-like activity. Cell, 65, 1281–1289.

Hatada, E.N., Nieters, A., Wulczyn, F.G., Naumann, M., Meyer, R., Nucifora, G., McKeithan, T.W. and Scheidereit, C. (1992). The ankyrin repeat domains of the NF-κB precursor p105 and the protooncogene *BCL3* act as specific inhibitors of NF-κB DNA binding. Proc. Natl Acad. Sci. USA, 89, 2489–2493.

Haury, M., Freitas, A., Hermitte, V., Coutinho, A. and Hibner, U. (1993). The physiology of *bcl-2* expression in murine B lymphocytes. Oncogene, 8, 1257–1262.

Hengartner, M.O., Ellis, R.E. and Howvitz, H.R. (1992). *Caenorhabditis elegans* gene *ced-9* protects cells from programmed cell death. Nature, 356, 494–499.

Hockenbery, D., Nunez, G., Milliman, C., Schreiber, R.D. and Korsmeyer, S.J. (1990). BCL2 is an inner mitochondrial membrane protein that blocks programmed cell death. Nature, 348, 334–336.

Hockenbery, D.M., Zutter, M., Hickey, W., Nahm, M. and Korsmeyer, S.J. (1991). BCL2 protein is topographically restricted in tissues characterized by apoptotic cell death. Proc. Natl Acad. Sci. USA, 88, 6961–6965.

Katsumata, M., Siegel, R.M., Louie, D.C., Miyashita, T., Tsujimoto, Y., Nowell, P.C., Greene, M.I. and Reed, J.C. (1992). Differential effects of BCL2 on T and B cells in transgenic mice. Proc. Natl Acad. Sci. USA, 89, 11376–11380.

Kerr, L.D., Duckett, C.S., Wamsley, P., Zhang, Q., Chiao, P., Nabel, G., McKeithanm, T.W., Baeurle, P.A. and Verma, I.M. (1992). The proto-oncogene *BCL3* encodes an IκB protein. Genes & Develop., 6, 2352–2363.

Keyomarsi, K. and Pardee, A.B. (1993). Redundant cyclin overexpression and gene amplification in breast cancer cells. Proc. Natl Acad. Sci. USA, 90, 1112–1116.

Lee, M.A. and Yates, J.L. (1992). BHRF1 of Epstein-Barr virus, which is homologous to human proto-oncogene *bcl*2, is not essential for transformation of B cells or for virus replication *in vitro*. J. Virol., 66, 1899–1906.

Levine, B., Huang, Q., Isaacs, J.T., Reed, J.C., Griffin, D.E. and Hardwick, J.M. (1993). Conversion of lytic to persistent alphavirus infection by the *bcl*-2 cellular oncogene. Nature, 361, 739–742.

Limpens, J., de Jong, D, van Krieken, J.H., Price, C.G., Young, B.D., van Ommen, G.J. and Kluin, P.M. (1991). BCL2/JH rearrangements in benign lymphoid tissues with follicular hyperplasia. Oncogene, 6, 2271–2276.

Lux, S.E., John, K.M. and Bennett, V. (1990). Analysis of cDNA for human erythrocyte ankyrin indicates a repeated structure with homology to tissue-differentiation and cell-cycle control proteins. Nature, 344, 36–42.

McDonnell, T.J., Deane, N., Platt, F.M., Nunez, G., Jaeger, U., McKearn, J.P. and Korsmeyer, S.J. (1989). *bcl-2*-immunoglobulin transgenic mice demonstrate extended B cell survival and follicular lympho-proliferation. Cell, 57, 79–88.

Matsushime, H., Roussel, M.F., Ashmun, R.A. and Sherr, C.J. (1991). Colony-stimulating factor 1 regulates novel cyclins during the G1 phase of the cell cycle. Cell, 65, 701–713.

Motokura, T., Bloom, T., Kim, H.G., Juppner, H., Ruderman, J.V., Kronenberg, H.M. and Arnold, A. (1991). A novel cyclin encoded by a *bcl*1-linked candidate oncogene. Nature, 350, 512–515.

Naumann, M., Wulczyn, F.G. and Scheidereit, C. (1993). The NF-κB precursor p105 and the proto-oncogene product bcl-3 are IκB molecules and control nuclear translocation of NF-κB. EMBO J., 12, 213–222.

Negrini, M., Silini, E., Kozak, C., Tsujimoto, Y. and Croce, C.M. (1987). Molecular analysis of *mBCL2*: structure and expression of the murine gene homologous to the human gene involved in follicular lymphoma. Cell, 49, 455–463.

Neri, A., Chang, C.-C., Lombardi, L., Salina, M., Corradini, P., Maiolo, A.T., Chaganti, R.S.K. and Dalla-Favera, R. (1991). B cell lymphoma-associated chromosomal translocation involves candidate oncogene *lyt*-10, homologous to NF-κBp50. Cell, 67, 1075–1087.

Nolan, G.P., Fujita, T., Bhatia, K., Huppi, C., Liou, H.-C., Scott, M.L. and Baltimore, D. (1993). The *bcl-3* proto-oncogene encodes a nuclear IκB-like molecule that preferentially interacts with NF-κB p50 and p52 in a phosphorylation-dependent manner. Mol. Cell. Biol., 13, 3557–3566.

Nunez, G., Hockenbery, D., McDonnell, T.J., Sorensen, C.M. and Korsmeyer, S.J. (1990). BCL2 maintains B cell memory. Nature, 353, 71–73.

Ohno, H., Takimoto, G. and McKeithan, T.W. (1990). The candidate proto-oncogene *BCL3* is related to genes implicated in cell lineage determination and cell cycle control. Cell, 60, 991–997.

Palmero, I., Holder, A., Sinclair, A.J., Dickson, C. and Peters, G. (1993). Cyclins D1 and D2 are differentially expressed in human B-lymphoid cell lines. Oncogene, 8, 1049–1054.

Pettersson, M., Jernberg-Wiklund, H., Larsson, L.G., Sundstrom, C., Givol, I., Tsujimoto, Y. and Nilsson, K. (1992). Expression of the *BCL2* gene in human multiple myeloma cell lines and normal plasma cells. Blood, 79, 495–502.

Pezzella, F., Tse, A.G.P., Cordell, J.L., Pulford, K.A.F., Gatter, K.C. and Mason, D.Y. (1990). Expression of the *BCL2* oncogene protein is not specific for the 14;18 chromosome translocation. Am. J. Pathol., 137, 225–232.

Pezzella, F., Jones, M., Ralfkiaer, E., Ersboll, J., Gatter, K.C. and Mason, D.Y. (1992). Evaluation of *BCL2* protein expression and 14;18 translocation as prognostic markers in follicular lymphoma. Brit. J. Cancer, 65, 87–89.

Proctor, A.J., Coombs, L.M., Cairns, J.P. and Knowles, M.A. (1991). Amplification at chromosome 11q13 in transitional cell tumours of the bladder. Oncogene, 6, 789–795.

Reed, J.C., Meister, L., Tanaka, S., Cuddy, M., Yum, S., Geyer, C. and Pleasure, D. (1991). Differential expression of *bcl2* protooncogene in neuroblastoma and other human tumor cell lines of neural origin. Cancer Res., 51, 6529–6538.

Sentman, C.L., Shutter, J.R., Hockenbery, D., Kanagawa, O. and Korsmeyer, S.J. (1991). *BCL2* inhibits multiple forms of apoptosis but not negative selection in thymocytes. Cell, 67, 879–888.

Seto, M., Jaeger, U., Hockett, R.D., Graninger, W., Bennett, S.B., Goldman, P. and Korsmeyer, S.J. (1988). Alternative promoters and exons, somatic mutation and deragulation of the *BCL2-Ig* fusion gene in lymphoma. EMBO J., 7, 123–131.

Seto, M., Yamamoto, K., Iida, Y., Utsumi, K.R., Kubonishi, I., Miyoshi, I., Ohtsuki, T., Yawata, Y., Namba, M., Motokura, T., Arnold, A., Takahashi, T. and Ueda, R. (1992). Gene rearrangement and over-expression of *PRAD1* in lymphoid malignancy with t(11;14)(q13;q32) translocation. Oncogene, 7, 1401–1406.

Strasser, A., Harris, A.W., Bath, M.L. and Cory, S. (1990). Novel primitive lymphoid tumours induced in transgenic mice by cooperation between *myc* and *bcl-2*. Nature, 348, 331–333.

Strasser, A., Harris, A.W. and Cory, S. (1991). *BCL2* transgene inhibits T cell death and perturbs thymic self-censorship. Cell, 67, 889–899.

Tanaka, S., Louie, D.C., Kant, J.A. and Reed, J.C. (1992). Frequent incidence of somatic mutations in trans-located BCL2 oncogenes of non-Hodgkin's lymphomas. Blood, 79, 229–237.

Tanaka, S., Saito, K. and Reed, J.C. (1993). Structure-function analysis of the Bcl-2 oncoprotein. J. Biol. Chem., 268, 10920–10926.

Tashiro, S., Takechi, M., Asou, H., Takauchi, K., Kyo, T., Dohy, H., Kikuchi, M., Kamada, N. and Tsuji-moto, Y. (1992). Cytogenetic 2;18 and 18;22 translocation in chronic lymphocytic leukemia with juxta-position of *BCL2* and immunoglobulin light chain genes. Oncogene, 7, 573–577.

Theillet, C., Adnane, J., Szepetowski, P., Simon, M.-P., Jeanteur, P., Birnbaum, D. and Gaudray, P. (1990). *BCL1* participates in the 11q13 amplification found in breast cancer. Oncogene, 5, 147–149.

Thompson, C.C., Brown, T.A. and McKnight, S.L. (1991). Convergence of Ets- and notch-related structural motifs in a heteromeric DNA binding complex. Science, 253, 762–768.

Tsujimoto, Y. and Croce, C. (1986). Analysis of the structure, transcripts, and protein products of *BCL2*, the gene involved in human follicular lymphoma. Proc. Natl Acad. Sci. USA, 83, 5214–5218.

Tsujimoto, Y. Yunis, J., Onorato-Showe, L., Erikson, J., Nowell, P.C. and Croce, C. (1984). Molecular clon-ing of the chromosomal breakpoint of B-cell lymphomas and leukemias with the t(11;14) chromosome translocation. Science, 224, 1403–1406.

Tsujimoto, Y. Finger, L.R., Yunis, J., Nowell, P.C. and Croce, C. (1986). Cloning of the chromosomal breakpoint of neoplastic B cells with the t(14;18) chromosome translocation. Science, 226, 1097–1099.

Vaux, D.L., Cory, S. and Adams, J.M. (1988). *Bcl-2* gene promotes haemopoietic cell survival and cooperates with c-*myc* to immortalize pre-B cells. Nature, 335, 440–442.

Villuendas, R., Piris, M.A., Orradre, J.L., Mollejo, M., Rodriguez, R. and Morente, M. (1991). Different *BCL2* protein expression in high-grade B-cell lymphomas derived from lymph node or mucosa-associated lymphoid tissue. Am. J. Pathol., 139, 989–993.

Weiss, L.M., Warnke, R.A., Sklar, J. and Cleary, M.L. (1987). Molecular analysis of the t(14;18) chromoso-mal translocation in malignant lymphomas. New Engl. J. Med., 317, 1185–1189.

Withers, D.A., Harvey, R.C., Faust, J.B., Melnyk, O., Carey, K. and Meeker, T.C. (1991). Characterization of a candidate *BCL1* gene. Mol. Cell. Biol., 11, 4846–4853.

Xiong, Y., Connolly, T., Futcher, B. and Beach, D. (1991). Human D-type cyclin. Cell, 65, 691–699.

Xiong, Y., Zhang, H. and Beach, D. (1992). D type cyclins associate with multiple protein kinases and the DNA replication and repair factor PCNA. Cell, 71, 505–514.

Yeh, T.M., Korsmeyer, S.J. and Teale, J.M. (1991). Skewed B cell VH family repertoire in *BCL2-Ig* transgenic mice. Int. Immunol., 3, 1329–1233.

Young, R.L. and Korsmeyer, S.J. (1993). A negative regulatory element in the *bcl-2* 5'-untranslated region inhibits expression from an upstream promoter. Mol. Cell. Biol., 13, 3686–3697.

CBL

v-*cbl* is the oncogene of the acutely transforming Cas NS-1 retrovirus (*Casitas B*-lineage *lymphoma*; Langdon *et al.*, 1989a).

Related genes

No homology with other known oncogenes. Sequence homology to the DNA binding and transcriptional activation domains of the yeast regulatory protein GCN4.

Cross-species homology

CBL: 93% identity (mouse and human).

Transformation

Cas NS-1 virus was generated from the ecotropic Cas-Br-M virus by sequential recombinations with endogenous retroviral sequences and a cellular onocogene. Isolated from an NFS/N mouse bearing a pre-B cell lymphoma induced by the Cas-Br-M murine leukaemia virus, it is an acutely transforming murine retrovirus that induces pre-B (sIg⁻, Lyb-2⁺, Ly-5 (B220⁺) and pro-B (Mac-1⁺) cell lymphomas and transforms fibroblasts, the *gag–onc* fusion protein appearing to be the responsible agent (Langdon *et al.*, 1989a). The oncogenes v-*cbl* and v-*abl* induce histologically and phenotypically similar tumours although for v-*cbl* there is longer latency and resistance in adult mice.

	CBL/Cbl	v-cbl
Nucleotides		
Human	2718	7400 (Cas NS-1 genome)
Chromosome		
Human	11q23.3-qter (*CBL2*)	
Mouse	6 (*Cbl-1*) and 9 (*Cbl-2*) *Cbl-1* may be a pseudogene The *Cbl-2* locus is in a region of chromosome 11 subject to translocations and is in close linkage to Thy-1.	
mRNA (kb)		
Human, mouse	11.0 3.5 (testis) 8.2/12.2 in WEHI-231 cells 3.5 in some other cell lines	3.4

	CBL/Cbl		v-*cbl*
Amino acids			
Human	906		
Mouse	896		390 (v-CBL)
Mass (kDa)			
(predicted)	100		
(expressed)	p135		p100$^{gag\text{-}cbl}$

Cellular location

CBL: Nuclear.
v-*CBL*: Nuclear.

Tissue location

Cbl is expressed in cells of the B, T, erythroid, myeloid and mast cell lineages and is most readily detectable in the thymus and testis (Langdon *et al.*, 1989b).

Protein function

v-CBL was generated by truncation of 60% of the C-terminus of CBL. This permits the *gag–cbl* fusion protein to enter the nucleus. v-CBL binds to DNA, whereas full-length CBL does not, and thus probably functions as a transcriptional activator (Blake *et al.*, 1991, 1993).

Sequences of human and mouse CBL

```
v-CBL        (1)                                   ASAGGGCRRGPSFSPGSIPSLAAERAPDPPLA

Human CBL    (1)    MAGNVKKSSGAGGGTGSGGSGSGGLIGLMKDAFQPHHHHHHHLSPHPPGTVDKKMVEKC
Mouse CBL    (1)    -------------- ------A------------------ ------C----------
v-CBL        (33)   ************** ****************************** *****************

Human CBL    (60)   WKLMDKVVRLCQNPKLALKNSPPYILDLLPDTYQHLRTILSRYEGKMETLGENEYFRVFM
Mouse CBL    (58)   -------------------------------------V--------------------
v-CBL        (90)   *********************************************************

Human CBL    (120)  ENLMKKTKQTISLFKEGKERMYEENSQPRRNLTKLSLIFSHMLAELKGIFPSGLFQGDTF
Mouse CBL    (118)  -----------------------------------------------------------
v-CBL        (150)  ***********************************************************

Human CBL    (180)  RITKADAAEFWRKAFGEKTIVPWKSFRQALHEVHPISSGLEAMALKSTIDLTCNDYISVF
Mouse CBL    (178)  -----------------------------------------------------------
v-CBL        (210)  ***********************************************************

Human CBL    (240)  EFDIFTRLFQPWSSLLRNWNSLAVTHPGYMAFLTYDEVKARLQKFIHKPGSYIFRLSCTR
Mouse CBL    (238)  -----------------------------------------------------------
v-CBL        (270)  ***********************************************************
```

```
Human CBL  (300)  LGQWAIGYVTADGNILQTIPHNKPLFQALIDGFREGFYLFPDGRNQNPDLTGLCEPTPQD
Mouse CBL  (298)  -----------------------------------------------------------
v-CBL      (330)  ***********************************************************HF

Human CBL  (360)  HIKVTQEQYELYCEMGSTFQLCKICAENDKDVKIEPCGHLMCTSCLTSWQESEGQGCPFC
Mouse CBL  (358)  ------                   -----------------------------------
v-CBL      (390)  S (390)

Human CBL  (420)  RCEIKGTEPIVVDPFDPRGSGSLLRQGAEGAPSPNYDDDDDERADDTLFMMKELAGAKVE
Mouse CBL  (401)  -----------------------------------------------------------
Human CBL  (480)  RPPSPFSMAPQASLPPVPPRLDLLPQRVCVPSSASALGTASKAASGSLHKDKPLPVPPTL
Mouse CBL  (461)  --S-------------------Q--AP--A-T-V-------------------------
Human CBL  (540)  DRLPPPPPPDRPYSVGAESRPQRRPLPCTPGDCPSRDKLPPVPSSRLGDSWLPRPIPKVP
Mouse CBL  (521)  -----------------T------------------------P-----S------
Human CBL  (600)  VSAPSSSDPWTGRELTNRHSLPFSLPSQMEPRPDVPRLGSTFSLDTSMSMNSSPLVGPEC
Mouse CBL  (581)  -AT-NPG---N-------------------A--------------T-----VA---S
Human CBL  (660)  DHPKIKPSSSANAIYSLAARPLPVPKLPPGEQCEGEEDTEYMTPSSRPL        RPL
Mouse CBL  (641)  E--------------------M--------G-S---------T---VGVQKPEPK---
Human CBL  (712)  DTSQSSRACDCDQQIDSCTYEAMYNIQSQAPSITESSTFGEGNLAAAHANTGPEESENED
Mouse CBL  (701)  EAT-----------------------L-VA-N-AS------T--TS----------
Human CBL  (772)  DGYDVPKPPVPAVLARRTLSDISNASSSFGWLSLDGDPTTNVTEGSQVPERPPKPFPRRI
Mouse CBL  (761)  -----------------------------------  --FN----------------
Human CBL  (832)  NSERKAGSCQQGSGPAASA ATA SPQLSSEIENLMSQGYSYQDIQKALVIAQNNLEMAK
Mouse CBL  (820)  ------S-Y-----AT-NPV---P---------R----------------H-------
Human CBL  (890)  NILREFVSISSPAHVAT (906)
Mouse CBL  (880)  ---------------- (896)
```

Dashes indicate identity with human CBL (>90%). * Indicates identity between mouse CBL and v-CBL. The putative nuclear localization signal and the leucine zipper sequence are underlined.

Protein structure

CBL has four potential *N*-linked glycosylation sites and many Ser/Thr stretches. v-CBL is a truncated form of CBL containing 355 N-terminal amino acids fused behind 32 non-cellular residues (Blake *et al.*, 1991). v-CBL has lost a C-terminal leucine zipper and a 208 residue proline-rich region that occur in CBL and are similar to the activation domains of some transcription factors. The N-terminal region is absolutely conserved in the generation of murine v-CBL and acquires only five changes in human v-CBL. The position of the oncogene junction is in the *gag* gene for p10 at a position that removes the terminal 24 *gag*-encoded amino acids.

A truncated form of *CBL* occurs in the cutaneous T cell lymphoma line HUT78 in which 259 C-terminal amino acids are removed: the 72 kDa protein produced lacks the leucine zipper region and part of the proline-rich domain (Blake and Langdon, 1992).

Databank file names and accession numbers

	GENE	EMBL	SWISSPROT	REFERENCES
Human	*CBL*	Hsccbl X57110		Blake *et al.*, 1991
Mouse	*Cbl*	Mmccbl X57111		Blake *et al.*, 1991
Mouse	*v-cbl*	Recasns1 J04169		Langdon *et al.*, 1989a
	(Cas NS-1 retrovirus)	GB:Casns1 J04169		

Papers

Blake, T.J. and Langdon, W.Y. (1992). A rearrangement of the c-cbl proto-oncogene in HUT78 T-lymphoma cells results in a truncated protein. Oncogene, 7, 757–762.

Blake, T.J., Shapiro, M., Morse, H.C. and Langdon, W.Y. (1991). The sequences of the human and mouse c-*cbl* proto-oncogenes show v-*cbl* was generated by a large truncation encompassing a proline-rich domain and a leucine zipper-like motif. Oncogene, 6, 653–657.

Blake, T.J., Heath, K.G. and Langdon, W.Y. (1993). The truncation that generated the v-*cbl* oncogene reveals an ability for nuclear transport, DNA binding and acute transformation. EMBO J., 12, 2017–2026.

Langdon, W.Y., Hartley, J.W., Klinken, S.P., Ruscetti, S.K. and Morse, H.C. (1989a). v-*cbl*, an oncogene from a dual-recombinant murine retrovirus that induces early B-lineage lymphomas. Proc. Natl Acad. Sci. USA, 86, 1168–1172.

Langdon, W.Y., Hyland, C.D., Grumont, R.J. and Morse, H.C. (1989b). The c-*cbl* proto-oncogene is preferentially expressed in thymus and testis tissue and encodes a nuclear protein. J. Virol., 63, 5420–5424.

v-*crk* (*CT*10 regulator of *k*inase) is the oncogene of avian sarcoma viruses CT10 (Mayer *et al.*, 1988) and ASV-1 (Tsuchie *et al.*, 1989).

Related genes

CRK proteins contain SH2 and SH3 domains homologous with those present in SRC, FPS/FES and ABL, RAS–GAP, the phosphatidylinositol-specific phospholipase C-Iγ isozymes, α-spectrin, the yeast actin binding protein ABP1p, myosin-I, p85α and p85β (Koch *et al.*, 1991; see **SRC**).

Cross-species homology

Human CRK-II: 95% homology with chicken CRK.

Transformation

IN VIVO

CT10 or ASV-1 cause rapid tumour formation in chickens (Mayer *et al.*, 1988; Tsuchie *et al.*, 1989).

IN VITRO

ASV CT10 transforms chick embryo fibroblasts which are then tumorigenic when injected into chickens (Mayer *et al.*, 1988). Cell lines expressing CRK-I are tumorigenic in nude mice. CRK-II does not transform cells *in vitro* and is non-tumorigenic (Matsuda *et al.*, 1992).

	CRK/Crk	v-*crk*
Nucleotides (bp)		2407
mRNA (kb)	4.2	
Amino acids	204 (human CRK-I)	440
	304 (human CRK-II)	
Mass (kDa) (expressed)	28 (CRK-I)	p47$^{gag-crk}$
	40/42 (CRK-II)	

Cellular location

Cytoplasmic.

Tissue location

CRK-I (p28) is expressed in human embryonic lung cells. CRK-II (p42) is present in the osteosarcoma cell line 143B, A431 cells and the T cell line H9. CRK-II (p40) is present in a wide variety of cell lines (Matsuda *et al.*, 1992).

Protein function

P47$^{gag\text{-}crk}$ causes tyrosine phosphorylation in CT10 infected chick embryo fibroblasts, notably of proteins in the 135–155 kDa range. P47 does not itself possess kinase activity and has thus been denoted CT10 regulator of kinase (Mayer *et al.*, 1988, 1989). P47$^{gag\text{-}crk}$ immunoprecipitates with a wide range of tyrosine phosphorylated proteins, including pp60$^{v\text{-}src}$ but association with the latter is prevented if autophosphorylation of Tyr416 is blocked (Matsuda *et al.*, 1990; Mayer and Hanafusa, 1990). Mutational studies indicate that the SH2 domain of P47$^{gag\text{-}crk}$ binds specifically to tyrosine phosphorylated regions of peptides (Matsuda *et al.*, 1991) and shows preferential affinity for binding to phosphotyrosine in the general motif pTyr–hydrophilic–hydrophilic–Ile/Pro (Songyang *et al.*, 1993).

Sequences of human CRK-I, CRK-II and P47$^{gag\text{-}crk}$

```
GAG-CRK    (1)    MEAVIKVISSACKTYCGKTSPSKKEIGAMLSLLQKEGLLMSPSDLYSPRSWDPITAALT
GAG-CRK    (60)   QRAMELGKSGELKTWGLVLGALEAAREEQEQVTSEQAKFWLGLGGGRVSPPGPECIEKPA
GAG-CRK    (120)  TERRIDKGEEVGETTVQRDAKMAPEETATPKTVGTSCYYCGAAIGCNCATASAPPPPYVG

CRK-II     (1)                                                          MAGN
GAG-CRK    (180)  SGLYPSLAGVGEQQGQGGDTPRGAEQPRAGRGAGHRGLRRPAGRGQRVRPAGGAAL---Q

CRK-II     (5)    FDSEERSSWYWGRLSRQEAVALLQGQRHGVFLVRDSSTSPGDYVLSVSENSRVSHYIINS
GAG-CRK    (240)  ----D-G---------GD--S--------T------GSI---F------S-------V--

CRK-II     (65)   SGPRPPVPPSPAQP PPGVSPSRLRIGDQEFDSLPALLEFYKIHYWDTTTLIEPVSRSRQ
GAG-CRK    (300)  L--AGGRRAGGEG-GA--LNPT-FL----V-----S---------L-------------

CRK-II     (124)  GSGVILRQEEAEYVRALFDFNGNDEEDLPFKKGDILRIRDKPEEQWWNAEDSEGKRGMIP
GAG-CRK    (360)  N--------V---------K---DG----------K------------MD-------

CRK-II     (184)  VPYVEKYRPASASVSALIGGNQEGSHPQPLGPPEPGPYAQPSVNTPLPNLQNGPIYARVI
CRK-I      (184)  -------------------R (204)
GAG-CRK    (420)  ------C--S-----T-T--R (440)

CRK-II     (244)  QKRVPNAYDKTALALEVGELVKVTKINVSGQWEGGCNGKRGHFPFTHVRLLDQQNPDEDFS (304)
```

v-CRK domains: GAG: 1–208; CRK: 209–437. Underlined: SH2 (CRK-II 11–104) and SH3 (CRK-II 133–184 and 238–290) domains. The termination codon for CRK-I is in the same position as that for v-CRK. CRK-I lacks a 170 bp sequence present in CRK-II: alternative splicing is presumed to remove this region, leaving a single SH3 domain in CRK-I.

Protein structure

The ASV CT10 genome (2407 bp; LTR: 521 bp) encodes the P47$^{gag\text{-}crk}$ transforming protein that comprises 440 amino acids commencing at the *gag* initiation codon. The 208 *gag*-encoded amino acids are fused to 232 novel residues presumed to be from a cellular proto-oncogene. The cellular sequence lacks start and stop codons so is presumed to be truncated at both ends. The last three amino acids and the stop codon are provided by viral sequences. The 3' recombination junction is identical to that of Rous sarcoma virus (Mayer *et al.*, 1988).

A member of the group of proteins of unrelated function that share homology with non-catalytic regions of *Src*, P47$^{gag\text{-}crk}$ contains *Src* homology regions 2 and 3 (SH2, SH3), transposed with respect to SRC. These regions also occur in phosphatidylinositol-specific phospholipase C-γ (Stahl *et al.*, 1988), where SH2 is duplicated, and P47*gag-crk* has strong homology with a 180 amino acid region of this protein.

Human CRK-I and CRK-II each contain one SH2 domain together with one and two SH3 domains, respectively (Matsuda *et al.*, 1992). The SH2 domain is approximately 100 amino acids long and commences at residue 11 in CRK-II. SH3 regions are approximately 50 amino acids long and commence at residue 133 and residue 238 in CRK-II. The B and C boxes of SH2, separated by a hinge region, coordinately form the functional phosphotyrosine binding domain (Matsuda *et al.*, 1993).

Chicken *Crk* contains an additional SH3 domain (Reichman *et al.*, 1992).

Databank file names and accession numbers

	GENE	*EMBL*	*SWISSPROT*	*REFERENCES*
ASV (strain CT10)	*gag–crk*	Reasv Y00302	GAGC_AVISC P05433	Mayer *et al.*, 1988
Human	*CRK*	Hscrk D10656		Matsuda *et al.*, 1992

Papers

Koch, C.A., Anderson, D., Moran, M.F., Ellis, C. and Pawson, T. (1991). SH2 and SH3 domains: elements that control interactions of cytoplasmic signaling proteins. Science, 252, 668–674.

Matsuda, M., Mayer, B.J., Fukui, Y. and Hanafusa, H. (1990). Binding of transforming protein p47*gag-crk* to a broad range of phosphotyrosine-containing proteins. Science, 248, 1537–1539.

Matsuda, M., Mayer, B.J. and Hanafusa, H. (1991). Identification of domains of the v-*crk* oncogene product sufficient for association with phosphotyrosine-containing proteins. Mol. Cell. Biol., 11, 1607–1613.

Matsuda, M., Tanaka, S., Nagata, S., Kojima, A., Kurata, T. and Shibuya, M. (1992). Two species of human *CRK* cDNA encode proteins with distinct biological activities. Mol. Cell. Biol., 12, 3482–3489.

Matsuda, M., Nagata, S., Tanaka, S., Nagashima, K. and Kurata, T. (1993). Structural requirement of *CRK* SH2 region for binding to phosphotyrosine-containing proteins. J. Biol. Chem., 268, 4441–4446.

Mayer, B.J. and Hanafusa, H. (1990). Association of the v-*crk* oncogene product with phosphotyrosine-containing proteins and protein kinase activity. Proc. Natl Acad. Sci. USA, 87, 2638–2642.

Mayer, B.J., Hamaguchi, M. and Hanafusa, H. (1988). A novel viral oncogene with structural similarity to phospholipase C. Nature, 332, 272–275.

Mayer, B.J., Hamaguchi, M. and Hanafusa, H. (1989). Characterization of P47*gag-crk*, a novel oncogene product with sequence similarity to a putative modulatory domain of protein-tyrosine kinases and phospholipase C. Cold Spring Harbor Symp. Quant. Biol., 53, 907–914.

Reichman, C.T., Mayer, B.J., Keshav, S. and Hanafusa, H. (1992). The product of the cellular crk gene consists primarily of SH2 and SH3 regions. Cell Growth Differ., 3, 451–460.

Songyang, Z., Shoelson, S.E., Chaudhuri, M., Gish, G., Pawson, T., Haser, W.G., King, F., Roberts, T., Ratnofsky, S., Lechleider, R.J., Neel, B.G., Birge, R.B., Fajardo, J.E., Chou, M.M., Hanafusa, H., Schaffhausen, B. and Cantley, L. (1993). SH2 domains recognize specific phosphopeptide sequences. Cell, 72, 767–778.

Stahl, M.L., Ferenz, C.R., Kelleher, K.L., Kriz, R.W. and Knopf, J.L. (1988). Sequence similarity of phospholipase C with the non-catalytic region of src. Nature, 332, 269–272.

Tsuchie, H., Chang, C.H.W., Yoshida, M. and Vogt, P.K. (1989). A newly isolated avian sarcoma virus, ASV-1, carries the *crk* oncogene. Oncogene, 4, 1281–1284.

v-*fms* is the transforming oncogene of the Susan McDonough (SM-FeSV; McDonough *et al.*, 1971) and Hardy–Zuckerman (HZ5-FeSV) strains of acutely transforming feline sarcoma virus (Besmer *et al.*, 1986).

CSF1R (*FMS*) encodes the receptor for colony stimulating factor-1 (CSF1 or M-CSF).

Related genes

FMS encodes a tyrosine-specific protein kinase most closely related to *KIT*, the two receptors for PDGF (Hampe *et al.*, 1984) and the product of the *FLT3/FLK2* gene (Rosnet *et al.*, 1991; Maroc *et al.*, 1993). Each has a distinctive pattern of cysteine spacing in the extracellular domain that includes sequences characteristic of the immunoglobulin (Ig) gene superfamily and in each the kinase domain is interrupted by a hydrophilic spacer of between 64 and 104 amino acids. Murine *Flt-3/Flk-2* encodes a 3.7 kb transcript expressed in the placenta and various adult tissues (brain, gonads and haematopoietic cells; Rosnet *et al.*, 1991; Lyman *et al.*, 1993; Maroc *et al.*, 1993). The *Fim-2* viral integration site in the mouse genome spans the *Fms* locus (see Table 2.2).

Human *FRT* (*fms*-related tyrosine kinase gene; Matsushime *et al.*, 1987) is also a member of this family.

FLT1 (*fms*-like tyrosine kinase, also *Flk-3*) encodes a receptor tyrosine kinase that is ~60% homologous to FMS (Shibuya *et al.*, 1990) but has a predicted seven Ig-like extracellular domains, compared to five in the members of the CSF1R/FMS family (de-Vries *et al.*, 1992). *FLK1* (human *KDR*, murine *Nyk* and rat TKr-III) and *FLT4* are the other members of the class of receptor tyrosine kinases with seven Ig-like loops (Galland *et al.*, 1993).

Cross-species homology

The feline v-*fms* and human *FMS* gene products are closely related, differing only by scattered amino acid substitutions. FMS: 80.5% identity (human and feline); 72% identity (human and mouse). Ligand binding domains: 75%; ATP binding and tyrosine kinase domains: 95% (human and feline).

Transformation

MAN

Activating mutations of *FMS* have been detected in 17% of patients with primary acute myeloblastic leukaemia (Ridge *et al.*, 1990).

ANIMALS

Inoculation of SM-FeSV-transformed NIH 3T3 fibroblasts or NRK cells into syngeneic animals or nude mice induces fatal tumours (McDonough *et al.*, 1971).

IN VITRO

SM-FeSV transforms NIH 3T3, MDCK, NRK, feline embryo fibroblasts and mink lung epithelial cells (Donner *et al.*, 1982). This requires tyrosine kinase activity, normal glycosylation and surface membrane expression. The presence of the complete ligand binding domain of CSF1 in v-FMS causes transformed cells to bind CSF1 specifically and CSF1 causes a further 2- to 3-fold increase in phosphotyrosine in gp140$^{v\text{-}fms}$, indicating further increase in the constitutive kinase activity of the transforming protein (Roussel *et al.*, 1987; Downing *et al.*, 1989). The expression of a constitutively activated tyrosine phosphatase suppresses transformation by v-*fms* (Zander *et al.*, 1993).

	FMS/Fms	*v-fms*
Nucleotides		
Human, feline	>30 kb	2969 8.2 kb (SM-FeSV genome)
Chromosome		
Human	5q33.3–34 13q12 (*FLT1*); 8p12 (*FLT2*) 5q35 (*FLT4*)	
Exons	22	
mRNA (kb)	3.7–5.0 2.2/3.0/7.5–8.0 (*FLT1*) 4.5/5.8 (*FLT4*)	8.2 (Donner *et al.*, 1982)
Amino acids		
Human	972	1437 (P180$^{gag\text{-}fms}$)
Human	1338 (FLT1) 1298 (FLT4)	(459 *gag*; 978 v-*fms* (SM-FeSV))
Feline	980	v-*fms* processed to 959 (SM-FeSV)
Murine	976	v-*fms* to 973 (HZ5-FeSV)
Mass (kDa)		
(predicted)	108	
(expressed)		gp180$^{gag\text{-}v\text{-}fms}$
Human	gp150 170 (FLT4)	p55^{gag} and p120$^{v\text{-}fms}$
Feline	gp170	gp140$^{v\text{-}fms}$ (SM-FeSV)
Murine	gp165	
Protein half-life (h)	2–3 (Rapid receptor-mediated endocytosis)	2–3

Cellular location

CSFR1/FMS encodes a transmembrane growth factor receptor that is localized at the cell surface. Immature forms of the protein occur in the endoplasmic reticulum and Golgi apparatus. The ectodomain may be released from cells (see also HER2, EGFR and IL2R; Downing *et al.*, 1991). v-FMS, unlike the oncogene product of v-*erbB*, retains normal ligand binding capacity.

Tissue location

CSF1R is normally only expressed on monocytes, macrophages and their precursors (Muller *et al.*, 1983a,b; Woolford *et al.*, 1985; Sherr, 1988) and at lower levels in normal and malignant B lymphocytes (Baker *et al.*, 1993) but is also detectable in the human and murine uteroplacental unit (Pampfer *et al.*, 1992; Regenstreif and Rossant, 1989) and in cell lines derived from human malignant placental trophoblasts (Rettenmier *et al.*, 1986). *FMS* is not expressed in normal vascular smooth muscle cells but is activated in intimal smooth muscle cells isolated from an experimental rabbit model of arteriosclerosis (Inaba *et al.*, 1992).

SM-FeSV-transformed NIH 3T3 cell surfaces express 5×10^4 gp140$^{v\text{-}fms}$ molecules/cell (Sacca *et al.*, 1986).

FLT1 is widely distributed in human and rat tissues but has not been detected in tumour cell lines (Shibuya *et al.*, 1990).

Protein function

CSF1R/FMS encodes the receptor for CSF1 (M-CSF) that cooperates with IL-2 or IL-3 to stimulate bone marrow cells during haematopoiesis (Stanley *et al.*, 1986). The enhanced expression of *Fms* in pregnant mice indicates a possible role in embryogenesis. *Fms* may also be involved in the induction of macrophage differentiation (Rohrschneider and Metcalf, 1989; Borzillo *et al.*, 1990). Expression of v-*fms* may cause haematopoietic disorders (Heard *et al.*, 1987).

FMS has intrinsic tyrosine kinase activity and the RAF protein is a substrate *in vitro*. In macrophages CSF1 activates the Na$^+$/K$^+$-ATPase, the Na$^+$/H$^+$ exchanger and *Fos* and *Myc* transcription. CSF1 also activates the *Src* family kinases SRC, FYN and YES and causes these proteins to associate with the CSF1R (Courtneidge *et al.*, 1993).

NIH 3T3 fibroblasts are mitogenically stimulated by CSF1 after transfection with the human *FMS* gene, but CSF1 causes barely detectable tyrosine phosphorylation of PLC-γ and no early (5 min) change in [Ca^{2+}]$_i$ (Downing *et al.*, 1989). It is possible that CSF1 activates other isoforms of PLC but it seems probable that, despite its structural similarity to the PDGF receptor, activation via FMS does not involve PtdIns(4,5)P_2 hydrolysis. CSF1 causes weak tyrosine phosphorylation of GAP (10% of that induced by PDGF-BB) and strongly tyrosine phosphorylates the GAP-associated proteins p62 and p190. Despite the contrast in effects on GAP, CSF1 and PDGF promote equivalent activation of p21^{ras}–GTP and stimulate mitogenesis to a similar extent in these cells (Heidaran *et al.*, 1992).

Substitution of Tyr809 in the human CSF1 receptor (equivalent to Tyr857 in the PDGFR) blocks ligand-dependent mitogenesis but does not inhibit the tyrosine kinase activity of the receptor nor its ability to associate with phosphatidylinositol 3-kinase and to induce *Fos* and *Jun* transcription (Roussel *et al.*, 1990) although it does decrease the binding and enzymatic activation of SRC, FYN and YES (Courtneidge *et al.*, 1993). Activated Phe809 mutant receptors do not, however, induce *Myc* expression but the co-expression of an exogenous *Myc* gene in cells expressing only the mutant form of the receptor restores the ability of the cells to proliferate in response to CSF1 (Roussel *et al.*, 1991). This implies the existence of an effector that interacts with the domain including Tyr809 that is required for *Myc* induction and CSF1-induced mitogenesis. Substitution of Glu582 with Lys and of Asp776 with Asn generates mutant proteins corresponding to the dominant negative W^{37} and W^{42} *Kit* alleles. These proteins have undetectable *in vitro* kinase activity and their expression does not transform rat-2 cells in the presence of exogenous CSF1 (Reith *et al.*, 1993). Their expression also inhibits the anchorage-independent growth mediated by the normal FMS receptor in the presence of CSF1 and the FMS-associated phosphatidylinositol 3-kinase activity.

Receptor-mediated endocytosis of FMS and v-FMS follows ligand binding but endocytosis of v-FMS does not require CSF1. The rapid internalization of the FMS receptor does not depend on the tyrosine kinase activity of the receptor or on the presence of the kinase insert region of the cytoplasmic domain although degradation requires both these regions (Carlberg *et al.*, 1991). The kinase insert region is also unnecessary for the growth-stimulating activity of the FMS kinase (Taylor *et al.*, 1989; Shurtleff *et al.*, 1990). The extracellular domain of FMS is rapidly cleaved following protein kinase C activation.

v-*fms*-Mediated transformation appears to be due to the sustained expression of CSF1-independent tyrosine kinase activity (Roussel *et al.*, 1987). In SM-FeSV-transformed mink lung epithelial cells PtdIns(4,5)P_2 hydrolysis and phosphatidylinositol kinase activities are increased (Jackowski *et al.*, 1986; Kaplan *et al.*, 1987).

The FMS-like tyrosine kinase FLT is a transmembrane receptor for vascular endothelial growth factor, also known as vascular permeability factor (VEGF-VPF), a factor that induces vascular permeability when injected in the guinea-pig skin and stimulates endothelial cell proliferation. Expression of *Flt* in *Xenopus laevis* oocytes induces calcium release in response to VEGF-VPF (de-Vries *et al.*, 1992).

The stimulation of HL-60 cell differentiation by vitamin D activates *FMS* expression as a component of the programme for monocytic differentiation (Rowley *et al.*, 1992).

Structure of feline leukaemia virus (FeLV) and the HZ5-FeSV and SM-FeSV proviral genomes and translation products

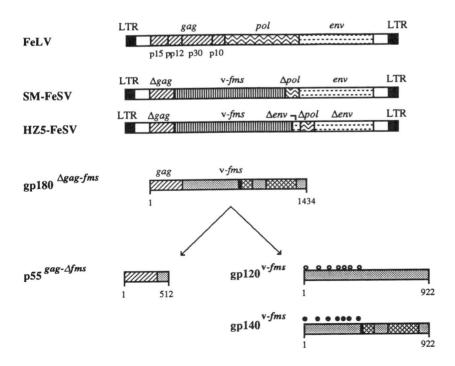

Cross-hatched box: *gag* sequences (encodes p15, pp12, p30 and p10 proteins: *gag–fms* includes p15, p12, p30 and the first 14 residues of p10).

The genomic organization of HZ5-FeSV is similar to that of SM-FeSV, identical portions of FeLV *gag* being retained. About 3 kb of cellular *Fms* sequence is transduced and combined with *gag*, deleting some p10^{gag} and most of *pol*. An 8 bp sequence homology region between *Fms* and the FeLV *gag* gene at the 5' recombination site that is identical in SM-FeSV and HZ5 may be a recombinational hot spot. The 3' recombination sites within *pol* differ, giving rise to different v-*fms* products (Hampe *et al.*, 1984; Guilhot *et al.*, 1987). The *gag* sequences of SM-FeSV and HZ5-FeSV are in frame with the 5' non-translated sequences of *Fms*, resulting in 34 amino acids being encoded between p10^{gag} and FMS, thereby retaining the N-terminal signal peptide of CSF1. The leader sequences are cleaved (19 N-terminal FMS residues and all of *gag* in v-FMS) so that the N-terminal regions of the final forms of feline FMS and SM- and HZ5-FeSV v-FMS are identical.

The primary product is P170$^{gag-fms}$; cleavage of the signal sequence coupled with co-translational N-linked glycosylation (open circles) yields gp180$^{gag-fms}$.

Proteolytic cleavage generates p55$^{gag-\Delta fms}$ (53 C-terminal v-*fms*-coded amino acids) and p120^{v-fms}: the latter is further post-translationally modified (closed circles) to gp140^{v-fms}. The two crossed boxes indicate the two kinase domains. The vertical bar represents a 26 amino acid transmembrane segment; thus the glycosylated N-terminus becomes the extracellular, ligand binding domain of the protein.

Structure of the human *FMS* gene

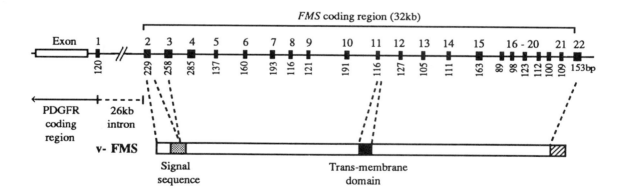

The overall gene structure and encoded amino acid sequence is similar to the PDGF receptor and the two genes may have arisen by duplication. Exon 1 (120 bp) encodes 112 nucleotides of *FMS* mRNA and is separated from exon 2 by a 26 kb intron. Exon 2 encodes part of the 5' untranslated sequence of *FMS* mRNA, the initiation codon and the signal peptide (Roberts *et al.*, 1988; Hampe *et al.*, 1989). The corresponding regions of the feline gene transduced by v-*fms* are indicated.

In the mouse, integration of Friend MuLV at the 5' end of *Fms* directly upstream of the region corresponding to exon 2 of the human gene induces transcription as a component of the development of myeloid leukaemia. Proviral insertion is head-to-head with respect to the direction of *Fms* transcription, indicating that the promoter may lie close to exon 2 (Gisselbrecht *et al.*, 1987).

Structures of FMS, v-FMS and SRC proteins

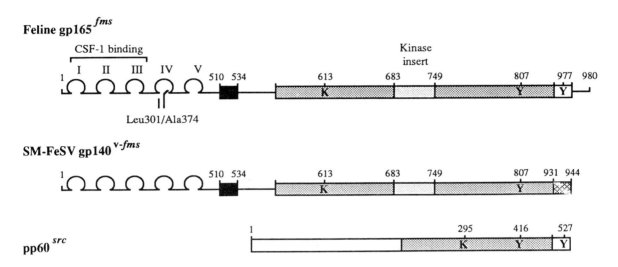

Black boxes: transmembrane domains. Shaded boxes: tyrosine kinase domains. Crossed box: 14 v-FMS amino acids that are not homologous to FMS (see below). Thus Tyr977 is eliminated in v-FMS. ATP binding sites: Lys613, 613 and 295 respectively. Autophosphorylation sites: Tyr807, 807 and 416. Negative regulatory phosphorylation sites: Tyr977 and 527.

FMS belongs to the immunoglobulin superfamily, containing five Ig-like loops that comprise the extracellular domain including the CSF1 binding region (Rohrschneider and Woolford, 1991; Rohrschneider, personal communication), the region undergoing conformational change leading to dimerization following CSF1 binding and which includes the activating point mutations in v-FMS (IV) and domain V that is involved in intracellular processing and transport (Lyman and Rohrschneider, 1987). In addition to these domains (comprised of 493 amino acids), FMS contains an N-terminal signal sequence (19 amino acids), a transmembrane region (26 amino acids) and a C-terminal tyrosine kinase domain (436 amino acids). The C-terminus is homologous to other tyrosine kinase receptors (see **SRC**). It contains a 68 residue "kinase insert" between the ATP binding site and the kinase domain that corresponds to but differs from those of the PDGFR and v-KIT.

Phosphatidylinositol 3-kinase binds to the CSF1 receptor via interaction of the two SH2 domains of the p85α subunit with phosphorylated Tyr721 in the kinase insert region (Reedijk *et al.*, 1992). Binding is independent of the phosphorylation of the other two tyrosine residues (Tyr697 and Tyr706) in the kinase insert region. Substitution of the extracellular and transmembrane domains with those of glycophorin generates a constitutively active tyrosine kinase that has increased associated phosphatidylinositol 3-kinase activity (Lee and Nienhuis, 1992). This suggests that oligomerization and activation of the normal FMS/CSF1 receptor may involve interactions between adjacent transmembrane domains.

Random mutagenesis of human *FMS* has revealed activating mutations within sequences separating the third and fourth immunoglobulin-like loops and within non-covalently stabilized loop 4 of the CSF1R extracellular domain, in addition to that previously identified at codon 301 (van Daalen-Wetters *et al.*, 1992).

There is extensive homology between FMS and v-FMS except for the 50 C-terminal amino acids of feline FMS that are unrelated to the final 14 residues of the truncated SM-FeSV v-FMS, encoded by a 3' untranslated region of feline *Fms* (Woolford *et al.*, 1988), or to the C-terminus of v-FMS HZ5-FeSV (Besmer *et al.*, 1986; Smola *et al.*, 1991). In v-FMS there are six point mutations in the extracellular domain and three in the 445 amino acid cytoplasmic domain by comparison with FMS (Hampe *et al.*, 1984; Woolford *et al.*, 1988). The mutations that appear critical for the activation of v-FMS (SM-FeSV) are the substitution of serine residues at positions 301 and 374 in the extracellular domain of feline FMS, together with the modification of the C-terminus (Roussel *et al.*, 1988). Transforming potential is further enhanced by replacement of Tyr969 with Phe in human FMS (Roussel *et al.*, 1987).

Differences between feline, human, murine and chicken FMS proteins and the two v-FMS isolates

Amino acid (feline FMS)	−16	11	91	301	304	374	399	461	499	505	554	587	711	C-terminus
SM-FeSV	Arg	Met	Arg	**Ser**	Thr	**Ser**	Pro	Tyr	Ser	Pro	Glu	Thr	Gly	Δ50aa
HZ5-FeSV	–	Val	Gln	Leu	**Ser**	Ala	**Ser**	His	Phe	Gln	Lys	Ala	Gly	Δ24aa
Feline	(Cys)	Val	Gln	Leu	Thr	Ala	Pro	His	Ser	Gln	Glu	Ala	Asp	
Human	(Trp)	Val	Leu	Leu	Ser	Ala	Pro	His	Ser	His	Glu	Ala	Gly	
Murine	(Pro)	Leu	Met	Leu	Thr	Ala	Pro	Asp	Ser	Gln	Glu	Ala	Gly	
Chicken	–	Leu	Asp	Val	Thr	Arg	Pro	Gln	Phe	Pro	Glu	Ala	Gly	

Differences between v-FMS proteins and feline FMS are shown, together with the corresponding residues in human, murine and chicken FMS. Differences causing activation are shown in bold type. Amino acids shown in brackets are not normally translated (Woolford *et al.*, 1988; Rohrschneider and Woolford, 1991).

Sequences of human, feline and mouse FMS and v-FMS (SM-FeSV)

```
v-FMS        (1)                              RMPSGPGHYGASAETPGPRPPLCPASSCCLPTEA

Human FMS    (1)   MGPGVLLLLLVATAWHGQGIPVIEPSVPELVVKPGATVTLRCVGNGSVEWDGPASPHWT
Feline FMS   (1)   ---RA--V--------A--V---Q--G-----E--T---------------I----N
Mouse FMS    (1)   -EL-PP-V--L--V-----A------G-----E--E---------------I--I--
v-FMS       (35)   ---RA--V--M-----A--V---Q--G-----E--T---------------I----N

Human FMS   (60)   LYSDGSSSILSTNNATFQNTGTYRCTEPGDPLGGSAAIHLYVKDPARPWNVLAQEVVVFE
Feline FMS  (60)   -DL-PP----T-----------H-----N-Q--N-T-----------K------T-L-
Mouse FMS   (60)   -DPESPG-T-T-S----K---------LE--MA--TT--------HS--------T-V-
v-FMS       (94)   -DL-P-----T-----------H-----N-R--N-T-----------K------T---

Human FMS  (120)   DQDALLPCLLTDPVLEAGVSLVRVRGRPLMRHTNYSFSPWHGFTIHRAKFIQSQDYQCSA
Feline FMS (120)   G------------A--------------VL-Q-------------K----ENHV-----
Mouse FMS  (120)   G-E-V----I---A-KDS---M-EG--QVL-K-V-F----R-SI-RK--VLD-NT-V-KT
v-FMS      (154)   G------------A--------------VL-Q-------------K----ENHV-----
```

```
Human FMS   (180)  LMGGRKVMSISIRLKVQKVIPGPPALTLVPAELVRIRGEAAQIVCSASSVDVNFDVFLQH
Feline FMS  (180)  RVD--T-T-MG-W-----D-S--AT---E-------Q-----------NI------S-R-
Mouse FMS   (180)  MVN--EST-TG-W--NR-H-E--QIK-E-SK---------------TNAE-G-N-I-KR
v-FMS       (212)  RVD--T-T-MG-W-----D-S--AT---E-------Q-----------NI------S- -

Human FMS   (240)  NNTKLAIPQQSDFHNNRYQKVLTLNLDQVDFQHAGNYSCVASNVQGKHSTSMFFRVVESA
Feline FMS  (240)  GD---T-S------D-----------H-S-QD------T-T-AW-N--A--V-------
Mouse FMS   (240)  GD---E--LN---QD-Y-K--RA-S-NA----D--I--------DV-TRTAT-N-Q----
v-FMS       (272)  GD---T-S------D-----------H-S--D------T-T-AW-N--A--V-------

Human FMS   (300)  YLNLSSEQNLIQEVTVGEGLNLKVMVEAYPGLQGFNWTYLGPFSDHQPEPKLANATTKDT
Feline FMS  (300)  ----T---S-L-------KVD-Q-K-------ES-----------Y-  D--DFVTI---
Mouse FMS   (300)  ----T---S-L---S--DS-I-T-HAD---SI-HY--------FED-  R--EFI-QRAI
v-FMS       (334)  -S--T---SLL-------KVD-Q-K-------ES-----------Y-  D--DFV-I---

Human FMS   (360)  YRHTFTLSLPRLKPSEAGRYSFLARNPGGWRALTFELTLRYPPEVSVIWTFINGSGTLLC
Feline FMS  (358)  --Y-S--------------------A--QN-------------R-TM-L----D----
Mouse FMS   (358)  --Y--K-F-N-V-A----Q-FLM-Q-KA--NNL-------------T-MPV---DV---
v-FMS       (392)  --Y-S-------R--S---------A--QN-------------R-TM-L----D----

Human FMS   (420)  AASGYPQPNVTWLQCSGHTDRCDEAQVLQVWDDPYPEVLSQEPFHKVTVQSLLTVETLEH
Feline FMS  (418)  E-------S--V--RS-------SAG- -LE-SHS-----V--E-I-H---AIG----
Mouse FMS   (418)  DV------S---ME-R---------A-HL-N-TH------K--D--II--Q-PIGP-K-
v-FMS       (452)  E-------S--V--RS-------SAG- -LE-SHS-----V--YE-I-H---AIG----

Human FMS   (480)  NQTYECRAHNSVGSGSWAFIPISAGAHTHPPDE*FLFTPVVVACMSIMALLLLLLLLLLYK*
Feline FMS  (477)  -R----T--F----NS-QT-W---I---QL---L-----LLT----------------
Mouse FMS   (478)  -M--F-KT-----NS-QY-RAV-L-QSKQL---S-----------V-S--V--------
v-FMS       (511)  -R------F----NS-QT-W---I----PL---L-----LLT----------------

Human FMS   (540)  YKQKPKYQVRWKIIESYEGNSYTFIDPTQLPYNEKWEFPRNNLQFGKT_LGAGAFGKV_VEA
Feline FMS  (537)  ------------------------------------------------------------
Mouse FMS   (538)  ------------------------------------------------------------
v-FMS       (571)  ----------------------------------------------------T---------

Human FMS   (600)  TAFGLGKEDAVLKVAV_K_MLKSTAHADEKEALMSELKIMSHLGQHENIVNLLGACTHGGPV
Feline FMS  (597)  ------------------------------------------------------------
Mouse FMS   (598)  ------------------------------------------------------------
v-FMS       (631)  ------------------------------------------------------------

Human FMS   (660)  LVITEYCCYGDLLNFLRRKAEAM_LGPSLSPGQDPEGGVYKNIHLEKKYVRRDSGFSSQG_
Feline FMS  (657)  -----------------Q----------V-----A-AG--------------D-----
Mouse FMS   (658)  -----------------------------S--DSS---------------
v-FMS       (691)  -----------------Q----P-----V-----A-AG--------------

Human FMS   (720)  _VDTYVEMRPVSTSS_NDSFSEQDLDKEDGRPLELRDLLHFSSQVAQGMAFLASKNCIHRDV
Feline FMS  (717)  --------------SN-----E--G-----------------------------------
Mouse FMS   (718)  --------------S ---FK------HS-----W-------------------------
v-FMS       (751)  --------------S------E--------------------------------------

Human FMS   (780)  AARNVLLTNGHVAKIGDFGLARDIMNDSN_Y_IVKGNARLPVKWMAPESIFDCVYTVQSDVW
Feline FMS  (777)  --------S-R-------------------------------------------------
Mouse FMS   (778)  --------S----------------V-----   --------------------
v-FMS       (812)  --------S-R-------------------------------------------------

Human FMS   (840)  SYGILLWEIFSLGLNPYPGILVNSKFYKLVKDGYQMAQPAFAPKNIYSIMQACWALEPTH
Feline FMS  (838)  ----------------------------------------------------------R
Mouse FMS   (837)  ---------------------N------------V-----------S--D----R
v-FMS       (872)  ----------------------------------------------------------R

Human FMS   (900)  RPTFQQICSFLQEQAQEDRRERDYTNLPSSSRSGGSGSSSSELEEESSSEHLTCCEQGDI
Feline FMS  (898)  ---------L--K-------VPN--------S-SS-S---CRTGSGGG-SSEPEE-SSSE
Mouse FMS   (897)  --------FL------LE--DQ--A-----GG-S--D-GGGSSGG ----PEEESSSEHL
v-FMS       (932)  ---------L--K-------VPN--------S-RLLRPWQRTPPVAR (978)
```

```
Human FMS    (960)  AQPLLQPNNYQFC (972)
Feline FMS   (958)  HLACCEQGDIAQPLLQPNNYQFC (980)
Mouse FMS    (956)  ACCEPGDIAQPLLQPNNYQFC (976)
```

The human FMS transmembrane region is shown in italics. The ATP binding regions (588–596 and 616) are underlined. The major *in vitro* autophosphorylation sites (murine 697 and 706) are underlined and in bold type, as are the two serine residues (335 and 408) critical for v-FMS activity (corresponding to Leu301 and Ala374 of feline FMS). There is a minor phosphorylation site at Tyr809 (human), Tyr807 (mouse) (Tapley *et al.*, 1990; van der Geer and Hunter, 1990). The human kinase insert region (683–749) is underlined. There are potential glycosylation sites at 45, 73, 153, 240, 302, 335, 353, 412, 428 and 480.

Amino acid numbering for v-FMS includes the 34 amino acid leader sequence that is cleaved. Thr973 (939) of v-FMS is phosphorylated by an unknown kinase in response to stimulation by CSF1 (Smola *et al.*, 1991).

C terminal homology in the FMS family

```
Feline FMS      (926)  SSSSSSSSSSSSCRTGSGGGSSSEPEEESSSEHLACCEQGDIAQPLLQPNNYQFC (980)
Human FMS       (928)  ---R-GG-G-              ----L---------T------------------- (972)
Mouse FMS       (925)  --GG--G-D-    GG--S--------------------P--------------- (976)
SM-FeSV v-FMS   (960)  -----RLLRPWQRTPPVAR (978)
HZ5-FeSV v-FMS  (960)  ----------- -----------------LL (991)
```

Dashes indicate identity with feline FMS. There is close homology between FMS proteins in this region: 14 amino acids are substituted in the terminal region of SM-FeSV and in HZ5-FeSV an 11 bp deletion substitutes two leucine residues before the termination codon. The sequences of SM-FeSV and HZ5-FeSV v-FMS are identical up to the 14 C-terminal residues of SM-FeSV (Besmer *et al.*, 1986).

Databank file names and accession numbers

	GENE	EMBL	SWISSPROT	REFERENCES
Human	CSF1R	Hscfms X03663	KFMS_HUMAN P07333	Coussens *et al.*, 1986
Human	FRT	Hsfrt D00133	KFRT_HUMAN P16057	Matsushime *et al.*, 1987
Human	FLT1	Hsflt X51602	KFLT_HUMAN P17948	Shibuya *et al.*, 1990
Human	FLT4			Galland *et al.*, 1993
Mouse	Fms	Mmfmscr X06368	KFMS_MOUSE P09581	Rothwell and Rohrschneider, 1987
				van der Geer and Hunter, 1990
Mouse	Flt-3	Mmflt3 X59398		Rosnet *et al.*, 1991
Feline	Fms	Fdfmsc J03149	KFMS_FELCA P13369	Woolford *et al.*, 1988
SM-FeSV	v-fms	Resmonc K01643	KFMS_FSVMD P00545	Hampe *et al.*, 1984, 1989
				Smola *et al.*, 1991

Reviews

Rohrschneider, L.R. and Woolford, J. (1991). Structural and functional comparison of viral and cellular *fms*. Seminars Virol., 2, 385–395.
Sherr, C.J. (1988). The *fms* oncogene. Biochim. Biophys. Acta, 948, 225–243.

Papers

Baker, A.H., Ridge, S.A., Hoy, T., Cachia, P.G., Culligan, D., Baines, P., Whittaker, J.A., Jacobs, A. and Padua, R.A. (1993). Expresion of the colony-stimulating factor 1 receptor in B lymphocytes. Oncogene, 8, 371–378.
Besmer, P., Lader, E., George, P.C., Bergold, P.J., Qui, F.-H., Zuckerman, E.E. and Hardy, W.D. (1986). A new acute transforming feline retrovirus with fms homology specifies a C-terminally truncated version of the c-*fms* protein that is different from SM-feline sarcoma virus v-*fms* protein. J. Virol., 60, 194–203.
Borzillo, G.V., Ashmun, R.A. and Sherr, C.J. (1990). Macrophage lineage switching of murine early pre-B lymphoid cells expressing transduced *fms* genes. Mol. Cell. Biol., 10, 2703–2714.
Carlberg, K., Tapley, P., Haystead, C. and Rohrschneider, L. (1991). The role of kinase activity and the kinase insert region in ligand-induced internalization and degradation of the c-*fms* protein. EMBO J., 10, 877–883.
Courtneidge, S., Dhand, R., Pilat, D., Twamley, G.M., Waterfield, M.D. and Roussel, M.F. (1993). Activation of Src family kinases by colony stimulating factor-1, and their association with its receptor. EMBO J., 12, 943–950.
Coussens, L., Van Beveren, C., Smith, D., Chen, E., Mitchell, R.L., Isacke, C.M., Verma, I.M. and Ullrich, A. (1986). Structural alteration of viral homologue of receptor proto-oncogene *fms* at carboxyl terminus. Nature 320, 277–280.
de-Vries, C., Escobedo, J.A., Ueno, H., Houck, K., Ferrara, N. and Williams, L.T. (1992). The *fms*-like tyrosine kinase, a receptor for vascular endothelial growth factor. Science, 255, 989–991.
Donner, L., Fedele, L.A., Garon, C.F., Anderson, S.J. and Sherr, C.J. (1982). McDonough feline sarcoma virus: characterization of the molecularly cloned provirus and its feline oncogene (v-*fms*). J. Virol., 41, 489–500.
Downing., J.R., Margolis, B.L., Zilberstein, A., Ashmun, R.A., Ullrich, A., Sherr, C.J. and Schlessinger, J. (1989). Phospholipase C-γ, a substrate for PDGF receptor kinase, is not phosphorylated on tyrosine during the mitogenic response to CSF-1. EMBO J., 8, 3345–3350.
Downing, J.R., Roussel, M.F. and Sherr, C.J. (1991). Ligand and protein kinase C downmodulate the colony-stimulating factor 1 receptor by independent mechanisms. Mol. Cell. Biol., 9, 2890–2896.
Galland, F., Karamysheva, A., Pebusque, M.-J., Borg, J.-P., Rottapel, R., Dubreuil, P., Rosnet, O. and Birnbaum, D. (1993). The *FLT4* gene encodes a transmembrane tyrosine kinase related to the vascular endothelial growth factor receptor. Oncogene, 8, 1233–1240.
Gisselbrecht, S., Fichelson, S., Sola, B., Bordereaux, D., Hampe, A., Andre, A., Galibert, F. and Tambourin, P. (1987). Frequent c-*fms* activation by proviral insertion in mouse myeloblastic leukemias. Nature, 329, 259–261.
Guilhot, S., Hampe, A., D'Auriol, L. and Galibert, F. (1987). Nucleotide sequence analysis of the LTRs and *env* genes of SM-FeSV and GA-FeSV. Virology, 161, 252–258.
Hampe, A., Gobet, M., Sherr, C.J. and Galibert, F. (1984). Nucleotide sequence of the feline retroviral oncogene v-*fms* shows unexpected homology with oncogenes encoding tyrosine specific protein kinases. Proc. Natl Acad. Sci. USA, 81, 85–89.
Hampe, A., Shamoon, B.-M., Gobet, M., Sherr, C.J. and Galibert, F. (1989). Nucleotide sequence and structure of the human *FMS* proto-oncogene. Oncogene Res., 4, 9–17.
Heard, J.M., Roussel, M.F., Rettenmier, C.W. and Sherr, C.J. (1987). Multilineage hematopoietic disorders induced by transplantation of bone marrow cells expressing the v-*fms* oncogene. Cell, 51, 663–673.
Heidaran, M.A., Molloy, C.J., Pangelinan, M., Choudhury, G.G., Wang, L.-M., Fleming, T.P., Sakaguchi, A.Y. and Pierce, J.H. (1992). Activation of the colony-stimulating factor 1 receptor leads to the rapid tyrosine phosphorylation of GTPase-activating protein and activation of cellular p21^{ras}. Oncogene, 7, 147–152.
Inaba, T., Yamada, N., Gotoda, T., Shimano, H., Shimada, M., Momomura, K., Kadowaki, T., Motoyoshi, K., Tsukada, T., Morisaki, N., Saito, Y., Yoshida, S., Takaku, F. and Yazaki, Y. (1992). Expression of M-CSF receptor encoded by c-*fms* on smooth muscle cells derived from arteriosclerotic lesion. J. Biol. Chem., 267, 5693–5699.
Jackowski, S., Rettenmier, C.W., Sherr, C.J. and Rock, C.O. (1986). A guanine nucleotide-dependent phos-

phatidylinositol-4,5-diphosphate phospholipase C in cells transformed by the v-*fms* and v-*fes* oncogenes. J. Biol. Chem., 261, 4978–4985.

Kaplan, D.R., Whitman, M., Schaffhausen, B., Pallas, D.C., White, M. Cantley, L. and Roberts, T.M. (1987). Common elements in growth factor stimulation and oncogenic transformation: 85kd phosphoprotein and phosphatidylinositol kinase activity. Cell, 50, 1021–1029.

Lee, A.W.-M. and Nienhuis, A.W. (1992). Functional dissection of structural domains in the receptor for colony-stimulating factor-1. J. Biol. Chem., 267, 16472–16483.

Lyman, S.D. and Rohrschneider, L.R. (1987). Analysis of functional domains of the v-*fms*-encoded protein of Susan McDonough strain feline sarcoma virus by linker insertion mutagenesis. Mol. Cell. Biol., 7, 3287–3296.

Lyman, S.D., James, L., Zappone, J., Sleath, P.R., Beckmann, M.P. and Bird, T. (1993). Characterization of the protein encoded by the flt3 (flk2) receptor-like tyrosine kinase gene. Oncogene, 8, 815–822.

McDonough, S.K., Larsen, S., Brodey, R.S., Stock, N.D. and Hardy, W.D. (1971). A transmissible feline fibrosarcoma of viral origin. Cancer Res., 31, 953–956.

Maroc, N., Rottapel, R., Rosnet, O., Marchetto, S., Lavezzi, C., Mannoni, P., Birnbaum, D. and Dubreuil, P. (1993). Biochemical characterization and analysis of the transforming potential of FLT3/FLK2 receptor tyrosine kinase. Oncogene, 8, 909–918.

Matsushime, H., Yoshida, M.C., Sasaki, M. and Shibuya, M. (1987). A possible new member of tyrosine kinase family, human *frt* sequence, is highly conserved in vertebrates and located on human chromosome 13. Jpn. J. Cancer Res., 78, 655–661.

Muller, R., Slamon, D.J., Adamson, E.D., Tremblay, J.M., Muller, D., Cline, M.J. and Verma, I.M. (1983a). Transcription of c-*onc* genes c-*ras*^{Ki} and c-*fms* during mouse development. Mol. Cell. Biol., 3, 1062–1069.

Muller, R., Tremblay, J.M., Adamson, E.D. and Verma, I.M. (1983b). Tissue and cell type-specific expression of two human c-*onc* genes. Nature, 304, 454–456.

Pampfer, S., Daiter, E., Barad, D. and Pollard, J.W. (1992). Expression of the colony-stimulating factor-1 receptor (c-*fms* proto-oncogene product) in the human uterus and placenta. Biol. Reprod., 46, 48–57.

Reedijk, M., Liu, X., van der Geer, P., Letwin, K., Waterfield, M.D., Hunter, T. and Pawson, T. (1992). Tyr721 regulates specific binding of the CSF-1 receptor kinase insert to PI 3'-kinase SH2 domains: a model for SH2-mediated receptor-target interactions. EMBO J., 11, 1365–1372.

Reith, A.D., Ellis, C., Maroc, N., Pawson, T., Bernstein, A. and Dubreuil, P. (1993). 'W' mutant forms of the fms receptor tyrosine kinase act in a dominant manner to suppress CSF-1 dependent cellular transformation. Oncogene, 8, 45–53.

Regenstreif, L.J. and Rossant, J. (1989). Expression of the c-*fms* proto-oncogene and of the cytokine, CSF-1, during mouse embryogenesis. Devel. Biol., 133, 284–294.

Rettenmier, C.W., Sacca, R., Furman, W.L., Roussel, M.F., Holt, J.T., Nienhuis, A.W., Stanley, E.R. and Sherr, C.J. (1986). Expression of the human c-*fms* proto-oncogene product (colony-stimulating factor-1 receptor) on peripheral blood monomuclear cells and choriocarcinoma cell lines. J. Clin. Invest., 77, 1740–1746.

Ridge, S.A., Worwood, M., Oscier, D., Jacobs, A. and Padua, R.A. (1990). *FMS* mutations in myelodysplastic, leukemic and normal subjects. Proc. Natl Acad. Sci. USA, 87, 1377–1380.

Roberts, W.M., Look, A.T., Roussel, M.F. and Sherr, C.J. (1988). Tandem linkage of human CSF-1 receptor (c-*fms*) and PDGF receptor genes. Cell, 55, 655–661.

Rohrschneider, L.R. and Metcalf, D. (1989). Induction of macrophage colony-stimulating factor-dependent growth and differentiation after introduction of the murine c-*fms* gene into FDC-P1 cells. Mol. Cell. Biol., 9, 5081–5092.

Rosnet, O., Marchetto, S., deLapeyriere, O. and Birnbaum, D. (1991). Murine Flt3, a gene encoding a novel tyrosine kinase receptor of the PDGF/CSF1R family. Oncogene, 6, 1641–1650.

Rothwell, V.M. and Rohrschneider, L.R. (1987). Murine c-*fms* cDNA: cloning, sequence analysis and retroviral expression. Oncogene Res., 1, 311–324.

Roussel, M.F., Dull, T.J., Rettenmier, C.W., Ralph, P. Ullrich, A. and Sherr, C.J. (1987). Transforming potential of the c-*fms* proto-oncogene (CSF-1 receptor). Nature, 325, 549–552.

Roussel, M.F., Downing, J.R., Rettenmier, C.W., and Sherr, C.J. (1988). A point mutation in the extracellular domain of the human CSF-1 receptor (c-*fms* proto-oncogene product) activates its transforming potential. Cell, 55, 979–988.

Roussel, M.F., Shurtleff, S.A., Downing, J.R. and Sherr, C.J. (1990). A point mutation at tyrosine-809 in the human colony-stimulating factor-1 receptor impairs mitogenesis without abrogating tyrosine kinase activity, association with phosphatidylinositol 3-kinase, or induction of c-*fos* and *junB* genes. Proc. Natl Acad. Sci. USA, 87, 6738–6742.

Roussel, M.F., Cleveland, J.L., Shurtleff, S.A. and Sherr, C.J. (1991). *Myc* rescue of a mutant CSF-1 receptor impaired in mitogenic signalling. Nature, 353, 361–363.

Rowley, P.T., Farley, B., Giuliano, R., LaBella, S. and Leary, J.F. (1992). Induction of the *fms* proto-oncogene product in HL-60 cells by vitamin D: a flow cytometric analysis. Leukemia Res., 16, 403–410.

Sacca, R., Stanley, E.R., Sherr, C.J. and Rettenmier, C.W. (1986). Specific binding of the mononuclear phagocyte colony-stimulating factor CSF-1 to the product of the v-*fms* oncogene. Proc. Natl Acad. Sci. USA, 83, 3331–3335.

Shibuya, M., Yamaguchi, S., Yamane, A., Ikeda, T., Tojo, A., Matsushime, H. and Sato, M. (1990). Nucleotide sequence and expression of a novel human receptor-type tyrosine kinase gene (*flt*) closely related to the *fms* family. Oncogene, 5, 519–524.

Shurtleff, S.A., Downing, J.R., Rock, C.O., Hawkins, S.A., Roussel, M.F. and Sherr, C.J. (1990). Structural features of the colony-stimulating factor 1 receptor that affect its association with phosphatidylinositol 3-kinase. EMBO J., 9, 2415–2421.

Smola, U., Hennig, D., Hadwiger-Fangmeier, A., Schutz, B., Pfaff, E., Niemann, H. and Tamura, T. (1991). Reassessment of the v-*fms* sequence: threonine phosphorylation of the COOH-terminal domain. J. Virol., 65, 6181–6187.

Stanley, E.R., Bartocci, A., Patinkin, D., Rosendaal, M. and Bradley, T.R. (1986). Regulation of very primitive, multipotent, hematopoietic cells by hemopoietin-1. Cell, 45, 667–674.

Tapley, P., Kazlaukas, A., Cooper, J.A. and Rohrschneider, L.R. (1990). Macrophage colony-stimulating factor-induced tyrosine phosphorylation of c-*fms* proteins expressed in FDC-P1 and BALB/c 3T3 cells. Mol. Cell. Biol., 10, 2528–2538.

Taylor, G.R., Reedijk, M., Rothwell, V., Rohrschneider, L. and Pawson, T. (1989). The unique insert of cellular and viral *fms* protein tyrosine kinase domains is dispensable for enzymatic and transforming activities. EMBO J., 8, 2029–2037.

van Daalen-Wetters, T., Hawkins, S.A., Roussel, M.F. and Sherr, C.J. (1992). Random mutagenesis of CSF-1 receptor (FMS) reveals multiple sites for activating mutations within the extracellular domain. EMBO J., 11, 551–557.

van der Geer, P. and Hunter, T. (1990). Identification of tyrosine 706 in the kinase insert as the major colony-stimulating factor 1 (CSF-1)-stimulated autophosphorylation site in the CSF-1 receptor in a murine macrophage cell line. Mol. Cell. Biol., 10, 2991–3002.

Woolford, J., Rothwell, V. and Rohrschneider, L.R. (1985). Characterization of the human c-*fms* gene product and its expression in cells of the monocyte-macrophage lineage. Mol. Cell. Biol., 5, 3458–3466.

Woolford, J., McAuliffe, A. and Rohrschneider, L.R. (1988). Activation of the feline c-*fms* proto-oncogene: multiple alterations are required to generate a fully transformed phenotype. Cell 55, 965–977.

Zander, N.F., Cool, D.E., Diltz, C.D., Rohrschneider, L.R., Krebs, E.G. and Fischer, E.H. (1993). Suppression of v-*fms*-induced transformation by overexpression of a truncated T-cell protein tyrosine phosphatase. Oncogene, 8, 1175–1182.

DBL

DBL (or *MCF2*) was identified by NIH 3T3 fibroblast transfection of DNA from a human *diffuse B cell lymphoma* (Fasano *et al.*, 1984; Eva and Aaronson, 1985).

Related genes

The central region of DBL has sequence homology with human BCR, VAV and RAS–GRF nucleotide exchange factor (Shou *et al.*, 1992).

Cross-species homology

The central region of DBL is 22% homologous to the corresponding regions of *Saccharomyces cerevisiae* CDC24 and CDC25 (see **ABL**).

Transformation

Expressed in Ewing's sarcoma (tumours of neuroectodermic origin; Vecchio *et al.*, 1989). Transforming potential enhanced 50- to 70-fold on substitution of 5′ sequences to form oncogenic *DBL* (Noguchi *et al.*, 1988). *DBL* does not induce neoplasia in transgenic mice but animals that express the DBL protein in their lenses develop cataracts. *DBL* therefore appears capable of interfering with the ability of lens epithelial cells to differentiate into lens fibre cells (Eva *et al.*, 1991).

	DBL/MCF2
Nucleotides (kb)	45
Chromosome	
Human	Xq27
Mouse	X
Exons	At least 6
mRNA (kb)	
Human	3.9 (testis, 5.3 (fetal brain)
Mouse	4.0, 4.5*
	2.8 (oncogenic)
Amino acids	925 (DBL)
	478 (oncogenic)
Mass (kDa) (predicted)	108
(expressed)	p115 (DBL)
	p66 (oncogenic)
Protein half-life (h)	1 (p115^{dbl})
	5–6 (p66)

*Alternative splicing of mouse *Mcf-2* can delete an exon (126 bp) encoding 42 amino acids that is not removed in man.

Cellular location

Cytoplasmic: associates with cytoskeletal actin (Graziani *et al.*, 1989).

Tissue location

Highly tissue specific: brain, adrenal glands, gonads.

Protein function

Unknown. Microinjection of DBL causes GVBD and activation of H1 histone kinase in oocytes (Graziani *et al.*, 1992). *In vitro* it acts as a guanine nucleotide exchange factor for CDC42Hs, the human homologue of the *S. cerevisiae* protein CDC42Sc (Hart *et al.*, 1992).

Sequence of human DBL

```
  (1)    MAEANPRRGKMRFRRNAASFPGNLHLVLVLRPTSFLQRTFTDIGFWFSQEDFMPKLPVVMLSSVSDLLTYIDDKQLTPE
 (80)    LGGTLQYCHSEWIIFRNAIENFALTVKEMAQMLQSFGTELAETELPDDIPSIEEILAIRAERYHLLKNDITAVTKEGKIL
(160)    LTNLEVPDTEGAVSSRLECHRQISGDWQTINKLLTQVHDMETAFDGFWEKHQLKMEQYLQLWKFEQDFQQLVTEVEFLLN
(240)    QQAELADVTGTIAQVKQKIKKLENLDENSQELLSKAQFVILHGHKLAANHHYALDLICQRCNELRYLSDILVNEIKAKRI
(320)    QLSRTFKMHKLLQQARQCCDEGECLLANQEIDKFQSKEDAQKALQDIENFLEMALPFINYEPETLQYEFDVILSPELK
                                                                                      ΔΔ
(398)    VQMKTIQLKLENIRSIFENQQAGFRNLADKHVRPIQFVVPTPENLVTSGTPFFSSKQGKKTWRQNQSNLKIEVVPDCQEK

(478)    RSSGPSSSLDNGNSLDVLKN HVLNELIQTERVYVRELYTVLLGYRAEMDNPEMFDLMPPLLRNKKDILFGNMAEIYEFH
                             Δ
(557)    NDIFLSSLENCAHAPERVGPCFLERKDDFQMYAKYCQNKPRSETIWRKYSECAFFQECQRKLKHRLRLDSYLLKPVQRIT
(637)    KYQLLLKELLKYSKDCEGSALLKKALDAMLDLLKSVNDSMHQIAINGYIGNLNELGKMIMQGGFSVWIGHKKGATKMKDL
(717)    ARFKPMQRHLFLYEKAIVFCKRRVESGEGSDRYPSYSFKHCWKMDEVGITEYVKGDNRKFEIWYGEKEEVYIVQASNVDV
(797)    KMTWLKEIRNILLKQQELLTVKKRKQQDQLTERDKFQISLQQNDEKQQGAFISTEETELEHTSTVVEVCEAIASVQAEAN
(877)    TVWTEASQSAEISEEPAEWSSNYFYPTYDENEEENRPLMRPVSEMALLY (925)
```

Regions of homology with CDC24 and BCR are underlined. There is N-terminal homology with vimentin and a 275 amino acid region of homology with VAV (Galland *et al.*, 1992). The MCF-2 (Δ) and DBL (ΔΔ) oncogene breakpoints are indicated (the DBL breakpoint lies within an *MCF2* exon).

Structure of DBL/MCF2, VAV and CDC24 proteins

DBL and *MCF2* represent two activated versions of the same proto-oncogene. Activation of the *DBL* oncogene occurs by 5′ fusion of 50 amino acids encoded by an unrelated human gene to 428 amino acids encoded by the 3′ portion of *DBL*, with the loss of the first 497 amino acids of DBL. There is only one (conservative) substitution in the C-terminal 428 amino acids of oncogenic DBL. The loss of the N-terminal 497 amino acids of DBL, rather than the properties of the N-terminus acquired by oncogenic DBL, is responsible for the transforming activity (Ron *et al.*, 1989). In MCF2 397 amino acids are removed.

Transfection of NIH 3T3 cells with DNA from a human nodular poorly differentiated lymphoma (NPDL) generates *NPDL–DBL* that is homologous to oncogenic *DBL*. This encodes a 3.5 kb mRNA and a 76 kDa protein (Eva *et al.*, 1987).

DBL

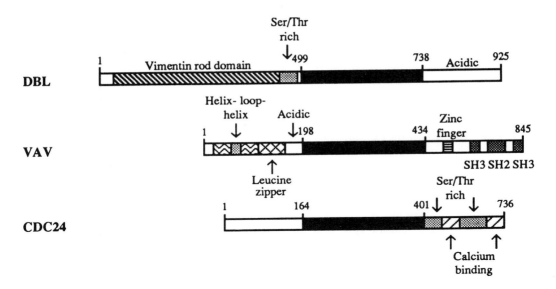

Amino acids 498–735 of DBL are 22–29% homologous to residues 163–400 and 501–755 of the CDC24 and BCR proteins respectively (Ron *et al.*, 1991). Small deletions within this region completely abolish the transforming activity of DBL. In yeast CLS4/CDC24 the region of DBL homology is important for Ca²⁺-modulated bud assembly (Miyamoto *et al.*, 1991). Cells transformed by *DBL* form multinucleated cells, as happens in *cdc*24 mutants arrested at the non-permissive temperature.

Databank file names and accession numbers

	GENE	EMBL	SWISSPROT	REFERENCES
Human	DBL	Hsdblpro X12556	DLB_HUMAN P10911	Ron *et al.*, 1988
			P14919	Eva *et al.*, 1988
				Noguchi *et al.*, 1988
Human	DBL	Hsdbltp J03639		Eva *et al.*, 1988
		Hsmcf2po X13230		
Mouse	Mcf-2	Mmmcf2po X57298		Galland *et al.*, 1991

Papers

Eva, A. and Aaronson, S.A. (1985). Isolation of a new human oncogene from a diffuse B-cell lymphoma. Nature, 316, 273–275.

Eva, A., Vecchio, G., Diamond, M., Tronick, S.R., Ron, D. and Aaronson, S.A. (1987). Independently activated *dbl* oncogenes exhibit similar yet distinct structural alterations. Oncogene, 1, 355–360.

Eva, A., Vecchio, G., Rao, C.D., Tronick, S.R. and Aaronson, S.A. (1988). The predicted DBL oncogene product defines a distinct class of transforming proteins. Proc. Natl Acad. Sci. USA, 85, 2061–2065.

Eva, A., Graziani, G., Zannini, M., Merin, L.M., Khillan, J.S. and Overbeek, P.A. (1991). Dominant dysplasia of the lens in transgenic mice expressing the *dbl* oncogene. New Biologist, 3, 158–168.

Fasano, O., Birnbaum, D., Edlund, L., Fogh, J., and Wigler, M. (1984). New human transforming genes detected by a tumorigenicity assay. Mol. Cell. Biol., 4, 1695–1705.

Galland, F., Pirisi, V., deLapeyriere, O. and Birnbaum, D. (1991). Restriction and complexity of *mcf2* proto-oncogene expression. Oncogene, 6, 833–839.

Galland, F., Katzav, S. and Birnbaum, D. (1992). The products of the *mcf-2* and *vav* proto-onocgenes and of the yeast gene *cdc*-24 share sequence similarities. Oncogene, 7, 585–587.

Graziani, G., Ron, D., Eva, A. and Srivastava, S.K. (1989). The human *dbl*-proto-oncogene product is a cytoplasmic phosphoprotein which is associated with the cytoskeletal matrix. Oncogene, 4, 823–829.

Graziani, G., Nebreda, A.R., Srivastava, S., Santos, E. and Eva, A. (1992). Induction of *Xenopus* oocyte meiotic maturation by the *dbl* oncogene product. Oncogene, 7, 229–235.

Hart, M.J., Eva, A., Evans, T., Aaronson, S.A. and Cerione, R.A. (1991). Catalysis of guanine nucleotide exchange on the CDC42Hs protein by the *dbl* oncogene product. Nature, 354, 311–314.

Miyamoto, S., Ohya, Y., Sano, Y., Sakaguchi, S., Iida-, H. and Anraku, Y. (1991). A DBL-homologous region of the yeast CLS4/CDC24 gene product is important for Ca^{2+}-modulated bud assembly. Biochem. Biophys. Res. Commun., 181, 604–610.

Noguchi, T., Galland, F., Batoz, M., Mattei, R.G. and Birnbaum, D. (1988). Activation of a *mcf*.2 oncogene by deletion of amino-terminal coding sequences. Oncogene, 3, 709–715.

Ron, D., Tronick, S.R., Aaronson, S.A. and Eva, A. (1988). Molecular cloning and characterization of the human *dbl* proto-oncogene: evidence that its overexpression is sufficient to transform NIH/3T3 cells. EMBO J., 7, 2465–2473.

Ron, D., Graziani, G., Aaronson, S.A. and Eva, A. (1989). The N-terminal region of proto-*dbl* down regulates its transforming activity. Oncogene, 4, 1067–1072.

Ron, D., Zannini, M., Lewis, M., Wickner, R.B., Hunt, L.T., Graziani, G., Tronick, S.R., Aaronson, S.A. and Eva, A. (1991). A region of proto-*dbl* essential for its transforming activity shows sequence similarity to a yeast cell cycle gene, CDC24, and the human breakpoint cluster gene, *bcr*. New Biologist, 3, 372–379.

Shou, C., Farnsworth, C.L., Neel, B.G. and Feig, L.A. (1992). Molecular cloning of cDNAs encoding a guanine-nucleotide-releasing factor for Ras p21. Nature, 358, 351–354.

Vecchio, G., Cavazzana, A., Triche, T., Ron, T., Reynolds, P. and Eva, A. (1989). Expression of the *dbl* proto-oncogene in Ewing's sarcomas. Oncogene, 4, 897–900.

DNA Tumour Viruses

The DNA tumour viruses are of considerable interest because in some of them genes have been identified which produce cell-transforming proteins; that is, the oncogene product has evolved to stimulate cells after viral infection. Thus the oncoproteins of papovaviruses (SV40 and polyoma), adenoviruses and papillomaviruses function at least in part by binding to and thus inhibiting the normal activity of the products of tumour suppressor genes (*P53* and retinoblastoma). However, even for these genes, demonstration of their transforming capacity depends critically on the experimental assay system employed. The Epstein–Barr herpesvirus carries one gene that is consistently expressed in Burkitt's lymphoma and another that is required for immortalization of primary B cells by EBV and is tumorigenic *in vitro*. For other DNA viruses (e.g. hepatitis B virus (HBV) and the herpesviruses HSV-1, HSV-2 and human cytomegalovirus) there is circumstantial evidence for their association with the development of a variety of human cancers and HBV is established as a causative agent in the vast majority of primary hepatocellular carcinomas that are responsible for up to 1 million deaths per annum worldwide (Harris, 1990; zur Hausen, 1991). However, the genomes of these viruses contain no known oncogenes, although the hepatitis B virus protein HBx *trans*-activates a variety of promoters commonly involved in transformation (Kekule *et al.*, 1993) and causes tumours in transgenic mice (Kim *et al.*, 1991).

Papers

Harris, C.C. (1990). Hepatocellular carcinogenesis: recent advances and speculations. Cancer Cells, 2, 146–148.
Kekule, A.S., Lauer, U., Weiss, L., Luber, B. and Hofschneider, P.H. (1993). Hepatitis B virus transactivator HBx uses a tumour promoter signalling pathway. Nature, 361, 742–745.
Kim, C.-M., Koike, K., Saito, I., Miyamura, T. and Jay, G. (1991). *HBx* gene of hepatitis B virus induces liver cancer in transgenic mice. Nature, 351, 317–320.
zur Hausen, H. (1991). Viruses in human cancers. Science, 254, 1167–1173.

Simian vacuolating virus 40 (SV40)

SV40 was first isolated from green monkey cells being used to prepare poliovirus vaccine. It was originally called vacuolating agent from the cytopathic effect observed in infected cells.

Genome

The genome consists of a 5227 base single circular DNA, which encodes six proteins; four of these are synthesized late in infection.

Related genes

The large T antigens of the human BK and JC papovaviruses have high structural and functional homology with SV40 T antigen. The T antigen sequence involved in p105^{RB} binding is conserved in adenovirus E1A, BK, JC and polyoma and HPV E7 (see **EBV** below).

Transformation

In vitro SV40 transforms cells of many non-permissive and semi-permissive species including mouse and human. A variety of human cells can be immortalized by SV40, including breast and trachial epithelial cells and foreskin keratinocytes. SV40 can also immortalize fibroblasts but more often these cells undergo senescence following infection. SV40-immortalized keratinocytes have been shown to retain the capacity to differentiate, with the viral genome being maintained in episomal form (Lechner and Laimins, 1991). Such cells may provide a model system for the study of human carcinomas, many of which are comprised of undifferentiated cells that can be established as immortal cell lines *in vitro* (Wu and Rheinwald, 1981). However, human cells may be described as semi-permissive for SV40 as infection occasionally leads to a lytic cycle with release of progeny virus.

Human BK and JC papovaviruses transform mammalian cells *in vitro* and are tumorigenic in rodents (Tavis *et al.*, 1990; Moens *et al.*, 1990; Marshall *et al.*, 1991).

Cells transfected with SV40 that are non-transforming may be rendered strongly tumorigenic by co-expression of *Hras* or *Nras* oncogenes (Fang *et al.*, 1992).

In transgenic mice SV40 T antigen under the control of its normal regulatory elements induces choroid plexus papillomas (Chen and van Dyke, 1991). Expression of high levels of T antigen in transgenic mice is correlated with the development of hepatocarcinoma in all animals and, in a small proportion (10%), of lung carcinoma (Dubois *et al.*, 1991). The human growth hormone-releasing factor (GRF) specifically directs expression of T antigen in thymic epithelial cells and the mice develop thymic hyperplasia (Moll *et al.*, 1992).

	Small t antigen	Large T antigen
Amino acids	174	708
Mass (kDa)		
(predicted)	20	82
(expressed)	17	90–100
Protein half-life	>4 h (nucleus); <30 min (plasma membrane)	

Cellular location

Small t antigen: Nucleus and cytoplasm.
Large T antigen: Nucleus (95%); plasma membrane (5%).

Protein structure

Small t antigen: N-terminal 82 amino acids identical to those of SV40 T antigen.
Large T antigen: Extensively post-translationally modified (phosphorylation, *O*-glycosylation, palmitoylation, poly-ADP-ribosylation, N-terminal acetylation, adenylation).

Protein function

T and t antigens are the first genes expressed after infection.

t ANTIGEN

Binds to protein phosphatase 2A, p32, p56 and tubulin. t Antigen has been shown to *trans*-activate polymerase II promoters but the effect is dependent on the type of assay system used, requiring the target gene to be transiently transfected (Rajan *et al.*, 1991).

T ANTIGEN

T Antigen is absolutely essential for replicative functions in the lytic infection of permissive cells but alone can transform a wide range of cell types. It is a potent transcriptional regulator activating expression of late viral genes and repressing transcription of early genes. AP-2-dependent transcription is reduced by T antigen binding to the transcription factor AP-2 (Mitchell *et al.*, 1987). T Antigen binds specifically to the SV40 origin of replication, whereupon its intrinsic DNA helicase and ATPase activities unwind the viral template. It forms a complex with DNA polymerase α which is presumed to lead to the synthesis of new DNA strands.

Primary mouse embryo fibroblasts are non-permissive for SV40 and infection causes immortalization of a small fraction of the cells. Immortalization correlates with the capacity of T antigen to bind p53 (Zhu *et al.*, 1991). The induction of transformed foci in normal human cell lines by SV40 is also dependent on the formation of stable complexes between T antigen and p53 (Lin and Simmons, 1991). The formation of hetero-oligomers with p53 (which inhibits T antigen association with DNA polymerase α) may also inhibit the anti-proliferative activity of p53 and the expression of wild-type p53 prevents SV40 transformation (Fukasawa *et al.*, 1991; Michael-Michalovitz *et al.*, 1991). In human endometrial stromal cells transfected with SV40, T antigen activates transcription of ornithine decarboxylase (Rinehart *et al.*, 1991).

In addition to associating with p53, T antigen also forms multimeric complexes with itself and with p105^{RB}, p68 and hsp70.

Structure, protein binding and phosphorylation sites of T antigen

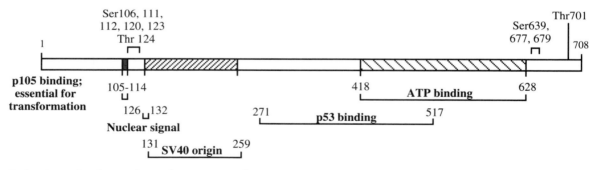

T Antigen (and its cleaved N-terminal region) are phosphorylated (Thr124) by p34^{cdc2} (McVey *et al.*, 1989) which decreases the extent of nuclear accumulation (Jans *et al.*, 1991). Phosphorylated T antigen binds much more tightly to the replication origin and becomes highly efficient at catalysing replication *in vitro*. Replication catalysed by T antigen is also stimulated by the action of protein phosphatase 2A (Cohen, 1989) which dephosphorylates serine residues in the protein (Virshup *et al.*, 1989). Both the large T and small t antigens of SV40 and polyoma associate with the catalytic and one of the regulatory (A) subunits of protein phosphatase 2A (Pallas *et al.*, 1990).

The rate of transport of T antigen to the nucleus is controlled by casein kinase II phosphorylation of Ser111 and Ser112 in the domain immediately flanking residues 126–132 that comprise the nuclear localization sequence (Rihs *et al.*, 1991). T Antigen binds to the human nuclear antigen, p68, an RNA-dependent ATPase (Iggo and Lane, 1989). p68 is one of a family of DEAD box proteins (sequence motif: Asp–Glu–Ala–Asp; Linder *et al.*, 1989) found in mammals, *Drosophila*, *Saccharomyces cerevisiae* and *E. coli* that are involved in translation, ribosome assembly, mitochondrial splicing, spermatogenesis and embryogenesis. This family includes eIF4-A, srmB,

MSS116 and *vasa* protein (Grifo *et al.*, 1984; Nishi *et al.*, 1988; Hay *et al.*, 1988; Seraphin *et al.*, 1989). The binding site for p68 on T antigen lies in the ATPase region, occupation of which by specific antibody blocks the replicative functions of large T.

Sequences of SV40 small t and large T antigens

```
t antigen   (1)    MDKVLNREESLQLMDLLGLERSAWGNIPLMRKAYLKKCKEFHPDKGGDEEKMKKMNTLY
T antigen   (1)    ----------------------------------------------------------

t antigen   (60)   KKMEDGVKYAHQPDFGGFWDATEVFASSLNPGVDAMYCKQWPECAKKMSANCICLLCLLR
T antigen   (60)   --------------------IPTYGTDEWEQWWNAFNEENLFCSEEMPSSDDEATAD

t antigen   (120)  MKHENRKLYRKDPLVWVDCYCFDCFRMWFGLDLCEGTLLLWCDIIGQTTYRDLKL  (174)
T antigen   (120)  SQHSTPPKKKRKVEDPKDFPSELLSFLSHAVFSNRTLACFAIYTTKEKAALLYKKIMEKY

T antigen   (180)  SVTFISRHNSYNHNILFFLTPHRHRVSAINNYAQKLCTFSFLICKGVNKEYLMYSALTRD
            (240)  PFSVIEESLPGGLKEHDFNPEEAEETKQVSWKLVTEYAMETKCDDVLLLLGMYLEFQYSF
            (300)  EMCLKCIKKEQPSHYKYHEKHYANAAIFADSKNQKTICQQAVDTVLAKKRVDSLQLTREQ
            (360)  MLTNRFNDLLDRMDIMFGSTGSADIEEWMAGVAWLHCLLPKMDSVVYDFLKCMVYNIPKK
            (420)  RYWLFKGPIDSGKTTLAAALLELCGGKALNVNLPLDRLNFELGVAIDQFLVVFEDVKGTG
            (480)  GESRDLPSGQGINNLDNLRDYLDGSVKVNLEKKHLNKRTQIFTPGIVTMNEFSVPKTLQA
            (540)  RFVKQIDFRAKDYLKHCLERSEFLLEKRIIQSGIALLLMLIWYRPVAEFAQSIQSRIVEW
            (600)  KERLDKEFSLSVYQKMKFNVAMGIGVLDWLRNSDDDDEDSQENADKNEDGGEKNMEDSGH
            (660)  ETGIDSQSQGSFQAPQSSQSVHDHNQPYHICRGFTCFKKPPTPPPEPET  (708)
```

The initial 82 residues of SV40 small t and large T antigens are encoded by the same nucleotide sequence. Underlined: T antigen nuclear location sequence.

Databank file names and accession numbers

GENE	EMBL	SWISSPROT	REFERENCES
SV40 t antigen	SV40xx V01380	TASM_SV40 P03081	Fiers *et al.*, 1978
	Papsv4cg J02400		Reddy *et al.*, 1978
SV40 T antigen	SV40xx V01380	TALA_SV40 P03070	Fiers *et al.*, 1978
	Papsv4cg J02400		Reddy *et al.*, 1978
			Kalderon *et al.*, 1984

Reviews

Butel, J.S. and Jarvis, D.L. (1986). The plasma membrane-associated form of SV40 large tumor antigen: biochemical and biological properties. Biochim. Biophys. Acta, 865, 171–195.
Challberg, M.D. and Kelly, T.J. (1989). Animal virus DNA replication. Annu. Rev. Biochem., 58, 671–717.
Cohen, P. (1989). The structure and regulation of protein phosphatases. Annu. Rev. Biochem., 58, 453–508.
Prives, C. (1990). The replication functions of SV40 T antigen are regulated by phosphorylation. Cell, 61, 735–738.

Papers

Chen, J.D. and van Dyke, T. (1991). Uniform cell-autonomous tumorigenesis of the choroid plexus by papovavirus large T antigens. Mol. Cell. Biol., 11, 5968–5976.

Dubois, N., Bennoun, M., Allemand, I., Molina, T., Grimber, G., Daudet-Monsac, M., Abelanet, R. and Briand, P. (1991). Time-course development of differentiated hepatocarcinoma and lung metastasis in transgenic mice. J. Hepatol., 13, 227–239.

Fang, X.J., Flowers, M., Keating, A., Cameron, R. and Sherman, M. (1992). *ras* transformation of simian virus 40-immortalized rat hepatocytes: an in vitro model of hepatocarcinogenesis. Cancer Res., 52, 173–180.

Fiers, W., Contreras, R., Haegeman, G., Rogiers, R., Van De Voorde, A., Van Heuverswyn, H., Van Herreweghe, J., Volckaert, G. and Ysebaert, M. (1978). Complete nucleotide sequence of SV40 DNA. Nature, 273, 113–120.

Fukasawa, K., Sakoulas, G., Pollack, R.E. and Chen, S. (1991). Excess wild-type p53 blocks initiation and maintenance of simian virus 40 transformation. Mol. Cell. Biol., 11, 3472–3483.

Grifo, J.A., Abramson, R.D., Satler, C.A. and Merrick, W.C. (1984). RNA-stimulated ATPase activity of eukaryotic initiation factors. J. Biol. Chem., 259, 8648–8654.

Hay, B., Jan, L.Y. and Jan, Y.N (1988). A protein component of *Drosophila* polar granules is encoded by *vasa* and has extensive sequence similarity to ATP-dependent helicases. Cell, 55, 577–587.

Iggo, R.D. and Lane, D.P. (1989). Nuclear protein p68 is an RNA-dependent ATPase. EMBO J., 8, 1827–1831.

Jans, D.A., Ackermann, M.J., Bischoff, J.R., Beach, D.H. and Peters, R. (1991). p34^{cdc2}-mediated phosphorylation at T^{124} inhibits nuclear import of SV-40 T antigen proteins. J. Cell Biol., 115, 1203–1212.

Kalderon, D., Roberts, B.L., Richardson, W.D. and Smith, A.E. (1984). A short amino acid sequence able to specify nuclear location. Cell, 39, 499–509.

Lechner, M.S. and Laimins, L.A. (1991). Human epithelial cells immortalized by SV40 retain differentiation capabilities in an *in vitro* raft system and maintain viral DNA extrachromosomally. Virology, 185, 563–571.

Lin, J.Y. and Simmons, D.T. (1991). The ability of large T antigen to complex with p53 is necessary for the increased life span and partial transformation of human cells by simian virus 40. J. Virol., 65, 6447–6453.

Linder, P., Lasko, P.F., Ashburner, M., Leroy, P., Nielsen, P.J., Nishi, K., Schnier, J. and Slonimiski, P.P. (1989). Birth of the D-E-A-D box. Nature, 337, 121–122.

Marshall, J., Smith, A.E. and Cheng, S.H. (1991). Monoclonal antibody specific for BK virus large-T antigen allows discrimination among the different papovaviral large-T antigens. Oncogene, 6, 1673–1676.

McVey, D., Brizuela, L., Mohr, I., Marshak, D.R., Gluzman, Y. and Beach, D. (1989). Phosphorylation of large tumour antigen by cdc2 stimulates SV40 DNA replication. Nature, 341, 503–507.

Michael-Michalovitz, D., Yehiely, F., Gottlieb, E. and Oren, M. (1991). Simian virus 40 can overcome the antiproliferative effect of wild-type p53 in the absence of stable large T antigen-p53 binding. J. Virol., 65, 4160–4168.

Mitchell, P.J., Wang, C. and Tijan, R. (1987). Positive and negative regulation of transcription *in vitro*: enhancer-binding protein AP-2 is inhibited by SV40 T antigen. Cell, 50, 847–861.

Moens, U., Sundsfjord, A., Flaegstad, T. and Traavik, T. (1990). BK virus early RNA transcripts in stably transformed cells: enhanced levels induced by dibutyryl cyclic AMP, forskolin and 12-O-tetradecanoyl-phorbol-13-acetate treatment. J. Gen. Virol., 71, 1461–1471.

Moll, J., Eibel, H., Botteri, F., Sansig, G., Regnier, C. and van der Putten, H. (1992). Transgenes encoding mutant simian virus 40 large T antigens unmask phenotypic and functional constraints in thymic epithelial cells. Oncogene, 7, 2175–2187.

Nishi, K., Morel-Deville, F., Hershey, J.W.B., Leighton, T. and Schnier, J. (1988). An eIF-4A-like protein is a suppressor of an *Esherichia coli* mutant defective in 50S ribosomal subunit assembly. Nature, 336, 496–498.

Pallas, D.C., Shahrik, L.K., Martin, B.L., Jaspers, S., Miller, T.B., Brautigan, D.L. and Roberts, T.M. (1990). Polyoma small and middle T antigen and SV40 small t antigen form stable complexes with protein phosphatase 2A. Cell, 60, 167–176.

Rajan, P. Dhamankar, V., Rundell, K. and Thimmapaya, B. (1991). Simian virus 40 small-t does not trans-activate RNA polymerase II promoters in virus infections. J. Virol., 65, 6553–6561.

Reddy, V.B., Thimmappaya, B., Dhar, R., Subramanian, K.N., Zain, B.S., Pan, J., Ghosh, P.K., Celma, M.L. and Weissman, S.M. (1978). The genome of simian virus 40. Science, 200, 494–502.

Rihs, H.-P., Jans, D.A., Fan, H. and Peters, R. (1991). The rate of nuclear cytoplasmic protein transport is determined by the casein kinase II site flanking the nuclear localization sequence of the SV40 T-antigen. EMBO J., 10, 633–639.

Rinehart, C.A., Haskill, J.S., Morris, J.S., Butler, T.D. and Kaufman, D.G. (1991). Extended life span of human endometrial stromal cells transfected with cloned, origin-defective, temperature-sensitive simian virus 40. J. Virol., 65, 1458–1465.

Seraphin, B., Simon, M., Boulet, A. and Faye, G. (1989). Mitochondrial splicing requires a protein from a novel helicase family. Nature, 337, 84–87.

Tavis, J.E., Frisque, R.J., Walker, D.L. and White, F.A. (1990). Antigenic and transforming properties of the DB strain of the human polyomavirus BK virus. Virology, 178, 568–572.

Virshup, D.M., Kauffman, M.G. and Kelly, T.J. (1989). Activation of SV40 DNA replication *in vitro* by cellular protein phosphatase 2A. EMBO J., 8, 3891–3898.

Wu, Y.-J. and Rheinwald, J.G. (1981). A new small (40kd) keratin filament protein made by some cultured human squamous cell carcinomas. Cell, 25, 627–635.

Zhu, J.Y., Abate, M., Rice, P.W. and Cole, C.N. (1991). The ability of simian virus 40 large T antigen to immortalize primary mouse embryo fibroblasts cosegregates with its ability to bind to p53. J.Virol., 65, 6872–6880.

Polyoma

Polyomavirus is a member of the Papovaviridae and was first isolated from mice.

Genome

The genome consists of a ~5.2 kbp single circular DNA, which encodes six proteins, four of which are synthesized late in infection. The pattern of polyoma transcription is essentially the same as that of SV40 but an additional early gene product (middle T antigen) is generated.

Transformation

In vitro mouse cells are permissive for polyoma replication and are thus killed. Middle T antigen (mT) transforms established cell lines of other species (Treisman *et al.*, 1981) and together with polyoma large T antigen it can transform primary cells (Mes and Hassell, 1982). *In vivo* polyomavirus is asymptomatic in mice but when injected at high titre into newborn or nude mice it causes epithelial and mesenchymal tumour formation (Dawe *et al.*, 1987; Talmage *et al.*, 1989; Berribi *et al.*, 1990).

In transgenic mice mT antigen regulated either by its own promoter or by that of the Moloney murine leukaemia virus causes disseminated endothelial tumours (Bautch *et al.*, 1987; Williams *et al.*, 1988), multiple neuroblastomas or carcinomas in neuronal or epithelial cells (Aguzzi *et al.*, 1990; Rassoulzadegan *et al.*, 1990) and induces mammary tumours when expressed from a mouse mammary tumour virus (MMTV) promoter (Guy *et al.*, 1992).

	t Antigen	Middle T (mT) antigen	T Antigen
Amino acids	195	421	785
Mass (kDa)			
(predicted)	23	48	88
(expressed)	22	55	100

Cellular location

t Antigen: Cytoplasm.

Middle T antigen: Plasma membrane.
T Antigen: Nucleus.

Protein structure

Phosphorylated and myristylated.

Protein function

t ANTIGEN

Binds to protein phosphatase 2A, p32 and p56 (Pallas *et al.*, 1990).

mT ANTIGEN

Binds to protein phosphatase 2A, SRC, YES, FYN, p61 and p81 (Walter *et al.*, 1990). Interaction with the tyrosine kinases causes their activation. In cells expressing more than one type of proto-oncogene tyrosine kinase, separate complexes are formed with mT antigen, suggesting that mT antigen simultaneously activates separate signalling pathways (Cheng *et al.*, 1990). Middle T antigen also increases the level of phosphorylation of RAF-1 kinase (Morrison *et al.*, 1988) and activates transcription of *Myc* and *JE* but not of *Fos* and *Jun* (Rameh and Armelin, 1991).

Elevated concentrations of phosphatidylinositol 3-kinase products (PtdIns(3,4)P_2 and PtdIns(3,4,5)P_3) are found in transformed and growth factor-activated cells. Phosphatidylinositol 3-kinase associates with mT antigen (Courtneidge and Hebner, 1987; Whitman *et al.*, 1985) and also with the activated receptors for PDGF, EGF, insulin and colony stimulating factor-1 (CSF1) and with the oncogene products of *Src*, *Fms*, *Yes* and *Crk*. Phosphatidylinositol 3-kinase activity increases five- to tenfold in lysates from cells stimulated by any of these growth factors or oncoproteins. Phosphatidylinositol 3-kinase contains 85 kDa and 110 kDa subunits: p85 occurs in the PDGFR and mT/pp60^{src} complexes phosphorylated on serine and tyrosine residues and is a direct substrate for pp60^{src} and the PDGFR. The interaction with pp60^{v-src} is mediated by the SH2 region (Fukui and Hanafusa, 1991). p85 contains two SH2 domains and one SH3 domain, one of the former probably associating with phosphorylated Tyr315 of mT: mutation of this residue to Phe reduces the association with phosphatidylinositol 3-kinase (see **SRC**).

Consensus sequence for a tyrosine kinase autophosphorylation site to which phosphatidylinositol 3-kinase can bind:

$$\begin{matrix} E & E & E & E \\ D & D & D & D \end{matrix} \ Y \ \begin{matrix} M \\ V \end{matrix} \ P \ M \ X \ X \qquad\qquad \text{X is a hydrophilic amino acid}$$

based on polyoma mT (Tyr315), human PDGFRB (Tyr751), mouse PDGFRB (Tyr750), human PDGFRA (Tyr 742), human KIT (Tyr721), Human CSF1R (Tyr721), human MET (Tyr1331), human insulin-R (Tyr1322), human ILGFR (Tyr 1346), rat ILGFR (Tyr1362) (Cantley *et al.*, 1991).

In lymphocytes transfected with a mT antigen expression vector, the tyrosine kinase activity of p59^{fyn} is increased threefold and immunoprecipitates of p59^{fyn} contain up to sixfold more phosphatidylinositol 3-kinase than those in non-transfected cells (Augustine *et al.*, 1991). Nevertheless, cells expressing mT antigen still require IL-2 for proliferation, indicating that the tyrosine kinase activity is insufficient to stimulate continuous growth.

Middle T antigen-induced transformation of rat-2 cells is reversed by co-expression of *Krev-1*, a dominant suppressor of *Kras* transformation (Jelinek and Hassell, 1992). *Krev-1* encodes a guanine nucleotide binding protein (p21^{rap1A} or SMG21) that may compete with p21^{ras} for RAS–GAP and its effect is consistent with a mechanism in which middle T antigen stimulates proliferation via p21^{ras}.

T ANTIGEN

Related to SV40 T antigen in both sequence and general properties, the T antigen of polyoma initiates DNA synthesis and regulates transcription. The observation that it binds p105^{RB} but not p53, distinguishes the T antigens of polyoma from those of SV40 and may account for the greater oncogenic potency of the latter.

Mutation of amino acids 144 (Cys) or 146 (Glu) to glycine and alanine, respectively, abolishes the interaction with p105^{RB} (Freund *et al.*, 1992). Either of these mutations abolishes the capacity of T antigen to immortalize primary rat embryo fibroblasts but the mutant viruses still transform both primary and established fibroblasts *in vitro* and are tumorigenic in mice, thus indicating that the action of middle T antigen is critical in the induction of tumours by polyoma virus.

Sequences of polyoma large T, middle T and small t antigens

```
T antigen   (1)    MDRVLSRADKERLLELLKLPRQLWGDFGRMQQAYKQQSLLLHPDKGGSHALMQELNSLW
mT antigen  (1)    ----------------------------------------------------------
small t     (1)    ----------------------------------------------------------

T antigen   (60)   GTFKTEVYNLRMNLGGTGFQGSPPRTAERGTEESGHSPLHDDYWSFSYGSKYFTREWNDF
mT antigen  (60)   -------------------VRRLHADGWNLSTKDTFGDRYYQRFCRMPLTCLVNVKYSS
small t     (60)   -------------------****************************************

T antigen   (120)  FRKWDPSYQSPPKTAESSEQPDLFCYEEPLLSPNPSSPTDTPAHTAGRRRNPCVAEPDDS
mT antigen  (120)  CSCILCLLRKQHRELKDKCDARCLVLG-CFCLECYMQWFG--TRDVLNLYADFI-SMPID
small t     (120)  ***********************************************************

T antigen   (180)  ISPDPPRTPVSRKRPRPAGATGGGGGGVHANGGSVFGHPTGGTSTPAHPPPYHSQGGSES
mT antigen  (180)  WLDLDVHSVYNPKRRSEELRRAATVHYTMTTGHSAMEASTSQGNGMISSESGTPATSRRL
small t     (180)  ***********RLSP (195)

T antigen   (240)  MGGSDSSGFAEGSFRSDPRCESENESYSQSCSQSSFNATPPKKAREDPAPSDFPSSLTGY
mT antigen  (240)  RLPSLLSNPTYSVMRSHSYPPTRVLQQIHPHILLEEDEILVLLSPMTAYPRTPPELLYPE

T antigen   (300)  LSHAIYSNKTFPAFLVYSTKEKCKQLYDTIGKFRPEFKCLVHYEEGGMLFFLTMTKHRVS
mT antigen  (300)  SDQDQLEPLEEEEEEYMPMEDLYLDILPGEQVPQLIPPPIIPRAGLSPWEG-ILRDLQRA

T antigen   (360)  AVKNYCSKLCRSFLMCKAVTKPMECYQVVTAAPFQLITENKPGLHQFEFTDEPEEQKAVD
mT antigen  (360)  HFDPILDASQ-MRATHR-ALRAHSMQRHLRRLGRT-LLVTFLAALLGICLMLFILI-RSR

T antigen   (420)  WIMVADFALENNLDDPLLIMGYYLDFAKEVPSCIKCSKEETRLQIHWKNHRKHAENADLF
mT antigen  (420)  HF (421)

T antigen   (480)  LNCKAQKTICQQAAASLASRRLKLVECTRSQLLKERLQQSLLRLKELGSSDALLYLAGVA
            (540)  WYQCLLEDFPQTLFKMLKLLTENVPKRRNILFRGPVNSGKTGLAAALISLLGGKSLNINC
            (600)  PADKLAFELGVAQDQFVVCFEDVKGQIALNKQLQPGMGVANLDNLRTTWNGSVKVNLEKK
            (660)  HSNKRSQLFPPCVCTMNEYLLPQTVWARFHMVLDFTCKPHLAQSLEKCEFLQRERIIQSG
            (720)  DTLALLLIWNFTSDVFDPDIQGLVKEVRDQFASECSYSLFCDILCNVQEGDDPLKDICDI
            (780)  AEYTVY (785)
```

Dashes indicate identity with large T antigen. * Indicates identity with middle T antigen. Underlined: mT antigen phosphatidylinositol 3-kinase binding sequence.

Databank file names and accession numbers

GENE	EMBL	SWISSPROT	REFERENCES
Polyoma T antigen (mouse: strain A2)	Papoa2 V01117	TALA_POVMA P03073	Soeda et al., 1980 Friedmann et al., 1979
Polyoma middle t antigen (mouse: strain A2)	Papoa2 V01117	TAMI_POVMA P03077	Soeda et al., 1980
Polyoma small t antigen (mouse: strain A2)	Papoa2 V01117	TASM_POVMA P03078	Soeda et al., 1980

Review

Cantley, L., Auger, K.R., Carpenter, C., Duckworth, B., Graziani, A., Kapeller, R. and Soltoff, S. (1991). Oncogenes and signal transduction. Cell, 64, 281–302.

Papers

Aguzzi, A., Wagner, E., Williams, R.L. and Courtneidge, S.A. (1990). Sympathetic hyperplasia and neuroblastomas in transgenic mice expressing polyoma middle T antigen. New Biol., 2, 533–543.
Augustine, J.A., Sutor, S.L. and Abraham, R.T. (1991). Interleukin 2- and polyomavirus middle T antigen-induced modification of phosphatidylinositol 3-kinase activity in activated T lymphocytes. Mol. Cell. Biol., 11, 4431–4440.
Bautch, V.L., Toda, S., Hassell, J.A. and Hanahan, D. (1987). Endothelial cell tumors develop in transgenic mice carrying polyoma virus middle T oncogene. Cell, 51, 529–538.
Berribi, M., Martin, P.M., Berthois, Y., Bernard, A.M. and Blangy, D. (1990). Estradiol dependence of the specific mammary tissue targeting of polyomavirus oncogenicity in nude mice. Oncogene, 5, 505–509.
Chang, S.H., Espino, P.C., Marshall, J.M., Harvey, R. and Smith, A.E. (1990). Stoichiometry of cellular and viral components in the polyomavirus middle-T antigen-tyrosine kinase complex. Mol. Cell. Biol., 10, 5569–5574.
Courtneidge, S.A. and Hebner, A. (1987). An 81 kDa protein complexed with middle T antigen and pp60^{c-src}: a possible phosphatidylinositol kinase. Cell, 50, 1031–1037.
Dawe, C.J., Freund, R., Mandel, G., Ballmer-Hoffer, K., Talmage, D.A. and Benjamin, T.L. (1987). Variations in polyomavirus genotype in relation to tumor induction in mice: characterization of wild type strains with widely differing tumor profiles. Am. J. Pathol., 127, 243–261.
Freund, R., Bronson, R.T. and Benjamin, T.L. (1992). Separation of immortalization from tumor induction with polyoma large T mutants that fail to bind the retinoblastoma gene product. Oncogene, 7, 1979–1987.
Friedmann, T., Esty, A., Laporte, P. and Deininger, P.L. (1979). The nucleotide sequence and genome organization of the polyoma early region: extensive nucleotide and amino acid homology with SV40. Cell, 17, 715–724.
Fukui, Y. and Hanafusa, H. (1991). Requirement of phosphatidylinositol-3 kinase modification for its association with p60^{src}. Mol. Cell. Biol., 11, 1972–1979.
Guy, C.T., Cardiff, R.D. and Muller, W.J. (1992). Induction of mammary tumors by expression of polyomavirus middle T oncogene: a transgenic mouse model for metastatic disease. Mol. Cell. Biol., 12, 954–961.

Jelinek, M.A. and Hassell, J.A. (1992). Reversion of middle T antigen-transformed rat-2 cells by *Krev-1*: implications for the role of p21^{c-ras} in polyomavirus-mediated transformation. Oncogene, 7, 1687–1698.

Mes, A.-M. and Hassell, J.A. (1982). Polyoma viral middle T-antigen is required for transformation. J. Virol., 42, 621–629.

Morrison, D.K., Kaplan, D.R., Rapp, U.R. and Roberts, T.M. (1988). Signal transduction from membrane to cytosol: growth factors and membrane-bound oncogene products increase raf-1 phosphorylation and associated protein kinase activity. Proc. Natl Acad. Sci. USA, 85, 8855–8859.

Pallas, D.C., Shahrik, L.K., Martin, B.L., Jaspers, S.L., Miller, T.B., Brautigan, D.L. and Roberts, T.M. (1990). Polyoma small and middle T antigens and SV40 small T antigen form stable complexes with protein phosphatase 2A. Cell, 60, 167–172.

Rameh, L.E. and Armelin, M.C.S. (1991). T antigens' role in polyomavirus transformation: c-*myc* but not c-*fos* or c-*jun* expression is a target for middle T. Oncogene, 6, 1049–1056.

Rassoulzadegan, M., Courtneidge, S.A., Loubiere, R., El Baze, P. and Cuzin, F. (1990). A variety of tumours induced by the middle T antigen of polyoma virus in a transgenic mouse family. Oncogene, 5, 1507–1510.

Soeda, E., Arrand, J.R., Smolar, N., Walsh, J.E. and Griffin, B.E. (1980). Coding potential and regulatory signals of the polyoma virus genome. Nature, 283, 445–453.

Talmage, D.A., Freund, R., Young, A.T., Dahl, J., Dawe, C.J. and Benjamin, T.L. (1989). Phosphorylation of middle T by pp60^{c-src}: a switch for binding of phosphatidylinositol 3-kinase and optimal tumorigenesis. Cell, 59, 55–65.

Treisman, R., Novak, U., Favaloro, J. and Kamen, R. (1981). Transformation of rat cells by an altered polyoma virus genome expressing only the middle-T protein. Nature, 292, 595–600.

Walter, G., Ruediger, C., Slaughter, C. and Mumby, M. (1990). Association of protein phosphatase 2A with polyoma virus medium tumor antigen. Proc. Natl Acad. Sci. USA, 78, 2521–2525.

Whitman, M., Kaplan, D.R., Schaffhausen, B., Cantley, L. and Roberts, T.M. (1985). Association of phosphatidylinositol kinase activity with polyoma middle T competent for transformation. Nature, 315, 239–242.

Williams, R.L., Risau, W., Zerwes, H.-G., Drexler, H., Aguzzi, A. and Wagner, E.F. (1988). Endothelioma cells expressing the middle T oncogene induce hemanginomas by host cell recruitment. Cell, 57, 1053–1063.

Adenovirus

The Adenoviridae are a large group of viruses first isolated from cultures of adenoid tissue.

Genome

The genome consists of ~35 kbp of linear double-stranded DNA encoding at least 35 proteins. Six early primary transcripts are converted to >17 early mRNAs with functions equivalent to the products of the early genes of SV40 and polyoma.

Transformation

There are at least 30 human adenovirus serotypes that range from highly oncogenic (serotypes 12, 18 and 31) to non-oncogenic (serotypes 1, 2, 5 and 6) in terms of tumour induction *in vivo*, but all can transform non-permissive cells *in vitro* and grow in permissive cells.

	E1A (243 R and 289R) (Adenovirus type 5)	E1B (Adenovirus type 5)
mRNA	12S, 13S	2.2 kb
Amino acids	243/289	176/496
Mass (kDa)	26 (243R); 32 (289R) (Two major differentially spliced mRNAs (12S, 243R and 13S, 289R))	20/58 (encoded by the same 2.2 kb mRNA utilizing different AUG codons)

Cellular location

E1A: Nucleus (some 243R in cytoplasm).
E1B: Membranes (p19); Nucleoplasm; cell–cell contacts (p55).

Protein function

E1A: Transcription factors. Complex with $p105^{RB}$, pRb2, p28, p40, p50, p60, p80, p90, p107, p130, p300, hsp70.

E1B: p55 binds and stabilizes p 53 (binding sites: amino acids 14–66 of p53 224–354 of E1B; Kao et al., 1990). p53 expression is increased in adenovirus-transformed cells.

Genes trans-activated by E1A: Other early adenovirus genes (E1B, E2A, E3 and E4), the major late promoter (MLP), HIV LTR promoter, human hsp70, β-tubulin, Fos, Jun and Myc. Type 5 E1A also induces Junb and Jund, in contrast to type 12 E1A that induces only Jun of this family (de Groot et al., 1991). The MLP binding site for major late transcription factor (MLTF) is identical to the MYC binding site: the same sequence occurs in the Nras promoter and MLTF also activates the mouse metallothionein and rat γ-fibrinogen genes.

Genes repressed by E1A: Viral SV40, polyoma and adenovirus E1A and the cellular immunoglobulin heavy chain, human metallothionein, MHC class I gene H-2K^b enhanson, estrogen and glucocorticoid receptors, insulin, cytochrome P-450, Myc, Neu, JE, MyoD, stromelysin and collagenase genes and yeast GAL4. E1A suppresses metastasis in Neu-transformed 3T3 fibroblasts. This range of targets suggests that E1A proteins can repress all trans-activator proteins that bind to enhancers (Rochette-Egly et al., 1990). The mechanisms involved are unknown although E1A proteins do not bind directly to DNA and it is probable that their effects on transcription factors are mediated indirectly, e.g., via phosphorylation.

Each of the E1B, E2A, E3 and E4 promoters contains an activating transcription factor (ATF) site (TTTCGCGC) that is the same as the cAMP response element (CRE) and CRE-BP1 mediates E1A trans activation of E4. E2 has two sites to which the E2F factor binds that share strong sequence similarity with elements in the human MYC P2 promoter, one of which mediates E1A-dependent trans activation from the MYC promoter.

The 12S E1A protein immortalizes quail cells (Guilhot et al., 1993). E1A and E1B (19 kDa or 55 kDa) cooperate to transform primary rodent cells. However, in addition to stimulating proliferation, E1A induces apoptosis and E1B 19 kDa or 55 kDa proteins or the human BCL2 gene product cooperate with E1A to transform primary cells through their capacity to suppress apoptosis (Rao et al., 1992). Both E1B 19 kDa and 55 kDa proteins inhibit apoptosis by eliminating p53 function (Debbas and White, 1993; Lowe and Ruley, 1993). The 55 kDa protein sequesters wild-type p53 into an inactive complex: the mechanism of E1B 19 kDa inactivation may be direct or indirect.

Structure and protein binding domains of adenovirus type 5 E1A 289R protein

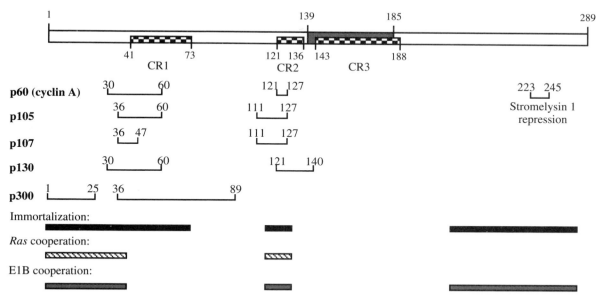

Three regions are highly conserved between adenovirus 5, 7 and 12 serotypes (CR1, CR2 and CR3; chequered boxes). In the 289R protein amino acids 1–138 and 186–289 are encoded by exon 1 and exon 2 respectively (open boxes): these regions are identical to the sequence of 243R. The shaded box indicates the 46 amino acid internal region unique to the 289R protein (residues 139–185). *Trans* activation maps to the unique 46 residue region of 289R. Mutation studies indicate that *trans* activation involves different transcription factors binding to the zinc finger region (147–177) and the carboxyl (183–188) region (Webster and Ricciardi, 1991). Transcriptional inhibition is principally regulated by the exon 1 region (1–139) and the repression of *MyoD* transcription correlates with the site of p300 association (Caruso *et al.*, 1993; Wang *et al.*, 1993), but repression of stromelysin 1 requires the region 223–245 (Linder *et al.*, 1992). Regions common to 289R and 243R (the N-terminal region, CR1 (40–60) and CR2 (120–140)) are required for transformation but not for *trans* activation.

The regions with which boxes are aligned have been defined as being required for immortalization and cooperation with *Ras* or E1B, as indicated, although these conclusions should be interpreted with caution as they are based on the effects of major deletions within the protein.

E1A binds directly to ATFa *trans*-activating proteins (ATFa1, ATFa2, ATFa3) and may interact with AP-1 (Maguire *et al.*, 1991; Chatton *et al.*, 1993).

Proteins associating with E1A

p300: nuclear phosphoprotein half-life 9 h; complexed with E1A: 16 h. Phosphorylated in quiescent and proliferating cells but is further modified to a lower electrophoretic mobility form during mitosis (Yaciuk and Moran, 1991).

p130: uncharacterized protein: the E1A region (127–140) to which it binds includes a potential casein kinase II phosphorylation site and lies within a region (124–145) of primary sequence and predicted β turn/α helix secondary structure that also occurs in SV40 T antigen and MYC. p60 (cyclin): associates with p34^{cdc2}, the expression of which is required for cell cycle progression from G_1 to S phase and from G_2 to mitosis. The region of E1A to which p60 binds is essential for transformation by E1A and distinct from that to which p105^{RB} binds (Giordano *et al.*, 1991; see **Tumour Suppressor Genes: RB**). Thus there may be a direct link between regulation of the normal cell growth cycle and neoplastic transformation caused by E1A.

Each of the E1A proteins can immortalize primary cells *in vitro*, although for neoplastic transformation both appear to be necessary together with the 20 kDa and 58 kDa E1B products. Studies with antisense E1A indicate that the continued expression of E1A is necessary to prevent senescence of immortalized cells (Quinlan, 1993). Several other oncogenes can complement E1A by substituting for E1B in transformation assays. Thus *Hras* or polyoma middle T antigen can cooperate with E1A and polyoma large T antigen, *Myc* or mutant *P53* can cooperate with E1B. For transformation in association with activated *Ras* the CR1 and CR2 regions are essential: deletion of either of these regions has little effect on *trans* activation by E1A. Transforming potential is linked to repression activity: mutations in CR1 that abolish transformation also prevent repression.

Sequence of human adenovirus type 5 E1A 289R

```
  (1)    MRHIICHGGVITEEMAASLLDQLIEEVLADNLPPPSHFEPPTLHELYDLDVTAPEDPNE
 (60)    EAVSQIFPDSVMLAVQEGIDLLTFPPAPGSPEPPHLSRQPEQPEQRALGPVSMPNLVPEV
(120)    IDLTCHEAGFPPSDDEDEEGEEFVLDYVEHPGHGCRSCHYHRRNTGDPDIMCSLCYMRTC
(180)    GMFVYSPVSEPEPEPEPEPEPARPTRRPKMAPAILRRPTSPVSRECNSSTDSCDSGPSNT
(240)    PPEIHPVVPLCPIKPVAVRVGGRRQAVECIEDLLNEPGQPLDLSCKRPRP (289)
```

Sequence of human adenovirus type 5 E1B large T antigen

```
  (1)    MERRNPSERGVPAGFSGHASVESGCETQESPATVVFRPPGDNTDGGAAAAAGGSQAAAA
 (60)    GAEPMEPESRPGPSGMNVVQVAELYPELRRILTITEDGQGLKGVKRERGACEATEEARNL
(120)    AFSLMTRHRPECITFQQIKDNCANELDLLAQKYSIEQLTTYWLQPGDDFEEAIRVYAKVA
(180)    LRPDCKYKISKLVNIRNCCYISGNGAEVEIDTEDRVAFRCSMINMWPGVLGMDGVVIMNV
(240)    RFTGPNFSGTVFLANTNLILHGVSFYGFNNTCVEAWTDVRVRGCAFYCCWKGVVCRPKSR
(300)    ASIKKCLFERCTLGILSEGNSRVRHNVASDCGCFMLVKSVAVIKHNMVCGNCEDRASQML
(360)    TCSDGNCHLLKTIHVASHSRKAWPVFEHNILTRCSLHLGNRRGVFLPYQCNLSHTKILLE
(420)    PESMSKVNLNGVFDMTMKIWKVLRYDETRTRCRPCECGGKHIRNQPVMLDVTEELRPDHL
(480)    VLACTRAEFGSSDEDTD (496)
```

Sequence of human adenovirus type 5 E1B 20 kDa protein

```
  (1)    MEAWECLEDFSAVRNLLEQSSNSTSWFWRFLWGSSQAKLVCRIKEDYKWEFEELLKSCG
 (60)    ELFDSLNLGHQALFQEKVIKTLDFSTPGRAAAAVAFLSFIKDKWSEETHLSGGYLLDFLA
(120)    MHLWRAVVRHKNRLLLLSSVRPAIIPTEEQQQQQEEARRRRQEQSPWNPRAGLDPRE(176)
```

Databank file names and accession numbers

GENE	EMBL	SWISSPROT	REFERENCES
E1A	Ad5001 X02996	E1A_ADE05 P03255	Van Ormondt *et al.*, 1980
(Human adenovirus type 5)			
E1B (55 kDa)	Ad5001 X02996	E1BL_ADE05	Bos *et al.*, 1981
(Human adenovirus type 5)			Van Ormondt *et al.*, 1980
E1B (20 kDa)	Ad5001 X02996	E1BS_ADE05 P03246	Bos *et al.*, 1981
(Human adenovirus type 5)			Van Ormondt *et al.*, 1980

Review

Nevins, J.R. (1989). Mechanisms of viral-mediated *trans*-activation of transcription. Adv. Virus Res., 37, 35–83.

Papers

Bos, J.L., Polder, L.J., Bernards, R., Schrier, P.I., Van den Elsen, P.J., Van der Eb A.J. and Van Ormondt, H. (1981). The 2.2 kb E1b mRNA of human Ad12 and Ad5 codes for two tumour antigens starting at different triplets. Cell, 27, 121–131.

Caruso, M., Martelli, F., Giordano, A. and Felsani, A. (1993). Regulation of myoD gene transcription and protein function by the transforming domains of the adenovirus E1A oncoprotein. Oncogene, 8, 267–278.

Chatton, B., Bocco, J.L., Gaire, M., Hauss, C., Reimund, B., Goetz, J. and Kedinger, C. (1993). Transcriptional activation by the adenovirus larger E1a product is mediated by members of the cellular transcription factor ATF family which can directly associate with E1a. Mol. Cell. Biol., 13, 561–570.

Debbas, M. and White, E. (1993). Wild-type p53 mediates apoptosis by E1A, which is inhibited by E1B. Genes Devel., 7, 546–554.

de Groot, R.P., Meijer, I., van den Brink, S., Mummery, C. and Kruijer, W. (1991). Differential regulation of *jun*B and *jun*D by adenovirus type 5 and 12 E1A proteins. Oncogene, 6, 2357–2361.

Giordano, A., McCall, C., Whyte, P. and Franza, B.R. (1991). Human cyclin A and the retinoblastoma protein interact with similar but distinguishable sequences in the adenovirus E1A gene product. Oncogene, 6, 481–485.

Guilhot, C., Benchaibi, M., Flechon, J.E. and Samarut, J. (1993). The 12S adenoviral E1A protein immortalizes avian cells and interacts with the avian RB product. Oncogene, 8, 619–624.

Kao, C.C., Yew, P.R. and Berk, A.J. (1990). Domains required for *in vitro* association between the cellular p53 and the adenovirus 2 E1B 55K proteins. Virology, 179, 806–814.

Linder, S., Popowicz, P., Svensson, C., Marshall, H., Bondesson, M. and Akusjarvi, G. (1992). Enhanced invasive properties of rat embryo fibroblasts transformed by adenovirus E1A mutants with deletions in the carboxy-terminal exon. Oncogene, 7, 439–443.

Lowe, S.W. and Ruley, H.R. (1993). Stabilization of the p53 tumor suppressor is induced by adenovirus 5 E1A and accompanies apoptosis. Genes Devel., 7, 535–545.

Maguire, K., Shi, X.-P., Horikoshi, N., Rappaport, J., Rosenberg, M. and Weinmann, R. (1991). Interactions between adenovirus E1A and members of the AP-1 family of cellular transcription factors. Oncogene, 6, 1417–1422.

Quinlan, M.P. (1993). Expression of antisencse E1A in 293 cells results in altered cell morphologies and cessation of proliferation. Oncogene, 8, 257–265.

Rao, L., Debbas, M., Sabbatini, P., Hockenbery, D., Korsmeyer, S. and White, E. (1992). The adenovirus E1A proteins induce apoptosis, which is inhibited by the E1B 19-kDa and bcl-2 proteins. Proc. Natl Acad. Sci. USA, 89, 7742–7746.

Rochette-Egly, C., Fromental, C. and Chambon, P. (1990). General repression of enhanson activity by the adenovirus-2 E1A proteins. Genes Devel., 4, 137–150.

Van Ormondt, H., Maat, J. and Van Beveren, C.P. (1980). The nucleotide sequence of the transforming early region E1 of adenovirus type 5 DNA. Gene, 11, 299–309.

Wang, H.-G.H., Rikitake, Y., Carter, M.G., Yacuik, P., Abraham, S.E., Zerler, B. and Moran, E. (1993). Identification of specific adenovirus E1A N-terminal residues critical to the binding of cellular proteins and to the control of cell growth. J. Virol., 67, 476–488.

Webster, L.C. and Ricciardi, R.P. (1991). *trans*-dominant mutants of E1A provide genetic evidence that the zinc finger of the *trans*-activating domain binds a transcription factor. Mol. Cell. Biol., 11, 4287–4296.

Yaciuk, P. and Moran, E. (1991). Analysis with specific polyclonal antiserum indicates that the E1A-associated 300-kDa product is a stable nuclear phosphoprotein that undergoes cell cycle phase-specific modification. Mol. Cell. Biol., 11, 5389–5397.

Papillomaviruses

There are over 60 human papillomavirus (HPV) genotypes (de Villiers, 1989) that colonize various stratified epithelia including the skin and oral and genital mucosa and induce the formation of self-limiting, benign tumours known as papillomas (warts) or condylomas. Viruses increase the division rate of infected stem cells in the epithelial basal layer and the viral genome replicates episomally in concert with the cell genome. As the keratinocytes terminally differentiate, synthesis of virally encoded late proteins causes cell death. Very infrequently this mechanism defaults and maligant tumours develop.

Genome

The genome consists of ~7.9 kbp of circular double-stranded DNA. It comprises "early" ORFs expressed in transformed cells (E1 to E8) and "late" ORFs (L1 and L2), the products of which are necessary for the production of virions that occurs only in differentiated cells.

Transformation

Eleven HPVs have been shown to be commonly associated with human tumours (Table 3.1). DNA sequences of HPV-16 or HPV-18 are expressed in ~90% of all cervical carcinomas and HPV-16 DNA is present in 50% of anal cancers. HPV types 6 and 11 are frequently present together with types 16 and 18 in genital infections but are rarely detected in cervical malignancies. Thus infection with certain types of HPV constitutes an increased risk of the onset of some cancers.

Table 3.1. Tumours associated with human papillomaviruses

HPV type	Cancer	References
5, 8	Epidermal carcinoma	Pfister *et al.*, 1983
16, 18	Cervical carcinoma	Durst *et al.*, 1987; Boshart *et al.*,
16	Anal carcinoma	1984
30	Laryngeal carcinoma	Schleurlen *et al.*, 1986a
33	Genital neoplasias	Kahn *et al.*, 1986
38	Melanoma	Beaudenon *et al.*, 1986
48	Skin carcinoma	Schleurlen *et al.*, 1986b
52	Cervical carcinoma	Muller *et al.*, 1989
54, 55	Buschke–Lowenstein tumour	Shimoda *et al.*, 1988
		Favre *et al.*, 1990

	E5	E6	E7
mRNA (bp)			
(type 16)	291 (249 coding)	492 (474 coding)	311 (294 coding)
(type 18)	240 (219 coding)	492 (474 coding)	396 (315 coding)

In carcinoma-derived cell lines E6, E7 and part of E1 are encoded in a variably spliced, 3.4 kb transcript (Schneider-Gaedicke and Schwarz 1986): 1.5, 2.3 and 4.5 kb mRNAs have also been detected (Smotkin and Wetstein, 1986).

	E5	E6	E7
Amino acids			
(type 16/18)	83/73	158/158	98/105
Mass (kDa)			
(predicted) (type 16/18)	9.4	19.2/18.8	11.0/11.9
(expressed)	44	18	20

Cellular location

E5: Plasma membrane (homodimers).
E6: Nucleus.
E7: Nucleus.

Protein function

E5: Activates receptors for PDGFB, EGF and CSF1.
E6: Binds p53.
E7: Binds p105^{RB}.

E6 AND E7

E6 and E7 DNAs are detectable in all HPV-associated tumours. E2 is usually interrupted or deleted and the late genes are often missing. In some classes of tumours (e.g. cervical carcinomas) the E1, E6 and E7 ORFs of HPV DNA are usually integrated into the host chromosome (the ORFs of E2, E3, E4 and E5 are lost) whereas in others (e.g. squamous cell carcinomas) they are present in extrachromosomal form (Cullen *et al.*, 1991). The expression of anti-sense

E6/E7 renders HPV-containing cervical carcinoma cells non-tumorigenic (von Knebel Doeberitz *et al.*, 1988).

HPV-16 E6 and E7 proteins cooperate to immortalize human fibroblasts, keratinocytes or mammary epithelial cells (McCance *et al.*, 1988; Watanabe *et al.*, 1989; Hawley-Nelson *et al.*, 1989; Band *et al.*, 1990; Hudson *et al.*, 1990). Prolonged growth *in vitro* produces malignant clones from such immortalized cells (Hurlin *et al.*, 1991). Alternatively, the co-expression of v-*ras* with E7 transforms primary cells (Durst *et al.*, 1989) and v-*ras* and E6 immortalize primary cells (Storey and Banks, 1993). E7 functions as an immortalizing oncogene in that there is a continued requirement for its expression, together with *Ras*, to maintain the transformed phenotype (Crook *et al.*, 1989). However, this does not imply that E6 functions as a RAS protein. Binding of E7 to the retinoblastoma protein is necessary but not sufficient for co-transformation (Banks *et al.*, 1990), although mutational analysis of the cottontail rabbit papillomavirus E7 protein indicates that its association with $p105^{RB}$ is not necessary for the viral induction of warts (Defeo-Jones *et al.*, 1993). E7 also associates with $p33^{CDK2}$ and cyclin A (Tommasino *et al.*, 1993). E7 is a weak mitogen for Swiss 3T3 fibroblasts in which its expression induces the appearance of the transcriptionally active form of E2F (Morris *et al.*, 1993).

Transformation of human keratinocytes by HPV and *Hras* activates expression of fibronectin and thrombospondin genes (Sheibani *et al.*, 1991).

HPV-16 and -18 E6 enhance the degradation rate of p53 via specific binding (see **Tumour Suppressor Genes: *P53***) and a fusion protein of the N-terminal half of HPV-16 E7 and full-length HPV-16 E6 promotes the degradation of $p105^{RB}$ (Scheffner *et al.*, 1992).

Immunization of mice with fibroblast cells expressing transfected HPV-16 E7 confers protection against challenge with HPV-16 E7 melanoma cells (Chen *et al.*, 1991). The E7 expressing cells elicit an immune response mediated by $CD8^+$ (cytotoxic) lymphocytes that is responsible for rejection of the tumour cells.

E5

Expression of the HPV-16 E5 gene transforms 3T3-A31 cells and enhances their tumorigenicity. The transcription of *Fos* in 3T3-A31 cells in response to EGF, PDGF or serum is increased by expression of E5 (Leechanachai *et al.*, 1992). This suggests that E5 may contribute to the early stages of tumorigenesis by enhancing proliferation in HPV-16-infected cells.

Regulation of HPV gene expression

The long control region (LCR) of HPV contains several repeats of the E2 binding sequence ($ACCGN_4CGGT$). HPVs found in skin lesions generally have the most proximal E2 binding sites >100 bp from the E6/E7 start site and occupancy of these sites promotes transcription (Guido *et al.*, 1993). Thus E2 has been shown to be necessary, together with E6 and E7, for immortalization of human cervical keratinocytes (Storey *et al.*, 1992). In all sequenced genital HPVs there are two proximal E2 binding sites just upstream from the E6/E7 TATA box, suggesting that, in genital carcinomas, continuous expression of E6 and E7 is incompatible with the presence of E2 protein.

The HPV-16 enhancer has binding sites for a variety of ubiquitous transcription factors (OCT-1, NFA, TEF-2, NF1 and AP-1). The epithelial cell specificity of HPV infection may, therefore, reside in cell-specific functional differences that lie outside the DNA binding domains of these factors (Chong *et al.*, 1991). In keratinocytes and cervical carcinoma cells transcriptional enhancer factor (TEF)-1, together with a "co-activator", binds to a 37 nt enhancer and their association is essential for E6 and E7 expression (Ishiji *et al.*, 1992). *Trans*-acting negative regulatory factors encoded by normal cellular genes can suppress transcription from HPV promoters (Rosl *et al.*, 1991).

The efficiency of HPV-16 transcription in primary human fibroblasts is correlated with a deletion in chromosome 11 and introduction of the normal allele into cervical carcinoma cells suppresses the tumorigenic phenotype (Koi *et al.*, 1989; Smits *et al.*, 1990). However, the best characterized tumour suppressor genes, *P53* and *RB1*, are not located on chromosome 11.

TGFB1 (TGFβ1)

TGFB1 inhibits the growth of normal and HPV-16-infected keratinocytes but has no effect on the growth of cervical carcinoma-derived cell lines (Braun *et al.*, 1990; Woodworth *et al.*, 1990). Carcinoma cells express TGFB1 receptors and TGFB1 activates *JUN* transcription in both normal and tumour cells. However, in non-tumour cells immortalized by HPV-16, TGFB1 suppresses transcription of both *MYC* and HPV-16 mRNA. The loss of responsiveness to the inhibitory signal of TGFB1 may therefore be associated with HPV malignancy.

Bovine papilloma virus 1 (BPV-1)

BPV-1 replicates episomally in fibroblasts *in vitro* and transforms the cells: replication with high efficiency requires the E1, E6 and E7 gene products. The E5 gene encodes a hydrophobic, 44 amino acid (7 kDa) protein that causes tumorigenic transformation of rodent fibroblasts (Schlegel *et al.*, 1986; Settleman *et al.*, 1989). In NIH 3T3 cells this involves activation of EGF and CSF1 receptors, independently of the presence of their ligands (Martin *et al.*, 1989). It is the smallest known oncoprotein and microinjection into the nucleus of the 13 C-terminal amino acids of E5 activates DNA synthesis. The 30 amino acid N-terminus contains two cysteine residues essential for homodimerization and biological activity. In two cell lines, E5 has been shown to form an activating complex with the PDGFRB and to stimulate DNA synthesis (Petti *et al.*, 1991; Petti and Dimaio, 1992) and activation of its transforming capacity may require association with a 16 kDa cellular protein (Goldstein and Schlegel, 1990).

The BPV-1 E2 protein has both *trans* activating and repressor functions and the loss of the latter when HPV DNA is integrated into the genome of a host cell may lead to transcriptional activation of E6 and E7 that promotes neoplastic transformation. Direct injection of BPV-1 E2 slows development of tumours caused by injection of cells derived from cervical neoplasms into nude mice.

Sequences of HPV and BPV-1 E5 proteins

```
HPV-16 E5    (1)    MTNLDTASTTLLACFLLCFCVLLCVCLLIRPLLLSVSTYTSLIILVLLLWITAASAFRC
HPV-18 E5    (1)    -LSLIFLFCFCVCMYVC-HVP--PSVCMCAYAWVL-FV-IVVITSPATAFTVYVFC-LL
BPV-1  E5    (1)    MPNLWFLLFLGLVAAMQLLLLLFLLLFFLVYWDHFECSCTGLPF (44)

HPV-16 E5   (60)    FIVYIIFVYIPLFLIHTHARFLIT(83)
HPV-18 E5   (60)    PMLLLHIHA-LSLQ(73)

HPV-16 E6    (1)    MHQKRTAMFQDPQERPRKLPQLCTELQTTIHDIILECVYCKQQLLRREVYDFAFRDLCI
HPV-18 E6    (1)      M-R-E--TR--Y---D-----N-SLQ--EIT-----TV-ELT--FE---K--FV

HPV-16 E6   (60)    VYRDGNPYAVCDKCLKFYSKISEYRHYCYSLYGTTLEQQYNKPLCDLLIRCINCQKPLCP
HPV-18 E6   (55)    ----SI-H-A-H--ID---R-R-L---SD-V--D---KLT-TG-YN-----LR-----N-
```

```
HPV-16 E6   (120)   HLNEKR       RFHNIAGHYRGQCHSCCNRARQERLQRRRETQV (158)
HPV-18 E6   (115)   AEK-R-EKQRHLDKKQ-----R-RWT-R-M---RSS-T       -----L (158)


HPV-16 E7    (1)    MHGDTPTLHEYMLDLQPETT DLYCYEQLNDSSEEE DEIDGPAGQAEPDRAHY
HPV-18 E7    (1)    ---PKA--QDIV-HLE-QNEIPV--L-H---S- ----N-----VNH-HL-A-RAEPQRH


HPV-16 E7   (53)    NIVTFCCKCDSTLRLCVQSTHVDIRTLEDLLMGTLGIVCPICSQKP (98)
HPV-18 E7   (60)    TMLCM----EARIK-V-E-SAD-L-AFQQ-FLN--SF---W-ASQQ (105)
```

p105^{RB} binds to E7 (HPV-16 residues 21–30; HPV-18 24–33 (underlined); Dyson *et al.*, 1989), as well as to E1A and SV40 T antigen (see **Tumour Suppressor Genes**). However, for E7 an additional domain (amino acids 60–98) appears necessary to inhibit complex formation between p105^{RB} and E2F (Huang *et al.*, 1993). Casein kinase II phosphorylates residues 31 and 32 (see **EBV**). Mutation in these regions inhibits transforming potential, although negative charge at these sites is not essential for p105^{RB} binding (Firzlaff *et al.*, 1991). The relative efficiency of p105^{RB} binding and CKII phosphorylation is lower in HPV-6 E7, correlating with the lower oncogenic activity of HPV-6 (Barbosa *et al.*, 1990). HPV-16 E7 shows significant sequence homology with E1A, T antigen, MYC and the yeast mitotic regulator *cdc*25.

Databank file names and accession numbers

GENE	EMBL	SWISSPROT	REFERENCES
HPV-16 E5	Pa16 K02718	VE5_HPV16 P06927	Seedorf *et al.*, 1985
			Bubb *et al.*, 1988
HPV-18 E5	Paphpv 18 X05015	VE5_HPV18 P06792	Cole and Danos, 1987
HPV-16 E6	Pa16 K02718	VE6_HPV16 P03126	Seedorf *et al.*, 1985
HPV-18 E6	Parhpv E6 X04354	VE6_HPV18 P06463	Cole and Danos, 1987
	Paphpv18 X05015		Matlashewski *et al.*, 1986
	Hshelb M20325		Inagaki *et al.*, 1988
	M26798; M26798		Schneider-Gaedicke and Schwarz, 1986
			Grossman and Laimins, 1989
HPV-16 E7	Pa16 K02718	VE7_HPV16 P03129	Seedorf *et al.*, 1985
			Phelps *et al.*, 1988
HPV-18 E7	Paphpv 18 X05015	VE7_HPV18 P06788	Cole and Danos, 1987
	Hshela M20324		Inagaki *et al.*, 1988
	Hshelb M20325		Schneider-Gaedicke and Schwarz, 1986
	M26798; M26798		
BPV-1 E5	Papabpv1 X02346	VE5_BPV1 P06928	Schlegel *et al.*, 1986
	Papppb2C M20219		Goldstein and Schlegel, 1990
			Petti *et al.*, 1991

Reviews

Campo, M.S. (1992). Cell transformation by animal papillomaviruses. J. Gen. Virol., 73, 217–222.

DiMaio, D. (1991). Transforming activity of bovine and human papillomaviruses in cultured cells. Adv. Cancer Res., 56, 133–159.

Galloway, D.A. and McDougall, J.K. (1989). Human papillomaviruses and carcinomas. Adv. Virus Res., 37, 125–171.

McBride, A.A., Romanczuk, H. and Howley, P.M. (1991). The papillomavirus E2 regulatory proteins. J. Biol. Chem., 266, 18411–18414.

Papers

Band, V., Zajchowski, D., Kulesa, V. and Sager, R. (1990). Human papillomavirus DNAs immortalize normal human mammary epithelial cells and reduce their growth factor requirements. Proc. Natl Acad, Sci. USA, 87, 463–467.

Banks, L., Edmonds, C. and Vousden, K.H. (1990). Ability of the HPV16 E7 protein to bind RB and induce DNA synthesis is not sufficient for efficient transformation. Oncogene, 5, 1383–1389.

Barbosa, M.S., Edmonds, C., Fisher, C., Schiller, J.T., Lowy, D.R. and Vousden, K.H. (1990). The region of the HPV E7 oncoprotein homologous to adenovirus E1a and SV40 large T antigen contains separate domains for Rb binding and casein kinase II phosphorylation. EMBO J., 9, 153–160.

Beaudenon, S., Kremsdorf, D., Croissant, O., Jablonska, S., Wain-Hobson, S. and Orth, G. (1986). A new type of human papillomavirus associated with genital neoplasms. Nature, 321, 246–249.

Boshart, M., Gissmann, L., Ikenberg, H., Kleinhertz, A., Schleurlen, W., and zur Hausen, H. (1984). A new type of papillomavirus DNA, its presence in genital cancer biopsies and in cell lines derived from cervical cancer. EMBO J., 3, 1151–1157.

Braun, L., Durst, M., Mikumo, R. and Gruppuso, P. (1990). Differential response of nontumorigenic and tumorigenic human papillomavirus type 16–positive epithelial cells to transforming growth factor β_1. Cancer Res., 50, 7324–7332.

Bubb, V., McCance, D.J. and Schlegel, R. (1988). DNA sequence of the HPV-16 E5 ORF and the structure conservation of its encoded protein. Virology, 163, 243–246.

Chen, L., Thomas, E.K., Hu, S.-L., Hellstrom, I. and Hellstrom, K.E. (1991). Human papillomavirus type 16 nucleoprotein E7 is a tumor rejection antigen. Proc. Natl Acad. Sci. USA, 88, 110–114.

Chong, T., Apt, D., Gloss, B., Isa, M. and Bernard, H.-U. (1991). The enhancer of human papillomavirus type 16: binding sites for the ubiquitous transcription factors oct-1, NFA, TEF-2, NF1 and AP-1 participate in epithelial cell-specific transcription. J. Virol., 65, 5933–5943.

Cole, S.T. and Danos, O. (1987). Nucleotide sequence and complete analysis of the human papillomavirus type 18 genome. J. Mol. Biol., 193, 599–608.

Crook, T., Morgenstern, J.P., Crawford, L. and Banks, L. (1989). Continued expression of HPV-16 E7 protein is required for maintenance of the transformed phenotype of cells co-transformed by HPV-16 plus EJ-ras. EMBO J., 8, 513–519.

Cullen, A.P., Reid, R., Campion, M. and Lorincz, A.T. (1991). Analysis of the physical state of different human papillomavirus DNAs in intraepithelial and invasive cervical neoplasm. J. Virol., 65, 606–612.

de Villiers, E.-M. (1989). Heterogeneity of the human papillomavirus group. J. Virol., 63, 4898–4903.

Defeo-Jones, D., Vuocolo, G.A., Haskell, K.M., Hanobik, M.G., Kiefer, D.M., McAvoy, E.M., Ivey-Hoyle, M., Brandsma, J.L., Oliff, A. and Jones, R.E. (1993). Papillomavirus E7 protein binding to the retinoblastoma protein is not required for viral induction of warts. J. Virol., 67, 716–725.

Durst, M., Croce, C.M., Gissmann, L., Schwarz, E. and Huebner, K. (1987). Papillomavirus sequences integrate near cellular oncogenes in some cervical carcinomas. Proc. Natl Acad. Sci. USA, 84, 1070–1074.

Durst, M., Gallahan, D., Jay, G. and Rhim, J.S. (1989). Glucocorticoid-enhanced neoplastic transformation of human keratinocytes by human papillomavirus type 16 and an activated ras oncogene. Virology, 173, 767–771.

Dyson, N., Howley, P.M., Munger, K. and Harlow, E. (1989). The human papillomavirus-16 E7 oncoprotein is able to bind to the retinoblastoma gene product. Science, 243, 934–937.

Favre, M., Kremsdorf, D., Jablonska, S., Obalek, S., Pehau-Arnaudet, G., Croissant, O. and Orth, G. (1990). Two new human papillomavirus types (HPV54 and HPV55) characterized from genital tumours illustrate the plurality of genital HPVs. Int. J. Cancer, 45, 40–46.

Firzlaff, J.M., Luscher, B. and Eisenman, R.N. (1991). Negative charge at the casein kinase II phosphorylation site is important for transformation but not for Rb protein binding by the E7 protein of human papillomavirus type 16. Proc. Natl Acad. Sci. USA, 88, 5187–5191.

Goldstein, D.J. and Schlegel, R. (1990). The E5 oncoprotein of bovine papillomavirus binds to 16 kd cellular protein. EMBO J., 9, 137–145.

Grossman, S.R. and Laimins, L.A. (1989). E6 protein of human papillomavirus type 18 binds zinc. Oncogene, 4, 1089–1093.

Guido, M.C., Zamorano, R., Garrido-Guerrero, E., Gariglio, P. and Garcia-Carranca, A. (1993). Early promoters of genital and cutaneous human papillomaviruses are differentially regulated by the bovine papillomavirus type 1 E2 gene product. J Gen Virol., 73, 1395–1400.

Hawley-Nelson, P., Vousden, K.H., Hubbert, N.L., Lowy, D.R. and Schiller, J.T. (1989). HPV16 E6 and E7 proteins cooperate to immortalize human foreskin keratinocytes. EMBO J., 8, 3905–3910.

Huang, P.S., Patrick, D.R., Edwards, G., Goodhart, P.J., Huber, H.E., Miles, L., Garsky, V.M., Oliff, A. and Heimbrook, D.C. (1993). Protein domains governing interactions between E2F, the retinoblastoma gene product, and human papillomvirus type 16 E7 protein. Mol. Cell. Biol., 13, 953–960.

Hudson, J.B., Bedell, M.A., McCance, D.J. and Laimins, L.A. (1990). Immortalization and altered differentiation of human keratinocytes in vitro by the E6 and E7 open reading frames of human papillomavirus type 18. J. Virol., 64, 519–526.

Hurlin, P.J., Kaur, P., Smith, P.P., Perez-Reyes, N., Blanton, R.A. and McDougall, J.K. (1991). Progression of human papillomavirus type 18-immortalized human keratinocytes to a malignant phenotype. Proc. Natl Acad, Sci. USA, 88, 570–574.

Inagaki, Y., Tsunokawa, Y., Takebe, N., Nawa, H., Nakanishi, S., Terada, M. and Sugimura, T. (1988). Nucleotide sequences of cDNAs for human papillomavirus type 18 transcripts in HeLa cells. J. Virol., 62, 1640–1646.

Ishiji, T., Lace, M.J., Parkkinen, S., Anderson, R.D., Haugen, T.H., Cripe, T.P., Xiao, J.-H., Davidson, I., Chambon, P. and Turek, L.P. (1992). Transcriptional enhancer factor (TEF)-1 and its cell-specific co-activator activate human papillomavirus-16 E6 and E7 oncogene transcription in keratinocytes and cervical carcinoma cells. EMBO J., 11, 2271–2281.

Kahn, T., Schwarz, E. and zur Hausen, H. (1986). Molecular cloning of the DNA of a new human papillomavirus (HPV 30) from a laryngeal carcinoma. Int. J. Cancer, 37, 61–65.

Koi, M., Morita, H., Yamada, H., Satoh, H., Barrett, J.C. and Oshimura, M. (1989). Normal human chromosome 11 suppresses tumorigenicity of human cervical tumor cell line SiHa. Mol. Carcinogen., 2, 12–21.

Leechanachai, P., Banks, L., Moreau, F. and Matlashewski, G. (1992). The E5 gene from human papillomavirus type 16 is an oncogene which enhances growth factor-mediated signal transduction to the nucleus. Oncogene, 7, 19–25.

Martin, P., Vass, W.C., Schiller, J.T., Lowy, D.R. and Velu, T.J. (1989). The bovine papillomavirus E5 transforming protein can stimulate the transforming activity of EGF and CSF-1 receptors. Cell, 59, 21–32.

Matlashewski, G., Banks, L., Wu-Liao, J., Spence, P., Pim, D., Crawford, L. (1986). The expression of human papillomavirus type 18 E6 protein in bacteria and the production of anti-E6 antibodies. J. Gen. Virol., 67, 1909–1916.

McCance, D.J., Kopan, R., Fuchs, E. and Laimins, L.A. (1988). Human papillomavirus type 16 alters human epithelial cell differentiation in vitro. Proc. Natl Acad, Sci. USA, 85, 7169–7173.

Morris, J.D.H., Crook, T., Bandara, L.R., Davies, R., LaThangue, N.B. and Vousden, K.H. (1993). Human papillomavirus type 16 E7 regulates E2F and contributes to mitogenic signalling. Oncogene, 8, 893–898.

Muller, M., Kelly, G., Fiedler, M. and Gissmann, L. (1989). Human papillomavirus type 48. J. Virol., 63, 4907–4908.

Petti, L., and DiMaio, D. (1992). Stable association between the bovine papillomavirus E5 transforming protein and activated platelet-derived growth factor receptor in transformed mouse cells. Proc. Natl Acad. Sci. USA, 89, 6736–6740.

Petti, L., Nilson, L.A. and DiMaio, D. (1991). Activation of the platelet-derived growth factor receptor by the bovine papillomavirus E5 transforming protein. EMBO J., 10, 845–856.

Pfister, H., Gassenmaier, A., Nurnberger, F. and Stuttgen, G. (1983). Human papillomavirus 5-DNA in case of an epidermodysplasia verruciformis patient infected with various human papillomavirus types. Cancer Res., 43, 1436–1441.

Phelps, W.C., Yee, C.L., Munger, K. and Howley, P.M. (1988). The human papillomavirus type 16 E7 gene encodes transactivation and transformation functions similar to those of adenovirus E1A. Cell, 53, 539–547.

Rosl, F., Achtstatter, T., Bauknecht, T., Hutter, K.-J., Futterman, G. and zur Hausen, H. (1991). Extinction of the HPV18 upstream regulatory region in cervical carcinoma cells after fusion with non-tumorigenic human keratinocytes under non-selective conditions. EMBO J., 10, 1337–1345.

Scheffner, M., Munger, K., Huibregtse, J.M. and Howley, P.M. (1992). Targeted degradation of the retinoblastoma protein by human papillomavirus E7-E6 fusion proteins. EMBO J., 11, 2425–2431.

Schlegel, R., Wade-Glass, M., Rabson, M.S. and Yang, Y.-C. (1986). The E5 transforming gene of bovine papillomavirus encodes a small, hydrophobic polypeptide. Science, 233, 464–467.

Schleurlen, W., Gissmann, L., Gross, G. and zur Hausen, H. (1986b). Molecular cloning of two new HPV types (HPV 37 and HPV 38) from a keratinoacanthoma and a malignant melanoma. Int. J. Cancer, 37, 505–510.

Schleurlen, W., Tremlau, A.S., Gissmann, L., Hohn, D., Zenner, H.-P. and zur Hausen, H. (1986a). Rearranged HPV 16 molecules in an anal and in a laryngeal carcinoma. Int. J. Cancer, 38, 671–676.

Schneider-Gaedicke, A. and Schwarz, E. (1986). Different human cervical carcinoma cell lines show similar transcription patterns of human papillomavirus type 18 early genes. EMBO J., 5, 2285–2292.

Seedorf, K., Krammer, G., Durst, M., Suhai, S. and Rowekamp, W.G. (1985). Human papillomavirus type 16 DNA sequence. Virology, 145, 181–185.

Settleman, J., Fazeli, A., Malicki, J., Horwitz, B.H. and DiMaio, D. (1989). Genetic evidence that acute morphologic transformation, induction of cellular DNA synthesis, and focus formation are mediated by a single activity of the bovine papillomavirus E5 protein. Mol. Cell. Biol., 9, 5563–5572.

Sheibani, N., Rhim, J.S. and Allen-Hoffmann, B.L. (1991). Malignant human papillomavirus type 16-transformed human keratinocytes exhibit altered expression of extracellular matrix glycoproteins. Cancer Res., 51, 5967–5975.

Shimoda, K., Lorincz, A.T., Temple, G.F. and Lancaster, W.D. (1988). Human papillomavirus type 52: a new virus associated with cervical neoplasia. J. Gen. Virol., 69, 2925–2928.

Smits, P.H.M., Smits, H.L., Jebbink, M.F. and ter Schegget, J. (1990). The short arm of chromosome 11 likely is involved in the regulation of the human papillomavirus type 16 early enhancer-promoter and in the suppression of the transforming activity of the viral DNA. Virology, 176, 158–165.

Smotkin, D. and Wetstein, F.O. (1986). Transcription of human papillomavirus type 16 early genes in a cervical cancer and a cancer-derived cell line and identification of the E7 protein. Proc. Natl Acad. Sci. USA, 83, 4680–4684.

Storey, A., Greenfield, I., Banks, L., Pim, D., Crook, T., Crawford, L. and Stanley, M. (1992). Lack of immortalizing activity of a human papillomavirus type 16 variant DNA with a mutation in the E2 gene isolated from normal human cervical keratinocytes. Oncogene, 7, 459–465.

Storey, A. and Banks, L. (1993). Human papillomavirus type 16 E6 gene cooperates with EJ-ras to immortalize primary mouse cells. Oncogene, 8, 919–924.

Tommasino, M., Adamczewski, J.P., Carlotti, F., Barth, C.F., Manetti, R., Contorni, M., Cavalieri, F., Hunt, T. and Crawford, L. (1993). HPV16 E7 protein associates with the protein kinase pp33^{CDK2} and cyclin A. Oncogene, 8, 195–202.

von Knebel Doeberitz, M., Oltersdorf, T., Schwarz, E. and Gissmann, L. (1988). Correlation of modified human papillomavirus early gene expression with altered growth properties in C4–1 cervical carcinoma cells. Cancer Res., 48, 3780–3786.

Watanabe, S., Kanda, T. and Yoshike, K. (1989). Human papillomavirus type 16 transformation of primary human embryonic fibroblasts requires expression of open reading frames E6 and E7. J. Virol., 63, 965–969.

Woodworth, C.D., Notario, V. and DiPaolo, J.A. (1990). Transforming growth factors beta 1 and 2 transcriptionally regulate human papillomavirus (HPV) type 16 early gene expression in HPV-immortalized human genital epithelial cells. J. Virol., 64, 4767–4775.

Epstein–Barr virus (EBV)

EBV is a herpesvirus of high incidence in humans that binds to the CR2 receptor for complement factor iC3b present only on B lymphocytes, follicular dendritic cells and B- and T-derived cell lines. After infection the viral genome circularizes through its terminal repeats and in immortalized cells is latently maintained as an episomal molecule. Approximately 11 genes are expressed in latent infections. Five regions of the genome encode latent polyadenylated transcripts and these give rise to six different nuclear proteins (Epstein–Barr nuclear antigens, EBNA1, 2, 3A, 3B and 3C and a leader protein, EBNA-LP) and three viral membrane proteins (latent membrane proteins, LMP1, 2A and 2B). The switch to expressing most of the other genes is mediated by the virally encoded transcription factor Z (also called BZLF1, EB1, ZEBRA or Zta). Z transcription can be enhanced by TPA, cross-linked cell surface Ig or by its own protein product. The Z protein has a basic DNA binding domain homologous to that of FOS that binds to AP-1 sites and activates transcription of the EBV early genes BSLF2 and BMLF1 in some cell types (e.g. HeLa cells) but not others (e.g. Jurkat cells). Z also has a coiled coil-like dimerization domain, shares homology with C/EBP and binds to the same CCAAT sequence as C/EBP (Kouzarides *et al.*, 1991). However, in Jurkat or Raji cells (an EBV⁺ B cell line), Z interacts synergistically with MYB to activate the BMRF1 promoter (Kenney *et al.*, 1992). Z–MYB binds through the interaction of Z with a 30 bp region containing an AP-1 consensus sequence. EBV also activates transcription from the HIV-1 LTR.

Genome

The genome consists of ~186 kbp; ~90 genes.

Transformation

EBV causes infectious mononucleosis (glandular fever) and is associated with Burkitt's lymphoma (BL), nasopharyngeal carcinoma (NPC) and Hodgkin's lymphoma. The endemic (African) form of BL is usually associated with Epstein–Barr virus, whereas the sporadic form is normally EBV⁻.

All BL tumours express only the EBNA1 EBV gene. High titres of antibodies directed against viral proteins precede the appearance of tumours by several months. The fully malignant phenotype requires the development of a BL clone and a chromosome translocation involving *MYC* (see **MYC**). NPCs always express EBNA1 and some (~65%) express LMP1 (Rowe *et al.*, 1987).

EBV infection of primary B cells *in vitro* causes little or no virus production but gives rise to an immortal lymphoblastoid cell line (LCL) that is not tumorigenic. LCL cells express six EBNAs, LMP1, LMP2A and LMP2B, two small RNAs (EBERs) and two terminal proteins (TP1 and TP2). LCLs are good targets for lysis by T cells, in contrast to BL cells (see below).

	EBNA1 (strain B95-8)	EBNA2 (strain B95-8)	LMP1 (strain B95-8)
mRNA (kb)	3.7	3.0	2.8
Amino acids	641	487	386
Mass (kDa)			
(predicted)	56	52.5	42
(expressed)	p80	p82	p58
Protein half-life (h)			2–5

Cellular location

EBNA1: Nucleus: free in nucleoplasm: some association with chromatin but little with the nuclear matrix.

EBNA2: Nuclear matrix.
LMP1: Transmembrane; localized in patches.

Protein function

EBNA1

EBNA1 does not have transforming capacity but is a *trans*-activating factor required for replication from the latency origin of replication (*oriP*) which is also an EBNA1-dependent enhancer. EBNA1 thus maintains replication of the EBV episome in the latent cycle. EBNA1 protein is inadequately processed for MHC class I recognition and thus escapes immune surveillance.

EBNA2

EBNA2 is a transcription factor involved in the latent cycle. It binds p105^{RB} and is phosphorylated by casein kinase II. EBNA2 is one of the first genes expressed after primary B cell infection *in vitro*. It *trans*-activates LMP1, LMP2A, LMP2B and a lymphoid-specific enhancer in the *Bam*H1 C promoter of EBV (Abbot *et al.*, 1990). EBNA2 also regulates *CD23*, *CD21* (Wang *et al.*, 1990) and *FGR* (Knutson, 1990).

EBNA2 is essential for EBV immortalization of human B cells and regulates transcription from several viral and cellular promoters. It has a region of partial homology (amino acids 463–473) with the p105^{RB} binding domain of adenovirus type 5 E1A, SV40 T antigen and HPV-16 E7 (Inoue *et al.*, 1991). Ser469 in EBNA2 corresponds to those in E7 and T antigen that are phosphorylated by casein kinase II.

Evidence that EBNA2 is required for transformation: (i) deletion of EBNA2 in the P3HR-1 or Daudi EBV genome is associated with the unique inability of these viruses to transform B cells; (ii) transformation-competent recombinants between P3HR-1 and another EBV genome have a restored EBNA2 coding region; and (iii) EBNA2 confers the ability of rat-1 cells to grow in media with low serum concentration (Sample *et al.*, 1986).

LMP1

LMP1 is a transforming protein, reducing serum dependency, contact inhibition and anchorage-dependent growth and increasing tumorigenicity in rodent fibroblasts (Wang *et al.*, 1985, 1988; Baichwal and Sugden, 1988). LMP1 expression is *trans*-activated by EBNA2 via a 142 bp *cis*-acting element (−234 to −92; Tsang *et al.*, 1991). The short half-life of the protein, its localized distribution on the cell surface and association with the cytoskeleton are necessary for its transforming function (Martin and Sugden, 1991). EBV transformation causes a major re-organization of intermediate filaments and microtubules and LMP1 appears in secondary lysosomes together with ubiquitin–protein conjugates and hsp70 (Laszlo *et al.*, 1991). Transient expression of LMP1 causes upregulation of *CD21*, *CD23*, *ICAM1* and *LFA1* and induces DNA synthesis in human B cells (Peng and Lundgren, 1992).

Human B cells are protected from apoptosis by the expression of LMP1 which activates transcription of *BCL2* (Henderson *et al.*, 1991). BCL2 protein is 25% identical to a 149 amino acid region encoded by the EBV immediate early *BHRF1* gene (Marchini *et al.*, 1991). BHRF1 is abundantly expressed early in the lytic life cycle but is not required for EBV-induced transformation of B lymphocytes *in vitro*. However, the *BHRF1* gene product may be essential for infected cell survival when *BCL2* is not induced by LMP1. In BL cells the *BCL2* and *BHRF1* gene products are equally effective in rescuing the cells from apoptosis (Henderson *et al.*, 1993).

LMPs are transcribed under the control of three adjacent promoters: a leftward LMP1 promoter initiating transcription at nucleotide 169 515, an adjacent rightward LMP2B promoter (initiating transcription at 169 734) and a rightward LMP2A promoter (166 498) downstream of the LMP gene (Tsang *et al.*, 1991).

LMP1 and LMP2A associate in the plasma membrane. LMP2A is phosphorylated and, in EBV-transformed B lymphocytes, forms a complex with the LYN tyrosine kinase (Burkhardt *et al.*, 1992).

Sequence of EBNA1 (strain B95–8)

```
  (1)   MSDEGPGTGPGNGLGEKGDTSGPEGSGGSGPQRRGGDNHGRGRGRGRGRGGGRPGAPGG
 (60)   SGSGPRHRDGVRRPQKRPSCIGCKGTHGGTHGGTGAGAGGAGAGGAGAGGGAGAGGGAGGAG
(120)   GAGGAGAGGGAGAGGGAGGAGGAGAGGGAGAGGGAGGAGAGGGAGGAGGAGAGGGAGAGG
(180)   GAGGAGAGGGAGGAGGAGAGGGAGAGGAGGAGGAGAGGGAGAGGGAGGAGGAGAGGAGAGG
(240)   AGAGGAGAGGAGGAGAGGAGGAGAGGGAGGAGAGGGAGGAGAGGAGGAGAGG
(300)   AGGAGAGGAGGAGAGGGAGAGGAGAGGGGRGRGGSGGRGRGGSGGRGRGGSGGRRGRGRE
(360)   RARGGSRERARGRGRGRGEKRPRSPSSQSSSSGSPPRRPPPGRRPFFHPVGEADYFEYHQ
(420)   EGGPDGEPDVPPGAIEQGPADDPGEGPSTGPRGQGDGGRRKKGGWFGKHRGQGGSNPKFE
(480)   NIAEGLRALLARSHVERTTDEGTWVAGVFVYGGSKTSLYNLRRGTALAIPQCRLTPLSRL
(540)   PFGMAPGPGPQPGPLRESIVCYFMVFLQTHIFAEVLKDAIKDLVMTKPAPTCNIRVTVCS
(600)   FDDGVDLPPWFPPMVEGAAAEGDDGDDGDEGGDGDEGEEGQE(641)
```

Sequence of EBNA2 (strain B95–8)

```
  (1)   MPTFYLALHGGQTYHLIVDTDSLGNPSLSVIPSNPYQEQLSDTPLIPLTIFVGENTGVP
 (60)   PPLPPPPPPPPPPPPPPPPPPPPPPPPPPPSPPPPPPPPPPPPPQRRDAWTQEPSPLDRDPLG
(120)   YDVGHGPLASAMRMLWMANYIVRQSRGDRGLILPQGPQTAPQARLVQPHVPPLRPTAPTI
(180)   LSPLSQPRLTPPQPLMMPPRPTPPTPLPPATLTVPPRPTRPTTLPPTPLLTVLQRPTELQ
(240)   PTPSPPRMHLPVLHVPDQSMHPLTHQSTPNDPDSPEPRSPTVFYNIPPMPLPPSQLPPPA
(300)   APAQPPPGVINDQQLHHLPSGPPWWPPICDPPQPSKTQGQSRGQSRGRGRGRGRGRGKGK
(360)   SRDKQRKPGGPWRPEPNTSSPSMPELSPVLGLHQGQGAGDSPTPGPSNAAPVCRNSHTAT
(420)   PNVSPIHEPESHNSPEAPILFPDDWYPPSIDPADLDESWDYIFETTESPSSDEDYVEGPS
(480)   KRPRPSIQ (487)
```

Underlined: p105^{RB} and casein kinase II recognition region.

Sequence homology between HPV-16, -17 and -6b E7, E1A, SV40 T antigen and EBV EBNA2 proteins in the RB and casein kinase II recognition regions

										31	32						
HPV–16 E7	21	D	L	Y	C	Y	E	Q	L	N	D	S	S	E	E	E	D E	37
HPV–18 E7	24	D	L	L	C	H	E	Q	L	S	D	S	E	E	E	N	D E	40
HPV–6b E7	22	G	L	H	C	Y	E	Q	L	V	D	S	S	E	D	E	V D	38
E1A	121	D	L	T	C	H	E	A	G	F	P	P	S	D	D	E	D E	137
T Antigen	102	N	L	F	C	S	E	E	M	P	S	S	D	D	E	A	T A	117
EBV EBNA2	458	W	D	Y	I	F	E	T	T	E	S	P	S	S	D	E	D Y	474

The expression of the EBNA genes is driven from one of two distal promoters (BWR1 (in multiple copies) and BCR2) near the left hand end of the viral genome but in BL cells EBNA1 is expressed from a third promoter (Schaefer *et al.*, 1991; Altiok *et al.*, 1992). EBV DNA in chronic lymphocytic leukaemia and in EBV-carrying BL cell lines is more highly methylated than EBV DNA from virally transformed normal diploid cells and lymphoblastoid cell lines, which may reflect suppressed expression (Lewin *et al.*, 1991).

The cumulative effect of the expression of the latent EBV proteins appears to be to activate growth-regulating pathways involved in normal B cell stimulation (Calender *et al.*, 1990), including the expression of a variety of surface antigens (the EBV receptor (C3d or CR2 (*CD21*)), *CD23*, LFA-1β (*CD18*) and LFA-3 (*CD58*)).

Fusion of BL cells and non-tumorigenic EBV-immortalized B-lymphoblastoid cells suppresses the malignant phenotype of the BL cell line, despite the fact that the hybrid cells contain EBV and express deregulated *MYC* (Wolf *et al.*, 1990). These observations may reflect the action of tumor necrosis factor (TNF) or a related protein. The synthesis of TNF by tumour cells correlates with reduced tumorigenicity and invasiveness (Vanhaesebroeck *et al.*, 1991). A TNF-like gene may be disrupted in BL with complementation occurring in the hybrid cells.

Sequences of latent membrane proteins (LMP1)

```
LMP1 (B95-8)    (1)    MEHDLERGPPGPRRPPRGPPLSSSLGLALLLLLLALLFWLYIVMSDWTGGALLVLYSFA

LMP1 (Raji)     (1)    -DL------------------------------------I--N----------A--

LMP1 (B95-8)    (60)   LMLIIIILIIFIFRRDLLCPLGALCILLLMITLLLIALWNLHGQALFLGIVLFIFGCLLV
LMP1 (Raji)     (60)   ---V----------------------L--------------------Y-------------

LMP1 (B95-8)    (120)  LGIWIYLLEMLWRLGATIWQLLAFFLAFFLDLILLIIALYLQQNWWTLLVDLLWLLLFLA
LMP1 (Raji)     (120)  ---------I-------------------------I------------------------

LMP1 (B95-8)    (180)  ILIWMYYHGQRHSDEHHHDDSLPHPQQATDDSGHESDSNSNEGRHHLLVSGAGDGPPLCS
LMP1 (Raji)     (180)  ------------------------------SNQ---------L--------------

LMP1 (B95-8)    (240)  QNLGAPGGGPDNGPQDPDNTDDNGPQDPDNTDDNGPHDPLPQDPDNTDDNGPQDPDNTDD
LMP1 (Raji)     (240)  ---------N----------------------------------------------

LMP1 (B95-8)    (300)  NGPHDPLPHSPSDSAGNDGGPPQLTEEVENKGGDQGPPLMTDGGGGHSHDSGHGGGDPHL
LMP1 (Raji)     (300)  ---------N------------------------------------D-I----

LMP1 (B95-8)    (360)  PTLLLGSSGSGGDDDDPHGPVQLSYYD (386)
LMP1 (Raji)     (360)  ------T------------------- (386)
```

Underlined regions indicate six potential transmembrane domains.

Sequences of membrane protein LMP2A/LMP2B

```
LMP2A                 (1)    MGSLEMVPMGAGPPSPGGDPDGYDGGNNSQYPSASGSSGNTPTPPNDEERESNEEPPPP
                      (60)   YEDPYWGNGDRHSDYQPLGTQDQSLYLGLQHDGNDGLPPPYSPRDDSSQHIYEEAGRGS
LMP2B (1)/LMP2A       (120)  MNPVCLPVIVAPYLFWLAAIAASCFTASVSTVVTATGLALSLLLLAAVASSYAAAQRKLL
                      (180)  TPVTVLTAVVTFFAICLTWRIEDPPFNSLLFALLAAAGGLQGIYVLVMLVLLILAYRRRW
                      (240)  RRLTVCGGIMFLACVLVLIVDAVLQLSPLLGAVTVVSMTLLLLAFVLWLSSPGGLGTLGA
                      (300)  ALLTLAAALALLASLILGTLNLTTMFLLMLLWTLVVLLICSSCSSCPLSKILLARLFLYA
                      (360)  LALLLLASALIAGGSILQTNFKSLSSTEFIPNLFCMLLLIVAGILFILAILTEWGSGNRT
                      (420)  YGPVFMCLGGGLLTMVAGAVWLTVMSNTLLSAWILTAGFLIFLIGFALFGVIRCCRYCCYY
                      (480)  CLTLESEERPPTPYRNTV(497)
```

Separate mRNAs (2.0 and 2.3 kb) are transcribed to give rise to two proteins, the shorter of which (LMP2B) lacks 119 N-terminal amino acids (Sample *et al.*, 1989). Underlined regions indicate 12 potential transmembrane domains.

Databank file names and accession numbers

GENE	EMBL	SWISSPROT	REFERENCES
EBNA1	EBV V01555	EBN1_EBV P03211	Baer *et al.*, 1984
	Hehs4NA1 M13941		Sample *et al.*, 1986
			Petti *et al.*, 1990
EBNA2	EBV V01555	EBN2_EBV P12978	Baer *et al.*, 1984
			Petti *et al.*, 1990
LMP1 (B95–8)	EBV V01555	LMP_EBV P03230	Baer *et al.*, 1984
			Baichwal and Sugden, 1988
			Moorthy and Thorley-Lawson, 1990
LMP1 (Raji)	HehS41mp M20868	LMP_EBVR P13198	Hatfull *et al.*, 1988
LMP2A/2B	EBV V01555	VTER_EBV P13285	Laux *et al.*, 1988
	EBVTERM Y00835		Sample *et al.*, 1989
	M24212		

Reviews

Chee, M. and Barrell, B. (1990). Herpesviruses: a study of parts. Trends Genet., 6, 86–91.
Middleton, T., Gahn, T.A., Martin, J.M.and Sugden, B. (1991). Immortalizing genes of Epstein-Barr virus. Adv. Virus Res., 40, 19–55.

Papers

Abbot, S.D., Rowe, M., Cadwallader, K., Ricksten, A., Gordon, J., Wang, F., Rymo, L. and Rickinson, A.B. (1990). Epstein-Barr virus nuclear antigen 2 induces expression of the virus-encoded latent membrane protein. J. Virol., 64, 2126–2134.
Altiok, E., Minarovits, J., Li-Fu, H., Contreras-Brodin, B., Klein, G. and Ernberg, I. (1992). Host-cell-phenotype-dependent control of the BCR2/BWR1 promoter complex regulates the expression of Epstein-Barr virus nuclear antigens 2–6. Proc. Natl Acad. Sci. USA, 89, 905–909.
Baer, R., Bankier, A.T., Biggin, M.D., Deininger,P.L., Farrell, P.J., Gibson, T.J., Hatfull, G., Hudson, G.S., Satchwell, S.C., Seguin, C., Tuffnell, P.S., and Barrell, B.G. (1984). DNA sequence and expression of the B95–8 Epstein-Barr virus genome. Nature, 310, 207–211.
Baichwal, V.R. and Sugden, B. (1988). Transfection of Balb 3T3 cells by the BNLF-1 gene of Epstein-Barr virus. Oncogene, 2, 461–467.
Burkhardt, A.L., Bolen, J.B., Kieff, E. and Longnecker, R. (1992). An Epstein-Barr virus transformation-associated membrane protein interacts with *src* family tyrosine kinases. J. Virol., 66, 5161–5167.
Calender, A., Cordier, M., Billaud, M. and Lenoir, G.M. (1990). Modulation of cellular gene expression in B lymphoma cells following *in vitro* infection by Epstein-Barr virus (EBV). Int. J. Cancer 46, 658–663.

Hatfull, G., Bankier, A.T., Barrell, B.G. and Farrell, P.J. (1988). Sequence analysis of the Raji Epstein-Barr virus DNA. Virology, 164, 334–340.

Henderson, S., Rowe, M., Gregory, C., Croom-Carter, D., Wang, F., Longnecker, R., Kieff, E. and Rickinson, A. (1991). Induction of bcl-2 expression by Epstein-Barr virus latent membrane protein 1 protects infected B cells from programmed cell death. Cell, 65, 1107–1115.

Henderson, S., Huen, D., Rowe, M., Dawson, C., Johnson, G. and Rickinson, A. (1993). Epstein–Barr virus-coded BHRF1 protein, a viral homologue of Bcl-2, protects human B cells from programmed cell death. Proc. Natl Acad. Sci. USA, in press.

Inoue, N., Harada, S., Honma, T., Kitamura, T. and Yanagi, K. (1991). The domain of Epstein–Barr virus nuclear antigen 1 essential for binding to oriP region has a sequence fitted for the hypothetical basic-helix–loop–helix structure. Virology, 182, 84–93.

Kenney, S.C., Holley-Guthrie, E., Quinlivan, E.B., Gutsch, D., Zhang, Q., Bender, T., Giot, J.-F. and Sergeant, A. (1992). The cellular oncogene c-myb can interact synergistically with the Epstein-Barr virus BZLF1 transactivator in lymphoid cells. Mol. Cell. Biol., 12, 136–146.

Knutson, J.C. (1990). The level of c-fgr RNA is increased by EBNA-2, an Epstein-Barr virus gene required for B-cell immortalization. J. Virol., 64, 2530–2536.

Kouzarides, T., Packham, G., Cook, A. and Farrell, P.J. (1991). The BZLF1 protein of EBV has a coiled coil dimerisation domain without a heptad leucine repeat but with homology to the C/EBP leucine zipper. Oncogene, 6, 195–204.

Laszlo, L., Tuckwell, J., Self, T., Lowe, J., Landon, M., Smith, S., Hawthorne, J.N. and Mayer, R.J. (1991). The latent membrane protein-1 in Epstein-Barr virus-transformed lymphoblastoid cells is found with ubiquitin-protein conjugates and heat-shock protein 70 in lysosomes oriented around the microtubule organizing centre. J. Pathol., 164, 203–214.

Laux, G., Perricaudet, M. and Farrell, P.J. (1988). A spliced Epstein-Barr virus gene expressed in immortalized lymphocytes is created by circularization of the linear viral genome. EMBO J., 7, 769–774.

Lewin, N., Minarovits, J., Weber, G., Ehlin-Hendriksson, B., Wen, T., Mellstedt, H., Klein, G. and Klein, E. (1991). Clonality and methylation status of the Epstein-Barr virus (EBV) genomes in in vivo-infected EBV-carrying chronic lymphocytic leukemia (CLL) cell lines. Int. J. Cancer, 48, 62–66.

Marchini, A., Tomkinson, B., Cohen, J.I. and Kieff, E. (1991). BHRF1, the Epstein-Barr virus gene with homology to bcl2, is dispensable for B-lymphocyte transformation and virus replication. J. Virol., 65, 5991–6000.

Martin, J. and Sugden, B. (1991). Transformation by the oncogenic latent membrane protein correlates with its rapid turnover, membrane localization, and cytoskeletal association. J. Virol., 65, 3246–3258.

Moorthy, R. and Thorley-Lawson, D.A. (1990). Processing of the Epstein-Barr virus-encoded latent membrane protein p63/LMP. J. Virol., 64, 829–837.

Peng, M. and Lundgren, E. (1992). Transient expression of the Epstein-Barr virus LMP1 gene in human primary B cells induces cellular activation and DNA synthesis. Oncogene, 7, 1775–1782.

Petti, L., Sample, C. and Kieff, E. (1990). Subnuclear localization and phosphorylation of Epstein-Barr virus latent infection nuclear proteins. Virology, 176, 563–574.

Rowe, M., Rowe, D.T., Gregory, C.D., Young, L.S., Farrell, P.J., Rupani, H. and Rickinson, A.B. (1987). Differences in B cell growth phenotype reflect novel patterns of Epstein-Barr virus latent gene expression in Burkitt's lymphoma cells. EMBO J., 6, 2743–2751.

Sample, J., Hummel, M., Braun, D., Birkenbach, M. and Kieff, E. (1986). Nucleotide sequences of mRNAs encoding Epstein-Barr virus nuclear proteins: a probable transcriptional initiation site. Proc. Natl Acad. Sci. USA, 83, 5096–5100.

Sample, J., Liebowitz, D. and Kieff, E. (1989). Two related Epstein-Barr virus membrane proteins are encoded by separate genes. J. Virol., 63, 933–937.

Schaefer, B.C. Woisetschlaeger, M., Strominger, J.L. and Speck, S.H. (1991). Exclusive expression of Epstein-Barr virus nuclear antigen 1 in Burkitt lymphoma arises from a third promoter, distinct from the promoters used in latently infected lymphocytes. Proc. Natl Acad. Sci. USA, 88, 6550–6554.

Tsang, S.-F., Wang, F., Izumi, K.M. and Kieff, E. (1991). Delineation of the cis-acting element mediating EBNA-2 transactivation of latent infection membrane protein expression. J. Virol., 65, 6765–6771.

Vanhaesebroeck, B., Mareel, M., Van Roy, F., Grooten, J. and Fiers, W. (1991). Expression of the tumor necrosis factor gene in tumor cells correlates with reduced tumorigenicity and reduced invasiveness in vivo. Cancer Res., 51, 2229–2238.

Wang, D., Liebowitz, D. and Kieff, E. (1985). An EBV membrane protein expressed in immortalized lymphocytes transforms established rodent cells. Cell, 43, 831–840.

Wang, D., Liebowitz, D. and Kieff, E. (1988). The truncated form of the Epstein-Barr virus latent-infection membrane protein expressed in virus replication does not transform rodent fibroblasts. J. Virol., 62, 2337–2346.

Wang, F., Gregory, C., Sample, C., Rowe, M., Liebowitz, D., Murray, R., Rickinson, A. and Kieff, E. (1990). Epstein-Barr virus latent membrane protein (LMP-1) and nuclear proteins 2 and 3C are effectors of phenotypic changes in B lymphocytes: EBNA-2 and LMP-1 cooperatively induce CD23. J. Virol., 64, 2309–2318.

Wolf, J., Pawlita, M., Bullerdiek, J. and zur Hausen, H. (1990). Suppression of the malignant phenotype in somatic cell hybrids between Burkitt's lymphoma cells and Epstein-Barr virus-immortalized lymphoblastoid cells despite deregulated c-*myc* expression. Cancer Res., 50, 3095–3100.

EPH

EPH (*EPHT*) is the prototype of a subfamily of tyrosine kinases, initially isolated from a human genomic library with a v-*fps* probe that is overexpressed in an *e*rythropoietin *p*roducing human *h*epatocellular (*EPH*) carcinoma cell line (Hirai *et al.*, 1987).

Related genes

EPH is related to *ELK* (eph-like kinase; Lhotak *et al.*, 1991); *EEK* (eph and elk-related kinase; Chan and Watt, 1991); *ECK* (epithelial cell kinase; Lindberg and Hunter, 1990); and *ERK* (elk-related kinase). Also related to murine *Nuk* (neural kinase) receptor kinase (Henkemeyer *et al.*, 1992), murine *Sek* (Gilardi-Hebenstreit *et al.*, 1992), murine *Mek-4* and chicken *Cek-4* (chicken embryo kinase 4; Sajjadi *et al.*, 1991), chicken *Cek-5* (Pasquale, 1991), chicken *Tyro-5* (Marcelle and Eichmann, 1992) and human *HEK* (Wicks *et al.*, 1992).

EEK is 69% and 57% identical in sequence to ELK and EPH, respectively. The ECK catalytic domain is 70% homologous with that of ELK and 60% with EPH but only between 34 and 43% homologous with those of SRC, ABL, FES, the EGFR and PDGFR.

Homology between *Eph* and v-*fps* in the kinase-coding domain is 43% (v-*abl* 44%, v-*erbB* 40%, v-*fms* 38%, v-*fgr* 45%, v-*kit* 37%, v-*ros* 41%, v-*src* 46%), compared with 70–80% between members of the *Src* family (*Src, Yes, Fgr, Lck, Fyn, Lyn, Hck*). This region is also 36–40% homologous with the corresponding regions of *Met, Trk, Ret* and *Ros*. The pattern of splicing points within the five exons of the kinase domain differ from those of other tyrosine kinases (*Src, Fps, Abl/Arg* and *HER2*), indicating that the *Eph* family represents the earliest evolutionary divergence within this group (Maru *et al.*, 1988).

Cross-species homology

Eph has been highly conserved during vertebrate evolution, being detectable by the same v-*fps* probe in man, mouse, rat and chicken. Human ERK: 90% identity with rat ELK; 74% with rat EEK.

Transformation

Eph is overexpressed in several carcinomas (Maru *et al.*, 1988). Overexpressed *Eph* renders NIH 3T3 cells tumorigenic (Maru *et al.*, 1990). *HEK* is expressed in cell lines derived from human lymphoid tumours (Wicks *et al.*, 1992).

	EPH/Eph	ECK/Eck	Elk (rat)	EEK	ERK*
Chromosome			1		
Human	7q32–q36	1		1	1
Mouse		4			
mRNA (kb)	3.5	~4.7	4.0		

	EPH/Eph	ECK/Eck	Elk (rat)	EEK	ERK*
Amino acids	984	976	984		
Mass (kDa)					
(predicted)	109		110		
(expressed)			130		

*ERK is distinct from the *Erk-1, -2* and *-3* family of serine/threonine kinases (Boulton *et al.*, 1991).

Tissue location

Eph: Kidney/testis, liver/lung.
Elk: Lung/skin, ovary/small intestine.
Eck: Brain/testis (rat).
Eek: Brain (rat).
Erk: Lung (rat).
Cek-4 (chicken), *Mek-4* (mouse) and *HEK* (human): Expressed in brain, testes.
Mek-4 and *Cek-4*: Highly expressed in mouse and chicken embryos, respectively. A cDNA encoding a putative secreted form of the *Mek-4* ligand binding domain has been isolated (Sajjadi *et al.*, 1991).
Cek-5 (chicken): Widely expressed in embryonic tissues; predominantly in the brain in adults (Pasquale, 1991).
Nuk: Brain, heart, liver (rat).
Sek: Developing hindbrain, heart and lung (mouse) (Gilardi-Hebenstreit *et al.*, 1992).

Protein function

EPH is the prototype class IV transmembrane tyrosine kinase receptor. The extracellular domain contains a putative immunoglobulin-like loop at the N-terminus, a single cysteine-rich region and two fibronectin type III repeats near to the transmembrane domain (Pasquale *et al.*, 1991). The kinase domain is uninterrupted. Ligand(s) unknown.

Sequences of EPH, ELK and ECK proteins

```
Human EPH    (1)    MERRWPLGLGLVLLLCAPLPPGA RAKEVTLMDTSKAQGELGWLLDPPKDGWSE QQQILN
Human ECK    (1)    MELQAARACFA-LWGCALPAAAA-QG---V-L-FAA-G------TH-YGK--DL M-N-M-
Rat ELK      (1)          MALDC--LFL-ASAVA-M-E-----RT-TA----TAN- AS--E-VSGYDE-

Human EPH    (60)   GTPLYMYQDCPMQGRRDTDHWLRSNWIYRGEEASRVHVELQFTVRDCKSFPGGAGPLGCK
Human ECK    (61)   DM-I---SV-NV MSG-Q-N---T--V---- -E-NNF--N------N------  SS--
Rat ELK      (52)   LNTIRT--V-NV FEPNQNN--LTTF-N-RG -H-IYT-MR------S-L-NVP GS--

Human EPH    (120)  ETFNLLYMESDQDVG    IQLRRPLFQKVTTVAADQSFTIRDLASGSVKLNVERCSLGR
Human ECK    (117)  -----Y-A---L---T   NFQKRL-T-ID-I-P-EITVSS-FEARH------ER-V-P
Rat ELK      (108)  -----Y-Y-T-SVIATKKSAFWSEAPYL--D-I---E--SQV-FGGRLM-V-T-VR-F-P

Human EPH    (176)  LTRRGLYLAFHNPGACVALVSVRVFYQRCPETLNGLAQFPDTLPGP  AGLVEVAGTCLP
Human ECK    (173)  ---K-F----QDI------L----Y-KK---L-Q---H--E-IA-SDAPS-AT-----VD
Rat ELK      (168)  ---N-F----QDY---MS-L-----FKK--SIVQNF-V--E-MT-AESTS--IAR---I-
```

```
Human EPH  (234)  HARASPRPSGAPRMHCSPDGEWLVPVGRCHCEPGYEEGGSGEACVACPSGSYRMDMDTPH
Human ECK  (233)  -- VV-PGGEE-----AV-------I-Q-L-QA---KVE  D--Q--SP-FFKFEASESP
Rat ELK    (228)  N-EEVDVP   IKLY-NG----M--I---T-KA---PENS V--K---A-TFKASQEAEG

Human EPH  (294)  CLTCPQQSTAESEGATICTCESGHYRAPGEGPQVACTGPPSAPRN LSFSASGTQLSLRW
Human ECK  (290)  --E--EHTLPSP----S-E--E-FF---QDPASMP--RP----HY -TAVGM-AKVE---
Rat ELK    (284)  -SH--SN-RSP--ASP----RT-Y---DFDP-E----SV--G---VI-IV NE-SII-E-

Human EPH  (353)  EPPADTGGRQDVRYSVRCSQCQGTAQDGGPCQPCGVGVHFSPGARGLTTPAVHVNGLEPY
Human ECK  (349)  T--Q-S---E-IV---T-E-- WPESGE-G--EAS-RY-EPPHG--RTS-T-SD---H
Rat ELK    (343)  H--RE----D--T-NII-KK- RADRRS-SR-DDN-EFV-RQLG--ECR-SISS-WAH

Human EPH  (413)  ANYTFNVEAQNGVSGLGSSGHAST SVSISMGHAESLSGLSLRLVKKEPRQLELTWAGSR
Human ECK  (406)  M----T---R------VT-RSFR-A---- NQT-PPKVRLQGRSTTSLSVSWSIPPPQQ
Rat ELK    (400)  TP---DIQ-I----SKSPFPPQHV --N-TTNQAAPSTVPIMHQ VSATMRSITLSWPQP

Human EPH  (472)  PRSPGANLTYELHVLNQDEERYQMVLEPRVLLT  ELQPDTTYIVRVRMLTPLGPGPF
Human ECK  (464)  SRLWKYEVT-RKKGDSNSYNVRRTEGFSVT-D  D-A-----L-Q-QAL-QE-Q-AG
Rat ELK    (458)  EQPN-II-D--IRYYEKEHNEFNSSMARSQTNTARIDG-R-GMV-V-Q--AR-VA-Y-K-

Human EPH  (528)  SPDHEFRT SPPVSRG  LTGGEIVAVIFGLLLGAALLLGILVFRSRRAQRQRQQRH
Human ECK  (519)  -KV---Q-L--EG-GN  -AVIGG---GVV---VL-G-GFFI HR--KNQRAR-SP
Rat ELK    (518)  -GKMC-Q-LTDDDYKSELREQ-PLIAGS-AAGVVFVVSLVAIS-VCS-K-AYSKEAVYSD

Human EPH  (582)  VTAPPMWIERTSCAEALCGTSRHTRTLHREPWTLPGGWSNFPSRELDPAWLMVDTVIGEG
Human ECK  (572)  EDVYFSK   -EQLKPLK-YVDPH-YEDPNQAVLKFTTEIHPSCV  TRQK---A-
Rat ELK    (578)  K   LQHYS-GRGSPGMKIYIDPF-YEDPNEAVREFAKEIDVSFV  KIEE---A-

Human EPH  (642)  EFGEVYRGTLRLPS QDCKTVAIKTLKDTSPGGQWWNFLREATIMGQFSHPHILHLEGVV
Human ECK  (623)  ------K-M-KTS-GKKEVP-------AGYTEK-RVD--G--G-------HN-IR----I
Rat ELK    (629)  ------K-R-K--G KREIY-------AGYSEK-RRD--S--S-----D--N-IR-----

Human EPH  (701)  TKRKPIMIITEFMENGALDAFLREREDQLVPGQLVAMLQGIASGMNYLSNHNYVHRDLAA
Human ECK  (683)  S-Y--M-----Y---G---K---EKDGEFSVL---G--R---QA--K--ANM--------
Rat ELK    (688)  --SR-V---------G---S---QNDGFQTVI---G--R---A--K---EM---------

                                              *
Human EPH  (761)  RNILVNQNLCCKVSDFGLTR LLDD FDGTYETQ GGKIPIRWTAPEAIAHRIFTTASDV
Human ECK  (743)  ------S--V--------S-V-E-- PEA--TTS --------------SY-K--S----
Rat ELK    (748)  ------S--V--------S-Y-Q--TSDP--TSSL-----V---------Y-K--S----

Human EPH  (818)  WSFGIVMWEVLSFGDKPYGEMSNQEVMKSIEDGYRLPPPVDCPAPLYELMKNCWAYDRAR
Human ECK  (801)  ----------MTY-ER--WEL--H----A-N--F---T-M---SAIYQ--MQ--QQE---
Rat ELK    (808)  --Y-------MS--ER--WD----D-INA--QD------M----A-HQ--LD--QK--NS

Human EPH  (878)  RPHFQKLQAHLEQLLANPHSLRTIANFDPRVTLRLPSLSGSDGIPYRTVSEWLESIRMKR
Human ECK  (861)  --K-ADIVSI-DK-IRA-D--K-L-D-----SI----T---E-V-F----------K-QQ
Rat ELK    (868)  --R-AEIVNT-DKMIR--A--K-V-TITAVPSQP-LDR-IP-FTAFT--DD--SA-K-VQ

Human EPH  (938)  YILHFHSAGLDTMECVLELTAEDLTQMGITLPGHQKRILCSIQGFKD (984)
Human ECK  (921)  -TE--MA--YTAI-K-VQM-ND-IKRI-VR-------AY-LL-LK-QVNTVGIPI (976)
Rat ELK    (928)  -RDS-LT--FTSLQL-TQM-S---LRI-V--A----K--S--HSMRVQMNQSPSVMA (984)
```

Dashes indicate identity with EPH. Signal sequences and transmembrane regions underlined.
* Indicates potential phosphorylation site (EPH Tyr789). EPH amino acids 24–547: extracellular; 548–568: transmembrane; 569–984: intracellular (catalytic); 638–646 and 664–664 ATP binding; and 414 and 478 are potential carbohydrate attachment sites. ECK: 534 extracellular N-terminal amino acids; 418: cytoplasmic tyrosine kinase domain.

Databank file names and accession numbers

	ONCOGENE	EMBL	SWISSPROT	REFERENCES
Human	EPH	Hstkr M18391	KEPH_HUMAN P21709	Hirai et al., 1987
Human	ECK	Hseck M36395		Lindberg and Hunter, 1990
Human	EEK	Hseekd2 X59291		Chan and Watt, 1991
Human	ERK	Hserkd23 X59292		Chan and Watt, 1991
Human	HEK	Hshek M83941		Wicks et al., 1992
Rat	Eek	Rneekr X59290		Chan and Watt, 1991
Rat	Elk	Rrelkf M59814		Lhotak et al., 1991
Mouse	Sek	Mmsek X65138		Gilardi-Hebenstreit et al., 1992

Papers

Boulton, T.G., Nye, S.H., Robbins, D.J., Ip, N.Y., Radziejewska, F., Morgenbesser, S.D., DePinho, R.A., Panayotatos, N., Cobb, M.H. and Yancopoulos, N. (1991). ERKs: a family of protein-serine/threonine kinases that are activated and tyrosine phosphorylated in response to insulin and NGF. Cell, 65, 663–675.

Chan, J. and Watt, V.M. (1991). *eek* and *erk*, new members of the *eph* subclass of receptor protein-tyrosine kinases. Oncogene, 6, 1057–1061.

Gilardi-Hebenstreit, P., Nieto, M.A., Frain, M., Mattei, M.-G., Chestier, A., Wilkinson, D.G. and Charnay, P. (1992). An eph-related receptor protein tyrosine kinase gene segmentally expressed in the developing mouse hindbrain. Oncogene, 7, 2499–2506.

Henkemeyer, M., McGlade, J., Greer, P. and Pawson, T. (1992). The murine receptor tyrosine kinase *nuk* is concentrated in a subset of cell–cell junctions during embryogenesis. J. Cell. Biochem., Suppl. 16F, 106.

Hirai, H., Maru, Y., Hagiwara, K., Nishida, J. and Takaku, F. (1987). A novel putative tyrosine kinase receptor encoded by the *eph* gene. Science, 238, 1717–1720.

Lhotak, V., Greer, P., Letwin, K. and Pawson, T. (1991). Characterization of elk, a brain-specific receptor tyrosine kinase. Mol. Cell. Biol., 11, 2496–2502.

Lindberg, R.A. and Hunter, T. (1990). cDNA cloning and characterization of *eck*, an epithelial cell receptor protein-tyrosine kinase in the *eph/elk* family of protein kinases. Mol. Cell. Biol., 10, 6316–6324.

Marcelle, C. and Eichmann, A. (1992). Molecular cloning of a family of protein kinase genes expressed in the avian embryo. Oncogene, 7, 2479–2487.

Maru, Y., Hirai, H. and Takaku, F. (1990). Overexpression confers an oncogenic potential upon the *eph* gene. Oncogene, 5, 445–447.

Maru, Y., Hirai, H., Yoshida, M.C. and Takaku, F. (1988). Evolution, expression and chromosomal location of a novel receptor tyrosine kinase gene, *eph*. Mol. Cell. Biol., 8, 3770–3776.

Pasquale, E.B. (1991). Identification of chicken embryo kinase 5, a developmentally regulated receptor-type tyrosine kinase of the *eph* family. Cell Regulation, 2, 523–534.

Sajjadi, F.G., Pasquale, E.B. and Subramani, S. (1991). Identification of a new *eph*-related receptor tyrosine kinase gene from mouse and chicken that is developmentally regulated and encodes at least two forms of the receptor. New Biologist, 3, 769–778.

Wicks, I.P., Wilkinson, D., Salvaris, E. and Boyd, A.W. (1992). Molecular cloning of HEK, the gene encoding a receptor tyrosine kinase expressed by human lymphoid tumor cell lines. Proc. Natl Acad. Sci. USA, 89, 1611–1615.

v-*ets* (*E t*wenty-six *s*pecific) and v-*myb* are the oncogenes of the acutely transforming avian erythroblastosis virus E26 (Ivanov *et al.*, 1962, 1964; Nedyalkov *et al.*, 1975; Nunn *et al.*, 1983; Leprince *et al.*, 1983).

Ets, *Erg* (ets-related gene), *Elf* (*E74-like factor 1*) and *Elk* encode transcription factors.

Related genes

PU.1/*Spi-1* (mouse), E1A enhancer binding protein, E1A-F (Higashino *et al.*, 1993), PEA3 (mouse; Xin *et al.*, 1992), E74A and E74B (*Xenopus*, sea urchin and *Drosophila*; Chen *et al.*, 1988; Burtis *et al.*, 1990; Thummel *et al.*, 1990), *FLI1* (Klemsz *et al.*, 1993), *Fli-1* (Ben-David *et al.*, 1991), mouse *Tpl-1* (see Table 2.2), *Drosophila* D-*elg* (Pribyl *et al.*, 1991; The *et al.*, 1992), *Drosophila elf-1* (Bray and Kafatos, 1991) and *yan* (Lai and Rubin, 1992), *Xenopus laevis ets-1* and *ets-2* (Wolff *et al.*, 1990, 1991). The α subunit of the heteromeric DNA binding protein GABP contains an 85 amino acid ETS domain (Thompson *et al.*, 1991). These lineages have arisen from primordial *Ets* genes via a minimum of five duplication events (Lautenberger *et al.*, 1992). SAP1 (Dalton and Treisman, 1992; see **FOS**) has three regions of homology with ETS proteins, including the ETS domain (see below).

The ETS binding domain sequence of FLI1 is 70% and 40% identical to those of ETS2 and PU.1, respectively. Human FLI1 is expressed in a subset of erythroleukaemic cell lines and binds to the ETS2 binding site (GACCGGAAGTG) but not to that of PU.1 (Klemsz *et al.*, 1993; Zhang *et al.*, 1993).

Cross-species homology

ETS1: >95% homology (human and chicken); 91% (human and mouse). Human and chicken ETS2 are also highly related (Lautenberger *et al.*, 1992).

Transformation

MAN

Chromosome 11q23 (*ETS1*) is involved in translocations associated with undifferentiated leukaemias and myelodysplastic syndrome (Ohyashiki *et al.*, 1990) and 21q22 (*ETS2* and *ERG*) is involved in the translocation (8;21)(q22;q22) that occurs in acute myelogenous leukaemia and Down's syndrome (Papas *et al.*, 1990). These translocations may result in activation of *ETS1* or *ERG*. ELK genes map close to the translocation breakpoint characteristic of synovial sarcoma [t(X;18)(p11.2;q11.2)] and the 14q32 breakpoints seen in ataxia telangiectasia and other T cell malignancies (Rowley 1983; Kocova *et al.*, 1985).

ETS1 is expressed in tumours of the peripheral nervous system (neuroblastomas and neuroepitheliomas) and in Ewing's sarcoma (Sacchi *et al.*, 1991).

ANIMALS

E26 and avian myeloblastosis virus (AMV) are the only two avian oncogenic viruses that cause acute leukaemias but do not transform chicken fibroblasts in culture. AMV has transduced v-*myb* and E26 has transduced two oncogenes, v-*myb* and v-*ets*, both of which encode transcription factors. In E26 these are expressed from a chimeric gene as a *gag–myb–ets* fusion protein.

The co-expression of non-fused v-*myb* and v-*ets* is only weakly leukaemogenic and the potent leukaemogenicity of E26 derives from the fusion of these two genes (Metz and Graf, 1991a, b).

E26 causes erythroblastosis and low level myeloblastosis in chickens. AMV causes only myeloblastosis. v-*ets* cooperates with v-*erbA* to cause avian erythroleukaemia (Metz and Graf, 1992).

IN VITRO

v-*myb* is responsible for myeloid cell transformation but either v-*myb* or v-*ets* can cause weak transformation of erythroid cells (Metz and Graf, 1991a). The *gag–myb–ets* fusion protein transforms immature erythroid cells that are almost totally inhibited from differentiating. However, when v-*myb* and v-*ets* are co-expressed separately from recombinant viruses they transform relatively mature erythroid cells that have a high capacity for spontaneous differentiation. The presence of both oncogenes increases the growth rate and the lifespan of transformed cells. The differing biological responses to the separate expression of the oncogenes (*trans*-cooperation) and the fusion protein (*cis*-cooperation) may reflect the generation of a functionally different transcription factor when MYB and ETS are expressed as a single protein.

In E26-transformed myeloid cells a point mutation in v-*ets* modulates the phenotype from that of immature myeloblasts (wt) to promyelocytes (Golay *et al.*, 1988).

Neither E26 nor AMV transform chick embryo fibroblasts (CEFs; Bister *et al.*, 1982) but E26 transforms quail fibroblasts and stimulates the proliferation of CEFs (Jurdic *et al.*, 1987), neuroretina cells (Amouyel *et al.*, 1989) and NIH 3T3 fibroblasts (Yuan *et al.*, 1989).

Ets-1 transforms NIH 3T3 fibroblasts (Seth and Papas, 1990).

	ETS1/Ets-1	ETS2/Ets-2	ERG, FLI1	ELK1	ELK2	v-ets
Nucleotides (kb)						
Human	60					5.7 (E26)
Chicken	80					2.46 (Δ*gag–myb–ets*)
Chromosome						
Human	11q23.3	21q22.3	21q22.3 11q23–24 (*FLI1*)	Xp11.2	14q32.3	
Mouse	9	16				
mRNA (kb)						1.5
Human	6.8[a]	2.7/3.2/4.7[b]	~3.4/5.0[c] 3.6 (*FLI1*)	3.1		
Chicken	1.5/2.0/7.5[d]	4.0				
Mouse	5.3[e]	3.5	3.4(*Fli1*)			
Exons	8	10				

	ETS1/Ets-1	ETS2/Ets-2	ERG, FLI1	ELK1	ELK2	v-ets
Amino acids						
Human	354/441 (p54)[a]	469	363 (ERG1) 462 (ERG2) 451 (FLI1)	428		491 (v-ets) 669 (Δgag–myb–ets)
Chicken	441 (p54)/485 (p68)[d]	479				
Mouse	440	468				
Mass (kDa)						
(predicted)						
Human	50/55	53/54	41/52	45		75
Chicken	48/55[d]	58/62	50 (FLI1)			
Mouse	50/51					p135[gag-myb-ets]
(expressed)						
Human	pp51/pp48[a] p42/p39	56	41/52[c] 55 (FLI1)			
Chicken	pp54/pp68[d]	58/64				
Mouse	pp60/pp62					
Protein half-life (min)		20				

[a]At least four transcripts generated by alternative splicing (see below).
[b]Transcripts differ in the length of their 3′ ends having three different polyadenylation sites: the coding regions are of the same length.
[c]Alternative splicing of ERG1 (5 kb mRNA) generates ERG2 in which a coding frameshift near the N-terminus results in a 99 amino acid insertion at the N-terminus (Reddy et al., 1987; Rao et al., 1987).
[d]Alternative splicing of chicken Ets-1 generates p54 that has 27 N-terminal amino acids in place of the 71 residues in p68. Chicken ETS2 (p58/p62) is phosphorylated on serine and threonine residues to give pp58/pp64 (Boulukos et al., 1988).
[e]Additional minor forms (2.0, 2.5, 4.0 kb) also occur (Bhat et al., 1989).

Cellular location

Nuclear.

Tissue location

ETS1

Human ETS1 expression is high in the thymus (Reddy and Rao, 1988), in endothelial cells differentiating or migrating during the development of blood vessels and in migrating neural crest cells (Desbiens et al., 1991). Abundantly expressed in fibroblasts and endothelial cells in invasive tumours.

Chicken p54[ets-1] and p68[ets-1] are highly expressed in the thymus and spleen, respectively (Chen, 1985; Ghysdael et al., 1986; Leprince et al., 1988, 1990).

Ets-1 is expressed in mature murine thymocytes (CD4+/CD8−; Bhat et al., 1989).

ETS2

Ets-2 is expressed in most tissues. In the mouse, post-natal expression precedes that of p54[ets-1] in the developing thymus and coincides with the appearance of CD4+/CD8+ and CD4−/CD8− cells (Bhat et al., 1989).

ERG

High levels of expression in human tumour-derived cell lines (Reddy *et al.*, 1987; Rao *et al.*, 1987).

ELK

Restricted to lung and testis (Rao *et al.*, 1989).

Protein function

The family of *ETS* genes encodes transcription factors that bind to the consensus sequence $^C/_AGGA^A/_T$ (Karim *et al.*, 1990). The sequence-specific DNA binding capacity resides in an 85 amino acid region, of similar sequence in ETS family members, designated the ETS domain (Reddy and Rao, 1990; Nye *et al.*, 1992). *ETS* gene products have been shown to interact with purine-rich motifs in the polyoma virus enhancer (Wasylyk *et al.*, 1990), Mo-MuSV LTR (Gunther *et al.*, 1990), E74 target sequences (Rao and Reddy, 1992a), the human T cell receptor (TCR) α-chain gene enhancer (Ho *et al.*, 1990), the *Mb-1* gene expressed in early B lymphocyte differentiation (Hagman and Grosschedl, 1992) and the class II major histocompatibility complex promoter (Klemsz *et al.*, 1990). Putative ETS binding sites are present in several T-cell-specific genes including interleukin-2 (IL-2), IL-3, granulocyte-macrophage colony stimulating factor (GM-CSF), CD2, CD3, TCRβ, TCRγ (Thompson *et al.*, 1992) and in human immunodeficiency virus type 2 (HIV-2) and the HTLV-1 LTR (Bosselut *et al.*, 1990; Gitlin *et al.*, 1991). Transcriptional activation of the HTLV-1 LTR requires the synergistic action of ETS1 and SP-1 and, in general, ETS proteins appear to function as components of transcription factor complexes to regulate the expression of viral and cellular genes (Gegonne *et al.*, 1993).

ETS1 and ETS2

These factors activate the stromelysin 1 and collagenase 1 genes (the expression of which is deregulated in transformed cells and tumours) via a distal region comprising a highly conserved palindrome with two strong binding sites for ETS1 (Wasylyk *et al.*, 1991; Fisher *et al.*, 1991; Woods *et al.*, 1992).

ETS1 binds to the enhancer sequence of the TCRα gene and may be specifically involved in the maturation of CD4$^+$ cells (Bhat *et al.*, 1989; Ho *et al.*, 1990). ETS1 is hyperphosphorylated in lymphocytes stimulated by the mitogen concanavalin A or by Ca^{2+} ionophore and in T cell lines during mitosis, and ETS2 is phosphorylated in Jurkat cells following activation of the TCR, suggesting that they have a role in cell proliferation (Pognonec *et al.*, 1988; Fujiwara *et al.*, 1990; Fleischman *et al.*, 1993).

Chicken p68^{ets-1} and p58^{ets-2} both contain two independent transcription activation domains (I and III, p68 amino acids 1–71 and 175–314; p58 amino acids 1–65 and 168–308). Domain I of p68^{ets-1} is deleted in p54^{ets-1} (Schneikert *et al.*, 1992).

Ets-2 expression is required for germinal vesicle breakdown in *Xenopus* oocytes (Chen *et al.*, 1990).

An 89 residue region adjacent to the DNA binding domains is conserved with 55% identity in ETS1 and ETS2 but does not occur in other members of the ETS family. This region inhibits DNA binding and activates transcription. The alternatively spliced form of human *ETS1*, lacking exon 7 (see below) does not have this inhibitory region and binds to DNA much more efficiently (Wasylyk *et al.*, 1992).

Expression in NIH 3T3 fibroblasts of the DNA binding and nuclear localization signal of ETS2 inhibits transformation by v-*ras* or by human colony-stimulating factor-1 (Langer *et al.*, 1992). In these cells CSF1 stimulates transcription of *Ets*-2, *Jun* and *Fos* but not of *Myc*. The overexpression of an exogenous *Myc* gene prevents the suppressive effect of ETS2. This suggests that ETS2 can regulate *Myc* expression and mediate CSF1R- and *Ras*-induced mitogenic signals.

ERG1 and ERG2

These transcription factors differ from ETS1 and ETS2 in their sequence specificity, binding weakly to the polyoma virus enhancer PEA3, Mo-MuSV LTR or PU box sequences, but strongly to E74 target sequences, although all of these regions contain a core GGAA motif (Reddy and Rao, 1991). In contrast to ETS1, ERG2 is phosphorylated by protein kinase C but not in response to Ca^{2+} ionophore (Murakami *et al.*, 1993).

ELK1

DNA sequence specificity similar to ETS1 and ETS2 (Rao and Reddy, 1992a) although it differs from other ETS proteins in having its ETS DNA binding domain located at the N-terminus of the protein (Reddy and Rao, 1990). ELK1 binds to the same DNA sequence (CAGGA) as $p62^{TCF}$, a component of the ternary complex that activates *Fos* transcription via the serum response element (SRE; see **FOS**; Hipskind *et al.*, 1991). The DNA binding domain of ELK1 is in the 76 amino acid ETS homology region, the C-terminal region of which contains the serum response factor (SRF) interaction domain (Rao and Reddy, 1992b). The truncated protein (residues 1–89) binds autonomously to SRE, unlike the full-length protein, indicating the presence of a negative regulatory domain within ELK1.

ELF1

The ELF1 DNA binding domain is nearly identical to that of *Drosophila* E74. ELF1 binds specifically to two potential ETS binding sites, EBS1 and EBS2, which are conserved in both the human and murine *IL2* enhancers. ETS1 and ETS2 do not, however, bind to these sites *in vitro* (Thompson *et al.*, 1992). In the human enhancer, EBS1 and EBS2 are essential for the formation of the NFAT-1 (nuclear factor of activated T cells) and NFIL-2B nuclear protein complexes. ELF1 also binds to the purine-rich region of HIV type 2 LTR to which NFAT also binds and which is required for inducible virus expression in response to signalling via the TCR (Li *et al.*, 1991).

Structure of the human *ETS1* gene

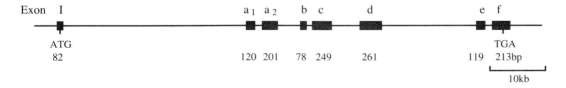

Exons (denoted I and a–f) are identical in size to those of chicken *Ets-1* (Jorcyk *et al.*, 1991). Alternative splicing generates human *ETS1* mRNAs lacking either exon a_2 and/or exon d (Jorcyk *et al.*, 1991). The absence of exon d causes smaller ETS1 proteins (p39/p42) to be synthesized. The principal proteins have been denoted as ETS1a (~50 kDa: 441 amino acids) and ETS1b

(~40 kDa: 354 amino acids) (Reddy and Rao, 1988). Scrambled splicing also occurs in which exon d or exon c splices with exon a_1, which normally splices 3′ with exon a_2 (Cocquerelle *et al.*, 1992).

The human *ETS1* gene promoter lacks a TATA or CAAT box but has a high GC content, six Sp-1 sites, one AP-1, one AP-2 consensus sequence and binding site motifs for PEA3 and OCT as well as a palindromic region resembling the *Fos* SRE and an ETS1 protein binding site (Oka *et al.*, 1991). Two negative regulatory elements (NRE1 and NRE2) are present 230 nt and 350 nt 5′ of the promoter respectively (Chen *et al.*, 1993). The human *ETS2* promoter contains a region (−159 to +141) that includes one Sp-1 site and a GC-rich region and is essential for transcription (Mavrothalassitis *et al.*, 1990).

Structure of the chicken *Ets-1* gene, avian myeloblastosis virus (AMV) E26 and their gene products

(a)

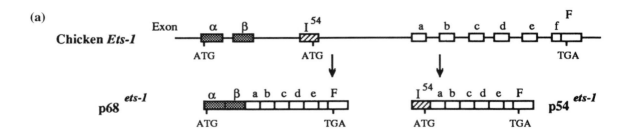

(b)

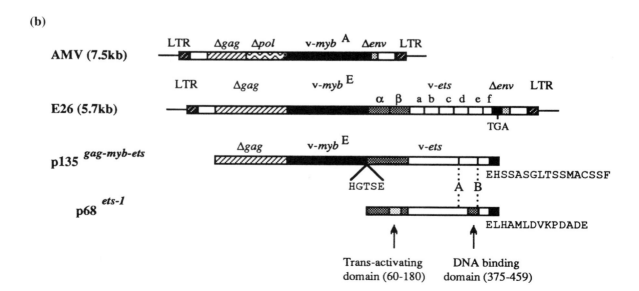

(a) Chicken *Ets-1* is encoded by a contiguous locus of two domains (6 and 18 kbp) separated by 40 kbp that includes the first coding exon of p54^{ets-1} (I^{54}). The 3' domain (18 kbp) contains six regions (a–f) of which five (a–e) are homologous between *Ets* and v-*ets* except for two point mutations. Alternative splicing generates two similar sized mRNAs (7.5 kb) that encode p54^{ets-1} or p68^{ets-1}. Exon a is a common cellular acceptor exon that can splice to either I^{54} (to yield p54 mRNA) or to the 5' exons α and β (to yield p68 mRNA). I^{54} encodes a hydrophilic N-terminus (27 amino acids) that is highly conserved among vertebrates. The the α and β exons encode a hydrophobic N-terminus (71 amino acids) that has *trans*-activating properties. Exons α and β have not been detected in mammals (Albagli *et al.*, 1992). Chicken *Ets-1* and *Ets-2* genes are contiguous (Leprince *et al.*, 1983; Rao *et al.*, 1987).

(b) AMV v-*myb* is designated v-*myb*^{A} and E26 v-*myb* is designated v-*myb*^{E} (Bister *et al.*, 1982; Nunn *et al.*, 1983). The erythroid leukaemogenicity of E26 derives from the presence of v-*ets* and the linkage of *myb*^{E} to Δ*gag*. Chicken p68^{ets-1} is the cellular progenitor of E26 v-*ets*, encoding a protein that is closely related to and co-linear with the v-*ets* domain of p135$^{Δgag-myb-ets}$ (Leprince *et al.*, 1990).

The 533 nucleotides at the 5' end of the E26 transforming gene are identical (except for nine nucleotide substitutions) to a region of AMV v-*myb*. E26 *myb–ets* is generated by aberrant splicing between a cryptic splice donor site in *Myb* exon 6 and the normal splice acceptor site of *Ets-1* exon α. The ORF created during this splicing event generates the additional N-terminal amino acids HGTSE shown in v-ETS from a non-coding *Ets-1* sequence. The 13 C-terminal residues of p68^{ets} (encoded by exon f) have been deleted during transduction and replaced in p135^{v-ets} by 16 C-terminal amino acids. At least 13 of these codons are specified by an inverted *Ets-1* sequence (Lautenberger and Papas, 1993). There are seven mutations in the nucleotide sequence (five conservative) and the two point mutations in the protein sequence that result are the conservative substitution of Ala and Ile by Val (A and B). The presence of *ets* extends the *myb* ORF by 491 amino acids (Leprince *et al.*, 1988). The C-terminal sequences of v-ETS and ETS are also shown.

Either p68^{ets-1} or v-ETS *trans*-activate transcription from a heterologous promoter linked to a polyoma PEA3 element. However, compared with v-ETS, p68^{ets-1} binds very weakly to an oligonucleotide containing PEA3 (Lim *et al.*, 1992). The C-terminus and a central region of the polypeptide sequence are involved in masking the ETS DNA binding domain in the full length protein. This is consistent with 13 C-terminal residues of p68^{ets-1} being replaced in the oncoprotein. A truncated form of p68^{ets-1} comprised of the C-terminal 311 amino acids (p35) does bind to the PEA3 motif (Leprince *et al.*, 1992). The introduction of mutations present in the homologous region of v-*ets* into p35 reduces sequence-specific DNA binding.

Human ETS1 and ETS2 are 98% and 95% homologous to the E26 viral ETS sequence and ELK1 is 82% homologous to the 3' end of v-ETS (Watson *et al.*, 1985). ERG has two domains that are 40% and 70% homologous to 5' and 3' regions of v-ETS.

Sequences of human ETS1 and ETS2

```
Human ETS1   (1)                           MKAAVDLKPTLTIIKTEKVDLELFP
Human ETS2   (1)    MNDFGIKNMDQVAPVANSYRGTLKRQPAFDTFDGSLF--FPSLNEEQTLQ-VPTGLDSI

             (26)   SPDMECADVPLLTPSSKEMMSQALKATFSGFTKEQQRLGIPKDPRQWTETHVRDWVMWAV
             (60)   -H-SANCEL-----C--AV-----------K---R------N-WL-S-QQ-CQ-LL--T

             (86)   NEFSLKGVDFQKFCMNGAALCALGKDCFLELAPDFVGDILWEHLEILQKEDVKPYQVNGV
            (120)   -----VN-NL-R-G---QM--N---ER----------------QMI--NQEKTEDQYE
```

```
(146)  NPAYPESRYTSDYFISYGIEHAQCVPPSEFSEPSFITESYQTLHPISSEELLSLKYENDY
(180)  ENSHLT-VPHWINSNTL-FGTE-APYGMQTQNYPKGGLLDSMCPASTPSV-S-EQEFQMF

(206)  PSVILRDPLQTDTLQNDYFAIKQEVVTPDNMCMGRTSRGKLGGQDSFESIESYDSCDRLT
(240)  -KSR-SSVSV-YCSVSQD-PGSNLNLLTN-SGTPKDHDSPEN-A-----  - --      -L

(266)  QSWSSQSSFNSLQRVPSYDSFDSEDYPAALPNHKPKGTFKDYVRDRADLNKD KPVIPAA
(294)  QSWNSQ--LLDV-----FE--EDDCSQSLCL-KPTMS ----IQE-S-PVEQG-------

(325)  ALAGYTGSGPIQLWQFLLELLTDKSCQSFISWTGDGWEFKLSDPDEVARRWGKRKNKPKM
(353)  V---F--------------S-----------------A------------------

(392)  NYEKLSRGLRYYYDKNIIHKTAGKRYVYRFVCDLQSLLGYTPEELHAMLDVKPDADE (441)
(420)  ---------------------S------------N---F-------I-G-Q--TED (469)
```

Underlined: ETS domains (ETS1: 331–415; ETS2: 359–443). There is ~65% identity between human ETS1 and ELK1, ETS2, ERG and v-ETS within the 80 amino acid C-terminal DNA binding domains.

Sequence of human ELK1, and SAP1a and SAP1b

```
Humn ELK1  (1)   MDPSVTLWQFLLQLLREQGNGHIISWTSRDGGEFKLVDAEEVARLWGLRKNKTNMNYDK
SAP1       (1)   --SAI----------QKPQ-K-M-C---M-- Q---LQ---------I----P------

           (60)  LSRALRYYYDKNIIRKVSGQKFVYKFVSYPEVAGCSTEDCPPQPEVSVTSTMPNVAPAAI
           (59)  ---------V----K--N-------------IL   NMD-MTVGRIEGDCESLNFSEV

          (120)  HAAPGDTVSGKPGTPKGAGMAGPGGLARSSRNEYMRSGLYSTFTIQSLQPQPPPHPRPAV
          (114)  SSSSK-VEN-    -KDKPPQP-AKT----D-IH-----S---LN--NSSNVKLFKLIK

          (180)  VLPNAAP AGAAAPPSGSRSTSPSPLEACLEAEEAGLPLQVILTPPEAPNLKSEELNVEP
          (168)  TENP-EKL-EKKSPQEPTP-VIKFVTTPSKKPPVEPVAATISIG-SIS-SSEETIQAL-T
          (239)  GLGRALPPEVKVEGPKEELE VAGERGFVPETTKAEPEVPPQEGVPARLPAVVMDTAGQA
          (228)  LVSPK--SLEAPTSASNVMTAF-TTPPISSIPPLQ--PRT-SPPLSS H-DIDT-IDSV-

          (298)  GGHAASSPEISQPQKGRKPRDLEL      PLSPSLL GGPGPERTPGSGSGSGLQAP
          (287)  SQPMELPENL-LEP-DQ-SVL--KDKVNNSRSKK-KF-FLA-TLVI-SSDP-PL-ILS-
```

```
ELK1    (349)  G     PALTPSLLPTHTLTPVLLTPSSLPPSIHFWSTLSPIAPRSPAKLS      FQFPSS
SAP1a   (347)  SLPTAS---AFFSQ    --II----P-LS----------V--L---R-QGANTL-----V
SAP1b   (361)         VACSLFMV  *****F*CPFKQIQNLYTQVCFL*LRFVLERLCVT*
```

```
ELK1    (420)  GSAQ      VHIPSISV      DGLSTPVVLSPGPQKP (428)
SAP1a   (404)  LNSHGPFTLSGWMDL--LAHFPQTYRRHN-C-CGMRE-RNEETDIQHDCI (453)
SAP1b   (405)  M (405)
```

Underlined: ETS domains (N-terminal). * Indicates identity between SAP1b and SAP1a (SRF-binding proteins: see *FOS*). The B box sequence involved in formation of a ternary complex at the *Fos* SRE is comprised of residues 148–168 (ELK1) and 136–156 (SAP1; Treisman *et al.*, 1992).

PERCENTAGE SEQUENCE HOMOLOGY WITH ETS1

Human ETS1: amino acids 331–415 (100%)
Human ETS2: amino acids 359–443 (96%)
Human ELK1: amino acids 3–86 (61%)
ERG (71%), PU.1 (38%), E74 (52%), D-*ets-2* (95%).

Sequences of chicken ETS1 (p68), ETS1 (p54), ETS2 and p135$^{gag\text{-}myb\text{-}ets}$

```
p135gag-myb-ets     (1)    NSTMRRKVEQEGYLQESSKAGLPSATTGFQKSSHLMAFAHNPPAGPLPGAGQAPLGSDYP
p135gag-myb-ets    (61)    YYHIAEPQNVPGQIPYPVALHVNIVNVPQPAAAAIQRHYNDEDPEKEKRIKELELLLMST
p135gag-myb-ets   (121)    ENELKGQQALPTQNHTANYPGWHSTTVADNTMTSGDNAPVSCLGEHHHCTPSPPVDHGTS

ETS1 (p68)          (1)    MMSYYMDTTIGSTGPYPLARPGVMQGASSCCEDPWMPCRLQSACCPPRSCCPPWDEAAI
ETS1 (p54)          (1)                                         MKAAVDLKPTLTIIK
ETS2                (1)                 MSEFAIRNMDQVAPVSNMYRGMLKRQPAFDTFDSSNSLF-GYF-SLNEDQTL
p135gag-myb-ets   (181)    E-----------------------------------------------------------

ETS1 (p68)         (60)    QEVPTGLEHYSTDMECADVPLLTPSSKEMMSQALKATFSGFAKEQQRLGIPKDPQQWTET
ETS1 (p54)         (16)    TEKVDIDLFPSP------------------------------------------------
ETS2               (53)    ------FDST-YESNNCEL-----C--AV------D-----T---C-----NN-WL---Q
p135gag-myb-ets   (241)    ------------------------------------------------------------

ETS1 (p68)        (120)    HVRDWVMWAVNEFSLKGVDFQKFCMNGAALCALGKECFLELAPDFVGDILWEHLEILQKE
ETS1 (p54)         (76)    ------------------------------------------R-----------------
ETS2              (113)    --CQ-LA--T-----AN-NIHQ-L-S-QD--N----R-------Y---------QMI-D
p135gag-myb-ets   (301)    ------------------------------------------------------------

ETS1 (p68)        (180)    EAKPYPANGVNAAYPESRYTSDYFISYGIEHAQCVPPSEFSEPSFITESYQTLHPISSEE
ETS1 (p54)        (136)    ------------------------------------------------------------
ETS2              (173)    SQEKTQDQY-ESSHLT-VPHWVNNN-LTVNVD-TPYGIQMPGYPKALSYPKPNLLSDICQ
p135gag-myb-ets   (361)    ------------------------------------------------------------

ETS1 (p68)        (240)    LLSLKYENDYPSVILRDPVQTDSLQTDYFTIKQEVVTPDNMCMGRASRGKLGGQDSFESI
ETS1 (p54)        (196)    ------------------------------------------------------------
ETS2              (233)    TSTGPNLLSPEQDFSLF-KTQVDAVSVNYCTVNQDF-RS-LNLLIDNS---REHE-S--G
p135gag-myb-ets   (421)    ------------------------------------------V-----------------

ETS1 (p68)        (300)    ESYDSCDRLTQSWSSQSSFQSLQRVPSYDSFDSEDYPAALPNHKPKGTFKDYVRDRADM
ETS1 (p54)        (256)    ------------------------------------------------------------
ETS2              (293)    A---E-S-SMLQ--N----LVD-------E--EDDCSQSLCMS--TMS----IQ--S-P
p135gag-myb-ets   (481)    ------------------------------------------------------------

ETS1 (p68)        (359)    NKDKPVIPAAALAGYTGSGPIQLWQFLLELLTDKSCQSFISWTGDGWEFKLSDPDEVAR
ETS1 (p54)        (315)    -----------------------------------------------------------
ETS2              (351)    VEQG-------I---F------------------------------------A------
p135gag-myb-ets   (540)    -----------------------------------------------------------

ETS1 (p68)        (418)    RWGKRKNKPKMNYEKLSRGLRYYYDKNIIHKTAGKRYVYRFVCDLQSLLGYTPEELHAML
ETS1 (p54)        (374)    ------------------------------------------------------------
ETS2              (412)    ---R-------------------------S-------------N-----A-------
p135gag-myb-ets   (599)    ----------D-------------V------------------------HSSAS

ETS1 (p68)        (478)    DVKPDADE (485)
ETS1 (p54)        (434)    -------- (441)
ETS2              (472)    G-Q--TED (479)
p135gag-myb-ets   (659)    GLTSSMACSSF (669)
```

The underlined residues in p135$^{gag\text{-}myb\text{-}ets}$ are those differing from chicken p68$^{ets\text{-}1}$. The ETS domains are also underlined: (p68$^{ets\text{-}1}$: 375–459; p54$^{ets\text{-}1}$: 331–415; ETS2: 369–453). Watson *et al.* (1988a) give Ala117 in p54$^{ets\text{-}1}$. The region between the DNA binding domain and the inhibitory region (373–379 p68$^{ets\text{-}1}$; 367–373 ETS2) is predicted to be particularly flexible.

Databank file names and accession numbers

	GENE	*EMBL*	*SWISSPROT*	*REFERENCES*
AEV-E26	*gag–myb–ets*	Reaev1 X00144	MYBE_AVILE P01105	Nunn *et al.*, 1983
Human	*ELK1*	M25269M25269	ELK_HUMAN P19419	Rao *et al.*, 1989

	GENE	EMBL	SWISSPROT	REFERENCES
Human	*ETS1*	Hscets1 X14798	ETS1_HUMAN P14921	Reddy and Rao, 1988
		Hsets1a J04101		Watson *et al.*, 1988b
Human	*ETS2*		ETS2_HUMAN P15036	Watson *et al.*, 1988b
Chicken	*Ets-1* (p54)	Ggcets1 M22462	ETSA_CHICK P13474	Duterque-Coquillaud *et al.*, 1988
		Ggcets X13026		Chen, 1988
		Ggetsc X13027		Watson *et al.*, 1988a
Chicken	*Ets-1* (p68)	Ggcetss9 M29515	ETSB_CHICK P15062	Watson *et al.*, 1988c
Chicken	*Ets-2*	Ggcets2 X07202	ETS2_CHICK P10157	Boulukos *et al.*, 1988
Mouse	*Ets-1*			Chen, 1990
Mouse	*Ets-2*	Mmets2 J04103	ETS2_MOUSE P15037	Watson *et al.*, 1988b
Human	*FLI1*	Hsfli1a M93255		Klemsz *et al.*, 1993
Mouse	*Fli-1*	Mmfli X59421	FLI1_MOUSE P26323	Ben-David *et al.*, 1991
Drosophila	E74A	DM74E X15087	E74A_DROME P20105	Burtis *et al.*, 1990
	E74B		E74B_DROME P11536	
Drosophila	D-*elg*			Pribyl *et al.*, 1991
				The *et al.*, 1992
Drosophila	*elf-1*			Bray and Kafatos, 1991
Xenopus	*ets-1A*	Xlcets1a X52692	ETSA_XENLA P18755	Stiegler *et al.*, 1990
Xenopus	*ets-2A*	Xlcets2a X51826	ETS2_XENLA P19102	Wolff *et al.*, 1990, 1991
		GB: M81683		Burdett *et al.*, 1992
Yeast	SAP-1			Dalton and Treisman, 1992

Papers

Albagli, O., Flourens, A., Crepieux, P., Begue, A., Stehelin, D. and Leprince, D. (1992). Phylogeny of the p68$^{c\text{-}ets\text{-}1}$ amino-terminal transactivating domain reveals some highly conserved structural features. Oncogene, 7, 1435–1439.

Amouyel, P., Laudet, V., Martin, P., Li, R., Quatannens, B., Stehelin, D and Saule, S. (1989). Two nuclear oncogene proteins, p135$^{gag\text{-}myb\text{-}ets}$ and p61/63^{myc}, cooperate to induce transformation of chicken neuro-retina cells. J. Virol., 63, 3382–3388.

Ben-David, Y., Giddens, E.B., Letwin, K. and Bernstein, A. (1991). Erythroleukemia induction by Friend murine leukemia virus: insertional activation of a new member of the *ets* gene family, *fli-1*, closely linked to c-*ets*-1. Genes Devel., 5, 908–918.

Bhat, N.K., Komschlies, K.L., Fujiwara, S., Fisher, R.J., Mathieson, B.J., Gregorio, T.A., Young, H.A., Kasik, J.W., Ozato, K. and Papas, T.S. (1989). Expression of *ets* genes in mouse thymocyte subsets and T cells. J. Immunol., 142, 672–678.

Bister, K., Nunn, M., Moscovici, C., Perbal, B., Baluda, M.A. and Duesberg, P.H. (1982). Acute leukemia viruses E26 and avian myeloblastosis virus have related transformation-specific RNA sequences but different genetic structures, gene products and oncogenic properties. Proc. Natl Acad. Sci. USA, 79, 3677–3681.

Bosselut, R., Duvall, J.F., Gegonne, A., Bailly, M., Hemar, A., Brady, J. and Ghysdael, J. (1990). The product of the c-*ets*-1 proto-oncogene and the related Ets2 protein act as transcriptional activators of the long terminal repeat of human T cell leukemia virus HTLV-1. EMBO J., 9, 3137–3144.

Boulukos, K.E., Pognonec, P., Begue, A., Galibert, F., Gesquiere, J.C., Stehelin, D. and Ghysdael, J. (1988). Identification in chickens of an evolutionarily conserved cellular *ets-2* gene (c-*ets-2*) encoding nuclear proteins related to the products of the c-*ets* proto-oncogene. EMBO J., 7, 697–705.

Bray, S.J. and Kafatos, F.C. (1991). Developmental function of Elf-1: an essential transcription factor during embryogenesis in *Drosophila*. Genes Devel., 5, 1672–1683.

Burdett, L.A., Qi, S., Chen, Z.-Q., Lautenberger, J.A. and Papas, T.S. (1992). Characterization of the cDNA sequences of two *Xenopus ets-2* proto-oncogenes. Nucleic Acids Res., 20, 371.

Burtis, K.C., Thummel, C.S., Jones, C.W., Karim, F.D. and Hogness, D.S. (1990). The *Drosophila* 74EF early puff contains E74, a complex ecdysone-inducible gene that encodes two *ets*-related proteins. Cell, 61, 85–99.

Chen, J.H. (1985). The proto-oncogene c-*ets* is preferentially expressed in lymphoid cells. Mol. Cell. Biol., 5, 2993–3000.

Chen, J.H. (1988). Complementary DNA clones of chicken proto-oncogene c-*ets*: sequence divergence from the viral oncogene v-*ets*. Oncogene Res., 2, 371–384.

Chen, J.H. (1990). Cloning, sequencing, and expression of mouse c-*ets*-1 cDNA in baculovirus expression system. Oncogene Res., 5, 277–285.

Chen, J.H., Jeha, S. and Oka, T. (1993). Negative regulatory elements in the human *ETS1* gene promoter. Oncogene , 8, 133–139.

Chen, Z.Q., Kan, N.C., Pribyl, L., Lautenberger, J.A., Moudrianakis, E. and Papas, T.S. (1988). Molecular cloning of the *ets* proto-oncogene of the sea urchin and analysis of its developmental expression. Devel. Biol., 125, 432–440.

Chen, Z.Q., Burdett, L.A., Seth, A.K., Lautenberger, J.A. and Papas, T.S. (1990). Requirement of *ets-2* expression for *Xenopus* oocyte maturation. Science, 250, 1416–1418.

Cocquerelle, C., Daubersies, P., Majerus, M.-A., Kerckaert, J.-P. and Bailleul, B. (1992). Splicing with inverted order of exons occurs proximal to large introns. EMBO J., 11, 1095–1098.

Dalton, S. and Treisman, R. (1992). Characterization of SAP-1, a protein recruited by serum response factor to the c-*fos* serum response element. Cell, 68, 597–612.

Desbiens, X., Queva, C., Jaffredo, T., Stehelin, D. and Vandenbunder, B. (1991). The relationship between cell proliferation and the transcription of the nuclear oncogenes c-*myc*, c-*myb* and c-*ets*-1 during feather morphogenesis in the chick embryo. Development, 111, 699–713.

Duterque-Coquillaud, M., Leprince, D., Flourens, A., Henry, C., Ghysdael, J., Debuire, B., Stehelin, D. (1988). Cloning and expression of chicken p54^{c-ets} cDNAs: the first p54^{c-ets} coding exon is located into the 40.0 kbp genomic domain unrelated to v-*ets*. Oncogene Res., 2, 335–344.

Fisher, R.J., Mavrothalassitis, G., Kondoh, A. and Papas, T.S. (1991). High-affinity DNA-protein interactions of the cellular ETS1 protein: the determination of the ETS binding motif. Oncogene, 6, 2249–2254.

Fleischman, L.F., Pilaro, A.M., Murakami, K., Kondoh, A.., Fisher, R.J. and Papas, T.S. (1993). c-*ets*-1 protein is hyperphosphorylated during mitosis. Oncogene, 8, 771–780.

Fujiwara, S., Koizumi, S., Fisher, R.J., Bhat, N.K. and Papas, T.S. (1990). Phosphorylation of the ETS-2 protein: regulation by the T-cell antigen receptor-CD3 complex. Mol. Cell. Biol., 10, 1249–1253.

Gegonne, A., Bosselut, R., Bailly, R.-A. and Ghysdael, J. (1993). Synergistic activation of the HTLV1 LTR Ets-responsive region by transcription factors Ets1 and Sp1. EMBO J., 12, 1169–1178.

Ghysdael, J., Gegonne, A., Pognonec, P., Dernis, D., LePrince, D. and Stehelin, D. (1986). Identification and preferential expression in thymic and bursal lymphocytes of a c-*ets* oncogene-encoded M$_r$ 54,000 cytoplasmic protein. Proc. Natl Acad. Sci. USA, 83, 1714–1718.

Gitlin, S.D., Bosselut, R., Gegonne, A., Ghysdael, J. and Brady, J.N. (1991). Sequence-specific interaction of the Ets1 protein with the long terminal repeat of the human T-lymphotropic virus type I. J. Virol., 65, 5513–5523.

Golay, J., Introna, M. and Graf, T. (1988). A single point mutation in the v-*ets* oncogene affects both erythroid and myelomonocytic cell differentiation. Cell, 55, 1147–1158.

Gunther, C.V., Nye, J.A., Bryner, R.S. and Graves, B.J. (1990). Sequence-specific DNA binding of the proto-oncogene *ets*-1 defines a transcriptional activator sequence within the long terminal repeat of the Moloney murine sarcoma virus. Genes Devel., 4, 667–679.

Hagman, J. and Grosschedl, R. (1992). An inhibitory carboxyl-terminal domain in ets-1 and ets-2 mediates differential binding of ETS family factors to promoter sequences of the *mb-1* gene. Proc. Natl Acad. Sci. USA, 89, 8889–8893.

Higashino, F., Yoshida, K., Fujinaga, Y., Kamio, K. and Fujinaga, K. (1993). Isolation of a cDNA encoding the adenovirus E1A enhancer binding protein: a new human member of the *ets* oncogene family. Nucleic Acids Res., 21, 547–553.

Hipskind, R.A., Rao, V.N., Mueller, C.G., Reddy, E.S. and Nordheim, A. (1991). Ets-related protein Elk-1 is homologous to the c-*fos* regulatory factor p62^{TCF}. (1991). Nature, 354, 531–534.

Ho, I.-C., Bhat, N.K., Gottschalk, L.R., Lindsten, T., Thompson, C.B., Papas, T.S. and Leiden, J.M. (1990). Sequence-specific binding of human ets-1 to the T cell receptor α gene enhancer. Science, 250, 814–818.

Ivanov, X., Mladenov, Z., Nedyalkov, S. and Todorov, T.G. (1962). Experimental investigations into avian leukosis. I. transmission experiments of certain diseases of the avian leukosis complex, found in Bulgaria. Bulgaria Acad. Sci. Bull. Inst. Pathol. Comp. Anim., 9, 5–36.

Ivanov, X., Mladenov, Z., Nedyalkov, S., Todorov, T.G. and Yakimov, M. (1964). Experimental investigations into avian leucoses. V. Transmission, haematology and morphology of avian myelocytomatosis. Izv. Inst. Pat. Zhivotnite Sofia, 10, 5–38.

Jorcyk, C.L., Watson, D.K., Mavrothalassitis and Papas, T.S. (1991). The human *ETS1* gene: genomic structure, promoter characterization and alternative splicing. Oncogene, 6, 523–532.

Jurdic, P., Benchaibi, M., Gandrillon, O. and Samarut, J. (1987). Transforming and mitogenic effects of avian leukemia virus E26 on chicken hematopoietic cells and fibroblasts, respectively, correlate with level of expression of the provirus. J. Virol., 61, 3058–3065.

Karim, F.D., Urness, L.D., Thummel, C.S., Klemsz, M.J., McKercher, S.R., Celada, A., van Beveren, C., Maki, R., Gunther, C.V., Nye, J.A. and Graves, B.J. (1990). The ETS-domain: a new DNA-binding motif that recognizes a purine-rich core DNA sequence. Genes Devel., 4, 1451–1453.

Klemsz, M.J., McKercher, S.R., Celada, A., Van Beveren, C. and Maki, R.A. (1990). The macrophage and B cell-specific transcription factor PU.1 is related to the *ets* oncogene. Cell, 61, 113–124.

Klemsz, M.J., Maki, R.A., Papayannopoulou, T., Moore, J., and Hromas, R. (1993). Characterization of the *ets* oncogene family member, *fli-1*. J. Biol. Chem., 268, 5769–5773.

Kocova, M., Kowalczyk, J.R. and Sandberg, A.A. (1985). Translocation 4;11 acute leukemia: three case reports and review of the literature. Cancer Genet. Cytogen., 16, 21–30.

Lai, Z.-C. and Rubin, G.M. (1992). Negative control of photoreceptor development in Drosophila by the product of the *yan* gene, an ETS domain protein. Cell, 70, 609–620.

Langer, S.J., Bortner, D.M., Roussel, M.F., Sherr, C.J. and Ostrowski, M.C. (1992). Mitogenic signaling by colony-stimulating factor 1 and *ras* is suppressed by the *ets*-2 DNA-binding domain and restored by *myc* overexpression. Mol. Cell. Biol., 12, 5355–5362.

Lautenberger, J.A. and Papas, T.S. (1993). Inversion of chicken *ets-1* proto-oncogene segment in avian leukemia virus E26. J. Virol., 67, 610–612.

Lautenberger, J.A., Burdett, L.A., Gunnell, M.A., Qi, S., Watson, D.K., O'Brien, S.J. and Papas, T.S. (1992). Genomic dispersal of the *ets* gene family during metazoan evolution. Oncogene, 7, 1713–1719.

Leprince, D., Gegonne, A., Coll, J., de Taisne, C., Schneeberger, A., Lagrou, C. and Stehelin, D. (1983). A putative second cell-derived oncogene of the avian leukemia retrovirus E26. Nature, 306, 395–397.

Leprince, D., Duterque-Coquillaud, M., Li, R.-P., Henry, C., Flourens, A., Debuire, B. and Stehelin, D. (1988). Alternative splicing within the chicken c-*ets*-1 locus: implications for transduction within the E26 retrovirus of the c-*ets* proto-oncogene. J. Virol., 62, 3233–3241.

Leprince, D., Gesquire, J.C. and Stehelin, D. (1990). The chicken cellular progenitor of the v-*ets* oncogene, p68$^{c-ets-1}$, is a nuclear DNA-binding protein not expressed in lymphoid cells of the spleen. Oncogene Res., 5, 255–265.

Leprince, D., Crepieux, P. and Stehelin, D. (1992). c-*ets*-1 DNA binding to the PEA3 motif is differentially inhibited by all the mutations found in v-*ets*. Oncogene, 7, 9–17.

Li, C., Lai, C., Sigman, D.S. and Gaynor, R.B. (1991). Cloning of a cellular factor, interleukin binding factor, that binds to NFAT-like motifs in the human immunodeficiency virus long terminal repeat. Proc. Natl Acad. Sci. USA, 88, 7739–7743.

Lim, F., Kraut, N., Framptom, J. and Graf, T. (1992). DNA binding by c-Ets-1, but not v-Ets, is repressed by an intramolecular mechanism. EMBO J., 11, 643–652.

Mavrothalassitis, G.J., Watson, D.K. and Papas, T.S. (1990). The human *ETS*-2 gene promoter: molecular dissection and nuclease hypersensitivity. Oncogene, 5, 1337–1342.

Metz, T. and Graf, T. (1991a). v-*myb* and v-*ets* transform chicken erythroid cells and cooperate both in *trans* and in *cis* to induce distinct differentiation phenotypes. Genes Devel., 5, 369–380.

Metz, T. and Graf, T. (1991b). Fusion of the nuclear oncoproteins v-*myb* and v-*ets* is required for the leukemogenicity of E26 virus. Cell, 66, 95–105.

Metz, T. and Graf, T. (1992). The nuclear oncogenes v-*erb*A and v-*ets* cooperate in the induction of avian erythroleukemia. Oncogene, 7, 597–605.

Murakami, K., Mavrothalassitis, G., Bhat, N.K., Fisher, R.J. and Papas, T.S. (1993). Human ERG-2 protein is a phosphorylated DNA-binding protein – a distinct member of the ets family. Oncogene, 8, 1559–1566.

Nedyalkov, St., Bozhkov, Sp. and Todorov, G. (1975). Experimental erythroblastosis in the Japanese quail (*Coturnix coturnix japonica*) induced by the E-26 leukosis strain. Acta Vet. (Brno), 44, 75–78.

Nunn, M.F., Seeburg, P.H., Moscovici, C. and Duesberg, P.H. (1983). Tripartite structure of the avain erythroblastosis virus E26 transforming gene. Nature 306, 391–395.

Nye, J.A., Petersen, J.M., Gunther, C.V., Jonsen, M.D. and Graves, B.J. (1992). Interaction of murine ets-1 with GGA-binding sites establishes the ETS domain as a new DNA-binding motif. Genes Devel., 6, 975–990.

Ohyashiki, K., Ohyashiki, J.M., Tauchi, T., Iwabuchi, H., Iwabuchi, A. and Toyama, K. (1990). *ETS1* gene in myelodysplastic syndrome with chromosome change at 11q23. Cancer Genet. Cytogenet., 45, 73–80.

Oka, T., Rairkar, A. and Chen, J.H. (1991). Structural and functional analysis of the regulatory sequences of the *ets*-1 gene. Oncogene, 6, 2077–2083.

Papas, T.S., Watson, D.K., Sacchi, N., Fujiwara, S., Seth, A.K., Fisher, R.J., Bhat, N.K., Mavrothalassitis, G., Koizumi, S., Jorcyk, C.L., Schweinfest, C.W., Kottaridis, S.D. and Ascione, R. (1990). ETS family of genes in leukemia and Down syndrome. Am. J. Med. Genet. Suppl., 7, 251–261.

Pognonec, P., Boulukos, K.E., Gesquire, J.C., Stehelin, D. and Ghysdael, J. (1988). Mitogenic stimulation of thymocytes results in the calcium-dependent phosphorylation of c-*ets*-1 protein. EMBO J., 7, 977–983.

Pribyl, L.J., Watson, D.K., Schulz, R.A. and Papas, T.S. (1991). D-*elg*, a member of the *Drosophila ets* gene family: sequence, expression and evolutionary comparison. Oncogene, 6, 1175–1183.

Rao, V.N. and Reddy, E.S.P. (1992a). A divergent *ets*-related protein, elk-1, recognises similar c-*ets*-1 proto-oncogene target sequences and acts as a transcriptional activator. Oncogene, 7, 65–70.

Rao, V.N. and Reddy, E.S.P. (1992b). *elk*-1 domains responsible for autonomous DNA binding, SRE:SRF interaction and negative regulation of DNA binding. Oncogene, 7, 2335–2340.

Rao, V.N., Papas, T.S. and Reddy, E.S.P. (1987). *erg*, a human *ets*-related gene on chromosome 21: alternative splicing, polyadenylation and translation. Science, 237, 635–653.

Rao, V.N., Huebner, K., Isobe, M., Ar-Rushdi, A., Croce, C.M. and Reddy, E.S.P. (1989). *elk*, tissue-specific *ets*-related genes on chromosomes X and 14 near translocation breakpoints. Science, 244, 66–70.

Reddy, E.S.P. and Rao, V.N. (1988). Structure, expression and alternative splicing of the human c-*ets*-1 proto-oncogene. Oncogene Res., 3, 239–246.

Reddy, E.S.P. and Rao, V.N. (1990). Localization and modulation of the DNA-binding activity of the human c-*ets*-1 protooncogene. Cancer Res., 50, 5013–5016.

Reddy, E.S.P. and Rao, V.N. (1991). *erg*, an *ets*-related gene, codes for sequence-specific transcriptional activators. Oncogene, 6, 2285–2289.

Reddy, E.S.P., Rao, V.N. and Papas, T.S. (1987). The *erg* gene: a human gene related to the *ets* gene. Proc. Natl Acad. Sci. USA, 84, 6131–6135.

Rowley, J.D. (1983). Human oncogene locations and chromosome aberrations. Nature, 301, 290–291.

Sacchi, N., Wendtner, C.M. and Thiele, C.J. (1991). Single-cell detection of *ets*-1 transcripts in human neuroectodermal cells. Oncogene, 6, 2149–2154.

Schneikert, J., Lutz, Y. and Wasylyk, B. (1992). Two independent activation domains in c-ets-2 and c-ets-2 located in non-conserved sequences of the *ets* gene family. Oncogene, 7, 249–256.

Seth, A. and Papas, T.S. (1990). The c-ets-1 proto-oncogene has oncogenic activity and is positively autoregulated. Oncogene, 5, 1761–1767.

Stiegler, P., Wolff, C.M., Baltzinger, M., Hirzlin, J., Senan, F., Meyer, D., Ghysdael, J., Stehelin, D., Befort, N. and Remy, P. (1990). Characterization of *Xenopus laevis* cDNA clones of the c-*ets*-1 proto-oncogene. Nucleic Acids Res., 18, 5298.

The, S.M., Xie, X., Smyth, F., Papas, T.S., Watson, D.K. and Schulz, R.A. (1992). Molecular characterization and structural organization of D-*elg*, an *ets* proto-oncogene-related gene of *Drosophila*. Oncogene, 7, 2471–2478.

Thompson, C.B., Wang, C.-Y., Ho, I.-C., Bohjanen, P.R., Petryniak, B., June, C.H., Miesfeldt, S., Zhang, L., Nabel, G.J., Karpinski, B. and Leiden, J.M. (1992). *cis*-acting sequences required for inducible interleukin-2 enhancer function bind a novel Ets-related protein, Elf-1. Mol. Cell. Biol., 12, 1043–1053.

Thompson, C.C., Brown, T.A. and McKnight, S.L. (1991). Convergence of Ets- and notch-related structural motifs in a heteromeric DNA binding complex. Science, 253, 762–768.

Thummel, C.S., Burtis, K.C. and Hogness, D.S. (1990). Spatial and temporal patterns of E74 transcription during *Drosophila* development. Cell, 61, 101–111.

Treisman, R., Marais, R. and Wynne, J. (1992). Spatial flexibility in ternary complexes between SRF and its accessory proteins. EMBO J., 11, 4631–4640.

Wasylyk, B.C., Wasylyk, C., Flores, P., Begue, A., Leprince, D. and Stehelin, D. (1990). The c-*ets* proto-oncogenes encode transcription factors that cooperate with c-*fos* and c-*jun* for transcriptional activation. Nature, 346, 191–193.

Wasylyk, C., Gutman, A., Nicholson, R. and Wasylyk, B. (1991). The c-Ets oncoprotein activates the stromelysin promoter through the same elements as several non-nuclear oncoproteins. EMBO J., 10, 1127–1134.

Wasylyk, C., Kerckaert, J.-P. and Wasylyk, B. (1992). A novel modulator domain of ets transcription factors. Genes Devel., 6, 965–974.

Watson, D.K., McWilliams, M.J., Nunn, M.F., Duesberg, P.H., O'Brien, S.J. and Papas, T.S. (1985). The *ets* sequence from the transforming gene of avian erythroblastosis virus, E26, has unique domains on human chromosomes 11 and 21: both loci are transcriptionally active. Proc. Natl Acad. Sci. USA, 82, 7294–7298.

Watson, D.K., McWilliams, M.J. and Papas, T.S. (1988a). A unique amino-terminal sequence predicted for the chicken proto-*ets* protein. Virology, 167, 1–7.

Watson, D.K., McWilliams, M.J., Lapis, P., Lautenberger, J.A., Schweinfest, C.W. and Papas, T.S. (1988b). Mammalian *ets-1* and *ets-2* genes encode highly conserved proteins. Proc. Natl Acad. Sci. USA, 85, 7862–7866.

Watson, D.K., McWilliams, M.J. and Papas, T.S. (1988c). Molecular organization of the chicken *ets* locus. Virology, 164, 99–105.

Wolff, C.M., Stiegler, P., Baltzinger, M., Meyer, D., Ghysdael, J., Stehelin, D., Befort, N. and Remy, P. (1990). Isolation of two different c-*ets-2* proto-oncogenes in *Xenopus laevis*. Nucleic Acids Res., 18, 4603–4604.

Wolff, C.M., Stiegler, P., Baltzinger, M., Meyer, D., Ghysdael, J., Stehelin, D., Befort, N. and Remy, P. (1991). Cloning, sequencing, and expression of two *Xenopus laevis* c-*ets-2* protooncogenes. Cell Growth Differ., 2, 447–456.

Woods, D.B., Ghysdael, J. and Owen, M.J. (1992). Identification of nucleotide preferences in DNA sequences recognised specifically by c-Ets-1 protein. Nucleic Acids Res., 20, 699–704.

Xin, J.H., Cowie, A., Lachance, P. and Hassell, J.A. (1992). Molecular cloning and characterization of PEA3, a new member of the *Ets* oncogene family that is differentially expressed in mouse embryonic cells. Genes Devel., 6, 481–496.

Yuan, C.C., Kan, N., Dunn, K.J., Papas, T.S. and Blair, D.G. (1989). Properties of a murine viral recombinant of avian acute leukemia virus E26: a murine fibroblast assay for v-*ets* function. J. Virol., 63, 205–215.

Zhang, L., Lemarchandel, V., Romeo, P.-H., Ben-David, Y., Greer, P. and Bernstein, A. (1993). The *Fli-1* proto-oncogene, involved in erythroleukemia and Ewing's sarcoma, encodes a transcriptional activator with DNA-binding specificities distinct from other Ets family members. Oncogene, 8, 1621–1630.

FGR

v-*fgr* is the oncogene of the acutely transforming Gardner–Rasheed feline sarcoma virus (GR-FeSV; Rasheed *et al.*, 1982).

FGR (formerly c-*src-2*) encodes a non-receptor tyrosine kinase.

Related genes

Fgr is a member of the *Src* tyrosine kinase family (*Blk, Fgr, Fyn, Hck, Lck/Tkl, Lyn, Src, Yes*). GR-FeSV has transduced portions of two distinct cellular genes, γ-actin and *Fgr*. The 128 amino acids upstream of v-*fgr* are 98% homologous to γ-actin: the 388 C-terminal residues are 80% homologous to v-*yes*, 74% to pp60^{src} and 39–41% to v-*abl*, v-*fes* and v-*fps*.

Cross-species homology

FGR: 86% identity (mouse and human). Amino acids 76–529 of human FGR (encoded by exons 3–12) are 74% homologous to the SRC equivalent region. The N-terminal 75 amino acids (exon 2) are only 15% homologous to the corresponding SRC sequence.

Transformation

MAN

Fifty-fold amplification of *FGR* occurs in B cells transformed by Epstein–Barr virus (Cheah *et al.*, 1986).

ANIMALS

GR-FeSV is highly infectious to cats, inducing differentiated fibrosarcomas and rhabdosarcomas in young animals (Rasheed *et al.*, 1982).

IN VITRO

FGR does not transform epithelial cells but transforms most mammalian fibroblasts including human (Rasheed *et al.*, 1982).

	FGR/Fgr	v-*fgr*
Nucleotides (kb)		4.6 (GR-FeSV)
Chromosome		
Human	1p36.2–p36.1	
Mouse	4 (*Fgr*)	
Exons	12	

	FGR/Fgr	v-*fgr*
mRNA (kb)	2.8/3.1	
Amino acids		663 (v-*fgr*)
Human	529	
Mouse	517	
Mass (kDa)		
(predicted)	55	72
(expressed)	p70	p70$^{gag\text{-}actin\text{-}fgr}$

Cellular location

Cytoplasmic: associates with plasma membrane. Present in the secondary granules of neutrophils. p70$^{gag\text{-}actin\text{-}fgr}$ is myristylated in the *gag* N-terminal region.

Tissue location

FGR expression is high in mature peripheral blood monocytes and granulocytes, alveolar and splenic macrophages, human natural killer cells and differentiating myelomonocytic HL-60 and U937 cells (Ley *et al.*, 1989; Katagiri *et al.*, 1991; Biondi *et al.*, 1991). It is not detectable in normal B cells but is induced by Epstein–Barr virus transformation (Cheah *et al.*, 1986). It is expressed only in the later stages of differentiation of myeloid leukaemia cells, in contrast to *Src* (Willman *et al.*, 1987, 1991).

Protein function

Tyrosine kinase. The γ-actin domain inhibits both the kinase activity and oncogenicity of GR-FeSV (Sugita *et al.*, 1989). In normal bone marrow-derived monocytic cells *Fgr* mRNA expression is transiently increased 20-fold by CSF1, GM-CSF or LPS (Yi and Willman, 1989) and agents that stimulate the differentiation of HL-60 cells also activate transcription and translation (Notario *et al.*, 1989).

Structures of the human FGR, murine *Lck* and chicken *Src* genes

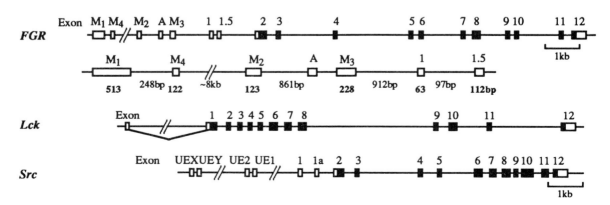

Open boxes: 5′ and 3′ untranslated regions. In the expanded diagram of the *FGR* promoter region the sizes of the exons (bp) are in bold type. In human myelomonocytes differential promoter utilization and alternative splicing gives rise to at least six distinct mRNAs that differ only in their 5′ untranslated regions (Link *et al.*, 1992).

The two predominant RNA species are *FGRA* (EBV-infected B cells) and *FGR4* (myelomonocytic cells). *FGRA* (2.8 kb) contains exon A linked to exon 1 and downstream exons and in *FGR4* exon M₄ is spliced to exon 1 and downstream exons (Gutkind *et al.*, 1991; Link *et al.*, 1992). Thus in EBV infection a cryptic exon A promoter is activated to regulate the expression of *FGR*, whereas the exon M_4 promoter is used exclusively in myelomoncytic cells. M_1 and M_2 are rarely utilized in mononuclear cells (monocytes, neutrophils and lymphocytes).

Exons 3–12 closely resemble those of avian *Src* and murine *Lck* (Nishizawa *et al.*, 1986). Upstream exons differ and the 5′ untranslated region of *FGR* has an extra intron. There is a cluster of transcriptional start sites upstream of exon 1a that is rich in GC regions but lacks a TATA box.

Structure of GR-FeSV

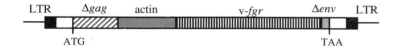

The GR-FeSV arose by recombination of the helper feline leukaemia virus (FeLV) with 1.7 kb of cellular sequence (essential for transformation of NIH 3T3 fibroblasts by the virus). Insertion of the cellular sequences caused partial deletion of *gag* and *env* (Naharro *et al.*, 1984). The v-*fgr* ORF codes for 663 amino acids (GR-gp70$^{gag-fgr}$). *gag* contributes 355 5′ nucleotides (118 amino acids), there are 151 amino acids of the N-terminus of feline non-muscle actin, 389 of feline FGR and *env* (FeLV) encodes the last 5 amino acids. The recombinatorial event occurred within *env*, altering the reading frame and creating a TAA (termination) codon. The region 269–657 is 80% homologous to avian p90^{v-yes}. v-FGR lacks 127 and 12 amino acids of the N- and C-termini respectively of p55^{fgr}.

Sequences of human FGR, mouse FGR and v-FGR

```
v-FGR        (1)                                          ARALCRPAVCRPRPLPPLPPTA

Human FGR    (1)    MGCVFCKKLEPVATAKEDAGLEGDFRSYGAADHYGPDPTKARPASSFAHIPNYSNFSSQ
Mouse FGR    (1)    ----------- AS ---V--------QT-EER-Y----QG-NS-V-PQ
v-FGR        (23)   RMEEEVAALVIDNGSGMCKAGFAGDDAPRAVFPSIVGPRHQGVMVGMGQKDSYVGDEAQS

Human FGR    (60)   AINPGFLDSGTIRGVSGIGVTLFIALYDYEARTEDDLTFTKGEKFHILNNTEGDWWEARS
Mouse FGR    (50)   PTS-A--NT-NM-SI--T---I-V---------G----------------Y-------
v-FGR        (83)   KRGILTLKYPIEH-IVTNWDDMEKIWHHTFYNELRVAPEEHPVLLTEAPLNPKANR-KMT

Human FGR    (120)  LSSGKTGCIPSNYVAPVDSIQAEEWYFGKIGRKDAERQLLSPGNPQGAFLIRESETTKGA
Mouse FGR    (110)  ----HR-YV--------------------S----------S-----------------
v-FGR        (143)  QIMFE-FN----------------------------------AR----V---------

Human FGR    (180)  YSLSIRDWDQTRGDHVKHYKIRKLDMGGYYITTRVQFNSVQELVQHYMEVNDGLCNLLIA
Mouse FGR    (170)  ----------N----I---------T--------A----İ-D-------------Y--T-
v-FGR        (203)  -------EA--------------T--------A------------V-------H--T-
```

```
Human FGR  (240)  PCTIMKPQTLGLAKDAWEISRSSITLERRLGTGCFGDVWLGTWNGSTKVAVKTLKPGTMS
Mouse FGR  (230)  ---TT-------------D-N--A------------------C--------------
v-FGR      (263)  A--T-----M---------------Q------------------------------

Human FGR  (300)  PKAFLEEAQVMKLLRHDKLVQLYAVVSEEPIYIVTEFMCHGSLLDFLKNPEGQDLRLPQL
Mouse FGR  (290)  ---------I-------------------------Y--------DR---N-M--H-
v-FGR      (323)  ---S-----I---------------P--------------E---DQ----T----

Human FGR  (360)  VDMAAQVAEGMAYMERMNYIHRDLRAANILVGERLACKIADFGLARLIKDDEYNPCQGSK
Mouse FGR  (350)  ------------------------------Y-I-----------E-N----Q--T-
v-FGR      (383)  ------------------------------V-----------E-N----R--A-

Human FGR  (420)  FPIKWTAPEAALFGRFTIKSDVWSFGILLTELITKGRIPYPGMNKREVLEQVEQGYHMPC
Mouse FGR  (410)  ----------------V----------------V------N--------H------
v-FGR      (443)  ------------------------S---V------N--------H------

Human FGR  (480)  PPGCPASLYEAMEQTWRLDPEERPTFEYLQSFLEDYFTSAEPQYQPGDQT (529)
Mouse FGR  (470)  -----------V---A----------------------T---------- (517)
v-FGR      (503)  ---------------------------------NGPQQN (545)
```

In human FGR amino acids 269–277 and 291 comprise the ATP binding site (257–265 and 279 in mouse), 412 is autophosphorylated (400 in mouse), and 82–134 (underlined) is the SH3 domain (70–122 in mouse). v-FGR domains: 23–157 actin homology; 151–539 homology with v-YES of avian sarcoma virus Y73; 292–300 and 314 ATP binding; 435 autophosphorylation; 82–134 SH3. Tyrosine 523 is equivalent to Tyr527 of p60^{src}. v-FGR is myristylated on p15^{gag}.

Databank file names and accession numbers

	ONCOGENE	EMBL	SWISSPROT	REFERENCES
Human	FGR (SRC2)	Hsfgr2 to Hsfgr7	KFGR_HUMAN P09769	Katamine et al., 1988
		M12719–M12724		Nishizawa et al., 1986
				Inoue et al., 1987
Mouse	Fgr	Mmcfgr X16440	KFGR_MOUSE P14234	Yi and Willman, 1989
GR-FeSV	v-fgr (src-2)	Refesv X00255	KFGR_FSVGR P00544	Naharro et al., 1984

Papers

Biondi, A., Paganin, C., Rossi, V., Benvestito, S., Perlmutter, R. M., Mantovani, A. and Allavena, P. (1991). Expression of lineage-restricted protein tyrosine kinase genes in human natural killer cells. Eur. J. Immunol., 21, 843–846.

Cheah, M.S.C., Ley, T.J., Tronick, S.R. and Robbins, K.C. (1986). fgr proto-oncogene mRNA induced in B lymphocytes by Epstein–Barr virus infection. Nature, 319, 238–240.

Gutkind, J.S., Link, D.C., Katamine, S., Lacal, P., Miki, T., Ley, T.J. and Robbins, K.C. (1991). A novel c-fgr exon utilized in Epstein–Barr virus-infected B lymphocytes but not in normal monocytes. Mol. Cell. Biol., 11, 1500–1507.

Inoue K., Ikawa, S., Semba, K., Sukegawa, J., Yamamoto, T. and Toyoshima, K. (1987). Isolation and sequencing of cDNA clones homologous to the v-fgr oncogene from a human B lymphocyte cell line, IM-9. Oncogene, 1, 301–304.

Katagiri, K, Katagiri, T., Koyama, Y., Morikawa, M., Yamamoto, T. and Yoshida, T. (1991). Expression of src family genes during monocytic differentiation of HL-60 cells. J. Immunol., 146, 701–707.

Katamine, S., Notario, V., Rao, C.D., Miki, T., Cheah, M.S., Tronick, S.R. and Robbins, K.C. (1988). Primary structure of the human *fgr* proto-oncogene product p55^{c-fgr}. Mol. Cell. Biol., 8, 259–266.

Ley, T.J., Connolly, N.L., Katamine, S., Cheah, M.S.C., Senior, R.M. and Robbins, K.C. (1989). Tissue-specific expression and developmental regulation of the human *fgr* proto-oncogene. Mol. Cell. Biol., 9, 92–99.

Link, D.C., Gutkind, S.J., Robbins, K.C. and Ley, T.J. (1992). Characterization of the 5′ untranslated region of the human c-*fgr* gene and identification of the major myelomonocytic c-*fgr* promoter. Oncogene, 7, 877–884.

Naharro, G., Robbins, K.C. and Reddy, E.P. (1984). Gene product of v-*fgr onc*: hybrid protein containing a portion of actin and a tyrosine-specific protein kinase. Science, 223, 63–66.

Nishizawa, M., Semba, K., Yoshida, M.C., Yamamoto, T., Saski, M. and Toyoshima, K. (1986). Structure, expression and chromosomal location of the human c-*fgr* gene. Mol. Cell. Biol., 6, 511–517.

Notario, V., Gutkind, J.S., Imaizumi, M., Katamine, S. and Robbins, K.C. (1989). Expression of the *fgr* protooncogene product as a function of myelomonocytic cell maturation. J. Cell Biol., 109, 3129–3136.

Patel, M., Leevers, S.J. and Brickell, P.M. (1990). Structure of the complete human c-*fgr* proto-oncogene and identification of multiple transcriptional start sites. Oncogene, 5, 201–206.

Rasheed, S., Barbacid, M., Aaronson, S. and Gardner, M.B. (1982). Origin and biological properties of a new feline sarcoma virus. Virology, 117, 238–244.

Sugita, K., Gutkind, J.S., Katamine, S., Kawakami, T. and Robbins, K.C. (1989). The actin domain of Gardner-Rasheed feline sarcoma virus inhibits tyrosine kinase and transforming activities. J. Virol., 63, 1715–1720.

Willman, C.L., Stewart, C.C., Griffith, J.K., Stewart, S.J. and Tomasi, T.B. (1987). Differential expression and regulation of c-*src* and c-*fgr* protooncogenes in myelomonocytic cells. Proc. Natl Acad. Sci. USA, 84, 4480–4484.

Willman, C.L., Stewart, C.C., Longacre, T.L., Head, D.R., Habbersett, R., Ziegler, S.F. and Perlmutter, R.M. (1991). Expression of the c-*fgr* and *hck* protein-tyrosine kinases in acute myeloid leukemic blasts is associated with early commitment and differentiation events in the monocytic and granulocytic lineages. Blood, 77, 726–734.

Yi, T.L. and Willman, C.L. (1989). Cloning of the murine c-*fgr* proto-oncogene cDNA and induction of c-*fgr* expression by proliferation and activation factors in normal bone marrow-derived monocytic cells. Oncogene 4, 1081–1087.

FOS

v-*fos* is the oncogene of the FBJ (Finkel, Biskis and Jinkins, 1966) and FBR (Finkel, Biskis and Reilly) murine osteosarcoma viruses (MuSV) and of the avian transforming virus NK24 (Nishizawa *et al.*, 1987). FBJ helper virus: FBJ-MuLV, ecotrophic, non-leukaemogenic, N-trophic virus, similar to AKR-MuLV. FBR helper virus: ecotrophic, B-trophic.

The *FOS* gene family encode transcription factors.

Related genes

Fra-1 and *Fra-2* (*Fos*-related *a*ntigens), *Fosb*, Δ*Fosb* (or *Fosb2*: *Fosb* minus 101 C-terminal amino acids) and r-*fos* (homologous to the third exon of *Fos*). Murine FOSB and FOS share 44% protein sequence identity: that between FOS, FOSB and FRA1 is 24%. Between FOS residues 124 and 205 there are 18 amino acids identical to those in the aligned sequences of FOSB, FRA1, JUN and JUNB (Zerial *et al.*, 1989). FOS and FOSB are 70% homologous.

The herpesvirus Marek disease virus (MDV) encodes a gene closely related to the *Fos*/*Jun* family that is expressed in MDV-transformed lymphoblastoid cells (Jones *et al.*, 1992).

Drosophila dFRA and dJRA (Perkins *et al.*, 1990).

The *Fos* family are members of the helix–loop–helix/leucine zipper superfamily (see ***JUN***).

Cross-species homology

FOS: 94% identity (human, mouse and rat); 79% (chicken and mouse). FRA1: 90% (human and rat). FRA2: 87% (human and chicken).

Transformation

MAN

FOS was overexpressed in 60% of one sample of human osteosarcomas (Wu *et al.*, 1990) and in a cell line derived from a pre-B cell acute lymphocytic leukaemia (Tsai *et al.*, 1991).

ANIMALS

In transgenic mice *Fos* expression activated by the FBJ-MuSV LTR causes bone tumours (Ruther *et al.*, 1989). FBJ- and FBR-MuSV induce sarcomas in animals (Van Beveren *et al.*, 1983, 1984). NK24 causes avian nephroblastoma (Nishizawa *et al.*, 1987).

IN VITRO

Fos: Overexpression of *FOS* does not transform human fibroblasts (Alt and Grassmann, 1993), but it does transform rat fibroblasts if (1) an LTR is present to enhance transcription and (2) an AT-rich region 500 bp downstream of the chain terminator and 150 bp upstream of the poly(A) addition signal in the 3′ UTR is removed. The AU sequence in many rapidly induced mRNAs is thought to mediate selective degradation. In *Fos* the removal of a 67 bp destabilizing element encompassing three conserved AUUUA motifs correlates with increased trans-forming potential (Meijlink *et al.*, 1985; Raymond *et al.*, 1989). A second region that regulates mRNA stability is present within the coding sequence. The 5′ end of this 0.32 kb "coding region determinant of mRNA instability" (CRDI) contains a 56 bp purine-rich region with which at least two protein factors associate to promote rapid degradation (Chen *et al.*, 1992).

Fosb: Fosb is a more potent transforming agent than *Fos* having a transforming capacity equival-ent to that of v-*fos* (Schuermann *et al.*, 1991). The C-terminal region appears to be responsible: the potential hairpin structure at the 3′ end of *Fos* is not present in *Fosb*, which may account for the observed increase in mRNA expression of the latter form. FOS also contains a consen-sus target sequence for a cAMP-dependent protein kinase (RKGSSS: 359–364), missing in FOSB, that may determine protein stability (Abate *et al.*, 1991).

FBJ- and FBR-MuSV: Both viruses transform cells *in vitro* but FBR-MuSV is the most effective. FBR-MuSV immortalizes murine cells in culture; FBJ-MuSV does not. FBR-MuSV v-*fos* trans-forms human epidermal keratinocyte cells *in vitro* (Lee *et al.*, 1993). The internal deletions in the C-terminal half of the FBR-MuSV oncogene are responsible for its transforming potential (removing the *trans*-repression domain, preventing binding to the promoter and hence consti-tutively activating the gene, see **Functional domains of human FOS, FOSB and FOSB2**, page 187) and a single mutation of Glu138 to Val138 activates the immortalizing capacity of p75$^{gag\text{-}fos\text{-}fox}$ (Jenuwein and Muller, 1987). p75 is therefore unusual among oncogenes in that both these activities appear to reside in one nuclear protein. v-*fos* transformation of fibroblasts induces the expression of a *Fos* transformation *effector* gene (*Fte-1*) that is a mammalian homologue of a yeast gene implicated in regulating protein import into mitochondria (Kho and Zarbl, 1992).

TRANSGENIC ANIMALS

Transgenic mice having a null mutation in *Fos* have low viability at birth (~40%). However, the homozygous mutants that survive have normal growth rates until severe osteopetrosis develops at approximately 11 days (Johnson *et al.*, 1992). Thus *Fos* is not essential for the growth of most cell types although null mutants show delayed or absent gametogenesis and in most animals there is a reduction of ~75% in the levels of circulating T and B lymphocytes.

	FOS/Fos	*FOSB/Fosb*	v-*fos* FBJ-MuSV	v-*fos* FBR-MuSV
Nucleotides (bp)	~3500	~4600	4026 (1639 from *Fos*)	3791 (709 *Fos*: 437 (*Fox*) from other cellular sequences)
Chromosome				
Human	14q24.3			
Mouse	12 [E–D]	7[A1–B1]		
Exons	4	4		
mRNA (kb)	2.2	5.0 (alternative splicing of exon 4 removes 140 bp to generate the short form of *Fosb* (*Fosb/sf* or *Fosb2*))	3.4	3.3

	FOS/Fos	FOSB/Fosb	v-fos FBJ-MuSV	v-fos FBR-MuSV
mRNA half-life	20–30 min Early response gene rapidly (~5 min) expressed in stimulated cells	10–15 min	>3 h	>3 h
Amino acids	380 (human, rat, mouse) 271 (human FRA1) 326 (human FRA2)	338 (human) 237 (FOSB2)	381	554
Mass (kDa)				
(predicted)	41.6 29 (FRA1) 35 (FRA2)	36	49.6	60
(expressed)	p55/pp62 (FOS) Anomalous mobility may be caused by the high proline (10%) content	p52 p37 (FOSB2)	pp55$^{v\text{-}fos}$	pp75$^{gag\text{-}fos\text{-}fox}$
pI	~4.6			
Protein half-life (min)	30 Transient expression (maximal ~2 h) in mitogenetically stimulated cells		120	120

Cellular location

Nuclear. FOS migrates to the cytoplasm in serum-starved fibroblasts (Vriz et al., 1992).

Tissue location

FOS: FOS expression is very low in most cell types: constitutive high expression in amnion, yolk sac, mid-gestation fetal liver, post-natal bone marrow and in one human pre-B leukaemic cell line but not others of similar origin (Muller et al., 1983; Gonda and Metcalf, 1984; Mason et al., 1985; Mitchell et al., 1985; Muller et al., 1985; Conscience et al., 1986; Kreipe et al., 1986; Panterne et al., 1992). Fos is an immediate early gene the expression of which is induced rapidly and transiently by growth factors and mitogens (Muller et al., 1984a). Fos mRNA is detectable within 5 min of stimulation: protein expression maximal after 90 min. Although in general *Fos* is barely detectable throughout the cell cycle it may be induced at any stage other than during mitosis (Bravo *et al.*, 1986). *Fos* expression is transiently activated in macrophages stimulated by CSF1 (Bravo *et al.*, 1987) or lipopolysaccharide (Tannenbaum *et al.*, 1988) and in myelomonocytic leukaemic cells induced to differentiate by TPA (Muller *et al.*, 1984b, 1985; Sariban *et al.*, 1985). *Fos* is also transiently expressed in interleukin-2- and IL-6-dependent mouse myeloma cell lines following withdrawal of growth factor and the onset of apoptosis (Colotta *et al.*, 1992).

FOSB: Expression of this immediate early gene is induced with kinetics similar to that of *Fos* (Zerial *et al.*, 1989).

FRA-1 and *FRA-2:* Expression is low in quiescent cells. It is induced rapidly (*FRA-1* detectable after 1 h, *FRA-2* after 2 h) and transiently following cell stimulation (Cohen and Curran, 1988; Matsui *et al.*, 1990; Nishina *et al.*, 1990; Yoshida *et al.*, 1993). After the initial activation period of serum-stimulated quiescent cells when FOS is the principal protein associated with JUN proteins (~3 h), FRA1 and FRA2 are the predominant partners in heterodimers with JUN proteins (Kovary and Bravo, 1992).

Protein function

FOS, FOSB, FRA1 and FRA2 form heterodimers with JUN proteins that function as positive or negative transcription factors by binding to specific DNA sequences via basic domains adjacent to the dimerizing helices (see **Transcriptional regulation of human *FOS* and *JUN***). The consensus DNA binding sequence for FOS heterodimers is the activation protein-1 (AP-1) site (also called the *cis*-acting TPA (12-*O*-tetradecanoylphorbol-13-acetate) response element (TRE)) TGA$^C/_G$TCA. The stability of dimers increases in the order FOS–FOS<JUN–JUN<FOS–JUN. The substitution of Glu168 by Lys enables FOS homodimers to bind to TRE (Nicklin and Casari, 1991). DNA bends of differing magnitude and orientation are induced by different combinations of FOS and JUN (Kerppola and Curran, 1991).

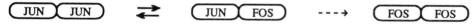

Rapid and transient FOS expression is almost invariably correlated with the stimulation of proliferation and also with the onset of differentiation. In Swiss 3T3 fibroblasts FOS and FOSB are mainly required during the G_0 to G_1 transition whereas FRA1 and FRA2 are involved in asynchronous growth (Kovary and Bravo, 1992). Nevertheless there is evidence, summarized below, that *Fos* expression is neither necessary nor sufficient to cause either of these processess. FOS interacts cooperatively with JUN to inhibit its own transcription. In pre-adipocytes FOS and JUN block expression of the adipocyte P2 lipid binding protein gene and in myocytes they inhibit atrial natriuretic factor transcription (McBride *et al.*, 1993). For human metallothionein IIA, collagenase, collagen α_1(III), transin, proenkephalin and SV40 genes, however, FOS–JUN dimers form a potent transcription activating complex. It seems probable that most cells in which FOS is expressed also activate the other genes in the *Fos* and *Jun* families (*Fra-1, Fra-2* and possibly *Fosb, Jun, Junb* and *Jund*). The expression of these genes is temporally distinct: together with the subtle factors that affect FOS–JUN binding to DNA (see *JUN*), a wide spectrum of transcription factor activities can be envisaged, our understanding of which is presently limited, as reflected by the apparent contradictions in the data summarized in the table at the end of this section.

The involvement of members of the *Fos/Jun* family in development is suggested by the observation that *Fos, Fosb* and *Fra-1* and *Jun, Junb* and *Jund* are differentially expressed during development and in adult tissues, consistent with their having distinct functions. In the newborn mouse a large transient (day 1) burst of *Fos* transcription occurs in all major tissues (Kasik *et al.*, 1987). The two *Drosophila* homologues, dFRA and dJRA, differ from *Fos* in that dFRA recognizes the AP-1 site on its own, although the affinity of the dFRA/dJFRA dimer is higher. Expression of dFRA mRNA is restricted in the developing *Drosophila* embryo, in contrast to that of dJFRA which is uniformly expressed (Perkins *et al.*, 1990).

Structures of FBJ-MuSV, cellular and FBR-MuSV *Fos* genes

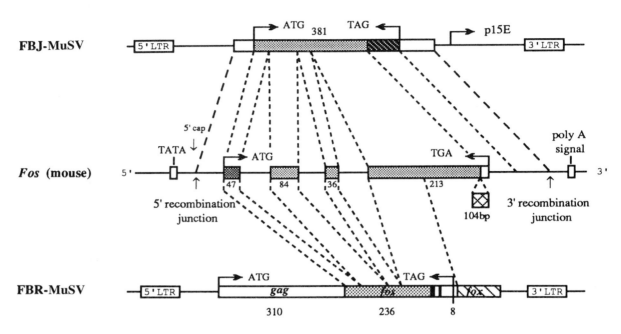

(From Ransone, L.J., and Verma, I.M. (1990). Nuclear proto-oncogenes FOS and JUN. Annu. Rev. Cell. Biol., 6, 539–557.)

FBJ-MuSV: The FBJ oncogene product has 332 N-terminal residues identical to FOS, save for five single amino acid changes but a deletion of 104 bp shifts the reading frame, giving rise to a different 49 residues at the C-terminus (cross-hatched).

Fos: Shaded boxes represent the four exons and the deletion from exon 4 occurring in p55$^{v\text{-}fos}$ (FBJ-MuSV) is represented by the crossed box. The termination codon is TGA (TAG in v-*fos*).

FBR-MuSV: Lines indicate sequences acquired from *Fos*: the two heavy bars indicate deletions from *Fos* in p75$^{gag\text{-}fos}$: FOS has lost 24 N-terminal amino acids (replaced by 310 from viral *gag*) and in the C-terminus there are in-frame internal deletions of 13 and 9 amino acids and replacement of the terminal 98 amino acids by 8 residues encoded by *fox* sequences. *Fox* is normal mouse DNA from a locus unrelated to *Fos* (Van Beveren *et al.*, 1983, 1984; Verma *et al.*, 1986). p75$^{gag\text{-}fos\text{-}fox}$ forms heterodimers with JUN (see below) that have decreased affinity for DNA *in vitro* compared with FOS–JUN dimers due to the N-terminal *gag* region: the FBR protein is myristylated at the N-terminal glycine and this appears to be responsible for the inhibition of *trans* activation of TRE-dependent transcription (Kamata *et al.*, 1991).

The FBJ-MuSV v-*fos* sequence is more closely related to murine than human *Fos* sequences. The deletion in the FBJ-MuSV v-*fos* oncogene relative to murine and human *Fos* proto-oncogenes that causes complete divergence of the C-terminal protein sequences corresponds to positions 3182–3285 inclusive of the human *FOS* sequence. The FBJ-MuSV v-*fos* coding sequence ends at a TAG stop codon corresponding to positions 2834–2836 of this sequence. A TATA box is located at positions 701–707 and two potential poly(A) signals are present in the 3′ untranslated region (see figures below).

The overall structure of the *Fosb* and *Fra-2* genes is very similar to that of *Fos* (Nishina *et al.*, 1990; Lazo *et al.*, 1992). The four exons of *Fosb* encode 42, 107, 36 and 153 amino acids, respectively and alternative splicing at nucleotide positions 4685 and 4825 generates the truncated FOSΔB form of 237 amino acids (Lazo *et al.*, 1992).

NK24 (avian transforming virus) expresses an unaltered FOS protein fused to the *gag* encoded sequence (Nishizawa *et al.*, 1987).

Transcriptional regulation of human *FOS*

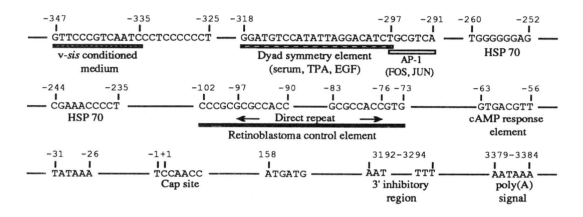

−56 to −63: Resembles the consensus for cAMP-regulated promoters (cAMP response element or CRE).

−76 and −90: Direct repeat (DR), required, with -56 to -63 for basal transcription.

−73 to −102: Retinoblastoma control element, through which transcriptional regulation by SV40 T antigen or E1A can also be mediated. $p105^{RB}$ represses *FOS* transcription following stimulation by serum and also lowers the concentration of *FOS* mRNA in cells growing in the presence of serum. Each of the two viral proteins stimulates transcriptional activity, probably by binding to $p105^{RB}$. Deletion of the putative leucine zipper region of $p105^{RB}$ abolishes transcriptional suppression.

−220 to −120: *Trans* activated by the hepatitis B virus (HBV) pX, which also modulates transcription through interactions with the SRE and AP-1 sites (Avantaggiati *et al.*, 1993).

−235 to −244 and −252 to −260: Contain homology with HSP 70 promoters.

−291 to −297: AP-1 binding site: FOS–JUN heterodimers bind to inhibit *FOS* transcription. FOS interacts cooperatively with JUN to activate other genes (e.g. human metallothionein IIA, collagenase, collagen α_1(III), transin (or stromeolysin, a metalloproteinase that degrades extracellular matrix), SV40) that contain the TRE element. FOS interacts with at least one other transcription factor in that it cooperates with NF-κB in activating HIV-1.

−297 to −318: A 20 bp dyad symmetry element (DSE) or serum response element (SRE) required for activation by serum, PDGF, TPA or EGF. Serum responsive factor ($p67^{SRF}$) in fibroblasts can interact with the SRE via the element CC(A/T)$_6$GG termed the CArG box. An additional factor, $p62^{TCF}$ that interacts directly with the 5′ region of the SRE, forms a ternary complex with the SRE and $p67^{SRF}$ and requires both DSE-bound $p67^{SRF}$ and sequences both within and outside the DSE for its interaction with DNA (Shaw *et al.*, 1989; Shaw, 1992; Sharrocks *et al.*, 1993). p67^{SRF} is also transcriptionally activated via its C-terminal half by HTLV-1 TAX1 (Fujii *et al.*, 1991, 1992). p67^{SRF} is phosphorylated by casein kinase II but this does not appear to be significant in the growth factor activation of *FOS* expression (Manak and Prywes, 1993). p62^{TCF} is phosphorylated *in vitro* by MAP kinase and this results in enhanced ternary complex formation (Gille *et al.*, 1992). ELK1 (see **ETS**) may be identical to p62^{TCF}; it binds to the same DNA region, indicating that members of the *Ets* family may regulate *Fos* expression (Hipskind *et al.*, 1991).

This sequence also confers inducibility on a heterologous promoter (the β globin promoter) but only in response to serum, not PDGF or TPA. This suggests that additional cooperative signals are required for transcriptional activation in response to PDGF or TPA. Sequences closely similar to that of SRE occur in other genes (e.g. actin and *Krox20*).

An additional SRF accessory protein (SAP) that occurs in two forms (SAP1a (52 kDa) and SAP1b (55 kDa)) has been isolated: SAP1 has similar DNA binding properties to p62 and is homologous to ELK1 (see **ETS**; Dalton and Treisman, 1992). These accessory proteins contact SRF via a conserved B box sequence (see **ETS**) and bind to DNA via an ETS motif ($^C/_A{}^C/_A$GGA$^A/_T$) that may vary in both its orientation and separation from the SRE (Treisman *et al.*, 1992).

The SRE contains multiple overlapping enhanson elements (Treisman, 1992) with which members of both the helix–loop–helix and the CCAAT/enhancer binding protein (C/EBP) transcription factor families (Metz and Ziff, 1991) and the zinc finger protein SRE-ZBP interact (Attar and Gilman, 1992). An additional SRE binding protein (SRE BP) is required for maximal serum induction of *FOS* (Boulden and Sealy, 1992). The binding site for SRE BP coincides with that for rNF-IL6 but the proteins are distinct (Metz and Ziff, 1991) and the SRE also includes binding sites for DBF/MAPF1 (Ryan *et al.*, 1989; Walsh, 1989), Phox1 (Grueneberg *et al.*, 1992) and E12 (Metz and Ziff, 1991).

Fos expression is greatly diminished during muscle cell differentiation and, consistent with this observation, the muscle-specific transcription factor MyoD binds to a region overlapping the SRE to function as a negative regulator of *Fos* transcription (Trouche *et al.*, 1993).

Overlapping enhanson elements within the SRE:

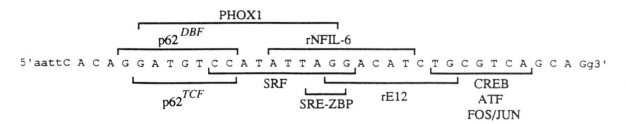

−325 to −339: Growth factor-inducible protein complex binding element (Hayes *et al.*, 1987).

−335 to −347: v-*sis*-conditioned medium inducible element (SIE). The SIE, DSE, DR and CRE can mediate *trans* activation by the HTLV-1 TAX protein (Wagner *et al.*, 1990; Alexandre and Verrier, 1991).

208 to 218 (palindrome): An additional *FOS* intragenic regulatory element (FIRE) at the end of exon 1 can cause premature termination of transcription. Intragenic regulation of transcription also occurs in the *Myc* and *Myb* genes (Lamb *et al.*, 1990).

Microinjection of an antisense oligomer to the SRE and part of the AP-1 site inhibits *FOS* production in serum-stimulated cells. In serum-starved cells, however, the microinjection of both anti-sense oligomers to SRE and FIRE is required for the induction of *FOS* synthesis.

Taken together, these observations indicate the existence of both positive and negative factors in the regulation of *FOS* expression.

The murine *Fosb* promoter contains SRE and AP-1 binding sites located in positions that are identical relative to those found in the *Fos* promoter and the activity of the *Fosb* promoter is downregulated by FOS or FOSB (Lazo *et al.*, 1992).

Sequences of v-FOS FBJ-MuSV, human FOS, mouse FOS and v-FOS FBR-MuSV

```
                                    +   gag  <----  -->  fos
                              *************************
v-FOS (FBJ-MuSV)  (1)         MMFSGFNADYEASSFRCSSASPAGDSLSYYHSPADSFSSMGSPVNTQDFCADLSVSSAN
FOS (human)                   MMFSGFNADYEASSSRCSSASPAGDSLSYYHSPADSFSSMGSPVNAQDFCTDLAVSSAN
FOS (mouse)                   MMFSGFNADYEASSSRCSSASPAGDSLSYYHSPADSFSSMGSPVNTQDFCADLSVSSAN
v-FOS (FBR-MuSV)              TQMPNEVNAAFPLERPDWDYTTPEDSLSYYHSPADSFSSMGSPVNTQDFCADLSVSSAN

                                *   +                                              +
v-FOS            (60)         FIPTVTATSTSPDLQWLVQPTLVSSVAPSQTRAPHPYGLPTQSAGAYARAEMVKTVSGGRAQSIGRRGKV
FOS (human)                  FIPTVTAISTSPDLQWLVQPALVSSVAPSQTRAPHPFGVPAPSAGAYSRAGVVKTMTGGRAQSIGRRGKV
FOS (mouse)                  FIPTVTAISTSPDLQWLVQPTLVSSVAPSQTRAPHPYGLPTQSAGAYARAGMVKTVSGGRAQSIGRRGKV
v-FOS                        FIPTETAISTSPDLQWLVQPTLVSSVAPSQTRAPHPYGLPTQSAGAYARAGMVKTVSGGRAQSIGRRGKV

                                *                                              +
v-FOS           (130)        EQLSPEEEEKRRIRRERNKMAAAKCRNRRRELTDTLQAETDQLEDKKSALQTEIANLLKEKEKLEFILAA
FOS (human)                 EQLSPEEEEKRRIRRERNKMAAAKCRNRRRELTDTLQAETDQLEDEKSALQTEIANLLKEKEKLEFILAA
FOS (mouse)                 EQLSPEEEEKRRIRRERNKMAAAKCRNRRRELTDTLQAETDQLEDEKSALQTEIANLLKEKEKLEFILAA
v-FOS                       EQLSPEEEVKRRIRRERNKMAAAKCRNRRRELTDTLQAETDQLEDEKSALQTEIANLLKEKEKLEFILAA

                                           ************          ********
v-FOS           (200)        HRPACKIPDDLGFPEEMSVASLDLTGGLPEASTPESEEAFTLPLLNDPEPKPSLEPVKSISNVELKAEPF
FOS (human)                 HRPACKIPDDLGFPEEMSVASLDLTGGLPEVATPESEEAFTLPLLNDPEPKPSVEPVKSISSMELKTEPF
FOS (mouse)                 HRPACKIPDDLGFPEEMSVASLDLTGGLPEASTPESEEAFTLPLLNDPEPKPSLEPVKSISNVELKAEPF
v-FOS                       HRPACKIPDDLGFPEEMSVASLDLTGGL          LPLLNDPEPKPSLEPVKS         SF

                            fos  <----  --> fox
                              **  |********                                       ++++++
v-FOS           (270)        DDFLFPASSRPSGSETSRSVPNVDLSGSFYAADWEPLHSNSLGMGPMVTELEPLCTPVVTCTPLLRLPEL
FOS (human)                 DDFLFPASSRPSGSETARSVPDMDLSGSFYAADWEPLHSGSLGMGPMATELEPLCTPVVTCTPSCTAYTS
FOS (mouse)                 DDFLFPASSRPSGSETSRSVPDVDLSGSFYAADWEPLHSNSLGMGPMVTELEPLCTPVVTCTPGCTTYTS
v-FOS                       DDFLFPASSGHSGFISMAGWQ

                                                                          <-- p55  v-fos
                            ++++++++++++++++++++++++++++++++ +++++
v-FOS           (340)        THAAGPVSSQRRQGSRHPDVPLPELVHYREEKHVFPQRFPST |
FOS (human)                 SFVFTYPEADSFPSCAAAHRKGSSSNEPSSDSLSSPTLLAL  |
FOS (mouse)                 SFVFTYPEADSFPSCAAAHRKGSSSNEPSSDSLSSPTLLAL  | <-- p55  fos
                                               ^         ^         ^
```

The amino acid sequences of mouse and human p55^*fos* are compared to those of the v-*fos*- and v-*fox*-encoded portions of the FBJ-MuSV p55^v-*fos* and FBR-MuSV p75^v-*fos* (van Straaten *et al.*, 1983). Underlined residues differ between FOS (human) and FOS (mouse). * Indicates differences between pp75^v-*fos* and FOS; + Indicates differences between p55^v-*fos* and mouse FOS. Principal phosphorylation sites are marked ^.

The 22 amino acid basic region 139–161 (KRRIRRERNKMAAAKCRNRRRL) is a nuclear targeting signal but is not essential for FOS nuclear localization (Tratner and Verma, 1991). Other FOS sequences that resemble known nuclear targeting signals are ineffective in directing pyruvate kinase to the nucleus: FOS may therefore contain a novel nuclear targeting sequence.

In FBJ-MuSV v-*fos* the central region of the protein alone (Met111 to Ile206) is both necessary and sufficient to transform chick embryo fibroblasts (Yoshida *et al.*, 1989).

Sequences of human FOS, FOSB, FRA1 and FRA2

```
FOS    (1)    MMFSGFNADYEA    SSSRCSSAS  PAGDSLSYYHSPADSFSSMGSPVNAQDFCTDLAV
FOSB   (1)    --QA-PG--     D-G-----SPSAESQY --SV     ---GSPPTAAAS-ECAGLGEM
FRA1   (1)    --RD-GE  PG   P--GNGGGYGG--QP        --A  AQAA   Q-K-HL
FRA2   (1)    *YQ    --**NFDT**RGSS*S  **HAESY       SSGGGG  ****RVD  M


FOS    (56)   SSANFIPTVTAISTSPDLQWLVQPALVSSVAPSQTRAPHPFGVPAPSAGA     YS
FOSB   (51)   PG-   -V------T--Q--------T-I--M-Q--GQPLASQPPAVDPYDMPGTS--T
FRA1   (38)       V-SINTM-G-QE---M---HFLGPSSYPRPLTYPQ              --PP
FRA2   (41)   PG-GSAF-*T**--T-**-*******TVITSM*N*Y*-S --          ***L


FOS    (108)            RAGVVKTMTGGRAQSIG RRGKVEQLSPEEEEKRRIRRERNK
FOSB   (107)  PGLSAYSTGGASGSGGPSTSTTTSGPVSA-PARARP--PRE-T-T--------V------
FRA1   (77)            QP-P--IRALGPPP     -V--RPC--I------R--V------
FRA2   (86)   PGL ASVPGHMAL     ******--I*TTV     * ***RD*********-**-******


FOS    (149)  MAAAKCRNRRRELTDTLQAETDQLEDEKSALQTEIANLLKEKEKLEFILAAHRPACKIPD
FOSB   (167)  L--------------R---------E---AE-ES---E-Q----R---V-V--K-G----
FRA1   (117)  L---------K---F------K------G--R--EE-Q-Q--R--LV-E----I---
FRA2   (136)  ***********-**EK*****EE**E******K**-****-**-**FM*V**G*V***S


FOS    (209)  DLGFPEEMSVASLDLT    GGLPEVATPESEEAFTLPLLNDPEPKPSVEPVKSISSME
FOSB   (226)     Y--GPGP        -P-A--RDLPGSTSAKEDGFGWLL-P-PPP-LPFQ--RD
FRA1   (175)    --GAKEGDTGS-     S-TSS              -PAPCR--PC-
FRA2   (195)    **-RRSPPAPGLQPMRS-*G*VG-VVVKQ-    --EE-SPSSSSAGLD-AQR-VI


FOS    (264)  LKTEPFDDFLFPASSRPSGSETARSVPDMDLSGSFYAADWEPLHSGSLGMGPMATELEPL
FOSB   (272)  APPNLTASLFTHSEVQ                                    VLGDPF
FRA1   (203)                                              --SP-- VL-P-A-
FRA2   (247)  KPISIA                        -G--GE                *-*


FOS    (324)  CTP VVTCTPSCTAYTSSFVFTYP   EADSF  PS  CAAAHRK GSSSNEPSSDSLSS
FOSB   (294)  - -- S -- ------L-C        - EV S-FAGAQRT-GS-QP--P-N-
FRA1   (216)  H--TLM- ---L-PF-P-L-----ST    - EP--S----SS---GD----P-G-
FRA2   (262)  ***I--*S**AV**G*-N*******VL-QE-PAS*S*S*SK*** R******Q***-*N*


FOS    (375)  PTLLAL (380)
FOSB   (333)  -S---- (338)
FRA1   (266)  ------ (271)
FRA2   (321)  ****** (326)
```

Dashes: identity with FOS. * Indicates identity between FRA2 and FRA1. Underlined: basic and leucine zipper motifs. Italics: N-terminal sequence (41–74) essential for the transforming activity of FOSB (Wisdom and Verma, 1993).

Structures of FOS proteins

The cross-hatched boxes in FOS represent regions deleted in p75$^{gag\text{-}fos}$. The C-terminal 49 amino acids of p55$^{v\text{-}fos}$ (black box) differ from those of FOS. v-FOS (FBR-MuSV) is myristylated at the N-terminus and this modification, together with its C-terminal mutation, causes loss of *trans*-repression activity (Kamata and Holt, 1992).

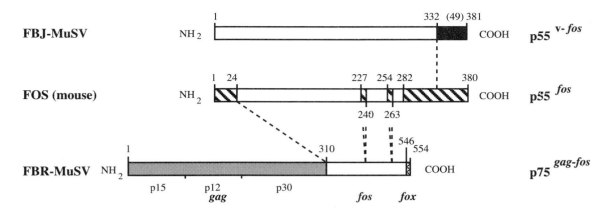

Functional domains of human FOS, FOSB and FOSB2

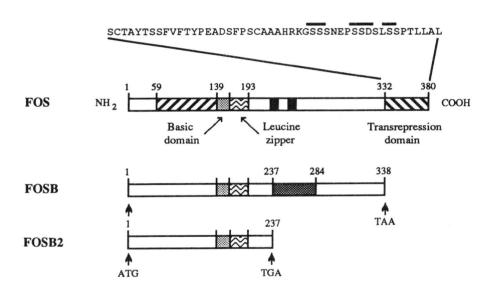

The two cross-hatched boxes represent regions encompassing phosphorylation sites. The bars mark the three groups of C-terminal serine residues in FOS (Ser362–364, Ser368, 369, 371 and Ser373–374). The N-terminal domain (59–139) is phosphorylated *in vitro* by protein kinase C, $p34^{cdc2}$ and a nuclear kinase: the C-terminal region by cAMP-dependent protein kinase and by $p34^{cdc2}$ (Abate *et al.*, 1991). In PC12 cells Ser362 is phosphorylated by a kinase selectively activated by NGF or EGF (Taylor *et al.*, 1993). FOSB (ORF: nucleotides 1202–2218) has a truncated C-terminus relative to FOS but retains the leucine zipper and basic DNA binding regions of FOS.

The alternative splicing event that generates FOSB2 removes 140 bp that are expressed in FOSB (nucleotides 1913–2052 of *Fosb*). This shifts the reading frame by −1 thereby creating a stop codon (TGA) after the leucine zipper, resulting in a loss of 101 C-terminal amino acids. The sequence of FOSB2 is identical to that of the first 237 amino acids of FOSB (Yen *et al.*, 1991).

Relationship between FOS and JUN

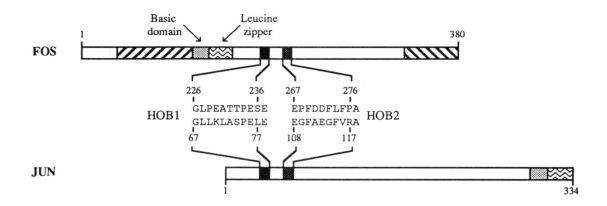

The two homology box regions (HOB1 and HOB2) of FOS lie within a *trans*-activating domain and are conserved in the A1 activation domain of JUN (Sutherland *et al.*, 1992). The FOS sequence is for rat, which is identical to that of human FOS except for the substitution of alanine and threonine by valine and alanine at positions 230 and 231. HOB1 and HOB2 regions also occur in C/EBP and they act cooperatively to stimulate transcription of reporter gene constructs. HOB1 contains a phosphorylation site for MAP kinase.

Transcriptional autoregulation by FOS–JUN dimers

The regulatory activity resides in the C-terminal region of the FOS proteins (mutated in the viral proteins of FBJ-MuSV and FBR-MuSV). One of the major post-translational modifications undergone by FOS is serine phosphoesterification in the C-terminus and the negative charge thus conferred on the molecule is crucial for suppression of transcription (Hunter and Karin, 1992). Mutant proteins containing acidic amino acids instead of Ser362–364 are as effective at suppressing promoter activity as wild-type FOS protein (Ofir *et al.*, 1990). Mutants that do not carry negative charge in this region, either due to phosphorylation or to the mutations described above, associate normally with JUN to activate transcription of promoters containing a TRE.

The truncated form of FOS, ΔFOSB (FOSB2), also retains the capacity to form dimers with JUN that bind to AP-1 sites but no longer activate transcription from AP-1-containing promoters or repress the *Fos* promoter (Nakabeppu and Nathans, 1991). The expression of FOSB2 suppresses transformation by v-*fos*, *Fos* or *Fosb*, presumably due to its interfering with *trans*-activation events required for transformation (Yen *et al.*, 1991). However, overexpression of *Fosb2* does not prevent normal cells from entering the cell cycle in response to serum, indicating that *Fosb2* is not a negative regulator of cell growth (Dobrzanski *et al.*, 1991). Transformation-defective FOS proteins that lack either the leucine zipper region or the N-terminal 110 amino acids inhibit transformation by either v-*fos* or *Ras* (Wick *et al.*, 1992).

The basic motif KCR (amino acids 153–155 in human FOS) is conserved in FOS, JUN and ATF/CREB family members and redox-regulation of the cysteine residue mediates DNA binding (Xanthoudakis *et al.*, 1992). Reduction of this cysteine by the ubiquitous nuclear redox factor REF-1 stimulates the DNA binding activity of FOS–JUN and JUN–JUN dimers, MYB, NF-κB and ATF/CREB proteins. Replacement of Cys154 by serine enhances the transforming activity of the FOS protein (Okuno *et al.*, 1993).

Sequence homology between FOS, FRA1, FRA2 and FOSB

FOS	(chicken)	14-22 60-79	123-208	308-334	344-367
FRA1	(rat)	11-13 39-58	93-179	217-242	251-275
FRA2	(chicken)	12-20 46-65	111-197	256-282	300-323
FOSB	(mouse)	11-19 54-73	142-227	285-309	315-338

The five homologous regions of the proteins are indicated by shaded boxes in the representation of FOS. The basic and leucine zipper regions occur between FOS residues 123 and 208. The aligned numbers below indicate the amino acids at the extremes of the corresponding regions in the other proteins (Nishina *et al.*, 1990).

Fos expression and control of the normal cell growth cycle

The evidence for or against an essential role in the $G_0/G_1/S$ transition can be summarized as follows:

FOR

1 All mitogens, physiological and non-physiological, stimulate rapid, transient *Fos* transcription.
2 RNA antisense oligonucleotides to *Fos* inhibit mitogenesis in 3T3 fibroblasts.
3 Microinjection of antibodies against FOS (or JUN) inhibits mitogenesis in 3T3 fibroblasts although antibodies against individual members of the FOS family (FOS, FOSB or FRA1) cause only ~30% inhibition whereas those against JUN, JUNB or JUND each cause 60–80% inhibition (Holt *et al.*, 1986; Nishikura and Murray, 1987; Riabowol *et al.*, 1988; Kovary and Bravo, 1991).

AGAINST

1 In Swiss 3T3 fibroblasts forskolin, prostaglandin E_1 or 8Br-cAMP cause only 10% of the increase in *Fos* due to bombesin, although each of these agents is fully mitogenic when added with insulin (Mehmet *et al.*, 1988). Furthermore, when protein kinase C is downregulated the bombesin/insulin *Fos* mRNA and protein responses are decreased by 90–97% although the mitogenic response is normal. The action of each mitogenic combination is, however, always correlated with large increases in *Myc* expression. These findings indicate that at most no more than 5% of the transient maximum concentration of FOS protein normally accumulated after stimulation may be necessary for progression through the cell cycle.
2 The ADP-ribosyltransferase (ADPRT) inhibitor 3-methoxybenzamide inhibits mitogenesis in human lymphocytes, blocking *Myc* transcription but having no effect on induced *Fos* expression (McNerney *et al.*, 1987). In fibroblasts 3-methoxybenzamide does not affect proliferation and super-induces both *Fos* and *Myc* expression. This suggests that *Fos* has a different role in the two cell types, even though it is normally an early response gene in both.
3 In embryonic stem cells that lack an intact *Fos* gene and do not synthesize FOS protein, cell viability, growth and differentiation are not impaired (Field *et al.*, 1992).

The fact that the *Fos* gene is activated by Ca^{2+} ionophores or phorbol esters suggests that its activation in mitogenically stimulated cells is a consequence of the rapid (<1 min) increases in $[Ca^{2+}]_i$ and protein kinase C activity that occur following the hydrolysis of $PtdIns(4,5)P_2$. The evidence from T lymphocytes, however, indicates that neither ionic signals nor protein kinase C are responsible for the activation of *Fos* (and *Myc*) expression caused by stimulation of the T cell receptor (Moore *et al.*, 1986, 1988) and it seems probable that the T cell receptor delivers an additional intracellular signal, which may be the activation of p59*fyn* tyrosine kinase.

Databank file names and accession numbers

	GENE	*EMBL*	*SWISSPROT*	*REFERENCES*
FBJ-MSV	v-*fos*	Remsv5 V01184	FOS_MSVFB P01102	Van Beveren *et al.*, 1983
		GB:FBJMUSV JO2084		
FBR-MSV	v-*fos*	GB:FBRMUSV KO2712		Van Beveren *et al.*, 1983
Human	*FOS*	Hscfos V01512	FOS_HUMAN P01100	van Straaten *et al.*, 1983
		GB:Humfos K00650 M16287		Treisman, 1985
				Verma *et al.*, 1986
Human	*FOSB*	Mmfosb X14897	FOSB_HUMAN P13346	Zerial *et al.*, 1989
		GB:Humfosb X14897		
Human	*FOS*-related antigen (*FRA1*)	Hsfra1m X16707	FRA1_HUMAN P15407	Matsui *et al.*, 1990
Human	*FOS*-related antigen 2 (*FRA2*)	Hsfra2m X16706	FRA2_HUMAN P15408	Matsui *et al.*, 1990
Mouse	*Fos*	Mmfos J00370	FOS_MOUSE P01101	Van Beveren *et al.*, 1983
		Mmcfos V00727		Meijlink *et al.*, 1985
		GB:Musfos J00370		Renz *et al.*, 1985
Mouse	*Fosb*	Mmfosb X14897		Zerial *et al.*, 1989
		GB: M7748		Lazo *et al.*, 1992
Rat	*Fos*	Rncfosr X06769	FOS_RAT P12841	Curran *et al.*, 1987
Rat	*Fos*-related antigen (*Fra-1*)	Rrfra1 M19651	FRA1_RAT P10158	Cohen and Curran, 1988
		GB:Ratfra1 M19651		
Chicken	*Fos*	Ggcfos M18043	FOS_CHICK P11939	Fujiwara *et al.*,1987
		Ggcfosa M37000		Molders *et al.*, 1987
		Ggcfos M18043		
		GB:Chkcfos		
Chicken	*Fos*-related antigen 2 (*Fra-2*)	Ggfra2a1 to Ggfra2a4 (D90104 to D90107)	FRA2_CHICK P18625	Nishina *et al.*, 1990
Drosophila	*fos*-related antigen (D-*fra*)		FRA_DROME P21525	Perkins *et al.*, 1990

Table 3.2. *Cellular activation of Fos mRNA expression*

Cell type	Agents	Comment
Fibroblasts	Serum, PDGF, EGF, bombesin, A23187, TPA, UV light, basic calcium phosphate crystals	Immediate early response gene rapidly (<5 min) and transiently (<1 h) expressed in quiescent cells undergoing mitogenic stimulation (Cochran *et al.*, 1984; Greenberg and Ziff, 1984; Liboi *et al.*, 1986; Moore *et al.*, 1986, 1988)
Lymphocytes	ConA, PHA, anti-TCR antibody, Thy-1 (mice), LPS, A23187, TPA	*Fosb* and *Fra-1* mRNA also accumulate transiently in stimulated fibroblasts but with a slight lag with respect to *Fos*
NIH 3T3 fibroblasts	Okadaic acid	Induces *Fos* mRNA (maximal after 4 h) and protein synthesis: the rate of transcription is increased and mRNA half-life extended (to 25 min). Okadaic acid acts synergistically with TPA but not with protein kinase A (cAMP). Thus expression of *Fos* is regulated by the serine/threonine-specific protein phosphatases 1 and 2A (Schonthal *et al.*, 1991a)
NIH 3T3 fibroblasts	Thapsigargin	Thapsigargin releases intracellular Ca^{2+} stores by inhibiting the endoplasmic reticulum Ca^{2+}-ATPase. It also induces rapid transcription of *Fos* and *Jun*. Thapsigargin does not activate protein kinase C in these cells: thus increase in $[Ca^{2+}]_i$ may be responsible for the transcriptional activation (Schonthal *et al.*, 1991b)
NIH 3T3 fibroblasts	Glucocorticoid-stimulated transcription	Glucocorticoid induction of gene expression is inhibited by FOS–JUN which binds to the glucocorticoid receptor. The effect on transcription is similar to that caused by *Hras*, v-*mos* or v-*src*, each of which activates *Fos* expression (Touray et al., 1991). The DNA binding domain of the glucocorticoid receptor differentially inhibits DNA binding by FOS–JUN and JUN–JUN dimers and may thus shift the occupancy of AP-1 sites (Kerppola *et al.*, 1993)
3T3 fibroblasts A431 epithelioid cells Mouse NB2a neuroblasts	Heat shock (1 h at 43°C), sodium arsenite	Transient *Fos*, hsp70 and *Myc* transcription (Gubits and Fairhurst 1988)
Pre-B cells (WEHI-231)	Lipopolysaccharide	Expression during differentiation to B cells
Neuronal cells	NGF, neurotransmitters, voltage-gated Ca^{2+} influx, pentylenetetrazole	Induce large and rapid (30 min) transcription of *Fos* and *Jun*. In rat hippocampus proenkephalin (*Enk*) transcription increases dramatically within 1 h of seizure induced by pentylenetetrazole: FOS–JUN complexes activate a regulatory 5′ region of the *Enk* gene (Sonnenberg *et al.*, 1989)
	N-methyl-D-aspartate, glutamate, morphine	Cause FOS protein accumulation *in vivo* and *in vitro*. *Fos* expression can be inhibited by anaesthetics. In spinal cord neurons nociceptive stimulation causes FOS synthesis in a subgroup of neurons that subsequently express prodynorphin
Rat spinal cord neurons *in vivo*	Injected Freund's adjuvant, hot water immersion	FOS protein synthesis and *Junb* transcription but not that of *Jun* or *Jund* stimulated within 3 h (Naranjo *et al.*, 1991)
Rat glioma cells (C6)	Neutrotrophic protein S100β	S100β stimulates *Fos* (30 min) and *Myc* (2 h) transcription prior to DNA synthesis (Selinfreund *et al.*, 1991)
Pheochromocytoma (PC12)	Nerve growth factor (NGF), EGF, dbcAMP, bFGF	Substantial accumulation of *Fos* and *Jun* mRNA during differentiation to neurons. Sustained *Fos* expression from transfected genes blocks differentiation (Ito *et al.*, 1989)
	Depolarization: (KCl or nicotine)	Activates transcription of *Fos* and *Junb* but not *Jun*, whereas growth factors activate all three (Bartel *et al.*, 1989). The increase in *Fos* and *Egr-1* transcription following depolarization by K^+ or ionomycin is blocked in protein kinase A-deficient cell lines (Ginty *et al.*, 1991)

Table 3.2. *Continued*

Cell type	Agents	Comment
	Barium ions	Ba^{2+} enters via Ca^{2+} channels, stimulating FOS expression. Effect blocked by putative protein kinase inhibitors (W7, trifluoperazine) (Curran and Morgan, 1986)
Monomyelocytes HL-60 (human)	TPA, vitamin D_3	*FOS* transcription is activated during differentiation to macrophages but is neither necessary nor sufficient for differentiation (Mitchell *et al.*, 1986). In U937s there is a progressive delay in reaching the maximum transcription rates of *FOS*, *FRA1* and *FRA2* (30, 60 and 120 min respectively; Matsui *et al.*, 1990)
U937	TPA	
Monomyelocytes (murine: WEHI-3B)	GM-CSF	*Fos* is expressed during differentiation to macrophages (Seyfert *et al.*, 1989)
Macrophages	Interferon-γ	IFN-γ inhibits the induction of *Fos* expression by lipopolysaccharide, TPA or A23187 by decreasing the mRNA half-life from ~37 min to ~27 min (Higuchi *et al.*, 1988; Radzioch and Varesio, 1991)
Erythroleukaemia cells (murine MEL)	DMSO, hypoxanthine, hexamethylenebisacetamide	There is a rapid decrease in *Fos* transcription after DMSO-induced differentiation. The constitutive expression of *Myc* blocks differentiation but does not prevent the modulation of *Fos* expression (Coppola *et al.*, 1989)
Murine myeloid leukaemic cell lines	Antisense *Fos* ODN	Constitutive expression of *Fos* stimulates differentiation and reduces the aggressiveness of the leukaemic phenotype. *Fos* antisense oligomers markedly reduce terminal differentiation (Lord *et al.*, 1993)
Transformed mast cells (P185 mastocytoma cells)	cAMP	Stimulates transcription five-fold. In t.s. mutants of P185, however, *Fos* expression not activated during differentiation (Goulding and Ralph, 1989)
S49	Adenovirus E1A + cAMP	Activates *Fos* and *Junb* transcription, suggesting interaction between E1A protein and the cAMP signalling system (Engel *et al.*, 1991)
Murine pre-adipocytes	Serum + insulin	The adipocyte P2 lipid binding protein gene (αP2) is only expressed in differentiated adipocytes. In pre-adipocytes FOS binds to the αP2 promoter repressing transcription; in differentiated cells it does not (Distel *et al.*, 1987)
Teratocarcinoma cells (murine F9)	cAMP + retinoic acid	Expressed during differentiation to parietal endoderm cells
TA1 adipogenic cell line	Tumour necrosis factor (TNF)	Induces *Fos* and *Jun* expression and the release of arachidonic acid (AA). AA induces *Fos* but not *Jun* in quiescent cells. Inhibitors of the lipoxygenase pathway block *Fos* but not *Jun* and the lipoxygenase metabolite 5-HPETE induces *Fos* but not *Jun* (Haliday *et al.*, 1991)
Macrophages	Fc- or C3b-mediated phagocytosis	*Fos* transcription activated by these physiological agents, not by latex beads (Collart *et al.*, 1989)
Thyroid follicular cell line (FRTL5)	Thyrotropin (TSH) or db-cAMP	*Fos* and *Myc* mRNA transiently increased (maximum after 30 and 60 min, respectively) (Colletta *et al.*, 1986; Tramontano *et al.*, 1986)
Rodent heart cells *in vivo*	Isoproterenol	β-Adrenergic agonists increase transcription: blocked by β-AR antagonists (e.g. propanolol) but not inhibited by Ca^{2+} channel blockers (Barka *et al.*, 1987)
Differentiated adrenal medulla cells	Insulin-induced hypoglycemia *in vivo*, angiotensin or nicotine *in vitro*	These non-mitogenic signals induce rapid synthesis of FOS, first detectable in the cytoplasm (Stachowiak *et al.*, 1990)
Vascular smooth muscle	Angiotensin II	Activates *Fos* transcription (Taubman *et al.*, 1989)
Rat uterus	Estrogen (*in vivo*)	*Fos* mRNA maximal 6 h after injection of estrogen. *Jun* and *Myc* also activated. These transcriptional activations are not sufficient to cause DNA synthesis (Papa *et al.*, 1991; Webb *et al.*, 1990)

Table 3.2. *Continued*

Cell type	Agents	Comment
Rat mesangial cells	Endothelin	Stimulates *Fos*, phospholipase C, Na$^+$/H$^+$ exchange and mitogenesis (Simonson *et al.*, 1989)
	EGF, TPA or vasopressin	Stimulate *Fos* and *Egr-1* transcription and DNA synthesis. Effects decreased by inhibitors of cytochrome P-450 monooxygenase and lipoxygenase systems (nordihydroguaiaretic acid, NDGA, S,K&F 525A or ketoconazole). Inhibition of cyclooxygenase or lipoxygenases alone has no effect (Sellmayer *et al.*, 1991)
Partial hepatectomy		Transcription of *Fos* (and the *Jun* family) transiently induced: maximal ~1 h after the operation (Morello *et al.*, 1990)
Disruption of hepatocytes	Collagenase, EDTA perfusion.	Transient *Fos*, sustained *Myc*, transcription (Etienne *et al.*, 1988)
Fetal lung fibroblasts	Ageing *in vitro*	Irreversible suppression of *Fos* induction by serum (Seshadri and Campisi, 1990). Serum still activates *Ras*, *Myc* and ODC (although the activity of the ODC enzyme is greatly reduced), suggesting that *Fos* is involved in proliferation but not terminal differentiation
Many	Cycloheximide, actinomysin	Inhibition of protein synthesis causes super-induction of *Fos* transcription
Human T cell leukaemia line (JURKAT)	p40^{tax} expression vector	HTLV-1 p40^{tax} causes transcription of *Fos* and (IL-2Rα expression) but not of *Jun*, *Myc* or *Myb* (Nagata *et al.*, 1989)

Reviews

Distel, R.J. and Spiegelman, B. (1990). Proto-oncogene c-*fos* as a transcription factor. Adv. Cancer Res., 55, 37–55.

Hunter, T. and Karin, M. (1992). The regulation of transcription by phosphorylation. Cell, 70, 375–387.

Kouzarides, T. and Ziff, E. (1989). Behind the fos and jun zipper. Cancer Cells, 1, 71–76.

Morgan, J.I. and Curran, T. (1989). Stimulus-transcription coupling in neurons: role of cellular immediate-early genes. Trends Neurosci., 12, 459–462.

Muller, R. (1986). Cellular and viral *fos* genes: structure, regulation of expression and biological properties of their encoded products. Biochim. Biophys. Acta, 823, 207–225.

Ransone, L.J. and Verma, I.M. (1990). Nuclear proto-oncogenes FOS and JUN. Annu. Rev. Cell Biol., 6, 539–557.

Treisman, R. (1992). The serum response element. Trends Biol. Sci., 17, 423–426.

Verma, I.M. (1986). Proto-oncogene *fos*: a multifaceted gene. Trends Genetics, 2, 93–96.

Papers

Abate, C., Marshak, D.R. and Curran, T. (1991). Fos is phosphorylated by p34^{cdc2}, cAMP-dependent protein kinase and protein kinase C at multiple sites clustered within regulatory regions. Oncogene, 6, 2179–2185.

Alexandre, C. and Verrier, B. (1991). Four regulatory elements in the human c-*fos* promoter mediate trans-activation by HTLV-1 Tax protein. Oncogene, 6, 543–551.

Alt, M. and Grassmann, R. (1993). Resistance of human fibroblasts to c-*fos* mediated transformation. Oncogene, 8, 1421–1427.

Attar, R.M. and Gilman, M.Z. (1992). Expression cloning of a novel zinc finger protein that binds to the c-*fos* serum response element. Mol. Cell. Biol., 12, 2432–2443.

Avantaggiati, M.L., Natoli, G., Balsano, C., Chirillo, P., Artini, M., De Marzio, E., Collepardo, D. and Levrero, M. (1993). The hepatitis B virus (HBV) pX transactivates the c-*fos* promoter through multiple *cis*-acting elements. Oncogene, 8, 1567–1574.

Barka, T., van der Noen, H. and Shaw, P.A. (1987). Proto-oncogene *fos* (c-*fos*) expression in the heart. Oncogene, 1, 439–443.

Bartel, D.P., Sheng, M., Lau, L.F. and Greenberg, M.E. (1989). Growth factors and membrane depolarization activate distinct programs of early response gene expression: dissociation of *fos* and *jun* induction. Genes Devel., 3, 304–315.

Boulden, A.M. and Sealy, L.J. (1992). Maximal serum stimulation of the c-*fos* serum response element requires both the serum response factor and a novel binding factor, SRE-binding protein. Mol. Cell. Biol., 12, 4769–4783.

Bravo, R., Burckhardt, J., Curran, T. and Muller, R. (1986). Expression of c-*fos* in NIH3T3 cells is very low but inducible throughout the cell cycle. EMBO J., 5, 695–700.

Bravo, R., Neuberg, M., Burckhardt, J., Almendral, J., Wallich, R. and Muller, R. (1987). Involvement of common and cell type-specific pathways in c-*fos* gene control: stabel induction by cAMP in macrophages. Cell, 48, 251–260.

Buscher, M., Rahmsdorf, H.J., Litfin, M., Karin, M. and Herrlich, P. (1988). Activation of the c-*fos* gene by UV and phorbol ester: different signal transduction pathways converge to the same enhancer element. Oncogene 3, 301–311.

Chen, C.-Y.A., You, Y. and Shyu, A.-B. (1992). Two cellular proteins bind specifically to a purine-rich sequence necessary for the destabilization function of a c-*fos* protein-coding region determinant of mRNA instability. Mol. Cell. Biol., 12, 5748–5757.

Cochran, B.H., Zullo, J., Verma, I.M. and Stiles, C.D. (1984). Expression of the c-*fos* gene and of an *fos*-related gene is stimulated by platelet-derived growth factor. Science, 226, 1080–1082.

Cohen, D.R. and Curran, T. (1988). *fra*-1: a serum-inducible, cellular immediate-early gene that encodes a *fos*-related antigen. Mol. Cell. Biol., 8, 2063–2069.

Collart, M.A., Belin, D., Briottet, C., Thorens, B., Vassalli, J.D. and Vassalli, P. (1989). Receptor-mediated phagocytosis by macrophages induces a calcium-dependent transient increase in c-*fos* transcription. Oncogene, 4, 237–241.

Colletta, G., Cirafici, A.M. and Vecchio, G. (1986). Induction of the c-*fos* oncogene by thyrotropic hormone in rat thyroid cells in culture. Science, 233, 458–460.

Colotta, F., Polentarutti, N., Sironi, M. and Mantovani, A. (1992). Expression and involvement of c-*fos* and c-*jun* protooncogenes in programmed cell death induced by growth factor deprivation in lymphoid cell lines. J. Biol. Chem., 267, 18278–18283.

Conscience, J.-F., Verrier, B. and Martin, G. (1986). Interleukin-3-dependent expression of the c-*myc* and c-*fos* proto-oncogenes in hemopoietic cell lines. EMBO J., 5, 317–323.

Coppola, J.A., Parker, J.M., Schuler, G.D. and Cole, M.D. (1989). Continued withdrawal from the cell cycle and regulation of cellular genes in mouse erythroleukemia cells blocked in differentiation by the c-*myc* oncogene. Mol. Cell. Biol., 9, 1714–1720.

Curran, T. and Morgan, J.I. (1986). Barium modulates c-*fos* expression and post-translational modification. Proc. Natl Acad. Sci. USA, 83, 8521–8524.

Curran, T., Gordon, M.B., Rubino, K.L. and Sambucetti, L.C. (1987). Isolation and characterization of the c-*fos*(rat) cDNA and analysis of post-translational modification *in vitro*. Oncogene 2, 79–84.

Dalton, S. and Treisman, R. (1992). Characterization of SAP-1, a protein recruited by serum response factor to the c-*fos* serum response element. Cell, 68, 597–612.

Distel, R.J., Ro, H.-S., Rosen, B.S., Groves, D.L. and Spiegelman, B.M. (1987). Nucleoprotein complexes that regulate gene expression in adipocyte differentiation direct participation of c-*fos*. Cell, 49, 835–844.

Dobrzanski, P., Noguchi, T., Kovary, K., Rizzo, C.A., Lazo, P.S. and Bravo, R. (1991). Both products of the *fos*B gene, fosB and its short form, fosB/SF, are transcriptional activators in fibroblasts. Mol. Cell. Biol., 11, 5470–5478.

Engel, D.A., Muller, U., Gedrich, R.W., Eubanks, J.S. and Shenk, T. (1991). Induction of c-fos mRNA and AP-1 DNA-binding activity by cAMP in cooperation with either the adenovirus 243- or the adenovirus 289-amino acid E1A protein. Proc. Natl Acad. Sci. USA, 88, 3957–3961.

Etienne, P.L., Baffet, G., Desvergne, B., Boisnard-Rissel, M., Glaise, D. and Guguen-Guillouzo, C. (1988). Transient expression of c-*fos* and constant expression of c-*myc* in freshly isolated and cultured normal adult rat hepatocytes. Oncogene Res., 3, 255–262.

Field, S.J., Johnson, R.S., Mortensen, R.M., Papaioannou, V.E., Spiegelman, B.M. and Greenberg, M.E. (1992). Growth and differentiation of embryonic stem cells that lack an intact c-*fos* gene. Proc. Natl Acad. Sci. USA, 89, 9306–9310.

Finkel, M.P., Biskis, B.O. and Jinkins, P B. (1966). Virus induction of osteosarcomas in mice. Science, 151, 698–701.

Fujii, M., Niki, T., Mori, T., Matsuda, T., Matsui, M., Nomura, N. and Seiki, M. (1992). HTLV-1 Tax induces expression of various immediate early serum responsive genes. Oncogene, 6, 1023–1029.

Fujii, M., Tsuchiya, H., Chuhjo, T., Akizawa, T. and Seiki, M. (1992). Interaction of HTLV-1 Tax1 with p67^{SRF} causes the aberrant induction of cellular immediate early genes through CArG boxes. Genes Devel., 6, 2066–2076.

Fujiwara, K.T., Ashida, K., Nishina, H., Iba, K., Miyajima, N., Nishizawa, M. and Kawai, S. (1987). The chicken c-*fos* gene: cloning and nucleotide sequence analysis. J. Virol., 61, 4012–4018.

Gille, H., Sharrocks, A.D. and Shaw, P.E. (1992). Phosphorylation of trancription factor p62^{TCF} by MAP kinase stimulates ternary complex formation at c-*fos* promoter. Nature, 358, 414–417.

Ginty, D.D., Glowacka, D., Bader, D.S., Hidaka, H. and Wagner, J.A. (1991). Induction of immediate early genes by Ca^{2+} influx requires cAMP-dependent protein kinase in PC12 cells. J. Biol. Chem., 266, 17454–17458.

Gonda, T.J. and Metcalf, D. (1984). Expression of *myb*, *myc* and *fos* proto-oncogenes during the differentiation of a murine myeloid leukemia. Nature, 310, 249–251.

Goulding, M.D. and Ralph, R.K. (1989). Cyclic-AMP-induced c-*fos* expression and its relevance to differentiation of a transformed cell line. Biochim. Biophys. Acta, 1007, 99–108.

Greenberg, M.E. and Ziff, E.B. (1984). Stimulation of 3T3 cells induces transcription of the c-*fos* proto-oncogene. Nature, 311, 433–438.

Greenberg, M.E., Hermanowski, A.L. and Ziff, E.B. (1986). Effect of protein synthesis inhibitors on growth factor activation of c-*fos*, c-*myc*, and actin gene transcription. Mol. Cell. Biol., 6, 1050–1057.

Grueneberg, D., Natesan, S., Alexandre, C. and Gilman, M.Z. (1992). Human and *Drosophila* homeodomain proteins that enhance the DNA-binding activity of serum response factor. Science, 257, 1089–1095.

Gubits, R.M. and Fairhurst, J.L. (1988). c-*fos* mRNA levels are increased by the cellular stressors, heat shock and sodium arsenite. Oncogene, 3, 163–168.

Haliday, E.M., Ramesha, C.S. and Ringold, G. (1991). TNF induces c-*fos* via a novel pathway requiring conversion of arachidonic acid to a lipoxygenase metabolite. EMBO J., 10, 109–115.

Hayes, T.E., Kitchen, A. M. and Cochran, B.H. (1987). Inducible binding of a factor to the c-*fos* regulatory region. Proc. Natl Acad. Sci. USA, 84, 1272–1276.

Hipskind, R.A., Rao, V.N., Mueller, C.G., Reddy, E.S. and Nordheim, A. (1991). Ets-related protein Elk-1 is homologous to the c-*fos* regulatory factor p62^{TCF}. (1991). Nature, 354, 531–534.

Higuchi, Y., Setoguchi, M., Yoshida, S., Akizuki, S. and Yamamoto, S. (1988). Enhancement of c-*fos* expression is associated with activated macrophages. Oncogene, 2, 515–521.

Holt, J.T., Gopal, V., Moulton, A.D. and Nienhuis, A.W. (1986). Inducible production of c-*fos* antisense RNA inhibits 3T3 cell proliferation. Proc. Natl Acad. Sci. USA, 83, 4794–4798.

Ito, E., Sonnenberg, J.L. and Narayanan, R. (1989). Nerve growth factor-induced differentiation in PC-12 cells is blocked by *fos* oncogene. Oncogene, 4, 1193–1199.

Jenuwein, T. and Muller, R. (1987). Structure-function analysis of *fos* protein: a single amino acid change activates the immortalising potential of v-*fos*. Cell, 48, 647–657.

Johnson, R.S., Spiegelman, B.M. and Papaioannou, V. (1992). Pleiotropic effects of a null mutation in the c-*fos* proto-oncogene. Cell, 71, 577–586.

Jones, D., Lee, L., Liu, J.-L., Kung, H.-J. and Tillotson, J.K. (1992). Marek disease virus encodes a basic-leucine zipper gene resembling the *fos/jun* oncogenes that is highly expressed in lymphoblastoid tumors. Proc. Natl Acad. Sci. USA, 89, 4042–4046.

Kamata, N. and Holt, J.T. (1992). Inhibitory effect of myristylation on transrepression by FBR (gag-fos) protein. Mol. Cell. Biol., 12, 876–882.

Kamata, N., Jotte, R.M. and Holt, J.T. (1991). Myristylation alters DNA-binding activity and transactivation of FBR (*gag-fos*) protein. Mol. Cell. Biol., 11, 765–772.

Kasik, J.W., Wan, Y.J. and Ozato, K. (1987). A burst of c-*fos* gene expression in the mouse occurs at birth. Mol. Cell. Biol., 7, 3349–3352.

Kerppola, T.K. and Curran, T. (1991). DNA bending by fos and jun: the flexible hinge model. Science, 254, 1210–1213.

Kerppola, T.K., Luk, D. and Curran, T. (1993). Fos is a preferential target of glucocorticoid receptor inhibition of AP-1 activity in vitro. Mol. Cell. Biol., 13, 3782–3791.

Kho, C.-J. and Zarbl, H. (1992). *Fte-1*, a v-*fos* transformation effector gene, encodes the mammalian homologue of a yeast gene involved in protein import into mitochondria. Proc. Natl Acad. Sci. USA, 89, 2200–2204.

Kovary, K. and Bravo, R. (1991). The *jun* and *fos* protein families are both required for cell cycle progression in fibroblasts. Mol. Cell. Biol., 11, 4466–4472.

Kovary, K. and Bravo, R. (1992). Existence of different fos/jun complexes during the G_0-to-G_1 transition and during exponential growth in mouse fibroblasts: differential role of fos protiens. Mol. Cell. Biol., 12, 5015–5023.

Kreipe, H., Radzun, H.J., Heidorn, K., Parwaresch, M., Verrier, B. and Muller, R. (1986). Lineage-specific expression of c-*fos* and c-*fms* in human hematopoietic cells: discrepancies with the *in vitro* differentiation of leukemia cells. Differentiation, 33, 56–60.

Lamb, N.J.C., Fernandez, A.F., Tourkine, N., Jeanteur, P. and Blanchard, J.-M. (1990). Demonstration in living cells of an intragenic negative regulatory element within the rodent c-*fos* gene. Cell, 61, 485–496.

Lazo, P.S., Dorfman, K., Noguchi, T., Mattei, M.-G. and Bravo, R. (1992). Structure and mapping of the *fos*B gene. FosB downregulates the activity of the *fos*B promoter. Nucleic Acids Res., 20, 343–350.

Lee, M.-S., Yang, J.-H., Salehi, Z., Arnstein, P., Chen, L.-S., Jay, G. and Rhim, J.S. (1993). Neoplastic transformation of a human keratinocyte cell line by the v-*fos* oncogene. Oncogene, 8, 387–393.

Liboi, E., Pelosi, E., Testa, U., Peschle, C. and Rossi, G.P. (1986). Proliferative response and oncogene expression induced by epidermal growth factor in EL2 rat fibroblasts. Mol. Cell. Biol., 6, 2275–2278.

Lord, K.A., Abdollahi, A., Hoffman-Liebermann, B. and Liebermann, D.A. (1993). Proto-oncogenes of the *fos/jun* family of transcription factors are positive regulators of myeloid differentiation. Mol. Cell. Biol., 13, 841–851.

McBride, K., Robitaille, L., Tremblay, S., Argentin, S. and Nemer, M. (1993). *fos/jun* repression of cardiac-specific transcription in quiescent and growth-stimulated myocytes is targeted at a tissue-specific *cis* element. Mol. Cell. Biol., 13, 600–612.

McNerney, R., Darling, D. and Johnstone, A. (1987). Differential control of proto-oncogene c-*myc* and c-*fos* expression in lymphocytes and fibroblasts. Biochem. J., 245, 605–608.

Manak, J.R. and Prywes, R. (1993). Phosphorylation of serum response factor by casein kinase II: evidence against a role in growth factor regulation of *fos* expression. Oncogene, 8, 703–711.

Mason, I., Murphy, D. and Hogan, B.L.M. (1985). Expression of c-*fos* in parietal endoderm, amnion and differentiating F9 teratocarcinoma cells. Differentiation, 30, 76–81.

Matsui, M., Tokuhara, M., Konuma, Y., Nomura, N. and Ishizaki, R. (1990). Isolation of human *fos*-related genes and their expression during monocyte-macrophage differentiation. Oncogene 5, 249–255.

Mehmet, H,. Sinnett-Smith, J., Moore, J.P., Evan, G.I. and Rozengurt, E. (1988). Differential induction of c-*fos* and c-*myc* by cyclic AMP in Swiss 3T3 cells: significance for the mitogenic response. Oncogene Res , 3, 281–286.

Meijlink, F., Curran, T., Miller, A.D. and Verma I.M. (1985). Removal of a 67-base-pair sequence in the noncoding region of protooncogene fos converts it to a transforming gene. Proc. Natl Acad. Sci. USA, 82, 4987–4991.

Metz, R. and Ziff, E. (1991). The helix-loop-helix protein rE12 and the C/EBP-related factor rNFIL-6 bind to neighboring sites within the c-*fos* serum response element. Oncogene, 6, 2165–2178.

Mitchell, R.L., Zokas, L., Schreiber, R.D. and Verma, I.M. (1985). Rapid induction of the expression of proto-oncogene fos during human monocytic differentiation. Cell, 40, 209–217.

Mitchell, R.L., Henning-Chubb, C., Huberman, E and Verma, I.M. (1986). C-*fos* expression is neither sufficient nor obligatory for differentiation of monomyelocytes to macrophages. Cell, 45, 497–504.

Molders, H., Jenuwein, T., Adamkiewicz, J. and Muller, R. (1987). Isolation and structural analysis of a biologically active chicken c-fos cDNA: identification of evolutionarily conserved domains in *fos* protein. Oncogene 1, 377–385.

Moore, J.P., Todd, J.A., Hesketh, T.R. and Metcalfe, J.C. (1986). c-*fos* and c-*myc* gene activation, ionic signals, and DNA synthesis in thymocytes. J. Biol. Chem., 261, 8158–8162.

Moore, J.P., Menzel, G.E., Hesketh, T.R. and Metcalfe, J.C. (1988).C-*fos* gene activation in murine thymocytes by a mechanism independent of protein kinase C or a Ca^{2+} signal. FEBS Letts., 233, 64–68.

Morello, D., Lavenu, A. and Babinet, C. (1990). Differential regulation and expression of *jun*, c-*fos* and c-*myc* proto-oncogenes during mouse liver regeneration and after inhibition of protein synthesis. Oncogene, 5, 1511–1519.

Muller, R., Verma, I.M. and Adamson, E.D. (1983). Expression of c-*onc* genes: c-*fos* transcripts accumulate to high levels during development of mouse placenta, yolk sac and amnion. EMBO J., 2, 679–684.

Muller, R., Bravo, R., Burckhardt, J. and Curran, T. (1984a). Induction of c-*fos* gene and protein by growth factors precedes activation of c-*myc*. Nature, 312, 716–720.

Muller, R., Muller, D. and Guilbert, L. (1984b). Differential expression of c-*fos* in hematopoietic cells: correlation with differentiation of monomyelocytic cells *in vitro*. EMBO J., 3, 1887–1890.

Muller, R., Curran, T., Muller, D. and Guilbert, L. (1985). Induction of c-*fos* during myelomonocytic differentiation and macrophage proliferation. Nature, 314, 546–548.

Muller, R., Bravo, R., Muller, D., Kurz, C. and Renz, M. (1987). Different types of modification in c-*fos* and its associated protein p39: modulation of DNA binding by phosphorylation. Oncogene Res, 2, 19–32.

Murakami, Y., Satake, M., Yamaguchi-Iwai, Y., Sakai, M., Muramatsu, M. and Ito, Y. (1991). The nuclear protooncogenes c-*jun* and c-*fos* as regulators of DNA replication. Proc. Natl Acad. Sci. USA, 88, 3947–3951.

Nagata, K., Ohtani, K., Nakamura, M. and Sugamura, K. (1989). Activation of endogenous c-*fos* proto-oncogene expression by human T-cell leukemia virus type I-encoded p40^{tax} protein in the human T-cell line, Jurkat. J. Virol., 63, 3220–3226.

Nakabeppu, Y. and Nathans, D. (1991). A naturally occurring truncated form of FosB that inhibits fos/jun transcriptional activity. Cell, 64, 751–759.

Naranjo, J.R., Mellstrom, B., Achaval, M., Lucas, J.J., Del-Rio, J. and Sassone-Corsi, P. (1991). Co-induction of *jun* B and c-*fos* in a subset of neurons in the spinal cord. Oncogene 6, 223–227.

Nicklin, M.J.H. and Casari, G. (1991). A single site mutation in a truncated *fos* protein allows it to interact with the TRE *in vitro*. Oncogene, 6, 173–179.

Nishikura, K. and Murray, J.M. (1987). Antisense RNA of proto-oncogene c-*fos* blocks renewed growth of quiescent 3T3 cells. Mol. Cell. Biol., 7, 639–649.

Nishina, H., Sato, H., Suzuki, T., Sato, M. and Iba, H. (1990). Isolation and characterization of *fra-2*, an additional member of the *fos* gene family. Proc. Natl Acad. Sci. USA, 87, 3619–3623.

Nishizawa, M., Goto, N. and Kawai, S. (1987). An avian transforming retrovirus isolated from a nephroblastoma that carries the *fos* gene as the oncogene. J. Virol., 61, 3733–3740.

Ofir, R., Dwarki, V.J., Rashid, D. and Verma, I.M. (1990). Phosphorylation of the C terminus of fos protein is required for transcriptional transrepression of the c-*fos* promoter. Nature, 348, 80–82.

Okuno, H., Akaahori, A., Sato, H., Xanthoudakis, S., Curran, T. and Iba, H. (1993). Escape from redox regulation enhances the transforming activity of fos. Oncogene, 8, 695–701.

Panterne, B., Hatzfeld, J., Blanchard, J.-M., Levesque, J.-P., Berthier, R., Ginsbourg, M. and Hatzfeld, A. (1992). c-*fos* mRNA constitutive expression by mature human megakaryocytes. Oncogene, 7, 2341–2344.

Papa, M., Mezzogiorno, V., Bresciani, F. and Weisz, A. (1991). Estrogen induces c-fos expression specifically in the luminal and glandular epithelia of adult rat uterus. Biochem. Biophys. Res. Commun., 175, 480–485.

Perkins, K.K., Admon, A., Patel, N. and Tjian, R. (1990). The *Drosophila fos*-related AP-1 protein is a developmentally regulated transcription factor. Genes Devel., 4, 822–834.

Radzioch, D. and Varesio, L. (1991). c-*fos* mRNA expression in macrophages is downregulated by interferon-γ at the posttranscriptional level. Mol. Cell. Biol., 11, 2718–2722.

Raymond, V., Atwater, J.A. and Verma, I.M. (1989). Removal of an mRNA destabilizing element correlates with the increased oncogenicity of proto-oncogene *fos*. Oncogene Res., 5, 1–12.

Renz, M., Neuberg, M., Kurz, C., Bravo, R. and Mueller, R. (1985). Regulation of c-fos transcription in mouse fibroblasts: identification of DNase I-hypersensitive sites and regulatory upstream sequences. EMBO J., 4, 3711–3716.

Riabowol, K.T., Vosatka, R.J. Ziff, E.B., Lamb, N.J. and Feramisco, J.R. (1988). Microinjection of *fos*-specific antibodies blocks DNA synthesis in fibroblast cells. Mol. Cell. Biol., 8, 1670–1676.

Robbins, P.D., Horowitz, J.M. and Mulligan, R.C. (1990). Negative regulation of human c-*fos* expression by the retinoblastoma gene product. Nature, 346, 668–671.

Ruther, U., Komitowski, D., Schubert, F.R. and Wagner, E.F. (1989). c-*fos* expression induces bone tumors in transgenic mice. Oncogene, 4, 861–865.

Ryan, W.A., Franza, B.R. and Gilman, M.Z. (1989). Two distinct cellular phosphoproteins bind to the c-*fos* serum response element. EMBO J., 8, 1785–1792.

Sariban, E., Mitchell, T. and Kufe, D. (1985). Expression of the c-*fms* proto-oncogene during human monocytic differentiation. Nature, 316, 64–66.

Schonthal, A., Tsukitani, Y. and Feramisco, J.R. (1991a). Transcription and post-transcriptional regulation of c-*fos* expression by the tumor promoter okadaic acid. Oncogene, 6, 423–430.

Schonthal, A., Sugarman, J., Brown, J.H., Hanley, M.R. and Feramisco, J.R. (1991b). Regulation of c-*fos* and c-*jun* protooncogene expression by the Ca^{2+}-ATPase inhibitor thapsigargin. Proc. Natl Acad. Sci. USA, 88, 7096–7100.

Schulam, P.G., Kuruvilla, A., Putcha, G., Mangus, L., Franklin-Johnson, J. and Shearer, W.T. (1991). Platelet-activating factor induces phospholipid turnover, calcium flux, arachidonic acid liberation, eicosanoid generation and oncogene expression in a human B cell line. J. Immunol., 146, 1642–1648.

Schuermann, M., Jooss, K. and Muller, R. (1991). *fos*B is a transforming gene encoding a transcription factor. Oncogene, 6, 567–576.

Selinfreund, R.H., Barger, S.W., Pledger, W.J. and Van-Eldik, L.J. (1991). Neurotrophic protein S100β stimulates glial cell proliferation. Proc. Natl. Acad. Sci. USA, 88, 3554–3558.

Sellmayer, A., Uedelhoven, W.M., Weber, P.C. and Bonventre, J.V. (1991). Endogenous non-cyclooxygenase metabolites of arachidonic acid modulate growth and mRNA levels of immediate-early response genes in rat mesangial cells. J. Biol. Chem., 266, 3800–3807.

Seshadri, T. and Campisi, J. (1990). Repression of c-*fos* transcription and an altered genetic progression in senescent human fibroblasts. Science, 247, 205–209.

Seyfert, V.L., Sukhatme, V.P. and Monroe, J.G. (1989). Differential expression of a zinc finger-encoding gene in response to positive versus negative signaling through receptor immunoglobulin in murine B lymphocytes. Mol. Cell. Biol., 9, 2083–2088.

Sharrocks, A.D., Gille, H. and Shaw, P.E. (1993). Identification of amino acids essential for DNA binding and dimerization in p67^{SRF}: implications for a novel DNA-binding motif. Mol. Cell. Biol., 13, 123–132.

Shaw, P.E. (1992). Ternary complex formation over the c-*fos* serum response element: p62^{TCF} exhibits dual component specificity with contacts to DNA and an extended structure in the DNA-binding domain of p67^{SRF}. EMBO J., 11, 3011–3019.

Shaw, P.E., Schroter, H. and Nordheim, A. (1989). The ability of a ternary complex to form over the serum response element correlates with serum inducibility of the human c-*fos* promoter. Cell, 56, 563–572.

Siegfried, Z. and Ziff, E.B. (1989). Transcription activation by serum, PDGF, and TPA through the c-*fos* DSE: cell type specific requirements for induction. Oncogene 4, 3–11.

Simonson, M.S., Wann, S., Mene, P., Dubyak, G.R., Nakazato, Y., Sedor, J.R. and Dunn, M.J. (1989). Endothelin stimulates phospholipase C, Na$^+$/H$^+$ exchange, c-*fos* expression and mitogenesis in rat mesangial cells. J. Clin. Invest., 83, 708–712.

Sonnenberg, J.L., Rauscher, F.J., Morgan, J.I. and Curran, T. (1989). Regulation of proenkephalin by fos and jun. Science, 246, 1622–1625.

Stachowiak, M,K, Sar, M., Tuominen, R.K, Jiang, H.K., An, S., Iadarola, M.J., Poisner, A.M., Hong, J.S. (1990). Stimulation of adrenal medullary cells *in vivo* and *in vitro* induces expression of c-*fos* proto-oncogene. Oncogene, 5, 69–73.

Sutherland, J.A., Cook, A., Bannister, A.J. and Kouzarides, T. (1992). Conserved motifs in fos and jun define a new class of activation domain. Genes Devel., 6, 1810–1819.

Tannenbaum, C.S., Koerner, T.J., Jansen, M.M. and Hamilton, T.A. (1988). Characterization of lipopolysaccharide-induced macrophage gene expression. J. Immunol., 140, 3640–3645.

Taubman, M.B., Berk, B.C., Izumo, S., Tsuda, T., Alexander, R.W. and Nadal-Ginard, B. (1989). Angiotensin II induces c-*fos* mRNA in aortic smooth muscle. J. Biol. Chem., 264, 526–530.

Taylor, L.K., Marshak, D.R. and Landreth, G.E. (1993). Identification of a nerve growth factor- and epidermal growth factor-regulated protein kinase that phosphorylates the protooncogene product c-fos. Proc. Natl Acad. Sci. USA, 90, 368–372.

Touray, M., Ryan, F., Jaggi, R. and Martin, F. (1991). Characterisation of functional inhibition of the glucocorticoid receptor by fos/jun. Oncogene, 6, 1227–1234.

Tramontano, D., Chin, W.W., Moses, A.C. and Ingbar, S.H. (1986). Thyrotropin and dibutyryl cyclic AMP increase levels of c-*myc* and c-*fos* mRNAs in cultured rat thyroid cells. J. Biol Chem., 261, 3919–3922.

Tratner, I. and Verma, I.M. (1991). Identification of a nuclear targeting sequence in the fos protein. Oncogene, 6, 2049–2053.

Treisman, R. (1985). Transient accumulation of c-fos RNA following serum stimulation requires a conserved 5' element and c-fos 3' sequences. Cell 42, 889–902.

Treisman, R., Marais, R. and Wynne, J. (1992). Spatial flexibility in ternary complexes between SRF and its accessory proteins. EMBO J., 11, 4631–4640.

Trouche, D., Grigoriev, M., Lenormand, J.L., Robin, P., Leibovitch, S.A., Sassone-Corsi, P. and Harel-Bellan, A. (1993). Repression of c-*fos* promoter by MyoD on muscle cell differentiation. Nature, 363, 79–82.

Tsai, L.-H., Nanu, L., Smith, R.G. and Ozanne, B. (1991). Overexpression of c-*fos* in a human pre-B cell acute lymphocytic leukemia derived cell line. Oncogene, 6, 81–88.

Van Beveren, C., van Straaten, F., Curran, T., Mu′ller, R. and Verma, I.M. (1983). Analysis of FBJ-MuSV provirus and c-*fos* (mouse) gene reveals that viral and cellular fos gene products have different carboxy termini. Cell 32, 1241–1255.

Van Beveren, C., Enami, S., Curran, T. and Verma, I.M. (1984). FBR murine osteosarcoma virus: II. Nucleotide sequence of the provirus reveals that the genome contains sequences acquired from cellular genes. Virology 135, 229–243.

van Straaten, F., Mueller, R., Curran, T., Van Beveren, C. and Verma, I.M. (1983). Complete nucleotide sequence of a human c-onc gene: Deduced amino acid sequence of the human c-*fos* protein. Proc. Natl Acad. Sci. USA, 80, 3183–3187.

Verma, I.M. and Sassone-Corsi, P. (1987). Proto-oncogene fos: complex but versatile regulation. Cell, 51, 513–514.

Verma, I.M., Deschamps, J., Van Beveren, C. and Sassone-Corsi, P. (1986). Human fos gene. Cold Spring Harb. Symp. Quant. Biol. 51, 949–958.

Vriz, S., Lemaitre, J.-M., Leibovici, M., Thierry, N. and Mechali, M. (1992). Comparative analysis of the intracellular localization of c-myc, c-fos, and replicative proteins during the cell cycle. Mol. Cell. Biol., 12, 3548–3555.

Wagner, B.J., Hayes, T.E., Hoban, C.J. and Cochran, B.H. (1990). The SIF binding element confers *sis*/PDGF inducibility onto the c-*fos* promoter. EMBO J., 9, 4477–4484.

Walsh, K. (1989). Cross-binding of factors to functionally different promoter elements in c-*fos* and skeletal actin genes. Mol. Cell. Biol., 9, 2191–2201.

Webb, D.K., Moulton, B.C. and Khan, S.A. (1990). Estrogen induced expression of the C-*jun* proto-oncogene in the immature and mature rat uterus. Biochem. Biophys. Res. Commun., 168, 721–726.

Wick, M., Lucibello, F.C. and Muller, R. (1992). Inhibition of fos- and ras-induced transformation by mutant fos proteins with structural alterations in functionally different domains. Oncogene, 7, 859–867.

Wisdom, R. and Verma, I.M. (1993). Proto-oncogene FosB: the amino terminus encodes a regulatory function required for transformation. Mol. Cell. Biol., 13, 2635–2643.

Wu, J.X., Carpenter, P.M., Gresens, C., Keh, R., Niman, H., Morris, J.W. and Mercola, D. (1990). The proto-oncogene c-*fos* is over-expressed in the majority of human osteosarcomas. Oncogene, 5, 989–1000.

Xanthoudakis, S., Miao, G., Wang, F., Pan. Y.-C.E. and Curran, T. (1992). Redox activation of fos-jun DNA binding activity is mediated by a DNA repair enzyme. EMBO J., 11, 3323–3335.

Yen, J., Wisdom, R.M., Tratner, I. and Verma, I.M. (1991). An alternative spliced form of *Fos*B is a negative regulator of transcriptional activation and transformation by *Fos* proteins. Proc. Natl Acad. Sci. USA, 88, 5077–5081.

Yoshida, T., Shindo, Y., Ohta, K., and Iba, H. (1989). Identification of a small region of the v-*fos* gene product that is sufficient for transforming potential and growth-stimulating activity. Oncogene Res., 5, 79–89.

Yoshida, T., Suzuki, T., Sato, H., Nishina, H. and Iba, H. (1993). Analysis of *fra*-2 gene expression. Nucleic Acids Res., 21, 2715–2721.

Zerial, M., Toschi, L., Ryseck, R.-P., Schuermann, M., Muller, R. and Bravo, R. (1989). The product of a novel growth factor activated gene, *fos* B, interacts with JUN proteins enhancing their DNA binding activity. EMBO J., 8, 805–813.

FPS/FES

v-*fps* (Fujinami-PRCII sarcoma) is the transforming gene of Fujinami sarcoma virus (FSV; Fujinami and Inamoto, 1914), an acutely transforming avian sarcoma virus that is defective in all three virion genes (Hanafusa *et al.*, 1980; Lee *et al.*, 1980). Four other retroviruses also carry v-*fps*: PRCII and PRCIV (Poultry Research Centre II and IV), UR1 (University of Rochester) and 16L). *fes* (feline sarcoma virus) is the cognate gene of *fps* present in three retroviruses (Snyder–Theilen (ST)-FeSV, Gardner–Arnstein (GA)-FeSV and Hardy–Zuckerman 1 (HZ1)-FeSV).

Members of the *FPS/FES* family encode non-receptor tyrosine kinases. Avian *Fps* and mammalian *Fes* are cognate cellular genes (MacDonald *et al.*, 1985). *FER* (human) is homologous to chicken *Fps* but has no known oncogene homologue.

Related genes

FER, human *FES/FPS*-related tyrosine kinase gene, is closely related in sequence and domain structure to *Fps/Fes* (Hao *et al.*, 1989; Morris *et al.*, 1990; Krolewski *et al.*, 1990). p94^{fer} has also been denoted as normal cellular protein (NCP) 92 or NCP94 (Feldman *et al.*, 1985; MacDonald *et al.*, 1985). *Flk* (fps/fes-like kinase) is the rat homologue of human *FER* (Letwin *et al.*, 1988; Pawson *et al.*, 1989). Other *Fps/Fes*-related genes are chicken p98^{fps}, also denoted as NCP98, murine *Fer*^{T} tyrosine kinase (Fischman *et al.*, 1990), and *Drosophila* d*fps*85D (chromosome position 85D10–13; Simon *et al.*, 1983; Katzen *et al.*, 1991).

The *Fps/Fes* family is homologous in the C-terminal region to *Src* and contains an SH2 domain located N-terminally with respect to the tyrosine kinase region. FER shares homology with TRK (49% identity between amino acids 715 and 752 in the FER tyrosine kinase domain (Morris *et al.*, 1991). The vesicular stomatitis virus L polymerase protein includes 377 amino acids that are 27% identical to the kinase domain of FPS/FES (McClure and Perrault, 1989). Sequences homologous to v-*fps* are present in the sea urchin genome (Mifflin and Robinson, 1988).

Cross-species homology

FPS/FES: 70% identity (human and chicken); 94% (human and feline); 70% (feline and chicken) (Roebroek *et al.*, 1987).

Transformation

MAN

FES/FPS expression is enhanced in some lung cancers and haematopoietic malignancies (Slamon *et al.*, 1984; Jucker *et al.*, 1992). *FER* is highly expressed in cell lines derived from human kidney carcinomas and glioblastomas (Hao *et al.*, 1989) and is frequently deleted from chromosome 5 in acute myeloid leukaemia and myelodysplastic syndromes (Morris *et al.*, 1990).

ANIMALS

FSV induces fibrosarcomas or myxosarcomas (Hanafusa *et al.*, 1980). PRCII is less oncogenic than FSV due to differences in the v-*fps* proteins encoded (see **Structures of gag–fps/fes-encoded** fusion proteins, page 204). Pre-neoplastic Chinese hamster lung fibroblasts transfected with v-*fps* cause rapidly growing tumours in nude mice that form pulmonary metastases (Sadowski *et al.*, 1988).

IN VITRO

Fps/Fes overexpression transforms NIH 3T3 fibroblasts and the effect is greatly potentiated by the presence of the tyrosine phosphatase inhibitor sodium vanadate (Feldman *et al.*, 1990). However, overexpression of human *FPS/FES* does not transform rat-2 fibroblasts (Greer *et al.*, 1988). Viruses carrying v-*fps* transform fibroblasts although the efficiency of PRCII is less than that of FSV (Hammond *et al.*, 1985). FSV transforms erythroid cells and FeSV transforms pre-B cells (Pierce and Aaronson, 1983; Kahn *et al.*, 1984). Rat-2 fibroblasts transfected with v-*fps* are tumorigenic and have metastatic potential (Dennis *et al.*, 1989). FSV transforms osteoblasts (Cogliano *et al.*, 1987; Birek *et al.*, 1988) and is a potent transforming agent for quail myogenic cells (Falcone *et al.*, 1985).

TRANSGENIC ANIMALS

Transgenic mice expressing v-*fps* have severe cardiac or neurological disorders and develop a variety of lymphoid or mesenchymal tumours (Pawson *et al.*, 1989; Chow *et al.*, 1991). Lymphoid tumours are monoclonal and appear between 2 and 12 months, indicating a requirement for other genetic changes in addition to the expression of v-*fps*.

	Fps/Fes	*v-fps/fes*
Nucleotides (kb)	13	5.3 (FSV genome)
		4.7 (ST-FeSV genome)
		6.5 (GA-FsSV genome)
Chromosome		
Human	15q25–q26 (*FES*)	
	5q21 (*FER*)	
Mouse	7 (*Fes*)	
Exons	19	
mRNA (kb)		
Human	~3.0 (*FES*)	4.462 (FSV)
Human	3.0/8.0 (*FER*)	2.283 (PRCII)
	(0.9kb in some lymphoid/lymphoma cell lines)	
Chicken	2.75–3.2	2.373 (ST-FeSV)
Rat	1.3/2.4/2.9 (*Flk*)	2.922 (Ga-FeSV)
Amino acids		
Human	822 (FES)	1182 (FSV)
	822 (FER)	887 (PRCII)
Cat	820	774 (ST-FeSV)
Chicken	875	957 (GA-FeSV)
Rat	323 (FLK)	

	Fps/Fes	*v-fps/fes*
Mass (kDa) (predicted)		
Human, chicken, mouse	94	
Cat	93	
(expressed)		
Human	p92*fes*	P130*gag-fps*, P140*gag-fps* (FSV) (P140 precipitated by anti-*gag* serum; P130 a mutated form from cloned FSV (DNA)
Human	p94*fer*	
Chicken	p98*fps*	P105*gag-fps* (PRCII)
Human	p17*fps/fes* (truncated protein transcribed from 0.9 kb mRNA (Jucker *et al.*, 1992))	P170*gag-fps* (PRCIV) P150*gag-fps* (UR1) P142*gag-fps* (16L) P85*gag-fps* (ST-FeSV) P110*gag-fps* (GA-FeSV) P100*gag-fps* (HZ1-FeSV)

Cellular location

FPS/FES: 60–90% cytosolic (Young and Martin, 1984).

P105*gag-fps*: Membrane associated but not attached to the plasma membrane.

P130*gag-fps*: Weakly associated with the plasma membrane (Moss *et al.*, 1984).

P140*gag-fps*: 60–80% membrane associated (Beemon and Mattingly, 1986).

ST-FeSV and GA-FeSV encoded proteins may bind to the plasma membrane.

FER occurs in the cytoplasm and in the nucleus associated with chromatin (Hao *et al.*, 1991).

Tissue location

FPS/FES is expressed in immature and differentiated haematopoietic cells of the myeloid lineage and in leukaemic myeloid cells (Feldman *et al.*, 1985; MacDonald *et al.*, 1985; Samarut *et al.*, 1985). It is not expressed in erythroid cells, with the exception of a human erythroleukaemia cell line that is able to differentiate into macrophage-like cells. In transgenic mice expression is particularly high in bone marrow macrophages (Greer *et al.*, 1990). Rat *Fps/Fes* is expressed in neonatal cardiac muscle but not in the adult tissue (Claycomb and Lanson, 1987).

FER is ubiquitously expressed and has been isolated in highly active form from HeLa cells (Feller and Wong, 1992). Multiple sizes of transcript have been detected (>9.5, 6.5, 4.6, 3.0 and 1.8 kb), presumably arising from alternative splicing (Krolewski *et al.*, 1990).

Rat *Flk* 2.9 kb mRNA is ubiquitous: in testes two different forms (1.3 and 2.4 kb) are expressed.

Protein function

FPS/FES genes encode cytoplasmic tyrosine kinases that phosphorylate exogenous substrates and are autophosphorylated. The tissue distribution of FPS/FES suggests that its normal role may be in the control of proliferation and differentiation of haematopoietic cells (Carmier and Samarut, 1986) and the introduction of human *FES* into cells can confer the capacity to undergo myeloid differentiation (Yu *et al.*, 1989).

In the human erythroleukaemia cell line TF-1 GM-CSF or IL-3 induce the tyrosine phosphorylation and kinase activity of p92^{FES} and GM-CSF causes FES to associate with the β chain of the GM-CSF receptor (Hanazono *et al.*, 1993).

The truncated protein (p17) expressed in some human leukaemic cell lines (Jucker *et al.*, 1992) lacks the ATP binding site and kinase activity but may function as a dominant suppressor of FPS/FES or other kinases.

In common with other viral tyrosine protein kinases, the expression of v-*fps* causes the phosphorylation of a number of cellular substrates and transformation by temperature-sensitive mutants of FSV is critically dependent on the expression of protein kinase activity by the v-*fps* gene product (Hanafusa *et al.*, 1981; Chen *et al.*, 1986). Nine proteins (36, 53, 58, 59, 60, 65, 80, 92 and 250 kDa) have been detected that are substrates for v-FPS and are also phosphorylated in response to v-*src*, v-*abl* or v-*fgr* (Kamps and Sefton, 1988a,b). v-FPS also causes tyrosine phosphorylation of the GAP-associated proteins p62 and p190, the extent of which correlates with transforming activity (Moran *et al.*, 1990) and v-*fps* expression causes phosphorylation on tyrosine residues of fibronectin receptor proteins (Hirst *et al.*, 1986).

In NIH 3T3 fibroblasts v-*fps* induces the expression of *Egr-1* via activation of repeated CArG box promoter sequences (CC(A/T)$_6$GG) that form the core of the serum response element (Alexandropoulos *et al.*, 1992). In rat fibroblasts v-*fps* induces expression of the *Ras*-related immediate early gene *RhoB* (Jahner and Hunter, 1991). *RhoB* is also activated by the PDGF and EGF receptor tyrosine kinases. The transformation-related 9E3 gene is also activated by v-*fps* via a G protein-regulated pathway that may involve protein kinase C (Spangler *et al.*, 1989; Barker and Hanafusa, 1990; Alexandropoulos *et al.*, 1991).

Cells transformed by *fps/fes* or by *src* have a similar phenotype. FPS/FES associates with p50 and p90, as does p60^{src} (Ziemiecki, 1986) but does not phosphorylate vinculin (Sefton *et al.*, 1981). Microinjection of anti-RAS antibody causes reversion of *fps/fes*-transformed cells (Smith *et al.*, 1986) and revertant cells derived from *Kras*-transformed cells are resistant to *fps/fes* transformation. The concentrations of PI(3)P, PI(3,4)P$_2$ and PI(3,4,5)P$_3$ are increased in v-*fps*-transformed fibroblasts (Fukui *et al.*, 1991; see **SRC**).

Transformation by v-*fps* enhances the uptake of cellular nutrients by rat-2 fibroblasts (Meckling-Gill and Cass, 1992) and in chick embryo fibroblasts increases the concentration of fructose 2,6-bisphosphate, a major regulator of glycolysis (Bosca *et al.*, 1986), as well as expression of the glucose transporter (Hiraki *et al.*, 1989).

Structures of cellular and viral *Fps/Fes* genes

Lines delineate regions containing homologous *Fps/Fes* exon sequences (Huang *et al.*, 1985).

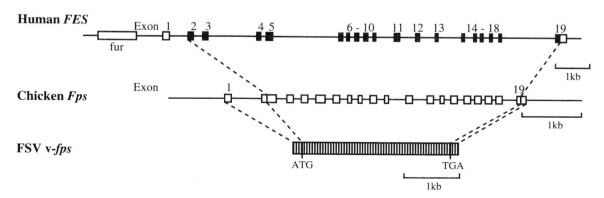

The truncated transcript detected in some human haematopoietic tumour cells initiates within exon 16 using a cryptic promoter (Jucker *et al.*, 1992). In the avian viruses the 5' junction of the *fps* sequence is in the middle of *gag* and the 3' junction lies in a non-coding sequence between *env* and the LTR U3 region. The *gag–fes* 5' junction is also in the middle of *gag* but the 3' *fes* junction is in the 3' end of *pol*.

A 9 kb upstream region (*FUR – fps/fes upstream region*) generates 4.5 kb transcripts in man and cats and encodes a 1498 bp putative ORF (499 amino acids) of unknown function (Roebroek *et al.*, 1986a, b).

Structures of *gag–fps/fes*-encoded fusion proteins (Hanafusa, 1988)

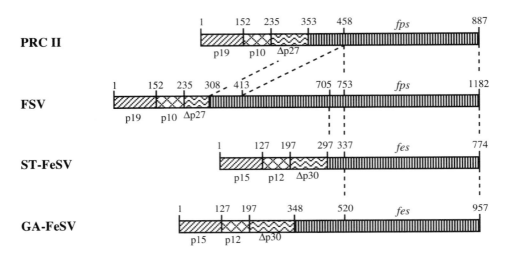

(Adapted from Hanafusa, H. (1988). In Curran, T., Reddy, E.P. and Skalka, A. (eds) The Oncogene Handbook: 42. Elsevier, Amsterdam.

Vertically lined boxes: *Fps/Fes*-derived sequences. Dashed lines delineate regions of homology.

P140$^{gag\text{-}fps}$ (FSV) contains 308 N-terminal amino acids of ALV p76^{gag} and 874 acquired from *Fps*. The C-terminal 429 residues in FSV and PRCII and 437 residues in ST-FeSV and GA-FeSV are identical (Carlberg *et al.*, 1984; Huang *et al.*, 1984). The 5' recombination sites are within p27^{gag} or p30^{gag} but differ for each virus. The 5' termini of *fps/fes* sequences are the same in PRCII and FSV but different in the other viruses: there are large internal deletions in *fps/fes* in PRCII (amino acids 413–753 of P140$^{gag\text{-}fps}$) and GA-FeSV and ST-FeSV (529–707 of P140$^{gag\text{-}fps}$).

The degree of homology of transduced sequences with FPS/FES is variable: in FSV 26 out of 874 amino acids are mutated: in PRCII there is complete identity between 533 amino acids.

The 280 C-terminal residues of FSV FPS are 40% homologous to pp60^{src}.

Antibodies against the kinase domain of p130$^{v\text{-}fps}$ also precipitate chicken p98^{fps} and human p94^{fer} proteins (Feldman *et al.*, 1985; MacDonald *et al.*, 1985).

An artificial, replication-competent virus (F36) expresses an active v-*fps* kinase (91 kDa) without *gag* and has *in vitro* and *in vivo* transforming activity: thus *gag* is not necessary for transformation by FSV. In the viral construct Fc51 substitution of v-*src* by *fps* produces a 98 kDa non-transforming kinase of low activity: addition of 5' *gag* sequences activates kinase, transforming and tumorigenic properties (Feldman *et al.*, 1987). Thus N-terminal *gag* substitution is sufficient to activate the oncogenic potential of *Fps/Fes* although the F36 data indicate that the scattered mutations occurring in v-*fps* can do likewise. However, v-*fps* is linked to N-terminal *gag* sequences in all spontaneously arising, *fps/fes*-containing transforming viruses (Foster *et al.*, 1985).

Sequences of human, mouse and chicken FES/FPS and v-FPS (GA-FeSV and FSV)

```
Chicken FPS      (1)                                                ASGQLHRPQPQEHTSTSAAAGTWRHTQASESRHRLPHCSAAP

Human FES        (1)         MGFSSELCSPQGHGVLQQMQEAELRLLEGMRKWMAQRVKSDREYAGLLHHMSLQDSGGQ    SRAISPDS
Mouse FPS        (1)         -------------AV-------------------------------------------    -WSSG---
(GA-FeSV)        (1)     AARADGT-------------AE----------------------------------------G--RGTG       -Y-
Ch FPS          (43)     SHQDHSA---GP--WC-K--SE-LRL-DS------L-K---S--A--------M----FS-LEKQEGLGHL--TDHS-
v-FPS (FSV)    (352)     *******************T*******************************************************

Human FES       (68)     PISQSWAEITSQTEGLSRLLRQHAEDLNSGPLSKLSLLIRERQQLRKTYSEQWQQLQQELTKTHSQDIEKLKSQYRAL
Mouse FPS       (68)     -V-----------N---V-------------------HS-----N-----------------------T---T-
(GA-FeSV)       (73)     --------------------------------G------------------------N------------
Ch FPS         (121)     Q-GE--WVLA----T--QT--R---E-AA--A---I--DK-----AF-------S--YAR-TQ-EM----A---S-
v-FPS (FSV)    (430)     ******************************************V*********W****V*************

Human FES      (146)     ARDSAQAKRKYQEASKDKDRDKAKDKYVRSLWKLFAHHNRYVLGVRAAQLHHQHHHQLLLPGLLRSLQDLHEEMACIL
Mouse FPS      (146)     V---T--R------------------------------------------H---RFM----Q-----------
(GA-FeSV)      (151)     -------R---------------  (174)
Ch FPS         (199)     V---T------------E-E---E---------Y-L--Q---A----A---H--Y-RA--T-HE--YS-QQ--VLV-
v-FPS (FSV)    (508)     **************************************S**********Q*********************

Human FES      (224)     KEILQEYLEISSLVQDEVVAIHREMAAAAARIQPEAEYQGFLRQYGSAPDVPPCVTFDESLLEEGEPLEPGELQLNEL
Mouse FPS      (224)     -D-------------D-AS----L----------F--L--------T-------------D--Q-----------
(GA-FeSV)        ()
Ch FPS(277)              ----G--CS------ED-L---Q-V-H-VEM-D-AT--SS-VQCHRYDSE---A----------T-S----------
v-FPS (FSV)    (586)     *********T***********K*************************************A-N**********

Human FES      (302)     TVESVQHTLTSVTDELAVATEMVFRRQEMVTQLQQELRNEEENTHPRERVQLLGKRQVLQEALQGLQVALCSQAKLQA
Mouse FPS      (302)     -L----------------KE-LS-----S---R--QS--Q-----------S---M----I----I-----D----
(GA-FeSV)        ()
Ch FPS         (355)     -I-----S---IEE--LASR-A-SSKEQR-WE--V---G--LALS-G---H------G----Q-Q--GLV-A------
v-FPS (FSV)    (664)     ******************K***************************R******************

Human FES      (380)     QQELLQTKLEHLGPGEPPPVLLLQDDRHSTSSSEQEREGGRTPTLEILKSHISGIFRPKFSLPPPLQLIPEVQKPLHE
Mouse FPS      (380)     ------S-M-Q--T----A-P-----------T-R-  ------------F----------------V-----Y-
(GA-FeSV)      (175)             --Q-----------------------------------------------V---------
Ch FPS         (433)     -RDM-AN--AE--SE----A-P--E--Q-VC-TD---S-V - A--TI-N------S-R------VP---------CQ
v-FPS (FSV)    (742)     *****************************AR******  GVT**K***********************

Human FES      (458)     QLWYHGAIPRAEVAELLVHSGDFLVRESQGKQEYVLSVLWDGLPRHFIIQSLDNLYRLEGEGFPSIPLLIDHLLSTQQ
Mouse FPS      (456)     ---------W--------T-T-----------------M--H----------------D---------T----S--
(GA-FeSV)      (245)     -------L---------T---------------------Q-------A-----P--D-A-----V----RS--
Ch FPS         (511)     -A--------S--Q---KC------------------------Q-------AA-------D---T--------QS--
v-FPS (FSV)    (818)     ****************Y****************************************D**L*************R
                                          #  #   #                          #

Human FES      (536)     PLTKKSGVVLHRAVPKDKWVLNHEDLVLGEQIGRGNFGEVFSGRLRADNTLVAVKSCRETLPPDLKAKFLQEARILKQ
Mouse FPS      (534)     ----------F---------K------------------------------------P-----------------
(GA-FeSV)      (323)     -------I-N--------------------------------------------I-------K----
Ch FPS         (589)     --I-R---I--T---L--------VL---R----------------P----------E------------
v-FPS (FSV)    (896)     ****************************************************************************

Human FES      (614)     YSHPNIVRLIGVCTQKQPIYIVMELVQGGDFLTFLRTEGARLRVKTLLQMVGDAAAGMEYLESKCCIHRDLAARNCLV
Mouse FPS      (612)     -N-----------------------------------------M-------------------------
(GA-FeSV)      (401)     -----------------------------------M---------------
Ch FPS         (667)     -N--------------------S---S--PH-KM-E-IK-MEN---------H-----------
v-FPS (FSV)    (974)     C*************************K*******K****************************************
```

```
Human FES   (692)  TEKNVLKISDFGMSREEADGVYAASGGLRQVPVKWTAPEALNYGRYSSESDVWSFGILLWETFSLGASPYPNLSNQQT
Mouse FPS   (690)  ------------------I---CS---------------------------------------------T----
(GA-FeSV)   (479)  ---------------A---I---------------------------------------------------------
Ch FPS      (745)  ----T---------Q-E----ST--MK-I-----------------------------A-----V--A-------
v-FPS (FSV)(1052)  *****************************************************W********************P*******
```

```
Human FES   (770)  REFVEKGGRLPCPELCPDAVFRLMEQCWAYEPGQRPSFSTIYQELQSIRKRHR  (822)
Mouse FPS   (768)  -------H-------------------------------IIC---H-------  (820)
(GA-FeSV)   (557)  -----------------------------------------A-----------  (609)
Ch FPS      (823)  --AI-Q-V--EP--Q--ED-Y---QR--E-D-RR----GAVH-D-IA------  (875)
v-FPS (FSV)(1130)  *****************************************H***************** (1182)
```

Dashes indicate amino acids indentical to human FES. * Indicates identity in FSV v-FPS with chicken FPS.

# Indicates ATP binding regions (human: 567–575 and 590, equivalent to p60^{SRC} Lys295; mouse 565–573 and 588; v-FPS 618–626 and 641). The autophosphorylation sites that are equivalent to SRC Tyr416 (human Tyr713; mouse Tyr711; v-FPS 764 (equivalent to Tyr1073 in P140$^{gag-fps}$)) are in underlined bold type.

FER is 51% homologous with human FES/FPS. FER Tyr714 is equivalent to SRC Tyr416. The FES/FPS residues equivalent to SRC Lys295 and Tyr416 are essential for kinase and transforming activity (Weinmaster *et al.*, 1984; Foster *et al.*, 1985).

v-FPS variants: 63 T –> S (clone TS); 251 H –> R (clone TS); 300 K –> E (clone TS); 343 N –> S (clone TS); 463 R –> C (clone TS); 716 E –> D (clone TS).

FLK (rat) is a distinct, N-terminally truncated form of FPS/FES. The sequence starts in the middle of the SH2 domain and is 65% identical to the human p92^{FES} and chicken p98$^{fps.}$

Protein structure

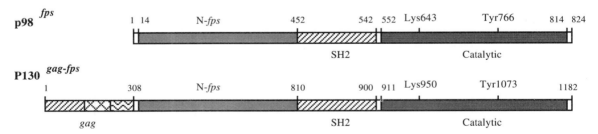

Cytoplasmic tyrosine kinases contain two adjacent regions of homology, the SH2 and kinase domains, flanked by structurally distinct N- and C-terminal regions. In p98^{fps} and the derived oncogene P130$^{gag-fps}$ the N-terminal domain adjacent to SH2 is comprised of ~250 amino acids (N*fps*).

FPS and *gag–fps*-encoded proteins contain an N-terminal potential myristylation site (Gly2), in common with members of the *Src* family, but, with the exception of the ST-FeSV and GA-FeSV proteins, do not appear to be myristylated (Beemon and Mattingly, 1986). This is consistent with the observation that, of this group, only P85$^{gag-fps}$ (ST-FeSV) and P110$^{gag-fps}$ (GA-FeSV) bind specifically to the plasma membrane.

The N*fps* region may determine the subcellular localization of FPS proteins. There is a deletion in N*fps* in P105$^{gag-fps}$ (PRCII) that may be responsible for the difference in distribution and oncogenicity between this protein and P130$^{gag-fps}$(FSV). Insertions or deletions in N*fps* do not affect kinase activity but greatly diminish transforming capacity (Ariizumi and Shibuya, 1985; Stone and Pawson, 1985). When the entire *gag*–N*fps* region of P130$^{gag-fps}$ is replaced by the N-terminal 14 amino acids of p60^{v-src} that are necessary and sufficient for myristylation and membrane association (see **SRC**), a potent transforming protein is generated (Brooks-Wilson *et* *al.*, 1989). However, the *gag–Nfps* domain confers weak transforming activity on non-myristylated v-SRC, indicating the importance of this region in mediating protein interactions essential for transformation.

The SH2 domain functions intramolecularly to stimulate the tyrosine kinase activity of v-*fps* and deletion of a conserved octapeptide from SH2 converts it to an inhibitory domain (Koch *et al.*, 1989). Mutation of the SH2 region by insertion of a dipeptide renders the transforming function of P130$^{gag\text{-}fps}$ both host- and temperature-dependent (DeClue *et al.*, 1987). The mutant protein no longer transforms rat-2 cells but still transforms chicken cells at the permissive temperature. v-*fps*-mediated tyrosine phosphorylation of the GAP-associated proteins p62 and p190 is also dependent on interaction via the SH2 domain (Moran *et al.*, 1990).

The two major phosphotyrosine residues and the major phosphoserine are in the C-terminal region of P130$^{gag\text{-}fps}$ (Weinmaster *et al.*, 1983). Tyr1073 is the major site of intermolecular *trans*-phosphorylation *in vitro*. Mutation of Tyr1073 decreases enzymatic activity and greatly slows the onset of NIH 3T3 cell transformation (Weinmaster and Pawson, 1986; Meckling-Hansen et al., 1987). The tyrosine kinase activities of the different v-*fps/fes* proteins are similar both *in vivo* and *in vitro* and are therefore largely unaffected by the deletions in PRCII, ST-FeSV and GA-FeSV with respect to FSV. Lys950 of FSV P130$^{gag\text{-}fps}$ is homologous to Lys295 in the ATP binding site of p60$^{v\text{-}src}$: mutation of Lys950 inhibits tyrosine kinase activity and renders the protein non-transforming (Weinmaster *et al.*, 1986). The second major site of tyrosine phosphorylation in P130$^{gag\text{-}fps}$ is Tyr836. When the kinase activity of P130$^{gag\text{-}fps}$ is activated by phosphorylation of Tyr1073, phosphorylation of Tyr836 is increased. However, substitution of Tyr836 by Phe does not inhibit either kinase activity or transforming capacity (Weinmaster *et al.*, 1988).

Databank file names and accession numbers

	GENE	*EMBL*	*SWISSPROT*	*REFERENCES*
Human	*FES/FPS*	Hsfesfps X06292	KFES_HUMAN P07332	Roebroek *et al.*, 1985
Human	*FER*	J03358		Hao *et al.*, 1989
Mouse	*Fes*	Mmfescr X12616	KFES_MOUSE P16879	Wilks and Kurban, 1988
Mouse	*Fer*^{T}	Mmfert M32054		Fischman *et al.*, 1990
Feline	*Fps/Fes*	Fcfes01–Fcfes19	KFES_FELCA P14238	Roebroek *et al.*, 1987
		M16665–M16674 and M16698–M16706		
Chicken	*Fps*	Ggcfpse1–Ggcfpse9		Huang *et al.*, 1985
		Ggcfps10–Ggcfps19		
Drosophila melanogaster	*Fps*	Dmfps8d X52844	KFPS_DROME P18106	Katzen *et al.*, 1991
SM-FeSV		M23025 M23025		
FSV	v-*fps*	Refsv J02194	KFPS_FUJSV P00530	Shibuya and Hanafusa, 1982
		Reacfts1 M14930		Chen *et al.*, 1986

	GENE	EMBL	SWISSPROT	REFERENCES
FSV	*fps*	Ncffps1; Ncffps2		
ASV-PRCII	v-*fps*	Regagfps K01690	KFES_AVISP P00541	Huang *et al.*, 1984
ST-FSV	v-*fps*	Restonc J02088	KFES_FSVST P00543	Hampe *et al.*, 1982
Feline	v-*fgr*	Fesvtp1 X14842		Kappes *et al.*, 1989
(TP1-FeSV)				
Rat	*Flk*	Rnflk X13412	KFLK_RAT P09760	Letwin *et al.*, 1988
GA-FSV	v-*fes*	Regaonc J02087	KFES_FSVGA P00542	Hampe *et al.*, 1982

Review

Hanafusa, H. (1988). The *fps/fes* oncogene. In Curran, T., Reddy, E.P. and Skalka, A. (eds) The Oncogene Handbook: 39–57. Elsevier, Amsterdam.

Papers

Alexandropoulos, K., Joseph, C.K., Spangler, R. and Foster, D.A. (1991). Evidence that a G-protein transduces signals initiated by the protein-tyrosine kinase v-*fps*. J. Biol. Chem., 266, 15583–15586.

Alexandropoulos, K., Qureshi, S.A., Rim, M., Sukhatme, V.P. and Foster, D.A. (1992). v-fps-responsiveness in the egr-1 promoter is mediated by serum response elements. Nucleic Acids Res., 20, 2355–2359.

Ariizumi, K. and Shibuya, M. (1985). Construction and biological analysis of deletion mutants of Fujinami sarcoma virus: 5'-*fps* sequence has a role in the transforming activity. J. Virol., 55, 660–669.

Barker, K. and Hanafusa, H. (1990). Expression of 9E3 mRNA is associated with mitogenicity, phosphorylation, and morphological alteration in chicken embryo fibroblasts. Mol. Cell. Biol., 10, 3813–3817.

Beemon, K. and Mattingly, B. (1986). Avian sarcoma virus *gag-fps* and *gag-yes* transforming proteins are not myristylated or palmitylated. Virology, 155, 716–720.

Birek, C., Pawson, T., McCulloch, C.A. and Tenenbaum, H.C. (1988). Neoplastic transformation of osteogenic cells: quantitative morphometric analysis of an *in vitro* model for osteosarcoma. Carcinogenesis, 9, 1785–1791.

Bosca, L., Mojena, M., Ghysdael, J., Rousseau, G.G. and Hue, L. (1986). Expression of the v-*src* or v-*fps* oncogene increases fructose 2,6-bisphosphate in chick-embryo fibroblasts. Novel mechanism for the stimulation of glycolysis by retroviruses. Biochem. J., 236, 595–599.

Brooks-Wilson, A.R., Ball, E. and Pawson, T. (1989). The myristylation signal of p60[v-src] functionally complements the N-terminal *fps*-specific region of P130[gag-fps]. Mol. Cell. Biol., 9, 2214–2219.

Carlberg, K., Chamberlin, M.E. and Beemon, K. (1984). The avian sarcoma virus PRCII lacks 1020 nucleotides of the *fps* transforming gene. Virology, 135, 157–167.

Carmier, J.F. and Samarut, J. (1986). Chicken myeloid stem cells infected by retroviruses carrying the v-*fps* oncogene do not require exogenous growth factors to differentiate *in vitro*. Cell, 44, 159–165.

Chen, L.H., Hatada, E., Wheatley, W. and Lee, W.H. (1986). Single amino acid substitution, from Glu1025 to Asp, of the *fps* oncogenic protein causes temperature sensitivity in transformation and kinase activity. Virology 155, 106–119.

Chow, L.H., Yee, S.P., Pawson, T. and McManus, B.M. (1991). Progressive cardiac fibrosis and myocyte injury in v-*fps* transgenic mice. A model for primary disorders of connective tissue in the heart? Lab. Invest., 64, 457–462.

Claycomb, W.C. and Lanson, N.A. (1987). Proto-oncogene expression in proliferating and differentiating cardiac and skeletal muscle. Biochem. J., 247, 701–706.

Cogliano, A., Mock, D., Birek, C., Pawson, A. and Tenenbaum, H.C. (1987). *In vitro* transformation of osteoblasts: putative formation of osteosarcoma *in vitro*. Bone, 8, 299–304.

DeClue, J.E., Sadowski, I., Martin, G.S. and Pawson, T. (1987). A conserved domain regulates interactions of the v-*fps* protein-tyrosine kinase with the host cell. Proc. Natl Acad. Sci. USA, 84, 9064–9068.

Dennis, J.W., Kosh, K., Bryce, D.M. and Breitman, M.L. (1989). Oncogenes conferring metastatic potential induce increased branching of Asn-linked oligosaccharides in rat2 fibroblasts. Oncogene, 4, 853–860.

Falcone, G., Tato, F. and Alema, S. (1985). Distinctive effects of the viral oncogenes *myc, erb, fps,* and *src* on the differentiation program of quail myogenic cells. Proc. Natl Acad. Sci. USA, 82, 426–430.

Feldman, R.A., Gabrilove, J.L., Tam, J.P., Moore, M.A.S. and Hanafusa, H. (1985). Specific expression of the human cellular *fps/fes*-encoded protein NCP92 in normal and leukemic myeloid cells. Proc. Natl Acad. Sci. USA, 82, 2379–2383.

Feldman, R.A., Vass, W.C. and Tambourin, P.E. (1987). Human cellular *fps/fes* cDNA rescued *via* retroviral shuttle vector encodes myeloid cell NCP92 and has transforming potential. Oncogene Res., 1, 441–458.

Feldman, R.A., Lowy, D.R. and Vass, W.C. (1990). Selective potentiation of c-*fps/fes* transforming activity by a phosphatase inhibitor. Oncogene Res., 5, 187–197.

Feller, S.M. and Wong, T.W. (1992). Identification and characterization of a cytosolic protein tyrosine kinase of HeLa cells. Biochemistry, 31, 3044–3051.

Fischman, K., Edman, J.C., Shackleford, G.M., Turner, J.A., Rutter, W.J. and Nir, U. (1990). A murine *fer* testis-specific transcript (*fer*[T]) encodes a truncated fer protein. Mol. Cell. Biol., 10, 146–153.

Foster, D.A., Shibuya, M. and Hanafusa, H. (1985). Activation of the transformation potential of the cellular *fps* gene. Cell, 42, 105–115.

Fujinami, A. and Inamoto, K. (1914). Uber Geschwulste bei japanischen Haushuhnern insbesondere uber einen transplantablen Tumor. Z. Krebsforschung, 14, 94–119.

Fukui, Y., Saltiel, A.R. and Hanafusa, H. (1991). Phosphatidylinositol-3 kinase is activated in v-*src*, v-*yes* and v-*fps* transformed chicken embryo fibroblasts. Oncogene, 6, 407–411.

Greer, P.A., Meckling-Hansen, K. and Pawson, T. (1988). The human c-*fps/fes* gene product expressed ectopically in rat fibroblasts is nontransforming and has restrained protein-tyrosine kinase activity. Mol. Cell. Biol., 8, 578–587.

Greer, P., Maltby, V., Rossant, J., Bernstein, A. and Pawson, T. (1990). Myeloid expression of the human c-*fps/fes* proto-oncogene in transgenic mice. Mol. Cell. Biol., 10, 2521–2527.

Guilhot, S., Hampe, A., D'Auriol, L. and Galibert, F. (1987). Nucleotide sequence analysis of the LTRs and *env* genes of SM-FeSV and GA-FeSV. Virology, 161, 252–258.

Hammond, C.I., Vogt, P.K. and Bishop, J.M. (1985). Molecular cloning of the PRCII sarcoma viral genome and the chicken proto-oncogene c-*fps*. Virology, 143, 300–308.

Hampe, A., Laprevotte, I., Galibert, F., Fedele, L.A. and Sherr, C.J. (1982). Nucleotide sequence of feline retroviral oncogenes (v-*fes*) provide evidence for a family of tyrosine-specific protein kinase genes. Cell, 30, 775–785.

Hanafusa, T., Wang, L.-H., Anderson, S.M., Karess, R.E., Hayward, W.S. and Hanafusa, H. (1980). Characterization of the transforming gene of Fujinami sarcoma virus. Proc. Natl Acad. Sci. USA, 77, 3009–3013.

Hanafusa, T., Mathey-Prevot, B., Feldman, R.A. and Hanafusa, H. (1981). Mutants of Fujinami sarcoma virus which are temperature sensitive for cellular transformation and protein kinase activity. J. Virol., 38, 347–355.

Hanazono, Y., Chiba, S., Sasaki, K., Mano, H., Miyajima, A., Arai, K.-I., Yazaki, Y. and Hirai, H. (1993). c-*fps/fes* protein-tyrosine kinase is implicated in a signaling pathway triggered by granulocyte-macrophage colony-stimulating factor and interleukin-3. EMBO J., 12, 1641–1646.

Hao, Q.L., Heisterkamp, N. and Groffen, J. (1989). Isolation and sequence analysis of a novel human tyrosine kinase gene. Mol. Cell. Biol., 9, 1587–1593.

Hao, Q.L., Ferris, D.K., White, G., Heisterkamp, N. and Groffen, J. (1991). Nuclear and cytoplasmic location of the FER tyrosine kinase. Mol. Cell. Biol., 11, 1180–1183.

Hiraki, Y., Garcia de Herreros, A. and Birnbaum, M.J. (1989). Transformation stimulates glucose transporter gene expression in the absence of protein kinase C. Proc. Natl Acad. Sci. USA, 86, 8252–8256.

Hirst, R., Horwitz, A., Buck, C. and Rohrschneider, L. (1986). Phosphorylation of the fibronectin receptor complex in cells transformed by oncogenes that encode tyrosine kinases. Proc. Natl Acad. Sci. USA, 83, 6470–6474.

Huang, C.-C., Hammond, C. and Bishop, M.J. (1984). Nucleotide sequence of v-*fps* in the PRCII strain of avian sarcoma virus. J. Virol., 50, 125–131.

Huang, C.-C., Hammond, C. and Bishop, M.J. (1985). Nucleotide sequence and topography of chicken c-*fps*: genesis of a retroviral oncogene encoding a tyrosine-specific protein kinase. J. Mol. Biol., 181, 175–186.

Jahner, D. and Hunter, T. (1991). The *ras*-related gene *rho*B is an immediate-early gene inducible by v-*fps*, epidermal growth factor, and platelet-derived growth factor in rat fibroblasts. Mol. Cell. Biol., 11, 3682–3690.

Jucker, M., Roebroek, A.J.M., Mautner, J., Koch, K., Eick, D., Diehl, V., Van de Ven, W.J.M. and Tesch,

H. (1992). Expression of truncated transcripts of the proto-oncogene c-*fps*/*fes* in human lymphoma and lymphoid leukemia cell lines. Oncogene, 7, 943–952.

Kahn, P., Adkins, B., Beug, H. and Graf, T. (1984). *src*- and *fps*-containing avian sarcoma viruses transform chicken erythroid cells. Proc. Natl Acad. Sci. USA, 81, 7122–7126.

Kamps, M.P. and Sefton, B.M. (1988a). Most of the substrates of oncogenic viral tyrosine protein kinases can be phosphorylated by cellular tyrosine protein kinases in normal cells. Oncogene Res., 3, 105–115.

Kamps, M.P. and Sefton, B.M. (1988b). Identification of multiple novel polypeptide substrates of the v-*src*, v-*yes*, v-*fps*, v-*ros*, and v-*erb*-B oncogenic tyrosine protein kinases utilizing antisera against phosphotyrosine. Oncogene, 2, 305–315.

Kappes, B., Ziemiecki, A., Mueller, R.G., Theilen, G.H., Bauer, H. and Barnekow, A. (1989). The TPI isolate of feline sarcoma virus encodes a *fgr*-related oncogene lacking γ-actin sequences. Oncogene 4, 363–372.

Katzen, A.L., Montarras, D., Jackson, J., Paulson, R.F., Kornberg, T. and Bishop, J.M. (1991). A gene related to the proto-oncogene *fps*/*fes* is expressed at diverse times during the life cycle of *Drosophila melanogaster*. Mol. Cell. Biol., 11, 226–239.

Koch, C.A., Moran, M., Sadowski, I. and Pawson, T. (1989). The common *src* homology region 2 domain of cytoplasmic signaling proteins is a positive effector of v-*fps* tyrosine kinase function. Mol. Cell. Biol., 9, 4131–4140.

Krolewski, J.J., Lee, R., Eddy, R., Shows, T.B. and Dalla-Favera, R. (1990). Identification and chromosomal mapping of new human tyrosine kinase genes. Oncogene, 5, 277–282.

Lee, W.-H., Bister, K., Pawson, A., Robins, T., Moscovici, C. and Duesberg, P.H. (1980). Fujinami sarcoma virus: an avian RNA tumor virus with a unique transforming gene. Proc. Natl Acad. Sci. USA, 77, 2018–2022.

Letwin, K., Yee, S.-P. and Pawson, T. (1988). Novel protein-tyrosine kinase cDNAs related to *fps*/*fes* and *eph* cloned using anti-phosphotyrosine antibody. Oncogene, 3, 621–627.

MacDonald, I., Levy, J. and Pawson, T. (1985). Expression of the mammalian c-*fes* protein in hematopoietic cells and identification of a distinct *fes*-related protein. Mol. Cell. Biol., 5, 2543–2551.

McClure, M.A. and Perrault, J. (1989). Two domains distantly related to protein-tyrosine kinases in the vesicular stomatitis virus polymerase. Virology, 172, 391–397.

Meckling-Gill, K.A. and Cass, C.E. (1992). Effects of transformation by v-*fps* on nucleoside transport in Rat-2 fibroblasts. Biochem. J., 282, 147–154.

Meckling-Hansen, K., Nelson, R., Branton, P. and Pawson, T. (1987). Enzymatic activation of Fujinami sarcoma virus *gag-fps* transforming proteins by autophosphorylation at tyrosine. EMBO J., 6, 659–666.

Mifflin, D. and Robinson, J.J. (1988). Proto-oncogene homologous sequences in the sea urchin genome. Biosci. Rep., 8, 415–419.

Moran, M.F., Koch, C.A., Anderson, D., Ellis, C., England, L., Martin, G.S. and Pawson, T. (1990). Src homology domains direct protein-protein interactions in signal transduction. Proc. Natl Acad. Sci. USA, 87, 8622–8626.

Morris, C., Heisterkamp, N., Hao, Q.L., Testa, J.R. and Groffen, J. (1990). The human tyrosine kinase gene (FER) maps to chromosome 5 and is deleted in myeloid leukemias with a del(5q). Cytogenet. Cell Genet., 53, 196–200.

Morris, C.M., Hao, Q.L., Heisterkamp, N., Fitzgerald, P.H. and Groffen, J. (1991). Localization of the TRK proto-oncogene to human chromosome bands 1q23–1q24. Oncogene, 6, 1093–1095.

Moss, P., Radke, K., Carter, V.C., Young, J., Gilmore, T. and Martin, G.S. (1984). Cellular localization of the transforming protein of wild-type and temperature-sensitive Fujinami sarcoma avirus. J. Virol., 52, 557–565.

Pawson, T., Letwin, K., Lee, T., Hao, Q.L., Heisterkamp, N. and Groffen, J. (1989). The FER gene is evolutionarily conserved and encodes a widely expressed member of the FPS/FES protein-tyrosine kinase family. Mol. Cell. Biol., 9, 5722–5725.

Pierce, J.H. and Aaronson, S.A. (1983). *In vitro* transformation of murine pre-B lymphoid cells by Snyder-Theilen feline sarcoma virus. J. Virol., 46, 993–1002.

Roebroek, A.J.M., Schalken, J.A., Verbeek, J.S., Van den Ouweland, A.M.W., Onnekink, C., Bloemers, H.P.J. and Van de Ven, W.J.M. (1985). The structure of the human c-*fes*/*fps* proto-oncogene. EMBO J., 4, 2897–2903.

Roebroek, A.J.M., Schalken, J.A., Bussemakers, M.J.G., van Heerikhuizen, H.P.J., Onnekink, C., Debruyne, F.M.J., Bloomers, H.P.J. and Van de Ven, W.J.M. (1986a). Characterization of human fes/fps reveals a new transcription unit (fur) in the immediate upstream region of the proto-oncogene. Mol. Biol. Rep., 11, 117–125.

Roebroek, A.J., Schalken, J.A., Leunissen, J.A., Onnekink, C., Bloemers, H.P. and Van de Ven, W.J. (1986b). Evolutionary conserved close linkage of the c-*fes*/*fps* proto-oncogene and genetic sequences encoding a receptor-like protein. EMBO J., 5, 2197–2202.

Roebroek, A.J.M., Schalken, J.A., Onnekink, C., Bloemers, H.P.J. and de Ven, W.J.M. (1987). Structure of the feline c-*fes/fps* proto-oncogene: Genesis of a retroviral oncogene. J. Virol. 61, 2009–2016.

Sadowski, I., Pawson, T. and Lagarde, A. (1988). v-*fps* protein-tyrosine kinase coordinately enhances the malignancy and growth factor responsiveness of pre-neoplastic lung fibroblasts. Oncogene, 2, 241–247.

Samarut, J., Mathey-Prevot, B. and Hanafusa, H. (1985). Preferential expression of the c-*fps* protein in chicken macrophages and granulocytic cells. Mol. Cell. Biol., 5, 1067–1072.

Sefton, B.M., Hunter, T., Ball, E.H. and Singer, S.J. (1981). Vinculin: a cytoskeletal target of the transforming protein of Rous sarcoma virus. Cell, 24, 165–174.

Shibuya, M. and Hanafusa, H. (1982). Nucleotide sequence of Fujinami sarcoma virus: evolutionary relationship of its transforming gene with transforming genes of other sarcoma viruses. Cell, 30, 787–795.

Simon, M.A., Kornberg, T.B. and Bishop, M.J. (1983). Three loci related to the *src* oncogene and tyrosine-specific protein kinase activity in *Drosophila*. Nature, 302, 837–839.

Slamon, D.J., deKernion, J.B., Verma, I.M. and Cline, M.J. (1984). Expression of cellular oncogenes in human malignancies. Science, 224, 256–262.

Smith, M.R., DeGudicibus, S.J. and Stacey, D.W. (1986). Requirement for c-*ras* proteins during viral oncogene transformation. Nature, 320, 540–543.

Spangler, R., Joseph, C., Qureshi, S.A., Berg, K.L. and Foster, D.A. (1989). Evidence that v-*src* and v-*fps* gene products use a protein kinase C-mediated pathway to induce expression of a transformation-related gene. Proc. Natl Acad. Sci. USA, 86, 7017–7021.

Stone, J.C. and Pawson, T. (1985). Correspondence between immunological and functional domains in the transforming protein of Fujinami sarcoma virus. J. Virol., 55, 721–727.

Weinmaster, G. and Pawson, T. (1986). Protein kinase activity of FSV (Fujinami sarcoma virus) P130$^{gag\text{-}fps}$ shows a strict specificity for tyrosine residues. J. Biol. Chem., 261, 328–333.

Weinmaster, G., Hinze, E. and Pawson, T. (1983). Mapping of multiple phosphorylation sites within the structural and catalytic domains of the Fujinami avian sarcoma virus transforming protein. J. Virol., 46, 29–41.

Weinmaster, G., Zoller, M.J., Smith, M., Hinze, E. and Pawson, T. (1984). Mutagenesis of Fujinami sarcoma virus: evidence that tyrosine phosphorylation of p130$^{gag\text{-}fps}$ modulates its biological activity. Cell, 37, 559–568.

Weinmaster, G., Zoller, M.J. and Pawson, T. (1986). A lysine in the ATP-binding site of P130$^{gag\text{-}fps}$ is essential for protein-tyrosine kinase activity. EMBO J., 5, 69–76.

Weinmaster, G.A., Middlemas, D.S. and Hunter, T. (1988). A major site of tyrosine phosphorylation within the SH2 domain of Fujinami sarcoma virus P130$^{gag\text{-}fps}$ is not required for protein-tyrosine kinase activity or transforming potential. J. Virol., 62, 2016–2025.

Wilks, A.F. and Kurban, R.R. (1988). Isolation and structural analysis of murine c-*fes* cDNA clones. Oncogene 3, 289–294.

Yee, S.P., Mock, D., Greer, P., Maltby, V., Rossant, J., Bernstein, A. and Pawson, T. (1989). Lymphoid and mesenchymal tumors in transgenic mice expressing the v-*fps* protein-tyrosine kinase. Mol. Cell. Biol., 9, 5491–5499.

Young, J.C. and Martin, G.S. (1984). Cellular localization of c-*fps* gene product NCP98. J. Virol., 52, 913–918.

Yu, G., Smithgall, T.E. and Glazer, R.I. (1989). K562 leukemia cells transfected with the human c-*fes* gene acquire the ability to undergo myeloid differentiation. J. Biol. Chem., 264, 10276–10281.

Ziemiecki, A. (1986). Characterization of the monomeric and complex-associated forms of the *gag-onc* fusion proteins of three isolates of feline sarcoma virus: phosphorylation, kinase activity, acylation and kinetics of complex formation. Virology, 151, 265–273.

FYN

FYN (formerly *SYN* (*src/yes*-related *novel gene*) or *SLK* (*src-like kinase*)) was originally cloned from an SV40-transformed human fibroblast library (Kawakami *et al.*, 1986; Semba *et al.*,1986). There is no naturally occurring *fyn*-containing retrovirus known.

Related genes

Fyn is a member of the *Src* tyrosine kinase family (*Blk*, *Fgr*, *Fyn*, *Hck*, *Lck/Tkl*, *Lyn*, *Src*, *Yes*) of which *Src*, *Yes* and *Fgr* have viral homologues. The encoded tyrosine kinases are between 505 and 543 amino acids in length, lack a transmembrane domain and are attached to the inner surface of the plasma membrane by a myristic acid molecule linked to their N-terminus. Each contains a highly conserved C-terminal kinase domain (~300 amino acids) joined to an extremely variable N-terminal region of ~70 amino acids.

FYN contains SH2 and SH3 domains and between amino acids 83 and 537 is 80% homologous to YES and 77% to SRC and FGR. The C-terminal 191 amino acids are 86% homologous to p60^{src}: the N-terminal 82 residues are 6% homologous.

Cross-species homology

Fyn has been highly conserved. Three domains (exon 2, exons 3–6 and exons 7–12) have evolved at different rates: amino acid similarity between human and *Xiphophorus* FYN is 84%, 91% and 95%, respectively in these domains.

Transformation

MAN

FYN is overexpressed in some human tumour cell lines (Kawakami *et al.*, 1986; Semba *et al.*, 1986; Kypta *et al.*, 1988).

ANIMALS

Chickens inoculated with a recombinant avian retrovirus expressing *fyn* develop fibrosarcomas that may arise from mutations in the kinase or SH2 domains of FYN (Semba *et al.*, 1990).

IN VITRO

Overexpression of normal *Fyn* transforms NIH 3T3 cells (Kawakami *et al.*, 1988). Substitution of the N-terminal two-thirds of FYN by the corresponding v-FGR region activates the FYN tyrosine kinase and transforming potential (Kawakami *et al.*, 1986).

TRANSGENIC ANIMALS

Mice that do not express FYN show no overt phenotype but are defective in signalling mechanisms from the thymocyte T cell receptor (Appleby *et al.*, 1992; Stein *et al.*, 1992).

	FYN/Fyn
Chromosome	
Human	6q21
Mouse	10
Exons	12
mRNA (kb)	3.3
	3.1/3.8 (oocytes)
Amino acids	537
Mass (kDa)	
(predicted)	p60
(expressed)	p59

Cellular location

Plasma membrane.

Tissue location

$p59^{fyn(B)}$ is mainly expressed in the brain but is detectable in most cell types other than epithelial cells (Kypta et al., 1988). In fetal rat brain $p59^{fyn(B)}$ is localized to axonal tracts and in the adult to subpopulations of neurons and glia (Bare et al., 1993). $p59^{fyn(T)}$ is mainly expressed in T cells. In the developing chick retina, $p59^{fyn(B)}$ is expressed in the ganglion and amacrine cells (Ingraham et al., 1992). The neuronal form of $pp60^{src}$ is also located in these cells. An additional form, $p72^{fyn}$, has been detected in transformed T cells and in in vitro translation systems (Espino et al., 1992). Fyn expression is also activated in HL-60 cells stimulated to differentiate by TPA (Katagiri et al., 1991) and in natural killer cells (Biondi et al., 1991).

Protein function

Fyn encodes a tyrosine kinase implicated in the control of cell growth. Its expression is activated by stimulation of the T cell receptor (TCR; Katagiri et al., 1989) and it may interact directly with CD3 after TCR activation (Samelson et al., 1990). FYN associates directly with the cytoplasmic domains of CD3ϵ, γ, ζ and η in chimeric proteins via a 10 amino acid region of its unique C-terminus (Gauen et al., 1992). CD2 and CD5 have each been shown to co-precipitate with FYN and may be tyrosine kinase substrates utilized during TCR activation (Bell et al., 1992; Burgess et al., 1992). The overexpression of $p59^{fyn(T)}$ in transgenic mice gives rise to T cells that are hyperstimulable, showing greatly enhanced phosphotyrosine accumulation and a twofold increase in $[Ca^{2+}]_i$ on activation by anti-CD3 or anti-Thy-1 antibodies or ConA (Cooke et al., 1991). The increased responsiveness is primarily in CD4$^+$/CD8$^+$ (relatively immature) cells. In thymocytes from Fyn$^-$ mice, increases in $[Ca^{2+}]_i$ and proliferation stimulated by activating the TCR or Thy-1 are markedly reduced, whereas the proliferative response of peripheral T cells remains essentially unaltered (Appleby et al., 1992; Stein et al., 1992).

The effects of $p59^{fyn(T)}$ are dependent on the kinase activity of the protein: mutation of Lys296 to Glu blocks enzymatic activity and prevents hyper-responsiveness. IL-2 secretion and DNA synthesis is also increased in T cells overexpressing p59$^{fyn(T)}$ in response to anti-CD3 antibody with TPA but not when ionomycin/TPA is the stimulus. Furthermore, overexpression of kinase-deficient p59$^{fyn(T)}$ inhibits the normal mitogenic response to anti-CD3/TPA. Overexpression of p56^{lck} or of the closely related p59^{hck} does not induce T cell hypersensitivity: p56^{lck} causes loss of surface CD3 and an increase in immature CD3$^-$4$^-$8^{lo} cells. These observations suggest a mimimal model in which FYN interacts directly with CD3 when the TCR is activated, leading to the phosphorylation and activation of phosphatidylinositol-PLC-γ_1 and subsequent cellular responses. The CD45 tyrosine phosphatase regulates the tyrosine kinase activity of FYN, which is reduced by 65% in CD45$^-$ T cells (Shiroo *et al.*, 1992). In CD45$^-$ cells, the TCR is uncoupled from protein tyrosine phosphorylation, PLC-γ_1 regulation, inositol phosphates accumulation, [Ca^{2+}]$_i$ responses, diacylglycerol production and protein kinase C activation, suggesting that FYN plays a critical role in coupling the activated TCR to these responses.

Activation of B lymphocytes causes the SRC family protein tyrosine kinases FYN, p53/56^{lyn} and p56^{lck} to associate with membrane Ig in spleen B cells and B cell lines and to undergo phosphorylation *in vitro* (Campbell and Sefton, 1992). In a mouse pro-B cell line IL-2 induces activation of FYN and its association with the IL-2R β chain (Kobayashi *et al.*, 1993).

In polyoma transformed cells, FYN forms complexes with middle T antigen (as does p60^{src} and p62^{yes}), an interaction mediated by the C-terminus of FYN (Kypta *et al.*, 1988; Cheng *et al.*, 1991). Following thrombin stimulation of platelets FYN, p53/56^{lyn} and p62^{yes} form complexes with GAP (Cichowski *et al.*, 1992).

In NIH 3T3 fibroblasts PDGF causes the association of FYN protein with the PDGF receptor and subsequent phosphorylation of FYN. This requires the SH2 domain of FYN (Twamley *et al.*, 1992).

Protein structure

FYN is myristylated; it is also phosphorylated on serine and tyrosine residues. Tyrosine kinase activity is negatively regulated by tyrosine phosphorylation. Tyr531 and Tyr420 are phosphorylated; mutation of Tyr531 to Phe does not activate the transforming capacity, in contrast to the effect of the equivalent mutation in pp60^{src} (Cheng *et al.*, 1991).

Two *Fyn* mRNAs (brain and thymus forms) arise by mutually exclusive splicing of alternative seventh exons: their products differ by 27 of the 51 amino acids encoded by the exon which is positioned at the beginning of the kinase domain and includes the presumptive nucleotide binding site (Cooke and Perlmutter, 1989).

Sequences of FYN, v-YES, SRC and FGR

```
Human FYN   (1)    MGCVQCK DKEATKLTEERDGSL NQSS GYRYGTD  PTPQHYPSFGVTSIPNYNNFHAAGG Q
v-YES       (277)  V--IKS-E--GPAMKYRTDNT PEPI--HVSH--S-SSQAT-SPAIK-SAVNF-SHSMTPF--PS
SRC         (1)    --  SS-S - P -DPSQ-RR--EPPDSTH HG-FPASQ--NKTAAPDTHRT- SRS-GTVA  T
FGR         (1)    ----F--KLEPVATAK-DAGLEGDFRSYGAADHYGPDPTKARPASSFAH  ----S--SS     -

Human FYN   (60)   GLTVFGGVNSS SHTGTLRTRG GT GVTLFVALYDYEARTEDDLSFHKGEKFQILNSSEGDWWE
v-YES       (341)  -M-P---AS--F-AVPSPYPST L-G-G-V----------T-----K---R---I-NT------
SRC         (57)   EPKL---F-T-DT VTSPQRA-ALAG---T--------S---T----K---RL--V-NT-----L
FGR         (60)       AINPGFLDSGTI--VSGI-----------------T-T-----H---NT------
```

```
Human FYN  (122)  ARSLTTGETGYIPSNYVAPVDSIQAEEWYFGKLGRKDAERQLLSFGNPRGTFLIRESETTKGAYS
v-YES      (405)  ---IA--K----------A-----------M-------L--NP--Q--I--V----------
SRC        (121)  -H-----Q----------S-----------IT-RES--L--NPE-------V---------C
FGR        (117)  ----SS-K--C-----------------I-----------P---Q-A-------------

Human FYN  (187)  LSIRDWDDMKGDHVKHYKIRKLDNGGYYITTRAQFETLQQLVQHYSERAAGLCCRLVVPCHKGMP
v-YES      (470)  -------EVR--N--------------------S--K--R-H-D---HK-TTV-PTV K
SRC        (186)  --VS-F-NA--LN---------S--F---S-T--SS-----AY--KH-D---H--TNV-PTS K
FGR        (182)  -------QTR-----------M---------V--NSV-E-----M-VND---NL-IA-- TI-K
                            #  #   #                            #
Human FYN  (252)  RLTDLSVKTKDVWEIPRESLQLIKRLGNGQFGEVWMGTWNGNTKVAIKTLKPGTMSPESFLEEAQ
v-YES      (534)  PQ- QGLA--A--------R-EVK--Q-C-----------T---------L---M--A--Q---
SRC        (250)  PQ- QGLA--A--------R-EVK--Q-C-----------T-R---------N----A--Q---
FGR        (246)  PQ- - GLA--A---S-S-IT-ER---T-C--D--L-----S----V---------KA------

Human FYN  (317)  IMKKLKHDKLVQLYAVVSEEPIYIVTEYMNKGSLLDFLKDGEGRALKLPNLVDMAAQVAAGMAYI
v-YES      (597)  -----R-----P---------------F-T---------E---KF----Q-------I-D-----
SRC        (313)  V----R-E-------------------S--------GEM-KY-R--Q-------I-S----V
FGR        (309)  V----R-------------------F-CH--------NP--QD-R--Q---------E----M

Human FYN  (382)  ERMNYIHRDLRSANILVGNGLICKIADFGLARLIEDNEYTARQGAKFPIKWTAPEAALYGRFTIK
v-YES      (662)  ----------A------DN-V------------------------------------------
SRC        (378)  -----V-----A------EN-V--V--------------------------------------
FGR        (374)  ----------A------ER-A-----------K-D--NPC--S------------F------

Human FYN  (447)  SDVWSFGILLTELVTKGRVPYPGMNNREVLEQVERGYRMPCPQDCPISLHELMIHCWKKDPEERP
v-YES      (727)  ----------------------V----------------G-E-----KL------D---
SRC        (443)  ------------T---------V-----D-----------PE--E---D--CQ--RR-----
FGR        (439)  ------------I----I------K-------Q--H----PG--A--Y-A-EQT-RL-----

Human FYN  (512)  TFEYLQSFLEDYFTATEPQYQPGENL (537)
v-YES      (792)  ----I----------A--SGY (812)
SRC        (508)  ------A-------S----------- (533)
FGR        (504)  -------------SA-------DQT (529)
```

Dashes indicate identity with FYN. Gly2 is the myristate attachment site. The SH3 domain (87–139) is underlined. # Indicates ATP binding sites (277–285 and 299). The autophosphorylated Tyr (420 in FYN) is shown in bold type.

Databank file names and accession numbers

	GENE	EMBL	SWISSPROT	REFERENCES
Human	*FYN*	Hscsyna M14333 Hsslk M14676	KFYN_HUMAN P06241	Semba *et al.*, 1986 Kawakami *et al.*, 1986 Peters *et al.*, 1990
Xenopus laevis	*Fyn*	Xlfync M27052	KFYN_XENLA P13406	Steele *et al.*, 1990
Xiphophorus helleri	*Fyn*	Xhcfyn X54971		Hanning *et al.*, 1991

Papers

Appleby, M.W., Gross, J.A., Cooke, M.P., Levin, S.D., Qian, X. and Perlmutter, R.M. (1992). Defective T cell receptor signaling in mice lacking the thymic isoform of p59^{fyn}. Cell, 70, 751–763.

Bare, D.J., Lauder, J.M., Wilkie, M.B. and Maness, P.F. (1993). p59^{fyn} in rat brain is localized in developing axonal tracts and subpopulations of adult neurons and glia. Oncogene, 8, 1429–1436.

Bell, G.M., Bolen, J.B. and Imboden, J.B. (1992). Association of src-like protein tyrosine kinases with the CD2 cell surface molecule in rat T lymphocytes and natural killer cells. Mol. Cell. Biol., 12, 5548–5554.

Biondi, A., Paganin, C., Rossi, V., Benvestito, S., Perlmutter, R. M., Mantovani, A. and Allavena, P. (1991). Expression of lineage-restricted protein tyrosine kinase genes in human natural killer cells. Eur. J. Immunol., 21, 843–846.

Burgess, K.E., Yamamoto, M., Prasad, K.V.S. and Rudd, C.E. (1992). CD5 acts as a tyrosine kinase substrate within a receptor complex comprising T-cell receptor ζ chain/CD3 and protein-tyrosine kinases p56^{lck} and p59^{fyn}. (1992). Proc. Natl Acad. Sci. USA, 89, 9311–9315.

Campbell, M.A. and Sefton, B.M. (1992). Association between B-lymphocyte membrane immunoglobulin and multiple members of the Src family of protein tyrosine kinases. Mol. Cell. Biol., 12, 2315–2321.

Cheng, S. H., Espino, P.C., Marshall, J., Harvey, R., Merrill, J. and Smith, A.E. (1991). Structural elements that regulate pp59^{c-fyn} catalytic activity, transforming potential, and ability to associate with polyoma-virus middle-T antigen. J. Virol., 65, 170–179.

Cichowski, K., McCormick, F. and Brugge, J.S. (1992). p21^{ras}GAP association with Fyn, Lyn, and Yes in thrombin-activated platelets. J. Biol. Chem., 267, 5025–5028.

Cooke, M.P. and Perlmutter, R.M. (1989). Expression of a novel form of the *fyn* proto-oncogene in hemato-poietic cells. New Biologist, 1, 66–74.

Cooke, M.F., Abraham, K.M., Forbush, K.A. and Perlmutter, R.M. (1991). Regulation of T cell receptor signaling by a *src* family protein-tyrosine kinase (p59^{fyn}). Cell, 65, 281–291.

Espino, P.C., Chou, W.-Y., Smith, A.E. and Cheng, S.H. (1992). The amino terminal half of pp59^{c-fyn} contains sequences necessary for formation of a 75 kDa form and also for repressive elements absent in pp60^{c-src}. Oncogene, 7, 317–322.

Gauen, L.K.T., Kong, A.-N.T., Samelson, L.E. and Shaw, A.S. (1992). p59^{fyn} tyrosine kinase associates with multiple T-cell receptor subunits through its amino-terminal domain. Mol. Cell. Biol., 12, 5438–5446.

Hannig, G., Ottilie, S. and Schartl. M. (1991). Conservation of structure and expression of the c-*yes* and *fyn* genes in lower vertebrates. Oncogene, 6, 361–369.

Ingraham, C.A., Cooke, M.P., Chuang, Y.-N., Perlmutter, R.M. and Maness, P.F. (1992). Cell type and developmental regulation of the *fyn* proto-oncogene in neural retina. Oncogene, 7, 95–100.

Katagiri, T., Urakawa, K., Yamanashi, Y., Semba, K., Takahashi, T., Toyoshima, K., Yamamoto, T. and Kano, K. (1989). Overexpression of *src* family gene for tyrosine-kinase p59^{fyn} in CD4⁻CD8⁻ T cells of mice with a lymphoproliferative disorder. Proc. Natl Acad. Sci. USA, 86, 10064–10068.

Katagiri, K, Katagiri, T., Koyama, Y., Morikawa, M., Yamamoto, T. and Yoshida, T. (1991). Expression of *src* family genes during monocytic differentiation of HL-60 cells. J. Immunol., 146, 701–707.

Kawakami, T., Pennington, C.Y. and Robbins, K.C. (1986). Isolation and oncogenic potential of a novel human *src*-like gene. Mol. Cell. Biol., 6, 4195–4201.

Kawakami, T., Kawakami, Y., Aaronson, S.A. and Robbins, K.C. (1988). Acquisition of transforming properties by *FYN*, a normal *SRC*-related human gene. Proc. Natl Acad. Sci. USA, 85, 3870–3874.

Kobayashi, N., Kono, T., Hatakeyama, M., Minami, Y., Miyazaki, T., Perlmutter, R.M. and Taniguchi, T. (1993). Functional coupling of the *src*-family protein tyrosine kinases p59^{fyn} and p53/56^{lyn} with the interleukin 2 receptor: Implications for redundancy and pleiotropism in cytokine signal transductions. Proc. Natl Acad. Sci. USA, 90, 4201–4205.

Kypta, R.M., Hemming, A. and Courtneidge, S.A. (1988). Identification and characterization of p59^{fyn} (a src-like protein tyrosine kinase) in normal and polyoma virus transformed cells. EMBO J., 7, 3837–3844.

Peters, D.J., McGrew, B.R., Perron, D.C., Liptak, L.M. and Laudano, A.P. (1990). *In vivo* phosphorylation and membrane association of the *fyn* proto-oncogene product in IM-9 human lymphoblasts. Oncogene, 5, 1313–1319.

Samelson, L.E., Phillips, A.F., Luong, E.T. and Klausner, R.D. (1990). Association of the fyn protein-tyrosine kinase with the T-cell antigen receptor. Proc. Natl Acad. Sci. USA, 87, 4358–4362.

Semba, K., Nishizawa, M., Miyajima, N., Yoshida, M.C., Sukegawa, J., Yamanashi, Y., Sasaki, M., Yamamoto, T., Toyoshima, K. (1986). *yes*-related protooncogene, *syn*, belongs to the protein-tyrosine kinase family. Proc. Natl Acad. Sci. USA, 83, 5459–5463.

Semba, K., Kawai, S., Matsuzawa, Y., Yamanashi, Y., Nishizawa, M. and Toyoshima, K. (1990). Transform-ation of chicken embryo fibroblast cells by avian retroviruses containing the human *fyn* gene and its mutated genes. Mol. Cell. Biol., 10, 3095–3104.

Shiroo, M., Goff, L., Biffen, M., Shivan, E. and Alexander, D. (1992). CD45 tyrosine phosphatase-activated p59^{fyn} couples the T cell antigen receptor to pathways of diacylglycerol production, protein kinase C activation and calcium influx. EMBO J., 11, 4887–4897.

Steele, R.E., Deng, J.C., Ghosn, C.R. and Fero, J.B. (1990). Structure and expression of *fyn* genes in *Xenopus laevis*. Oncogene, 5, 369–376.

Stein, P.L., Lee, H.-M., Rich, S. and Soriano, P. (1992). pp59^{fyn} mutant mice display differential signaling in thymocytes and peripheral T cells. Cell, 70, 741–750.

Twamley, G.M., Kypta, R.M., Hall, B. and Courtneidge, S.A. (1992). Association of fyn with the activated platelet-derived growth factor receptor: requirements for binding and phosphorylation. Oncogene, 7, 1893–1901.

HCK

HCK (hematopoietic cell kinase) encodes an Src-family protein tyrosine kinase detected in human cells with v-src and murine Lck probes (Klemsz et al., 1987; Quintrell et al., 1987; Ziegler et al., 1987).

Related genes

Hck is a member of the Src tyrosine kinase family (Blk, Fgr, Fyn, Hck, Lck/Tkl, Lyn, Src, Yes). Murine gene Bmk (B cell/myeloid kinase: Holtzman et al., 1987) is related. Hck-2 and Hck-3 are the murine homologues of LYN and LCK, respectively (Siracusa et al., 1989).

Cross-species homology

HCK: 97.6% identity (mouse and rat) (Okano et al., 1991). Murine BMK: 70% homology with human LYN (see Table 2.5 Supplement); 65% with murine LCK; 57% with chicken SRC.

Transformation

HCK expression is detectable in several human leukaemia cell lines (Ziegler et al., 1987; Quintrell et al., 1987; Perlmutter et al., 1988). Transgenic male mice that are hemizygous for the Hck transgene are sterile, indicating that the gene may be important in spermatogenesis (Magram and Bishop, 1991).

	HCK/Hck
Nucleotides (kb)	
Human	>30
Mouse	>50
Chromosome	
Human	20q11
Mouse	2 (Hck-1)
	4 (Hck-2/Lyn)
	4 (Hck-3/Lck)
Exons	
Human	12
Mouse	13 (1st non-coding)
mRNA (kb)	
Human, mouse	2.2
mRNA half-life (h)	>4

	HCK/Hck
Amino acids	
Human	505
Mouse, rat	503
Mass (kDa)	
(predicted) Human, mouse	57
(expressed)	p56, p59

Cellular location

Membrane fraction: p56 and p59. Cytosol: p59 alone.

Tissue location

Expression restricted to haematopoietic cells, predominantly in cells of the myeloid and B-lymphoid lineages (Ziegler *et al.*, 1987; Quintrell *et al.*, 1987). *Hck* is expressed when acute myeloid leukaemic cells are induced to differentiate *in vitro* to cells with monocytic characteristics (Willman *et al.*, 1991). Transcript is present in normal bone marrow-derived monocytic cells: transcription is enhanced by LPS or interferon-γ (Yi and Willman, 1989; Boulet *et al.*, 1992). Detectable in human lung (Holtrich *et al.*, 1991).

Protein function

HCK may be involved in the differentiation of monocytes and granulocytes.

Structure of the human and murine *Hck* genes

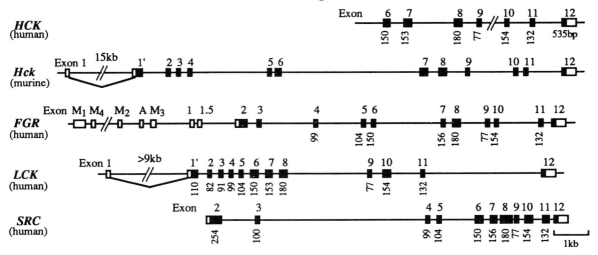

The organization of the genes is compared with that of other *Src* family genes. Black boxes represent coding exons. The sizes of *Hck* exons 6 to 12 (Hradetzky *et al.*, 1992) are compared with the corresponding exons of *FGR*, *LCK* and *SRC*.

The murine *Hck* promoter has no TATA or CAAT elements but contains GC-rich regions, three Sp-1 and two AP-2 consensus binding sites and an LPS-responsive element (Ziegler *et al.*, 1991; Lichtenberg *et al.*, 1992).

p59 is generated by translation from a CTG codon that is 21 codons 5' of the ATG used to generate p56 (Lock *et al.*, 1991).

Sequences of human and mouse HCK

```
Human HCK    (1)   MGSMKSKFLQVGGNTFSKTETSASPHCPVYVPDPTSTIKPGPNSHNSNTPGIREAGSED
Mouse HCK    (1)   --CV-----RD-SKA ----P--NQKG---------SS-L---NS--MP--FV- ----

            (60)   IIVVALYDYEAIHHEDLSFQKGDQMVVLEESGEWWKARSLATRKEGYIPSNYVARVDSLE
            (58)   T-----------R---------------A----------K------------N---

           (120)   TEEWFFKGISRKDAERQLLAPGNMLGSFMIRDSETTKGSYSLSVRDYDPRQGDTVKHYKI
           (118)   ---------------H---------------------------F--QH---------

           (180)   RTLDNGGFYISPRSTFSTLQELVDHYKKGNDGLCQKLSVPCMSSKPQKPWEKDAWEIPRE
           (178)   ----S-----------S-----L-----K----------V-P---------------
                           # #  #                       #
           (240)   SLKLEKKLGAGQFGEVWMATYNKHTKVAVKTMKPGSMSVEAFLAEANVMKTLQHDKLVKL
           (238)   --QM---------------------------------------L--S---------

           (300)   HAVVTKEPIYIITEFMAKGSLLDFLKSDEGSKQPLPKLIDFSAQIAEGMAFIEQRNYIHR
           (298)   ----SQ---F-V--------------E----------------S-------------

           (360)   DLRAANILVSASLVCKIADFGLARVIEDNEYTAREGAKFPIKWTAPEAINFGSFTIKSDV
           (358)   ----------------------------I----------------------------

           (420)   WSFGILLMEIVTYGRIPYPGMSNPEVIRALERGYRMPRPENCPEELYNIMMRCWKNRPEE
           (418)   ----------------------------H-------D---------I---------

           (480)   RPTFEYIQSVLDDFYTATESQYQQQP (505)
           (478)   ------------------------- (503)
```

Underlined: SH3 domains (human 61–111). Italics: SH2 (human 112–223). # Indicates ATP binding region. Catalytic domain 224–488.

Databank file names and accession numbers

	GENE	EMBL	SWISSPROT	REFERENCES
Human	HCK	Hshcka and Hshckb M16591 and M16592	KHCK_HUMAN P08631	Quintrell *et al.*, 1987 Ziegler *et al.*, 1987
Human	HCK	X59741, X59742, X59743		Hradetzky *et al.*, 1992
Mouse	Hck	Mmhck Y00487	KHCK_MOUSE P08103	Holtzman *et al.*, 1987 Klemsz *et al.*, 1987
Rat	Hck	Rnhctk M83666 Rrhckmr X62345		Okano *et al.*, 1991

Papers

Boulet, I., Ralph, S., Stanley, E., Lock, P., Dunn, A.R., Green, S.P. and Phillips, W.A. (1992). Lipopolysaccharide- and interferon-gamma-induced expression of *hck* and *lyn* tyrosine kinases in murine bone marrow-derived macrophages. Oncogene, 7, 703–710.

Holtrich, U., Brauninger, A., Strebhardt, K. and Rubsamen-Waigmann, H. (1991). Two additional protein-tyrosine kinases expressed in human lung: fourth member of the fibroblast growth factor receptor family and an intracellular protein-tyrosine kinase. Proc. Natl Acad. Sci. USA, 88, 10411–10415.

Holtzman, D.A., Cook, W.D. and Dunn, A.R. (1987). Isolation and sequence of a cDNA corresponding to a src-related gene expressed in murine hemopoietic cells. Proc. Natl Acad. Sci. USA, 84, 8325–8329.

Hradetzky, D., Strebhardt, K. and Rubsamen-Waigmann, H. (1992). The genomic locus of the human hemopoietic-specific cell protein tyrosine kinase (PTK)-encoding gene (*HCK*) confirms conservation of exon-intron structure among human PTKs of the *src* family. Gene, 113, 275–280.

Klemsz, M.J., McKercher, S.R. and Maki, R.A. (1987). Nucleotide sequence of the mouse *hck* gene. Nucleic Acids Res., 15, 9600.

Lichtenberg, U., Quintrell, N. and Bishop, M.J. (1992). Human protein-tyrosine kinase gene *HCK*: expression and structural analysis of the promoter region. Oncogene, 7, 849–858.

Lock, P., Ralph, S., Stanley, E., Boulet, I., Ramsay, R. and Dunn, A.R. (1991). Two isoforms of murine *hck*, generated by utilization of alternative translational initiation codons, exhibit different patterns of subcellular localization. Mol. Cell. Biol., 11, 4363–4370.

Magram, J. and Bishop, J.M. (1991). Dominant male sterility in mice caused by insertion of a transgene. Proc. Natl Acad. Sci. USA, 88, 10327–10331.

Okano, Y., Sugimoto, Y., Fukuoka, M., Matsui, A., Nagata, K. and Nozawa, Y. (1991). Identification of rat cDNA encoding *hck* tyrosine kinase from megakaryocytes. Biochem. Biophys. Res. Commun., 181, 1137–1144.

Perlmutter, R.M., Marth, J.D., Ziegler, S.F., Garvin, A.M., Pawar, S., Cooke, M.P. and Abraham, K.M. (1988). Specialized protein tyrosine kinase proto-oncogenes in hematopoietic cells. Biochim. Biophys. Acta, 948, 245–262.

Quintrell, N., Lebo, R., Varmus, H., Bishop, J.M., Pettenati, M.J., LeBeau, M.M., Diaz, M.O. and Rowley, J.D. (1987). Identification of a human gene (*HCK*) that encodes a protein-tyrosine kinase and is expressed in hemopoietic cells. Mol. Cell. Biol., 7, 2267–2275.

Siracusa, L.D., Buchberg, A.M., Copeland, N.G. and Jenkins, N.A. (1989). Recombinant inbred strain and interspecific backcross analysis of molecular markers flanking the murine *agouti* coat color locus. Genetics, 122, 669–679.

Willman, C.L., Stewart, C.C., Longacre, T.L., Head, D.R., Habbersett, R., Ziegler, S.F. and Perlmutter, R.M. (1991). Expression of the c-*fgr* and *hck* protein-tyrosine kinases in acute myeloid leukemic blasts is associated with early commitment and differentiation events in the monocytic and granulocytic lineages. Blood, 77, 726–734.

Yi, T.L. and Willman, C.L. (1989). Cloning of the murine c-*fgr* proto-oncogene cDNA and induction of c-*fgr* expression by proliferation and activation factors in normal bone marrow-derived monocytic cells. Oncogene 4, 1081–1087.

Ziegler, S.F., Marth, J.D., Lewis, D.B. and Perlmutter, R.M. (1987). Novel protein-tyrosine kinase gene (*hck*) preferentially expressed in cells of hematopoietic origin. Mol. Cell. Biol., 7, 2276–2285.

Ziegler, S.F., Pleiman, C.M. and Perlmutter, R.M. (1991). Structure and expression of the murine *hck* gene. Oncogene, 6, 283–288.

HSTF1/Hst-1 and INT2

HSTF1 (*heparan secretory transforming protein 1*) is a human transforming gene originally detected by NIH 3T3 fibroblast transfection with DNA from *human stomach tumours* (Sakamoto *et al.*, 1986) that has no homology with known viral oncogenes. *HST2* is a close homologue of *HSTF1* that was cloned by cross-hybridization with *HSTF1* probes (Sakamoto *et al.*, 1988).

Murine *Int-2* was initially identified as a frequent target for activation by proviral insertion of mouse mammary tumour virus (Peters *et al.*, 1983; see Chapter 2, Table 2.2). Human *INT2* was detected by cross-hybridization with mouse *Int-2* probes (Casey *et al.*, 1986).

The *HSTF1/Hst-1* and *INT2/Int-2* oncogenes are members of the fibroblast growth factor (FGF) family (Dickson and Peters, 1987; Moore *et al.*, 1986).

Related genes

THE FGF FAMILY

This family includes seven proteins: acidic fibroblast growth factor (*FGFA*, aFGF, HBGF-1 or FGF1), basic FGF (*FGFB*, bFGF, HBGF-2 or FGF2) and the oncogenes *INT2* (FGF3), *HSTF1* (*Hst-1*/Kaposi-FGF/K-FGF or FGF4), *FGF5*, *HST2/Hst-2* (*FGF6*) (Coulier *et al.*, 1991; Iida *et al.*, 1992) and keratinocyte growth factor, KGF (FGF7; Rubin *et al.*, 1989). FGFA occurs in three forms generated by N-terminal processing of the same precursor protein.

HSTF1 is homologous to FGFA (38%), FGFB (43%) and mouse INT2 (40%). Murine FGF6 is 66% identical to murine HST1/K-FGF and 39% identical to INT2 (de Lapeyriere *et al.*, 1990).

THE FIBROBLAST GROWTH FACTOR RECEPTOR (FGFR) FAMILY

There are both low-affinity receptors (heparan sulfate proteoglycans) and high-affinity receptors (110–150 kDa) for FGFA and FGFB. The FGFBR family are class IV receptors, closely related to but distinct from the class III receptor family (*FMS*, *FLT3/FLK2*, *KIT*, *PDGFRA*, *PDGFRB*), that have three (rather than five) extracellular immunoglobulin-like domains, the N-terminal pair being separated by a hydrophilic acidic motif, and an insert in the intracellular tyrosine kinase region (Lee *et al.*, 1989).

There are four families of human FGF receptor genes: *FGFR1/FLG*, *FGFR2/BEK*, *FGFR3* (Keegan *et al.*, 1991) and *FGFR4* (see *UFO*, Table 2.5 supplement). *BEK* (bacterial expressed kinase; Kornbluth *et al.*, 1988) and *FLG* (*Fms*-like gene, also *Flt2*; Ruta *et al.*, 1988) were originally cloned from human and murine cDNA libraries. The four genes encode distinct tyrosine kinase cell surface receptors of class IV that include a kinase insert region.

FGFR1/FLG is the high-affinity receptor for FGFB; however, FGFR1/FLG and one form of BEK bind FGFA and FGFB with equal, high affinity. Murine FGFR1/FLG also binds HST1/FGF4 equally well. FGFR4 (TKF: tyrosine kinase related to FGF) binds FGFA but not FGFB (Partanen *et al.*, 1991). FGFR transcripts undergo extensive alternative splicing. For *FGFR1/FLG* this results in four classes of variant receptors (FLG1, FLG2, H2, H4) with the following features: (1) two Ig domains, (2) truncated tyrosine kinase domains, (3) loss of the signal sequence, and (4) generation of a secreted protein (Champion-Arnaud *et al.*, 1991; Eisemann *et al.*, 1991; Hou *et al.*, 1991). Sixteen isoforms of *FLG* have been characterized (Xu *et al.*, 1992). FLG2 is 68% and 64% identical to BEK and FLG1 respectively (Avivi *et al.*, 1991).

The *BEK* family comprises *BEK, TK14, TK25, K-SAM* (tumour) and K-*SAM* (kerat) that is expressed in a keratinocyte cell line (Hattori *et al.*, 1990). Murine BEK with three Ig-like domains is the high-affinity receptor for FGFA, FGFB and HST1/FGF4 (Mansukhani *et al.*, 1992). In murine keratinocytes an alternatively spliced form of *FGFR2/Bek* that lacks the N-terminal Ig-like domain and the acidic motif binds FGFA and KGF with high affinity but binds FGFB with much lower affinity (Miki *et al.*, 1991). Variants of human FGFR2/BEK lacking the N-terminal Ig-like domain and the hydrophilic motif bind FGFA and FGFB equally well, however, although this form differs from the murine variant in the Ig-like domain adjacent to the membrane (Crumley *et al.*, 1991). The murine BEK and FLG receptors and also the TEK receptor (Raz *et al.*, 1991) require interaction with heparan sulfate proteoglycans to facilitate ligand binding (Mansukhani *et al.*, 1992). *Flg* and *Bek* have different patterns of spatial expression during development (Orr-Urtreger *et al.*, 1991; Peters *et al.*, 1992) that presumably reflects difference in their promoter sequences (Avivi *et al.*, 1992; Saito *et al.*, 1992).

Cross-species homology

Human HSTF1 and mouse HST1: 81% overall identity; the C-terminal 150 residues are 90% identical. Human and mouse INT2: 89% identity up to the C-terminus in which 22 amino acids of human INT2 are replaced by 27 unrelated residues in the mouse protein (Brookes *et al.*, 1989a). Human HSTF1: ~40% identity with mouse INT2 in selected regions (see **Protein structure** below). Human HST2: 93% identity with mouse FGF6 (de Lapeyriere *et al.*, 1990).

Chicken *Bek* encodes a 4 kb mRNA and a predicted 824 amino acid (92 kDa) protein tyrosine kinase related to the FGF receptor (Sato *et al.*, 1991). Chicken *Cek-1, Cek-2, Cek-3, Cek-4* and *Cek-5* (chick embryo kinase) form a closely related family of tyrosine kinases (Pasquale and Singer, 1989; Pasquale, 1990). *Cek-1* is the chicken FGFB receptor. *Cek-2* (also called *Brk* (Bek-related kinase) and *Cek-3* are related to *Bek*. *Cek-4* and *Cek-5* are homologous to *Eph*. A *Cek-2/Brk*-related protein (120 kDa) is expressed in human lung tissue.

Transformation

MAN

FGFs have oncogenic potential: they can induce blood vessel formation and are synthesized by many tumour cells (Burgess and Maciag, 1989; Goldfarb, 1990).

HSTF1, together with *INT2* and *BCL1*, is amplified in up to 22% of human breast carcinomas (Tsuda *et al.*, 1989a; Theillet *et al.*, 1990). Although the frequency of *INT2* amplification in breast carcinomas is relatively low, one study has detected polymorphism of *INT2* in 61% of lymph-node positive patients (Meyers *et al.*, 1990). *HSTF1, INT2* and anionic glutathione-S-transferase are co-amplified in ~30% of breast carcinomas (Saint-Ruf *et al.*, 1991). However, there is no evidence that the HSTF1 or INT2 proteins are expressed in breast tumours. Co-amplification of *HSTF1/INT2* occurs in up to 47% of esophageal carcinomas (Tsuda *et al.*, 1989b; Kitagawa *et al.*, 1991; Wagata *et al.*, 1991) and *HSTF1* is expressed together with *KIT* in some testicular germ cell tumours (Strohmeyer *et al.*, 1991). *HSTF1* has also been identified in human DNA from gastric cancers, hepatomas, colon carcinomas (Yoshida *et al.*, 1987, 1991), melanoma (Adelaide *et al.*, 1988), osteosarcoma (Zhan *et al.*, 1987) and in Kaposi's sarcoma (Delli-Bovi *et al.*, 1987).

INT2 is frequently amplified in squamous cell carcinomas (SCC) of the head and neck. Co-amplification of *INT2* and *EGFR* has been detected in a laryngeal SCC and an SCC metastatic to the neck (Somers *et al.*, 1990).

HST2 mRNA has been detected in some human leukaemia cell lines (Iida *et al.*, 1992). K-*SAM* is the *KATO*-III cell-derived *s*tomach cancer *am*plified gene; Hattori *et al.*, 1990). *FGF5* is expressed in some human tumour cell lines (Zhan *et al.*, 1988).

The human *FGFA* gene is localized to 5q31.3–33.2. In 10–20% of acute non-lymphocytic leukaemias there is a deletion in the long arm of chromosome 5. The deletion does not affect the *FGFA* gene (Wang *et al.*, 1991) but may affect nearby genes encoding the growth factors macrophage colony stimulating factor-1 (CSF1) and granulocyte-macrophage colony stimulating factor (GM-CSF) and the receptors for CSF1, PDGF, adrenergic drugs, glucocorticoids and dopamine.

FGFR4/TKF is expressed (3.3 kb mRNA) in some gastrointestinal tumours (Strebhardt *et al.*, 1992).

FGFR1/FLG and *FGFR2/BEK* are amplified in ~10% of human breast tumours. There is evidence that *BEK* expression may correlate with that of *MYC* and expression of *FGFR1/FLG* with *HSTF1/INT2/BCL1* (Adnane *et al.*, 1991).

ANIMALS

Hst-1 may be activated by MMTV proviral insertion on either side of the gene: some insertions activate both *Hst-1* and the 17 kb distant *Int-2* gene (Peters *et al.*, 1989). *Hst-1* may be involved in tumour progression from a non-metastatic to a metastatic phenotype in the mouse mammary tumour system (Murakami *et al.*, 1990).

Hst-1 expressed by retrovirally mediated gene transfer is angiogenic in rat neural transplants but is not oncogenic (Brustle *et al.*, 1992). The MFS virus, isolated from a mouse fibrosarcoma, encodes an *env–HSTF1* fusion protein derived by recombination *in vivo* between a retroviral construct carrying human *HSTF1* and MoMuLV. MFS induces diffuse meningeal tumours and soft-tissue fibrosarcomas and its tumorigenic capacity appears to reflect the oncogenic potential of *HSTF1* (Talarico *et al.*, 1993).

Int-2 is a frequent target for activation by MMTV proviral insertion. In spontaneously arising murine mammary tumours *Int-2* may be activated together with other *Int* genes, for example, *Wnt-1* (Peters *et al.*, 1986).

Transfectants of MCF-7 human breast cancer cells with FGF4 are tumorigenic and metastatic when injected into mice (Kurebayashi *et al.*, 1993).

IN VITRO

HSTF1 or *FGF5* genomic and cDNA sequences transfected into NIH 3T3 cells induce morphological transformation, anchorage-independent growth and tumorigenicity (Delli-Bovi *et al.*, 1987; Taira *et al.*, 1987; Sakamoto *et al.*, 1988; Wellstein *et al.*, 1990; Fuller-Pace *et al.*, 1991; Talarico and Basilico, 1991).

HST2 does not transform NIH 3T3 cells in a normal assay but does induce foci in medium lacking PDGF and FGF (Yoshida *et al.*, 1991).

The secreted form of FGFA transforms NIH 3T3 cells and renders them tumorigenic in nude mice (Forough *et al.*, 1993). FGFB causes de-regulated cell growth and transformation (Neufeld *et al.*, 1988; Rogelj *et al.*, 1988) and is a melanocyte mitogen (Halaban *et al.*, 1988). Contrary to earlier reports, the high-affinity FGF receptor is not required for herpes simplex virus type 1 (HSV-1) infection (Mirda *et al.*, 1992). FGFB DNA does not transform NIH 3T3 cells unless expressed at high levels or with an added signal sequence (Rogelj *et al.*, 1988). However, *Int-2*

transforms NIH 3T3 cells with very low efficiency (Goldfarb *et al.*, 1991) b
FGFB in some cell lines (Venesio *et al.*, 1992).

FGF5 is expressed in exponentially growing fibroblasts and induced as an ε
(<4 h) by serum, PDGF, EGF or TGFα (Werner *et al.*, 1991). It is a mitogen
vascular smooth muscle cells (Zhan *et al.*, 1988). FGF6 (*Hst-2*) transforms NIl
(Iida *et al.*, 1992).

Antisense oligodeoxynucleotides inhibiting the expression of *FGFR1/FLG* prev
ation of normal human melanocytes and malignant melanoma cells *in vitro* (Beck   ., ⌐992).
They also disrupt morphology in regions of cell–cell contact, and expression of *FGFR1* may be
necessary for the prevention of terminal differentiation in these cells.

TRANSGENIC ANIMALS

In mice the *Int-2* transgene causes mammary hyperplasia and in some males prostatic hyperplasia, although induction of tumours is rare (Muller *et al.*, 1990; Ornitz *et al.*, 1991). Thus *Int-2*
acts as a potent growth factor in these epithelial cells. In double transgenic mice *Int-2* and *Wnt-
1* cooperate in the induction of mammary tumours (see *WNT1/WNT3*) and in *Wnt-1* transgenic
mice infected with MMTV *Int-2* and *Hst-1* can cooperate with *Wnt-1* (Shackleford *et al.*, 1993).

	HSTF1/Hst-1	*HST2/Hst-2*	*INT2/Int-2*
Nucleotides (kb)	11		
Chromosome			
Human	11q13.3	12p13 (Marics *et al.*, 1989)	11q13
Mouse	7	6 (de Lapeyriere *et al.*, 1990)	7
Exons	3 (coding)		3
mRNA (kb)			
Human	1.7/3.0 (Strohmeyer *et al.*, 1991)	5.7/8.6/12.0/15.0	
Mouse	3.0 (Peters *et al.*, 1989)	0.85/0.95/1.5/4.8 (de Lapeyriere *et al.*, 1990)	1.6/1.8/2.7/2.9 (at least 6 mRNAs: different promoters and poly(A) signals (Smith *et al.*, 1988; Mansour and Martin, 1988))
Amino acids			
Human	206 (encoded by 1.2 kb mRNA)	198	239
Mouse	202		245
Mass (kDa)			
(predicted)	22		27
(expressed)	p22		27.5–31.5 (Dixon *et al.*, 1989)

...ar location

...ST1: HST1 is glycosylated and secreted, the secreted protein being stabilized by heparin (Delli-Bovi *et al.*, 1988). Cleavage of 58 N-terminal amino acids yields a 17.5 kDa protein (Miyagawa *et al.*, 1991).

INT2: NIH 3T3 cells transformed by mouse *Int-2* cDNA express a series of INT2-related proteins. The use of different initiation codons gives rise to proteins located in the endoplasmic reticulum, the Golgi apparatus or the nucleus (Acland *et al.*, 1990). In highly transformed clonal lines INT2 proteins undergo further post-translational processing and are secreted, becoming associated with the cell surface and the extracellular matrix (Dixon *et al.*, 1989; Kiefer *et al.*, 1991).

Tissue location

HSTF1/Hst-1: This is expressed in undifferentiated embryonal carcinoma cell lines and at a limited stage of embryonal development. It is also detectable in other types of testicular germ cell tumours including teratocarcinoma, choriocarcinoma and seminoma (Strohmeyer *et al.*, 1991). In the mouse embryo *Hst-1* is expressed in the apical ectodermal ridge (Suzuki *et al.*, 1992).

Hst-2: This is only detectable in leukaemic cell lines (Iida *et al.*, 1992).

Int-2: In addition to its activation in MMTV-induced tumours in mice (see Table 2.2), *Int-2* is expressed in embryos and in some teratocarcinomas (Jakobovits *et al.*, 1986). Murine mRNA expression occurs in specific tissues during gastrulation and neurulation and subsequently is restricted to Purkinje cells in the cerebellum, to regions of the developing retina and to the mesenchyme of the developing teeth and sensory regions of the inner ear (Wilkinson *et al.*, 1988, 1989). It is rarely detected in adult tissues.

The use of KDEL mutants indicates that transformation by K-FGF is due to autocrine activation via a surface receptor (Talarico and Basilico, 1991). The receptors for FGFA and FGFB are present on many types of cell: receptors for other members of the FGF family are more restricted. FGF proteins are tightly associated with proteoglycans in the extracellular matrix.

Protein function

The members of the FGF family appear to act as paracrine or autocrine growth factors. FGFA and FGFB may function in both cell growth and in differentiation and have been implicated in cell transformation, angiogenesis and embryonic development (Burgess and Maciag, 1989). HST1 and INT2 induce mesoderm formation in *Xenopus laevis* animal pole cells (Paterno *et al.*, 1989).

The complex pattern of murine expression suggests multiple roles for INT2 during fetal development. INT2 secreted by highly transformed cells can be displaced from the cell surface by glycosaminoglycans and the addition of excess heparin causes the cells to revert to normal morphology (Dixon *et al.*, 1989; Kiefer *et al.*, 1991).

Gene structure

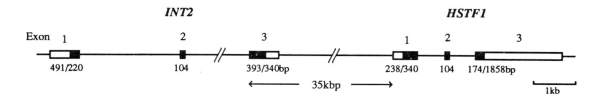

Black boxes: coding regions. The members of the FGF family have a common genomic organization and each member has a conserved 104 bp exon encoding the central 35 amino acids. Human *INT2* and *HSTF1* are in the same transcriptional orientation, as are the related mouse genes, *Int-2* and *Hst-1*, that are within 17 kbp of one another on chromosome 7 (Yoshida *et al.*, 1991). In the mouse *Int-2* gene transcription can initiate at multiple sites within three separate promoter domains and terminate distal to one of two polyadenylation signals (Smith *et al.*, 1988; Mansour and Martin, 1988). An alternative non-coding first exon (exon 1a) occurs in minor classes of *Int-2* mRNA. Homology between murine *Int-2* and human *INT2* extends throughout the promoter domains, although there is no evidence for the use of exon 1a in *INT2* (Brookes *et al.*, 1989a).

The *HSTF1* promoter contains a TATA box and three putative Sp-1 binding sites. The 5' non-coding region and exon 1 are GC-rich regions, a characteristic of housekeeping genes (Yoshida *et al.*, 1987). Expression of *HSTF1* may be regulated by protein factor(s) binding to an enhancer located in the third exon of the gene (Sasaki *et al.*, 1991).

Protein structure

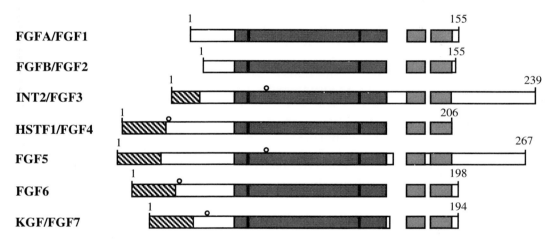

FGF family proteins contain two major regions of homology (heavy and light shading) and there are two absolutely conserved cysteine residues indicated by the vertical bars (see below). The cross-hatched boxes indicate N-terminal signal sequences, circles potential *N*-glycosylation sites. The human proteins are represented, with the exception of FGF6 for which the structure of the mouse protein is shown.

Sequences of human HSTF1, HST2, FGF5, FGFB, FGFA, KGF, INT2 and mouse INT2

```
Human HSTF1/FGF4   (1)          MSGPGTAAVALLPAVLLALLAPWAGRGGAAAPTAPNGTLEAELERRWESLVALSLARLP
Human HST2/FGF6    (1)                MSRG-GR-QGTLWALVFL-ILVGMVVPSPAGTRANNTLLDSRGWGTLLSR
Human FGF5         (1)      MSLSFLLLLLFFSHLILS-WAHGEKRLAPKGQPGPAATDRNPRGSSSRQSSSSAMSSSSASSSP
FGFB (FGF2)        (1)                                                                 MAA
FGFA (FGF1)        (1)                                                                   M
KGF (FGF7)         (1)              MHKWILTWILPTLLYRSCFHIICLVGTISLACNDMTPEQM
Human INT2/FGF3    (1)                           MGLIWLLLLS-LEPGWPAAG
Mouse INT2         (1)                           ************S**TTG
```

```
Human HSTF1    (60)   VAA QPKEAAVQSGAGDYLLG IKRLRRLYCNVGIGFHLQALPDGRIGGAHADTRDSL LELS
Human HST2     (51)   SR-GLAGEIAGVNWESG--V- ---Q--------------V------S-T-EENPY-- --I-
Human FGF5     (64)   A-SLGSQGSGLEQSSFQWS-- A-TGS---R--------IY---KVN-S-EANML-V --IF
FGFB          (4)    GSITTLPALPEDG-S-AFPP-HF-DPK----KN- --F-RIH----VD-VREKSDPHIK-Q-Q
FGFA          (2)    AEGEITTFT-LTEKFNL PP-NY-KPKL---SN- -HF-RI---TVD-TRDRSDQHIQ-Q--
KGF            (41)   ATNVNCSSPERHTRSYD-ME-GDI-V---F-R TQWY-RIDKR-KVK-TQEMKNNYNIM-IR
Human INT2     (22)   PG-R ARRD-GVRGGVYEH--GAP-R-K--- ATKY---LH-S--VN-SLENSAY-I --IT
Mouse INT2     (22)   **T* L****G********************* ************************** ****


Human HSTF1    (120)  PVERGVVSIFGVASRFFVAMSSKGKLYGSPFFTDECTFKEILLPNNYNAYES
Human HST2     (112)  T-------L---R-AL---N---R--AT-S-QE--K-R-T-----------
Human FGF5     (124)  A-SQ-I-GIR--F-NK-L---K----H--AK---D-K-R-RFQE-S--T-A-A
FGFB          (66)   AE-------K--CANRYL--KED-R-LA-KCV----F-F-R-ES----T-R
FGFA          (63)   AESV-E-Y-KSTETGQYL--DTD-L---SQTPNE--L-L-R-EE-H--T-LR
KGF            (102)  T-AV-I-AIK---E-EFYL--NKE-K-YAKKECNED-N-K-LI-E-H--T-A-A
Human INT2     (80)   A--V-I-A-R-LF-GRYL--NKR-R--A-EHYSA--E-V-RIHELG--T-A-RLYRTVSSTP
Mouse INT2     (80)   *****V***K********************D**N*********************G**G*


Human HSTF1    (172)     YKYPGMFIALSKNGKTKKG NRVSPTMKVTHFLPRL (206)
Human HST2     (164)     DL-Q-TY-----Y-RV-R- SK---I-T-------I (198)
Human FGF5     (177)  IHRTEKTGREWYV--N-R-KA-R-CSP--K-QHIS------FKQSEQPELSFTVTVPEKKN
FGFB          (118)  RKYTSWYV--KRT-QY-L- SKTG-GQ-AIL---MSAKS (155)
FGFA          (114)     KKHAEKNW-VG-K---SC-R- P-THYGQ-AIL---LPVSSD (155)
KGF            (155)  KWTHNGGEMFV--NQK-IPVR- KKKTKKEQKTA----MAIT (194)
Human INT2     (142)  GARRQPSAERLWYVSVNGK-RPRR- FKTRRTQKSSL----VLDHRDHEMVRQLQSGLPRP
Mouse INT2     (142)  **Q***G*Q*P************* ****************G*K******L***SQ**A


Human FGF5     (238)  PPSPIKSKIPLSAPRKNTNSVKYRLKFRFG (267)
Human INT2     (202)  PGKGVQPRRRRQKQSPDNLEPSHVQASRLGSQLEASAH (239)
Mouse INT2     (202)  **E*S***Q****KQSPGDHGKMETL*TRATPSTQLHTGGLAVA (245)
```

Dashes indicate amino acid identity with HSTF1. * Indicates identity between mouse and human INT2. Underlined: N-terminal signal sequences. Underlined and italicized regions in FGFB: heparin binding sites (27–31 and 116–119). Underlined region in FGFB: cell attachment site (44–47). ^ Indicates the conserved cysteine residues (88 and 155 in HSTF1 (FGF4)).

Sequences of human FLG2, FLG and BEK

```
FLG2  (1)    MVVPACVLVFCVAVVAGATSEPPG  PEQRVVRRAAEVPGPEPSQQEQVAFGSGDTVEL
BEK   (1)    --SWGRFICLV-VTM-TLSLAR-SFSLV-DTTLEPEEPPTKYQI--P-VYVAAP-ESL-V
FLG   (1)    -WSWK-L-FWA-L-T-TLCTAR-SPTL  PEQAQ-WGA-VEV-SFLVHP--LLQ-
                 C                                              C
FLG2  (58)   SCHPPGGAPTGPTVWAKDGTGLVASHRILVGPQRLQVLNASHEDAGVYSCQHRLTR RVL
BEK   (61)   R-LLKDA-VIS  -T---VH-GPNN-TVLIGEY--IKG-TPR-S-L-A-TASR-V DSE
FLG   (54)   R-RLRDDVQ SIN-LR--VQ-AE-N-TRITGEEVE-QDSVPA-S-L-A-VTSSPSGSDT
FLG2  (117)  C HFSVRVTDA PSSGDDEDGEDVAED          TGAPYWTRPERMDKKLLAVPA
BEK   (117)  TWY-M-N---- I-------DT-G---FVSENSNN    KR-----NT-K-E-R-H----
FLG   (112)  T Y---N-S--L---E--D-DD-SSSEEKETDNTKPNRMPV-----S--K-E---H----
                 C                                              C
FLG2  (163)  ANTVRFRCPAAGNPTPSISWLKNGKEFRGQHRIGGIKLRHQQWSLVMESVVPSDRGNYTC
BEK   (172)  ----K-----G---M-TMR--------KQE-----Y-V-N-H---I-------K-----
FLG   (171)  -K--K-K--SS-T-N-TLR--------KPD-----Y-V-YAT--II-D------K-----
                                                              C
FLG2  (223)  VVENKFGSIRQTYTLDVLERSPHRPILQAGLPANQTAILGSDVEFHCKVYSDAQPHIQWL
BEK   (232)  ----EY---NH-H---V---------------ASTVV-G----V-------------I
FLG   (231)  I---EY---NH--Q---V---------------K-VA---N---M------P-------
                                                              C
FLG2  (283)  KHVEVNGSKVGPDGTPYDTVLKTAGANTTDKELEVLSLHNVTFEDAGEYTCLAGNSIGFS
BEK   (292)  ----K----Y----L--LK---A--V------I---YIR-------------I-
FLG   (291)  --I------I---NL--VQI-----V------M---H-R--S--------------L-
```

```
FLG2   (343)  HHSAWLVVLPAEEELMETDEAGSVYAGVLSYGVVFFLFILVVAAVILCRLRSPPKK GLG
BEK    (352)  F-----T----PGREK-I T-SPD-LEIAI-CIGV--IACM-VT-----MKNTT--PDFS
FLG    (351)  ------T--E-L-- RPAVMTSPL-LEIII-CTGA--ISCM-GS--VYKMK-GT--SDFH

FLG2   (402)  S PTVHKVS RFPLKRQ  VSLESNSSMNSNTPLVRI ARLSS GEGPVLANVSELELPA
BEK    (411)  -Q-A---LTK-I-R--VT--A--S------------TT----TADT-M--G---Y---E
FLG    (410)  -QMA---LAKSI-R--VT--AD-SA----GVL---P S----S-TP M--G---Y---E

                                # #   #                              #
FLG2   (456)  DPKWELSRTRLTLGKPLGEGCFGQVVMAEAIGIDKDRTAKPVTVAVKMLKDDATDKDLSD
BEK    (471)  -----FP-DK-------------------V-----KPKEA------------E-----
FLG    (468)  --R---P-D--V-------------L-----L---KPNRVTK-------S---E-----

FLG2   (516)  LVSEMEMMKMIGKHKNIINLLGACTQGGPLYVLVEYAAKGNLREFLRARRPPGMDYSFDA
BEK    (531)  -----------------------D-----I----S------Y---------E--Y-I
FLG    (528)  -I---------------------D-----I----S------Y-Q------LE-CYNP

FLG2   (576)  CRLPEEQLTCKDLVSCAYQVARGMEYLASQKCIHRDLAARNVLVTEDNVMKIADFGLARD
BEK    (591)  N-V----M-F------T--L----------------------N------------
FLG    (588)  SHN-----SS-----------------K-----------------------------

FLG2   (636)  VHNLDYYKKTTNGRLPVKWMAPEALFDRVYTHQSDVWSFGVLLWEIFTLGGSPYPGIPVE
BEK    (651)  IN-I--------------------------------M----------------
FLG    (648)  I-HI--------------------I------------------------V---

FLG2   (696)  ELFKLLKEGHRMDKPASCTHDLYMIMRECWHAVPSQRPTFKQLVEDLDRILTVTSTDEYL
BEK    (711)  ---------------N--NE---M--D---------------------L-TNE---
FLG    (708)  --------------SN--NE---M--D---------------------VAL--NQ---

FLG2   (756)  DLSVPFEQYSPGGQDTPSS SSSGDDSVFTHDL        LPPGPPSNGGPRT (800)
BEK    (771)  ---Q-L-----SYP--R-- C--------SP-PMPYEPC   --QY-HI--SVK- (821)
FLG    (768)  ---M-LD----SFP--R--TC---E----S-EPLPEEPCLPRH- AQLA---LKRR (822)
```

Dashes indicate identical amino acids to FLG2. Underlined: signal sequences. Underlined and italic: transmembrane regions. C Indicates cysteines in the immunoglobulin loops. # Indicates conserved ATP binding sites. Italics: inter-kinase region.

Structure and sequence homology of FGF receptors

See page 230 for diagram. Two FGFR2/BEK variants are shown on the left hand side: a potentially secreted form comprising only the signal sequence (open box), the N-terminal Ig-like domain and the acidic motif (black box) and BEK lacking the first Ig-like domain and the acidic motif. Figures at the left of the full-length BEK structure denote the number of amino acids in each domain (Avivi et al., 1991).

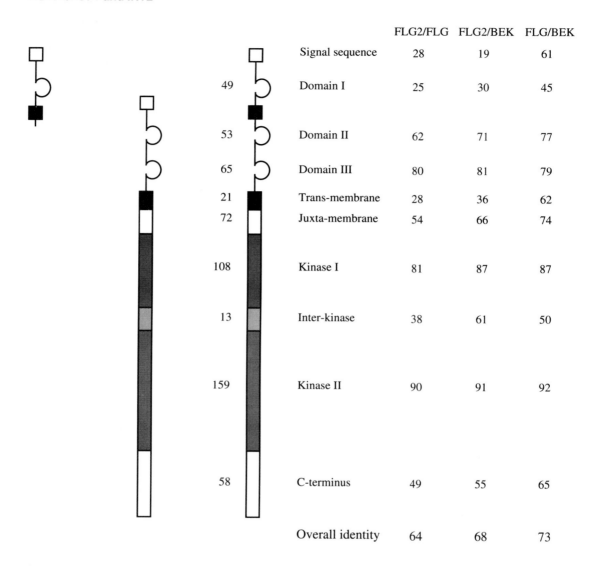

	FLG2/FLG	FLG2/BEK	FLG/BEK
Signal sequence	28	19	61
Domain I	25	30	45
Domain II	62	71	77
Domain III	80	81	79
Trans-membrane	28	36	62
Juxta-membrane	54	66	74
Kinase I	81	87	87
Inter-kinase	38	61	50
Kinase II	90	91	92
C-terminus	49	55	65
Overall identity	64	68	73

Databank file names and accession numbers

	GENE	EMBL	SWISSPROT	REFERENCES
Human	HSTF1 (FGF4) (or HST or KS3)	Hshst J02986 Hsksgfa M17446	HBG4_HUMAN P08620	Yoshida *et al.*, 1987 Taira *et al.*, 1987 Delli-Bovi *et al.*, 1987
Human	INT2 (FGF3)	Hsint2 X14445	HBG3_HUMAN P11487	Brookes *et al.*, 1989a
Human	FGF5	Hsfgf51 M23534 Hsfgf53 M23536	HBG5_HUMAN P12034 Hsfgf52 M23535	Zhan *et al.*, 1988

	GENE	EMBL	SWISSPROT	REFERENCES
Human	FGF6	Hsfgf6E1 X14071 Hsfgf6E2 X14072 Hsfgf6E3 X14073	HBG6_HUMAN P10767	Marics *et al.*, 1989
Human	KGF	Hskgf M60828	HBG7_HUMAN P21781	Finch *et al.*, 1989 Rubin *et al.*, 1989

Human	FGFA	Hsecgfb M13361
		Hshpgfl X51943
		Hsfgfa1/2/3
		  M30490/1/2
		Hsafgfa/b
		  M60515/6
		Hshbgf2/3
		  M23086/7
			HBG1_HUMAN
			P05230; P07502
				Wang *et al.*, 1991

Human	FGFB	Hsgfbf M17599 Hsfgfg1/2/3 X04431/2/3 Hsfgfb M27968	HBG2_HUMAN P09038	Sommer *et al.*, 1987 Kurokawa *et al.*, 1987
Human	BEK	Hsfgfrbe X52832		Dionne *et al.*, 1990
Human	FLG	Hsfgfrfl X52833		Dionne *et al.*, 1990
Human	FLG (FMS-like gene)	Hsflgmr Y00665	FGR1_HUMAN P11362	Ruta *et al.*, 1988
Human	FLG2	Daily:Hsfg12 X58255		Avivi *et al.*, 1991
	BEK K-SAM	M23362 M23362 GB M35718		Kornbluth *et al.*, 1988 Hattori *et al.*, 1990
Mouse	Int-2 (FGF-3)	Mmint2 Y00848	HBG3_MOUSE P05524	Moore *et al.*, 1986 Smith *et al.*, 1988
Mouse	Hst-1	Mmkfgf X14849 Mmfgfb M30642	HBG4_MOUSE P11403; P15657	Brookes *et al.*, 1989b Hebert *et al.*, 1990
Mouse	Fms-like gene (Flg)	Mmfgf X51893		Safran *et al.*, 1990
Chicken	Bek			Sato *et al.*, 1991
Chicken	Cek-1	Ggcek M24637	FGR1_CHICK P21804	Pasquale and Singer, 1989 Pasquale, 1990
Human	FLG2	Hsfg12 X58255		Avivi *et al.*, 1991

Reviews

Burgess, W.H. and Maciag, T. (1989). The heparin binding (fibroblast) growth factor family of proteins. Annu. Rev. Biochem., 58, 575–606.
Goldfarb, M. (1990). The fibroblast growth factor family. Cell Growth Differ., 1, 439–445.
Peters, G. (1991). Inappropriate expression of growth factor genes in tumors induced by mouse mammary tumor virus. Seminars Virol., 2, 319–328.

Papers

Acland, P., Dixon, M., Peters, G. and Dickson, C. (1990). Subcellular fate of the *int*-2 oncoprotein is determined by choice of initiation colon. Nature, 343, 662–665.

Adelaide, J., Mattei, M.-G., Marics, F., Raybaud, J., Planche, O., De Lapeyriere, O. and Birnbaum, D. (1988). Chromosomal localization of the *hst* oncogene and its co-amplification with the int.2 oncogene in a human melanoma. Oncogene, 2, 413–416.

Adnane, J., Gaudray, P., Dionne, C.A., Crumley, G., Jaye, M., Schlessinger, J., Jeanteur, P., Birnbaum, D. and Theillet, C. (1991). *BEK* and *FLG*, two receptors to members of the FGF family, are amplified in subsets of human breast cancers. Oncogene, 6, 659–663.

Avivi, A., Zimmer, Y., Yayon, A., Yarden, Y. and Givol, D. (1991). Flg-2, a new member of the family of fibroblast growth factor receptors. Oncogene, 6, 1089–1092.

Avivi, A., Skorecki, K., Yayon, A., and Givol, D. (1992). Promoter region of the murine fibroblast growth factor receptor 2 (*bek*/KGFR) gene. Oncogene, 7, 1957–1962.

Becker, D., Lee, P.L., Rodeck, U. and Herlyn, M. (1992). Inhibition of the fibroblast growth factor receptor 1 (FGFR-1) gene in human melanocytes and malignant melanomas leads to inhibition of proliferation and signs indicative of differentiation. Oncogene, 7, 2303–2313.

Brookes, S., Smith, R., Casey, G., Dickson, C. and Peters, G. (1989a). Sequence organization of the human *int*-2 gene and its expression in teratocarcinoma cells. Oncogene, 4, 429–436.

Brookes, S., Smith, R., Thurlow, J., Dickson, C. and Peters, G. (1989b). The mouse homologue of *hst*/k-FGF: sequence, genome organization and location relative to *int*-2. Nucleic Acids Res., 17, 4037–4045.

Brustle, O., Aguzzi, A., Talarico, D., Basilico, C., Kleihues, P. and Wiestler, O.D. (1992). Angiogenic activity of the K-fgf/hst oncogene in neural transplants. Oncogene, 7, 1177–1183.

Casey, G., Smith, R., McGillivray, D., Peters, G. and Dickson, C. (1986). Characterization and chromosome assignment of the human homolog of *int*-2, a potential proto-oncogene. Mol. Cell. Biol., 6, 502–510.

Champion-Arnaud, P., Ronsin, C., Gilbert, E., Gesnel, M.C., Houssaint, E. and Breathnach, R. (1991). Multiple mRNAs code for proteins related to the BEK fibroblast growth factor receptor. Oncogene, 6, 979–987.

Coulier, F., Batoz, M., Marics, I., de Lapeyriere, O. and Birnbaum, D. (1991). Putative structure of the *FGF6* gene product and role of the signal peptide. Oncogene, 6, 1437–1444.

Crumley, G., Bellot, F., Kaplow, J.M., Schlessinger, J., Jaye, M. and Dionne, C.A. (1991). High-affinity binding and activation of a truncated FGF receptor by both aFGF and bFGF. Oncogene, 6, 2255–2262.

de Lapeyriere, O., Rosnet, O., Benharroch, D., Raybaud, F., Marchetto, S., Planche, J., Galland, F., Mattei, M.G., Copeland, N.G., Jenkins, N.A, Coulier, F. and Birnbaum, D. (1990). Structure, chromosome mapping and expression of the murine *fgf*-6 gene. Oncogene, 5, 823–831.

Delli-Bovi, P., Curatola, A.M., Kern, F, G., Greco, A. Ittmann, M. and Basilico, C. (1987). An oncogene isolated by transfection of Kaposi's sarcoma DNA encodes a growth factor that is a member of the FGF family. Cell 50, 729–737.

Delli-Bovi, P., Curatola, A.M., Newman, K.M., Sato, Y., Moscaltelli, D., Hewick, R.M., Rifkin, D.B. and Basilico, C. (1988). Processing, secretion, and biological properties of a novel growth factor of the fibroblast growth factor family with oncogenic potential. Mol. Cell. Biol., 8, 2933–2941.

Dickson, C. and Peters, G. (1987). Potential oncogene product related to growth factors, Nature, 326, 833.

Dionne, C.A., Crumley, G.R., Bellot, F., Kaplow, J.M., Searfoss, G., Ruta, M., Burgess, W.H., Jaye, M. and Schlessinger, J. (1990). Cloning and expression of two distinct high-affinity receptors cross-reacting with acidic and basic fibroblast growth factors. EMBO J., 9, 2685–2692.

Dixon, M., Deed, R., Acland, P., Moore, R., Whyte, A., Peters, G. and Dickson, C. (1989). Detection and characterization of the fibroblast growth factor-related oncoprotein INT-2. Mol. Cell. Biol., 9, 4896–4902.

Eisemann, A., Ahn, J.A., Graziani, G., Tronick, S.R. and Ron, D. (1991). Alternative splicing generates at least five different isoforms of the human basic-FGF receptor. Oncogene, 6, 1195–1202.

Finch, P.W., Rubin, J.S., Miki, T., Ron, D. and Aaronson, S.A. (1989). Human KGF is FGF-related with properties of a paracrine effector of epithelial cell growth. Science, 245, 752–755.

Forough, R., Zhan, X., MacPhee, M., Friedman, S., Engleka, K.A., Sayers, T., Wiltrout, R.H. and Maciag, T. (1993). Differential transforming abilities of non-secreted and secreted forms of human fibroblast growth factor-1. J. Biol. Chem., 268, 2960–2968.

Fuller-Pace, F., Peters, G. and Dickson, C. (1991). Cell transformation by kFGF requires secretion but not glycosylation. J. Cell. Biol., 115, 547–555.

Goldfarb, M., Deed, R., MacAllan, D., Walther, W., Dickson, C. and Peters, G. (1991). Cell transformation by *int*-2 - a member of the fibroblast growth factor family. Oncogene, 6, 65–71.

Halaban, R., Langdon, R., Birchall, N., Cuono, C., Baird, A., Scott, G., Moellmann, G. and McGuire, J. (1988). Basic fibroblast growth factor from human keratinocytes is a natural mitogen for melanocytes. J. Cell Biol., 107, 1611–1619.

Hattori, Y., Odagiri, H., Nakatani, H., Miyagawa, K., Naito, K., Sakamoto, H., Katoh, O., Yoshida, T.,

Sugimura, T. and Terada, M. (1990). K-*sam*, an amplified gene in stomach cancer, is a member of the heparin-binding growth factor receptor genes. Proc. Natl Acad. Sci. USA, 87, 5983–5987.

Hebert, J.M., Basilico, C., Goldfarb, M., Haub, O. and Martin, G.R. (1990). Isolation of cDNAs encoding four murine fibroblast growth factor family members and characterization of their expression patterns. Devel. Biol., 138, 454–463.

Hou, J.Z., Kan, M.K., McKeehan, K., McBride, G., Adams, P. and McKeehan, W.L. (1991). Fibroblast growth factor receptors from liver vary in three structural domains. Science, 251, 665–668.

Iida, S., Yoshida, T., Naito, K., Sakamoto, H., Katoh, O., Hirohashi, S., Sato, T., Onda, M., Sugimura, T. and Terada, M. (1992). Human *hst*-2 (FGF-6) oncogene: cDNA cloning and characterization. Oncogene, 7, 303–310.

Jakobovits, A., Shackleford, G.M., Varmus, H.E. and Martin, G.R. (1986). Two protooncogenes implicated in mammary carcinogenesis, int-1 and int-2, are independently regulated during mouse development. Proc. Natl Acad. Sci. USA, 83, 7806–7810.

Keegan, K., Meyer, S. and Hayman, M.J. (1991). Structural and biosynthetic characterization of the fibroblast growth factor receptor 3 (FGFR-3) protein. Oncogene, 6, 2229–2236.

Kiefer, P., Peters, G. and Dickson, C. (1991). The *int*-2/*fgf*-3 oncogene product is secreted and associates with extracellular matrix: implications for cell transformation. Mol. Cell. Biol., 11, 5929–5936.

Kitagawa, Y., Ueda, M., Ando, N., Shinozawa, Y., Shimizu, N. and Abe, O. (1991). Significance of int-2/*hst*-1 coamplification as a prognostic factor in patients with esophageal squamous carcinoma. Cancer Res., 51, 1504–1508.

Kornbluth, S., Paulson, K.E. and Hanafusa, H. (1988). Novel tyrosine kinase identified by phosphotyrosine antibody screening of cDNA libraries. Mol. Cell. Biol., 8, 5541–5544.

Kurebayashi, J., McLeskey, S.W., Johnson, M.D., Lippman, M.E., Dickson, R.B. and Kern, F.G. (1993). Quantitative demonstration of spontaneous metastasis by MCF-7 human breast cancer cells cotransfected with fibroblast growth factor 4 and *lacZ*. Cancer Res., 53, 2178–2187.

Kurokawa, T., Sasada, R., Iwane, M. and Igarashi, K. (1987). Cloning and expression of cDNA encoding human basic fibroblast growth factor. FEBS Letts., 213, 189–194.

Lee, P.L., Johnson, D.E., Cousens, L.S., Fried, V.A. and Williams, L.T. (1989). Purification and complementary DNA cloning of a receptor for basic fibroblast growth factor. Science, 245, 57–60.

Mansour, S.L. and Martin, G.R. (1988). Four classes of mRNA are expressed from the mouse *int*-2 gene, a member of the FGF gene family. EMBO J., 7, 2035–2041.

Mansukhani, A., Dell'Era, P., Moscatelli, D., Kornbluth, S., Hanafusa, H. and Basilico, C. (1992). Characterization of the murine BEK fibroblast growth factor (FGF) receptor: activation by three members of the FGF family and requirement for heparin. Proc. Natl Acad. Sci. USA, 89, 3305–3309.

Marics, I., Adelaide, J., Raybaud, F., Mattei, M.-G., Coulier, F., Planche, J., de Lapeyriere, O. and Birnbaum, D. (1989). Characterization of the *HST*-related *FGF.6* gene, a new member of the fibroblast growth factor gene family. Oncogene, 4, 335–340.

Meyers, S.L., O'Brien, M.T., Smith, T. and Dudley, J.P. (1990). Analysis of the *int-1*, *int-2*, c-*myc*, and *neu* oncogenes in human breast carcinomas. Cancer Res., 50, 5911–5918.

Miki, T., Fleming, T.P., Bottaro, D.P., Rubin, J.S., Ron, D. and Aaronson, S.A. (1991). Expression cloning of the KGF receptor by creation of a transforming autocrine loop. Science, 251, 72–75.

Mirda, D.P., Navarro, D., Paz, P., Lee, P.L., Pereira, L. and Williams, L.T. (1992). The fibroblast growth factor receptor is not required for herpes simplex virus type 1 infection. J. Virol., 66, 448–457.

Miyagawa, K., Kimura, S., Yoshida, T., Sakamoto, H., Takaku, F., Sugimura, T. and Terada, M. (1991). Structural analysis of a mature *hst*-1 protein with transforming growth factor activity. Biochem. Biophys. Res. Commun., 174, 404–410.

Moore, R., Casey, G., Brookes, S., Dixon, M., Peters, G. and Dickson, C. (1986). Sequence, topography and protein coding potential of mouse *int*-2: a putative oncogene activated by mouse mammary tumour virus. EMBO J., 5, 919–924.

Muller, W.J., Lee, F.S., Dickson, C., Peters, G., Pattengale, P. and Leder, P. (1990). The *int*-2 gene product acts as an epithelial growth factor in transgenic mice. EMBO J., 9, 907–913.

Murakami, A., Tanaka, H. and Matsuzawa, A. (1990). Association of *hst* gene expression with metastatic phenotype in mouse mammary tumors. Cell Growth Differ., 1, 225–231.

Neufeld, G., Mitchell, R., Ponte, P. and Gospodarowicz, D. (1988). Expression of human basic fibroblast growth factor cDNA in baby hamster kidney-derived cells results in autonomous cell growth. J. Cell Biol., 106, 1385–1394.

Ornitz, D.M., Moreadith, R.W. and Leder, P. (1991). Binary system for regulating transgene expression in mice: targeting int-2 gene expression with yeast GAL4/UAS control elements. Proc. Natl Acad. Sci. USA, 88, 698–702.

Orr-Urtreger, A. Givol, D., Yayon, A., Yarden, Y. and Lonai, P. (1991). Developmental expression of two murine fibroblast growth factor receptors, *flg* and *bek*. Development, 113, 1419–1434.

Partanen, J., Makela, T.P., Eerola, E., Korhonen, J., Hirvonen, H., Claessin-Welsh, L. and Alitalo, K. (1991). FGFR-4, a novel acidic fibroblast growth factor receptor with a distinct expression pattern. EMBO J., 10, 1347–1354.

Pasquale, E. (1990). A distinctive family of embryonic protein-tyrosine kinase receptors. Proc. Natl Acad. Sci. USA, 87, 5812–5816.

Pasquale E.B. and Singer S.J. (1989). Identification of a developmentally regulated protein tyrosine kinase using a novel general method for the detection of tyrosine kinases. Proc. Natl Acad. Sci. USA, 86, 5449–5453.

Paterno, G.D., Gillespie, L.L., Dixon, M.S., Slack, J.M. and Heath, J.K. (1989). Mesoderm-inducing properties of INT-2 and kFGF: two oncogene-encoded growth factors related to FGF. Development, 106, 79–83.

Peters, G., Brookes, S., Smith, R. and Dickson, C. (1983). Tumorigenesis by mouse mammary tumor virus: evidence for a common region for provirus integration in mammary tumors. Cell, 33, 369–377.

Peters, G., Lee, A.E. and Dickson, C. (1986). Concerted activation of two potential proto-oncogenes in carcinomas induced by mouse mammary tumour virus. Nature, 320, 628–631.

Peters, G., Brookes, S., Smith, R., Placzek, M. and Dickson, C. (1989). The mouse homolog of the *hst/k-FGF* gene is adjacent to *int-2* and is activated by proviral insertion in some virally induced mammary tumors. Proc. Natl Acad. Sci. USA, 86, 5678–5682.

Peters, K.G., Werner, S., Chen, G. and Williams, L.T. (1992). Two fibroblast growth factor receptor genes are differentially expressed in epithelial and mesenchymal tissues during limb formation and organogenesis in the mouse. Development, 114, 233–243.

Raz, V., Kelman, Z., Avivi, A., Neufeld, G., Givol, D. and Yarden, Y. (1991). PCR-based identification of new receptors: molecular cloning of a receptor for fibroblast growth factors. Oncogene, 6, 753–760.

Rogelj, S., Weinberg, R.A., Fanning, P. and Klagsbrun, M. (1988). Basic fibroblast growth factor fused to a signal peptide transforms cells. Nature, 331, 173–175.

Rubin, J.S., Osada, H., Finch, P.W., Taylor, W.G., Rudikoff, S. and Aaronson, S.A. (1989). Purification and characterization of a newly identified growth factor specific for epithelial cells. Proc. Natl Acad. Sci. USA, 86, 802–806.

Ruta, M., Howk, R., Ricca, G., Drohan, W., Zabelshansky, M., Laureys, G., Barton, D.E., Francke, U., Schlessinger, J. and Givol, D. (1988). A novel protein tyrosine kinase gene whose expression is modulated during endothelial cell differentiation. Oncogene, 3, 9–15.

Safran, A., Avivi, A., Orr-Urtereger, A., Neufeld, G., Lonai, P., Givol, D. and Yarden, Y. (1990). The murine *flg* gene encodes a receptor for fibroblast growth factor. Oncogene, 5, 635–643.

Saint-Ruf, C., Malfoy, B., Scholl, S., Zafrani, B. and Dutrillaux, B. (1991). GSTπ gene is frequently coamplified with INT2 and HSTF1 proto-oncogenes in human breast cancers. Oncogene, 6, 403–406.

Saito, H., Kouhara, H., Kasayama, S., Kishimoto, T. and Sato, B. (1992). Characterization of the promoter region of the murine fibroblast growth factor receptor 1 gene. Biochem. Biophys. Res. Commun., 183, 688–693.

Sakamoto, H., Mori, M., Taira. M., Yoshida, T., Matsukawa, S., Shimizu, K., Sekiguchi, M., Terada, M. and Sugimura, T. (1986). Transforming gene from human stomach cancers and a noncancerous portion of stomach mucosa. Proc. Natl Acad. Sci. USA, 83, 3997–4001.

Sakamoto, H., Yoshida, T., Nakakuki, M., Odagiri, H., Miyagawa, K., Sugimura, T. and Terada, M. (1988). Cloned *hst* gene from normal human leukocyte DNA transforms NIH3T3 cells. Biochem. Biophys. Res. Commun., 151, 965–972.

Sasaki, A., Kubo, M., Hasan, S., Yano, Y. and Kakinuma, M. (1991). Regulation of human *hst* expression by an enhancer element residing in the third exon. Jpn J. Cancer Res., 82, 1191–1195.

Sato, M., Kitazawa, T., Iwai, T., Seki, J., Sakato, N., Kato, J.-Y. and Takeya, T. (1991). Isolation of chicken-*bek* and a related gene: identification of structural variation in the ligand-binding domains of the FGF-receptor family. Oncogene, 6, 1279–1283.

Shackleford, G.M., MacArthur, C.A., Kwan, H.C. and Varmus, H.E. (1993). Mouse mammary tumor virus infection accelerates mammary carcinogenesis in *Wnt-1* transgenic mice by insertional activation of *int-2/Fgf-3* and *hst/Fgf-4*. Proc. Natl Acad. Sci. USA, 90, 740–744.

Smith, R., Peters, G. and Dickson, C. (1988). Multiple RNAs expressed from the *int-2* gene in mouse embryonal carcinoma cell lines encode a protein with homology to fibroblast growth factors. EMBO J., 7, 1013–1022.

Somers, K.D., Cartwright, S.L. and Schechter, G.C. (1990). Amplification of the *int-2* gene in human head and neck squamous cell carcinomas. Oncogene, 5, 915–920.

Sommer, A., Brewer, M.T., Thompson, R.C., Moscatelli, D., Presta, M. and Rifkin, D.B. (1987). A form of human basic fibroblast growth factor with an extended amino terminus. Biochem. Biophys. Res. Commun., 144, 543–550.

Strebhardt, K., Brauninger, A., Holtrich, U. and Rubsamen-Waigmann, H. (1992). The role of a new FGF-receptor in the development of human lung tumors. J. Cell. Chem., Suppl. 16F, 17.

Strohmeyer, T., Peter, S., Hartmann, M., Munemitsu, S., Ackermann, R., Ullrich, A. and Slamon, D.J. (1991). Expression of the *hst*-1 and c-*kit* protooncogenes in human testicular germ cell tumors. Cancer Res., 51, 1811–1816.

Suzuki, H.R., Sakamoto, H., Yoshida, T., Sugimura, T., Terada, M. and Solursh, M. (1992). Localization of *hst*I transcripts to the apical ectodermal ridge in the mouse embryo. Devel. Biol., 150, 219–222.

Taira, M., Yoshida, T., Miyagawa, K., Sakamoto, H., Terada, M. and Sugimura, T. (1987). cDNA sequence of human transforming gene *hst* and identification of the coding sequence required for transforming activity. Proc. Natl Acad. Sci. USA, 84, 2980–2984.

Talarico, D. and Basilico, C. (1991). The K-*fgf/hst* oncogene induces transformation through an autocrine mechanism that requires extacellular stimulation of the mitogenic pathway. Mol. Cell. Biol., 11, 1138–1145.

Talarico, D., Ittmann, M.M., Bronson, R. and Basilico, C. (1993). A retrovirus carrying the K-*fgf* oncogene induces diffuse meningeal tumors and soft-tissue fibrosarcomas. Mol. Cell. Biol., 13, 1998–2010.

Theillet, C., Adnane, J., Szepetowski, P., Simon, M.-P., Jeanteur, P., Birnbaum, D. and Gaudray, P. (1990). *BCL-1* participates in the 11q13 amplification found in breast cancer. Oncogene, 5, 147–149.

Tsuda, H., Hirohashi, S., Shimosato, Y., Hirota, T., Tsugane, S., Yamamoto, H., Miyajima, N., Toyoshima, K., Yamamoto, T., Yokota, J., Yoshida, T., Sakamoto, H., Terada, M. and Sugimura, T. (1989a). Correlation between long-term survival in breast cancer patients and amplification of two putative oncogene-coamplification units: *hst*-1/*int*-2 and c-*erb*B-2/*ear*-1. Cancer Res., 49, 3104–3108.

Tsuda, T., Tahara, E., Kajiyama, G., Sakamoto, H., Terada, M. and Sugimura, T. (1989b). High incidence of coamplification of *hst*-1 and *int*-2 genes in human esophageal carcinomas. Cancer Res., 49, 5505–5508.

Venesio, T., Taverna, D., Hynes, N.E., Deed, R., MacAllan, D., Ciardiello, F., Valverius, E.M., Salomon, D.S., Callahan, R. and Merlo, G. (1992). The *int*-2 gene product acts as a growth factor and substitutes for basic fibroblast growth factor in promoting the differentiation of a normal mouse mammary epithelial cell line. Cell Growth Differen., 3, 63–71.

Wagata, T., Ishizaki, K., Imamura, M., Shimada, Y., Ikenaga, M. and Tobe, T. (1991). Deletion of 17p and amplification of the *int*-2 gene in esophageal carcinomas. Cancer Res., 51, 2113–2117.

Wang, W.-P., Quick, D., Balcerzak, S.P., Needleman, S.W. and Chiu, I.-M. (1991). Cloning and sequence analysis of the human acidic fibroblast growth factor gene and its preservation in leukemia patients. Oncogene, 6, 1521–1529.

Wellstein, A., Lupu, R., Zugmaier, G., Flamm, S.L., Cheville, A.L., Dello Bovi, P., Basilico, C., Lippman, M. and Kern, F.G. (1990). Autocrine growth stimulation by secreted Kaposi fibroblast growth factor but not by endogenous basic fibroblast growth factor. Cell Growth Differ., 1, 63–71.

Werner, S., Roth, W.K., Bates, B., Goldfarb, M. and Hofschneider, P.H. (1991). Fibroblast growth factor 5 proto-oncogene is expressed in normal human fibroblasts and induced by serum growth factors. Oncogene, 6, 2137–2144.

Wilkinson, D.G., Peters, G., Dickson, C. and McMahon, A.P. (1988). Expression of the FGF-related proto-oncogene *int*-2 during gastrulation and neurulation in the mouse. EMBO J., 7, 691–695.

Wilkinson, D.G., Bhatt, S. and McMahon, A.P. (1989). Expression pattern of the FGF-related proto-oncogene *int*-2 suggests multiple roles in fetal development. Development, 105, 131–136.

Xu, J., Nakahara, M., Crabb, J.W., Shi, E., Matuo, Y., Fraser, M., Kan, M., Hou, J. and McKeehan, W.L. (1992). Expression and immunochemical analysis of rat and human fibroblast growth factor receptor (flg) isoforms. J. Biol. Chem., 267, 17792–17803.

Yoshida, T., Miyagawa, K., Odagiri, H., Sakamoto, H., Little, P.F., Terada, M. and Sugimura, T. (1987). Genomic sequence of *hst*, a transforming gene encoding a protein homologous to fibroblast growth factors and the *int*-2-encoded protein. (published erratum appears in Proc. Natl Acad. Sci. USA, (1988), 85, 1967). Proc. Natl Acad. Sci. USA, 84, 7305–7309.

Yoshida, T., Miyagawa, K., Sakamoto, H., Sugimura, T. and Terada, M. (1991). Identification and characterization of fibroblast growth factor-related transforming gene *hst*-1. Methods Enzymol., 198, 124–138.

Zhan, X., Culpepper, A., Reddy, M., Loveless, J. and Goldfarb, M. (1987). Human oncogenes detected by a defined medium culture assay. Oncogene, 1, 369–376.

Zhan, X., Bates, B., Hu, X. and Goldfarb, M. (1988). The human FGF-5 oncogene encodes a novel protein related to fibroblast growth factors. Mol. Cell. Biol., 8, 3487–3495.

v-*jun* is the oncogene of avian sarcoma virus 17 (ASV 17) isolated from a spontaneous chicken sarcoma (Maki *et al.*, 1987). It is specifically responsible for the oncogenicity of ASV 17 (*ju-nana* is Japanese for the number 17).

The *Jun* gene family encode nuclear transcription factors.

Related genes

Human JUN is 44% identical to JUNB and 45% identical to JUND. The JUN family bind to the same consensus DNA sequence as the transcription factors PEA1 (mouse) and GCN4 (yeast). In the mouse an additional *Jund* gene (*Jund-2*) has been detected on chromosome 2 that probably represents a processed pseudogene (Shapiro and Kozak, 1991). Murine *Jund* shows close genetic linkage to *Junb* and *Mel* (Howard *et al.*, 1991).

Cross-species homology

JUN, JUNB: 98% identity (human and mouse); 45% (chicken and mouse). JUNB: 95.3% (human and rat); 99.5% (mouse and rat). JUND: 77% (human and mouse); 71% (chicken and mouse) (Ryder *et al.*, 1988; Schutte *et al.*, 1989b; Nomura *et al.*, 1990; Hartl *et al.*, 1991; Kawakami *et al.*, 1992).

Transformation

MAN

JUN is overexpressed between 4- and 12-fold in 40% of small-cell lung cancers and 20% of non-small-cell lung cancers (Schuette *et al.*, 1988). *JUND* loci may be involved in chromosome translocations that occur in some cases of acute lymphocytic leukaemia (ALL) and acute non-lymphocytic leukaemia (19;11 and 19;1)(Mattei *et al.*, 1990).

ANIMALS

Viruses carrying v-*jun* or a recombinant between v-*jun* and *Jun* induce tumours when injected into the wing web of chicks (Wong *et al.*, 1992). Embryonic stem (ES) cells induce teratocarcinomas when subcutaneously injected into syngeneic mice: however, the tumorigenicity of ES cells is drastically reduced when both copies of the *Jun* gene have been inactivated by homologous recombination, indicating that JUN may be necessary for efficient tumour growth (Hilberg and Wagner, 1992).

IN VITRO

THRA (*ErbA*), the thyroid hormone receptor, and *Jun* are the first examples of transcription factor genes that can acquire tumorigenic properties. As occurs with *Src*, the cellular gene (*Jun*) placed in an appropriate retroviral vector is able by itself to transform immortalized rat fibroblasts and, in cooperation with *Hras*, primary rat fibroblasts (Schutte *et al.*, 1989a). *Jun* and *Hras* transform more effectively than *Junb* and *Hras*, and *Junb* inhibits *Jun/Ras* transformation (Schutte *et al.*, 1989a), consistent with the differential DNA affinities of JUN and JUNB.

v-*jun* transformation potential in chick embryo fibroblasts is increased 10^3-fold relative to *Jun* by deletion of the δ region and further increased by loss of the 3′ untranslated region (Bos *et al.*, 1990; Vogt and Bos, 1990).

Transformation by *Jun* of chick embryo fibroblasts is prevented (or reversed) by the expression of a synthetic *Fos* gene lacking a DNA binding domain (Okuno *et al.*, 1991), the mutant FOS protein forming heterodimers with JUN that are inactive as transcription factors.

TRANSGENIC ANIMALS

In mice carrying v-*jun* in the germ line, wounding is a prerequisite for tumorigenesis, following which ~25% of animals homozygous for the transgene develop dermal fibrosarcomas. v-*jun* transgenic cells require TNFα or IL-1 to become anchorage-independent for *in vitro* growth, indicating that these agents may act as cofactors in wound-induced carcinogenesis (Vanhamme *et al.*, 1993).

	JUN/Jun	*JUNB/Junb*	*JUND/Jund*	v-*jun*
Nucleotides (bp)	3622	2136		930 3.5 (ASV 17)
Chromosome				
Human	1p32–p31	19p13.2	19p13.2	
Mouse	4	8	8 (*Jund-1*)	
Exons				
Human and chicken	1	1	1	
mRNA (kb)	2.7/3.4	2.1	1.8	3.5
mRNA half-life (min)	30	30	30	
Amino acids				296
Human	331	347	303	
Chicken	310		323	
Mouse	334	344	341	
Mass (kDa)				
(predicted)	35.7	36		32(v-*jun*)
(expressed)	39	35	40–50 (chicken)	65$^{gag\text{-}jun}$

Cellular location

Nuclear.

Tissue location

Jun: Early response gene undergoing strong, transient activation when quiescent cells are stimulated by growth factors (Quantin and Breathnach, 1988; Ryder and Nathans, 1988; Ryseck *et* al., 1988). mRNA expression in the mouse is maximal in the lung, ovary and heart and is very low in the intestine and liver (Kovary and Bravo, 1991; Mollinedo *et al.*, 1991). *Jun* is also transiently expressed in interleukin-2- and IL-6-dependent mouse myeloma cell lines following withdrawal of growth factor and the onset of apoptosis (Colotta *et al.*, 1992).

Junb: Early response gene induced by serum (Ryder *et al.*, 1988). Induction of *Junb* and *Jun* by serum is attenuated in cells transformed by tyrosine kinase oncoproteins (Yu *et al.*, 1993). Murine *Junb* expression is ubiquitous but is particularly high in the testis where *Jun* and *Jund* are barely detectable.

Jund: mRNA is 5- to 10-fold more abundant than *Jun* mRNA and occurs in most tissues, being maximal in the intestine and thymus (Ryder *et al.*, 1989). It is present in serum-starved cells and is not significantly induced by the addition of serum (Hirai *et al.*, 1989).

JUN, JUNB and *JUND* are all expressed in human peripheral blood granulocytes (Mollinedo *et al.*, 1991).

Protein function

Jun transcription, like that of *Fos*, is rapidly activated in mitogenically stimulated fibroblasts and two other genes closely related to *Jun*, *Junb* and *Jund*, are also members of the group of "early response genes", although *Jund* is significantly expressed in quiescent cells. Bovine papilloma virus transgenic mice develop dermal fibrosarcoma and the enhanced expression of *Jun* and *Junb* but not of *Jund* or *Fos* correlates with the onset of an intermediate stage of tumour development (Bossy-Wetzel *et al.*, 1992).

JUN forms heterodimers with FOS and with FOS-related antigens (FRA1, FRA2) that bind with high affinity to the AP-1 consensus site (the *cis*-acting TPA response element TRE, 5'-TGA^C/$_G$TCA-3'). Human JUN was originally termed AP-1 (PEA1 in mice; Bohmann *et al.*, 1987) and was first identified by its selective binding to enhancer elements in the *cis* control regions of SV40 and human metallothionein IIA. AP-1 is a complex of polypeptides (39–47 kDa) comprised predominantly of heterodimers of members of the JUN and FOS families. Material precipitated by anti-JUN antibody is generally denoted as JUN/AP-1 (p39; Chiu *et al.*, 1988). The AP-1 complex binds to the same consensus sequence as GCN4 and in artificial constructs both v-JUN and JUN activate transcription via AP-1 binding sites.

JUN homodimers also bind to AP-1 sites with high affinity, to which JUNB and JUND bind very weakly (Ryseck and Bravo, 1991) and JUN and JUND *trans*-activate the human *MYB* promoter via an AP-1-like sequence (Nicolaides *et al.*, 1992). However, JUN affinity depends on the flanking sequences (ATGACTCAPy>>ATGACTCAPu: for the sequence CTGACTCAT, more distant nucleotides may confer high or low affinity). Proteins of the FOS family enhance JUN binding to AP-1 in the order FOSB>FRA1>FOS and also confer significant affinity for DNA on JUNB and JUND, increasing the half-lives of the JUN–FOS/DNA complexes. JUN–JUN and JUN–FOS complexes also bind to CRE-containing nucleotides but with affinities that depend on the flanking sequences. The FOS–JUN and ATF–CREB families of transcription factors form selective cross-family heterodimers having distinct DNA binding specificities (see **Introduction**, page 13; Hai and Curran, 1991).

JUN and JUND but not JUNB also form complexes with OCT-1 that activate transcription from an element in the IL-2 promoter (Ullman *et al.*, 1993). This mechanism of transcriptional activation occurs during T cell stimulation and is Ca^{2+}-sensitive and inhibited by cyclosporin A.

The protein IP-1 (30–40 kDa, labile, located both in the nucleus and cytoplasm) specifically blocks AP-1 complex and FOS–JUN binding to DNA when unphosphorylated but not after PKA-mediated phosphorylation (Auwerx and Sassone-Corsi, 1991). AP-1 DNA binding is increased in cells treated with A23187 or dibutyryl cAMP, consistent with an inhibition of IP-1 activity by phosphorylation (Auwerx and Sassone-Corsi, 1992; de Groot and Sassone-Corsi, 1992).

In mitogenically stimulated fibroblasts essentially all JUN protein exists as JUN–FOS heterodimers, which presumably facilitates binding to the region of dyad symmetry that comprises the AP-1 consensus sequence. JUN shares approximately 44% sequence homology in its C-terminal 70 amino acids with GCN4, the yeast protein that stimulates the transcription of several unlinked genes by binding to upstream regulatory regions, and JUN can function as a transcriptional regulator in GCN4-deficient yeast strains. JUN, JUNB, JUND and GCN4 can all form homodimers that bind to DNA, but the heterodimeric forms have greatly increased affinity and efficacy as transcriptional activators (Nakabeppu et al., 1988; Chiu et al., 1988).

Structure of the ASV 17 provirus and mouse *Jun*

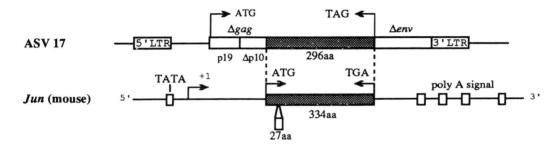

220 residues encoding viral *gag* p19 and p10 are joined in-frame to 296 *Jun*-encoded amino acids. v-*jun* also lacks an extensive 3' non-translated region of *Jun* mRNA. The 27 amino acid δ region is missing from v-JUN.

Transcriptional regulation

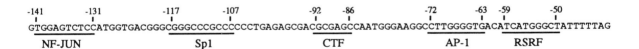

Jun genes (human and chicken) contain a potential AP-1 binding site, to which JUN itself binds to confer positive autoregulation of its own transcription, and NF-JUN, Sp-1, CTF and RSRF binding sites within the same −60 to −142 region (Angel et al., 1988b). The RSRF (related to serum response factor) site is sufficient for EGF, serum or TPA induction when assayed using a heterologous promoter and a number of factors in nuclear extracts of HeLa cells bind to RSRF (Han et al., 1992). There is >70% homology between the human and mouse promoters in the region between −142 and −441 with a second AP-1 site between −183 and −192. The region between −142 and −711 is responsible for mediating TPA-induced *Jun* transcription (Unlap et al., 1992).

Part of the DNA binding domain of the JUN–AP-1 complex is very similar in sequence to a region of the 43 kDa cAMP responsive element (CRE; consensus sequence: TGACGTCA) binding protein (CREB; Bohmann et al., 1987; Angel et al., 1988b). Furthermore, the transcriptional activity of the *Jun* promoter is repressed by CREB so that in NIH 3T3 cells that express CREB,

Jun is no longer induced by serum. The murine protein mXBP/CRE-BP2 (>99% identical to human CRE-BP1 but missing 94 N-terminal amino acids and internal residues 150–247) binds specifically to CRE. mXBP–JUN dimers bind with high affinity to the CRE but not to the TPA response element (TRE; Ivashkiv *et al.*, 1990). When phosphorylated, however, CREB does not bind to the AP-1 site, and this is promoted by the action of protein kinase A following forskolin addition. Thus, depending on its phosphorylation state, CREB can act as an inhibitor or an activator of *Jun* transcription. There is a range of CREB proteins, some but not all of which form heterodimers with JUN (Benbrook and Jones, 1990; Macgregor *et al.*, 1990; Dwarki *et al.*, 1990). JUN–AP-1 itself can undergo phosphorylation via the action of protein kinase C.

Nuclear factor JUN (NF-JUN), present in human myeloid leukaemia cells but not in monocytes, granulocytes, T cells or lung fibroblasts, is activated by TNFα or TPA and causes transcriptional induction of *Jun* (Brach *et al.*, 1992). NF-JUN contains 55 and 125 kDa subunits and has features in common with NF-κB, including the capacity to translocate from the cytoplasm to the nucleus.

The E1A 13S RNA product directly activates *Fos*, *Jun* and *Junb* promoters, inducing JUN–AP-1 binding to a TRE. E1A *trans* activation is mediated by the JUN2 TRE (TTACCTCA) sequence to which JUN–ATF-2 heterodimers bind (van Dam *et al.*, 1993). E1A 12S RNA expression alone does not activate via TRE but, together with JUN does so: this activation is, in turn, blocked by expression of FOS (de Groot *et al.*, 1991a). Thus FOS modulates the dominance of E1A 12S or 13S products.

Junb transcription is specifically stimulated by the expression of v-SRC, the tyrosine kinase activity of which modulates binding of factors to a 121 bp region encompassing the CCAAT and TATAA elements (Apel *et al.*, 1992).

Relationship between JUN and v-JUN and the origin of the ASV 17 open reading frame

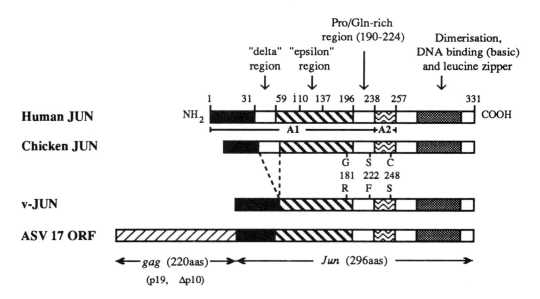

Region A1 (activator domain, amino acids 5–196) confers transcriptional activity when fused to a heterologous DNA binding domain (e.g. Sp-1 or GAL4). Residues 67–77 and 108–117 constitute the two homology box regions (HOB1 and HOB2) that are conserved in FOS and C/EBP (see **FOS**). Amino acids 92–110 (the a1 region) function as an activation domain (Baichwal *et al.*, 1992). Amino acids 1–87 of this domain mediate repression of the muscle creatine kinase enhancer (Li *et al.*, 1992: see Table 3.3).

The ε region (amino acids 110–137) together with the δ region, interacts with a cell-type-specific repressor protein (Baichwal *et al.*, 1992).

Region A2 (activation domain, amino acids 238–257) is essential for *in vivo* activity. The δ domain (amino acids 28–54 in chicken JUN), missing in v-JUN, stabilizes the interaction of a cell-specific transcriptional inhibitor with A1 (Baichwal and Tjian, 1990). The inhibitor occurs in HeLa TK⁻ cells but not in the human hepatoma cell line HepG2, F9 cells or *Drosophila* Schneider (SL2) cells. Expression of v-SRC or oncogenic RAS disrupts the JUN–inhibitor complex by interacting with the A1 domain, increasing transcriptional activity (Baichwal *et al.*, 1991). For v-SRC this appears to require the SH2 domain.

Amino acids 190–224 form a Pro/Gln-rich *Jun* ancilliary DNA binding domain (Abate *et al.*, 1991).

The C-terminal ~110 amino acids is the DNA binding domain, comprising a basic region and a leucine zipper, highly conserved within the JUN family. This region, together with the transactivation domain, is essential for *Jun*-induced oncogenic transformation (Morgan *et al.*, 1992).

In v-JUN there is a 27 amino acid deletion (the "δ region") in the N-terminal region of JUN and three non-conservative substitutions in the C-terminal half (Gly181, Ser222 and Cys248), two of which are in the DNA binding domain (Nishimura and Vogt, 1988). The Ser222 to Phe mutation prevents the phosphorylation *in vitro* of the negative regulatory site by glycogen synthase kinase-3 (see **Phosphorylation of JUN**, below) and the mutation Cys248 to Ser may disrupt a regulatory mechanism involving the reversible oxidation of Cys248 which can inactivate DNA binding to AP-1 sites *in vitro* (Frame *et al.*, 1991).

Sequences of human JUN, JUNB and JUND

```
JUN    (1)    MTAKMETTFYDD ALNASFLPSESGPYGYSNPKILKQSMTLNLADPVGSLK
JUNB   (1)    -CT---QP--H-DSYT-TGYGRAP-GLSLHDY-L--P-LAV-----YR---APGARGPG
JUND   (1)            MKKDALTLSLSEQVAAALKPAAAPPPTPLRA

                       *              *
JUN   (51)    PHLRAKNSDLLTSPDVGLLKLASPELERLIIQSSNGHITTTPTPTQFLCPKNVTDEQE
JUNB  (60)    PEGGGGGSYFSGQG-DTGAS-----S------VPN---VI------PGQYFYPRGGGSGG
JUND  (32)    DGAPSA-PPDG--A---L---------------  --LV-----SS---Y--VAAS-EQ

JUN  (109)    GFAEGFVRALAELHSQNTLPSVTSAAQPVNGAGMVAPAVASVAGGSGSGGFSASLHSEPP
JUNB (120)    -AGGAGGGVTE-QEGFADGFVKALDDLHKMNHVTPPNVSLGAT--PPA-PGGVYAGP---
JUND  (93)    E------K--ED--K--Q-GAGAA--AAAAA--GPSGTATGS-PPGELAPAA-APEAPVY

JUN  (169)    VYANLSNFNPGALSSGGGAPSYGAAGLAFPAQPQQQQQQPPHHLPQ   QMPVQHPRLQAL
JUNB (180)    PVYTNLSSYSP-SA-S---GAAVGT-SSY-TTTISYLPHAPPFAGGHPAQLGLGRGASTF
JUND (151)    ANLSSYAGGA-GAGGAATVAFAAEPVPFP-PP-PGALG--RLAALKDEPQT-PDVPSF

                     *         *   *      *
JUN  (226)    KEEPQTVPEMP  GETPPLSPIDMESQERIKAERKRMRNRIAASKCRKRKLERIARLEEK
JUNB (240)    ---------ARSRDA---V---N--D-----V----L---L--T-------------
JUND (209)             --S--------DT----------L------------------S-----

JUN  (284)    VKTLKAQNSELASTANMLREQVAQLKQKVMNHVNSGCQLMLTQQLQTF (331)
JUNB (300)    ------E-AG-S---GL------------T--SN----L-GVKGHA- (347)
JUND (256)    ----_S--T-_---SL------------LS-------LPQH-VPAY (303)
```

Dashes indicate positions in JUNB and JUND that are identical to those in JUN. The three JUN proteins are 50% homologous in sequence and each has six domains separated by segments of variable length and sequence. The basic and leucine zipper regions are underlined. * Indicates residues in JUN phosphorylated by MAP kinase (Ser63, Ser73), casein kinase II (Thr231, Ser249) and glycogen synthase kinase-3 (Thr239, Ser243, Ser249).

Sequences of chicken JUN and v-JUN

```
Chicken JUN   (1)                                           MEPTFYEDALNASFAPP
v-JUN         (1)                               VPPLRGLCSMSAK----------------

              (18)   ESGGYGYNNAKVLKQSMTLNLSDAASSLKPHLRNKNADILTSPDVGLLKLASPELERLII
              (31)   ----------                            ---------------------

              (78)   QSSNGLITTTPTPTQFLCPKNVTDEQEGFAEGFVRALAELHNQNTLPSVTSAAQPVSGGM
              (91)   ------------------------------------------------------------

              (138)  APVSSMAGGGSFNTSLHSEPPVYANLSNFNPNALNSAPNYNANGMGYAPQHHINPQMPVQ
              (144)  ------------------------------------------R-----------------

              (198)  HPRLQALKEEPQTVPEMPGETPPLSPIDMESQERIKAERKRMRNRIAASKCRKRKLERIA
              (190)  ----------------------F-----------------------S---------

              (258)  RLEEKVKTLKAQNSELASTANMLREQVAQLKQKVMNHVNSGCQLMLTQQLQTF  (310)
              (248)  ---------------------------------------------------- (296)
```

Phosphorylation of JUN

In resting human epithelial cells and fibroblasts JUN is phosphorylated on five sites (serine and threonine): three of these (phosphorylated *in vitro* by glycogen synthase kinase-3) are just upstream of the DNA binding domain (residues 227–252). Activation of protein kinase C causes dephosphorylation of one or more of these residues leading to increased binding to the AP-1 promoter site (Boyle *et al.*, 1991; Hunter and Karin, 1992). Mutation of Ser243 to Phe blocks phosphorylation of all three sites *in vitro* and increases the *trans*-activation capability of JUN by tenfold. In v-JUN this serine residue is not present and v-JUN binds to the AP-1 site to activate constitutively transcription of the gene. Ser249 may also be phosphorylated by the DNA-dependent protein kinase or by casein kinase II, dependent on the cellular location of JUN (Bannister *et al.*, 1993).

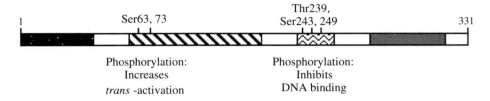

Transforming oncogenes, including *Hras*, stimulate AP-1 activity: in rat embryo fibroblasts *Hras* increases JUN synthesis by 4.5-fold but causes a 35-fold increase in JUN phosphorylation particularly at Ser63 and Ser73 in the N-terminus (Binetruy *et al.*, 1991; Smeal *et al.*, 1991). Similar increases in the phosphorylation state of serines 63 and 73 are caused by v-SIS, v-SRC and RAF-1 (Smeal *et al.*, 1992). The N-terminal sites are phosphorylated *in vitro* and in U937 cells by

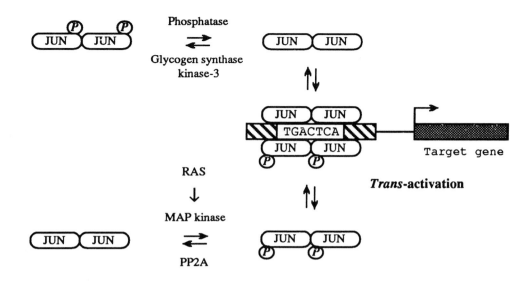

mitogen-activated protein kinases (MAP kinases; Pulverer *et al.*, 1991, 1993). *Hras* also affects the overall phosphorylation state of the C-terminus, producing under-phosphorylated forms of JUN that bind to DNA (similar to the effect of TPA). These effects may underlie the cooperativity between *Ras* and *Jun* in transforming these cells.

Phosphorylation of sites in the N-terminal region of JUN is reversed by protein phosphatase 2A (PP2A), to which v-JUN is insensitive (Black *et al.*, 1991). A possible PP2A-sensitive site (Ser48) lies in the δ domain, deleted from v-JUN, but other sites have not yet been mapped.

Chicken JUN is efficiently phosphorylated *in vitro* by p34^{cdc2}, ERK1 (p44^{mapk}), protein kinase C or casein kinase II (Baker *et al.*, 1992). The major sites of phosphorylation are serines 63, 73 and 246 but, in contrast to the observations summarized above, the phosphorylation state of these residues does not affect FOS–JUN dimerization, DNA binding or *in vitro* transcription activity.

In unstimulated cells JUN mainly exists as a phosphorylated, inactive form in equilibrium with a hypophosphorylated form that is competent to bind to DNA. The equilibrium is maintained by a specific protein kinase and a phosphatase and shifted to the right by agents stimulating JUN-mediated transcription from AP-1 sites. The equilibrium is also shifted to the right in cells transfected so as to increase the number of AP-1 binding sites, which raises the concentration of bound dimer and causes a net dephosphorylation of JUN (Papavassiliou *et al.*, 1992).

Leucine zippers

The homology between the DNA binding regions of JUN and CREB includes the leucine zipper motif involved in the interaction of JUN–AP-1 and FOS (Landschulz *et al.*, 1988; Kouzarides and Ziff, 1988). Leucine zippers are amphipathic α helices that contain four or five leucine residues separated by six other amino acids (Busch and Sassone-Corsi, 1990). This distribution gives approximate alignment of the leucine resides on the surface of an α helix and dimerization is thought to occur via hydrophobic interaction between their sidechains, specificity being conferred by the intervening sequences. Eight amino acids comprising the heptad repeat region from FOS and from JUN are sufficient to mediate preferential heterodimer formation (Schuermann *et al.*, 1991; O'Shea *et al.*, 1992).

In addition to the JUN and FOS families, the oncoproteins RAF and MET, the intermediate

                    L1   L2   L3   L4   L5

FOS (136) EEEKRRIRRERNKMAAAKCRNRRRELTDTLQAETDQLEDEKSALQTEIANLLKEKEKLE (194)
FOSB (154) EEEKRRVRRERNKLAAAKCRNRRRELTDRLQAETDQLEEEKAELESEIAELQKEKERLE (212)
FRA1 (104) EEERRRVRRERNKLAAAKCRNRRKELTDFLQAETDKLEDEKSGLQREIEELQKQKERLE (162)
                          *

JUN (254) ERIKAERKRMRNRIAASKCRKRKLERIARLEEKVKTLKAQNSELASTANMLREQVAQL (311)
JUNB (270) ERIKVERKRLRNRLAATKCRKRKLERIARLEDEKVKTLKAENAGLSSTAGLLREQVAQL (328)
JUND (225) ERIKAERKRLRNRIAASKCRKRKLERISRLEEKVKTLKSQNTELASTASLLREQVAQL (283)

GCN4   SSDPAALKRARNTEAARRSRARKLQRMKQLEDKVEELLSKNYHLENEVARLKKLVGER
CREB   AARKREVRLMKNREAARECRKKKKEYVKCLENRVAVLENQNKTLIEELKALKDLYCHK

                    L1   L2   L3   L4

MYC (345) PRSSDTEENVKRRTHNVLERQRRNELKRSFFALRDQIPELENNEKAPKVVILKKATAYILSVQAEEQKLISEEDLLRKRREQLKHKLEQLRNSCA (439)
MYCN (372) PRNSDSEDSERRRNHNILERQRRNDLRSSFLTLRDHVPELVKNEKAAKVVILKKATEYVHSLQAEEHQLLLEKEKLQARQQQLLKKIEHARTC (464)
MYCL (272) PVSSDTEDVTKRKNHNFLERKRRNDLRSRFLALRDQVPTLASCSKAPKVVILSKALEYLQALVGAEKRMATEKRQLRCRQQQLQKRIAYLSGY (364)

MYOD1   ACKRKTTNADRRKAATMRERRRLSKVNEAFETLKRCTSSNPNQ-RLPKVEILRNAIRYIEGLQALLR
E12   PEQKAEREKERVANNARERLRVRDINEAFKELGRMCQLHLNSEKPQTKLLILHQAVSVILNLEQQVR
E47   LEEKDLRDRERRMANNARERVRVRDINEAFRELGRMCQMHLKSDKAQTKLLELQQAVQVILGLEQQV

Sequences of leucine zipper and helix–loop–helix transcription factors. Solid bars indicate basic regions; L1-L5 leucine zipper motifs. Numbers indicate amino acid position in the complete sequence. * Indicates the cysteine residue conserved in the FOS, JUN and ATF/CREB families that regulates DNA binding (see *FOS*).

filament protein vimentin (Capetanaki *et al.*, 1990), the transcription factors C/EBP (Landschulz *et al.*, 1988), CREB, GCN4 and the yeast factor yAP-1 all contain leucine zippers, although in CREB and GCN4 the fifth leucine is replaced by arginine and lysine respectively and in yAP-1 Leu 3 has become an asparagine. The leucine zipper motif in these proteins is closely adjacent to a DNA binding domain comprised of two clusters of basic amino acids separated by a short spacer region. This structure constitutes a third type of potential DNA binding domain in addition to the α helix/β turn/α helix motif contained in each subunit of some proteins that bind to target sequences as dimers and the zinc finger motif in which coordinate binding of zinc atoms via cysteine or histidine residues promotes the affinity for DNA. A subgroup of the leucine zipper family contains the MYC family of oncoproteins (MYC, MYCL and MYCN), the octamer binding protein OCT2, the κ enhancer binding proteins E12 and E47 and the products of the *Drosophila* genes *daughterless*, *twist* and *achaete scute* (Prendergast and Ziff, 1989), together with the myogenic proteins MyoD, myogenin, Myf-5 and herculin (Miner and Wold, 1990) that regulate the progression from multipotential mesodermal stem cell to fully differentiated multinucleated myotube. This group contains fewer leucine residues in the zipper region and a low content of adjacent basic amino acids but has a basic region nearer the C-terminus, giving rise to an amphipathic helix–loop–helix motif. In artificial constructs both the leucine zipper and basic domains have been shown to be essential for DNA binding and to be functionally interchangeable between FOS, JUN and GCN4 (Ransone *et al.*, 1989). There is evidence that the basic regions take up a stable α-helical structure when bound to a specific DNA site (Sauer, 1990). Id is another member of the helix–loop–helix group but this protein lacks the basic region essential for DNA binding. Id specifically binds to MyoD, E12 and E47 thereby diminishing their affinity for DNA (Benezra *et al.*, 1990).

Table 3.3 *Cellular Jun mRNA expression*

Cell type	Agents	Comments
Human fibroblasts (WI-38)	Serum	In addition to the early (1 h) transient expression of *JUN* and *JUNB* mRNA, transient *JUN* transcription (but not *JUNB*) also occurs in the G_1/S period (27–35 h). Increased AP-1 occurs at both times but the complexes involved are different: anti-FOS antibody decreases binding in early G_1 but not at the S phase border (Carter *et al.*, 1991)
NIH 3T3 fibroblasts	Serum, dexamethasone	Dexamethasone inhibits *Jun* transcription, consistent with interaction between the glucocorticoid hormone receptor (GHR) and the AP-1 complex regulating *Jun* expression, as occurs in the inhibition of collagenase transcription by GHR (Lee *et al.*, 1991)
Skeletal muscle myoblasts	10% serum ± ASV 17	*Jun* or v-*jun* inhibits differentiation of myoblasts into myotubes. v-*jun* inhibits the expression of the muscle-specific proteins desmin, myosin and creatine phosphokinase and the cells continue to replicate (Su *et al.*, 1991). Constitutive expression of JUN inhibits *trans* activation of the *MyoD* promoter and JUN, JUNB or FOS inhibits *trans* activation of the muscle creatine kinase enhancer by myogenin or *MyoD* (Li *et al.*, 1992). JUND, however, which is constitutively expressed in muscle cells, does not inhibit *trans* activation by myogenin. MyoD protein suppresses the *trans* activation by JUN of genes linked to an AP-1 site. These effects reflect the fact that MyoD and JUN proteins physically associate in normal myoblasts (Bengal *et al.*, 1992)

Table 3.3 *Continued*

Cell type	Agents	Comments
Differentiated BC3H1 myocytes	TGFβ	TGFβ causes de-differentiation: accompanied by rapid (15 min), transient transcription of *Junb* (20-fold above the level in unstimulated cells) and a much smaller increase (2.5-fold) in *Jun* (Li *et al.*, 1990). A third member of the *Jun* family is constitutively expressed in these cells and is not regulated by TGFβ
Rat aortic smooth muscle cells	Angiotensin II	Transient increase in *Jun* transcription: maximal at 1 h (Naftilan *et al.*, 1990)
Human breast cancer cell line MCF-7	Overexpression of *JUN*, *FOS*, *JUNB*	Suppresses estrogen-dependent transcription of an ERE-containing reporter gene. *JUND* expression is without effect. Repression is dependent on amino acids 147–220 in JUN (Doucas *et al.*, 1991)
Chicken oviduct and liver	Tamoxifen	The anti-estrogen tamoxifen increases *Jun* mRNA levels in oviduct (2.5-fold in 4 h) and blocks *Jun* expression in the liver (Lau *et al.*, 1991)
HeLa and CV-1	Retinoic acid (RA)-activated RA receptors	Activated RA receptors (α, β or γ) repress AP-1-mediated induction of gene expression. This suggests that the receptor may form a non-activating complex with JUN. This could explain the inhibitory effects of RA on cell growth and transformation (Schule *et al.*, 1991)
HeLa cells	*ErbA*, v-*erbA*	Transcription of reporter constructs expressing AP-1 and TRE sites was stimulated by JUN/ERBA protein interaction, whereas v-ERBA represses the JUN response. In constructs expressing only the AP-1 site, however, v-ERBA co-activates transcription with JUN (Sharif and Privalsky, 1992)
Human embryo lung cells	Human cytomegalovirus (HCMV) infection	HCMV infection causes DNA synthesis preceded by a transient increase in *FOS*, *JUN* (40 min) and *MYC* transcription (Boldogh *et al.*, 1991)
Human B cell line (SKW6.4: EBV-transformed)	Platelet activating factor (PAF)	Stimulates *JUN* and *FOS* transcription (90 min) together with other "early" responses (phosphotidylinositol and phosphotidylcholine turnover, increase in $[Ca^{2+}]_i$ and arachidonic acid release; Schulam *et al.*, 1991)
Human T cell line JPX-9 (Jurkat-derived)	HTLV-1 TAX1 (TAX1 expression plasmid)	TAX1 *trans*-activates the expression of immediate early genes (*JUN, JUNB, JUND, FOS, FRA1, EGR1* and *EGR2*). Consistent with the increase in binding to TPA response elements (TREs) observed in HTLV-1-infected T cells (Fujii *et al.*, 1991)
Mouse fibroblasts	Polyomavirus middle T antigen	Expression of middle T antigen strongly activates *Jun* transcription as a result of increased AP-1 transcription factor activity (Schontal *et al.*, 1992). The extent of *Jun* activation correlates with the transforming efficiency of polyoma mutants
Mouse embryonal carcinoma cell line F9	DNA replication assay	Overexpression of *Fos* and *Jun* strongly stimulates DNA replication from the polyoma virus origin of replication, acting via the AP-1 site. The effect requires AP-1 to be adjacent to the origin core sequence: when AP-1 is inverted and placed ~ 2.3 kb from the origin and early mRNA promoter, FOS–JUN activates transcription but not replication (Murakami *et al.*, 1991)

Table 3.3 *Continued*

Cell type	Agents	Comments
Embryonal carcinoma cell line PC19	Adenovirus E1A	Type 5 E1A induces *Jun, Junb* and *Jund* transcription. Type 12 E1A induces only *Jun* (as does retinoic acid) and type 12 E1A (but not type 5 E1A) causes complete differentiation (de Groot *et al.*, 1991b)
Chinese hamster ovary cells	Amino acid derivation	Removal of a single amino acid activates *Jun, Myc* and ornithine decarboxylase transcription (Pohjanpelto and Holta, 1990)
Hamster insulinoma (HIT) cells	Glucose deprivation	Removal of glucose activates *Jun* transcription and JUN represses the human insulin promoter when it is expressed in HIT cells, acting via cAMP response elements (Inagaki *et al.*, 1992)
Hamster tracheal epithelial (HTE) and rat pleural mesothelial (RPM) cells	Asbestos	A 2 h exposure causes a progressive increase in both *Fos* and *Jun* expression in RPM cells and of *Jun* in HTE cells (Heintz *et al.*, 1993)

Databank file names and accession numbers

	GENE	*EMBL*	*SWISSPROT*	*REFERENCES*
ASV 17	v-*jun*	Reacsjun M16266	TJUN_AVIS1 P05411	Maki *et al.*, 1987
Human	*JUN*	Hsjuna J04111	TAP1_HUMAN P05412	Bohmann *et al.*, 1987 Hattori *et al.*, 1988
Human	*JUNB*	Hsjuncaa M29039 Hsjunb X51345	TABP_HUMAN P17275	Nomura *et al.*, 1990 Schutte *et al.*, 1989b
Human	*JUND*	Hsjund X51346	TAPD_HUMAN P17535	Nomura *et al.*, 1990 Berger and Shaul, 1991
Human	*JUN*	(promoter region)		Unlap *et al.*, 1992
Mouse	*Jun*	Mmjun X12761 Mmjunc X12740 Mmcjun J04115 Hscjunu X59744	TAP1_MOUSE P05627	Lamph *et al.*, 1988 Ryder *et al.*, 1988 Ryseck *et al.*, 1988
Mouse	*Junb*	Mmjunba J03236	TABP_MOUSE P09450	Ryder *et al.*, 1988
Mouse	*Jund*	Mmjund J04509 Mmjunda X15358 Mmjundr J05205	TAPD_MOUSE P15066	Ryder *et al.*, 1989 Hirai *et al.*, 1989 Berger and Shaul, 1991
Rat	*Jun*	Rsjunap1 X17163 Rnrjg9 X17215	TAP1_RAT P17325	Sakai *et al.*, 1989 Kitabayashi *et al.*, 1990
Rat	*Junb*	Rnpjunb X54686	TABP_RAT P24898	Kawakami *et al.*, 1992
Chicken	*Jun*	Ggjun M57467	TAP1_CHICK P18870	Nishimura and Vogt, 1988
Chicken	*Jund*	Gdjundg X60063		Hartl *et al.*, 1991
Japanese quail	*Jun*	Ccjun X15547	TAP1_COTJA P12981	Brun *et al.*, 1989
Drosophila	D-*jun*	Dmjun M36181	TAP1_DROME P18289	Zhang *et al.*, 1990 Perkins *et al.*, 1990

Reviews

Busch, S.J. and Sassone-Corsi, P. (1990). Dimers, leucine zippers and DNA-binding domains. Trends Genet., 6, 36–40.

Hunter, T. and Karin, M. (1992). The regulation of transcription by phosphorylation. Cell, 70, 375–387.

Kouzarides, T. and Ziff, E. (1989). Behind the fos and jun zipper. Cancer Cells, 1, 71–76.

Prendergast, G.C. and Ziff, E.B. (1989). DNA-binding motif. Nature, 341, 392.

Sauer, R.T. (1990). Scissors and helical forks. Nature, 347, 514–515.

Vogt, P.K. and Bos, T.J. (1990). *jun*: oncogene and transcription factor. Adv. Cancer Res., 55, 1–35.

Papers

Abate, C., Luk, D. and Curran, T. (1991). Transcriptional regulation by *Fos* and *Jun in vitro*: interaction among multiple activator and regulatory domains. Mol. Cell. Biol., 11, 3624–3632.

Adunyah, S.E., Unlap, T.M., Wagner, F. and Kraft, A.S. (1991). Regulation of c-jun expression and AP-1 enhancer activity by granulocyte-macrophage colony-stimulating factor. J. Biol. Chem., 266, 5670–5675.

Angel, P., Allegretto, E.A., Okino, S.T., Hattori, K., Boyle, W.J., Hunter, T. and Karin, M. (1988a). Oncogene *jun* encodes a sequence-specific *trans*-activator similar to AP-1. Nature, 332, 166–171.

Angel, P., Hattori, K., Smeal, T. and Karin, M. (1988b). The *jun* proto-oncogene is positively autoregulated by its product, Jun/AP-1. Cell, 55, 875–885.

Apel, I., Yu, C.-L., Wang, T., Dobry, C., van Antwerp, M.E., Jove, R. and Prochownik, E.V. (1992). Regulation of the *jun*B gene by v-*src*. Mol. Cell. Biol., 12, 3356–3364.

Auwerx, J. and Sassone-Corsi, P. (1991). IP-1: a dominant inhibitor of fos/jun whose activity is modulated by phosphorylation. Cell, 64, 983–993.

Auwerx, J. and Sassone-Corsi, P. (1992). AP-1 (fos-jun) regulation by IP-1: effect of signal transduction pathways and cell growth. Oncogene, 7, 2271–2280.

Baichwal, V.R. and Tjian, R. (1990). Control of c-jun activity by interaction of a cell-specific inhibitor with regulatory domain δ: differences between v- and c-jun. Cell, 63, 815–825.

Baichwal, V.R., Park, A. and Tjian, R. (1991). v-src and EJ ras alleviate repression of c-jun by a cell-specific inhibitor. Nature, 352, 165–168.

Baichwal, V.R., Park, A. and Tjian, R. (1992). The cell-type-specific activator region of c-*jun* juxtaposes constitutive and negatively regulated domains. Genes Devel., 6, 1493–1502.

Baker, S.J., Kerppola, T.K., Luk, D., Vandenberg, M.T., Marshak, D.R., Curran, T. and Abate, C. (1992). Jun is phosphorylated by several protein kinases at the same sites that are modified in serum-stimulated fibroblasts. Mol. Cell. Biol., 12, 4694–4705.

Bannister, A.J., Gottlieb, T.M., Kouzarides, T. and Jackson, S.P. (1993). c-Jun is phosphorylated by the DNA-dependent protein kinase *in vitro*: definition of the minimal kinase recognition motif. Nucleic Acids Res., 21, 1289–1295.

Benbrook, D.M. and Jones, N.C. (1990). Heterodimer formation between CREB and JUN proteins. Oncogene 5, 295–302.

Benezra, R., Davis, R.L., Lockshon, D., Turner, D.L. and Weintraub, H. (1990). The protein Id: a negative regulator of helix-loop-helix DNA binding proteins. Cell, 61, 49–59.

Bengal, E., Ransone, Scharfmann, R., Dwarki, V.J., Tapscott, S.J., Weintraub, H. and Verma, I.M. (1992). Functional antagonism between c-jun and myoD proteins: a direct physical association. Cell, 68, 507–519.

Berger, I. and Shaul, Y. (1991). Structure and function of human *jun*-D. Oncogene, 6, 561–566.

Binetruy, B., Smeal, T. and Karin, M. (1991). Ha-*Ras* augments c-*Jun* activity and stimulates phosphorylation of its activation domain. Nature, 351, 122–127.

Black, E.J., Street, A.J. and Gillespie, D.A.F. (1991). Protein phosphatase 2A reverses phosphorylation of c-*jun* specified by the delta domain *in vitro*: correlation with oncogenic activation and deregulated transactivation activity of v-*jun*. Oncogene, 6, 1949–1958.

Bohmann, D., Bos, T.J., Admon, A., Nishimura, T. Vogt, P.K. and Tijan, R. (1987). Human proto-oncogene c-*jun* encodes a DNA binding domain with structural and functional properties of transcription factor AP-1. Science, 238, 1386–1392.

Boldogh, I., AbuBakar, S., Deng, C.Z. and Albrecht, T. (1991). Transcriptional activation of cellular oncogene fos, jun, and myc by human cytomegalovirus. J. Virol., 65, 1568–1571.

Bos, T.J., Monteclaro, F.S., Mitsunobu, F., Ball, A.R., Chang, C.H.W., Nishimura, T. and Vogt, P.K. (1990). Efficient transformation of chicken embryo fibroblasts by c-jun requires structural modification of coding and noncoding sequences. Genes Devel., 4, 1677–1687.

Bossy-Wetzel, E., Bravo, R. and Hanahan, D. (1992). Transcription factors junB and c-jun are selectively up-regulated and functionally implicated in fibrosarcoma development. Genes Devel., 6, 2340–2351.

Boyle, W.J., Smeal, T., Defize, L.H.K., Angel, P., Woodgett, J.R., Karin, M. and Hunter, T. (1991). Activation of protein kinase C decreases phosphorylation of c-jun at sites that negatively regulate its DNA-binding activity. Cell, 64, 573–584.

Brach, M.A., Herrmann, F., Yamada, H., Bauerle, P.A. and Kufe, D.W. (1992). Identification of NF-jun, a novel inducible transcription factor that regulates c-*jun* expression. EMBO J., 11, 1479–1486.

Brun, G., La Vista, N., Dangy, J.P. and Castellazzi, M. (1989). Nucleotide sequence of the quail c-*Jun* protooncogene. Nucleic Acids Res., 17, 6393.

Capetanaki, Y,. Kuisk, I., Rothblum, K. and Starnes, S. (1990). Mouse vimentin: structural relationship to *fos*, *jun*, CREB and *tpr*. Oncogene, 5, 645–655.

Carr, M.D. and Mott, R.F. (1991). The transcriptional control proteins c-*Myb* and v-*Myb* contain a basic region DNA binding motif. FEBS Letts., 282, 293–294.

Carter, R., Cosenza, S.C., Pena, A., Lipson, K., Soprano, D.R. and Soprano, K.J. (1991). A potential role for c-*jun* in cell cycle progression through late G1 and S. Oncogene, 6, 229–235.

Chiu, R., Boyle, W.J., Meek, J., Smeal, T., Hunter, T. and Karin, M. (1988). The c-*fos* protein interacts with c-*jun*/AP-1 to stimulate transcription of AP-1 responsive genes. Cell, 54, 541–552.

Colotta, F., Polentarutti, N., Sironi, M. and Mantovani, A. (1992). Expression and involvement of c-*fos* and c-*jun* protooncogenes in programmed cell death induced by growth factor deprivation in lymphoid cell lines. J. Biol. Chem., 267, 18278–18283.

de Groot, R.P. and Sassone-Corsi, P. (1992). Activation of jun/AP-1 by protein kinase A. Oncogene, 7, 2281–2286.

de Groot, R., Foulkes, N., Mulder, M., Kruijer, W. and Sassone-Corsi, P. (1991a). Positive regulation of *jun*/AP-1 by E1A. Mol. Cell Biol., 11, 192–201.

de Groot, R.P., Meijer, I., van den Brink, S., Mummery, C. and Kruijer, W. (1991b). Differential regulation of *jun*B and *jun*D by adenovirus type 5 and 12 E1A proteins. Oncogene, 6, 2357–2361.

Doucas, V., Spyrou, G. and Yaniv, M. (1991). Unregulated expression of c-*Jun* or c-*Fos* proteins but not *Jun* D inhibits oestrogen receptor activity in human breast cancer derived cells. EMBO J., 10, 2237–2245.

Dwarki, V.J., Montminy, M. and Verma, I.M. (1990). Both the basic region and the 'leucine zipper' domain of the cyclic AMP response element binding (CREB) protein are essential for transcriptional activation. EMBO J., 9, 225–232.

Frame, M.C., Wilkie, N.M., Darling, A.J., Chudleigh, A., Pintzas, A., Lang, J.C. and Gillespie, D.A.F. (1991). Regulation of AP-1/DNA complex formation *in vitro*. Oncogene, 6, 205–209.

Fujii, M., Niki, T., Mori, T., Matsuda, T., Matsui, M., Nomura, N. and Seiki, M. (1991). HTLV-1 Tax induces expression of various immediate early serum responsive genes. Oncogene, 6, 1023–1029.

Hai, T. and Curran, T. (1991). Cross-family dimerization of transcription factors fos/jun and ATF/CREB alters DNA binding specificity. Proc. Natl Acad. Sci. USA, 88, 3720–3724.

Han, T.-H., Lamph, W.W. and Prywes, R. (1992). Mapping of epidermal growth factor-, serum-, and phorbol ester-responsive sequence elements in the c-*jun* promoter. Mol. Cell. Biol., 12, 4472–4477.

Hartl, M., Hutchins, J.T. and Vogt, P.K. (1991). The chicken *jun*D gene and its product. Oncogene, 6, 1623–1631.

Hattori, K., Angel, P., Le Beau, M.M. and Karin M. (1988). Structure and chromosomal localization of the functional intronless human JUN protooncogene. Proc. Natl Acad. Sci. USA, 85, 9148–9152.

Heintz, N.H., Janssen, Y.M. and Mossman, B.T. (1993). Persistent induction of c-*fos* and c-*jun* expression by asbestos. Proc. Natl Acad. Sci. USA, 90, 3299–3303.

Hilberg, F. and Wagner, E.F. (1992). Embryonic stem (ES) cells lacking functional c-*jun*: consequences for growth and differentiation, AP-1 activity and tumorigenicity. Oncogene, 7, 2371–2380.

Hirai, S.-I., Ryseck, R.-P., Mechta, F., Bravo, R. and Yaniv, M. (1989). Characterization of *jun*-D: a new member of the *jun* proto-oncogene family. EMBO J., 8, 1433–1439.

Howard, T.A., Rochelle, J.M., Saunders, A.M. and Seldin, M.F. (1991). A linkage map of mouse chromosome 8: further definition of homologous linkage relationships between mouse chromosome 8 and human chromosomes 8, 16 and 19. Genomics, 10, 207–213.

Huang, T.S., Lee, S.C. and Lin, J.K. (1991). Suppression of c-*Jun*/AP-1 activation by an inhibitor of tumor promotion in mouse fibroblast cells. Proc. Natl Acad. Sci. USA, 88, 5292–5296.

Inagaki, N., Maekawa, T., Sudo, T., Ishii, S., Seino, Y. and Imura, H. (1992). c-jun represses the human insulin promoter activity that depends on multiple cAMP response elements. Proc. Natl Acad. Sci. USA, 89, 1045–1049.

Ito, E., Sweterlitsch, L.A., Tran, P.B., Rauscher, F.J. and Narayanan, R. (1990). Inhibition of PC-12 cell differentiation by the immediate early gene *fra*-1. Oncogene, 5, 1755–1760.

Ivashkiv, L.B., Liou, H.-C., Kara, C.J., Lamph, W.W., Verma, I.M. and Glimcher, L.H. (1990). mXBP/CRE-

BP2 and c-jun form a complex which binds to the cyclic AMP, but not the 12-*O*-tetradecanoylphorbol-13-acetate, response element. Mol. Cell. Biol., 10, 1609–1621.

Kawakami, Z., Kitabayashi, I., Matsuoka, T., Cachelin, G. and Yokoyama, K. (1992). Conserved structural motifs among mammalian *junB* genes. Nucleic Acids Res., 20, 914.

Kitabayashi, I., Saka, F., Gachelin, G. and Yokoyama K. (1990). Nucleotide sequence of rat c-*jun* proto-oncogene. Nucleic Acids Res., 18, 3400.

Kouzarides, T. and Ziff, E. (1988). The role of the leucine zipper in the *fos-jun* interaction. Nature, 336, 646–656.

Kovary, K. and Bravo, R. (1991). Expression of different *Jun* and *Fos* proteins during the G_0-to-G_1 transition in mouse fibroblasts: *in vitro* and *in vivo* associations. Mol. Cell. Biol., 11, 2451–2459.

Lamph, W.W., Wamsley, P., Sassone-Corsi, P. and Verma I.M. (1988). Induction of proto-oncogene JUN/AP-1 by serum and TPA. Nature, 334, 629–631.

Landschulz, W.H., Johnson, P.F. and McKnight, S.L. (1988). The leucine zipper: a hypothetical structure common to a new class of DNA binding proteins. Science, 240, 1759–1764.

Lau, C.K., Subramaniam, M., Rasmussen, K. and Spelsberg, T.C. (1991). Rapid induction of the c-*jun* proto-oncogene in the avian oviduct by the antiestrogen tamoxifen. Proc. Natl Acad. Sci. USA, 88, 829–833.

Lee, H., Shaw, Y.-T., Chiou, S.-T., Chang, W.-C. and Lai, M.-D. (1991). The effects of glucocorticoid hormone on the expression of c-*jun*. FEBS Letts., 280, 134–136.

Li, L., Hu, J.-S. and Olson, E.N. (1990). Different members of the *jun* proto-oncogene family exhibit distinct patterns of expression in response to type β transforming growth factor. J. Biol. Chem., 265, 1556–1562.

Li, L., Chambard, J.-C., Karin, M. and Olson, E.N. (1992). Fos and jun repress transcriptional activation by myogenin and myoD: the amino terminus of jun can mediate repression. Genes Devel., 6, 676–689.

Macgregor, P.F., Abate, C. and Curran, T. (1990). Direct cloning of leucine zipper proteins: Jun binds cooperatively to the CRE with CRE-BP1. Oncogene, 5, 451–458.

Maki, Y., Bos, T.J., Davis, C., Starbuck, M. and Vogt, P.K. (1987). Avian sarcoma virus 17 carries the *jun* oncogene. Proc. Natl Acad. Sci. USA, 84, 2848–2852.

Mattei, M.G., Simon-Chazottes, D., Hirai, S., Ryseck, R.P., Galcheva-Gargova, Z., Guenet, J.-L., Mattei, J.F., Bravo, R. and Yaniv, M. (1990). Chromosomal localization of the three members of the *jun* proto-oncogene family in mouse and man. Oncogene, 5, 151–156.

Miner, J.H. and Wold, B. (1990). Herculin, a fourth member of the *myoD* family of myogenic regulatory genes. Proc. Natl Acad. Sci. USA, 87, 1089–1093.

Mollinedo, F., Vaquerizo, M.J. and Naranjo, J.R. (1991). Expression of c-*jun*, *jun* B and *jun* D proto-oncogenes in human peripheral-blood granulocytes. Biochem. J., 273, 477–479.

Morgan, I.M., Ransone, L.J., Bos, T.J., Verma, I.M. and Vogt, P.K. (1992). Transformation by jun: requirement for leucine zipper, basic region and transactivation domain and enhancement by fos. Oncogene, 7, 1119–1125.

Murakami, Y., Satake, M., Yamaguchi-Iwai, Y., Sakai, M., Muramatsu, M. and Ito, Y. (1991). The nuclear protooncogenes c-*jun* and c-*fos* as regulators of DNA replication. Proc. Natl Acad. Sci. USA, 88, 3947–3951.

Naftilan, A.J., Gilliland, G.K., Eldridge, C.S. and Kraft, A.S. (1990). Induction of the proto-oncogene c-*jun* by angiotensin II. Mol. Cell. Biol., 10, 5536–5540.

Nakabeppu, Y., Ryder, K. and Nathans, D. (1988). DNA binding activities of three murine *jun* proteins: stimulation by *fos*. Cell, 55, 907–915.

Nicolaides, N.C., Correa, I., Casadevall, C., Travali, S., Soprano, K.J. and Calabretta, B. (1992). The jun family members, c-jun and junD, transactivate the human c-*myb* promoter via an AP-1-like element. J. Biol. Chem., 267, 19665–19672.

Nishimura, T. and Vogt, P.K. (1988). The avian cellular homolog of the oncogene *jun*. Oncogene, 3, 659–663.

Nomura, N., Ide, M., Sasamoto, S., Matsui, M., Date, T. and Ishizaki R. (1990). Isolation of human cDNA clones of *jun*-related genes, *jun*-B and *jun*-D. Nucleic Acids Res., 18, 3047–3048.

O'Shea, E.K., Rutkowski, R. and Kim, P.S. (1992). Mechanism of specificity in the fos–jun oncoprotein heterodimer. Cell, 68, 699–708.

Okuno, H., Suzuki, T., Yoshida, Y., Curran, T. and Iba, H. (1991). Inhibition of *jun* transformation by a mutated *fos* gene: design of an anti-oncogene. Oncogene, 6, 1491–1497.

Papavassiliou, A.G., Chavrier, C. and Bohmann, D. (1992). Phosphorylation state and DNA-binding activity of c-jun depend on the intracellular concentration of binding sites. Proc. Natl Acad. Sci. USA, 89, 11562–11565.

Perkins, K.K., Admon, A., Patel, N. and Tjian, R. (1990). The *Drosophila fos*-related AP-1 protein is a developmentally regulated transcription factor. Genes Devel., 4, 822–834.

Pohjanpelto, P. and Holta, E. (1990). Deprivation of a single amino acid induces protein synthesis-dependent increases in c-*jun*, c-*myc* and ornithine decarboxylase mRNAs in Chinese hamster ovary cells. Mol. Cell. Biol., 10, 5814–5821.

Pulverer, B.J., Kyriakis, J.M., Avruch, J., Nikolakaki, E. and Woodgett, J.R. (1991). Phosphorylation of c-*jun* mediated by MAP kinases. Nature, 353, 670–674.

Pulverer, B.J., Hughes, K., Franklin, C.C., Kraft, A.S., Leevers, S.J. and Woodgett, J.R. (1993). Co-purification of mitogen-activated protein kinases with phorbol ester-induced c-jun kinase activity in U937 leukemic cells. Oncogene, 8, 407–415.

Quantin, B. and Breathnach, R. (1988). Epidermal growth factor stimulates transcription of the c-*jun* proto-oncogene in rat fibroblasts. Nature, 334, 538–539.

Ransone, I.J. Visvader, J., Sassone-Corsi, P. and Verma, I. (1989). Fos-Jun interactions: mutational analysis of the leucine zipper domain of both proteins. Genes Devel., 3, 770–781.

Ryder, K. and Nathans, D. (1988). Induction of protooncogene c-*jun* by serum growth factors. Proc. Natl Acad. Sci. USA, 85, 8464–8467.

Ryder, K., Lau, L.F. and Nathans, D. (1988). A gene activated by growth factors is related to the oncogene v-*jun*. Proc. Natl Acad. Sci. USA, 85, 1487–1491.

Ryder, K., Lanahan, A., Perez-Albuerne, E. and Nathans, D. (1989). *Jun*-D: A third member of the *Jun* gene family. Proc. Natl Acad. Sci. USA, 86, 1500–1503.

Ryseck, R.-P. and Bravo, R. (1991). c-JUN, JUN B, and JUN D differ in their binding affinities to AP-1 and CRE consensus sequences: effect of FOS proteins. Oncogene, 6, 533–542.

Ryseck, R.P., Hirai, S.I., Yaniv, M. and Bravo, R. (1988). Transcriptional activation of c-*jun* during the G_0/G_1 transition in mouse fibroblasts. Nature, 334, 535–537.

Sakai, M., Okuda, A., Hatayama, I., Sato, K., Nishi, S. and Muramatsu, M. (1989). Structure and expression of the rat c-*jun* messenger RNA: tissue distribution and increase during chemical hepatocarcinogenesis. Cancer Res., 49, 5633–5637.

Schontal, A., Srinivas, S. and Eckhart, W. (1992). Induction of c-*jun* protooncogene expression and transcription factor AP-1 activity by the polyoma virus middle-sized tumor antigen. Proc. Natl Acad. Sci. USA, 89, 4972–4976.

Schuermann, M., Hunter, J.B., Hennig, G. and Muller, R. (1991). Non-leucine residues in the leucine repeats of fos and jun contribute to the stability and determine the specificity of dimerization. Nucleic Acids Res., 19, 739–746.

Schule, R., Rangarajan, P., Yang, N., Kliewer, S., Ransone, L.J., Bolado, J., Verma, I.M. and Evans, R.M. (1991). Retinoic acid is a negative regulator of AP-1-responsive genes. Proc. Natl Acad. Sci. USA, 88, 6092–6096.

Schulam, P.G., Kuruvilla, A., Putcha, G., Mangus, L., Franklin-Johnson, J. and Shearer, W.T. (1991). Platelet-activating factor induces phospholipid turnover, calcium flux, arachidonic acid liberation, eicosanoid generation, and oncogene expression in a human B cell line. J. Immunol., 146, 1642–1648.

Schutte, J., Nau, M., Birrer, M., Thomas, F., Gazdar, A. and Minna, J. (1988). Constitutive expression of multiple mRNA forms of the c-*jun* oncogene in human lung cancer cell lines. Proc. Am. Assoc. Cancer Res., Art. 1808, 455.

Schutte, J., Minna, J.D. and Birrer, M.J. (1989a). Deregulated expression of human c-*jun* transforms primary rat embryo cells in cooperation with an activated c-Ha-*ras* gene and transforms Rat-1a cells as a single gene. Proc. Natl Acad. Sci. USA, 86, 2257–2261.

Schutte, J., Viallet, J., Nau, M., Segal, S., Fedorko, J. and Minna, J. (1989b). *jun*-B inhibits and c-*fos* stimulates the transforming and trans-activating activities of c-*jun*. Cell, 59, 987–997.

Shapiro, M. and Kozak, C.A. (1991). Genetic mapping in the mouse of four loci related to the *jun* family of transcriptional activators. Somatic Cell Mol. Genet., 17, 341–347.

Sharif, M. and Privalsky, M.L. (1992). v-*erb*A and c-*erb*A proteins enhance transcriptional activation by c-*jun*. Oncogene, 7, 953–960.

Smeal, T., Binetruy, B., Mercola, D.A., Birrer, M. and Karin, M. (1991). Oncogenic and transcriptional cooperation with Ha-*ras* requires phosphorylation of c-*jun* on serine-63 and serine-73. Nature, 354, 494–496.

Smeal, T., Binetruy, B., Mercola, D.A., Grover-Bardwick, A., Heidecker, G., Rapp, U.R. and Karin, M. (1992). Oncoprotein-mediated signalling cascade stimulates c-jun activity by phosphorylation of serines 63 and 73. Mol. Cell. Biol., 12, 3507–3513.

Su, H., Bos, T.J., Monteclaro, F.S. and Vogt, P.K. (1991). *Jun* inhibits myogenic differentiation. Oncogene, 6, 1759–1766.

Trejo, J. and Brown, J.H. (1991). c-*fos* and c-*jun* are induced by muscarinic receptor activation of protein kinase C but are differentially regulated by intracellular calcium. J. Biol. Chem., 266, 7876–7882.

Ullman, K.S., Northrop, J.P., Admon, A. and Crabtree, G.R. (1993). Jun family members controlled by a calcium-regulated, cyclosporin A-sensitive signaling pathway in activated T lymphocytes. Genes Devel., 7, 188–196.

Unlap, T., Franklin, C.C., Wagner, F. and Kraft, A.S. (1992). Upstream regions of the c-*jun* promoter regulate phorbol ester-induced transcription in U937 leukemic cells. Nucleic Acids Res., 20, 897–902.

van Dam, H., Duyndam, M., Rottier, R., Bosch, A., de Vries-Smits, L., Herrlich, P., Zantema, A., Angel, P. and van der Eb, A.J. (1993). Heterodimer formation of cjun and ATF-2 is responsible for induction of c-*jun* by the 243 amino acid adenovirus E1A protein. EMBO J., 12, 479–487.

Vanhamme, L., Marshall, G.M., Schuh, A.C., Breitman, M.L. and Vogt, P.K. (1993). Tumor necrosis factor α and interleukin 1α induce anchorage independence in v-*jun* transgenic murine cells. Cancer Res., 53, 615–621.

Wong, W.-Y., Havarstein, L.S., Morgan, I.M. and Vogt, P.K. (1992). c-jun causes focus formation and anchorage-independent growth in culture but is non-tumorigenic. Oncogene, 7, 2077–2080.

Yu, C.-L., Prochownik, E.V., Imperiale, M.J. and Jove, R. (1993). Attenuation of serum inducibility of immediate early genes by oncoproteins in tyrosine kinase signaling pathways. Mol. Cell. Biol., 13, 2011–2019.

Zhang, K., Chaillet, J.R., Perkins, L.A., Halazonetis, T.D. and Perrimon N. (1990). *Drosophila* homolog of the mammalian *jun* oncogene is expressed during embryonic development and activates transcription in mammalian cells. Proc. Natl Acad. Sci. USA, 87, 6281–6285.

v-*kit* is the oncogene of the Hardy–Zuckerman 4 strain of acutely transform
virus (HZ4-FeSV) (Besmer *et al.*, 1986).

KIT encodes a membrane tyrosine kinase receptor.

Related genes

KIT is a member of receptor tyrosine kinase subclass III which also includes *KDR/Flk-1*, *Flk-2/Flt-3*, *PDGFRA*, *PDGFRB*, and *CSF1R*, each encoding five Ig-like loops in an extracellular domain and a cytoplasmic region containing a 60–100 residue tyrosine kinase insert region (77 amino acids in KIT). It has 58% homology with the tyrosine-specific protein kinase family (v-FMS) and low sequence homology with other tyrosine kinases (v-ABL, v-FES, v-FGR and v-SRC and human EGF and insulin receptors; Hampe *et al.*, 1984).

There is close genetic linkage between the murine genes of the *Kit/Fms/Pdgfra/Flk-1* family (Matthews *et al.*, 1991a) and *Kit* is physically linked to *Pdgfra* (Vandenbark *et al.*, 1992).

There are two *KIT* isoforms in both mice and humans distinguished by the differential splicing of a 12 bp exon immediately upstream of the region encoding the transmembrane domain. The inclusion of this exon gives rise to *KitA*$^+$ (Hayashi *et al.*, 1991; Reith *et al.*, 1991).

Mouse *Flk-1* (*fetal liver kinase 1*) is 24% identical to *Kit* in the extracellular domain and the two are highly homologous in the intracellular kinase domains (Matthews *et al.*, 1991a). Mouse *Flk-2/Flt-3* is also related to *Kit* (Matthews *et al.*, 1991b).

Cross-species homology

KIT: 82% identity (human and mouse). Mouse KIT: 95% identity with feline v-KIT.

Transformation

MAN

KIT and its ligand are highly expressed in small-cell lung cancer (Hibi *et al.*, 1991; Sekido *et al.*, 1991) and in a significant proportion of testicular germ cell tumours (Strohmeyer *et al.*, 1991). The level of expression of *KIT* declines during the progression of cutaneous melanoma (Natali *et al.*, 1992).

ANIMALS

HZ4-FeSV induces fibrosarcomas in the domestic cat but does not cause tumours in kittens.

IN VITRO

v-*kit* transforms NIH 3T3 cells (Besmer *et al.*, 1986). Tumour cells bearing HZ4-FeSV transform feline embryo fibroblasts and CCL64 mink cells (Hampe *et al.*, 1984; Besmer *et al.*, 1986).

Mice expressing the dominant negative W^{42} mutation show effects on pigmentation and the number of tissue mast cells that are characteristic of some W phenotypes. Germ cell development and erythropoiesis are not affected (Ray *et al.*, 1991).

	KIT/Kit	v-kit
Nucleotides	80 kb	1110 2370 (HZ4-FeSV genome)
Chromosome		
Human	4q11–q21	
Mouse	5	
Exons		
Human	21	
mRNA (kb)		
Human, mouse	5	4.5
Amino acids		370 (v-KIT)
Human	976	
Mouse	975	
Mass (kDa)		
(predicted)	109	
(expressed)	gp124/gp160	p81$^{gag\text{-}kit}$

Cellular location

Plasma membrane, myristylated, receptor-like tyrosine kinase (Yarden *et al.*, 1987; Nocka *et al.*, 1990b).

Tissue location

KIT mRNA and protein are present in normal human neonatal and adult melanocytes and in the early stages of erythroid and myeloid cell differentiation (Andre *et al.*, 1989; Nocka *et al.*, 1989) but are not detectable in most human melanoma-derived cell lines (Lassam and Bickford, 1992).

Murine *Kit* is expressed in neural crest-derived melanocytes, primordial germ cells, in the brain and spinal cord (Manova *et al.*, 1990; Orr-Urtreger *et al.*, 1990; Motro *et al.*, 1991) and in most haematopoietic precursor cells but not on B-lineage cells (Keshet *et al.*, 1991). Expression of the KIT receptor and its ligand occurs in complementary tissues throughout the body from the early presomite stage to the mature adult. For example, the ligand (*steel*) is expressed in the follicular cells of the ovary and in Sertoli cells of the testes, the layers immediately surrounding the germ cells that express *Kit* (Matsui *et al.*, 1990; Motro *et al.*, 1991; Keshet *et al.*, 1991). *Kit* is also expressed on cultured primary mast cells (Fujita *et al.*, 1989; Nocka *et al.*, 1989).

Protein function

In humans KIT is the receptor for stem cell factor (SCF, also called mast cell growth factor, MGF; Anderson *et al.*, 1990; Huang *et al.*, 1990; Martin *et al.*, 1990; Nocka *et al.*, 1990a; Williams *et al.*, 1990; Zsebo *et al.*, 1990a).

The KIT receptor in mice is encoded by the dominant white spotting (*W*) locus. The ligand, KL (or SCF or MGF), is a growth factor encoded by the mouse *steel* (*Sl*) locus (Copeland *et al.*, 1990; Huang *et al.*, 1990; Zsebo *et al.*, 1990b; Brannan *et al.*, 1991). The phenotypes of *W* and *Sl* mutant mouse strains that bear germ line loss of function mutations in *Kit* and its ligand, respectively, clearly demonstrate roles for *Kit* in haematopoiesis, melanogenesis and germ cell development (Russell, 1979; Silvers, 1979; Chabot *et al.*, 1988; Geissler *et al.*, 1988; Nocka *et al.*, 1990b; Reith *et al.*, 1990; Tan *et al.*, 1990). Furthermore, SCF acts synergistically with other cytokines to stimulate *in vitro* growth of a number of committed haematopoietic precursors (Bernstein *et al.*, 1991; Briddell *et al.*, 1991; Broxmeyer *et al.*, 1991; McNeice *et al.*, 1991; Metcalf and Nicola, 1991; Migliaccio *et al.*, 1991). These activities can be blocked by antibodies directed against KIT (Ogawa *et al.*, 1991) or by antisense oligodeoxynucleotides that block *Kit* expression (Ratajczak *et al.*, 1992). Anti-KIT antibodies also block melanoblast migration and prevent melanocyte activation in post-natal mice (Nishikawa *et al.*, 1991). SCF promotes germ cell survival *in vitro* (Dolci *et al.*, 1991; Godin *et al.*, 1991) and anti-KIT antibodies inhibit survival and/or proliferation of mature type-A spermatogonia, whereas primitive type A spermatogonia or spermatogenic stem cells appear to proliferate independently of *Kit* expression (Yoshinaga *et al.*, 1991).

The interaction of the ligand KL with its receptor causes receptor dimerization (Lev *et al.*, 1992) that leads to enhanced KIT tyrosine autophosphorylation and association with phosphatidylinositol 3-kinase and PLC-γ though not detectably with GAP. Activated KIT also transiently associates with the tyrosine phosphatase haematopoietic cell phosphatase (HCP or PTP1C) that can dephosphorylate KIT *in vitro* (Yi and Ihle, 1993). The low constitutive levels of autophosphorylation and association with phosphatidylinositol 3-kinase and PLC-γ shown by KIT expressed in COS cells in the absence of exogenous *steel* factor are not detectable for *KitA*$^+$ although both isoforms are stimulated by the ligand (Reith *et al.*, 1991). Activation of KIT also increases the cellular concentration of GTP.p21^{ras} (Duronio *et al.*, 1992). Studies of a chimeric protein of the extracellular domain of the EGFR and the transmembrane and cytoplasmic domains of KIT have shown that activated KIT binds to phosphatidylinositol kinase, causes the tyrosine phosphorylation of PLC-γ and the serine phosphorylation of RAF1, although it does not induce inositol phosphate formation (Lev *et al.*, 1991). In transformed mast cells, KIT is constitutively autophosphorylated and binds phosphatidylinositol 3-kinase in the absence of ligand (Rottapel *et al.*, 1991). In the human cell lines M07E and TF-1 SCF causes rapid (<2 min), heavy tyrosine phosphorylation of p95^{vav} although KIT does not appear to interact directly with the VAV protein (Alai *et al.*, 1992).

In mice *Kit* is functionally required during mid-gestation for the proliferation of melanocyte precursors and in post-natal life for melanocyte activation during the hair cycle (Nishikawa *et al.*, 1991). KL occurs either as a secreted or as a transmembrane protein due to alternative splicing (Flanagan *et al.*, 1991). Mutations in either gene cause impaired development of neural crest-derived melanocytes, germ cells and hepatopoietic cells. Exogenous expression of *Kit* rescues the defective proliferative response to *steel* factor in cells from both W/W^v (viable) and W/W (lethal) mutant mice (Alexander *et al.*, 1991).

Structure of the HZ4-FeSV proviral genome

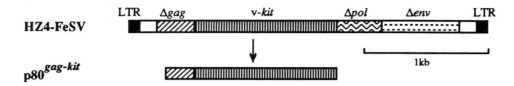

v-*gag–kit–pol* lacks the transmembrane and extracellular domains and 49 C-terminal amino acids of KIT. The 5′ end of v-*kit* recombines near the 3′ end of *gag* in the same ORF. Initiation of translation may be at the 5′ end of p15^{gag} (i.e. p15, p12 and 144 amino acids of p30 are translated). The termination codon is 18 nucleotides 3′ of the recombination site in *pol*. p80$^{gag-kit-pol}$ comprises 414 amino acids from FeLV *gag*, 370 from KIT and 6 from *pol* (Besmer *et al.*, 1986).

Structure of the human *KIT* gene

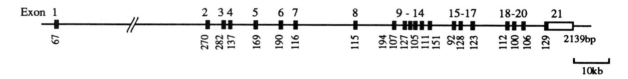

Boxes represents exons with the sizes shown beneath (Vandenbark *et al.*, 1992; Andre *et al.*, 1992; Giebel *et al.*, 1992). Exon 21 contains a 3′ untranslated region of 2139 bp. The overall structure closely resembles that of *FMS* including the large first intron (30 kb) and identical exon/intron boundaries in their two kinase domains. The two *KIT* isoforms arise from alternative splicing of the final 12 nucleotides of exon 9 (Vandenbark *et al.*, 1992). The structure of murine *Kit* is similar (Hayashi *et al.*, 1991; Gokkel *et al.*, 1992).

Structure of mouse KIT

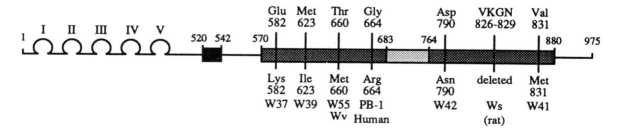

Loops: five extracellular immunoglublin-like repeats. Black box: transmembrane region. Dark shaded boxes: ATP binding and phosphotransferase domains. Light shaded box: kinase insert domain. Point mutations and deletions occurring in mutated *Kit* alleles are shown below the diagram.

The third immunoglobulin domain is essential for rodent SCF binding whereas the major binding determinant for human SCF is the second domain (Lev *et al.*, 1993). In mouse, W^{55} and

W^v arise from the same substitution in independent alleles giving identical phenotypes. The W^{42} mutation, which is particularly severe in its effects in both the homozygous and heterozygous states, arises from a missense mutation that replaces Asp790 with Asn (Tan *et al.*, 1990). The original *W* mutant bears a 234 bp deletion encoding the transmembrane domain and part of the kinase domain, a consequence of a point mutation in the 5′ splice donor site of exon 10 (Hayashi *et al.*, 1991). The product of this gene is not expressed at the cell surface, kinase activity is lost and the homozygous mutation is lethal. For the other mutations indicated in the diagram immunoprecipitable KIT protein is synthesized: its kinase activity is reduced in W^{39}, W^{55}, W^v and W^{41} mutants and abolished in W^{37} and W^{42} mutants (Nocka *et al.*, 1990b; Reith *et al.*, 1990; Tan *et al.*, 1990). The W^v, W^{41} and W^{42} mutations also differentially affect the binding of p145^{kit} to PLC-γ, GTPase-activating protein and the p85 subunit of phosphatidylinositol 3′-kinase (Herbst *et al.*, 1992).

PB-1 refers to a substitution at Gly664 in the human sequence detected in a case of piebaldism, a condition similar to the dominant white spotting (*W*) disorder in mice (Giebel and Spritz, 1991). *Ws* refers to a mutant rat strain having a four amino acid deletion in the conserved phosphotransferase region (Tsujimura *et al.*, 1991).

Sequences of human and mouse KIT, v-KIT and the cytoplasmic domain of v-FMS

```
Human KIT  (1)    MRGARGAWDFLCVLLLLLRVQTGSSQPSVSPGEPSPPSIHPGKSDLIVRVGDEIRLLCT
Mouse KIT  (1)    ---------L-----V---G--AT----A-----------AQ-E---EA--TLS-T-I

           (60)   DPGFVKWTFEILDE TNENKQNEWITEKAEATNTGKYTCTNKHGLSNSIYVFVRDPAKLF
           (60)   --D--R---KTYFNEMV---K----Q------R--T---S-SN--TS-----------

           (119)  LVDRSLYGKEDNDTLVRCPLTDPEVTNYSLKGCQGKPLPKDLRFIPDPKAGIMIKSVKRA
           (120)  --GLP-F----S-A---------Q-S----IE-D--S---T--T-V-N-----T--N----

           (179)  YHRLCLHCSVDQEGKSVLSEKFILKVRPAFKAVPVVSVSKASYLLREGEEFTVTCTIKDV
           (180)  -----VR-AAQRD-TWLH-D--T----E-I--I-----PET-H--KK-DT---V------

           (239)  SSSVYSTWKRENSQTKL QEKYNSWHHGDFNYERQATLTISSARVNDSGVFMCYANNTF
           (240)  -T--N-M-LKM-P-PQHIA-V-H------------E---------D-------------

           (297)  GSANVTTTLEVVDKGFINIFPMINTTVFVNDGENVDLIVEYEAFPKPEHQQWIYMNRTFT
           (300)  ---------K--E------S-VK------T-------V-----Y-------------SA

           (357)  DKWEDYPKSENESNIRYVSELHLTRLKGTEGGTYTFLVSNSDVNAAIAFNVYVNTKPEIL
           (360)  N-GK--V--D-K------NQ-R------------------AS-SVT-----------

           (417)  TYDRLVNGMLQCVAAGFPEPTIDWYFCPGTEQRCSASVLPVDVQTLNSSGPPFGKLVVQS
           (420)  -----I--------E-----------T-A----TTP-S-----VQ-V-VS--------

           (478)  SIDSSAFKHNGTVECKAYNDVGKTSAYFNFAFKGNNKEQIHPHTLFTPLLIGFVIVAGMM
           (480)  -----V-R---------S-----S--F------     ---QA-----------VA----

Human KIT  (537)  CIIVMILTYKYLQKPMYEVQWKVVEEINGNNYVYIDPTQLPYDHKWEFPRNRLSFGKTLG
Mouse KIT  (536)  G----V------------------------------------------------------
v-KIT      (1)                 -------  ------------------------
v-FMS      (569)  YKYKQKPKYQVRWKIIESY-G-SYTF -------NE-------N-Q------

Human KIT  (597)  AGAFGKVVEATAYGLIKSDAAMTVAVKMLKPSAHLTEREALMSELKVLSYLGNHMNIVNL
Mouse KIT  (595)  ------------------------------------------------------------
v-KIT      (35)   ------------------------------------------------------------
v-FMS      (622)  T----------F--G-E--VLK-------ST--AD-K--------IM-H--Q-E-----
```

```
Human KIT  (657)  LGACTIGGPTLVITEYCCYGDLLNFLRRKRDSFICSKQEDHAEAALYKNLLHSKESSCSD
Mouse KIT  (656)  -----V-------------------------F----EQ-----------T-P-- -
v-KIT       (95)  -----V------------------------------------V-------Q------N-
v-FMS      (681)  -----H---V----------------QAEAMPGPSLSVGQDPEAGAGYKNIHLEKKYV

Human KIT  (717)  STNEYMDMKPGVSYVVPTKADKRRSVRIGSYIERDVTPAIMEDDELALDLEDLLSFSYQV
Mouse KIT  (715)  -S---------------T-----A--D--------------------D---------
v-KIT      (155)  -----------------A--------------G----------------
v-FMS      (741)  RRDSGFSSQ --DTY-EM   -PVSTSS-NDSFSEEDLGK---RP -E-R---H--S--

Human KIT  (777)  AKGMAFLASKNCIHRDLAARNILLTHGRITKICDFGLARDIKNDSNYVVKGNARLPVKWM
Mouse KIT  (775)  --A-------------------------------------------------------
v-KIT      (215)  ----------------------------------------------------------
v-FMS      (794)  -Q-------------V----V---S--VA--G--------M-----I-----------

Human KIT  (837)  APESIFNCVYTFESDVWSYGIFLWELFSLGSSPYPGMPVDSKFYKMIKEGFRMLSPEHAP
Mouse KIT  (835)  ------S----------------------------------------------V-----
v-KIT      (275)  ----------------------------------------------------------
v-FMS      (962)  ------D----VQ--------L---I----LN----IL-N-----LV-D-YQ-AQ-AF--

Human KIT  (897)  AEMYDIMKTCWDADPLKRPTFKQIVQLIEKQISESTNHIYSNLANCSPNRQKPVV DHSV
Mouse KIT  (895)  -----V----------------V---------D--K---------N--PEN---V----
v-KIT      (335)  ---------------------------KNKNE (370)
v-FMS      (915)  KNI-S--QA--ALE-TR----Q--CS-LQ--AQEDRRVPNYTNLPS961SSSSRLLRPWRGPPL (975)

Human KIT  (956)  RINSVGSTASSSQPLLVHDDV (976)
Mouse KIT  (955)  -V-----S---T------E-A (975)
```

Dashes indicate identity with human KIT. The transmembrane region is italicized. The nucleotide binding and phosphorylation domains of the human sequence are underlined. ATP binding: human amino acids 596–601 and 623. There are 10 *N*-linked glycosylation sites. The insertion in murine *KitA*[+] encodes Gly–Asn–Asn–Lys between amino acids 512 and 513 (Reith *et al.*, 1991): this insert is also present in human KIT. v-KIT contains the ATP-binding consensus sequence GXGXXG (residue 374) and Lys402. v-*kit* appears to be oncogenically activated by the removal of the extracellular and transmembrane domains, together with 50 amino acids from the C-terminus of KIT (Qiu *et al.*, 1988).

Databank file names and accession numbers

	GENE	EMBL	SWISSPROT	REFERENCES
HZ4-FeSV	v-*kit*	Refeskit X03711	KKIT_FSVHZ P04048	Besmer *et al.*, 1986
Human	*KIT*	Hskitcr X06182	KKIT_HUMAN P10721	Yarden *et al.*, 1987 Vandenbark *et al.*, 1992 Giebel *et al.*, 1992
Mouse	*Kit*	Mmckit Y00864	KKIT_MOUSE P05532	Qui *et al.*, 1988 Tan *et al.*, 1990
Mouse	*Flk-1*	Mmflk1 X59397		Matthews *et al.*, 1991a

Review

Russell, E.S. (1979). Hereditary anemias of the mouse: a review for geneticists. Adv. Genetics, 20, 357–459.

Papers

Alai, M., Mui, A.L.-F., Cutler, R.L., Bustelo, X.R., Barbacid, M. and Krystal, G. (1992). Steel factor stimulates the tyrosine phosphorylation of the proto-oncogene product, p95^{vav}, in human hemopoietic cells. J. Biol. Chem., 267, 18021–18025.

Alexander, W.S., Lyman, S.D. and Wagner, E.F. (1991). Expression of functional c-kit receptors rescues the genetic defect of *W* mutant mast cells. EMBO J., 10, 3683–3691.

Anderson, D.M., Lyman, S.D., Baird, A., Wignall, J.M., Eisenman, J., Rauch, C., March, C.J., Boswell, H.S., Gimpel, S.D., Cosman, D. and Williams, D.E. (1990). Molecular cloning of mast cell growth factor, a hematopoietin that is active in both membrane bound and soluble forms. Cell, 63, 235–243.

Andre, C., d'Auriol, L., Lacombe, C., Gisselbrecht, S. and Galibert, F. (1989). c-*kit* mRNA expression in human and murine hematopoietic cell lines. Oncogene, 4, 1047–1049.

Andre, C., Martin, E., Cornu, F., Hu, W.X., Wang, X.P. and Galibert, F. (1992). Genomic organization of the human c-*kit* gene: evolution of the receptor tyrosine kinase subclass III. Oncogene, 7, 685–691.

Bernstein, I.D., Andrews, R.G. and Zsebo, K.M. (1991). Recombinant human stem cell factor enhances the formation of colonies by CD34$^+$ and CD34$^-$lin$^-$ cells, and the generation of colony-forming cell progeny from CD34$^+$lin$^-$ cells cultured with interleukin-3, granulocyte colony-stimulating factor, or granulocyte-macrophage colony-stimulating factor. Blood, 77, 2316–2321.

Besmer, P., Murphy, J.E., George, P.C., Qiu, F., Bergold, P.J., Lederman, L., Snyder, H.W., Brodeur, D., Zuckerman, E.E. and Hardy, W.D. (1986). A new acute transforming feline retrovirus and relationship of its oncogene v-*kit* with the protein kinase gene family. Nature, 320, 415–421.

Brannan, C.I., Lyman, S.D., Williams, D.E., Eisenman, J., Anderson, D.M., Cosman, D., Bedell, M.A., Jenkins, N.A. and Copeland, N.G. (1991). Steel-Dickie mutation encodes c-kit ligand lacking transmembrane and cytoplasmic domains. Proc. Natl Acad. Sci. USA, 88, 4671–4674.

Briddell, R.A., Bruno, E., Cooper, R.J., Brandt, J.E. and Hoffman, R. (1991). Effect of c-*kit* ligand on in vitro human megakaryocytopoiesis. Blood, 78, 2854–2859.

Broxmeyer, H.E., Cooper, S., Lu, L., Hangoc, G., Anderson, D., Cosman, D., Lyman, S.D. and Williams, D.E. (1991). Effect of murine mast cell growth factor (c-*kit* proto-oncogene ligand) on colony formation by human marrow hematopoietic progenitor cells. Blood, 77, 2142–2149.

Chabot, B., Stephenson, D., Chapman, V., Besmer, P. and Bernstein, A. (1988). The proto-oncogene c-kit encoding a transmembrane tyrosine kinase receptor maps to the mouse *W* locus. Nature, 335, 88–89.

Copeland, N.G., Gilbert, D.J., Cho, B.C., Donovan, P.J., Jenkins, N.A., Cosman, D., Anderson, D., Lyman, S.D. and Williams, D.E. (1990). Mast cell growth factor maps near the Steel locus on mouse chromosome 10 and is deleted in a number of Steel alleles. Cell, 63, 175–183.

Dolci, S., Williams, D.E., Ernst, M.K., Resnick, J.L., Brannan, C.I., Lock, L.F., Lyman, S.D., Boswell, H.S. and Donovan, P.J. (1991). Requirement for mast cell growth factor for primordial germ cell survival in culture. Nature, 352, 809–811.

Duronio, V., Welham, M.J., Abraham, S., Dryden, P. and Schrader, J.W. (1992). p21^{ras} activation via hemopoietin receptors and c-kit requires tyrosine kinase activity but not tyrosine phosphorylation of p21^{ras} GTPase-activating protein. Proc. Natl Acad. Sci. USA, 89, 1587–1591.

Flanagan, J.G., Chan, D.C. and Leder, P. (1991). Transmembrane form of the *kit* ligand growth factor is determined by alternative splicing and is missing in the *Sl^d* mutant. Cell, 64, 1025–1035.

Fujita, J., Oncoue, H., Ebi, Y., Makayama, H. and Kanakura, Y. (1989). *In vitro* duplication and *in vivo* cure of mast cell deficiency of *Sl/Sl^d* mutant mice by cloned 3T3 fibroblasts. Proc. Natl Acad. Sci. USA, 86, 2888–2891.

Geissler, E., Ryan, M. and Housman, D. (1988). The dominant white spotting (*W*) locus of the mouse encodes the c-*kit* proto-oncogene. Cell, 55, 185–192.

Giebel, L.B. and Spritz, R.A. (1991). Mutation of the KIT (mast/stem cell growth factor receptor) proto-oncogene in human piebaldism. Proc. Natl Acad. Sci. USA, 88, 8696–8699.

Giebel, L.B., Strunk, K.M., Holmes, S.A. and Spritz, R.A. (1992). Organization and nucleotide sequence of the human KIT (mast/stem cell growth factor receptor) proto-oncogene. Oncogene, 7, 2207–2217.

Godin, I., Deed, R., Cooke, J., Zsebo, K., Dexter, M. and Wylie, C.C. (1991). Effects of the steel gene product on mouse primordial germ cells in culture. Nature, 352, 807–809.

Gokkel, E., Grossman, Z., Ramot, B., Yarden, Y. and Givol, D. (1992). Structural organization of the murine c-*kit* proto-onocgene. Oncogene, 7, 1423–1429.

Hampe, A., Gobet, M., Sherr, C.J. and Galibert, F. (1984). Nucleotide sequence of the feline retroviral oncogene v-*fms* shows unexpected homology with oncogenes encoding tyrosine specific protein kinases. Proc. Natl Acad. Sci. USA, 81, 85–89.

Hayashi, S.-I., Kunisada, T., Ogawa, M., Yamaguchi, K. and Nishikawa, S.-I. (1991). Exon skipping by mutation of an authentic splice site of c-*kit* gene in *W/W* mouse. Nucleic Acids Res., 19, 1267–1271.

Herbst, R., Shearman, M.S., Obermeier, A., Schlessinger, J. and Ullrich, A. (1992). Differential effects of *W* mutations on p145^{c-kit} tyrosine kinase activity and substrate interaction. J. Biol. Chem., 267, 13210–13216.

Hibi, K., Takahashi, T., Sekido, Y., Ueda, R., Hida, T., Ariyoshi, Y., Takagi, H. and Takahashi, T. (1991). Coexpression of the stem cell factor and the c-*kit* genes in small-cell lung cancer. Oncogene, 6, 2291–2296.

Huang, E., Nocka, K., Beier, D.R., Chu, T.-Y., Buck, J., Lahm, H.-W., Wellner, D., Leder, P. and Besmer, P. (1990). The hematopoietic growth factor KL is encoded by the *Sl* locus and is the ligand of the c-*kit* receptor, the gene product of the *W* locus. Cell, 63, 225–233.

Keshet, E., Lyman, S.D., Williams, D.E., Anderson, D.M., Jenkins, N.A., Copeland, N.G. and Parada, L.F. (1991). Embryonic RNA expression patterns of the c-*kit* receptor and its cognate ligand suggest multiple functional roles in mouse development. EMBO J., 10, 2425–2435.

Lassam, N. and Bickford, S. (1992). Loss of c-*kit* expression in cultured melanoma cells. Oncogene, 7, 51–56.

Lev, S., Givol, D. and Yarden, Y. (1991). A specific combination of substrates is involved in signal transduction by the *kit*-encoded receptor. EMBO J., 10, 647–654.

Lev, S., Yarden, Y. and Givol, D. (1992). Dimerization and activation of the kit receptor by monovalent and bivalent binding of the stem cell factor. J. Biol. Chem., 267, 15970–15977.

Lev , S., Blechman, J., Nishikawa, S.-I., Givol, D. and Yarden, Y. (1993). Interspecies molecular chimeras of kit help define the binding site of the stem cell factor. Mol. Cell. Biol., 13, 2224–2234.

McNeice, I.K., Langley, K.E. and Zsebo, K.M. (1991). Recombinant human stem cell factor synergises with GM-CSF, G-CSF, IL-3 and Epo to stimulate human progenitor cells of the myeloid and erythroid lineages. Exp. Hematol., 19, 226–231.

Manova, K., Nocka, K., Besmer, P. and Bachvarova, R.F. (1990). Gonadal expression of c-kit encoded at the *W* locus of the mouse. Development, 110, 1057–1069.

Martin, F.H., Suggs, S.V., Langley, K.E., Lu, H.S., Ting, J., Okino, K.H., Morris, C.F., McNiece, I.K., Jacobsen, F.W., Mendiaz, E.A., Birkett, N.C., Smith, K.A., Johnson, M.J., Parker, V.P., Flores, J.C., Patel, A.C., Fisher, E.F., Erjavec, H.O., Herrera, C.J., Wypych, J., Sachdev, R.K., Pope, J.A., Leslie, I., Wen, D., Lin, C.-H., Cupples, R.L. and Zsebo, K.M. (1990). Primary structure and functional expression of rat and human stem cell factor DNAs. Cell, 63, 203–211.

Matsui, Y., Zsebo, K.M. and Hogan, B.L.M. (1990). Embryonic expression of a haematopoietic growth factor encoded by the *Sl* locus and the ligand for c-*kit*. Nature, 347, 667–669.

Matthews, W., Jordan, C.T., Gavin, M., Jenkins, N.A., Copeland, N.G. and Lemischka, I.R. (1991a). A receptor tyrosine kinase cDNA isolated from a population of enriched primitive hematopoietic cells and exhibiting close genetic linkage to c-*kit*. Proc. Natl Acad. Sci. USA, 88, 9026–9030.

Matthews, W., Jordan, C.T., Wiegand, G.W., Pardoll, D. and Lemischka, I.R. (1991b). A receptor tyrosine kinase specific to hematopoietic stem and progenitor cell-enriched populations. Cell, 65, 1143–1152.

Metcalf D. and Nicola, N.A. (1991). Direct proliferative actions of stem cell factor on murine bone marrow cells *in vitro*: effects of combination with colony-stimulating factors. Proc. Natl Acad. Sci. USA, 88, 6239–6243.

Migliaccio, G., Migliaccio, A.R., Valinsky, J., Langley, K., Zsebo, K., Visser, J.W.M. and Adamson, J.W. (1991). Stem cell factor induces proliferation and differentiation of highly enriched murine hematopoietic cells. Proc. Natl Acad. Sci. USA, 88, 7420–7424.

Motro, B., van der Kooy, D., Rossant, J., Reith, A. and Bernstein, A. (1991). Contiguous patterns of c-*kit* and *steel* expression: analysis of mutations at the *W* and *Sl* loci. Development, 113, 1207–1222.

Natali, P.G., Nicotra, M.R., Winkler, A.B., Cavaliere, R., Bigotti, A. and Ullrich, U. (1992). Progression of human cutaneous melanoma is associated with loss of expression of c-*kit* proto-oncogene receptor. Int. J. Cancer, 52, 197–201.

Nishikawa, S., Kusakabe, M., Yoshinaga, K., Ogawa, M., Hayashi, S.-I., Kunisada, T., Era, T., Sakakura, T. and Nishikawa, S.-I. (1991). *In utero* manipulation of coat color formation by a monoclonal anti-c-*kit* antibody: two distinct waves of c-*kit*-dependency during melanocyte development. EMBO J., 10, 2111–2118.

Nocka, K., Majumder, S., Chabot, B., Ray, P., Cervone, M., Bernstein, A. and Besmer, P. (1989). Expression of c-*kit* gene products in known cellular targets of *W* mutations in normal and *W* mutant mice. Genes Devel., 3, 816–826.

Nocka, K., Buck, J., Levi, E. and Besmer, P. (1990a). Candidate ligand for the c-kit transmembrane receptor: KL, a fibroblast derived growth factor stimulates mast cells and erythroid progenitors. EMBO J., 9, 3287–3294.

Nocka, K., Tan, J.C., Chiu, E., Chu, T.Y., Ray, P., Traktman, P. and Besmer, P. (1990b). Molecular basis of down regulation and loss of function mutations at the murine c-kit/white spotting locus: W^{37}, W^v, W^{41} and W. EMBO J., 9, 1805–1813.

Ogawa, M., Matsuzaki, Y., Nishikawa, S., Hayashi, S.-I., Kunisada, T., Sudo, T., Kina, T., Nakauchi, H. and Nishikawa, S.-I. (1991). Expression and function of c-kit in hemopoietic progenitor cells. J. Exp. Med., 174, 63–71.

Orr-Urtreger, A., Avivi, A., Zimmer, Y., Givol, D., Yarden, Y and Lonai, P. (1990). Developmental expression of c-kit, a proto-oncogene encoded by the W locus. Development, 109, 911–923.

Qiu, F., Ray, P., Brown, K., Barker, P.E., Jhanwar, S., Ruddle, F.H. and Besmer, P. (1988). Primary structure of c-kit: relationship with the CSF-1/PDGF receptor kinase family – oncogenic activation of v-kit involves deletion of extracellular domain and C terminus. EMBO J., 7, 1003–1011.

Ratajczak, M.Z., Luger, S.M., DeRiel, K., Abrahm, J., Calabretta, B. and Gewirtz, A.M. (1992). Role of the KIT protooncogene in normal and malignant human hematopoiesis. Proc. Natl Acad. Sci. USA, 89, 1710–1714.

Ray, P., Hoggins, K.M., Tan, J.C., Chu, T.Y., Yee, N.S., Nguyen, H., Lacy, E and Besmer, P. (1991). Ectopic expression of a c-kit^{W42} minigene in transgenic mice: recapitulation of W phenotypes and evidence for c-kit function in melanoblast progenitors. Genes Devel., 5, 2265–2273.

Reith, A.D., Rottapel, R., Giddens, E., Brady, C., Forrester, L. and Bernstein, A. (1990). W mutant mice with mild or severe developmental defects contain distinct point mutations in the kinase domain of the c-kit receptor. Genes Devel., 4, 390–400.

Reith, A.D., Ellis, C., Lyman, S.D., Anderson, D.M., Williams, D.E., Bernstein, A. and Pawson, T. (1991). Signal transduction by normal isoforms and W mutant variants of the kit receptor tyrosine kinase. EMBO J., 10, 2451–2459.

Rottapel, R., Reedijk, M., Williams, D.E., Lyman, S.D., Anderson, D.M., Pawson, T. and Bernstein, A. (1991). The steel/W transduction pathway: kit autophosphorylation and its association with a unique subset of cytoplasmic signaling proteins is induced by the steel factor. Mol. Cell. Biol., 11, 3043–3051.

Sekido, Y., Obata, Y., Ueda, R., Hida, T., Suyama, M., Shimokata, K., Ariyoshi, Y. and Takahashi, T. (1991). Preferential expression of c-kit protooncogene transcripts in small cell lung cancer. Cancer Res., 51, 2416–2419.

Silvers, W.K. (1979). Dominant spotting, patch, and rump-white. In The Coat Colors of Mice: a Model for Mammalian Gene Action and Interaction: 206–241. Springer-Verlag, New York.

Strohmeyer, T., Peter, S., Hartmann, M., Munemitsu, S., Ackermann, R., Ullrich, A. and Slamon, D.J. (1991). Expression of the hst-1 and c-kit protooncogenes in human testicular germ cell tumors. Cancer Res., 51, 1811–1816.

Tan, J.C., Nocka, K., Ray, P., Traktman, P. and Besmer, P. (1990). The dominant W^{42} spotting phenotype results from a missense mutation in the c-kit receptor kinase. Science, 247, 209–212.

Tsujimura, T., Hirota, S., Nomura, S., Niwa, Y., Yamazaki, M., Tono, T., Morii, E., Kim, H.-M., Kondo, K., Nishimune, Y. and Kitamura, Y. (1991). Characterization of Ws mutant allele of rats: a 12 base deletion in tyrosine kinase domain of c-kit gene. Blood, 78, 1942–1946.

Vandenbark, G.R., deCastro, C.M., Taylor, H., Dew-Knight, S. and Kaufman, R.E. (1992). Cloning and structural analysis of the human c-kit gene. Oncogene, 7, 1259–1266.

Williams, D.E., Eisenman, J., Baird, A., Rauch, C., van Ness, K., March, C.J., Park, L.S., Martin, U., Mochizuki, D.Y., Boswell, H.S., Burgess, G.S., Cosman, D. and Lyman, S.D. (1990). Identification of a ligand for the c-kit proto-oncogene. Cell, 63, 167–174.

Yarden, Y., Kuang, W.J., Yang-Feng, T., Coussens, L., Munemitsu, S., Dull, T.J., Chen, E., Schlessinger, J., Francke, U. and Ullrich, A. (1987). Human proto-oncogene c-kit: a new cell surface receptor tyrosine kinase for an unidentified ligand. EMBO J., 6, 3341–3351.

Yi, T. and Ihle, J.N. (1993). Association of hematopoietic cell phosphatase with c-Kit after stimulation with c-Kit ligand. Mol. Cell. Biol., 13, 3350–3358.

Yoshinaga, K., Nishikawa, S., Ogawa, M., Hayashi, S.-I., Kunisada, T., Fujimoto, T. and Nishikawa, S.-I. (1991). Role of c-kit in mouse spermatogenesis: identification of spermatogonia as a specific site of c-kit expression and function. Development, 113, 689–699.

Zsebo, K.M., Wypych, J., McNiece, I.K., Lu, H.S., Smith, K.A., Karkare, S.B., Sachdev, R.K., Yuschenkoff, V.N., Birkett, N.C., Williams, L.R., Satyagal, V.N., Tung, W., Bosselman, R.A., Mendiaz, E.A. and Langley, K.E. (1990a). Identification, purification, and biological characterization of hematopoietic stem cell factor from buffalo rat liver-conditioned medium. Cell, 63, 195–201.

Zsebo, K.M., Williams, D.A., Geissler, E.N., Broudy, V.C., Martin, F.H., Atkins, H.L., Hsu, R.-Y., Birkett, N.C., Okino, K.H., Murdock, D.C., Jacobsen, F.W., Langley, K.E., Smith, K.A., Takeishi, T., Cattanach, B.M., Galli, S.J. and Suggs, S.V. (1990b). Stem cell factor is encoded at the *Sl* locus of the mouse and is the ligand for the c-*kit* tyrosine kinase receptor. Cell, 63, 213–224.

LCK

Lck encodes a cellular tyrosine kinase (formerly *lsk*[T] *or tck*), one of eight members of the *Src* family, detected originally in the LSTRA murine lymphoma cell line derived from MuLV-induced thymomas (Casnellie *et al.*, 1982; Marth *et al.*, 1985).

Related genes

Lck is a member of the *Src* tyrosine kinase family (*Blk, Fgr, Fyn, Hck, Lck/Tkl, Lyn, Src* and *Yes*). A *Lck*-related gene is expressed in murine eggs (Mori *et al.*, 1992).

Cross-species homology

LCK: 96.5% identity (human and mouse).

Tkl is the avian cellular *tyrosine kinase* homologue of *Lck. Tkl* encodes a 457 amino acid ORF 81.7% identical in sequence to LCK (Strebhardt *et al.*, 1987). The N-terminus is 68% identical to that of LCK (Chow *et al.*, 1992).

Transformation

MAN

LCK is expressed in B cells from patients with chronic lymphocytic leukaemia (CLL) though not in normal B cells (Abts *et al.*, 1991). A translocation breakpoint within the first *LCK* intron has been detected in a T cell acute lymphoblastic leukaemia (T cell ALL) cell line with a t(1;7)(p34;q34). This separates the two *LCK* promoters (see below) and juxtaposes the constant region of the T cell receptor (TCR) β chain to the proximal promoter and protein-coding region of the *LCK* gene (Burnett *et al.*, 1991).

ANIMALS

The phenotype of LSTRA murine lymphoma cells appears to be due to the enhanced expression of p56[lck] caused by promoter insertion (Marth *et al.*, 1985). Substitution of Phe for Tyr505 increases the apparent kinase activity and causes p56[lck] to transform NIH 3T3 cells (Marth *et al.*, 1988). The overexpression of p56[lck] promotes tumorigenesis in otherwise normal thymocytes (Abraham *et al.*, 1991).

A significant proportion (14%) of primary tumours induced in rats by Moloney murine leukaemia virus have a proviral insertion upstream of *Lck* that increases *Lck* transcription, generating three different hybrid transcripts (Shin and Steffen, 1993).

TRANSGENIC ANIMALS

Transgenic mice that do not express p56[lck] show considerable thymic atrophy with a marked decrease in the number of CD4[+]/CD8[+] thymocytes (Molina *et al.*, 1992). Transgenic mice expressing high levels of a catalytically inactive form of p56^{lck} are defective in the production of virtually all T lymphocytes (Levin *et al.*, 1993).

	LCK/Lck	*Tkl* (chicken)
Nucleotides (kb)	2.2	
Chromosome		
Human	1p35–p32	14q32
Exons	5	
mRNA (kb)	~2.2	4.0/3.5
Amino acids		457
Human	509	
Mouse	509	
Mass (kDa)		
(predicted)	58	
(expressed)	56 (phosphorylated by protein kinase C on at least three sites between residues 14 and 261: this gives rise to pp60 and pp64	56

Cellular location

Cytoplasmic face of the plasma membrane.

Tissue location

p56^{lck}, *Fgr*, *Lyn* and *Hck* are expressed only in haematopoietic cells and *Lck* is found specifically only in lymphoid cells, T cells, NK cells and some B cells. T cells also express the *Src* family members *Fyn* and *Yes*: *Yes* has a wide tissue distribution but one of the isoforms of p59^{fyn}, *fyn(T)*, like p56^{lck}, occurs primarily in lymphocytes.

Chicken *Tkl* is abundantly expressed in the thymus; lesser expression in the spleen (Chow *et al.*, 1992).

Protein function

p56^{lck} is a lymphocyte-specific tyrosine kinase associated with the cytoplasmic domains of CD4 and CD8α (CD8 can exist as αα or αβ dimers) that bind to class II and class I MHC molecules respectively (i.e. it co-immunoprecipitates with CD4 or CD8). In human T cells phosphatidylinositol 3-kinase co-precipitates with CD4/p56^{lck} (Thompson *et al.*, 1992) and p56^{lck} also associates in immunoprecipitates with the IL-2R β chain (Hatakeyama *et al.*, 1991), CD5 (Burgess *et al.*, 1992) and with CD2 (Bell *et al.*, 1992). The interaction is between a short region of the C-termini of the CD4/CD8 receptors and an N-terminal region of p56^{lck} not conserved in other protein tyrosine kinases (Hatakeyama *et al.*, 1991).

Stimulation of the TCR activates p56^{lck} and antibodies against CD4 or CD8 block T cell activation via the TCR. The expression of mutant forms of CD4 in T cell lines that are CD4-dependent but lack endogenous CD4 indicates that association of p56^{lck} with the CD4 cytoplasmic domain is essential for activation via the TCR (Glaichenhaus *et al.*, 1991). However, activation by antibodies to the TCR causes *FYN* tyrosine kinase but not *LCK* or *YES* to co-precipitate with the TCR (Samelson *et al.*, 1990). Furthermore, T cells from p56^{lck}-deficient mice proliferate in response to activation of the TCR or to IL-2 (Molina *et al.*, 1992). Nevertheless, the stimulation by IL-2 of proliferation in IL-2-dependent T cells is accompanied by the association of p56^{lck} with the IL-2 receptor β chain (Minami *et al.*, 1993) and activation of p56^{lck} (a significant proportion migrating as p59–p60^{lck}; Horak *et al.*, 1991), indicating that different tyrosine kinases may be activated during the course of mitogenesis (see *FYN* for discussion of the roles of *Fyn* and *Lck* in T cell activation). Cross-linking CD4 enhances the autophosphorylation of p56^{lck}, which may cause the phosphorylation of the ζ-chain of the CD3/TCR complex, although ζ has only been shown to be a direct substrate *in vitro*. The serine–threonine kinase RAF1 is a substrate for CD4-activated p56^{lck} (Thompson *et al.*, 1991) and a RAF1-related protein (p110) associates with the CD4–p56^{lck} complex but is phosphorylated mainly on serine residues (Prasad and Rudd, 1992).

The mitogen-activated protein (MAP) kinase p42^{mapk} is a substrate of p56^{lck} (Ettehadieh *et al.*, 1992). p42^{mapk} is tyrosyl phosphorylated and activated in the murine T lymphoma cell line 171CD4^{+} after stimulation of the TCR. *In vitro* p56^{lck} also phosphorylates and activates the serine/threonine phosphotransferase activity of p44^{mpk}, a MAP kinase isoform from sea star oocytes. Thus MAP kinases may be directly regulated by LCK and other members of the SRC family and participate in cell signalling cascades that may activate substrates such as ribosomal S6 kinases (RSKs).

An alternative role for p56^{lck} may be in regulating T cell maturation and differentiation: it is expressed before CD4/CD8 in developing T cells and is present in complexes with CD4 and CD8 in immature CD4^{+}/CD8^{+} cells. The expression in transgenic mice of a catalytically inactive form of p56^{lck} that functions in a dominant negative manner indicates that normal p56^{lck} plays a critical role in thymocyte development for which FYN cannot substitute (Levin *et al.*, 1993). However, this role may be independent of association between LCK and CD4 or CD8 as CD4^{-} or CD8^{-} mice have normal numbers of thymocytes.

In LSTRA cells that overexpress p56^{lck} (by retroviral promoter insertion), GAP and the GAP-associated proteins p62 and p190 are tyrosine phosphorylated (Ellis *et al.*, 1991) and GAP also binds to p56^{lck} *in vitro* (Amrein *et al.*, 1992). Interaction between GAP and tyrosine phosphorylated p62 is mediated by the GAP SH2 domain. In NIH 3T3 fibroblasts tyrosine phosphorylation of GAP complexes requires activated and myristylated p56^{lck} and correlates with *Lck* transforming activity. Overexpression of p56^{lck} in developing thymocytes inhibits the process of Vβ–Dβ rearrangement that normally leads to the expression of a single functional β chain gene (Anderson *et al.*, 1992).

The stimulation of B lymphocytes with antibodies to membrane immunoglobulin causes the receptor to associate with *Src* family protein tyrosine kinases including p56^{lck} (Campbell and Sefton, 1992) and p56^{lck} expression is specifically upregulated (Taieb *et al.*, 1993).

p56^{tkl} is associated with avian CD4 and CD8 via a cysteine motif at positions 20 and 23 (Chow *et al.*, 1992) and appears to be functionally equivalent to p56^{lck}.

Structure of the *LCK* gene

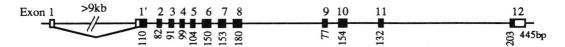

The structures of the human and murine *LCK* genes are closely similar. They have identical exon sizes except for the untranslated region of exon 12 which is 407 bp in the mouse gene (Rouer *et al.*, 1989). There are at least two *LCK* mRNAs expressed in human and mouse cells, types I and II (Garvin *et al.*, 1988). These have different 5' untranslated regions arising from the use of different promoters (Adler *et al.*, 1988). The type I promoter in Jurkat cells and in the colon carcinoma cell line SW620 contains an ETS-binding element that is essential for its activity (Leung *et al.*, 1993). Type II *LCK* transcripts initiate from a promoter ~9 kb from the downstream promoter and create an alternative 5' UTR by splicing five nucleotides 5' to the initiation ATG codon. The sequence between −584 and +37 with respect to the proximal promoter transcription start site directs tissue-specific and temporally appropriate transcription of p56^{lck} (Allen *et al.*, 1992). The type II promoter is used in both normal, mature T cells and in transformed T cells and an alternatively spliced transcript utilizing this promoter is also expressed in both types of cell (Rouer and Benarous, 1992). In this type IIB mRNA the deletion of exon 1' results in the use of a different AUG codon in exon 1, located 35 bp upstream from the normal initiation codon in exon 1'. In the type IIB translation product 10 residues encoded by exon 1 replace the first 35 residues encoded by exon 1'.

In LSTRA cells elevated expression of *Lck* results from Moloney murine leukaemia virus promoter insertion: the proviral sequence is truncated and rearranged with a 554 cellular base sequence flanking either end, 962 bp upstream of the start site for type I *Lck* (Takadera *et al.*, 1989). LSTRA cell *Lck* mRNA comprises the 5' untranslated region of Moloney murine leukaemia virus genome and the complete *Lck* coding sequence. The fused gene directs synthesis of p56^{lck} identical to that of normal cells but increased translation efficiency gives rise to 40-fold more p56^{lck} in LSTRA cells than in normal T cells.

Structure of p56^{lck}

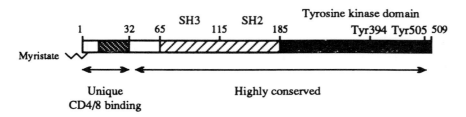

There is a high degree of similarity within the SRC family: all contain Gly2 (including type IIB) which becomes myristylated and contributes to membrane anchoring of the proteins; all share sequences throughout sequence homology (SH) domains 1, 2 and 3. p56^{lck} has 65% sequence homology to SRC in the C-terminal 450 amino acids: the N-termini are unrelated. It contains an ATP binding site (Lys273), tyrosine kinase domain and a regulatory C-terminus (Bolen and Veillette, 1989). Deletion of the SH2 or SH3 domains increases p56^{lck} tyrosine kinase activity and phosphorylation of the autophosphorylation site Tyr394 (Reynolds *et al.*, 1992). The structure of the SH2 domain of p56^{lck} complexed with an 11 amino acid peptide derived from hamster polyoma middle T antigen has been analysed by high-resolution crystallography (Eck *et al.*, 1993).

The regulatory site, phosphorylated in resting T cells, is Tyr505 (equivalent to Tyr527 in SRC). Site-directed mutagenesis of Tyr505 activates the oncogenic potential of p56^{lck}, as does deletion of the C-terminal region containing Tyr505 (Adler and Sefton, 1992). The SH2 but not the SH3 domain is required for full oncogenic activity in p56^{lck} from which Tyr505 has been removed (Veillette *et al.*, 1992). Tyr505 is specifically phosphorylated by the human p50^{csk} tyrosine kinase which thus negatively regulates that activity of p56^{lck} (Bergman *et al.*, 1992).

Tyr505 is dephosphorylated by the tyrosine phosphatase activity of CD45 when cells are activated via surface receptors, thus permitting the phosphorylation of Tyr394 which represents the switch to the activated enzyme form. (Tyr394 is equivalent to Tyr416 in SRC). Physical association between p56^{lck} and CD45 occurs independently of the TCR (Koretzky *et al.*, 1993). In CD45$^-$ Jurkat human leukaemia cells the activation of p56^{lck} after CD2 stimulation requires the expression of exogenously introduced CD45 (Danielian *et al.*, 1992). A subclone of Jurkat cells that is defective in the expression of p56^{lck} and CD45 requires TPA for optimal growth, suggesting that the stimulation of protein kinase C may compensate for the loss of the tyrosine kinase activity of p56^{lck} (Tchou-Wong and Weinstein, 1992). The expression of *Lck* cDNA in these cells restores responsiveness to stimulation via the TCR (Straus and Weiss, 1992).

Sequences of human and mouse p56^{lck}, chicken SRC and v-YES

```
Human LCK    (1)    MGCGCSSHPEDDWMENIDVCENCHYPIVPLDGKGTLLIRNGSEVRDPLVTYEGSNPPASP
Mouse LCK    (1)    ---V---------------------------S-ISLP----------------L-----
SRC          (21)   PDSTHHGGFPASQTPNKTAAPDT-RTPSRSF-TVATEPKLFGGFNTSDTVTSPQRAG-LA
v-YES        (29)   *EHYGSDSSQ*T*S*AIKGSAVNFNSH*MTPFGGPSGMTP***ASS*FSAVPSPYPST*T

Human LCK    (61)   LQDNLVIALHSYEPSHDGDLGFEKGEQLRILEQS GEWWKAQSLTTGQEGFIPFNFVAKA
Mouse LCK    (61)   -------------------------------------- -------------------
SRC          (81)   GGVTTFV--YD--SRTET--S-K---R-Q-VNNTE-D--L-H------T-Y--S-Y--PS
v-YES        (89)   ****V********A**TD********F**I*******E*R*IA**K**********A

Human LCK    (120)  NSLEPEPWFFKNLSRKDAERQLLAPGNTHGSFLIRESESTAGSFSLSVRDFDQNQGEVVK
Mouse LCK    (120)  -----------------------------------------------------------
SRC          (141)  DSIQAEE-Y-GKIT-RES--L--N-E-PR-T---V----T-K-AYC---S--NAK-LN--
v-YES        (149)  ***E********MG*KDA******G*Q**I************S**IR*W*EVR*D***

Human LCK    (180)  HYKIRNLDNGGFYISPRITFPGLHELVRHYTNASDGLCTRLSRPCQTQKPQKPWWE DEW
Mouse LCK    (180)  ----------------------D-------------K---------------- ---
SRC          (201)  -----K--S----ITS-TQ-SS-QQ--AY-SKHA----H--TNV-PTS---TQGLAK-A-
v-YES        (209)  ********N**Y***TRA**E***K**KH*RE*******K**T****V***********
                                   # #  #                     #

Human LCK    (239)  EVPRETLKLVERLGAGQFGEVWMGYYNGHTKVAVKSLKQGSMSPDAFLAEANLMKQLQHQ
Mouse LCK    (239)  ----------------------------------------------VP----------P
SRC          (261)  -I---S-R-EVK--Q-C-------TW--T-R--I-T--P-N---E---Q--QV--K-R-E
v-YES        (269)  *****************************K******L*T*M*********I*****D

Human LCK    (299)  RLVRLYAVVTQEPIYIITEYMENGSLVDFLKTPSGIKLTINKLLDMAAQIAEGMAFIEER
Mouse LCK    (299)  --------------------------------NV-----------------Q
SRC          (321)  K--Q-----SE-----V----SK---L----GEM-KY-RLPQ-V-------S---YV-RM
v-YES        (329)  ***P**********F*T*********EGE**F*************D***I***

Human LCK    (359)  NYIHRDLRAANILVSDTLSCKIADFGLARLIEDNEYTAREGAKFPIKWTAPEAINYGTFT
Mouse LCK    (359)  -----------------------------------------------------------
SRC          (381)  --V----------GEN-V--V----------------Q-------------AL--R--
v-YES        (389)  **I***********D*****I***********************************
```

```
Human LCK  (419) IKSDVWSFGILLTEIVTHGRIPYPGMTNPEVIQNLERGYRMVRPDNCPEELYQLMRLCWK
Mouse LCK  (419) ---------------------------------------------------------H--M----
SRC        (441) --------------LT-K--V-----V-R--LDQV------PC-PE---S-HD--CQ--R
v-YES      (449) ****************V*****************E**********QG*****E**KL**K

Human LCK  (479) ERPEDRPTFDYLRSVLEDFFTATEGQYQPQP (509)
Mouse LCK  (479) ---------------D-------------- (509)
SRC        (501) RD--E----E--QAF---Y--S--P----GENL (533)
v-YES      (509) K*PD*******I*S*******AA**SGY (529)
```

* Indicates identity between v-YES and SRC. Dashes indicate identity between SRC and p56*lck*. Underlined: SH3 domain (65–115). Italics: SH2. # Indicates ATP binding region. p56*lck* domains: Gly2, myristate attachment site; 232–493 catalytic; 251–259 and 273 ATP binding; 394 autophosphorylation; 505 potential phosphorylation site. Sequence conflicts: 87 Q –> P (Perlmutter *et al.*, 1988); 206–212 VRHYTNA –> ASAITPIA (Koga *et al.*, 1986); 258–267 EVWMGYYNGH –> RCGWGTTTGT (Koga *et al.*, 1986); 282–286 PDAFL –> AGRLP (Koga *et al.*, 1986); 375–375 T –> A (Trevillyan *et al.*, 1986); 472–472 L –> H (Veillette *et al.*, 1987); 504–509 QYQPQP –> STA (Koga *et al.*, 1986). See **SRC** for the sequence of TKL.

Databank file names and accession numbers

	GENE	EMBL	SWISSPROT	REFERENCES
Human	*LCK*	Hslckb X13529 Hsptkjur X04476 Hslck3 X14055 Hslck X06369 Hstcptk X05027 Hslcka M21510	KLSK_HUMAN P06239; P07100	Perlmutter *et al.*, 1988 Koga *et al.*, 1986 Rouer *et al.*, 1989 Trevillyan *et al.*, 1986 Veillette *et al.*, 1987
Mouse	*Lck*	Mmlckaa M21511		Garvin *et al.*, 1988
Chicken	*Tkl*	Ggtkl J03579		Strebhardt *et al.*, 1987 Chow *et al.*, 1992

Reviews

Bolen, J.B. and Veillette, A. (1989). A function for the *lck* proto-oncogene. Trends Biochem. Sci., 14, 404–407.

Sefton, B.M. (1991). The *lck* tyrosine protein kinase. Oncogene, 6, 683–686.

Papers

Abraham, K.M., Levin, S.D., Marth, J.D., Forbush, K.A. and Perlmutter, R.M. (1991). Thymic tumorigenesis induced by overexpression of p56*lck*. Proc. Natl Acad. Sci. USA, 88, 3977–3981.

Abts, H., Jucker, M., Diehl, V. and Tesch, H (1991). Human chronic lymphocytic leukemia cells regularly express mRNAs of the protooncogenes *lck* and c-*fgr*. Leukemia Res., 15, 987–997.

Adler, H.T. and Sefton, B.M. (1992). Generation and characterization of transforming variants of the *lck* tyrosine protein kinase. Oncogene, 7, 1191–1199.

Adler, H.T., Reynolds, P.J., Kelly, C.M. and Sefton, B.M. (1988). Transcriptional activation of *lck* by retrovirus promoter insertion between two lymphoid-specific promoters. J. Virol., 62, 4113–4122.

Allen, J.M., Forbush, K.A. and Perlmutter, R.M.. (1992). Functional dissection of the *lck* proximal promoter. Mol. Cell. Biol., 12, 2758–2768.

Amrein, K.E., Flint, N., Panholzer, B. and Burn, P. (1992). Ras GTPase-activating protein: a substrate and a potential binding protein of the protein-tyrosine kinase p56*lck*. Proc. Natl Acad. Sci. USA, 89, 3343–3346.

Anderson, S.J., Abraham, K.M., Nakayama, T., Singer, A. and Perlmutter, R.M. (1992). Inhibition of T-cell receptor β-chain gene rearrangement by overexpression of the non-receptor protein tyrosine kinase p56*lck*. EMBO J., 11, 4877–4886.

Bell, G.M., Bolen, J.B. and Imboden, J.B. (1992). Association of src-like protein tyrosine kinases with the CD2 cell surface molecule in rat T lymphocytes and natural killer cells. Mol. Cell. Biol., 12, 5548–5554.

Bergman, M., Mustelin, T., Oetken, C., Partanen, J., Flint, N.A., Amrein, K.E., Autero, M., Burn, P. and Alitalo, K. (1992). The human p50*csk* tyrosine kinase phosphorylates p56*lck* at Tyr-505 and down regulates its catalytic activity. EMBO J., 11, 2919–2924.

Burgess, K.E., Yamamoto, M., Prasad, K.V.S. and Rudd, C.E. (1992). CD5 acts as a tyrosine kinase substrate within a receptor complex comprising T-cell receptor ζ chain/CD3 and protein-tyrosine kinases p56*lck* and p59*fyn*. (1992). Proc. Natl Acad. Sci. USA, 89, 9311–9315.

Burnett, R.C., David, J.C., Harden, A.M., Le-Beau, M.M., Rowley, J.D. and Diaz, M.O. (1991). The LCK gene is involved in the t(1;7)(p34;q34) in the T-cell acute lymphoblastic leukemia derived cell line, HSB-2. Genes Chromosomes & Cancer, 3, 461–467.

Campbell, M.A. and Sefton, B.M. (1992). Association between B-lymphocyte membrane immunoglobulin and multiple members of the *src* family of protein tyrosine kinases. Mol. Cell. Biol., 12, 2315–2321.

Casnellie, J.E., Harrison, M.L., Pike, L.J., Hellstrom, K.E. and Krebs, E.G. (1982). Phosphorylation of synthetic peptides by a tyrosine protein kinase from the particulate fraction of a lymphoma cell line. Proc. Natl Acad. Sci. USA, 79, 282–286.

Chow, L.M.L., Ratcliffe, M.J.H. and Veillette, A. (1992). *tkl* is the avian homolog of the mammalian *lck* tyrosine protein kinase gene. Mol. Cell. Biol., 12, 1226–1233.

Cooke, M.F., Abraham, K.M., Forbush, K.A. and Perlmutter, R.M. (1991). Regulation of T cell receptor signaling by a *src* family protein-tyrosine kinase (p59*fyn*). Cell, 65, 281–291.

Danielian, S., Alcover, A., Polissard, L., Stefanescu, M., Acuto, O., Fischer, S. and Fagard, R. (1992). Both T cell receptor (TcR)–CD3 complex and CD2 increase the tyrosine kinase activity of p56*lck*. CD2 can mediate TcR–CD3-independent and CD45-dependent activation of p56*lck*. Eur. J. Immunol., 22, 2915–2921.

Eck, M.J., Shoelson, S.E. and Harrison, S.C. (1993). Recognition of a high-affinity phosphotyrosyl peptide by the Src homology-2 domain of p56*lck*. Nature, 362, 87–91.

Ellis, C., Liu, X., Anderson, D., Abraham, N., Veillette, A. and Pawson, T. (1991). Tyrosine phosphorylation of GAP and GAP-associated proteins in lymphoid and fibroblast cells expressing *lck*. Oncogene, 6, 895–901.

Ettehadieh, E., Sanghera, J.S., Pelech, S.L., Hess-Bienz, D., Watts, J., Shastri, N. and Aebersold, R. (1992). Tyrosyl phosphorylation and activation of MAP kinases by p56*lck*. Science, 255, 853–855.

Garvin, A.M., Pawar, S., Marth, J.D. and Perlmutter, R.M. (1988). Structure of the murine *lck* gene and its rearrangement in a murine lymphoma cell line. Mol. Cell. Biol. 8, 3058–3064.

Glaichenhaus, N., Shastri, N., Littman, D.R. and Turner, J.M. (1991). Requirement for association of p56*lck* with CD4 in antigen-specific signal transduction in T cells. Cell, 64, 511–529.

Hatakeyama, M., Kono, T., Kobayashi, N., Kawakara, A., Levin, S.D., Perlmutter, R.M. and Taniguchi, T. (1991). Interaction of the IL-2 receptor with the *src*-family kinase p56*lck*: identification of novel intermolecular association. Science, 252, 1523–1528.

Horak, I.D., Gress, R.E., Lucas, P.J., Horak, E.M., Waldmann, T.A. and Bolen, J.B. (1991). T-lymphocyte interleukin 2-dependent tyrosine protein kinase signal transduction involves the activation of p56*lck*. Proc. Natl Acad. Sci. USA, 88, 1996–2000.

Koga, Y., Caccia, N., Toyonaga, B., Spolski, R., Yanagi, Y., Yoshikai, Y. and Mak, T.W. (1986). A human T cell-specific cDNA clone (YT16) encodes a protein with extensive homology to a family of protein-tyrosine kinases. Eur. J. Immunol., 16, 1643–1646.

Koretzky, G.A., Kohmetscher, M. and Ross, S. (1993). CD45-associated kinase activity requires *lck* but not T cell receptor expression in the Jurkat T cell line. J. Biol. Chem., 268, 8958–8964.

Leung, S., McCracken, S., Ghysdael, J. and Miyamoto, N.G. (1993). Requirement of an ETS-binding element for transcription of the human *lck* type I promoter. Oncogene, 8, 989–997.

Levin, S.D., Anderson, S.J., Forbush, K.A. and Perlmutter, R.M. (1993). A dominant negative transgene defines a role for p56*lck* in thymopoiesis. EMBO J., 12, 1671–1680.

Louie, R.R., King, C.S., MacAuley, A., Marth, J.D., Perlmutter, R.M., Eckhart, W. and Cooper, J.A. (1988). p56*lck* protein-tyrosine kinase is cytoskeletal and does not bind to polyomavirus middle T antigen. J. Virol., 62, 4673–4679.

Marth, J.D., Peet, R., Krebs, E.G. and Perlmutter, R.M. (1985). A lymphocyte-specific protein-tyrosine kinase gene is rearranged and overexpressed in the murine T cell lymphoma LSTRA. Cell, 43, 393–404.

Marth, J.D., Cooper, J.A., King, C.S., Ziegler, S.F., Tinker, D.A., Overell, R.W., Krebs, E.G. and Perlmutter, R.M. (1988). Neoplastic transformation induced by an activated lymphocyte-specific protein tyrosine kinase (pp56^{lck}). Mol. Cell. Biol., 8, 540–550.

Minami, Y., Kono, T., Yamada, K., Kobayashi, N., Kawahara, A., Perlmutter, R.M. and Taniguchi, T. (1993). Association of p56^{lck} with IL-2 receptor β chain is critical for the IL-2-induced activation of p56^{lck}. EMBO J., 12, 759–768.

Molina, T.J., Kishihara, K., Siderovski, D.P., van Ewijk, W., Narendran, A., Timms, E., Wakeham, A., Paige, C.J., Hartmann, K.-U., Veillette, A., Davidson, D. and Mak, T.W. (1992). Profound block in thymocyte development in mice lacking p56^{lck}. Nature, 357, 161–164.

Mori, T., Gou, M.W., Yoshida, H., Saito, S. and Mori, E. (1992). Expression of the signal transducing regions of CD4-like and lck genes in murine egg. Biochem. Biophys. Res. Commun., 182, 527–533.

Perlmutter, R.M., Marth, J.D., Lewis, D.B., Peet, R., Ziegler, S.F. and Wilson, C.B. (1988). Structure and expression of *lck* transcripts in human lymphoid cells. J. Cell. Biochem., 38, 117–126.

Prasad, K.V.S. and Rudd, C.E. (1992). A raf-1-related p110 polypeptide associates with the CD4–p56^{lck} complex in T cells. Mol. Cell. Biol., 12, 5260–5267.

Reynolds, P.J., Hurley, T.R. and Sefton, B.M. (1992). Functional analysis of the SH2 and SH3 domains of the *lck* tyrosine protein kinase. Oncogene, 7, 1949–1955.

Rouer, E. and Benarous, R. (1992). Alternative splicing in the human *lck* gene leads to the deletion of exon 1′ and results in a new type II *lck* transcript. Oncogene, 7, 2535–2538.

Rouer, E., Van Huynh, T., Lavareda de Souza, S., Lang, M.C., Fischer, S. and Benarous, R. (1989). Structure of the human *lck* gene: differences in genomic organisation within *src*-related genes affect only N-terminal exons. Gene, 84, 105–113.

Samelson, L.E., Phillips, A.F., Luong, E.T. and Klausner, R.D. (1990). Association of the *fyn* protein-tyrosine kinase with the T-cell antigen receptor. Proc. Natl Acad. Sci. USA, 87, 4358–4362.

Shin, S. and Steffen, D.L. (1993). Frequent activation of the *lck* gene by promoter insertion and aberrant splicing in murine leukemia virus-induced rat lymphomas. Oncogene, 8, 141–149.

Straus, D.B. and Weiss, A. (1992). Genetic evidence for the involvement of the lck tyrosine kinase in signal transduction through the T cell antigen receptor. Cell, 70, 585–593.

Strebhardt, K., Mullins, J.I., Bruck, C. and Ruebsamen-Waigmann H. (1987). Additional member of the protein-tyrosine kinase family: The *src*- and *lck*-related protooncogene c-*tkl*. Proc. Natl Acad. Sci. USA, 84, 8778–8782.

Taieb, J., Vitte-Mony, I., Auffredou, M.T., Dorseuil, O., Gacon, G., Bertoglio, J. and Vazquez, A. (1993). Regulation of p56^{lck} kinase expression and control of DNA synthesis in activated human B lymphocytes. J. Biol. Chem., 268, 9169–9171.

Takadera, T., Leung, S., Gernone, A., Koga, Y., Takihara, Y., Miyamoto, N.G. and Mak, T.K. (1989). Structure of the two promoters of the human *lck* gene: differential accumulation of two classes of *lck* transcripts in T cells. Mol. Cell. Biol., 9, 2173–2180.

Tchou-Wong, K.-M. and Weinstein, I.B. (1992). Altered expression of protein kinase C, lck, and CD45 in a 12-O-tetradecanoylphorbol-13-acetate-dependent leukemic T-cell variant that expresses a high level of interleukin-2 receptor. Mol. Cell. Biol., 12, 394–401.

Thompson, P.A., Ledbetter, J.A., Rapp, U.R. and Bolen, J.B. (1991). The *raf*-1 serine-threonine kinase is a substrate for the p56^{lck} protein tyrosine kinase in human T-cells. Cell Growth Differ., 2, 609–617.

Thompson, P.A., Gutkind, J.S., Robbins, K.C., Ledbetter, J.A. and Bolen, J.B. (1992). Identification of distinct populations of PI-3 kinase activity following T-cell activation. Oncogene, 7, 719–725.

Trevillyan, J.M., Lin, Y., Chen, S.J., Phillips, C.A., Canna, C. and Linna, T.J. (1986). Human T lymphocytes express a protein-tyrosine kinase homologous to p56LSTRA. Biochim. Biophys. Acta, 888, 286–295.

Veillette, A., Foss, F.M., Sausville, E.A., Bolen, J.B. and Rosen, N. (1987). Expression of the *lck* tyrosine kinase gene in human colon carcinoma and other non-lymphoid human tumor cell lines. Oncogene Res., 1, 357–374.

Veillette, A., Caron, L., Fournel, M. and Pawson, T. (1992). Regulation of the enzymatic function of the lymphocyte-specific tyrosine protein kinase p56^{lck} by the non-catalytic SH2 and SH3 domains. Oncogene, 7, 971–980.

MAS

MAS is a human transforming gene having no homology with known viral oncogenes that was originally detected by NIH 3T3 fibroblast transfection of DNA from an epidermoid carcinoma (Young *et al.*, 1986).

Related genes

Rat t*horacic* a*orta* (*Rta*): 34% sequence identity between RTA and MAS proteins (Ross *et al.*, 1990).

Human *mas*-related gene (*MRG*): 35% identity between MRG and MAS proteins (Monnot *et al.*, 1991).

There is close structural similarity and a similar hydrophobicity pattern predicting seven transmembrane domains in MAS and a number of transmitter and hormone receptors including the visual opsins, α_2, β_1 and β_2 adrenergic receptors, M1 and M2 muscarinic acetylcholine receptors and substance K receptor.

Transformation

MAS renders NIH 3T3 fibroblasts tumorigenic in nude mice and has a weak focus-inducing activity in NIH 3T3 cells (Young *et al.*, 1986). Oncogenic rearrangement of non-coding regions accelerates tumorigenesis by an unknown mechanism.

	MAS/Mas
Nucleotides (kb)	Not fully mapped
Chromosome	
Human	6q24–q27
Mouse	17
	(Cebra-Thomas *et al.*, 1992)
Exons	ORF contained in a single exon
mRNA (kb)	2.5 (957 bp ORF)
Amino acids	
Human	325
Mouse, rat	324
Mass (kDa)	
(predicted)	37
(expressed)	45

Cellular location

Transmembrane cell surface protein.

Tissue location

Rat *Mas* is strongly expressed in the hippocampus and cerebral cortex (Young *et al.*, 1988; Bunnemann *et al.*, 1990). The related RTA protein is significantly expressed in the gut, vas deferens, uterus and aorta (Ross *et al.*, 1990). *MRG* expression has not been detected (Monnot *et al.*, 1991).

Protein function

MAS is a neuronal type angiotensin III receptor. Its action is mediated by G proteins that activate PIP_2 hydrolysis causing increase in $[Ca^{2+}]_i$ (Jackson *et al.*, 1988).

Sequences of human and rat MAS

```
Human MAS    (1)   MDGSNVTSFVVEEPTNISTGRNASVGNAHRQIPIVHWVIMSISPVGFVENGILLWFLCF
Rat MAS      (1)   --Q--M---AE-KAM-T- S----L-TS-PP------------L--------------

            (60)   RMRRNPFTVYITHLSIADISLLFCIFILSIDYALDYELSSGHYYTIVTLSVTFLFGYNTG
            (59)   ----------------------------------------------------------

           (120)   LYLLTAISVERCLSVLYPIWYRCHRPKYQSALVCALLWALSCLVTTMEYVMCIDREEESH
           (119)   ------------------------H---F--------------------SG----

           (180)   SRNDCRAVIIFIAILSFLVFTPLMLVSSTILVVKIRKNTWASHSSKLYIVIMVTIIIFLI
           (179)   -QS-------------------------------------------------------

           (240)   FAMPMRLLYLLYYEYWSTFGNLHHISLLFSTINSSANPFIYFFVGSSKKKRFKESLKVVL
           (239)   ------V---------------------------------------------------

           (300)   TRAFKDEMQPRRQKDNCNTVTVETVV(325)
           (299)   ------------EGNG---SI----(324)
```

Putative domains: 1–30 extracellular; 31–61, 66–97, 105–135, 150–172, 186–214, 225–250, 258–286 seven transmembrane; 62–65, 136–149, 215–224, 287–325 cytoplasmic; 98–104, 173–185, 251–257 extracellular; 5, 16, 22 potential carbohydrate attachment sites.
   Rat: Putative domains: 1–329 extracellular; 30–60, 65–96, 104–134, 149–171, 185–213, 224–249, 257–285 transmembrane; 61–64, 135–148, 214–223, 286–324 cytoplasmic; 97–103, 172–184, 250–256 extracellular; 5, 16, 21 potential carbohydrate attachment sites.

Databank file names and accession numbers

	GENE	EMBL	SWISSPROT	REFERENCES
Human	*MAS*	Hsmas M13150	TMAS_HUMAN P04201	Young *et al.*, 1986 Jackson *et al.*, 1988
Rat	*Mas*	Rnmas01 J03823	TMAS_RAT P12526	Young *et al.*, 1988

Papers

Bunnemann, B., Fuxe, K., Metzger, R., Mullins, J., Jackson, T.R., Hanley, M.R. and Ganten, D. (1990). Autoradiographic localization of *mas* proto-oncogene mRNA in adult rat brain using in situ hybridization. Neurosci. Lett., 114, 147–153.

Cebra-Thomas, J.A., Tsai, J.-Y., Pilder, S.H., Copeland, N.G., Jenkins, N.A. and Silver, L.M. (1992). Localization of the *Mas* proto-oncogene to a densely marked region of mouse chromosome 17 associated with genomic imprinting. Genomics, 13, 444–446.

Jackson, T.R., Blair, L.A., Marshall, J., Goedert, M. and Hanley, M.R. (1988). The *mas* oncogene encodes an angiotensin receptor. Nature, 335, 437–440.

Monnot, C., Weber, V., Stinnakre, J., Bihoreau, C., Teutsch, B., Corvol, P. and Clauser, E. (1991). Cloning and functional characterization of a novel *mas*-related gene, modulating intracellular angiotensin II actions. Mol. Endocrinol., 5, 1477–1487.

Ross, P.C., Figler, R.A., Corjay, M.H., Barber, C.M., Adam, N., Harcus, D.R. and Lynch, K.R. (1990). RTA, a candidate G protein-coupled receptor: cloning, sequencing and tissue distribution. Proc. Natl Acad. Sci. USA, 87, 3052–3056.

Young, D., Waitches, G., Birchmeler, C., Fasano, O. and Wigler, M. (1986). Isolation and characterization of a new cellular oncogene encoding a protein with multiple potential transmembrane domains. Cell, 45, 711–719.

Young, D., O'Neill, K., Jessell, T. and Wigler, M. (1988). Characterization of the rat *mas* oncogene and its high-level expression in the hippocampus and cerebral cortex of rat brain. Proc. Natl Acad. Sci. USA, 85, 5339–5342.

MET

MET was identified as an activated oncogene in an *N*-methyl-*N'*-nitrosoguanidine-treated human osteosarcoma cell line (MNNG-HOS; Cooper *et al.*, 1984; Park *et al.*, 1986). It was activated as an oncogene by the formation of a chimeric gene generated by chromosomal rearrangement fusing the *TPR* gene (*t*ranslocated *p*romoter *r*egion) to the N-terminally truncated *MET* kinase domain.

Related genes

TPR has weak homology in α-helical regions to tropomyosin, spectrin, laminin B1, myosin heavy chain and *Drosophila glued* protein (Mitchell and Cooper, 1992a) and to vimentin (Capetanaki *et al.*, 1990). The C-terminus of the larger TPR protein (TPR-L) is homologous to *Drosophila engrailed* protein, *E. coli* RNA polymerase sigma subunit and nucleolin (Mitchell and Cooper, 1992b).

MET has homology with v-*sea* (Smith *et al.*, 1989). MET has 63% overall identity with RON (1400 amino acids).

Cross-species homology

MET: 91% identity (human and mouse). TPR: N-terminus highly conserved (human and rat).

Transformation

MAN

MET mRNA and protein concentrations are increased in some human carcinomas and in epithelial tumour cell lines (Di Renzo *et al.*, 1991). In colorectal carcinomas *MET* is overexpressed by sixfold, although other tyrosine kinase receptors (EGFR and HER2) are not significantly overexpressed (Liu *et al.*, 1992). In thyroid papillary carcinomas MET protein concentration is increased by 100-fold (Di Renzo *et al.*, 1992) but it is not detectably overexpressed in breast carcinomas. *MET* is amplified and overexpressed in cell lines from human tumours of non-haematopoietic origin, particularly gastric tumours (Soman *et al.*, 1991). The *MET*-related *RON* gene maps to human chromosome 3p21, a region frequently deleted in small-cell carcinoma of the lung and in renal cell carcinoma (Ronsin *et al.*, 1993).

IN VITRO

Transforms NIH 3T3 fibroblasts when expressed from *Met*-SV40 promoter constructs (Cooper *et al.*, 1984) and NIH 3T3 cells overexpressing mouse *Met* are highly tumorigenic in nude mice (Rong *et al.*, 1992).

	MET/Met	TPR/Tpr	TPR–MET
Chromosome			
Human	7q31	1	
Mouse	6		
mRNA (kb)	3.0, 5.0, 7.0 and 8.0 Two 8 kb RNA generated by alternative splicing encode 170 kDa and 190 kDa isoforms (Rodrigues *et al.*, 1991). 6.0/7.0 (HOS and MNNG-HOS cells) 7.0 (Calu I human epithelial cell line)	8.5–10.0	5.0
Amino acids			
Human	1408	726 (TPR-S) 2094 (TPR-L)	1361
Mouse	1379	810	
Mass (kDa)			
(predicted) (expressed)	155.5 gp190 (p50$^\alpha$/p145$^\beta$ disulfide-linked, heterodimer synthesized as a single 170 kDa precursor) gp140 (p50$^\alpha$/p85$^\beta$) gp130 (p50$^\alpha$/p75$^\beta$) (Prat *et al.*, 1991)	84 (726) A 30 bp deletion extends the ORF to 2094 amino acids	p65$^{TPR\text{-}MET}$

Cellular location

MET β subunit (p145): Transmembrane growth factor tyrosine kinase receptor.
MET α subunit (p50): Extracellular, autophosphorylated.
Multimeric forms of the α/β heterodimer occur, suggesting that the receptors exist as patches on the cell surface (Faletto *et al.*, 1992).
TPR–MET: Probably cytosolic (Cooper, 1992).

Tissue location

High levels of *MET* mRNA occur in liver, gastrointestinal tract, thyroid and kidney. Low levels are expressed in normal colorectal mucosa (Iyer *et al.*, 1990; Liu *et al.*, 1992). Both gp190 and the truncated form gp140 are present in the microglial cells of the human CNS (Di Renzo *et al.*, 1993).

TPR is expressed in tumour cell lines of epithelial and mesenchymal origin and in T and B cell neoplasia (Park *et al.*, 1986). The alternatively spliced *TPR-L* (9 kb) is expressed in rat testis, lung, thymus and spleen (Mitchell and Cooper, 1992b).

Protein function

MET is a tyrosine kinase receptor that binds hepatocyte growth factor (HGF, also called scatter factor; Bottaro *et al.*, 1991; Naldini *et al.*, 1991c; Hartmann *et al.*, 1992). The activity of MET may be greatly enhanced by autophosphorylation of the cytoplasmic domain (Naldini *et al.*, 1991a). HGF causes rapid tyrosine phosphorylation of the β subunit of MET and a fragment of HGF can be cross-linked to MET (Bottaro *et al.*, 1991; Naldini *et al.*, 1991b). HGF is a potent mitogen for hepatocytes *in vitro* and is an hepatotrophic factor possibly involved in liver regeneration (Vande Woude, 1992). In the epithelial cell A549 HGF stimulates the RAS guanine nucleotide exchanger and increases the proportion of RAS-GTP (Graziani *et al.*, 1993).

HGF (scatter factor) was originally discovered as an activity that causes MDCK epithelial cells to change shape and become motile (Stoker and Perryman, 1985) and invasive in *in vitro* assays (Rosen *et al.*, 1991). HGF exerts similar effects on NIH 3T3 cells transfected to express p190^{MET} (Giordano *et al.*, 1993). Responses to HGF are cell-dependent and it can exert mitogenic, motogenic or morphogenic effects (Vande Woude, 1992). HGF is a co-mitogen for normal human melanocytes, acting synergistically with basic fibroblast growth factor (FGFB) or mast cell growth factor (MGF). Melanocytes express the MAP2 kinases ERK1 and ERK2, the latter being phosphorylated in response to HGF (Halaban *et al.*, 1992). NIH 3T3 fibroblasts that overexpress the human *MET* (*MET*^{hu}) proto-oncogene are only weakly tumorigenic in nude mice but cells co-transfected with *MET*^{hu} and *HGF*^{hu} are highly tumorigenic, indicating that an autocrine transformation mechanism occurs (Rong *et al.*, 1992).

TPR is a protein of unknown function with high α-helical content that contains a domain rich in the leucine zipper repeat motif (Mitchell and Cooper, 1992a).

TPR activates the oncogenic potential of both *MET*, *RAF* and *TRK* (Testa *et al.*, 1990). The *TPR–MET* oncogene appears to be activated by an insertion of chromosome 1 (*TPR*) DNA into the *MET* locus on chromosome 7, both upstream and downstream portions of *MET* being conserved. This is similar to the mechanism of activation of *RAF* by *TPR* (Ishikawa *et al.*, 1987). Both *TPR–MET* and *TPR–RAF* rearrangements occur within introns but there is no sequence homology between the sites.

A second *MET* allele is rearranged in the chemically treated human cell line MNNG-HOS. der(7)t(1;7)(q23;q32) represents a deletion of the N-terminus of the MET extracellular ligand binding domain but the rearranged allele also includes sequences derived from chromosome 2 (Testa *et al.*, 1990).

In the human gastric carcinoma cell line GTL-16 *MET* is amplified and overexpressed but is not rearranged with *TPR* sequences: a point mutation is presumed to activate MET kinase in these cells. In contrast to the normal location of *MET* (chromosome 7 in proximity to the cystic fibrosis (CFTR) gene), the amplification unit is located on another chromosome in GTL-16 cells, together with the *CFTR* and *IRP* genes, the latter encoding a putative growth factor, and neither *CFTR* nor *IRP* are transcribed (Ponzetto *et al.*, 1991).

Sequences of human and mouse MET

```
Human MET    (1)    MKAPAVLAPGILVLLFTLVQRSNGECKEALAKSEMNVNMKYQLPNFTAETPIQNVILHE
Mouse MET    (1)    ----T----------LS-----H-------V----------------------V--G

            (60)    HHIFLGATNYIYVLNEEDLQKVAEYKTGPVLEHPDCFPCQDCSSKANLSGGVWKDNINMA
            (61)    --IY----------DK-----S-F-----------L--R-------S-----------

           (120)    LVVDTYYDDQLISCGSVNRGTCQRHVFPHNHTADIQSEVHCIFSPQIEEPSQCPDCVVSA
           (120)    -L---------------------------L-PDNS---------M---E --SG--------
```

```
 (180)  LGAKVLSSVKDRFINFFVGNTINSSYFPDHPLHSISVRRLKETKDGFMFLTDQSYIDVLP
 (179)  ------L-E---------------P-GYS-----------Q---K-----------

 (240)  EFRDSYPIKYVHAFESNNFIYFLTVQRETLDAQTFHTRIIRFCSINSGLHSYMEMPLECI
 (239)  --L-------I---------------K----------------VD-------------

 (300)  LTEKRKKRSTKKEVFNILQAAYVSKPGAQLARQIGASLNDDILFGVFAQSKPDSAEPMDR
 (299)  -----R----RE---------------N--K-----PS----------------VN-

 (360)  SAMCAFPIKYVNDFFNKIVNKNNVRCLQHFYGPNHEHCFNRTLLRNSSGCEARRDEYRTE
 (359)  --V---------------------------------------------S------

 (420)  FTTALQRVDLFMGQFSEVLLTSISTFIKGDLTIANLGTSEGRFMQVVVSRSGPSTPHVNF
 (419)  ------------RLNQ-------------------------L--TAHL------

 (480)  LLDSHPVSPEVIVEHTLNQNGYTLVITGKKITKIPLNGLGCRHFQSCSQCLSAPPFVQCG
 (479)  ---------------PS-------V--------------G------------Y-I---

 (540)  WCHDKCVRSEECLSGTWTQQICLPAIYKVFPNSAPLEGGTRLTICGWDFGFRRNNKFDLK
 (539)  ---NQ---FD--P------E-----V-----T--------V----------K-----R

 (600)  KTRVLLGNESCTLTLSESTMNTLKCTVGPAMNKHFNMSIIISNGHGTTQYSTFSYVDPVI
 (599)  --K---------------T-----------SE---V-V----SRE-----A--------

 (660)  TSISPKYGPMAGGTLLTLTGNYLNSGNSRHISIGGKTCTLKSVSNSILECYTPAQTISTE
 (659)  -----R---Q----------K----------------------D-----------T-D-

 (720)  FAVKLKIDLANRETSIFSYREDPIVYEIHPTKSFISTWWKEPLNIVSFLFCFASGGSTIT
 (719)  -P------------S-------V------------                 ------

 (780)  GVGKNLNSVSVPRMVINVHEAGRNFTVACQHRSNSEIICCTTPSLQQLNLQLPLKTKAFF
 (761)  -I--T-----L-KL--D---V-V-Y------------------K--G----------

 (840)  MLDGILSKYFDLIYVHNPVFKPFEKPVMISMGNENVLEIKGNDIDPEAVKGEVLKVGNKS
 (821)  L-------H---T-------E---------------V-----N--------------Q-

 (900)  CENIHLHSEAVLCTVPNDLLKLNSELNIEWKQAISSTVLGKVIVQPDQNFTGLIAGVVSI
 (881)  --SL-W--G-------S----------------V---------------A---I-A---

 (960)  STALLLLLGFFLWLKKRKQIKDLGSELVRYDARVHTPHLDRLVSARSVSPTTEMVSNESV
 (941)  -VVV---S-L---MR--- H-------------------------------------

(1020)  DYRATFPEDQFPNSSQNGSCRQVQYPLTDMSPILTSGDSDISSPLLQNTVHIDLSALNPE
(1000)  -----------------A---------L----------------------------

(1080)  LVQAVQHVVIGPSSLIVHFNEVIGRGHFGCVYHGTLLDNDGKKIHCAVKSLNRITDIGEV
(1060)  ---------------------------------------------------E--

(1140)  SQFLTEGIIMKDFSHPNVLSLLGICLRSEGSPLVVLPYMKHGDLRNFIRNETHNPTVKDL
(1120)  ----------------------------------------------------

(1200)  IGFGLQVAKAMKYLASKKFVHRDLAARNCMLDEKFTVKVADFGLARDMYDKEYYSVHNKT
(1180)  --------G-----------------------------------------------

(1260)  GAKLPVKWMALESLQTQKFTTKSDVWSFGVVLWELMTRGAPPYPDVNTFDITVYLLQGRR
(1240)  -------------------------L--------------------I-------

(1320)  LLQPEYCPDPLYEVMLKCWHPKAEMRPSFSELVSRISAIFSTFIGEHYVHVNATYVNVKC
(1300)  ---------A----------------------S-------------------

(1380)  VAPYPSLLSSEDNADDEVDTRPASFWETS (1408)
(1360)  --------PSQ--I-G-GN- (1379)
```

Human protein domains: signal sequence (1–24); extracellular (25–950); transmembrane (951–973); nucleotide binding (1102–1110 and 1028); potential carbohydrate attachment sites: 45, 106, 149, 202, 399, 405, 607, 635, 803, 897, 948. 1027/1028: breakpoint for the translocation to form TPR–MET.

Sequence of human TPR

```
  (1)   MAAVLQQVLERTELNKLPKSVQNKLEKFLADQQSEIDGLKGRHEKFKVESEQQYFEIEKRLSHSQERLV
 (70)   NETRECQSLRLELEKLNNQLKALTEKNKELEIAQDRNIAIQSQFTRTKEELEAEKRDLIRTNERLSQELE
(140)   YLTEDVKRLNEKLKESNTTKGELQLKLDELQASDVSVKYREKRLEQEKELLHSQNTWLNTELKTKTDELL
(210)   ALGREKGNEILELKCNLENKKEEVSRLEEQMNGLKTSNEHLQKHVEDLLTKLKEAKEQQASMEEKFHNEL
(280)   NAHIKLSNLYKSAADDSEAKSNELTRAVEELHKLLKEAGEANKAIQDHLLEVEQSKDQMEKEMLEKIGRL
(350)   EKELENANDLLSATKRKGAILSEEELAAMSPTAAAVAKIVKPGMKLTELYNAYVETQDQLLLEKLENKRI
(420)   NKYLDEIVKEVEAKAPILKRQREEYERAQKAVASLSVKLEQAMKEIQRLQEDTDKANKQSSVLERDNRRM
(490)   EIQVKDLSQQIRVLLMELEEARGNHVIRDEEVSSADISSSEVISQHLVSYRNIEELQQQNQRLLVALRE
(560)   LGETREREEQETTSSKITELQLKLESALTELEQLRKSRQHQMQLVDSIVRQRDMYRILLSQTTGVAIPLH
(630)   ASSLDDVSLASTPKRPSTSQTVSTPAPVPVIESTEAIEAKAALKQLQEIFENYKKEKAENEKIQNEQLEK
(700)   LQEQVTDLRSQNTKISTQLDFASKRYL (726)
                                EMLQDNVEGYRREITSLHERNQKLTATTQKQEQIINTMTQDLRG
(770)   ANEKLAVAEVRAENLKKEKEMLKLSEVRLSQQRESLLAEQR (810)
```

The 30 bp deletion that extends the ORF to 810 amino acids causes the deletion of the C-terminal leucine from p84^{TPR} and the substitution of 85 amino acids.

Protein structure

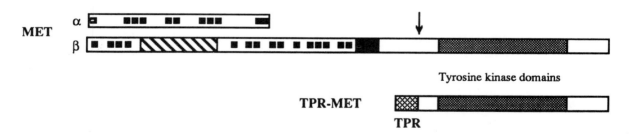

Black box: transmembrane region. The sequence Lys–Arg–Arg–Lys–Arg–Ser approximately 300 amino acids from the N-terminus of the MET precursor (190 kDa) may be cleaved to release the α subunit which then associates with the membrane-bound β subunit. The 170 kDa alternative form of MET is also expressed as a membrane tyrosine kinase but does not undergo cleavage to yield α and β subunits. In TPR–MET the tyrosine kinase domain of MET is fused to 140 N-terminal amino acids of TPR. The arrow indicates the breakpoint involved in the formation of TPR–MET.

Databank file names and accession numbers

	GENE	EMBL	SWISSPROT	REFERENCES
Human	*MET*	Hsmetpoa J02958	KMET_HUMAN P08581	Park *et al.*, 1987 Chan *et al.*, 1987 Dean *et al.*, 1985 Bottaro *et al.*, 1991
Mouse	*Met*	Mmmetonc Y00671	KMET_MOUSE P16056	Chan *et al.*, 1988
Human	*TPR-S*	Hstprmr X63105		Mitchell and Cooper, 1992a
Human	*TPR-L*	Hstpra M15326; X66397		Mitchell and Cooper, 1992b

Review

Cooper, C.S. (1992). The *met* oncogene: from detection by transfection to transmembrane receptor for hepatocyte growth factor. Oncogene, 7, 3–7.

Vande Woude, G. (1992). Hepatocyte growth factor: mitogen, motogen, and morphogen. Jpn J. Cancer Res., 83, cover article.

Papers

Bottaro, D.P., Rubin, J.S., Faletto, D.L., Chan, A.M.-L., Kmiecik, T.E., Vande Woude, G.F. and Aaronson, S.A. (1991). Identification of the hepatocyte growth factor receptor as the c-*met* proto-oncogene product. Science, 251, 802–804.

Capetanaki, Y., Kuisk, I., Rothblum, K. and Starnes, S. (1990). Mouse vimentin: structure relationship to *fos*, *jun*, CREB and *tpr*. Oncogene, 5, 645–655.

Chan, A.M.L., King, H.W.S., Tempest, P.R., Deakin, E.A., Cooper, C.S. and Brookes, P. (1987). Primary structure of the *met* protein tyrosine kinase domain. Oncogene, 1, 229–233.

Chan, A.M.L., King, H.W.S., Deakin, E.A., Tempest, P.R., Hilkens, J., Kroezen, V., Edwards, D.R., Wills, A.J., Brookes, P. and Cooper, C.S. (1988). Characterization of the mouse *met* proto-oncogene. Oncogene, 2, 593–599.

Cooper, C.S., Park, M., Blair, D., Tainsky, K., Huebner, C.M., Croce, C.M. and Vande Woude, G.F. (1984). Molecular cloning of a new transforming gene from a chemically transformed human cell line. Nature, 311, 29–33.

Daar, I.O., White, G.A., Schuh, S.M., Ferris, D.K. and Vande Woude, G.F. (1991). *tpr-met* oncogene product induces maturation-promoting factor activation in *Xenopus* oocytes. Mol. Cell. Biol., 11, 5985–5991.

Dean, M., Park, M., LeBeau, M.M., Robins, T.S., Diaz, M.O., Rowley, J.D., Blair, D.G. and Vande Woude, G.F. (1985). The human *met* oncogene is related to the tyrosine kinase oncogenes. Nature, 318, 385–388.

Di Renzo, M.F., Narsimhan, R.P., Olivero, M., Bretti, S., Giordano, S., Medico, E., Gaglia, P., Zara, P. and Comoglio, P.M. (1991). Expression of the met/HGF receptor in normal and neoplastic human tissues. Oncogene, 6, 1997–2003.

Di Renzo, M.F., Olivero, M., Ferro, S., Prat, M., Bongarzone, I., Pilotti, S., Belfiore, A., Costantino, A., Vigneri, R., Pierotti, M.A. and Comoglio, P.M. (1992). Overexpression of the c-*MET*/HGF receptor gene in human thyroid carcinomas. Oncogene, 7, 2549–2553.

Di Renzo, M.F., Bertolotto, A., Olivero, M., Putzolu, P., Crepaldi, T., Schiffer, D., Pagni, C.A. and Comoglio, P.M. (1993). Selective expression of the *met*/HGF receptor in human central nervous system microglia. Oncogene, 8, 219–222.

Faletto, D.L., Tsarfaty, I., Kmiecik, T.E., Gonzatti, M., Suzuki, T. and Vande Woude, G.F. (1992). Evidence for non-covalent clusters of the c-*met* proto-oncogene product. Oncogene, 7, 1149–1157.

Giordano, S., Zhen, Z., Medico, E., Gaudino, G., Galimi, F. and Comoglio, P.M. (1993). Transfer of motogenic and invasive response to scatter factor/hepatocyte growth factor by transfection of human *MET* protooncogene. Proc. Natl Acad. Sci. USA, 90, 649–653.

Graziani, A., Gramaglia, D., dalla Zonca, P. and Comoglio, P.M. (1993). Hepatocyte growth factor/scatter factor stimulates the Ras-guanine nucleotide exchanger. J. Biol. Chem., 268, 9165–9168.

Halaban, R., Rubin, J.S., Funasaka, Y., Cobb, M., Boulton, T., Faletto, D., Rosen, E., Chan, A., Yoko, K., White, W., Cook, C. and Moellmann, G. (1992). Met and hepatocyte growth factor/scatter factor signal transduction in normal melanocytes and melanoma cells. Oncogene, 7, 2195–2206.

Hartmann, G., Naldini, L., Weidner, K.M., Sachs, M., Vigna, E., Comoglio, P.M. and Birchmeier, W. (1992). A functional domain in the heavy chain of scatter factor/hepatocyte growth factor binds the c-*met* receptor and induces cell dissociation but not mitogenesis. Proc. Natl Acad. Sci. USA, 89, 11574–11578.

Ishikawa, F., Takaku, F., Nagao, M. and Sugimura, T. (1987). Rat c-*raf* oncogene activation by a rearrangement that produces a fused protein. Mol. Cell. Biol., 7, 1226–1232.

Iyer, A., Kmiecik, T.E., Park, M., Daar, I., Blair, D., Dunn, K.J., Sutrave, P., Ihle, J.N., Bodescot, M., and Vande Woude, G.F. (1990). Structure, tissue-specific expression and transforming activity of the mouse *met* proto-oncogene. Cell Growth Differ., 1, 87–95.

King, H.W.S., Tempest, P.R., Merrifield, K.R. and Rance, A.J. (1988). *tpr* homologues activate *met* and *raf*. Oncogene, 2, 617–619.

Liu, C., Park, M. and Tsao, M.-S. (1992). Overexpression of c-*met* proto-oncogene but not epidermal growth factor receptor or c-*erb*B-2 in primary human colorectal carcinomas. Oncogene, 7, 181–185.

Mitchell, P.J. and Cooper, C.S. (1992a). Nucleotide sequence analysis of human *tpr* cDNA clones. Oncogene, 7, 383–388.

Mitchell, P.J. and Cooper, C.S. (1992b). The human *tpr* gene encodes a protein of 2094 amino acids that has extensive coiled-coil regions and an acidic C-terminal domain. Oncogene, 7, 2329–2333.

Naldini, L., Vigna, E., Ferracini, R., Longati, P., Gandino, L., Prat, M and Comoglio, P.M. (1991a). The tyrosine kinase encoded by the *MET* proto-oncogene is activated by autophosphorylation. Mol. Cell. Biol., 11, 1793–1803.

Naldini, L., Vigna, E., Narsimhan, R.P., Gaudino, G., Zarnegar, R., Michalopoulos, G.K. and Comoglio, P.M. (1991b). Hepatocyte growth factor (HGF) stimulates the tyrosine kinase activity of the receptor encoded by the proto-oncogene c-*MET*. Oncogene, 6, 501–504.

Naldini, L., Weidner, K.M., Vigna, E., Gaudino, G., Bardelli, A., Ponzetto, C., Narsimhan, R.P., Hartmann, G., Zarnegar, R., Michalopoulos, G.K., Birchmeier, W. and Comoglio, P.M. (1991c). Scatter factor and hepatocyte growth factor are indistinguishable ligands for the *MET* receptor. EMBO J., 10, 2867–2878.

Park, M., Dean, M., Cooper, C.S., Schmidt, M., O'Brien, S.J., Blair, D.G. and Vande Woude, G.F. (1986). Mechanism of *met* oncogene activation. Cell, 45, 895–904.

Park, M., Dean, M., Kaul, K., Braun, M.J., Gonda, M.A. and Vande Woude, G. (1987). Sequence of *MET* protooncogene cDNA has features characteristic of the tyrosine kinase family of growth-factor receptors. Proc. Natl Acad. Sci. USA, 84, 6379–6383.

Ponzetto, C., Giordano, S., Peverali, F., Valle, G.D., Abate, M.L., Vaula, G. and Comoglio, P.M. (1991). c-*met* is amplified but not mutated in a cell line with an activated met tyrosine kinase. Oncogene, 6, 553–559.

Prat, M., Crepaldi, T., Gandino, L., Giordano, S., Longati, P. and Comoglio, P.M. (1991). C-terminal truncated forms of met, the hepatocyte growth factor receptor. Mol. Cell. Biol., 11, 5954–5962.

Rodrigues, G.A., Naujokas, M.A. and Park, M. (1991). Alternative splicing generates isoforms of the *met* receptor tyrosine kinase which undergo differential processing. Mol. Cell. Biol., 11, 2962–2970.

Rong, S., Bodescot, M., Blair, D., Dunn, J., Nakamura, T., Mizuno, K., Park, M., Chan, A., Aaronson, S. and Vande Woude, G.F. (1992). Tumorigenicity of the met proto-oncogene and the gene for hepatocyte growth factor. Mol. Cell. Biol., 12, 5152–5158.

Ronsin, C., Muscatelli, F., Mattei, M.-G. and Breathnach, R. (1993). A novel putative receptor protein tyrosine kinase of the met family. Oncogene, 8, 1195–1202.

Rosen, E.M., Knesel, J. and Goldberg, I.D. (1991). Scatter factor and its relationship to hepatocyte growth factor and *met*. Cell Growth Differ., 2, 603–607.

Smith, D.R., Vogt, P.K. and Hayman, M.J. (1989). The v-*sea* oncogene of avian erythroblastosis retrovirus S13: another member of the protein-tyrosine kinase gene family. Proc. Natl Acad. Sci. USA, 86, 5291–5295.

Soman, N.R., Correa, P., Ruiz, B.A. and Wogan, G.N. (1991). The *TPR-MET* oncogenic rearrangement is present and expressed in human gastric carcinoma and precursor lesions. Proc. Natl Acad. Sci. USA, 88, 4892–4896.

Stoker, M. and Perryman, M. (1985). An epithelial scatter factor released by embryo fibroblasts. J. Cell. Sci., 77, 209–223.

Testa, J.R., Park, M., Blair, D.G., Kalbakji, A., Arden, K. and Vande Woude, G.F. (1990). Analysis by pulsed field gel electrophoresis reveals complex rearrangements in two *MET* alleles in a chemically-treated human cell line, MNNG-HOS. Oncogene, 5, 1565–1571.

v-*mil* is the oncogene of avian retrovirus Mill-Hill-2 (MH2), which also carries v-*myc* (Saule *et al.*, 1983; Kan *et al.*, 1983; Coll *et al.*, 1983; Jansen *et al.*, 1983). MH2 is a defective leukaemia virus. v-*Rmil* is the oncogene of the IC10 and IC11 retroviruses generated during *in vitro* passaging of RAV-1 in chicken NR cells (Felder *et al.*, 1991).

Related genes

Mil is an evolutionarily conserved gene that is the avian homologue of mammalian *Raf*. v-*Rmil* is the avian homologue of human *RAFB1* (Koenen *et al.*, 1988; Dozier *et al.*, 1991; Eychene *et al.*, 1992).

Mil has homology with *Src*, *Fes*, *Fms*, *Mos*, *Yes*, *Fps*, *ErbB*, the catalytic subunit of cAMP-dependent protein kinase and protein kinase C.

Transformation

ANIMALS

MH2 induces monocytic leukaemias and liver tumours in chickens. Deletion mutants lacking either v-*mil* or v-*myc* do not (Graf *et al.*, 1986).

IN VITRO

MH2 rapidly transforms chick haematopoietic cells (macrophages) and fibroblasts (Graf *et al.*, 1986). In contrast to its mammalian homologue v-*raf*, v-*mht/mil* alone does not fully transform avian primary fibroblasts, probably because v-*mht/mil* contains an extra 5' segment relative to v-*raf* that affects substrate recognition (Kan, 1991).

	Mil	*Rmil*	v-*mil*
Nucleotides			1154 (MH2 genome)
Exons	11 (homologous to v-*mil*)		
mRNA (bk)			5.5 (*gag–mil*)
Chicken	4.0 2 differentially expressed forms from splicing of a 60nt exon (E7a) at the junction of exons 7 and 8	>10.0 Alternative splicing includes an exon upstream of the kinase domain	
Amino acids	647	767/807	379
Mass (kDa)			
(predicted)	73		42.8
(expressed)	71/73	93.5/95	p100$^{gag-mil}$

Cellular location

Mil: Unknown.
p100^{gag-mil}: Cytoplasmic (Bunte *et al.*, 1983).

Tissue location

In most chicken tissues *Mil* mRNA lacking exon 7a is expressed: mRNA containing E7a occurs only in heart, skeletal muscle and brain (Dozier *et al.*, 1991). *Rmil* is expressed at much higher levels in neural cells, neuroretinas and brain than in other embryonic tissues.

Protein function

MIL is a serine/threonine kinase belonging to the RAF–MOS subfamily of unknown function (Moelling *et al.*, 1984). It is phosphorylated *in vivo* (Patschinsky *et al.*, 1986). p100^{gag-mil} binds RNA and DNA *in vitro* (Bunte *et al.*, 1983).

In MH2-infected macrophages v-*myc* stimulates proliferation while v-*mil* induces synthesis of chicken myelomonocytic growth factor (Graf *et al.*, 1986). However, quail macrophages are transformed by MH2 *mil*⁻/*myc*⁺ viruses (Biegalke and Linial, 1987).

gag–mil (*gag–mht*) has only weak transforming capacity but it abolishes the growth factor dependence of avian macrophages transformed by other oncogenes. RMIL contains N-terminal sequences not present in other MIL/RAF proteins (Eychene *et al.*, 1992).

Sequences of chicken MIL and v-MIL (MH2)

```
Chicken MIL   (1)     MEHIQGAWKTISNGFGLKDSVFDGPNCISPTIVQQFGYQRRASDDGKISDTSKTSNTIR
              (60)    VFLPNKQRTVVNVRNGMTLHDCLMKALKVRGLQPECCAVFRLVTEPKGKKVRLDWNTDAA
              (120)   SLIGEELQVDFLDHVPLTTHNFARKTFLKLAFCDICQKFLLNGFRCQTCGYKFHEHCSTK
              (180)   VPTMCVDWSNIRQLLLFPNSNISDSGVPALPPLTMRRMRESVSRIPVSSQHRYSTPHVFT

MIL           (240)   FNTSNPSSEGTLSQRQRSTSTPNVHMVSTTMPVDSRIIEDAIRNHSESASPSALSGSPNN
v-MIL         (1)     -----------------------S------

MIL           (300)   MSPTGWSQPKTPVPAQRERAPGTNTQEKNKIRPRGQRDSSYYWEIEASEVMLSTRIGSGS
v-MIL         (33)    --------------------------------------------------L---------

MIL           (360)   FGTVYKGKWHGDVAVKILKVVDPTPEQFQAFRNEVAVLRKTRHVNILLFMGYMTKDNLAI
v-MIL         (93)    ------------------------------------------------------------

MIL           (420)   VTQWCEGSSLYKHLHVQETKFQMFQLIDIARQTAQGMDYLHAKNIIHRDMKSNNIFLHEG
v-MIL         (153)   ------------------------------------------------------------

MIL           (480)   LTVKIGDFGLATVKSRWSGSQQVEQPTGSILWMAPEVIRMQDSNPFSFQSDVYSYGIVLY
v-MIL         (213)   ------------------------------------------------------------

MIL           (540)   ELMTGELPYSHINNRDQIIFMVGRGYASPDLSKLYKNCPKAMKRLVADCLKKVREERPLF
v-MIL         (273)   ------------------------------------------------------------

MIL           (600)   PQILSSIELLQHSLPKINRSASEPSLHRASHTEDINSCTLTSTRLPVF (647)
v-MIL         (333)   ------------------------------------------------ (379)
```

Databank file names and accession numbers

	GENE	EMBL	SWISSPROT	REFERENCES
Chicken	*Mil*	Ggcmil X07017	KMIL_CHICK P05625	Koenen *et al.*, 1988
Chicken	*Mil* exon E7a	Ggmil7b X55430		Dozier *et al.*, 1991
Quail	*Mil* exon E7a	Cjmil7a X55431		Dozier *et al.*, 1991
Quail	*Rmil*			Eychene *et al.*, 1992
Mouse	*Mil* exon E7a	Mmraf X55432		Dozier *et al.*, 1991
MH2	v-*mil* (or v-*mht*)	Rear01 X00534	KMIL_AVIMH P00531	Sutrave *et al.*, 1984 Kan *et al.*, 1984

Papers

Biegalke, B. and Linial, M. (1987). Retention or loss of v-*mil* sequences after propagation of MH2 virus in vivo or in vitro. J. Virol., 61, 1949–1956.

Bunte, T., Greiser-Wilke, I. and Moelling, K. (1983). The transforming protein of the MC29-related virus CMII is a nuclear DNA-binding protein whereas MH2 codes for a cytoplasmic RNA–DNA binding polyprotein. EMBO J., 2, 1087–1092.

Coll, J., Righi, M., de Taisne, C., Dissous, C., Gegonne, A. and Stehelin, D. (1983). Molecular cloning of the avian transforming retrovirus MH2 reveals a novel cell-derived sequence (v-*mil*) in addition to the *myc* oncogene. EMBO J., 2, 2189–2194.

Dozier, C., Ansieau, S., Ferreira, E., Coll, J. and Stehelin, D. (1991). An alternatively spliced c-*mil*/*raf* mRNA is predominantly expressed in chicken muscular tissues and conserved among vertebrate species. Oncogene, 6, 1307–1311.

Eychene, A., Barnier, J.V., Dezelee, P., Marx, M., Laugier, D., Calogeraki, I. and Calothy, G. (1992). Quail neuroretina c-R*mil*(B-*raf*) proto-oncogene cDNAs encode two proteins of 93.5 and 95 kDa resulting from alternative splicing. Oncogene, 7, 1315–1323.

Felder, M.-P., Eychene, A., Barnier, J.V., Calogeraki, I., Calothy, G. and Marx, M. (1991). Common mechanism of retrovirus activation and transduction of c-*mil* and c-R*mil* in chicken neuroretina cells infected with Rous-associated virus type 1. J. Virol., 65, 3633–3640.

Graf, T., von Weizsacker, F., Grieser, S., Coll, J., Stehelin, D., Patschinsky, T., Bister, K., Bechade, C., Calothy, G. and Leutz, A. (1986). v-*mil* induces autocrine growth and enhanced tumorigenicity in v-*myc*-transformed avian macrophages. Cell, 45, 357–364.

Jansen, H.W., Ruckert, B., Lurz, R. and Bister, K. (1983). Two unrelated cell-derived sequences in the genome of avian leukemia and carcinoma inducing retrovirus MH2. EMBO J., 2, 1969–1975.

Kan, N.C. (1991). Mutagenesis of the v-*mht*/*mil* oncogene in avian carcinoma virus MH2. Avian Dis., 35, 941–949.

Kan, N.C., Flordellis, C.S., Garon, C.F., Duesberg, P.H. and Papas, T.S. (1983). Avian carcinoma virus MH2 contains a transformation-specific sequence, *mht*, and shares the *myc* sequence with MC29, CMII, and OK10 viruses. Proc. Natl Acad. Sci. USA, 80, 6566–6570.

Kan, N.C., Flordellis, C.S., Mark, G.E., Duesberg, P.H. and Papas, T.S. (1984). A common *onc* gene sequence transduced by avian carcinoma virus MH2 and by murine sarcoma virus 3611. Science, 223, 813–816.

Koenen, M., Sippel, A.E., Trachmann, C. and Bister, K. (1988). Primary structure of the chicken c-*mil* protein: identification of domains shared with or absent from the retroviral v-*mil* protein. Oncogene, 2, 179–185.

Moelling, K., Heimann, B., Beimling, P., Rapp, U.R. and Sander, T. (1984). Serine- and threonine-specific protein kinase activities of purified gag-mil and gag-raf protein. Nature, 312, 558–561.

Morrison, D.K., Kaplan, D.R., Escobedo, J.A., Rapp, U.R., Roberts, T.M. and Williams, L.T. (1989). Direct activation of the serine/threonine kinase activity of raf-1 through tyrosine phosphorylation by the PDGF β-receptor. Cell, 58, 649–657.

Patschinsky, T., Schroeer, B. and Bister, K. (1986). Protein product of proto-oncogene c-*mil*. Mol. Cell. Biol., 6, 739–744.

Saule, S., Coll, J., Righi, M., Lagrou, C., Raes, M.B. and Stehelin, D. (1983). Two different types of transcription for the myelocytomatosis viruses MH2 and CMII. EMBO J., 2, 805–809.

Sutrave, P., Bonner, T.I., Rapp, U.R., Jansen, H.W., Patschinsky, T. and Bister, K. (1984). Nucleotide sequence of avian retroviral oncogene v-*mil*: homologue of murine retroviral oncogene v-*raf*. Nature, 309, 85–88.

MOS

v-*mos* is the oncogene of the acutely transforming murine *Moloney* sarcoma virus (Mo-MuSV). Isolated from a rhabdosarcoma in BALB/c mice infected with Moloney murine leukaemia virus (Mo-MuLV; Moloney, 1966).

Related genes

Mos is a member of the *Raf–Mos* subfamily and has homology with *Src* but is not a tyrosine kinase.

Murine *Mos, Lyn, Jun, Lmyc, Lck, Fgr* and *Dsi-1* genes map to the same region of chromosome 4 (Ceci *et al.*, 1989).

Cross-species homology

MOS: 97% identity (human and monkey) (Paules *et al.*, 1988); 91% (mouse and rat); 77% (human and mouse); 62% (human, mouse and chicken) (Schmidt *et al.*, 1988); 53% (human and *Xenopus*) (Sagata *et al.*, 1988; Freeman *et al.*, 1989).

Transformation

MAN

MOS and the flanking regions of its gene are mutated in some benign pleomorphic adenomas of the salivary glands (Stenman *et al.*, 1991).

ANIMALS

Mos causes fibrosarcomas in mice following Mo-MuSV infection and can also cause osteosarcomas in other species (Fefer *et al.*, 1967; Fujinaga *et al.*, 1970). Activation of *Mos* by insertion of an endogenous intracisternal A-particle has been detected in some mouse plasmacytomas (Canaani *et al.*, 1983; Horowitz *et al.*, 1984).

IN VITRO

Mos/LTR or v-*mos*/LTR hybrid genes transform NIH 3T3 fibroblasts (Oskarsson *et al.*, 1980; Blair *et al.*, 1981; Wood *et al.*, 1984; Freeman *et al.*, 1989).

TRANSGENIC ANIMALS

Transgenic mice expressing *Mos* develop pheochromocytomas and medullary C-cell carcinomas of the thyroid resembling the human syndrome multiple endocrine neoplasia type II (Schulz *et al.*, 1992).

	MOS/Mos	v-mos
Nucleotides (kb)	1.2	>1.2
Chromosome		
Human	8q11	
Mouse	4	
Exons	Transcripts not processed	
mRNA (kb)		3.9, 5.2, 6.3 (HT1 MuSV)
Human	~1 (testes)	
Mouse	1.4 (ovaries); 1.7 (testes) (Propst and Vande Woude, 1985)	
Rat	1.7; 3.6 (Leibovitch *et al.*, 1990)	
Amino acids		
Human	346	374 (MuSV HT1 and clone 124)
Mouse	343	376 (MuSV M1)
Chicken	349	
Rat	339	
Xenopus	359	
Mass (kDa)		
(predicted) Human, chicken, mouse	38	41
(expressed)	39 (Paules *et al.*, 1989) p24, p29, p42 and p44 detected in transformed NIH 3T3 cells (Paules *et al.*, 1992)	$p37/39^{env-mos}$ $p85^{gag-mos}$
Protein half-life (min)	30	

Cellular location

Mos: Cytoplasm.
v-*mos*: Mainly nuclear.

Tissue location

Human *MOS* is expressed at low levels in normal T and B lymphocytes and in neuroblastoma and cervical carcinoma cell lines (Li *et al.*, 1993). *MOS* mRNA is only detectable in germ cells in testes (Propst and Vande Woude, 1985) and ovaries (Keshet *et al.*, 1987; Goldman *et al.*, 1988). The mouse transcript size varies with tissue suggesting tissue-specific regulation. In *Xenopus* and mouse oocytes pp39^{mos} is expressed specifically during meiotic maturation (Sagata *et al.*, 1988; Paules *et al.*, 1989). The *Mos* gene product has been reported to be expressed in other tissues (Herzog *et al.*, 1989; Leibovitch *et al.*, 1991).

Protein function

pp39^{mos} is a serine/threonine kinase. pp39^{mos} from *Xenopus* eggs exhibits autophosphorylation activity *in vitro* (Watanabe *et al.*, 1989). *Mos* expression is sufficient to cause meiosis I (Yew *et al.*, 1992), is required for meiosis II (Kanki and Donoghue, 1991; Daar *et al.*, 1991a) and is an active component of cytostatic factor (Sagata *et al.*, 1989a,b), an activity responsible for arrest in metaphase at the end of meiosis II (Lorca *et al.*, 1991). Therefore MOS directly or indirectly activates and/or stabilizes maturation promoting factor (MPF (p34^{cdc2} and cyclin)). Proteins other than MOS contribute to cytostatic factor and are not required for meiosis I (Yew *et al.*, 1992). MOS is an upstream activator of mitogen-activated protein (MAP) kinase and may directly phosphorylate MAP kinase during *Xenopus* oocyte entry into meiosis (Posada *et al.*, 1993; Nebreda and Hunt, 1993).

Immune complexes of pp39^{mos} from unfertilized eggs or transformed cells contain stoichiometric amounts of the p34^{cdc2} isoform p35^{cdk} and of tubulin, which is a substrate for MOS kinase activity *in vitro* (Zhou *et al.*, 1991a,b, 1992; Bai *et al.*, 1992a,b). MOS polymerizes with tubulin *in vitro* and co-localizes with tubulin in the spindle pole region during metaphase and in asters and the midbody during telophase (Zhou *et al.*, 1991a, b). These and other observations imply that MOS promotes the re-organization of microtubules that leads to meiotic spindle formation (Zhou *et al.*, 1991a, b). Microinjection of anti-MOS antibody interferes with meiotic spindle formation (Zhao *et al.*, 1990). The *Mos* proto-oncogene functions specifically during M phase and at a major cell cycle control point. Its transforming capacity (Yew *et al.*, 1992) probably derives from expression of its M phase activity during interphase (Sagata *et al.*, 1988, 1989a,b; Daar *et al.*, 1991b) and altered morphology and loss of contact inhibition phenotypes could be explained by this inappropriate expression.

MOS has unexplained ATP-dependent DNA binding activity (Seth *et al.*, 1987) and a major portion of the oncogene product is localized in the nucleus (Zhou *et al.*, 1991b). Cyclin B2 has been proposed as a substrate of MOS kinase *in vitro* (Roy *et al.*, 1990) but does not influence meiotic maturation *in vivo* (Freeman *et al.*, 1991).

MOS and v-MOS are equally effective in inducing meiotic maturation and cell cycle arrest and as transforming agents (Yew *et al.*, 1991).

The p85$^{gag-mos}$ protein increases in kinase activity by twofold as cells pass from G_0/G_1 to S and M phases. p85$^{gag-mos}$ is also hyperphosphorylated during mitosis and, *in vitro*, is phosphorylated in its N-terminal region (Ser47) by the mitotic form of p34^{cdc2} (Bai *et al.*, 1991). The G_1 phase expression of *Mos* is crucial for transformation, in contrast to cytostatic factor activity that is required for the normal G_2–M transition (Okazaki *et al.*, 1992).

v-MOS, v-HRAS or v-SRC inhibits glucocorticoid receptor (GR) function. In transfected NIH 3T3 cells v-MOS or v-FOS impairs transcription from two glucocorticoid responsive promoters. Activation of v-*mos* (or v-*Hras*) transiently stimulates *Fos* transcription and the co-expression of antisense *Fos* prevents the inhibition by v-*mos* of transcription from GR promoters (Touray *et al.*, 1991). This suggests that v-*mos*-induced expression of *Fos* mediates GR function.

Sequences of *Xenopus* MOS, human MOS, chicken MOS, mouse MOS and v-MOS (clone 124)

```
                                       .  . . .              . .   .                   .    .
Xenopus MOS   (1)    MPSPIPVERFLPRDLSPSIDLRPCSSPLELSHR   KLPGGLPACSGRRRLLPPRLAWCSIDWEQV
Human MOS     (1)    ----LALRPY-RSEF---V-A------S--P    A--LL-  -TLP-APR--R-----------
Chicken MOS   (1)    ------FNS---LE----A--------VVIPGKDG-AFL-G  TP-P-T-R-----------DRL
Mouse MOS     (1)    ----LSLC-Y---E----V-S-S---I--VAPRKAG--FL-  TTPP-APG--R----F-------
v-MOS         (1)    ***************************************  ***********************
```

```
                           . . . .             . .  .                   .     .
Xenopus MOS   (64)   LLLEPLGSSGGFGSVYRATYRGETVALKKVKRSTKNSLASKQSFWAELNAARLRHPHVVRVVAASA
Human MOS     (61)   C--QR--A-------K----QVP--I_Q-NKC---R---RR-------V-----DNI------T
Chicken MOS   (65)   C--Q--------A--K---H-V---V_Q--K-S--R---R--------V---Q-DN-------T
Mouse MOS     (64)   C-MHR---------K---H-VP--I_Q-NKC--DLR--QR-------I-----DNI------T
v-MOS         (64)   *****************************************G***********
                           ‾‾‾‾‾‾‾‾‾‾                 ‾
```

```
                       . . .            . ......          .  .
Xenopus MOS   (129)  SCPGDPGCPGTIIMEYTGTGTLHQRIYG  RS P     PLGA        EICMRYARHVADGL
Human MOS     (126)  RT-AGSNSL------FG-NV----V---AAGH -EGDAGE-HCRTGGQLSLGK-LK-SLD-VN--
Chicken MOS   (130)  CA-ASQNSL-------V-NV---HV--- T-DAWRQGEEEEG-CGRKALSMAEAVC-SCDIVT--
Mouse MOS     (129)  RT-E-SNSL------FG-NV----V---AT-- -E      --SC REQLSLGK-LK-SLD-VN--
v-MOS         (129) ************************D**** **      ******K****************
```

```
                       . . .       . . . ..        . .
Xenopus MOS   (178)  RFLHRDGVVHLDLKPANVLLAPGDLCKIGDFGCSQRLREGDEAAGGEPCCTQLRHVGGTYTHRAP
Human MOS     (190)  L---SQSI---------I-ISEQ-V---S-----EK-EDL   LCFQ-PSYPL---------
Chicken MOS   (194)  A---SQ-I---------I-ITEHGA-----------E--    LSQSHHVCQQ---------
Mouse MOS     (187)  L---SQSIL--------I-ISEQ-V---S------K-QDL   RCRQASPH-I------Q--
v-MOS         (187) ***********************************G*****P**********
```

```
                       . .      . . . . .        . .
Xenopus MOS   (243)  ELLKGEPVTAKADIYSFAITLWQMVSRELPYTGDRQCVLYAVVAYDLRPEM GPLFSHTEEGRAA
Human MOS     (249)  ------G--P-------------TTKQA--S-E--HI-----------SLSAAV-EDSLP-QRL
Chicken MOS   (253)  ------R--------------I-M--Q--L-E--Y--------N---PLAAAI-HESAV-QRL
Mouse MOS     (246)  -I----IA-P-------G------TT--V--S-EP-Y-Q------N---SLA-AV-TASLT-KTL
v-MOS         (246) ****************************************************A*
```

```
                       . .            .
Xenopus MOS   (307)  RTIVQSCWAARPQERPNAEQLLERLEQECAMCTGGPPSCSPESNAPPPLGTGL (359)
Human MOS     (314)  GDVI-R--RPSAAQ--S-RL--VD-TSLK-ELG (346)
Chicken MOS   (318)  -S-ISC--K-DVE--LS-A---PS-RALKENL (349)
Mouse MOS     (311)  QN-I----E--ALQ--G--L-QRD-KAFRGALG (343)
v-MOS         (311) **********G***S**************T** (374)
```

Dashes indicate identity with *Xenopus* MOS (Sagata *et al.*, 1988). * Indicates identity with mouse MOS. ATP binding sites underlined. Dots above the sequence indicate common amino acids that are conserved among members of the SRC family.

Protein structure

v-MOS from the earliest Mo-MuSV isolated (HT1 Mo-MuSV) is identical in amino acid sequence to MOS (Seth *et al.*, 1985). The *gag* protein (p65) is encoded in many Mo-MuSV strains (but not in HT1 Mo-MuSV). Five N-terminal *env* amino acids precede the v-*mos* ORF (the remainder of *env* being deleted in all Mo-MuSVs). The transforming properties of Mo-MuSVs are dependent on the presence of an LTR, LTR⁻ constructs being 4000-fold less effective (Wood *et al.*, 1983). A number of other MuSV isolates show some sequence changes in transduced v-*mos* (11 in MuSV-124 (van Beveren, 1982; Reddy *et al.*, 1981); 8 C-terminal in M1 Mo-MuSV; (Brow *et al.*, 1984)).

Transcription of *Mos* in mouse oocytes is directed by a simple promoter (consensus PyPyCAPyPyPyPyPy) comprised of sequences within 20 bp of the transcription start site (Pal *et al.*, 1991).

A negative regulatory region between 400 and 500 bp upstream from the *Mos* ATG inhibits transcription in somatic cells (Zinkel *et al.*, 1992). In rat and mouse a 200 bp region 1651–1835 bp upstream of the *Mos* exon has *cis*-inhibitory activity (e.g. can block the transforming activity of v-*mos*). The region contains two poly(A) signals and when located downstream of a gene causes termination of transcription (McGeady *et al.*, 1986).

Databank file names and accession numbers

	GENE	*EMBL*	*SWISSPROT*	*REFERENCES*
Human	*MOS*	Hscmos J00119	KMOS_HUMAN P00540	Watson *et al.*, 1982
Mouse	*Mos*	Mmrcmos J00620	KMOS_MOUSE P00536	van Beveren *et al.*, 1981 Rechavi *et al.*, 1982
Chicken	*Mos*		KMOS_CHICK P10741	Schmidt *et al.*, 1988
Rat	*Mos*	Rncmos X00422 Rncmoso X52952	KMOS_RAT P00539	van der Hoorn and Firzlaff, 1984 Leibovitch *et al.*, 1990
Green monkey	*Mos*	Camosc X12449	KMOS_CERAE P10650	Paules *et al.*, 1988
Xenopus laevis	pp39*mos*	Xlcmosa M25366 Xlp39mos X13311	KMOS_XENLA P12965	Freeman *et al.*, 1989 Sagata *et al.*, 1988
Mo-MuSV (strain HT1)	v-*mos*		KMOS_MSVMH P07331	Seth *et al.*, 1985
Mo-MuSV (strain M1)	v-*mos*	Remosml K02728	KMOS_MSVMM P00537	Brow *et al.*, 1984
	v-*mos*	Remsymos M15424	KMOS_MSVTS P10421	Friel *et al.*, 1987
(Myeloproliferative sarcoma virus clone TS159)				
Mo-MuSV (clone 124)	v-*mos*		KMOS_MSVMO P00538	van Beveren *et al.*, 1982 Reddy *et al.*, 1981

(Reddy *et al.*, 1981, found an additional C residue causing a frameshift and adding 409 amino acids to the sequence.)

Papers

Bai, W., Singh, B., Karshin, W.L., Shonk, R.A. and Arlinghaus, R.B. (1991). Phosphorylation of v-*mos* ser 47 by the mitotic form of p34^{cdc2}. Oncogene, 6, 1715–1723.

Bai, W., Singh, B., Yang, Y., Ramagli, L.S., Nash, M., Herzog, N.K. and Arlinghaus, R.B. (1992a). The physical interactions between p37$^{env-mos}$ and tubulin structures. Oncogene, 7, 493–500.

Bai, W., Singh, B., Yang, Y. and Arlinghaus, R.B. (1992b). Evidence for interaction between v-mos and a p34^{cdc2} isoform, p35^{cdk}. Oncogene, 7, 1757–1763.

Blair, D.G., Oskarsson, M., Wood, T.G., McClements, W.L., Fischinger, P.J. and Vande Woude, G.F. (1981). Activation of the transforming potential of a normal cellular sequence: a molecular model for oncogenesis. Science, 212, 941–943.

Brow, M.A., Sen, A. and Sutcliffe, J.G. (1984). Nucleotide sequence of the transforming gene of m1 murine sarcoma virus. J. Virol., 49, 579–582.

Canaani, E., Dreazen, O., Klar, A., Rechavi, G., Ram, D., Cohen, J.B. and Givol, D. (1983). Activation of the c-*mos* oncogene in a mouse plasmacytoma by insertion of an endogenous intracisternal A-particle genome. Proc. Natl Acad. Sci. USA, 80, 7118–7122.

Ceci, J.D., Siracusa, L.D., Jenkins, N.A. and Copeland, N.G. (1989). A molecular genetic linkage map of mouse chromosome 4 including the localization of several proto-oncogenes. Genomics, 5, 699–709.

Daar, I., Paules, R.S. and Vande Woude, G.F. (1991a) A characterization of cytostatic factor activity from *Xenopus* eggs and c-*mos*-transformed cells. J. Cell Biol., 114, 329–335.

Daar, I., Nebreda, A.R., Yew, N., Sass, P., Paules, R., Santos, E., Wigler, M. and Vande Woude, G.F. (1991b). The *ras* oncoprotein and M-phase activity. Science, 253, 74–76.

Donoghue, D.J. (1982). Demonstration of biological activity and nucleotide sequence of an *in vitro* synthesized clone of the Moloney murine sarcoma virus *mos* gene. J.Virol., 42, 538–546.

Fefer, A., McCoy, J.L. and Glynn, J.P. (1967). Induction and regression of primary Moloney sarcoma virus-induced tumors in mice. Cancer Res., 27, 1626–1631.

Freeman, R.S., Pickham, K.M., Kanki, J.P., Lee, B.A., Pena, S.V. and Donoghue, D.J. (1989). *Xenopus* homolog of the *mos* protooncogene transforms mammalian fibroblasts and induces maturation of *Xenopus* oocytes. Proc. Natl Acad. Sci. USA, 86, 5805–5809.

Freeman, R.S., Ballantyne, S.M. and Donoghue, D.J. (1991). Meiotic induction by *Xenopus* cyclin B is accelerated by co-expression with *mos*^{xe}. Mol. Cell. Biol., 11, 1713–1717.

Friel, J., Stocking, C., Stacey, A. and Ostertag, W. (1987). A temperature-sensitive mutant of the myeloproliferative sarcoma virus, altered by a point mutation in the *mos* oncogene, has been modified as a selectable retroviral vector. J. Virol., 61, 889–897.

Fujinaga, S., Poel, W.E. and Dmochowski, L. (1970). Light and electron microscope studies of osteosarcomas induced in rats and hamsters by Harvey and Moloney sarcoma viruses. Cancer Res., 30, 1698–1708.

Goldman, D.S., Kiessling, A.A., Millette, C.F. and Cooper, G.M. (1988). Expression of c-*mos* RNA in germ cells of male and female mice. Proc. Natl Acad. Sci. USA, 84, 4509–4513.

Herzog, N.K., Ramagli, L.S. and Arlinghaus, R.B. (1989). Somatic cell expression of the c-*mos* protein. Oncogene, 4, 1307–1315.

Horowitz, M., Luria, S., Rechavi, G. and Givol, D. (1984). Mechanism of activation of the mouse c-*mos* oncogene by the LTR of an intracisternal A-particle gene. EMBO J., 3, 2937–2941.

Kanki, J.P. and Donoghue, D.J. (1991). Progression from meiosis I to meiosis II in *Xenopus* oocytes requires *de novo* translation of the *mos*^{xe} protooncogene. Proc. Natl Acad. Sci. USA, 88, 5794–5798.

Keshet, E., Rosenberg, M., Mercer, J.A., Propst, F., Vande Woude, G.F., Jenkins, N.A. and Copeland, N.G. (1987). Developmental regulation of ovarian-specific *mos* expression. Oncogene, 2, 234–240.

Leibovitch, S.A., Lenormand, J.-L., Leibovitch, M.-P., Guillier, M., Mallard, L. and Harel, J. (1990). Rat myogenic c-*mos* cDNA: cloning sequence analysis and regulation during muscle development. Oncogene, 5, 1149–1157.

Leibovitch, S.A., Guillier, M., Lenormand, J.-L. and Leibovitch, M.-P. (1991). Accumulation of the c-*mos* protein is correlated with post-natal development of skeletal muscle. Oncogene, 6, 1617–1622.

Li, C.-C.H., Chen, E., O'Connell, C.D. and Longo, D.L. (1993). Detection of c-*mos* proto-oncogene expression in human cells. Oncogene, 8, 1685–1691.

Lorca, T., Galas, S., Fesquet, D., Devault, A., Cavadore, J.-C. and Doree, M. (1991). Degradation of the proto-oncogene product p39^{mos} is not necessary for cyclin proteolysis and exit from meiotic metaphase: requirement for a Ca^{2+}-calmodulin dependent event. EMBO J., 10, 2087–2093.

McGeady, M.L., Wood, T.G., Maizel, J.V. and Vande Woude, G.F. (1986). Sequences upstream to the mouse c-*mos* oncogene may function as a transcription termination signal. DNA, 5, 289–298.

Moloney, J.B. (1966). A virus induced rhabdomyosarcoma of mice. Natl Cancer Inst. Monogr., 22, 139–142.

Nebreda, A.R. and Hunt, T. (1993). The c-*mos* proto-oncogene protein kinase turns on and maintains the activity of MAP kinase, but not MPF, in cell-free extracts of *Xenopus* oocytes and eggs. EMBO J., 12, 1979–1986.

Okazaki, K., Nishizawa, M., Furuno, N., Yasuda, H. and Sagata, N. (1992). Differential occurrence of CSF-like activity and transforming activity of mos during the cell cycle in fibroblasts. EMBO J., 11, 2447–2456.

Oskarsson, M., McClements, W.L., Blair, D.G., Maizel, J.V. and Vande Woude, G.F. (1980). Properties of a normal mouse cell DNA sequence (sarc) homologous to the src sequence of Moloney sarcoma virus. Science, 207, 1222–1224.

Pal, S.K., Zinkel, S.S., Kiessling, A.A. and Copper, G.M. (1991). c-*mos* expression in mouse oocytes is controlled by initiator-related sequences immediately downstream of the transcription initiation site. Mol. Cell. Biol., 11, 5190–5196.

Paules, R.S., Propst, F., Dunn, K.J., Blair, D.G., Kaul, K., Palmer, A.E. and Vande Woude, G.F. (1988). Primate c-*mos* proto-oncogene structure and expression: transcription initiation both upstream and within the gene in a tissue-specific manner. Oncogene, 3, 59–68.

Paules, R.S., Buccione, R., Moschel, R.C., Vande Woude, G.F. and Eppig, J.J. (1989). Mouse *mos* protooncogene product is present and functions during oogenesis. Proc. Natl Acad. Sci. USA, 86, 5395–5399.

Paules, R.S., Resnick, J., Kasenally, A.B., Ernst, M.K., Donovan, P. and Vande Woude, G.F. (1992). Characterization of activated and normal mouse *mos* gene in murine 3T3 cells. Oncogene, 7, 2489–2498.

Posada, J., Yew, N., Ahn, N.G., Vande Woude, G.F. and Cooper, J.A. (1993). Mos stimulates MAP kinase in *Xenopus* oocytes and activates MAP kinase kinase in vitro. Mol. Cell. Biol., 13, 2546–2553.

Propst, F. and Vande Woude, G.F. (1985). Expression of c-*mos* proto-oncogene transcripts in mouse tissues. Nature, 315, 516–518.

Rechavi, G., Givol, D. and Canaani, E. (1982). Activation of a cellular oncogene by DNA rearrangement: possible involvement of an IS-like element. Nature, 300, 607–611.

Reddy, E.P., Smith, M.J. and Aaronson, S.A. (1981). Complete nucleotide sequence and organization of the Moloney murine sarcoma virus genome. Science, 214, 445–450.

Roy, L.M., Singh, B., Gautier, J., Arlinghaus, R.B., Nordeen, S.K. and Maller, J.L. (1990). The cyclin B2 component of MPF is a substrate for the c-*mos*^{xe} proto-oncogene product. Cell, 61, 825–831.

Sagata, N., Oskarsson, M., Copeland, T., Brumbaugh, J. and Vande-Woude, G.F. (1988). Function of c-*mos* proto-oncogene product in meiotic maturation in *Xenopus* oocytes. Nature, 335, 519–525.

Sagata, N., Daar, I., Oskarsson, M., Showalter, S. and Vande Woude, G.F. (1989a). The product of the *mos* proto-oncogene as a candidate "initiator" for oocyte maturation. Science, 245, 643–646.

Sagata, N., Watanabe, N., Vande-Woude, G.F. and Ikawa, Y. (1989b). The c-*mos* proto-oncogene product is a cytoskeletal factor responsible for meiotic arrest in vertebrate eggs. Nature, 342, 512–518.

Schmidt, M., Oskarsson, M.K., Dunn, J.K., Blair, D.G., Hughes, S., Propst, F. and Vande-Woude, G.F. (1988). Chicken homolog of the *mos* proto-oncogene. Mol. Cell. Biol., 8, 923–929.

Schulz, N., Propst, F., Rosenberg, M.P., Linnoila, R.I., Paules, R.S., Kovatch, R. Ogiso, Y. and Vande Woude, G.F. (1992). Pheochromocytomas and C-cell thyroid neoplasms in transgenic c-*mos* mice: a model system for the human multiple endocrine neoplasia type 2 syndrome. Cancer Res., 52, 450–455.

Seth, A. and Vande-Woude, G.F. (1985). Nucleotide sequence and biochemical activities of the Moloney murine sarcoma virus strain HT-1 *mos* gene. J. Virol., 56, 144–152.

Seth, A., Priel, E. and Vande Woude, G.F. (1987). Nucleoside triphosphate-dependent DNA-binding properties of *mos* protein. Proc. Natl Acad. Sci. USA, 84, 3560–3564.

Stenman, G., Sahlin, P., Mark, J. and Landys, D. (1991). Structural alterations of the c-*mos* locus in benign pleomorphic adenomas with chromosome abnormalities of 8q12. Oncogene, 6, 1105–1108.

Touray, M., Ryan, F., Saurer, S., Martin, F. and Jaggi, R. (1991). *mos*-induced inhibition of glucocorticoid receptor function is mediated by Fos. Oncogene, 6, 211–217.

van Beveren, C. (1982). Complete nucleotide sequence of Moloney murine sarcoma virus, clone 124, integrated circular DNA containing two LTRs. Cold Spring Harbor Monogr. Ser. 10C, 1357–1375.

van Beveren, C., van Straaten, F., Galleshaw, J.A. and Verma, I.M. (1981). Nucleotide sequence of the genome of a murine sarcoma virus. Cell, 27, 97–108.

van der Hoorn, F.A. and Firzlaff, J. (1984). Complete c-*mos* (rat) nucleotide sequence: presence of conserved domains in c-*mos* proteins. Nucleic Acids Res., 12, 2147–2156.

Watanabe, N., Vande Woude, G.F., Ikawa, Y. and Sagata, N. (1989). Specific proteolysis of the c-*mos* proto-oncogene product by calpain upon fertilization of *Xenopus* eggs. Nature, 342, 505–511.

Watson, R., Oskarsson, M. and Vande Woude, G.F. (1982). Human DNA sequence homologous to the transforming gene (*mos*) of Moloney murine sarcoma virus. Proc. Natl Acad. Sci. USA, 79, 4078–4082.

Wood, T.G., McGeady, M.L., Blair, D.G. and Vande Woude, G.F. (1983). Long terminal repeat enhancement of v-*mos* transforming activity: identification of essential regions. J. Virol., 46, 726–736.

Wood, T.G., McGeady, M.L., Baroudy, B.M., Blair, D.G. and Vande Woude, G.F. (1984). Mouse c-*mos* oncogene activation is prevented by upstream sequences. Proc. Natl Acad. Sci. USA, 81, 7817–7821.

Yew, N., Oskarsson, M., Daar, I., Blair, D.G. and Vande Woude, G.F. (1991). *mos* gene transforming efficiencies correlate with oocyte maturation and cytostatic factor activities. Mol. Cell. Biol., 11, 604–610.

Yew, N., Mellini, M.L. and Vande Woude, G.F. (1992). Meiotic initiation by the *mos* protein in *Xenopus*. Nature, 355, 649–652.

Zhao, X., Batten, B., Singh, B. and Arlinghaus, R.B. (1990). Requirement of the c-*mos* protein kinase for murine meiotic maturation. Oncogene, 5, 1727–1730.

Zhao, X., Singh, B. and Batten, B.E. (1991). The role of c-*mos* proto-oncoprotein in mammalian meiotic maturation. Oncogene, 6, 43–49.

Zhou, R., Oskarsson, M., Paules, R.S., Schulz, N., Cleveland, D. and Vande Woude, G.F. (1991a). Ability of the c-*mos* product to associate with and phosphorylate tubulin. Science, 251, 671–675.

Zhou, R., Shen, R., Pinto da Silva, P. and Vande Woude, G.F. (1991b). *In vitro* and *in vivo* characterization of pp39^{mos} association with tubulin. Cell Growth Differ., 2, 257–265.

Zhou, R., Daar, I., Ferris, D.K., White, G., Paules, R.S. and Vande Woude, G.F. (1992). pp39^{mos} is associated with p34^{cdc2} kinase in c-*mos*^{xe}-transformed NIH 3T3 cells. Mol. Cell. Biol., 12, 3583–3589.

Zinkel, S.S., Pal, S.K., Szeberenyi, J. and Cooper, G.M. (1992). Identification of a negative regulatory element that inhibits c-*mos* transcription in somatic cells. Mol. Cell. Biol., 12, 2029–2036.

MYB

v-*myb* is the oncogene of the acutely transforming avian myeloblastosis virus (AMV; Hall *et al.*, 1941) and E26 leukaemia virus (Ivanov *et al.*, 1964; Nedyalkov *et al.*, 1975).

The *MYB* gene family encodes DNA binding proteins.

Related genes

Related genes include human *MYBA* and *MYBB* (Nomura *et al.*, 1988) and *MYB*-like genes *MYBL1* (8q22) and *MYBL2* (Xq13); chicken *B-myb* (Foos *et al.*, 1992). MYB-related proteins occur in *Xenopus laevis* (Bouwmeester *et al.*, unpublished results), *Drosophila melanogaster* (Katzen *et al.*, 1985; Peters *et al.*, 1987; England *et al.*, 1992), yeast (BAS1, REB1: Tice-Baldwin *et al.*, 1989; Ju *et al.*, 1990), *D. discoideum* (Stober-Grasser *et al.*, 1992), *Zea mays* (Paz-Ares *et al.*, 1987), barley (Marocco *et al.*, 1989) and *Arabidopsis thaliana* (Oppenheimer *et al.*, 1991). The most highly conserved regions between all these genes are the N-terminal 50–53 amino acid repeats of the DNA binding domain (see **Structural domains of the p75^{myb} protein,** page 300).

Cross-species homology

Myb is highly conserved between mammalian species. The homology between subregions of mouse and avian genes ranges from 45% to 100%. MYB: 99.5%, 96% and 82% identity between residues 1–200, 261–410 and 71–444 (human and mouse); 82% (human and chicken). *MYBB*: 84% identity (human and mouse); 74% (human and chicken) (Lam *et al.*, 1992; Foos *et al.*, 1992).

Transformation

MAN

Amplification of *MYB* has been detected in acute myeloblastic leukaemia (AML), chronic myelogenous leukaemia (CML), acute lymphoblastic leukaemia (ALL), T cell leukaemias, colon carcinomas and melanomas (Alitalo *et al.*, 1984; Balaban *et al.*, 1984; Pellici *et al.*, 1984; Slamon *et al.*, 1984; Griffin and Baylin, 1985; Barletta *et al.*, 1987; Melani *et al.*, 1991; Tesch *et al.*, 1992). The stability of *MYB* and *MYC* mRNAs is increased in the cells of some AML patients (Baer *et al.*, 1992). Malignant haematopoietic colony forming units can be removed from the cells of CML patients by exposure to *MYB* antisense oligodeoxynucleotides (Ratajczak *et al.*, 1992).

MYB mRNA (3.8 kb) is detectable in some ovarian cancers and derived cell lines: it is not expressed in normal ovary tissue (Barletta *et al.*, 1992). *MYB* amplification is detected in some breast carcinomas in which its expression is inversely correlated with that of *HER2* and thus constitutes a good prognostic factor (Guerin *et al.*, 1990).

ANIMALS

AMV induces acute myeloid leukaemia in chickens (Baluda and Goetz, 1961). E26 causes avian erythroleukaemias and (in a minor population of cells) myeloid leukaemia (Sotirov, 1981;

Moscovici *et al.*, 1981; Radke *et al.*, 1982). Expression of the product of the chimeric *myb–ets* gene is necessary for the leukaemogenicity of E26 (Metz and Graf, 1991b).

The recombinant avian leukosis virus (ALV) EU-8, injected into chicken embryos, induces a high incidence of B cell lymphomas (Kanter *et al.*, 1988). These are caused by proviral integration of EU-8 in the *Myb* locus. A similar metastatic lymphoma develops when chicken embryos are infected with the RAV-1 isolate of ALV (Pizer and Humphries 1989). The induction of lymphomas following infection of embryos, rather than the classic lymphoid leukosis caused by ALV in adult animals, implies that the target cells in which *Myb* is activated occur only in embryos.

Injection of pristane together with Abelson virus and helper virus (Mo-MuLV) causes Abelson virus-induced myeloid lymphosarcomas (ABMLs) in BALB/c mice. Mo-MuLV alone induces similar tumours (MMLs: Mo-MuLV-induced myeloid leukaemias; Shen-Ong *et al.*, 1984, 1986; Gonda *et al.*, 1987). There is substantial expression of *Myb* mRNA in murine pre-B cell lymphomas and significantly lower expression in B cell lymphomas and plasmacytomas (Catron *et al.*, 1992).

Chemically induced rat colon tumours have frequent rearrangements, insertions or deletions in the *Myb* and *Hras* loci (Alexander *et al.*, 1992).

IN VITRO

AMV transforms macrophage precursors (monoblasts) *in vivo* and *in vitro*, chicken bone marrow cells and avian yolk-sac cells. It does not transform fibroblasts and may be a unique oncogene in this respect. E26 transforms fibroblasts (quail) and erythroid or myeloid cells. Erythroid cell transformation is due to the presence in E26 of v-*ets* which has a cooperative effect with v-*myb* in this lineage (Metz and Graf, 1991a). The "erythroid" cells transformed by the *gag–myb–ets* fusion protein are more immature than those transformed by the separate proteins (see **ETS**) and are also multipotent, differentiating into myeloblasts and eosinophilic cells following super-infection with viruses expressing either kinase-type oncogenes (v-*erbB*, v-*mil*, v-*sea*, v-*src*) or *ras* (Graf *et al.*, 1992). The intact v-*ets* gene of E26 is necessary for erythroid cell transformation but neither the DNA binding domain nor the *trans*-activating domain of v-*myb* is required (Domenget *et al.*, 1992).

In E26-transformed myeloid cells a point mutation in v-*ets* modulates the phenotype from that of immature myeloblasts to promyelocytes (Golay *et al.*, 1988).

v-*myb* appears to block differentiation (Patel *et al.*, 1993) and, in normal or v-*myc*-transformed macrophages, AMV or E26 cause "de-differentiation", inducing changes characteristic of immature cells (Ness *et al.*, 1987).

The *in vitro* survival and proliferation of *myb*-transformed myeloid cells requires haematopoietic growth factors, for example, IL-3 or cMGF (Weinstein *et al.*, 1986). The requirement for an exogenous growth factor is relieved by the expression of v-*src*, v-*fps*, v-*yes*, v-*ros*, v-*mil* or v-*erbB* (Adkins *et al.*, 1984; Sterneck *et al.*, 1992). These oncogenes cause autocrine growth stimulation via the action of a myeloid cell-specific transcription factor.

E26 stimulates the proliferation of chicken neuroretina cells, as does AMV in the presence of basic fibroblast growth factor (Garrido *et al.*, 1992).

TRANSGENIC ANIMALS

Homozygous *Myb* mutant mice appear normal at day 13 of gestation but by day 15 are severely anaemic. Embryonic erythropoiesis is not impaired but adult-type erythropoiesis is greatly diminished (Mucenski *et al.*, 1991). This indicates that *Myb* is not essential for early development but may be required to maintain the proliferative state of haematopoietic progenitor cells.

	MYB/Myb	v-myb
Nucleotides	>25 kb	7139 (AMV genome)
		5700 (E26 genome)
Chromosome		
Human	6q22–q23	
Chicken	3	
Mouse	10	
Exons	15	
mRNA (kb)		
Human	3.4–4.5	2.0 and 7.0 (AMV)
Chicken	3.8	2.46 (E26 p135$^{gag-myb-ets}$)
Mouse	3.6/4.0	5.3 (in ABML; Mushinski *et al.*, 1983)
Alternative splicing can generate 3.9/5.3 kb murine *Myb* mRNAs (Ramsay *et al.*, 1989)		
Human	5.0 (*MYBA*)	
	2.6 (*MYBB*)	
mRNA half-life (h)	1–3	
Amino acids		
Human	640	382 (AMV v-*myb*)
Chicken	641/699	669 (E26 p135$^{gag-myb-ets}$)
Mouse	636	
Human	745 (MYBA)	
	700 (MYBB)	
Mouse	704 (MYBB)	
Chicken	686 (MYBB)	
Mass (kDa)		
(predicted)	72.5	43^{v-myb}
		75$^{gag-myb-ets}$
(expressed)	p75	p48^{v-myb} (AMV)
	p90	p135$^{gag-myb-ets}$ (E26)
Protein half-life (min)	~30 (MYB)	~30
	3–4 h (MYBB; Foos *et al.*, 1992)	

Cellular location

Nuclear (Klempnauer *et al.*, 1984; Boyle *et al.*, 1984).

Tissue location

Myb is expressed in immature cells of the lymphoid, erythroid and myeloid lineages (Gonda and Metcalf, 1984; Sheiness and Gardinier, 1984; Duprey and Boettiger, 1985). It is also strongly expressed in the thymus in CD4+ T cells and induced in T lymphocytes by mitogen or antigen stimulation (Thompson *et al.*, 1986). *Myb* is co-expressed with *Mim-1* during granulopoiesis in the chicken pancreas and spleen (Queva *et al.*, 1992). *Myb* expression decreases dramatically as cells differentiate to more mature forms (Westin et al., 1982; Thompson *et al.*, 1986; Thiele *et al.*, 1988).

MYB mRNA is detectable in human neuroblastoma (Thiele *et al.*, 1988) and teratocarcinoma cell lines (Janssen *et al.*, 1986), vascular smooth muscle cells (Brown *et al.*, 1992; Simons and Rosenberg, 1992) and in fibroblasts after serum stimulation (Thompson *et al.*, 1986).

MYBA and *MYBB* are expressed in a variety of human haematopoietic cell lines and also in carcinoma and sarcoma-derived cell lines (Nomura *et al.*, 1988).

Protein function

MYB contains DNA binding, transcriptional activation and negative regulatory domains and binds directly to double-stranded DNA (Sakura *et al.*, 1989). The consensus binding site is $YAAC^G/_TG$; most commonly: CCTAACTG (Biedenkapp *et al.*, 1988) or $YAAC^{T}/(C)_{/G}GYCA$ (Weston, 1992), from which intact MYB or v-MYB activates transcription. Of the seven cysteine residues in v-MYB, Cys65, conserved in all MYB-related proteins, is essential for *trans* activation of transcription and for transformation of myeloid cells (Grasser *et al.*, 1992). Binding of v-MYB and MYB is decreased by CpG methylation of the binding motif (Klempnauer, 1993).

High *Myb* expression is generally associated with immature cells of haematopoietic lineage and *Myb* is essential for normal haematopoiesis. In differentiated cells there is evidence that *Myb* expression is associated with cell proliferation and in lymphoid cells that the appearance of *Myb* mRNA correlates with the interaction of IL-2 with its receptor. Transformed cells increase *Myb* expression as the cells enter the cycle: avian thymocytes express high levels of *Myb* in G_0 or G_1 and throughout the cycle. Differentiation is accompanied by suppression of *Myb* expression but this does not seem to be necessary for the initiation of differentiation. Thus *Myb* is probably an important regulator of cell differentiation and the generation in normal cells of multiple isoforms of *Myb* by alternative splicing and/or alternative initiation indicates that the protein products may have differing, tissue-specific roles (Ramsay *et al.*, 1989; see Table 3.4). However, transgenic mice that do not express *Myb* develop normally until day 13 but then rapidly become anaemic (Mucenski *et al.*, 1991). Embryonic erythropoiesis is unaffected but adult erythropoiesis, which first occurs in the liver, is greatly diminished, suggesting that the function of *Myb* is unique to haematopoiesis.

There is a dramatic increase in *Myb* expression (30- to 60-fold) associated with generalized autoimmune diseases, which appears to occur in the greatly expanded population of CD4⁻8⁻ cells. Studies in MRL-*lpr/lpr* mice, which carry the same defect, indicate the existence of specific nuclear DNA binding proteins that regulate *Myb* expression (Mountz and Steinberg, 1989). *lpr* cells lack mature T cell surface markers (Lyt-2 and L3T4), express high levels of *Myb* mRNA and are generally unresponsive to T cell mitogens. Induction of differentiation (by TPA + A23187) depresses *Myb* and activates IL-2R transcription (Yokota *et al.*, 1987).

Myb may be critically involved in the proliferation of smooth muscle cells. The expression of antisense phosphorothiolate oligodeoxynucleotides against *Myb* or non-muscle myosin heavy chain reversibly suppresses growth of these cells (Simons and Rosenberg, 1992; Simons *et al.*, 1992). Antisense *Myb* oligonucleotides also inhibit the twofold increase in the concentration of intracellular free calcium that normally occurs at the G_1/S phase interface in rat vascular smooth muscle cells (Simons *et al.*, 1993). The MYB-dependent rise in $[Ca^{2+}]_i$ is dependent on extracellular Ca^{2+} but is not mediated by L type channels (i.e. is nifedipine-insensitive) or T type channels (which are not normally present in vascular smooth muscle cells).

REGULATION OF GENE EXPRESSION BY MYB

Mim-1: Mim-1 (Myb induced myeloid protein-1) encodes a 326 residue protein with an 18 residue hydrophobic, N-terminal putative signal peptide (Ness *et al.*, 1989). *Mim-1* has three MYB binding sites in its regulatory region and is the only cellular gene that is known to be a direct target of MYB. *Mim-1* is activated by p135$^{myb\text{-}ets}$ in myeloid cells but not in erythroid or other non-haematopoietic cell types. MYB is a poor activator of the *Mim-1* promoter but co-expression of ETS2 with MYB greatly enhances *trans* activation (Dudek *et al.*, 1992). In promyelocytes and in the yolk sac of the chick embryo *Mim-1* is efficiently transcribed in the absence of MYB (Queva *et al.*, 1992). Thus, although *Mim-1* is *trans* activated by the truncated v-MYB protein, its expression is also activated by other transcription factors, including the combination of ETS2 and MYB and members of the C/EBP transcription factor family (Burk *et al.*, 1993).

MYB: The region of the human *MYB* gene between nucleotides −616 and −575 upstream from the cap site contains putative MYB binding sites that confer MYB-inducible expression when linked to a reporter gene (Nicolaides *et al.*, 1991). Mutation of the putative binding sites inhibits *trans* activation by MYB and also reduces the binding of MYB protein to the sites. Thus human MYB may exert a positive regulatory effect on transcription of its own gene during proliferation and/or differentiation.

MYC: Eight MYB binding sites occur in the regulatory region of human *MYC* although the highest binding affinity is to the palindromes AACXGTT or AACGTT, rather than the above consensus sequence (Zobel *et al.*, 1991). In co-transfection assays both MYB and MYBB strongly activate transcription from the human *MYC* promoter (Nakagoshi *et al.*, 1992). In murine T cells (CTLL-2) expression of high levels of MYB strongly activates transcription of *Myc* but not of *Fos* (Evans *et al.*, 1990).

CD4: Maximum activation of the promoter of the T-cell-specific CD4 gene requires MYB (Siu *et al.*, 1992).

DNA polymerase α: There are six MYB binding sites in the promoter of this gene and in T cells the inhibition of proliferation by *MYB* antisense oligodeoxynucleotide correlates with down regulation of DNA polymerase α expression. However, MYB does not directly *trans*-activate the promoter (Sudo *et al.*, 1992).

Epstein–Barr virus (EBV) transcription factor Z (BZLF1): MYB interacts synergistically with Z to activate the EBV early promoter BMRF1 in Jurkat or Raji cells (Kenney *et al.*, 1992; see **DNA Tumour Viruses**).

HIV-1: HIV-1 LTR contains a high-affinity *MYB* binding site and at least two low-affinity binding sites and MYB *trans*-activates the HIV-1 LTR (Dasgupta *et al.*, 1990).

HTLV-1: Six specific binding sites for MYB are present in the human T cell lymphotropic virus type 1 (HTLV-1) LTR and HTLV-1 LTR chloramphenicol acetyl transferase reporter plasmids are specifically *trans*-activated by MYB (Bosselut *et al.*, 1992; Dasgupta *et al.*, 1992).

Insulin-like growth factor I (IGF-I): When expressed in BALB/c 3T3 cells, MYB activates transcription of both IGF-I and IGF-I receptor. When co-expressed with *Myc*, *Myb* promotes growth in the absence of any exogenous factors (Reiss *et al.*, 1991; Travali *et al.*, 1991a).

Ribonuclease A-related gene: In co-transfection experiments with a reporter construct, the promoter of the ribonuclease A-related gene is regulated by v-MYB although it does not contain a MYB-specific binding sequence (Nakano and Graf, 1992).

SV40: MYB binds to SV40 DNA at two sites (MBS-I, residues 246–264; MBS-II, residues 128–146 and 184–202; Nishina *et al.*, 1989; Mizuguchi *et al.*, 1990). MYBB binds with high affinity to MBS-I and to the MBS-BI site to which MYB binds only weakly, but does not bind to MBS-II.

Chicken B-MYB contains an N-terminal DNA binding domain corresponding to that of MYB and specifically recognizes v-MYB binding sites *in vitro* (Foos *et al.*, 1992). However, B-MYB represses v-MYB and MYB *trans* activation via a number of promoters including that of *Mim-1* and may function as an inhibitory member of the MYB family. In contrast to MYB, murine B-MYB does not *trans*-activate the SV40 early promoter although truncation of the B-MYB C-terminus enables the protein to bind to the MBS-I motif (Watson *et al.*, 1993).

The inhibition of *Mybb* expression in BALB/c 3T3 fibroblasts by transfection of a vector expressing antisense oligodeoxynucleotide correlates with inhibition of proliferation (Sala and Calabretta, 1992). Constitutive expression of *Mybb* is accompanied by activation of cyclin D1 and *cdc*2 transcription and the suppression of cyclin D1 has an antiproliferative effect.

Structure of the chicken *Myb* gene: proviral insertion

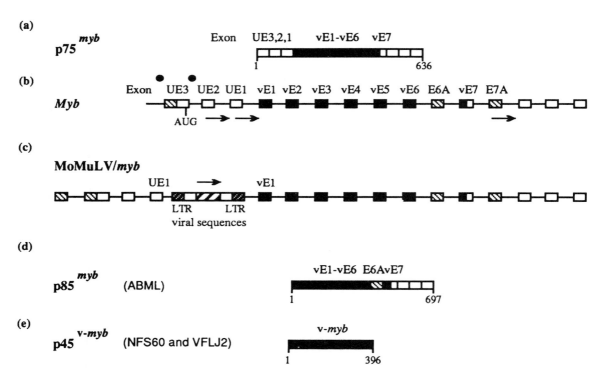

UE3, 2 and 1: upstream exons 5′ to the *Myb* exons that are homologous to v-*myb* (vE1–vE7). Black boxes: exons containing AMV v-*myb* sequences. Open boxes: *Myb* exons not found in v-*myb*. Hatched boxes: exons occurring in alternatively spliced forms of *Myb*. Viral insertions occur in the regions shown by the arrows in murine myeloid tumour cells and by the dots in chicken B lymphoid tumours.

(a) p75^(myb), thought to be translated from the major *Myb* mRNA containing UE3, UE2, UE1 and vE1–vE7.

(b) The *Myb* gene. Alternative splicing generates a larger mRNA (~10% of the total RNA) encoding p90^(myb) by the inclusion of the additional vE6A 363 nucleotide exon (also called exon 9a) that encodes 121 amino acids (Rosson *et al.*, 1987; Sheng-Ong, 1987; Shen-Ong *et al.*, 1989). An alternative initiation site generates *Mbm-2* encoding a protein commencing 20 residues downstream from the normal MYB N-terminus. Insertion of a 122 bp cryptic sixth exon leads to premature translational termination. *Mbm-2* p75*myb* contains DNA binding and nuclear location sequences but not transcription regulating regions (Westin *et al.*, 1990).

(c) Proviral insertion of Moloney murine leukaemia virus (Mo-MuLV) 5' of the first *Myb* exon that is expressed in v-*myb*. In ABMLs *Myb* is rearranged as a result of the integration of the Mo-MuLV genome in a 1.5 kb region of DNA upstream of the first *Myb* exon present in v-*myb* and in the same orientation as *myb* (i.e. in intron 3 of *Myb*). Mo-MuLV alone causes a similar disruption and induces ABML-like MML tumours. These proviral insertions give rise to translation products lacking either UE3 and UE2 or UE3, UE2 and UE1. Proviral insertion may also cause alternative splicing and the expression of vE6A in p85*myb*. Other gene products (p50, p72, p87) have been detected in myeloid leukaemic cells as a result of viral integration (Ramsay *et al.*, 1989).

(d) p85*myb* translated from the alternatively spliced mRNA in ABML tumours (see below). v-MYB corresponds to amino acids 72–636 of MYB, although some tumours have a more 5' insertion point and express residues 48–636 of MYB.

(e) p45*v-myb* arising from the integration of the Cas-Br Mo-MuLV genome in NFS mice. In the NFS-60 line derived from these animals, viral insertion has occurred towards the 3' end of the *Myb* locus and residues 1–414 of MYB are expressed. Residues 204–254 of p45*v-myb* linked to the yeast transcriptional activator GAL4 activate transcription of genes linked in *cis* to a GAL4 binding site (Weston and Bishop, 1989) but there is evidence that *trans* activation by v-*myb* also requires the highly conserved N-terminal DNA binding domain and that this correlates with transformation potency (Lane *et al.*, 1990).

The organization of *Myb* sequences is not completely resolved. In the chicken, 15 exons of *Myb* span 35 kb of genomic DNA on chromosome 3. An additional exon (E_T) located on chromosome 17q25 and specifically expressed in thymus cells has also been reported (Vellard *et al.*, 1991). The complete gene is expressed as the result of an intermolecular recombination process and a putative splicing factor (PR264) is encoded by the opposite strand of the *Myb trans*-spliced exon (Vellard *et al.*, 1992). As E_T bears 85% homology to the equivalent human and mouse exons and human E_T maps to a different chromosome to that carrying the remainder of *MYB* (6q22–q24), it seems probable that the complex organization of the chicken gene reflects a general property of mammalian *Myb*.

Proviral genomes and translation products of AMV and E26

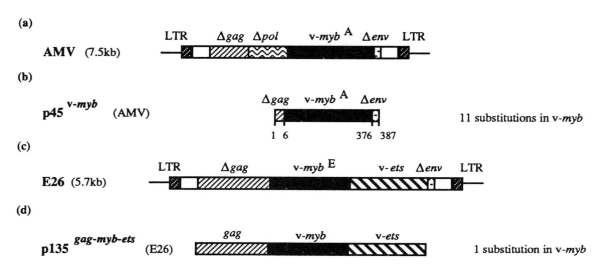

(a)

AMV (7.5kb)   LTR   Δ*gag* Δ*pol*   v-*myb* A Δ*env*   LTR

(b)

p45 v-*myb* (AMV)   Δ*gag*   v-*myb* A   Δ*env*   11 substitutions in v-*myb*
1 6   376 387

(c)

E26 (5.7kb)   LTR   Δ*gag*   v-*myb* E   v-*ets* Δ*env*   LTR

(d)

p135 gag-myb-ets (E26)   *gag*   v-*myb*   v-*ets*   1 substitution in v-*myb*

(a) Structure of the avian myeloblastosis virus (AMV) genome. v-*myb* is designated v-*myb*^A *in AMV and* v-*myb*^E *in E26* (Nunn *et al.*, 1983).

(b) AMV p45^v-*myb* is derived via extensive 5′ and 3′ deletions of p75^*myb*, generating *myb*^A (lacking 71 N-terminal amino acids and 198 C-terminal amino acids of MYB, and with 11 point mutations). v-*myb* replaces 26 codons of the 3′ end of *pol* and most of *env*. There are six *gag*-encoded amino acids and 33 bp of *env* give rise to 11 C-terminal amino acids, up to TAG (Klempnauer *et al.*, 1983).

(c) Structure of the E26 leukaemia virus genome.

(d) E26 v-*myb* (*myb*^E): lacks 80 N-terminal and 278 C-terminal amino acids of p75^*myb*, has one point mutation and is expressed as p135^*gag-myb-ets*. v-*ets* is derived from *Ets-1* (see *ETS*).

Transcriptional regulation

The promoters of chicken and mouse *Myb* contain GC-rich upstream regions with no TATA box (mouse) or with a TATA box that is not associated with a CAAT box (chicken). In murine *Myb* a positive intragenic regulatory mechanism operates via two tandem repeats of AP-1 sites in the first intron (Reddy and Reddy, 1989; see also *FOS* and *MYC*). Thus the decrease in the level of *Myb* mRNA that accompanies differentiation of mouse erythroleukaemic cells correlates with a decrease in sequence-specific protein binding to this region. Transcriptional attenuation is also the major mechanism of regulation of human *MYB* during retinoic acid- or vitamin D3-induced differentiation of HL-60 cells (Boise *et al.*, 1992). However, DMSO or phorbol ester regulate *Myb* expression by an additional, post-translational mechanism that, for DMSO, requires continuous transcription. This latter mechanism may involve activation of an AUUUA-binding protein, six such elements being present in the 3′ untranslated region of *Myb* mRNA.

Structural domains of the p75^*myb* protein

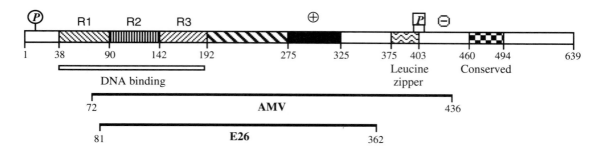

$\textcircled{P}$: Serines 11 and 12: casein kinase II phosphorylation sites which, when phosphorylated, reduce MYB binding to DNA (Luscher *et al.*, 1990).

38–192: R1, R2 and R3: 51–52 amino acid repeats. R2 and R3 (23% basic amino acids) are essential for MYB binding to the MYB-recognition element (pyAAC^G/$_T$G): deletion of five residues from R3 abolishes DNA binding (Howe *et al.*, 1990; Oehler *et al.*, 1990). R1 is deleted from v-*myb*. R1, R2 and R3 contain a conserved motif of three tryptophans separated by 18 or 19 amino acids (see also *ETS*). Each MYB repeat consists of three α helices surrounding a hydrophobic core that includes the three highly conserved tryptophan residues (amino acids 6, 26 and 45 in each R unit). The C-terminal helix of each repeat unit forms part of the helix–turn–helix motif that can be positioned in the major groove of B-form DNA (Frampton *et al.*,

1989, 1991; Gabrielsen *et al.*, 1991). Removal of the C-terminus of MYB (amino acids 193–639) enhances the affinity for DNA of this N-terminal region by sevenfold (Ramsay *et al.*, 1992).

275–325 ⊕: Transcription activation domain that interacts with the MYB response element (MRE: Weston and Bishop, 1989; Sakura *et al.*, 1989). MREs occur in the promoters of *Myc* and *Mim-1* (Evans *et al.*, 1990; Zobel *et al.*, 1991; see **MYC**). The DNA binding domain juxtaposed to the transcription activation domain is sufficient to block differentiation of murine erythroleukaemia cells (Cuddihy *et al.*, 1993).

326–500 ⊖: Domain that normally represses transcriptional activation by MYB (Sakura *et al.*, 1989; Dubendorff *et al.*, 1992). Removal of the C-terminus up to and including the negative regulatory domain increases transforming capacity: the *trans*-activation domain (amino acids 241–325) is essential for transformation (Yu *et al.*, 1991). The 136 C-terminal residues (503–639) are necessary for optimal *trans* activation of *Myc* (Nakagoshi *et al.*, 1992).

383–403: Leucine zipper domain, lying beyond the DNA binding region, that is not transduced by E26 but is a component of the negative regulatory domain (Kanei-Ishii *et al.*, 1992). Mutations in this region increase both the *trans*-activating and transforming capacities of MYB. This domain interacts with cellular proteins and it is probable that an inhibitory protein can associate with the leucine zipper of MYB to suppress *trans* activation.

P̄: Region containing several phosphorylation sites. MYB is phosphorylated on serine and threonine residues in intact cells by p34^{cdc2} (Luscher and Eisenman, 1992).

460–494: Domain conserved between mammalian and *Drosophila* MYB.

N-terminal 200 amino acids: Dispersed nuclear localization signal.

Sequences of human MYB and chicken MYB

```
Human MYB    (1)    MARRPRHSIYSSDEDDEDFEMCDHDYDGLLPKSGKRHLGKTRWTREEDEKLKKLVEQNGT
Chicken MYB  (1)    ------------D----V--Y---------A-----------------------------

             (61)   DDWKVIANYLPNRTDVQCQHRWQKVLNPELIKGPWTKEEDQRVIELVQKYGPKRWSVIAK
             (61)   E------SF---------------------------------------------------

             (121)  HLKGRIGKQCRERWHNHLNPEVKKTSWTEEEDRIIYQAHKRLGNRWAEIAKLLPGRTDNA
             (121)  ------------------------------------------------------------

             (181)  IKNHWNSTMRRKVEQEGYLQESSKASQPAVATSFQKNSHLMGFAQAPPTAQLPATGQPTV
             (181)  ----------------------GL-SAT-G---S----A--HN--AGP--GA--APL

             (241)  NNDYSYYHISEAQNVSSHVPYPVALHVNIVNVPQPAAAAIQRHYNDEDPEKEKRIKELEL
             (241)  GS--P----A-P---PGQI-----------------------------------------

             (301)  LLMSTENELKGQQVLPTQNHTCSYPGWHSTTIADHTRPHGDSAPVSCLGEHHSTPSLPA.
             (301)  -------------A-------AN--------V--N--TS--N----------HCTPS-PV

             (360)  DPGSLPEESASPARCMIVHQGTILDNVKNLLEFAETLQFIDSFLNTSSNHENSDLEMPSL
             (361)  -H-C--------------SN---------------L-------------LN-DN-A-

             (420)  TSTPLIGHKLTVTTPFHRDQTVKTQKENTVFRTPAIKRSILESSPRTPTPFKHALAAQEI
             (421)  ----VC---MS---------PF------H-----------------------N-------

             (480)  KYGPLKMLPQTPSHLVEDLQDVIKQESDESGFVAEFQENGPPLLKKIKQEVESPTDKSGN
             (481)  -----------T-------------E--AI--GLH-S-----------------A--

             (540)  FFCSHHWEGDSLNTQLFTQTSPVRDAPNILTSSVLMAPASEDEDNVLKAFTVPKNRSLAS
             (541)  -F--N----EN-------HA-TME-V-------I-KM-V--E-GSFH---A-----P---

             (600)  PLQPCSSTWEPASCGKMEEQMTSSSQARKYVNAFSARTLVM   (640)
             (601)  -M-HLNNA--S-----T-D--ALTD-----MA--PT-----   (641)
```

Dashes: identical amino acids. The underlined region of chicken MYB indicates the 371 amino acid region (72–442) incorporated in AMV v-MYB p135*gag–myb–ets*. Bold type: conserved tryptophan residues in the R1, R2 and R3 domains. Cys130 in the chicken sequence is also shown in bold type; the reduction of this cysteine residue is essential for MYB to bind to DNA (Guehmann *et al.*, 1992). The equivalent amino acid in v-MYB (Cys65) is essential for the transcription factor activity of v-MYB. The italicized leucine residues (383, 389, 396, 403) are those comprising the leucine zipper (Kanei-Ishii *et al.*, 1992).

Sequence of p135*gag-myb-ets*

```
  (1)  NSTMRRKVEQEGYLQESSKAGLPSATTGFQKSSHLMAFAHNPPAGPLPGAGQAPLGSDYP
 (61)  YYHIAEPQNVPGQIPYPVALHVNIVNVPQPAAAAIQRHYNDEDPEKEKRIKELELLLMST
(121)  ENELKGQQALPTQNHTANYPGWHSTTVADNTMTSGDNAPVSCLGEHHHCTPSPPVDHGTS
(181)  EMMSYYMDTTIGSTGPYPLARPGVMQGASSCCEDPWMPCRLQSACCPPRSCCPPWDEAAI
(241)  QEVPTGLEHYSTDMECADVPLLTPSSKEMMSQALKATFSGFAKEQQRLGIPKDPQQWTET
(301)  HVRDWVMWAVNEFSLKGVDFQKFCMNGAALCALGKECFLELAPDFVGDILWEHLEILQKE
(361)  EAKPYPANGVNAAYPESRYTSDYFISYGIEHAQCVPPSEFSEPSFITESYQTLHPISSEE
(421)  LLSLKYENDYPSVILRDPVQTDSLQTDYFTIKQEVVTPDNMCMGRVSRGKLGGQDSFESI
(481)  ESYDSCDRLTQSWSSQSSFQSLQRVPSYDSFDSEDYPAALPNHKPKGTFKDYVRDRADMN
(541)  KDKPVIPAAALAGYTGSGPIQLWQFLLELLTDKSCQSFISWTGDGWEFKLSDPDEVARRW
(601)  GKRKNKPKMDYEKLSRGLRYYYDKNVIHKTAGKRYVYRFVCDLQSLLGYTPEEHSSASGL
(660)  TSSMACSSF (669)
```

The underlined region is homologous to chicken MYB (amino acids 186–363) with the substitution of Met152 (p135) for Arg337 (MYB).

Sequences of human MYBA and MYBB

```
Human MYBA   (1)  MAKRSRSEDEDDDLQYADHDYEVPQQKGLKKLWNRVKWTRDEDDKLKKLVEQHGTDDWTL
Human MYBB   (1)  -SR-T-C--L-ELHYQDTDSDVPE-RDSKC-      ----HE--EQ-RA--R-FGQQ--KF

            (61)  IASHLQNRSDFQCQHRWQKVLNPELIKGPWTKEEDQRVIELVQKYGPKRWSLIAKHLKGR
            (57)  L---FP--T-Q--QY--LR----D-V---------K-----K---T-Q-T---------

           (121)  IGKQCRERWHNHLNPEVKKSSWTEEEDRIIYEAHKRLGNRWAEIAKLLPGRTDNSIKNHW
           (117)  ------------------C---------C----V----------M-------AV----

           (181)  NSTMRRKVEQEGYLQDGIKSERSSSKLQHKPCAAMDHMQTQNQFYIPVQIPGYQYVSPEG
           (176)  ---IK---DTG-F-SESKDCKPPVYLLLELEDKDGLQSAQPTEGQGSLLTNWPSVPPTIK

           (241)  NCIEHVQPTSAFIQQPFIDEDPDKEKKIKELEMLLMSAENEVRRKRIPSQPGSFSSWSGS
           (237)  EEENSEEELAAATTSKEQEPIGTDLDAVRTPEPLEEFPKREDQEGSPPETSLPYKWVVEA

           (301)  FLMDDNMSNTLNSLDEHTSEFYSMDENQPVSAQQNSPTKFLAVEANAVLSSLQTIPEFAE
           (297)  ANLLIPAVGSSLSEALDLIESDPDAWCDLSKFDLPEEPSAEDSINNSLVQLQASHQQQVL

           (361)  TLELIESDPVAWSDVTSFDISDAAASPIKSTPVKLMRIQHNEGAMECQFNVSLVLEGKKN
           (357)  PPRQPSALVPSVTEYRLDGHTISDLSRSSRGELIPISPSTEVGGSGIGTPPSVLKRQRKR

           (421)  TCNGGNSEAVPLTSPNIAKFSTPPAILRKKRKMRVGHSPGSELRDGSLNDGGNMALKHTP
           (417)  RVALSPVTENSTSLSFLDSCNSLTPKSTPVKTLPFSPSQFLNFWNKQDTLELESPSLTST

           (481)  LKTLPFSPSQFFNTCPGNEQLNIENPSFTSTPICGQKALITTPLHKETTPKDQKENVGFR
           (477)  PVCSQKVVVTTPLHRDKTPLHQKHAAFVTPDQKYSMDNTPHTPTPFKNALEKYGPLKPLP

           (541)  TPTIRRSILGTTPRTPTPFKNALAAQEKKYGPLKIVSQPLAFLEEDIREVLKEETGTDLF
```

```
(537)   QTPHLEEDLKEVLRSEAGIELIIEDDIRPEKQKRKPGLRRSPIKKVRKSLALDIVDEDVK

(601)   LKEEDEPAYKSCKQENTASGKKVRKSLVLDNWEKEESGTQLLTEDISDMQSENRFTTSLL
(597)   LMMSTLPKSLSLPTTAPSNSSSLTLSGIKEDNSLLNQGFLQAKPEKAAVAQKPRSHFTTP

(661)   MIPLLEIHDNRCNLIPEKQDINSTNKTYTLTKKKPNPNTSKVVKLEKNLQSNCEWETVVY
(657)   APMSSAWKTVACGGTRDQLFMQEKARQLLGRLKPSHTSRTLILS (700)

(721)   GKTEDQLIMTEQARRYLSTYTATSS (745)
```

MYBA and MYBB are highly homologous to MYB, particularly in their DNA binding and negative regulatory domains. MYBB has similar DNA binding capacity to MYB (Mizuguchi *et al.*, 1990).

Table 3.4. *Cellular Myb mRNA expression*

Cell type	Agent	Comment
Proliferation		
Chick embryo fibroblasts; chicken T cells	Serum	*Myb* mRNA increases transiently in late G_1 and S phases (maximal between 4 h and 8 h). mRNA stabilized by cycloheximide. Normal thymocytes (quiescent or proliferating) express high concentrations of *Myb* mRNA (Thompson *et al.*, 1986)
BHK fibroblasts (temperature-sensitive) transfected with *Myb* plasmid	Serum	At the restrictive temperature (39.6°C) these cells arrest in G_1. Expression of *Myb* drives cells through one round of DNA replication with the expression of proliferating cell nuclear antigen (PCNA) and histone H3 mRNA (Travali *et al.*, 1991b)
T helper cell clones	IL-1α	*Myb* (and *Myc*) transcription activated (Zubiaga *et al.*, 1991)
Human T cells and T cell clones	PHA or ConA, IL-2	PHA or ConA stimulate *FOS*, IL-2 stimulates *MYB* and each agent stimulates *MYC* transcription (Reed *et al.*, 1987; Kelly and Siebenlist, 1988)
Human T cells	IL-2	*MYB* transcription maximal 5 h after IL-2 addition (Stern and Smith, 1986; Pauza, 1987)
Mouse T helper cell clones	Anti-CD3-antibody, IL-2	Activate *Myc* and *Myb* transcription (Bohjanen *et al.*, 1990)
Human megakaryoblastic cell line	IL-3	IL-3-dependent proliferation does not correlate with enhanced expression of *MYC*, ODC, *P53*, or *MYB* but only of the "late genes" PCNA, TK and histone H3 transcription (Avanzi *et al.*, 1991)
Murine haematopoietic cells	IL-2, IL-3 (CTLL-2-derived lines)	*Pim* and *Myb* transcription stimulated by IL-2 or IL-3. In mature cells IL-2 induces *Myb*: in immature cells *Myb* is continuously highly expressed and is not further increased by IL-2, although the cells are still growth factor-dependent (Dautry *et al.*, 1988)

Table 3.4. *Continued*

Cell type	Agent	Comment
Human bone marrow cells	Antisense ODN to *MYB* (18mer starting from 2nd codon)	Decreases haematopoiesis (Gewirtz and Calabretta, 1988)
T cells	IL-2 Antisense ODN to *Myb/Myc*	*Myb* transcription correlates with IL-2 responsiveness (i.e., IL-2/IL-2R interaction). *Myc* is also activated by IL-2 (maximal by 4 h and sustained for up to 9 days). Antisense *Myc* or *Myb* blocks IL-2-stimulated DNA synthesis (Churilla *et al.*, 1989)
Human T cells	Antisense ODN to *MYB*	Blocks *MYB* mRNA and protein synthesis, histone H3 transcription, the mitogen-stimulated increase in p34^{cdc2} mRNA (Furukawa *et al.*, 1990) and progression to S phase. Does not block IL-2R expression (Gewirtz *et al.*, 1989)
Human colon cancer cell lines	Antisense ODN to *MYB*	In human colon carcinoma cell lines that express significant *MYB*, the ODN inhibits proliferation (Melani *et al.*, 1991)
Human promyelocytic leukaemia cell line (HL-60)	Antisense ODN to *MYB*	Inhibits cell proliferation (Citro *et al.*, 1992)
Myeloid leukaemia cell lines	Antisense ODN to *Myb*	Proliferation is inhibited (Anfossi *et al.*, 1989)
Mouse spleen	Regenerating *in vivo*	T cells have high *Myb* and *Myc* mRNA levels (Sihvola *et al.*, 1989)
Differentiation		
Human neuroblastoma cell lines	Retinoic acid	Decreased transcription of *MYB* during differentiation (Thiele *et al.*, 1988)
Human T cell leukaemia line (Jurkat)	TPA	TPA inhibits proliferation and stimulates the terminal differentiation of Jurkat cells. This correlates with the induction of transcription of *FOS*, *JUN* and *EGR1*, followed by that of IL-2R. TPA also reduces the high levels of *MYC*, *NRAS* and *BCL2* mRNAs present in proliferating in Jurkat cells. However, transcription of *MYB*, *RAF1*, *LCK*, *FYN* and *FGR* is unchanged (Makover *et al.*, 1991)
Promyelocytic leukaemia cell line (HL-60)	DMSO, retinoic acid	Downregulates *MYB* (Westin *et al.*, 1982)
Chicken myelomonocytic transformed by v-*myc* (MC29 virus)	E26 mutant temperature-sensitive in v-*myb*	When transformed by v-*myc* these cells resemble mature macrophages, whereas v-*myb* or v-*myb*–*ets* induce an immature phenotype. Cells transformed by both v-*myc* and either v-*myb* or v-*myb*–*ets* are indistinguishable from those transformed by v-*myb* or v-*myb*–*ets* alone. Thus v-*myb* is dominant over v-*myc*. v-*myc* induces cell proliferation without affecting differentiation whereas in the same cells v-*myb* causes both proliferation and inhibition or reversal of differentiation (Ness *et al.*, 1987)

Table 3.4. *Continued*

Cell type	Agent	Comment
Chicken myelomonocytic cells	E26 mutant temperature-sensitive in v-*myb*	Cells transformed at the permissive temperature can be induced to differentiate into macrophages by shift to the non-permissive temperature. This process is partly reversible, the cells gradually acquiring an immature phenotype and proliferative capacity when shifted back to 37°C (Beug *et al.*, 1987)
Chicken myelomonocytic cells	Point mutants in v-*myb*	Myelomonocytic cells transformed by AMV resemble monoblasts and do not express *Mim-1*. Point mutations in the DNA binding domain that restore the MYB structure transform cells resembling promyelocytes (Introna *et al.*, 1990). AMV mutant-transformed promyelocytes express eight genes that are silent in AMV-transformed monoblasts, the most abundant being the *Myb*-regulated *Mim-1* gene (Nakano and Graf, 1992)
Chicken macrophage cell line (MC29-transformed)	Estrogen-dependent v-*myb* expression	v-*myb* expression induces an immature state of myeloid differentiation and inhibits phagocytosis. A novel gene, MD-1, is also expressed (Burk and Klempnauer, 1991)
Murine myeloid leukaemia cell line (WEH1-3B)	G-CSF and actinomycin D	Decrease in *Myb* (and *Myc*) transcription occurs only at a late stage of differentiation to macrophages. Thus *Myb* may be necessary for proliferation but not to control myeloid differentiation. *Fos* mRNA is increased (Gonda and Metcalf, 1984)
Murine erythroleukaemia cells (SKT6)	Erythropoietin, DMSO	Erythropoietin normally downregulates *Myb*. As in WEH1-3B cells, the inhibition of differentiation by *Myb* occurs very late in the process (Danish *et al.*, 1992)
	Myb plasmid or *Fos* plasmid	Sustained (via plasmid activation) *Myb* (or *Fos*) expression blocks erythropoietin-induced differentiation and partially blocks the effect of DMSO. Thus chemically and erythropoietin-induced differentiation mechanisms may differ. Sustained expression of *Fos* causes sustained *Myb* expression after erythropoietin addition (Todokoro *et al.*, 1988)
Murine erythroleukaemia cells (MELC DS19-sc9)	HMBA	Downregulates *Myb* (and *Myc*) during first 4 h; *Myb* expression remains suppressed (but not that of *Myc*). *Fos* mRNA is increased (Ramsay *et al.*, 1986)
Murine erythroleukaemia cells (MEL-745-C19)	HMBA and *Myb* plasmid	Downregulation of *Myb* is required for differentiation but is necessary only after the first 2 days (McClinton *et al.*, 1990)
Friend erythroleukaemia cells	DMSO and *Mbm-2* plasmid	Sustained expression of *Mbm-2* (the alternatively spliced form of *Myb*) accelerates differentiation whereas *Myb* inhibits (Weber *et al.*, 1990)
Friend erythroleukaemia cells	DMSO and pSV40-*Myb*	Sustained expression of *Myb* blocks differentiation (Clarke *et al.*, 1988)

Table 3.4. *Continued*

Cell type	Agent	Comment
Myeloblastic leukaemia cell line (M1)	IL-6, leukaemia inhibitory factor (LIF)	IL-6 or LIF induce terminal differentiation of M1 cells. They transiently stimulate *Myc* but after 12 h both *Myc* and *Myb* expression are suppressed. Sustained expression of *Myc* from a transfected vector blocks terminal differentiation (Hoffman-Liebermann and Liebermann, 1991). Sustained expression of *Myb* inhibits differentiation independently of *Myc*. Suppression of *Myb* is not essential to suppress growth (Selvakumaran *et al.*, 1992)
Myeloid leukaemia cell line (NFS-60)	IL-3	These cells express truncated MYB and IL-3 does not cause them to differentiate (Weinstein *et al.*, 1986)
Murine teratocarcinoma cells (F9)	Retinoic acid, db-cAMP	*Myb* transcription is undetectable after 24 h (Fukuda *et al.*, 1987; Lockett and Sleigh, 1987)
Erythroid precursor cells	Antisense *MYB*	Inhibits erythroid progenitor cell differentiation (Valtieri *et al.*, 1991)

Databank file names and accession numbers

	GENE	*EMBL*	*SWISSPROT*	*REFERENCES*
Chicken (AMV)	v-*myb*	Reonvmyb J02012	MYB_AVIMB P01104	Klempnauer *et al.*, 1982 Rushlow *et al.*, 1982
Chicken (AEV E26)	v-*myb*–*ets*	Reaev1 X00144	MYBE_AVILE P01105	Nunn *et al.*, 1983
Human	*MYB*	Hscmybla M15014	MYB_HUMAN P10242	Majello *et al.*, 1986 Slamon *et al.*, 1986
Human	*MYBB*	Hsbmyb X13293		Nomura *et al.*, 1988
Human	*MBM2*	Hscmyba1/Hscmyba2 X52125/X52126		Westin *et al.*, 1990
Human	*MYBA*	Hsamyb X13294	MYBA_HUMAN P10243	
	MYBB	Hsbmyb X13293	MYBB_HUMAN P10244	Nomura *et al.*, 1988
Chicken	*Myb*	Ggmybpo M14129		Gerondakis and Bishop, 1986
		Ggcmybl L00052; J02011		Klempnauer *et al.*, 1982
Chicken	*B-myb*	Ggbmyb X67505		Foos *et al.*, 1992
Mouse	*Myb*	Mmmyba M16449		Rosson *et al.*, 1987 Bender and Kuehl, 1986
Mouse	*Myb* (Cas-BR-M insertion site)	Mmmybmlv M13138		Shen-Ong *et al.*, 1986

	GENE	EMBL	SWISSPROT	REFERENCES
Mouse	Mybb			Lam et al., 1992
Bovine	Myb	Btcmybpo M82978		Brown et al., 1992
Drosophila	D-myb	Dmmybdr X05939	MYB_DROME P04197	Katzen et al., 1985
		Dmmybc M11281		Peters et al., 1987
Drosophila	Adf-1			England et al., 1992
Yeast	REB1	Screb1 M58728; M36598	REB1_YEAST P21538	Ju et al., 1990
Zea mays	cl	Zmmybaa M37153	MYB1_MAIZE P20024	Paz-Ares et al., 1987
Zea mays	Factor P	Zmppra M73029; M62879 Zmppr M73028; M62878		Grotewold et al., 1991
Arabidopsis thaliana	myb	Atmybo M79448		Oppenheimer et al., 1991
Dictyostelium discoideum	myb	Ddmybbd Z11534 (DNA-Binding domain)		Stober-Grasser et al., 1992 Biedenkapp et al., 1988
Xenopus laevis	myb-1	Xlmybrp1 M75870		Bouwmeester et al., unpublished
Xenopus laevis	myb-2	Xlmybrp2 M75871		Bouwmeester et al., unpublished

Reviews

Graf, T. (1992). Myb: a transcriptional activator limiting proliferation and differentiation in hematopoietic cells. Curr. Opin. Genetics Devel., 2, 249–255.
Luscher, B. and Eisenman, R.N. (1990). New light on myc and myb. Part II. Myb. Genes Devel., 4, 2235–2241.
Shen-Ong, G.L.C. (1990). The myb oncogene. Biochim. Biophys. Acta, 1032, 39–52.

Papers

Adkins, B., Leutz, A. and Graf, T. (1984). Autocrine growth induced by src-related oncogenes in transformed chicken myeloid cells. Cell, 39, 439–445.
Alexander, R.J., Buxbaum, J.N. and Raicht, R.F. (1992). Oncogene alterations in rat colon tumors induced by N-methyl-N-nitrosourea. Am. J. Med. Sci., 303, 16–24.
Alitalo, K., Winquist, R., Lin, C.C., De la Chapelle, A., Schwab, M. and Bishop, M.J. (1984). Aberrant expression of an amplified c-myb oncogene in two cell lines from a colon carcinoma. Proc. Natl Acad. Sci. USA, 81, 4534–4538.
Anfossi, G., Gewirtz, A.M. and Calabretta, B. (1989). An oligomer complementary to c-myb-encoded mRNA inhibits proliferation of human myeloid leukemia cell lines. Proc. Natl Acad. Sci. USA, 86, 3379–3383.
Avanzi, G.C., Porcu, P., Brizzi, M.F., Ghigo, D., Bosia, A. and Pegoraro, L. (1991). Interleukin 3-dependent proliferation of the human Mo-7e cell line is supported by discrete activation of late G_1 genes. Cancer Res., 51, 1741–1743.
Baer, M.R., Augustinos, P. and Kinniburgh, A.J. (1992). Defective c-myc and c-myb RNA turnover in acute myeloid leukemia cells. Blood, 79, 1319–1326.
Balaban, G.B., Herlyn, M., Guerry, D., Bartolo, R., Koprowski, H., Clark, W.H. and Nowell, P.C. (1984). Cytogenetics of human malignant melanoma and premalignant lesions. Cancer Genet. Cytogenet., 11, 429–439.

Baluda, M.A. and Goetz, I.E. (1961). Morphological conversion of cell cultures by avian myeloblastosis virus. Virology, 15, 185–199.

Barletta, C., Pellici, P., Kenyon, L., Smith, S.D. and Dalla-Favera, R. (1987). Relationship between c-*myb* locus and the 6q-chromosomal aberration in leukemias and lymphomas. Science, 235, 1064–1067.

Barletta, C., Lazzaro, D., Prosperi-Porta, R., Testa, U., Grignani, F., Ragusa, R.M., Leone, R., Patella, A, Carenza, L. and Peschle, C. (1992). C-MYB activation and the pathogenesis of ovarian cancer. Eur. J. Gynaecol. Oncol., 13, 53–59.

Bender, T.P. and Kuehl, W.M. (1986). Murine *myb* protooncogene mRNA: cDNA sequence and evidence for 5' heterogeneity. Proc. Natl Acad. Sci. USA, 83, 3204–3208.

Beug, H., Blundell, P.A. and Graf, T. (1987). Reversibility of differentiation and proliferative capacity in avian myelomonocytic cells transformed by *ts*E26 leukemia virus. Genes Devel., 1, 277–286.

Biedenkapp, H., Borgmeyer, U., Sippel, A.E. and Klempnauer, K.-H. (1988). Viral *myb* oncogene encodes a sequence-specific DNA-binding activity. Nature, 335, 835–837.

Bohjanen, P.R., Okajima, M. and Hodes, R.J. (1990). Differential regulation of interleukin 4 and interleukin 5 gene expression: a comparison of T-cell gene induction by anti-CD3 antibody or by exogenous lymphokines. Proc. Natl Acad. Sci. USA, 87, 5283–5287.

Boise, L.H., Gorse, K.M. and Westin, E.H. (1992). Multiple mechanisms of regulation of the human c-*myb* gene during myelomonocytic differentiation. Oncogene, 7, 1817–1825.

Bosselut, R., Lim, F., Romond, P.C., Frampton, J., Brady, J. and Ghysdael, J. (1992). Myb protein binds to multiple sites in the human T cell lymphotropic virus type 1 long terminal repeat and transactivates LTR-mediated expression. Virology, 186, 764–769.

Bouwmeester T., Guehmann S., El-Baradi T., Kalkbrenner F., Wijk D., Moelling K., Pieler T. Molecular cloning, expression and *in vitro* functional characterization of *myb* related proteins in *Xenopus*. Unpublished.

Boyle, W.J., Lampert, M.A., Lipsick, J.S. and Baluda, M.A. (1984). Avian myeloblastosis virus and E26 virus oncogene products are nuclear proteins. Proc. Natl Acad. Sci. USA, 81, 4265–4269.

Brown, K.E., Kindy, M.S. and Sonenshein, G.E. (1992). Expression of the c-*myb* proto-oncogene in bovine vascular smooth muscle cells. J. Biol. Chem., 267, 4625–4630.

Burk, O. and Klempnauer, K.-H. (1991). Estrogen-dependent alterations in differentiation state of myeloid cells caused by a v-*myb*/estrogen receptor fusion protein. EMBO J., 10, 3713–3719.

Burk, O., Mink, S., Ringwald, M. and Klempnauer, K.-H. (1993). Synergistic activation of the chicken *mim*-1 gene by v-*myb* and C/EBP transcription factors. EMBO J., 12, 2027–2038.

Catron, K.M., Purkerson, J.M., Isakson, P.C. and Bender, T.P. (1992). Constitutive versus cell cycle regulation of c-*myb* mRNA expression correlates with developmental stages in murine B lymphoid tumors. J. Immunol., 148, 934–942.

Churilla, A.M., Braciale, T.J. and Braciale, V.L. (1989). Regulation of T lymphocyte proliferation. Interleukin 2-mediated induction of c-myb gene expression is dependent on T lymphocyte activation state. J. Exp. Med., 170, 105–121.

Citro, G., Perrotti, D., Cucco, C., D'Agnano, I., Sacchi, A., Zupi, G. and Calabretta, B. (1992). Inhibition of leukemia cell proliferation by receptor-mediated uptake of c-*myb* antisense oligodeoxynucleotides. Proc. Natl Acad. Sci. USA, 89, 7031–7035.

Clarke, M.F., Kukowska-Latallo, J.F., Westin, E., Smith, M. and Prochownik, E.V. (1988). Constitutive expression of a c-*myb* DNA blocks Friend murine erythroleukemia cell differentiation. Mol. Cell. Biol., 8, 884–892.

Cuddihy, A.E., Brents, L.A., Aziz, N., Bender, T.P. and Kuehl, W.M. (1993). Only the DNA binding and transactivation domains of c-myb are required to block terminal differentiation of murine erythroleukemia cells. Mol. Cell. Biol., 13, 3505–3513.

Danish, R., El-Awar, O., Weber, B.L., Langmore, J., Turka, L.A., Ryan, J.J. and Clarke, M.F (1992). c-*myb* effects on kinetic events during MEL cell differentiation. Oncogene, 7, 901–907.

Dasgupta, P., Saikumar, P., Reddy, C.D. and Reddy, E.P. (1990). Myb protein binds to human immunodeficiency virus 1 long terminal repeat (LTR) sequences and transactivates LTR-mediated transcription. Proc. Natl Acad. Sci. USA, 87, 8090–8094.

Dasgupta, P., Reddy, C.D., Saikumar, P. and Reddy, E.P. (1992). The cellular proto-oncogene product *myb* acts as transcriptional activator of the long terminal repeat of human T-lymphotropic virus type I. J. Virol., 66, 270–276.

Dautry, F., Weil, D., Yu, J. and Dautry-Varsat, A. (1988). Regulation of *pim* and *myb* mRNA accumulation by interleukin 2 and interleukin 3 in murine hematopoietic cell lines. J. Biol. Chem., 263, 17615–17620.

Domenget, C., Leprince, D., Pain, B., Peyrol, S., Li, R.P., Stehelin, D. and Jurdic, P. (1992). The various domains of v-*myb* and v-*ets* oncogenes of E26 retrovirus contribute differently, but cooperatively, in transformation of hematopoietic lineages. Oncogene, 7, 2231–2241.

Dubendorff, J.W., Whittaker, L.J., Eltman, J.T. and Lipsick, J.S. (1992). Carboxyl-terminal elements of c-myb negatively regulate transcriptional activation in *cis* and in *trans*. Genes Devel., 6, 2524–2535.

Dudek, H., Tantravahi, R.V., Rao, V.N., Reddy, E.S.P. and Reddy, E.P. (1992). myb and ets proteins cooperate in transcriptional activation of the *mim-1* promoter. Proc. Natl Acad. Sci. USA, 89, 1291–1295.

Duprey, S.P. and Boettiger, D. (1985). Developmental regulation of c-*myb* in normal myeloid progenitor cells. Proc. Natl Acad. Sci. USA, 82, 6937–6941.

England, B.P., Admon, A. and Tjian, R. (1992). Cloning of *Drosophila* transcription factor Adf-1 reveals homology to myb oncoproteins. Proc. Natl Acad. Sci. USA, 89, 683–687.

Evans, J.L., Moore, T.L., Kuehl, W.M., Bender, T. and Ting, J.P. (1990). Functional analysis of c-*Myb* protein in T-lymphocytic cell lines shows that it trans-activates the c-*myc* promoter. Mol. Cell. Biol., 10, 5747–5752.

Foos, G., Grimm, S. and Klempnauer, K.-H. (1992). Functional antagonism between members of the *myb* family: B-*myb* inhibits v-*myb*-induced gene activation. EMBO J., 11, 4619–4629.

Frampton, J., Leutz, A., Gibson, T.J. and Graf, T. (1989). DNA-binding domain ancestry. Nature, 342, 134.

Frampton, J., Gibson, T.J., Ness, S.A., Doderlein, G. and Graf, T. (1991). Proposed structure for the DNA-binding domain of the *myb* oncoprotein based on model building and mutational analysis. Protein Engin., 4, 891–901.

Fukuda, M., Ikuma, S., Setoyama, C. and Shimada, K. (1987). Decrease in the c-*myb* transcript during differentiation of mouse teratocarcinoma stem cells. Biochem. International, 15, 73–79.

Furukawa, Y., Piwnica-Worms, H., Ernst, T.J., Kanakura, Y. and Griffin, J.D. (1990). *cdc2* gene expression at the G_1 to S transition in human T lymphocytes. Science, 250, 805–808.

Gabrielsen, O.D., Sentenac, A. and Fromageot, P. (1991). Specific DNA binding by c-*myb*: evidence for a double helix–turn–helix-related motif. Science, 253, 1140–1143.

Garrido, C., Leprince, D., Lipsick, J.S., Stehelin, D., Gospodarowicz, D. and Saule, S. (1992). Definition of functional domains in P135$^{gag-myb-ets}$ and p48^{v-myb} proteins required to maintain the response of neuro-retina cells to basic fibroblast growth factor. J. Virol., 66, 160–166.

Gerondakis, S. and Bishop, J.M. (1986). Structure of the protein encoded by the chicken proto-oncogene c-*myb*. Mol. Cell. Biol. 6, 3677–3684.

Gewirtz, A.M. and Calabretta, B. (1988). A c-*myb* antisense oligodeoxynucleotide inhibits normal human hematopoiesis *in vitro*. Science, 243, 1303–1306.

Gewirtz, A.M., Anfossi, G., Venturelli, D., Valpreda, S., Sims, R. and Calabretta, B. (1989). G_1/S transition in normal human T-lymphocytes requires the nuclear protein encoded by c-*myb*. Science, 245, 180–183.

Golay, J., Introna, M. and Graf, T. (1988). A single point mutation in the v-*ets* oncogene affects both erythroid and myelomonocytic cell differentiation. Cell, 55, 1147–1158.

Gonda, T.J. and Metcalf, D. (1984). Expression of *myb*, *myc* and *fos* proto-oncogenes during the differentiation of a murine myeloid leukemia. Nature, 310, 249–251.

Gonda, T.J., Cory, S., Sobieszczuk, P., Holtzman, D. and Adams, J.M. (1987). Generation of altered transcripts by retroviral insertion within the c-*myb* gene in two murine monocytic leukemias. J. Virol., 61, 2754–2763.

Graf, T., McNagny, K., Brady, G. and Frampton, J. (1992). Chicken "erythroid" cells transformed by the gag-myb-ets-encoding E26 leukemia virus are multipotent. Cell, 70, 1–20.

Grasser, F.A., LaMontagne, K., Whittaker, L., Stohr, S. and Lipsick, J.S. (1992). A highly conserved cysteine in the v-myb DNA-binding domain is essential for transformation and transcriptional *trans*-activation. Oncogene, 7, 1005–1009.

Griffin, C.A. and Baylin, S.B. (1985). Expression of c-*myb* oncogene in human small cell lung carcinoma. Cancer Res., 45, 272–275.

Grotewold E., Athma P. and Peterson T. (1991). Alternatively spliced products of the maize P gene encode proteins with homology to the DNA-binding domain of *myb*-like transcription factors. Proc. Natl Acad. Sci. USA, 88, 4587–4591.

Guehmann, S., Vorbrueggen, G., Kalkbrenner, F. and Moelling, K. (1992). Reduction of a conserved Cys is essential for myb DNA-binding. Nucleic Acids Res., 20, 2279–2286.

Guerin, M., Sheng, Z.-M., Andrieu, N. and Riou, G. (1990). Strong association between c-*myb* and oestrogen-receptor expression in human breast cancer. Oncogene, 5, 131–135.

Hall, W.J., Bean, C.W. and Pollard, M. (1941). Transmission of fowl leucosis through chick embryos and young chicks. Am. J. Vet. Res., 2, 272–279.

Hoffman-Liebermann, B. and Liebermann, D.A. (1991). Interleukin-6- and leukemia inhibitory factor-induced terminal differentiation of myeloid leukemia cells is blocked at an intermediate stage by constitutive c-*myc*. Mol. Cell. Biol., 11, 2375–2381.

Howe, K.M., Reakes, C.F.L. and Watson, R.J. (1990). Characterization of the sequence-specific interaction of mouse c-*myb* protein with DNA. EMBO J., 9, 161–169.

Introna, M., Golay, J., Frampton J., Nakano, T., Ness, S.A. and Graf, T. (1990). Mutations in v-*myb* alter the differentiation of myelomonocytic cells transformed by the oncogene. Cell, 63, 1287–1297.

Ivanov, X., Mladenov, Z., Nedyalkov, S., Todorov, T.G. and Yakimov, M. (1964). Experimental investigations into avian leucoses. V. Transmission, haematology and morphology of avian myelocytomatosis. Izv. Inst. Pat. Zhivotnite Sofia, 10, 5–38.

Janssen, J.W.G., Vernole, P., de Boer, P.A.J., Oosterhuis, J.W. and Collard, J.G. (1986). Sublocalisation of c-*myb* to 6q21–q23 by in situ hybridization and c-*myb* expression in a human teratocarcinoma with 6q rearrangements. Cytogenet. Cell. Genet., 41, 129–135.

Ju, Q., Morrow, B. and Warner, J.R. (1990). REB1, a yeast DNA-binding protein with many targets, is essential for cell growth and bears some resemblance to the oncogene myb. Mol. Cell. Biol., 10, 5226–5234.

Kanei-Ishii, C., MacMillan, E.M., Nomura, T., Sarai, A., Ramsay, R.G., Aimoto, S., Ishii, S. and Gonda, T.J. (1992). Transactivation and transformation by *myb* are negatively regulated by a leucine-zipper structure. Proc. Natl Acad. Sci. USA, 89, 3088–3092.

Kanter, M.R., Smith, R.E. and Hayward, W.S. (1988). Rapid induction of B-cell lymphomas: insertional activation of c-*myb* by avian leukosis virus. J. Virol., 62, 1423–1432.

Katzen, A.L., Kornberg, T.B. and Bishop, M.J. (1985). Isolation of the proto-oncogene c-*myb* from D. melanogaster. Cell, 41, 449–456.

Kelly, K. and Siebenlist, U. (1988). Mitogenic activation of normal T cells leads to increased initiation of transcription in the c-*myc* locus. J. Biol. Chem., 263, 4828–4831.

Kenney, S.C., Holley-Guthrie, E., Quinlivan, E.B., Gutsch, D., Zhang, Q., Bender, T., Giot, J.-F. and Sergeant, A. (1992). The cellular oncogene c-*myb* can interact synergistically with the Epstein–Barr virus BZLF1 transactivator in lymphoid cells. Mol. Cell. Biol., 12, 136–146.

Klempnauer, K.-H. (1993). Methlation-sensitive DNA binding by v-*myb* and c-*myb* proteins. Oncogene, 8, 111–115.

Klempnauer, K.-H., Gonda, T.J. and Bishop, M.J. (1982). Nucleotide sequence of the retroviral leukemia gene v-*myb* and its cellular progenitor c-*myb*: the architecture of a transduced oncogene. Cell, 31, 453–463.

Klempnauer, K.-H., Ramsay, G., Bishop, M.J., Moscovici, G.M., Moscovici, C., McGrath, J.P. and Levinson, A.D. (1983). The product of the retroviral transforming gene v-*myb* is a truncated version of the protein encoded by the cellular oncogene c-*myb*. Cell, 33, 345–355.

Klempnauer, K.-H., Symonds, G., Evan, G.I. and Bishop, M.J. (1984). Subcellular localization of proteins encoded by oncogenes of avian myeloblastosis virus and avian leukemia virus E26 and by the chicken c-*myb* gene. Cell, 37, 537–547.

Lam, E.W.-F., Robinson, C. and Watson, R.J. (1992). Characterization and cell cycle-reguleted expression of mouse B-*myb*. Oncogene, 7, 1885–1890.

Lane, T., Ibanez, C., Garcia, A., Graf, T. and Lipsick, J. (1990). Transformation by v-*myb* correlates with trans activation of gene expression. Mol. Cell. Biol., 10, 2591–2598.

Lockett, T.J. and Sleigh, M.J. (1987). Oncogene expression in differentiated F9 mouse embryonic carcinoma cells. Exp. Cell Res., 173, 370–378.

Luscher, B. and Eisenman, R.N. (1992). Mitosis-specific phosphorylation of the nuclear oncoproteins Myc and Myb. J. Cell. Biol., 118, 775–784.

Luscher, B., Christenson, E., Litchfield, D.W., Krebs, E.G. and Eisenman, R.N. (1990). Myb DNA binding inhibited by phosphorylation at a site deleted during oncogenic activation. Nature, 344, 517–522.

McClinton, D., Stafford, J., Brents, L., Bender, T.P. and Kuehl, W.M. (1990). Differentiation of mouse erythroleukemia cells is blocked by late up-regulation of a c-*myb* transgene. Mol. Cell. Biol., 10, 705–710.

Majello B., Kenyon L.C., Dalla-Favera R. (1986). Human c-*myb* protooncogene: Nucleotide sequence of cDNA and organization of the genomic locus. Proc. Natl Acad. Sci. USA, 83, 9636–9640.

Makover, D., Cuddy, M., Yum, S., Bradley, K., Alpers, J., Sukhatme, V. and Reed, J.C. (1991). Phorbol ester-mediated inhibition of growth and regulation of proto-oncogene expression in the human T cell leukemia line JURKAT. Oncogene, 6, 455–460.

Marocco, A., Wissenbach, M., Becker, D., Paz-Ares, J., Saedler, H., Salamini, F. and Rohde, W. (1989). Multiple genes are transcribed in *Hordeum vulgare* and *Zea mays* that carry the DNA binding domain of the *myb* oncoproteins. Mol. Gen. Genet., 216, 183–187.

Melani, C., Rivoltini, L., Parmiani, G., Calabretta, B. and Colombo, M.P. (1991). Inhibition of proliferation by c-*myb* antisense oligodeoxynucleotides in colon adenocarcinoma cell lines that express c-*myb*. Cancer Res., 51, 2897–2901.

Metz, T. and Graf, T. (1991a). v-*myb* and v-*ets* transform chicken erythroid cells and cooperate both in *trans* and in *cis* to induce distinct differentiation phenotypes. Genes Devel., 5, 369–380.

Metz, T. and Graf, T. (1991b). Fusion of the nuclear oncoproteins v-*myb* and v-*ets* is required for the leukemogenicity of E26 virus. Cell, 66, 95–105.

Mizuguchi, G., Nakagoshi, H., Nagase, T., Nomura, N., Date, T., Ueno, Y. and Ishii, S. (1990). DNA binding activity and transcriptional activator function of the human B-*myb* protein compared with c-MYB. J. Biol. Chem., 265, 9280–9284.

Moscovici, C. and Vogt, P.K. (1968). Effects of genetic cellular resistance on cell transformation and virus replication in chicken hematopoietic cell cultures infected with avian myeloblastosis virus (BAI-A). Virology, 35, 487–497.

Moscovici, C., Samarut, J., Gazzolo, L. and Moscovici, M.G. (1981). Myeloid and erythroid neoplastic responses to avian defective leukemia viruses in chickens and in quail. Virology, 113, 765–768.

Mountz, J.D. and Steinberg, A.D. (1989). Studies of c-*myb* gene regulation in MRL-*lpr/lpr* mice. Identification of a 5' c-*myb* nuclear protein binding site and high levels of binding factors in nuclear extracts of lpr/lpr lymph node cells. J. Immunol., 142, 328–335.

Mucenski, M.L., McLain, K., Kier, A.B., Swerdlow, S.H., Schreiner, C.M., Miller, T.A., Peitryga, D.W., Scott, W.J. and Potter, S.S. (1991). A functional c-*myb* gene is required for normal murine fetal hepatic hematopoiesis. Cell, 65, 677–689.

Mushinski, J.F., Potter, M., Bauer, S.R. and Reddy, E.P. (1983). DNA rearrangement and altered RNA expression of the c-*myb* oncogene in mouse plasmacytoid lymphosarcomas. Science, 220, 795–798.

Nakagoshi, H., Kanei-Ishii, C., Sawazaki, T., Mizuguchi, G. and Ishii, S. (1992). Transcriptional activation of the c-*myc* gene by the c-*myb* and B-*myb* gene products. Oncogene, 7, 1233–1239.

Nakano, T. and Graf, T. (1992). Identification of genes differentially expressed in two types of v-*myb*-transformed avian myelomonocytic cells. Oncogene, 7, 527–534.

Nedyalkov, St., Bozhkov, Sp. and Todorov, G. (1975). Experimental erythroblastosis in the Japanese quail (*Coturnix coturnix japonica*) induced by the E-26 leukosis strain. Acta Vet. (Brno), 44, 75–78.

Ness, S.A., Beug, H. and Graf, T. (1987). v-*myb* dominance over v-*myc* in doubly transformed chick myelo-monocytic cells. Cell, 51, 41–50.

Ness, S.A., Marknell, A. and Graf, T. (1989). The v-*myb* oncogene product binds to and activates the promyelocyte-specific *mim-1* gene. Cell, 59, 1115–1125.

Nicolaides, N.C., Gualdi, R., Casadevall, C., Manzella, L. and Calabretta, B. (1991). Positive autoregulation of c-*myb* expression via myb binding sites in the 5' flanking region of the human c-*myb* gene. Mol. Cell. Biol., 11, 6166–6176.

Nishina, Y., Nakagoshi, H., Imamoto, F., Gonda, T.J. and Ishii, S. (1989). *Trans*-activation by the c-*myb* proto-oncogene. Nucleic Acids Res., 17, 107–117.

Nomura, N., Takahashi, M., Matsui, M., Ishii, S., Date, T., Sasamoto, S. and Ishizaki, R. (1988). Isolation of human cDNA clones of *myb*-related genes A-*myb* and B-*myb*. Nucleic Acids Res., 16, 11075–11090.

Nunn, M.F., Seeburg, P.H., Moscovici, C. and Duesberg, P.H. (1983). Tripartite structure of the avian erythroblastosis virus transforming gene. Nature, 306, 391–395.

Oehler, T., Arnold, H., Biedenkapp, H. and Klempnauer, K.-H. (1990). Characterization of the v-*myb* DNA binding domain. Nucleic Acids Res., 18, 1703–1710.

Oppenheimer D.G., Herman P.L., Sivakumaran S., Esch J., Marks M.D. (1991). A *myb* gene required for leaf trichome differentiation in Arabidopsis is expressed in stipules. Cell, 67, 483–493.

Patel, G., Kreider, B., Rovera, G. and Reddy, E.P. (1993). v-*myb* blocks granulocyte colony-stimulating factor-induced myeloid cell differentiation but not proliferation. Mol. Cell. Biol., 13, 2269–2276.

Pauza, C.D. (1987). Regulation of human T-lymphocyte gene expression by interleukin 2: immediate-response genes include the proto-oncogene c-*myb*. Mol. Cell. Biol., 7, 342–348.

Paz-Ares, J., Ghosal, D., Wienand, U., Peterson, P.A. and Saedler, H. (1987). The regulatory *c1* locus of *Zea mays* encodes a protein with homology to *myb* proto-oncogene products and with structural similarities to transcription activators. EMBO J., 6, 3553–3558.

Pellici, P.G., Lanfrancone, L., Brathwaite, M.D., Wolman, S.R. and Dalla-Favera, R. (1984). Amplification of the c-*myb* oncogene in a case of human acute myelogenous leukemia. Science, 224, 1117–1121.

Peters, C.W.B., Sippel, A.E., Vingron, M. and Klempnauer, K.-H. (1987). *Drosophila* and vertebrate *myb* proteins share two conserved regions, one of which functions as a DNA-binding domain. EMBO J., 6, 3085–3090.

Pizer, E. and Humphries, E.H. (1989). RAV-1 insertional mutagenesis: disruption of the c-*myb* locus and development of avian B-cell lymphomas. J. Virol., 63, 1630–1640.

Queva, C., Ness, S.A., Grasser, F.A., Graf, T., Vandenbunder, B. and Stehelin, D. (1992). Expression patterns of c-*myb* and of v-*myb* induced myeloid-1 (*mim*-1) gene during the development of the chick embryo. Development, 114, 125–133.

Radke, K., Beug, H., Kornfeld, S. and Graf, T. (1982). Transformation of both erythroid and myeloid cells by E26, an avian leukemia virus that contains the *myb* gene. Cell, 31, 643–653.

Ramsay, R.G., Ikeda, K., Rifkind, R.A. and Marks, P.A. (1986). Changes in gene expression associated with induced differentiation of erythroleukemia: protooncogenes, globin genes, and cell division. Proc. Natl Acad. Sci. USA, 83, 6849–6853.

Ramsay, R.G., Ishii, S., Nishina, Y., Soe, G. and Gonda, T.J. (1989). Characterization of alternate and truncated forms of murine c-*myb* proteins. Oncogene Res., 4, 259–269.

Ramsay, R.G., Ishii, S. and Gonda, T.J. (1992). Interaction of the *myb* protein with specific DNA binding sites. J. Biol. Chem., 267, 5656–5662.

Ratajczak, M.Z., Hijiya, N., Catani, L., DeRiel, K., Luger, S.M., McGlave, P. and Gewirtz, A.M. (1992). Acute- and chronic-phase chronic myelogenous leukemia colony-forming units are highly sensitive to the growth inhibitory effects of c-*myb* antisense oligodeoxynucleotides. Blood, 79, 1956–1961.

Reddy, C.D. and Reddy, E.P. (1989). Differential binding of nuclear factors to the intron 1 sequences containing the transcriptional pause site correlates with c-*myb* expression, Proc. Natl Acad. Sci. USA, 86, 7326–7330.

Reed, J.C., Alpers, J.D., Scherle, P.A., Hoover, R.G., Nowell, P.C. and Prystowsky, M.B. (1987). Protooncogene expression in cloned T lymphocytes: mitogens and growth factors induce different patterns of expression. Oncogene, 1, 223–228.

Reiss, K., Ferber, A., Travali, S., Porcu, P., Phillips, P.D. and Baserga, R. (1991). The protooncogene c-*myb* increases the expression of insulin-like growth factor 1 and insulin-like growth factor 1 receptor messenger RNAs by a transcriptional mechanism. Cancer Res., 51, 5997–6000.

Rosson, D., Dugan, D. and Reddy E.P. (1987). Aberrant splicing events that are induced by proviral integration: Implications for *myb* oncogene activation. Proc. Natl Acad. Sci. USA, 84, 3171–3175.

Rushlow, K.E., Lautenberger, J.A., Papas, T.S., Baluda, M.A., Perbal, B., Chirikjian, J.G. and Reddy, E.P. (1982). Nucleotide sequence of the transforming gene of avian myeloblastosis virus. Science, 216, 1421–1423.

Sakura, H., Kanei-Ishii, C., Nagase, T., Nakagoshi, H., Gonda, T.J. and Ishii, S. (1989). Delineation of three functional domains of the transcriptional activator encoded by the c-*myb* protooncogene. Proc. Natl Acad. Sci. USA, 86, 5758–5762.

Sala, A. and Calabretta, B. (1992). Regulation of BALB/c 3T3 fibroblast proliferation by B-myb is accompanied by selective activation of cdc2 and cyclin D1 expression. Proc. Natl Acad. Sci. USA, 86, 10415–10419.

Selvakumaran, M., Liebermann, D.A. and Hoffman-Liebermann, B. (1992). Deregulated c-*myb* disrupts interleukin-6- or leukemia inhibitory factor-induced myeloid differentiation prior to c-*myc*: role in leukemogenesis. Mol. Cell. Biol., 12, 2493–2500.

Sheiness, D. and Gardinier, M. (1984). Expression of a proto-oncogene (proto-*myb*) in hemopoietic tissues of mice. Mol. Cell. Biol., 4, 1206–1212.

Shen-Ong, G.L.C. (1987). Alternative internal splicing in c-*myb* RNAs occurs commonly in normal and tumor cells. EMBO J., 6, 4035–4039.

Shen-Ong, G.L.C., Potter, M., Mushinski, J.F., Lavu, S. and Reddy, E.P. (1984). Activation of the c-*myb* locus by viral insertional mutagenesis in plasmacytoid lymphosarcomas. Science, 226, 1077–1080.

Shen-Ong, G.L.C., Morse, H.C., Potter, M. and Mushinski, J.F. (1986). Two modes of c-*myb* activation in virus-induced mouse myeloid tumors. Mol. Cell. Biol., 6, 380–392.

Shen-Ong, G.L.C., Luscher, B. and Eisenman, R.N. (1989). A second c-*myb* protein is translated from an alternative spliced mRNA expressed from normal and 5'-disrupted *myb* loci. Mol. Cell. Biol., 9, 5456–5463.

Sihvola, M., Sistonen, L., Alitalo, K. and Hurme, M. (1989). Mechanism of T cell proliferation in vivo: analysis of IL-2 receptor expression and activation of c-*myc* and c-*myb* oncogenes during lymphatic regeneration. Biochem. Biophys. Res. Commun., 160, 181–188.

Simons, M. and Rosenberg, R.D. (1992). Antisense nonmuscle myosin heavy chain and c-myb oligonucleotides suppress smooth muscle cell proliferation *in vitro*. Circ. Res., 70, 835–843.

Simons, M., Edelman, E.R., DeKeyser, J.-L., Langer, R. and Rosenberg, R.D. (1992). Antisense c-*myb* oligonucleotides inhibit arterial smooth muscle cell accumulation *in vivo*. Nature, 359, 67–70.

Simons, M., Morgan, K.G., Parker, C., Collins, E. and Rosenberg, R.D. (1993). The proto-oncogene c-*myb* mediates an intracellular calcium rise during the late G_1 phase of the cell cycle. J. Biol. Chem., 268, 627–632.

Siu, G., Wurster, A.L., Lipsick, J.S. and Hedrick, S.M. (1992). Expression of the CD4 gene requires a myb transcription factor. Mol. Cell. Biol., 12, 1592–1604.

Slamon, D.J., deKernion, J.B., Verma, I.M. and Cline, M.J. (1984). Expression of cellular oncogenes in human malignancies. Science, 224, 256–262.

Slamon, D.J., Boone, T.C., Murdock, D.C., Keith, D.E., Press, M.F., Larson, R.A. and Souza, L.M. (1986). Studies of the human c-*myb* gene and its product in human acute leukemias. Science, 233, 347–351.

Sotirov, N. (1981). Histone H5 in the immature blood cells of chickens with leukosis induced by avian leukosis virus strain E26. J. Natl Cancer Inst., 66, 1143–1147.

Stern, J.B. and Smith, K.A. (1986). Interleukin-2 induction of T-cell G_1 progression and c-*myb* expression. Science, 233, 203–206.

Sterneck, E., Muller, C., Katz, S. and Leutz, A. (1992). Autocrine growth induced by kinase type oncogenes in myeloid cells requires AP-1 and NF-M, a myeloid specific, C/EBP-like factor. EMBO J., 11, 115–126.

Stober-Grasser, U., Brydolf, B., Bin, X., Grasser, F., Firtel, R.A. and Lipsick, J.S. (1992). The *myb* DNA-binding domain is highly conserved in *Dictyostelium discoideum*. Oncogene, 7, 589–596.

Sudo, T., Miyazawa, H., Hanaoka, F. and Ishii, S. (1992). The c-*myb* proto-oncogene product binds to but does not activate the promoter of the DNA polymerase α gene. Oncogene, 7, 1999–2006.

Tesch, H., Michels, M., Jucker, M., Pahl, I., Klein, S., Bading, H., Moelling, K. and Diehl, V. (1992). Heterogeneous expression of c-*myb* protein in human leukemia detected by simultaneous two color flow cytometric analysis. Leukemia Res., 16, 265–274.

Thiele, C.J., Cohen, P.S. and Israel, M.A. (1988). Regulation of c-*myb* expression in human neuroblastoma cells during retinoic acid-induced differentiation. Mol. Cell. Biol., 8, 1677–1683.

Thompson, C.B., Challoner, P.B., Neiman, P.E. and Groudine, M. (1986). Expression of the c-*myb* proto-oncogene during cellular proliferation. Nature, 319, 374–380.

Tice-Baldwin, K., Fink, G.R. and Arndt, K.T. (1989). BAS1 has a *myb* motif and activates *HIS4* transcription only in combination with BAS2. Science, 246, 931–935.

Todokoro, K., Watson, R.J., Higo, H., Amanuma, H., Kuramochi, S., Yanagisawa, H. and Ikawa, Y. (1988). Down-regulation of c-*myb* gene expression is a prerequisite for erythropoietin-induced erythroid differentiation. Proc. Natl Acad. Sci. USA, 85, 8900–8904.

Travali, S., Reiss, K., Ferber, A., Petralia, S., Mercer, W.E., Calabretta, B. and Baserga, R. (1991a). Constitutively expressed c-*myb* abrogates the requirement for insulinlike growth factor 1 in 3T3 fibroblasts. Mol. Cell. Biol., 11, 731–736.

Travali, S., Ferber, A., Reiss, K., Sell, C., Koniecki, J., Calabretta, B. and Baserga, R. (1991b). Effect of the *myb* gene product on expression of the PCNA gene in fibroblasts. Oncogene, 6, 887–894.

Valtieri, M., Venturelli, D., Care, A., Fossati, C., Pelosi, E., Labbaye, C., Mattia, G., Gewirtz, A.M., Calabretta, B. and Peschle, C. (1991). Antisense *myb* inhibition of purified erythroid progenitors in development and differentiation is linked to cycling activity and expression of DNA polymerase alpha. Blood, 77, 1181–1190.

Vellard, M., Soret, J., Viegas-Pequignot, E., Galibert, F., van Cong, N., Dutrillaux, B. and Perbal, B. (1991). c-*myb* proto-oncogene: evidence for intermolecular recombination of coding sequences. Oncogene, 6, 505–514.

Vellard, M., Sureau, A., Soret, J., Martinerie, C. and Perbal, B. (1992). A potential splicing factor is encoded by the opposite strand of the trans-spliced c-*myb* exon. Proc. Natl Acad. Sci. USA, 89, 2511–2515.

Watson, R.J., Robinson, C. and Lam, E.W.-F. (1993). Transcription regulation by murine B-*myb* is distinct from that by c-*myb*. Nucleic Acids Res., 21, 267–272.

Weber, B.L., Westin, E.H. and Clarke, M.F. (1990). Differentiation of mouse erythroleukemia cells enhanced by alternatively spliced c-*myb* mRNA. Science, 249, 1291–1293.

Weinstein, Y., Ihle, J.N., Lavu, S. and Reddy, E.P. (1986). Truncation of the c-*myb* gene by a retroviral integration in an interleukin 3-dependent myeloid leukemia cell line. Proc. Natl Acad. Sci. USA, 83, 5010–5014.

Westin, E.H., Gallo, R.C., Arya, S.K., Eva, A., Souza, L.M., Baluda, M.A., Aaronson, S.A. and Wong-Staal, F. (1982). Differential expression of the *amv* gene in human hematopoietic cells. Proc. Natl Acad. Sci. USA, 79, 2194–2198.

Westin, E.H., Gorse, K.M. and Clarke, M.F. (1990). Alternative splicing of the human c-*myb* gene. Oncogene, 5, 1117–1124.

Weston, K. (1992). Extension of the DNA binding consensus of the chicken c-myb and v-myb proteins. Nucleic Acids Res., 20, 3043–3049.

Weston, K. and Bishop, M.J. (1989). Transcriptional activation by the v-*myb* oncogene and its cellular progenitor, c-*myb*. Cell, 58, 85–93.

Yokota, S., Yuan, D., Katagiri, T., Eisenberg, R.A., Cohen, P.L. and Ting, J.P. (1987). The expression and regulation of c-*myb* transcription in B6/*lpr* Lyt-2⁻, L3T4⁻ T lymphocytes. J. Immunol., 139, 2810–2817.

Yu, Y., Ramsay, R.G., Kanei-Ishii, C., Ishii, S. and Gonda, T.J. (1991). Transformation by carboxyl-deleted *myb* reflects increased *trans*-activating capacity and disruption of a negative regulatory domain. Oncogene, 6, 1549–1553.

Zobel, A., Kalkbrenner, F., Guehmann, S., Nawrath, M., Vorbrueggen, G. and Moelling, K. (1991). Interaction of the v- and c*myb* proteins with regulatory sequences of the human c-*myc* gene. Oncogene, 6, 1397–1407.

Zubiaga, A.M., Munoz, E. and Huber, B.T. (1991). Production of IL-1a by activated Th type 2 cells. Its role as an autocrine growth factor. J. Immunol., 146, 3849–3856.

MYC

The v-*myc* oncogene was originally derived from avian *myelocytomatosis* virus MC29 (Sheiness and Bishop, 1979). There are four MC29 group acutely transforming avian retroviruses (MC29, CMII, OK10, MH2 and FH3) that cause myeloid leukaemias, sarcomas and carcinomas (Bister and Jansen, 1986; Chen *et al.*, 1989).

MYC, MYCN, MYCL1 (murine *Myc*, *Nmyc* and *Lmyc*) encode transcription factors.

Related genes

The *Myc* gene family contains at least seven closely related genes, *Myc*, *Nmyc*, *Lmyc*, *Pmyc*, *Rmyc*, *Smyc* and *Bmyc* (together with *Lmyc*Ψ, an inactive pseudogene) detected by cross-hybridization of amplified sequences to an oncogene probe (DePinho *et al.*, 1991; Ingvarsson *et al.*, 1988). *MYCL2* (chromosome Xq22–q28) is closely related to *MYCL* (*MYCL1* (1p32) and to *MYCLK1*; Morton *et al.*, 1989). In the mouse two probable pseudogenes (*Lmyc-2* and *Nmyc-2*) map to chromosomes 12 and 5, respectively (Adolph *et al.*, 1987; Campbell *et al.*, 1989).

Also related are maize *Lc* gene (Ludwig *et al.*, 1989) and northern sea star, *Asterias vulgaris*, pAv-*myc* (Walker *et al.*, 1992).

Cross-species homology

MYC: 70–90% (all species); exon 1: 70%; coding exons >90% (human and mouse). The two coding exons (2 and 3) are highly conserved between species. Thus, the invertebrate pAv-*myc* encodes a protein with ~30% identity to human MYC (Walker *et al.*, 1992). There is no significant homology between exon 1 (mammals and chicken) (Bernard *et al.*, 1983). *Myc*, *Nmyc* and *Lmyc*: no significant exon 1 homology. Exon 2 of *Nmyc* and *Lmyc* contains two regions (40 and 60 nucleotides) of high homology with *Myc* exon 2 (this feature defines "*Myc* box proteins"). *Xenopus Myc* genes are highly related to the mammalian forms: two distinct copies of the *Xenopus Myc* gene (xc-*myc* I, xc-*myc* II) have been isolated (Vriz *et al.*, 1989).

Transformation

MAN

MYC: *MYC* is amplified in many tumours, particularly small-cell-lung carcinoma (SCLC: Gazdar *et al.*, 1985), breast (Guerin *et al.*, 1988; Mariani-Costantini *et al.*, 1988; Tsuda *et al.*, 1989) and cervical carcinomas (Ocadiz *et al.*, 1987). Genomic rearrangement may also occur (Alitalo *et al.*, 1986; Alitalo and Schwab, 1986). Enhanced transcription arising from translocation of *MYC* occurs in some but not all Burkitt's lymphomas. There is infrequent amplification of *MYC* (or *MYCN*) in pediatric gliomas (Wasson *et al.*, 1990). The stability of *MYC* and *MYB* mRNAs is increased to >75 min in the cells of some patients with acute myeloid leukaemia (AML; Baer *et al.*, 1992). *MYC* is constitutively overexpressed in lymphoblastoid cells lines derived from individuals with the cancer-prone condition Bloom's syndrome (Sullivan *et al.*,

1989) and there is evidence that *MYC* de-regulation may be involved in the early stages of mammary carcinogenesis (Escot *et al.*, 1993). All human tumour cells that have been examined show abnormal regulation of *MYC* in that removal of serum or growth factors does not cause the rapid repression of transcription and degradation of *MYC* mRNA and protein characteristic of normal cells.

MYCN: *MYCN* is frequently amplified in neuroblastomas (Schwab *et al.*, 1983), retinoblastomas and SCLC. Expression correlates with appearance of the more severe forms of cervical intra-epithelial carcinoma (CIN Types II and III) and with increased metastasis in the advanced stages of neuroblastoma. Increased expression usually correlates with gene amplification but in Wilms' tumour it occurs from single copies (Shaw *et al.*, 1988; Babiss and Friedman, 1990).

MYCL1: *MYCL1* is amplified in small-cell lung carcinoma (Little *et al.*, 1983). Approximately 40% of SCLC cell lines have one *MYC* gene amplified: amplification of more than one *MYC* gene within one cell line has not been detected. In primary SCLC tumours, however, the incidence of *MYC* amplification is much lower than in tumour-derived cell lines (up to 12%; Saksela, 1987; Yokota *et al.*, 1988). Increased expression usually correlates with gene amplification although in some SCLC cell lines it occurs from single copies. In two SCLC cell lines an intrachromosomal rearrangement at 1p32 results in the production of a chimeric mRNA containing 5' sequences from the *RLF* gene and the second and third exons of *MYCL1* (Makela *et al.*, 1991). The fusion protein has 79 RLF amino acids joined to 3 amino acids from the non-coding *MYCL1* sequences attached to the N-terminus of *MYCL1*.

ANIMALS

In chickens MC29, CMII or FH3 cause myelocytomatosis. MC29, MH2 or OK10 cause liver and kidney carcinomas. Proviral integration (see **Introduction**, page 6, and below) of non-defective retroviruses may cause activation of *Myc*. Thus avian retroviruses may induce B cell lymphomas, adenocarcinoma or T-lymphoma in chickens that are associated with activation of *Myc* (Hayward *et al.*, 1981; Payne *et al.*, 1982; Swift *et al.*, 1987). *Myc* may also be activated by murine leukaemia viruses (Corcoran *et al.*, 1984; Selten *et al.*, 1984; O'Donnell *et al.*, 1985; Mucenski *et al.*, 1987) and feline leukaemia virus (Forrest *et al.*, 1987) that cause T-lymphomas, intracisternal A-particle (Greenberg *et al.*, 1985) and retroposon insertion (Katzir *et al.*, 1985).

Nmyc is frequently activated by proviral insertion of murine leukaemia viruses (Dolcetti *et al.*, 1989; van Lohuizen *et al.*, 1989).

IN VITRO

MC29, CMII, OK10, MH2 or FH3 transform immature macrophages or fibroblasts, although FH3 does not completely transform the latter (Chen *et al.*, 1989). MH2, which also carries the v-*mil* (or v-*mht*: see **Mil**) oncogene, but not MC29, CMII, OK10 or FH3, causes growth factor (CSF)-independent proliferation of fibroblasts and macrophages (Heaney *et al.*, 1986).

Primary fibroblasts are immortalized by *Myc*, *Nmyc* or v-*myc* but are rendered tumorigenic only when activated *Ras* is also expressed (Schreiber-Agus *et al.*, 1993a). Fibroblast cell lines, however, show reduced growth factor requirements and are tumorigenic when transfected with *Myc* alone. *Lmyc* also co-transforms primary cells with an activated *Ras* gene but is <10% as effective as *Myc*, a difference that reflects the relative potencies of the activation domains of the MYC proteins (Barrett *et al.*, 1992).

Myc is amplified 4- to 16-fold in NIH 3T3 (but not Swiss 3T3) fibroblasts transformed by v-*abl*: *Fos* and *P53* are not amplified in these cells (Colledge *et al.*, 1989).

Normal B cells are fully transformed by infection with Epstein–Barr virus followed by transfection with *Myc* (see **DNA Tumour Viruses**).

Co-transformation by *Myc* and oncogenic *Ras* of rat embryo cells is inhibited by expression of *Bmyc* (Resar *et al.*, 1993). *Bmyc* encodes a protein of 168 amino acids that is highly homologous to the N-terminal region encoded by *Myc*. *Bmyc* thus lacks the basic/helix–loop–helix/leucine zipper DNA binding domain of other MYC proteins (see below) and may therefore be an indirect regulator of MYC function.

TRANSGENIC MICE

When linked to the MMTV LTR, *Myc* can cause mammary carcinomas in transgenic mice (Sinn *et al.*, 1987), and mice carrying a transgene of the *Myc* coding region and the 5′ regulatory sequences of Wap (whey acidic protein, hence the Wap–*myc* transgene is expressed in lactating mice) have an 80% incidence of mammary adenocarcinomas (Schoenenberger *et al.*, 1988). Nevertheless, excessive expression of *Myc* in transgenic mice does not prevent normal development and mammary tumours and lymphomas develop in a stochastic manner, indicating that overexpression of *Myc* is necessary but not sufficient for tumorigenesis. The additional expression of an MMTV–v-*Hras* transgene causes a synergistic increase in the incidence of tumours but their monoclonal and stochastic nature remains.

Transgenic mice bearing the *Myc* (or *Nmyc*) gene coupled to the Igμ enhancer (Eμ) overexpress MYC and rapidly develop B cell lymphomas (Adams *et al.*, 1985; Rosenbaum *et al.*, 1989). This may seem to imply that activating the *Myc* gene is sufficient to cause lymphoid neoplasia, a conclusion consistent with the *in vivo* potency of acutely transforming retroviruses (e.g. carrying v-*myc*). However, in the transgenic mice the latency period is variable and a pre-neoplastic state occurs in which no malignancy arises following the transplantation of lymphoid cells from young animals.

These observations are generally consistent with *in vitro* data indicating that alteration in the *Myc* content of cells, rather than mutation, activates its oncogenic potential and that transformation probably requires cooperation between MYC and other oncogene products including RAS.

In Eμ transgenics B cell tumour formation is accelerated by retroviral infection (Moloney murine leukaemia virus, Mo-MuLV). Identification of loci occupied by the integrated provirus (*Pim-1*, *Pim-2*, *Bmi-1*, *Pal-1*, *Bla-1* and *Emi-1*, see Table 2.2 and supplement) shows that *Bmi-1* may cooperate with *Myc* in as many as 50% of tumours formed (van Lohuizen *et al.*, 1991; Haupt *et al.*, 1991). *Pim-1*, which encodes a cytoplasmic protein serine/threonine kinase, synergizes strongly with *Myc* in the generation of tumours. Thus in double transgenic mice, *Myc*/ *Pim-1* animals develop pre-B cell leukaemia prenatally (Verbeek *et al.*, 1991): *Nmyc/Pim-1* and *Lmyc/Pim-1* double transgenics develop lymphoid malignancies with mean latency periods of 36 and 94 days respectively (Moroy *et al.*, 1991).

Mice that express fusion transgenes comprised of the HTLV-1LTR positioned to drive *Myc* and the Ig promoter/enhancer driving the HTLV-1 *tax* gene develop CD4+ T cell lymphomas and brain tumours (Benvenisty *et al.*, 1992a). The rate at which these tumours develop is similar to that observed in *Myc/Pim-1* bigenic animals and suggests that the *tax* gene product activates other transforming events in addition to *Myc* transcription.

Homozygous deletion of *Nmyc* results in embryonic lethality (Sawai *et al.*, 1991; Moens *et al.*, 1992). In these animals the lung airway epithelium is underdeveloped and death results from inability to oxygenate their blood.

	MYC/Myc	MYCN/Nmyc	MYCL/Lmyc	v-*myc*
Nucleotides (kb)				
Human	6–7	6–7	6–7	5.7 (MC29) 6.0 (CMII) 8.6 (OK10) 5.7 (MH2)
Chromosome				
Human	8q24	2p24.1	1p32 (*MYCL1*) 7p15 (*MYCLK1*)	
Mouse	15	12 (*Nmyc-1*)	4 (*Lmyc-1*)	
Exons	3	3 (Exon 1: non- coding)	3	
mRNA (kb)	2.3–2.5 (human, mouse, chicken)	3.0	2.2/3.6/3.8 (SCLC cells (U1690): the 2.2 kb mRNA lacks exon 3 and is more stable than the 3.8 kb mRNA)	5.4 (MC29) 7.5 (OK10) 5.2 (MH2) 7.5–8.0 (FH3)
mRNA half-life (min)	20–30	60	120	20–30
Amino acids	439/454 (chicken: 416)	464	364	875 (MC29) 699 (CMII) 427 (OK10) 423 (MH2) 1079 (FH3)
Mass (kDa)				
(predicted)	49	49.5	40	96 (MC29) 75 (CMII) 47 (OK10) 46 (gag–myc, MH2) 118 (FH3)
(expressed)	pp64/pp67	pp66	pp60/pp66/pp68	pP110$^{\Delta gag-myc}$ (MC29) pP90$^{\Delta gag-myc}$ (CMII) P200$^{gag-\Delta pol-myc}$ P58$^{\delta gag-myc}$ (OK10) P100$^{\Delta gag-mht}$ P57$^{\delta gag-myc}$ (MH2) P145$^{gag-myc}$ (FH3)
Protein half-life (min)	20–30 >3 h after heat shock (Luscher and Eisenman, 1988)	60–75	90–150	15–40*

*P200$^{gag-\Delta pol-myc}$ (OK10) >90 min; P145$^{gag-myc}$ (FH3) 60–70 min (Chen *et al.*, 1989).

Cellular location

Nuclear (van Straaten and Rabbitts, 1987; Koskinen *et al.*, 1991; Bond and Wold, 1993). P200$^{gag-\Delta pol-myc}$ (OK10): nuclear and cytoplasmic; P100$^{\Delta gag-mht}$ (MH2): cytoplasmic. MYC is detectable in the cytoplasm of serum-starved fibroblasts (Vriz *et al.*, 1992).

Tissue location

MYC protein is present in a wide variety of adult tissues and at all stages of during embryonal development. It is also expressed in non-dividing differentiated keratinocytes and in *Xenopus* oocytes. *Nmyc* and *Lmyc* expression is generally restricted to embryonic brain, kidney and lung, suggesting their possible involvement in differentiation (Zimmerman *et al.*, 1986). MYCN is also expressed during final stages of neuroblastomas.

The MYC protein content (Moore *et al.*, 1987; Waters *et al.*, 1991) of cell lines derived from the following sources is shown in brackets as molecules per cell: quiescent human MRC-5 fibroblasts and Swiss 3T3 fibroblasts (undetectable); serum-stimulated fibroblasts (3000–6000 transiently between 3 and 5 h: thereafter declining to 1000–3000 in sub-confluent cells and to undetectable levels in confluent cells); normal human fibroblasts (750); lymphoblastoid cells from patients with Bloom's syndrome (48 000); Burkitt's lymphoma (62 000–104 000); colon carcinoma (124 000).

Protein function

MYC, MYCN and MYCL are helix–loop–helix/leucine zipper proteins that form sequence-specific (CACGTG), DNA binding heterodimers with MAX (Blackwood and Eisenman, 1991; see page 330). NMYC also binds to asymmetric (CATGTG) sequences (Ma *et al.*, 1993). Both the leucine zipper domain and the helix–loop–helix motif of MYC contribute to specific heterodimer formation (Davis and Halazonetis, 1993). The binding of MYC–MAX dimers causes a change in the conformation of DNA (Wechsler and Dang, 1992). The members of the MYC family possess common functional elements: thus, *trans*-activation-incompetent mutants of one member can act in *trans* to suppress dominantly the co-transformation activities of all three MYC proteins (Mukherjee *et al.*, 1992). Truncated MYC that retains the basic, helix–loop–helix and leucine zipper domains binds to the sequence GGGCAC^G/$_A$TGCCC (Kato *et al.*, 1992). MYC proteins do not appear to dimerize with other helix–loop–helix/leucine zipper proteins (e.g. FOS, JUN, MyoD or E12), although a point mutation in the basic domain of MyoD confers the capacity to bind to a *Myc* DNA site with high affinity (van Antwerp *et al.*, 1992).

Myc is implicated in the control of normal proliferation, transformation and differentiation. Expression of *Myc* in untransformed cells is growth factor dependent and essential for progression through the cell cycle. High levels of expression accelerate growth. *Myc* (and *Fos*) expression is transiently activated in the rabbit aorta following injury to the arterial wall by balloon angioplasty (Bauters *et al.*, 1992) and cultured human atherosclerotic plaque smooth muscle cells overexpress *MYC* (Parkes *et al.*, 1991). Downregulation of *Myc* expression usually correlates with the onset of differentiation and constitutive expression interferes with normal differentiation. However, the following examples illustrate exceptions to this simple correlation in normal cells:

1 A variety of types of rapidly proliferating embryonic cells show little or no *Myc* expression (Jaffredo *et al.*, 1989; Downs *et al.*, 1989) and it is not expressed in dividing germ cells (Stewart *et al.*, 1984).

2 In *Xenopus* high levels of cytoplasmic MYC protein are present during oogenesis (i.e. in non-dividing cells) but on fertilization MYC is transported to the nucleus and has been degraded by the gastrula stage (Gusse *et al.*, 1989).

3 In keratinocytes the levels of *Fos* and *Myc* mRNA remain high during Ca^{2+}-induced differentiation (Dotto *et al.*, 1986).

4 In haematopoietic cells sustained expression of *Myc* accelerates apoptosis (Askew *et al.*, 1991; Williams, 1991). Thus, in the IL-3-dependent myeloid cell line 32D, withdrawal of IL-3 inhibits *Myc* transcription and causes the cells to arrest in G_1. Cells constitutively expressing *Myc*, however, do not arrest in G_1 but within 6 h show morphological changes characteristic of apoptosis. In immature T cells and in some T cell hybridomas activation of the T cell receptor causes apoptosis that is dependent on the sustained expression of *Myc* (Shi *et al.*, 1992). In rat-1 fibroblasts constitutive *Myc* expression also causes apoptosis when proliferation is inhibited by the absence of serum (Evan *et al.*, 1992). The regions of MYC protein that are essential for apoptosis are identical to those required for co-transformation, auto-suppression and inhibition of differentiation, namely part of the N-terminus (amino acids 7–91 and 106–143), the helix–loop–helix region (371–412) and the leucine zipper (414–433; see **Structure of human MYC**, page 325). These results suggest that genes that are known to cooperate with *MYC* in transformation, e.g. *Pim-1* (expressed in 32D cells), *BCL2*, *HRAS* and v-*raf*, may maintain cell viability without being directly mitogenic: in the absence of any of these gene products MYC may accelerate programmed cell death.

De-regulation of *MYC* expression correlates with the occurrence of many types of tumours. No amino acid mutations are required to render MYC oncogenic although these may enhance pathogenicity (Symonds *et al.*, 1989). The most clearly understood example of a mechanism by which the oncogenicity of *MYC* may be activated is the transcriptional activation that occurs following translocation of the gene to the vicinity of the immunoglobulin enhancer (see below).

v-MYC has been reported to associate with MYC-associated protein (MYAP, 500 kDa; Gillespie and Eisenman, 1989). MYC associates with the retinoblastoma protein p105^{RB}: microinjection of p105^{RB} reversibly arrests cell cycle progression in G_1 and this effect is antagonized by the co-injection of MYC (Goodrich and Lee, 1992).

Genes shown to be regulated directly or indirectly by highly expressed MYC or MYCN include the following:

Trans activation:

- Cyclins A and E (Jansen-Durr *et al.*, 1993)
- Human heat shock protein (hsp70) promoter (Kaddurah-Daouk *et al.*, 1987)
- Adenovirus E4 promoter (via the E1A activation region) (Onclercq *et al.*, 1988)
- α-Prothymosin and serum-inducible genes (Schweinfest *et al.*, 1988; Eilers *et al.*, 1991)
- *mr1* (plasminogen activator inhibitor-1) and *mr2* fibroblast genes (Prendergast *et al.*, 1990)
- *ECA39*: expressed during embryonic stem cell development (Benvenisty *et al.*, 1992b)

Trans repression:

- MHC class I antigens (also repressed by E1A; Bernards *et al.*, 1986; Lenardo *et al.*, 1989)
- Lymphocyte function-related antigen-1 (LFA-1; Versteeg *et al.*, 1989; Inghirami *et al.*, 1990)
- Neural cell adhesion molecule (N-CAM; Akeson and Bernards, 1990)
- Collagen genes (Yang *et al.*, 1991).
- Mouse metallothionein I promoter (Jin and Ringertz, 1990)

Transient or stable overexpression of either MYC or v-MYC but not NMYC protein induces translocation of hsp70 from cytoplasm to nucleus (Koskinen *et al.*, 1991).

Plasmids containing the 5' region of human *MYC* have been shown to replicate episomally in HeLa cells (McWhinney and Leffak, 1988). The 5′ flanking region of *MYC* may contain a putative *ori* sequence and there is controversial evidence that MYC can drive plasmid replication *in vitro* and substitute for SV40 T antigen to initiate replication from SV40 *ori* sequences. This sequence may function as a transcriptional enhancer within the *MYC* gene and thus MYC protein may stimulate transcription of its own gene (Iguchi-Ariga *et al.*, 1988). These results have not been completely reproduced in other laboratories, however, and it may be that, other than at very high concentrations when low-affinity homodimers are formed, normal MYC does not bind directly to DNA.

MYCN expression correlates with metastatic potential (Bernards *et al.*, 1986), consistent with the repressive effects of MYC on genes coding for MHC class I antigens and N-CAM. In polyomavirus-induced murine tumour cell lines the downregulation of MHC class I antigens does not correlate with tumorigenicity (Dahllof, 1990). *MYCN* expression in neuroblastoma cells suppresses the expression of MHC class I antigens and one isoform of protein kinase C (PK-Cδ) and induces PK-Cζ (Bernards, 1991). MHC class I expression is suppressed by reduction of the binding of an H2TF1-like factor to the gene enhancer A. The H2TF1-like factor itself contains the p50 subunit of NF-κB and transcription of p50 mRNA is suppressed by MYCN (Van't Veer *et al.*, 1993). After *Nmyc* transfection, phorbol ester no longer activates *Fos* or the transcription factor NF-κB.

Structure of the human *MYC* gene

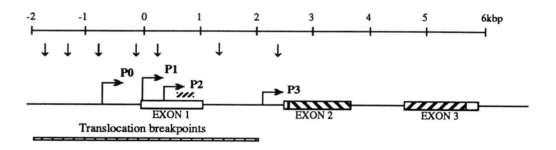

Exon 1 (non-coding) includes two major transcriptional initiation sites (TATAA boxes), P1 and P2. P1 is separated by 161 bp (164 bp in the mouse) from the downstream promoter P2 near the 5′ end of exon 1. Two minor promoters, P0 (550–650 bp upstream of P1) and P3 (near the 3′ end of intron 1) lack TATAA boxes. The cross-hatched regions of the boxes represent translational reading frames (within exons 2 and 3) that are between 70% and 90% identical between species. The shaded bar represents the major region encompassing translocation breakpoints. The vertical arrows indicate DNAase hypersensitive sites. The cross-hatched bar represents the sequence upstream of +47 relative to the P2 initiation site that is the site of the conditional block to transcriptional elongation (Krumm *et al.*, 1992).

When *MYC* is undergoing rapid transcription three regions of the gene in the vicinity of the promoters form Z-DNA. This may be caused by the generation of positive supercoils downstream of the RNA polymerase and negative supercoiling upstream (Wittig *et al.*, 1992).

Transcriptional regulation

```
      -2329   P1 and P2 ⊕   -1257  P1 and P2 ⊕   -353   -343        AP-1          -318
                                                                  (FOS, JUN) ⊖
        |              |        |           |      |      |       ‾‾‾‾‾‾‾‾‾‾‾        |
      AGCT ▮▮▮▮▮▮▮ GAATCGA ▮▮▮▮▮▮▮ GGGC ——— GCCTGCGATGATTTATACTCACAGGA ———
        |                      |                  |      |    ············          |
        1                    1072              1976   1986   ACTAAATATG          2011
                                                                 OCT


   -142      PuF/RNP ⊕/⊖          -115  -90   TCE ⊖        -68  -49    AP-2 ⊕      -28  -24
     |                              |    |                  |    |                  |    |
  — CCTTCCCCACCCTCCCCACCCTCCCCAT — GCAGAGGGCGTGGGGGAAAAGAA — AATCTCCGCCCACCGGCCCTTTATAA —
       GGGTGGG  GGGTGGG  |          |    |                        |    |                  |
       ········          2186    2213  2238                    2260 2279              2304


        ┌→ P1           -67   E2F ⊕  -57       T1A       MBP-1 ⊖        T1B      ┌→ P2
     -1│1                                    -38  -30  -26      -10 -7 -4  -1│1
     │ │             │             │           │    │    │        │   │  │  │ │
  —  GAGGACCC ——————— TGGCGGGAAAA ——————— CGCGCTGAGTATAAAAGCCGGTTTTCGGGGCTTTATCTAACTC ———
       |                 |           |        |         |             |       |
     2327             2423        2433      2452      2464          2480    2489
```

The numbers above the sequences denote the nucleotide separation from the human P1 promoter, except for the E2F and MBP-1 binding sites and the second TATAA box which are relative to P2. The black bars (−2329 to −1257 and −1257 to −353) represent positive transcriptional control elements essential for full activity of both promoters. Nuclear factor 1 (NF1) binds to sites within these regions (TGGAAGGCAGCCAA: −1338 to −1351 and TGGAGGTATCCAA: −696 to −709) and may exert negative control over transcription (Siebenlist *et al.*, 1984).

−343 to −318: Negative element that includes an AP-1 site to which FOS–JUN dimers bind; the negative strand contains an octamer binding protein region (consensus: ATTAAACGTA).

−142 to −115: PuF binds to this purine-rich region (specifically to GGGTGGG repeats in the negative strand) and a ribonucleoprotein also binds to this element so that transcription may be positively or negatively modulated (Spencer and Groudine, 1990). The negative strand in this region contains sequence homologous to the mouse ME1a1 binding site (GGAGGGGAGGGATC), which is required for maximal initiation of transcription at P2 but is also one of the *cis*-acting elements necessary for transcriptional block (Dufort *et al.*, 1993). The murine P2 promoter elements ME1a2, E2F and ME1a1 have been mapped at −85, −64 and −46, respectively (Moberg *et al.*, 1992). Different types of mouse cells growing in culture show differential occupancy of ME1a2, E2F and ME1a1 (Plet *et al.*, 1992). However, the occupancy of ME1a2 and E2F in Friend erythroleukaemic cells does not alter when they are induced to differentiate by DMSO, indicating that other factors are involved in the complete block of transcriptional elongation that accompanies the onset of differentiation. The transcription factor MAZ (MYC-associated zinc finger protein) binds to ME1a1 (Bossone *et al.*, 1992).

Murine *Myc* has two NF-κB sites (−1101 to −1081 (URE) and +440 to 459 (IRE)) relative to P1 (Kessler *et al.*, 1992). In Jurkat or HeLa cells constructs containing URE or IRE are transcriptionally activated by human T cell leukaemia virus type 1 TAX protein (Duyao *et al.*, 1992).

The element 400–1200 bp upstream of murine P1 has been shown to exert negative control in a CAT transfection assay (Remmers *et al.*, 1986). Murine MYC–PRF (−270 to −295) and MYC–CF1 (common factor 1: −252 to −261) interact to repress transcription in plasmacytoma cells and may therefore be involved in negative regulation of *Myc* in terminally differentiated B cells (Kakkis *et al.*, 1989).

−90 to −68: A TGFβ control element (TCE) mediating repression of *MYC* transcription in proliferating human keratinocytes by binding $TGF\beta_1$ or $p105^{RB}$ (Pietenpol *et al.*, 1991).

−49 to −28: AP-2 site through which protein kinase C- or cAMP-mediated transcriptional activation occurs (Imagawa *et al.*, 1987).

−67 to −57 (relative to P2): Binding site for the ubiquitous transcription factor E2F. E2F binding is necessary for *MYC trans* activation by E1A (Hiebert *et al.*, 1991) and p55, present in HeLa and MEL cells, also binds to this region (Parkin and Sonenberg, 1989). The homologous region is necessary and sufficient for transcription from P2 in *Xenopus* oocytes.

−10 to −38: *MYC*-binding protein 1 (MBP-1; 40 kDa) binds immediately upstream of the P2 promoter to repress transcription (Ray and Miller, 1991).

−4 to −39: This region contains T1A and T1B, two termination sites for a significant proportion of transcripts initiated at the P1 promoter (Roberts *et al.*, 1992). The binding of a terminator-binding factor (TBF I) to a 28 base sequence including T1A correlates with transcriptional termination at T1A.

Eight binding sites for v-MYB or MYB proteins occur in the regions +615 to +798, −1061 to −1256 and −1698 to −1846 (see **MYB**). MYB can induce transcription from both the murine P1 and P2 promoters (Cogswell *et al.*, 1993).

The transcription factors Sp-1, NF1 and CCAAT-binding protein (CBP) bind to regulatory regions within 131 bp 5′ of the first major P0 RNA start (Lang *et al.*, 1991).

A transcriptional inhibitor binds to a 20 bp region (AGAGTAGTTATGGTAACTGG) 119 bp into intron 1 (Zajac-Kaye *et al.*, 1988); point mutations that abolish binding occur in some Burkitt lymphomas. Intragenic regulatory regions also occur in the *Fos* and *Myb* genes but the sequence in *Myc* is unrelated to the FIRE sequence of *Fos* (Tourkine *et al.*, 1989).

The rapid increase in fibroblast mRNA from very low levels in G_0 cells that occurs on stimulation with EGF is due to relief of a block to transcriptional elongation, as evidenced by the high concentration of RNA polymerase II in the exon 1 region in G_0 cells. *In vitro* studies have defined a 95 bp 5′ region of exon 1 of the human *MYC* gene that specifies premature termination (Kerppola and Kane, 1988; Strobl and Eick, 1992). The efficiency of premature termination sites declines markedly when they are placed >~400 bp from the start site (Roberts and Bentley, 1992).

In contrast to the effect of EGF, serum stimulation (which causes up to 40-fold elevation of RNA level) increases initiation by stabilizing mRNA (Nepveu *et al.*, 1987). *Myc* mRNA instability is due to untranslated regions of exons 1 and 3, principally three copies of AUUUA at the 3′ end of exon 3 (see also **FOS**).

A human T cell leukaemia-derived cell line carries a translocation 24 nucleotides 5′ of the first poly(A) addition signal of *MYC*. This replaces a 61 bp AU-rich region with sequences derived from chromosome 2 and causes a fivefold increase in *MYC* expression due to enhanced mRNA stability. The hybrid gene transforms rat fibroblasts to a tumorigenic phenotype (Aghib and Bishop, 1991). This *MYC* rearrangement contrasts with those discussed below in that it does not involve T cell receptor or immunoglobulin loci.

Two regions within *Myc* mRNA regulate the half-life of the molecule: one is within the 3′ untranslated region and the other is the C-terminal portion of the coding region (Wisdom and Lee, 1991; Bernstein *et al.*, 1992). Two proteins (37 kDa and 40 kDa) bind to AU-rich regions in the 3′-UTR of *Myc* and other unstable mRNAs and increase the *in vitro* rate of RNA degradation. A 75 kDa binds to the C-terminal coding region of *Myc* mRNA and appears to confer stability on the transcript.

In both normal and transformed mouse cells RNA polymerase II-directed transcription of *Myc* occurs in both the sense and antisense direction (Nepveu and Marcu, 1986). Regions upstream of the first exon, within the first intron and in introns 2 and 3 have high levels of antisense transcription that is not co-regulated with transcription of the sense strand. Transcription on the antisense strand also occurs in human cells where it is restricted to upstream of P1. Approximately equal sense and antisense transcription also occurs in *Nmyc* exon 1 (Krystal *et al.*, 1990) and in the human colon cancer cell line COLO 320, under conditions of polyamine depletion, antisense transcription of intron 2 is inversely proportional to expression of sense *MYC* RNA (Celano *et al.*, 1992). The role of antisense transcription is unknown.

The general genomic organization of *Nmyc* and *Lmyc* is similar to *Myc* but *Nmyc* transcription is initiated from sites around two promoters (Stanton and Bishop, 1987), that of *Lmyc* from a single 5′ site (Kaye *et al.*, 1988). *Nmyc* transcription is regulated by three promoter regions: −680 to −1000 regulates tissue-specific expression, +90 to −220 controls the basal level of transcription and the 3′ end of exon 1 and/or part of the first intron appears to mediate tissue-specific downregulation of *Nmyc* (Hiller *et al.*, 1991; Wada *et al.*, 1992).

Myc transcripts from the P0 promoter undergo differential splicing: two forms of *Nmyc* mRNA occur, differing in their 5′ ends: a range of *Lmyc* transcripts occurs due to differential splicing and multiple polyadenylation signals (De Greve *et al.*, 1988).

Transcription and translation products arising from the use of different *Myc* promoters

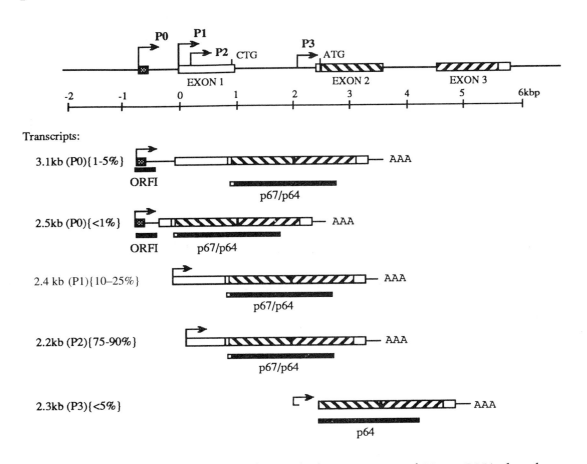

Transcript sizes are shown (left) together with the percentage of *Myc* mRNA that they contribute (Spencer and Groudine, 1990). The product of ORF I (114 amino acids) obtained *in vitro* is not detected in intact cells. The significance of the minor promoters, P0 and P3, is unknown.

In addition to initiation at the first AUG codon in exon 2 (p67, MYC1), translation may also occur from an unconventional CUG codon (p64, MYC2) at the 3' end of exon 1 (Hann *et al.*, 1988). Lymphoblastic cell lines (LCLs) immortalized by Epstein–Barr virus (see **DNA Tumour Viruses**) that do not have a rearranged *MYC* locus synthesize p64 MYC2 and low amounts of p67 MYC1. Burkitt lymphoma cell lines produce no detectable p67 MYC1 and normal or increased amounts of p64 MYC2. In lymphoid, erythroid and embryo fibroblast cells *in vitro* there is a large induction of MYC1 synthesis on deprivation of methionine (Hann *et al.*, 1992). Translation of MYC may be inhibited by the formation of secondary structure in the mRNA, sequestering AUG in a loop flanked by double-stranded RNA (Saito *et al.*, 1983).

Nmyc translation (p66) is initiated from two AUG codons 24 bp apart: the variants of *Lmyc* (pp60, pp66, pp68) arise by differential phosphorylation of p59 and p65 derived from translational initiation at a CUG in exon 1 or AUG in exon 2 (Dosaka-Akita *et al.*, 1991).

Structures of proviral genomes and the major translation products

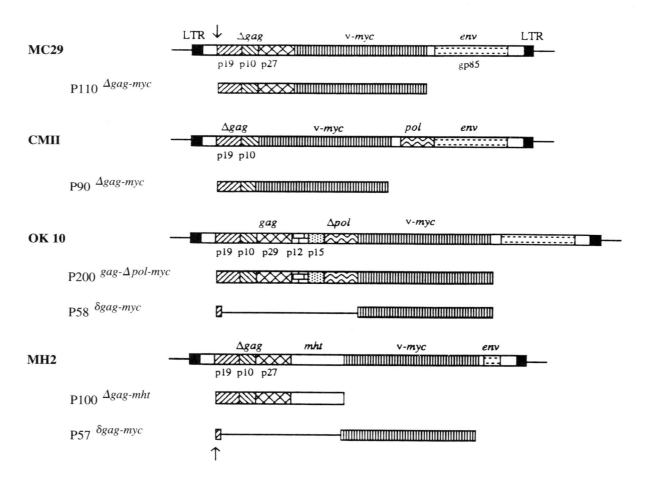

Boxes represent domains of the proviral genomes and corresponding protein products. Vertical arrows mark translation initiation sites. The chicken *Myc* sequences in MC29 that encode a 47 kDa protein start in intron 1 and contain all the coding sequences plus 296 bp of 3' exon 3

that is non-coding in *Myc*. Only eight bases of the transduced sequences differ from the normal gene. The other MC29 group v-*myc* sequences are all highly homologous but have acquired variable amounts of intron 1 and non-coding exon 3 sequences (see below).

MC29: The 5' junction between v-*myc* (1600 bp) and the viral structural genome lies within the *gag* region: the *gag* termination codon is deleted and the p27 *gag* 3' sequence is truncated. Recombination using the splice acceptor site at the 5' end of *Myc* inserts five alanines between *gag* and the initiating MYC methionine (this also occurs in CMII and FH3) and four additional amino acids are inserted 5' of the alanines. *pol* and the N-terminus of gp85^{env} are also deleted. P110$^{gag-myc}$: 875 amino acids (453 *gag*; 422 v-*myc*). Mutants of MC29 (P110$^{\Delta gag-myc}$) with deleted phosphorylation sites in MYC transform fibroblasts but not macrophages and are no longer tumorigenic (Ramsay *et al.*, 1980). MC29-HB1 is a back mutant that has regained the MYC sequence and transforming capacity of the original mutant (Hayman, 1983).

CMII: The 5' junction lies 516 bp 5' of that in MC29. Not all of *pol* is deleted and there is some truncation of *env*. v-*myc* lacks 12 bases on the 3' end of MC29. P90$^{\Delta gag-myc}$: 699 amino acids (278 *gag*; 421 v-*myc*).

OK10: *gag* is complete: 348 bp of 3' *pol* and 1076 bp of 5' *env* are deleted. v-*myc* contains 50 additional bases from intron 1 and 37 fewer from the 3' non-coding region than MC29 v-*myc*. p58$^{\delta gag-myc}$ translated from spliced (3.5 kb) mRNA; P200$^{gag-\Delta pol-myc}$ from genomic RNA. OK10 is a unique retrovirus in that both P58 and P200 possess autonomous transforming activity (Pfaff and Duesberg, 1988).

MH2: 3' *gag*, all of *pol* and most of *env* deleted. Carries the unique *Mht* (or *Mil*) sequence (1154 nucleotides), derived from *Mil*, homologous to v-*raf*. v-*myc* has ~177 bases from exon 1 that are not present in MC29 but has lost ~250 bases of 3' non-coding sequence (Coll *et al.*, 1983; Kan *et al.*, 1983; Sutrave *et al.*, 1984a,b). P57$^{\delta gag-myc}$: 423 amino acids (6 *gag*, 417 v-*myc*). P100$^{\Delta gag-v-mil}$ contains 514 *gag* amino acids and 380 of v-*mil*.

FH3: The C-terminal 43 amino acids of p15^{gag} are deleted. Recombination occurs at the splice acceptor site at the 5' end of *Myc* exon 2, which inserts five alanines between the end of the *gag* sequences and the initiating MYC methionine. The 3' end of MYC is intact and FH3 also contains *pol*, *env* and U3 helper virus sequences (Chen *et al.*, 1989). P145$^{gag-myc}$: 1079 amino acids (658 *gag*; 421 *Myc*).

Evidence from artificial viral constructs indicates that the *gag* modification of v-*myc* is not essential for transformation (Rapp *et al.*, 1985; Tikhonenko *et al.*, 1993) and in FH3 the C-terminal region of the *gag* sequence suppresses the fibroblast-transforming activity of v-*myc* (Tikhonenko and Linial, 1992).

Structure of human MYC

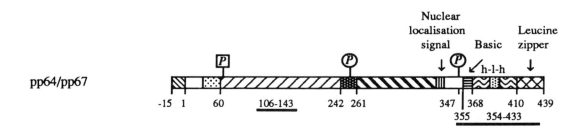

−15−1: Additional 15 amino terminal residues in pp64 due to CUG initiation codon in exon 1 (Hann *et al.*, 1988).

40−60: Proline/glutamine-rich region (exon 2) that may cause the anomalous electrophoretic mobility of MYC proteins.

1−143: The three segments that make up this N-terminal region, when fused to the DNA binding domain and nuclear localization signal of the yeast transcription factor GAL4, each activate transcription of a reporter gene linked to GAL4 binding sites (Kato *et al.*, 1990; Seth *et al.*, 1991). The phosphorylation of Thr58 and Ser62 is necessary for high levels of *trans* activation by MYC (Gupta *et al.*, 1993).

P : MAP kinase phosphorylation site (Ser62). Ser62 is phosphorylated by MAP kinases (ERK, ERT (*EGF Receptor Thr669*) and MAP2 protein kinase, activated by Thr/Tyr phosphorylation). The consensus sequence is Pro–Leu–Ser/Thr–Pro, found also in the EGFR (Thr669) and rat JUN (Ser246) that are also substrates for ERT (Alvarez *et al.*, 1991). Ser62 is within a p34^{cdc2} kinase recognition motif but MYC is not phosphorylated by p34^{cdc2} *in vitro* (Luscher and Eisenman, 1992). Ser62 lies in a proline-rich region that is highly conserved in the MYC family and carries transcriptional activation capacity.

106−143 and 354−433 (bars): Regions essential for autoregulation of *Myc* expression and co-transformation with *Ras*. Deletion of 106−143 domain dominantly inhibits the cooperation of normal MYC with oncogenic *Ras* to transform rat embryo fibroblasts (Ueno *et al.*, 1988; Dang *et al.*, 1989).

242−261: Central acidic region resembling those of transcriptional activators. Deletions in this region have little effect on MYC–RAS co-transformation but do influence the transforming host range of v-*myc* retroviruses.

P : Casein kinase II phosphorylation: major site in the central acidic domain (MYC is hyperphosphorylated during mitosis due to casein kinase II). NMYC is also phosphorylated by casein kinase II in the central acidic region and in the C-terminal region (Hamann *et al.*, 1991).

290−318: Non-specific DNA binding region.

320−328: Major nuclear localization signal.

364−374: Incomplete nuclear localization signal: highly conserved between MYC, NMYC and LMYC and essential for oncogenicity.

355−439: The C-terminus of MYC contains a basic region (355−368) followed by a helix–loop–helix motif (368−410) and a leucine zipper (410−439): this domain is essential for DNA binding. Other transcription factors also contain this combination of motifs (TFE3, TFEB, USF and AP-4; Beckman *et al.*, 1990; Carr and Sharp, 1990; Gregor *et al.*, 1990; Hu *et al.*, 1990).

Sequences of human MYCN, MYC and MYCL1

```
MYCN   (1)    .MPSCSTST**GMICKNP...**EF**L**C**P**DD..**FGGPD*T..**G..************
MYC    (1)    .........MPLNVSFTNRNYDLDYDSVQPYFYCDEEEN.FYQQQQQSELQPPAPSEDIWKKFELLPTP
MYCL1  (1)    ....................M*****Y*H***DYDCGED**R....*T....************V*S*


MYCN   (60)   ******GFAEH*SEP**W..**EML.................**N..**WGSPAEEDAFGLGG***LTP
MYC    (60)   PLSPSRRSGLCS...PSYVAVTPFSLRGDNDGGGGSFSTADQLEMVTEL.............LGGDMV
MYCL1  (40)   *T**PWGL*PGAGD.................................PAPGIGPPEPWP**CTG


MYCN   (108)  NPV.....................*L**********RE**ERA*****QHGRGPPTAGSTAQ**G
MYC    (112)  *QSFICDPDDETFIKN..........IIIQDCMWSGFSAAAKL...VSEKLASYQAARKDSG...SPN
MYCL1  (71)   ........**AESRGHSKGWGRNYAS**RR********RER*ERAV*DR**.............*G
```

```
MYCN    (152)  AGAAS**G***GGAAGAGRAGAALP*ELAHP**.**V**A****F*V*KREPAPVP*APA*APAAGPAV
MYC     (164)  .....PA.RGHSVCSTSSLYLQDLSA.....AASECIDPSVVFPYPLNDSSSPKSCASQDSSAFSPSSD
MYCL1   (117)  APRGN*PKAS...................**PD*T.**LEAGN*...............APAA*CPL


MYCN    (220)  ASGAGIAAPAGAPGVAPPRPGGRQTSGGDHKALS**GEDTL***DD*DD*E**E********T****RSS
MYC     (222)  SLLSSTESSPQGSPEPLVLHEETPP........TTS.....SDSE.E..EQED.EEEIDVVSVEKRQA.
MYCL1   (149)  GEPKTQAC*GSE**............................****N.........******T****SL


MYCN    (289)  SNTKAVTTFTITVRPKNAALG**RAQS**LI................****LPIH.....Q*******S
MYC     (273)  ...................PGKR..SESGSPSAGGHSKPPHSPLVLKRCHVST.....HQHNYAAPP
MYCL1   (182)  GIRKPVT...ITVRAD.............................**DPCMK*FHISIHQ.Q******RF


MYCN    (337)  PYVESED*P...........................PQ*KI*SEASPRPLK**IPPKAK*L.....*
MYC     (314)  STRKDYPAA................................KRVKLD......SVRVLRQISNNRKCTS
MYCL1   (219)  PP.ESCSQEEASERGPQEEVLERDAAGEKEDEEDEEIVSPPP*ESEAAQSCH.....PKPV*.......


MYCN    (372)  **N**S*DSER**N**I*******D*RS**LT***HV***VK****A*********E*VH*L*.***H.
MYC     (345)  PRSSDTEENVKRRTHNVLERQRRNELKRSFFALRDQIPELENNEKAPKVVILKKATAYILSVQ.AEEQK
MYCL1   (275)  ...****DVT**KN**F***K***D*RSR*L****V*TLASCS********S**LE*LQALVG**KRM


MYCN    (439)  ..............**LLEKE**QARQQ**LKKIEHARTC (464)
MYC     (413)  LISEEDLLRKRREQLKH...KLE....QLRNSCA (439)
MYCL1   (341)  ATE......KR..QLRC.......RQQQLQKRIAYLSGY (364)
```

* Indicates identity with MYC. Basic and leucine zipper regions in MYC are underlined. MYC amino acids 105–143 and 320–439 are essential for *ras* complementation in transforming normal rat embryo cells: these domains are conserved in MYCN and MYCL1 (MYC box proteins). Underlined in MYCN: casein kinase II phosphorylation sites (Hamann *et al.*, 1991).

MYC contains PEST sequences (as do FOS, JUN, v-MYB, p53 and E1A) the presence of which has been correlated with increased susceptibility of the protein to degradation (Rogers *et al.*, 1986). The major MYC PEST sequence is HEETPPTTSSDSEEEQEDEEEIDVVSVEK (241–269) but deletions in this region do not affect MYC stability.

Sequences of chicken MYC and v-MYC (MC29, CMII, OK10 and MH2E21)

```
MYC      (1)           MPLSASLPSKNYDYDYDSVQPYFYFEEEEENFYLAAQQRGSELQPPAPS
MC29     (1)      QAAAAA------------------------------------------
CMII     (1)       AAAAA------------------------------------------
OK10     (1)            ------------------------------------------
MH2E21   (1)    MEAVIKAAAAA----V------------------------------------------


MYC      (50)  EDIWKKFELLPTPPLSPSRRSSLAAASCFPSTADQLEMVTELLGGDMVNQSFICDPDDES
MC29     (56)  ----------M-------------------------------------------------
CMII     (55)  ------------------------------------------------------------
OK10     (50)  -----------A------------------------------------------------
MH2E21   (61)  -----------A------C--N-----------------------------S--------


MYC      (110)  FVKSIIIQDCMWSGFSAAAKLEKVVSEKLATYQASRREGGPAAASRPGPPPSGPPPPPAG
MC29     (116)  ----------------------------------Q-------------------------
CMII     (115)  ------------------------------------------------------------
OK10     (110)  ------------------------------------------------------------
MH2E21   (121)  -------R-----------------------K----------------------------
```

```
MYC     (170)  PAASAGLYLHDLGAAAADCIDPSVVFPYPLSERAPRAAPPGANPAALLGVDTPPTTSSDS
MC29    (176)  -----------------------------------------------------------
CMII    (175)  -----------------------------------------------------------
OK10    (170)  -----------------------------------------------------------
MH2E21  (181)  ----------------G--GS-----C--GR-G-PG-  -  --------A---AGGG-


MYC     (230)  EEEQEEDEEIDVVTLAEANESESSTESSTEASEEHCKPHHSPLVLKRCHVNIHQHNYAAP
MC29    (236)  -----------------------------------------------------------
CMII    (235)  -----------------------------------------------------------
OK10    (230)  -----------------------------------------------------------
MH2E21  (237)  --------------------------------------------E--------------


MYC     (290)  PSTKVEYPAAKRLKLDSGRVLKQISNNRKCSSPRTSDSEENDKRRTHNVLERQRRNELKL
MC29    (296)  -------------------------------------L---------------------
CMII    (295)  -----------------------------------------------------------
OK10    (290)  --------------------------------------------M--------------
MH2E21  (297)  ---------------------V--------------V----------------------


MYC     (350)  SFFALRDQIPEVANNEKAPKVVILKKATEYVLSIQSDEHRLIAEKEQLRRRREQLKHKLEQLRNSRA  (416)
MC29    (356)  R-----------------------------L-----K---------------N-------         (422)
CMII    (355)  -----------------------------------------------------------------   (421)
OK10    (350)  -----------------------------------------------------------------   (416)
MH2E21  (357)  -----------------------------------------------------------------   (423)
```

Dashes indicate identity with chicken MYC. MC29, MH2 and OK10 are all mutated at amino acid 61 relative to MYC. Artificial mutation of Thr61 enhances MYC oncogenicity (Frykberg et al., 1987).

The basic, helix–loop–helix and leucine zipper domains of human MYC and MAX proteins

The helix I and leucine zipper domains may be regions within one continuous helix. Solid bars indicate basic regions: L1–L5 leucine zipper motifs. Numbers indicate amino acid position in the complete sequence.

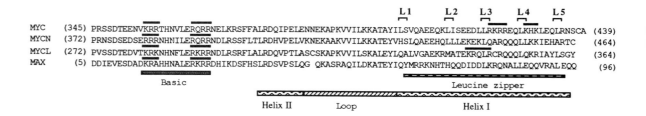

	MAX/Myn
Nucleotides	
Chromosome	
Human	14q22–q24
Mouse *Myn*	12.D1–D3
	(Gilladoga *et al.*, 1992)
Exons	2
mRNA (kb)	
Human	2.3 (major)
	1.9, 3.0, 3.5 (minor)
Mouse *Myn*	2.0
	In human, mouse and rat genomic DNA a 101 bp insert in *MAX* derived from an alternatively spliced exon introduces an in-frame termination codon giving rise to a truncated MAX protein, ΔMAX (Makela *et al.*, 1992)
Amino acids	151/160 (MAX)
	94/103 (ΔMAX)
Mass (kDa)	
(predicted)	17
(expressed)	21/22
	16.5 (ΔMAX)
	A variant of MAX (p22) contains a 9 amino acid N-terminal insertion. ΔMAX has also two alternative forms, with or without the 9 amino acid N-terminal insert
Protein half-life (h)	>24 (cf. MYC, 20–30 min)
	~20 min (3.5 kb encoded ΔMAX)

Cellular location

Nuclear; translocation from the cytosol is dependent on association with MYC. The steady state concentration of MAX is constant throughout the cell cycle (Blackwood *et al.*, 1992) and intracellular MYC is always complexed with MAX.

Tissue location

MAX and MYN, its murine homologue to which human MYCN also binds, occur in many cell types of diverse origin: MAX has been detected in NIH 3T3 fibroblasts, HeLa cells and neuroblastoma-derived cell lines. The ratio of MAX to ΔMAX is cell-line specific (Makela *et al.*, 1992).

Protein function

MAX is a helix–loop–helix protein that forms sequence-specific (CACGTG), DNA binding heterodimers with MYC (Blackwood and Eisenman, 1991). The leucine zipper domain is critical to the formation of heterodimers with MAX (Reddy *et al.*, 1992). Unlike MYC, MAX can homo-dimerize efficiently to bind to the same DNA sequence as the MYC–MAX heterodimer. X-ray structural analysis of the MAX homodimer has revealed a symmetrical, parallel, left-handed, four-helix bundle in which each monomer contributes two α-helical segments separated by a loop (Ferre-D'Amare *et al.*, 1993). Phosphorylation of the N-terminus of MAX by casein kinase II inhibits DNA binding of the homodimer *in vitro* but does not affect that of MYC–MAX heterodimers (Berberich and Cole, 1992).

The basic/helix–loop–helix/leucine zipper proteins MAD (Ayer *et al.*, 1993) and MXI1 (Zervos *et al.*, 1993) are distinct from MAX but form heterodimers with MAX that bind efficiently to the MYC–MAX consensus sequence to repress transcription. Thus the relative abundance of these binding partners may determine the extent of formation of the transcriptionally active MYC–MAX complex.

The promoters listed above are potential targets for MYC–MAX complexes, but no direct evidence for targets has yet been reported. In Chinese hamster ovary cells, GAL4–MAX fusion proteins do not activate transcription, indicating that MAX lacks a transcriptional activation domain (Kato *et al.*, 1992). In *S. cerevisiae* MAX homodimers do not *trans*-activate and they antagonize MYC–MAX function (Amati *et al.*, 1992). Thus MAX may act as a transcriptional activator when complexed with MYC or function by itself as a repressor. Repression requires the DNA binding domain of MAX and is relieved by overexpression of MYC through its dimeriz-ation and transcription activating domains (Kretzner *et al.*, 1992).

In neuroblastoma cells MAX (p20) and a structurally related 22 kDa protein form hetero-oligomeric complexes with MYCN (Wenzel *et al.*, 1991).

Co-transfection assays indicate that MAX decreases the number of transformed foci in rat embryo fibroblasts caused by *Myc* and *Hras*, whereas ΔMAX enhances transformation (Makela *et al.*, 1992; Prendergast *et al.*, 1992). This is consistent with the fact that ΔMAX retains the capacity to form heterodimers with MYC that bind to the CACGTG motif but lacks the putative regulatory domain of MAX.

Transcriptional regulation by MYC and MAX

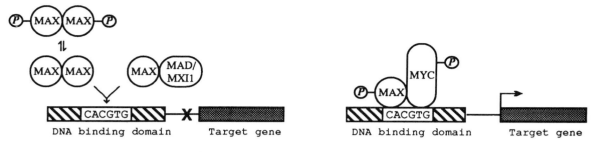

Trans-repression   **Trans-activation**

MAX homodimers phosphorylated by casein kinase II do not interact with binding domains. Unphosphorylated MAX homodimers repress transcription of genes that are targets for MYC, for example, in quiescent cells in which the concentration of MYC is low. Phosphorylated MAX–MYC heterodimers *trans*-activate target genes, for example, in proliferating cells (Berberich and Cole, 1992).

Structures of MYC, MAX and ΔMAX proteins

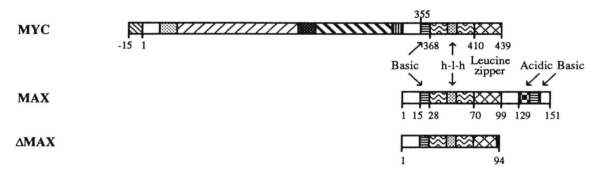

Human MAX contains basic (15–28) and helix–loop–helix (28–70) motifs, a hydrophobic sequence including three leucines spaced seven residues apart (70–99), a nuclear localization sequence (PQSRKKLR, amino acids 140–147), an acidic region (129–139) and a basic region (141–147). The helix–loop–helix/leucine zipper domain mediates the interaction between MYC and MAX and these regions are critical for transforming potential, autoregulation of *Myc* expression and inhibition of differentiation (Penn *et al.*, 1990b; Crouch *et al.*, 1990). An artificially generated form of MAX that lacks 37 N-terminal amino acids forms a non-DNA binding complex with MYC that inhibits the reduction in MHC class I antigens and protein kinase Cδ caused by expression of MYCN in neuroblastoma cells, thus acting as a dominant-negative mutant of MAX (Billaud *et al.*, 1993).

Both MYC and MAX are phosphorylated *in vivo* by casein kinase II.

Sequence of human MAX and ΔMAX

```
maX     (1)   MSDNDDIEVESD (EEQPRFQSA) ADKRAHHNALERKRRDHIKDSFHSLRDSVPSLQGEKAS
ΔMAX    (1)   ----------- (-------) ----------------------------------------
```

```
                                           GEHPSSWGSWPCCAPARSGFGTW
MAX    (60)  RAQILDKATEYIQYMRRKNHTHQQDIDDLKRQNALLEQQVRALGKARSS
ΔMAX   (60)  ---------------------------------------GESES (94/103)

             ACRVRASHGVCAQ (125/134)
MAX   (100)  AQLQTNYPSSDNSLYTNAKGSTISAFDGGSDSSSESEPEEPQSRKKLRMEAS (151/160)
```

The sequence in brackets is the 9 amino acid insertion in p22. Helix I and helix II of the basic helix–loop–helix region are underlined. The hydrophobic heptad repeat is in bold, underlined type. ΔMAX differs from MAX only in the replacement of the C-terminal 62 amino acids by GESES. The sequence in italics is the 36 residue C-terminus predicted to be encoded in the 3.5 kb mRNA form by the 5′ region of the first intron of *MAX* (Vastrik *et al.*, 1993). Bold type: potential casein kinase II phosphorylation sites. Underlined italics: nuclear localization signal (Prendergast *et al.*, 1992).

Activation of *MYC*

MYC may be activated to become a transforming gene by (1) proviral insertion, (2) chromosomal translocation, (3) gene amplification. In general, the result is to elevate expression of *MYC*, rather than to change the structure of the protein itself.

(1) PROVIRAL INSERTION

The natural helper virus for the MC29 group of defective viruses is the avian leukosis virus (ALV). ALV itself is a major cause of leukaemias in chickens and the first direct evidence that proto-oncogenes are activated in tumour cells came from the demonstration that ALV was integrated into the *Myc* locus in virally induced B cell lymphomas (Hayward *et al.*, 1981). There is no known sequence specificity that governs proviral DNA insertion, hence insertion next to a specific gene is a rare event. The proviral sequences integrated in this random manner become defective during insertion (Varmus, 1984).

When ALV-induced chicken bursal lymphomas arise, over 90% of the ALV insertions occur in intron 1 or exon 1 of *Myc*. The effect is to separate *Myc* coding regions from their normal promoters by inserted viral sequences. Insertion can also occur 5′ to the *Myc* coding domains but in the opposite transcriptional orientation or 3′ of exon 3.

Sites of ALV proviral insertion in chicken bursal lymphomas

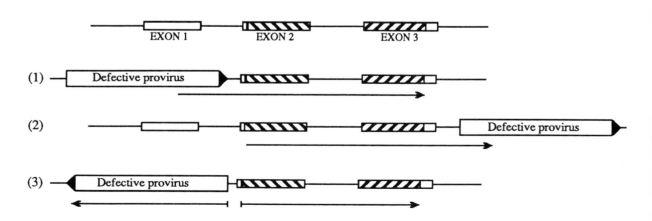

Top: Basic structure of *Myc* gene. ALV insertion: (1) 5′ to *Myc* in same orientation. (2) 3′ to *Myc* in same orientation. (3) 5′ to *Myc* in opposite transcriptional orientation. Arrowheads indicate sites and transcriptional orientation of ALV provirus. Arrows indicate transcriptional patterns (Payne *et al.*, 1982). In (1) promoter insertion causes initiation of *Myc* transcription, usually from the 3′ LTR promoter. Frequently deletions occur next to the 5′ LTR: this may impair its function and enhance the promoter activity of the remaining LTR for adjacent sequences (Cullen *et al.*, 1984). In (2) and (3) the ALV LTR appears to exert *cis*-acting enhancer effects on the normal *Myc* promoters.

Other retroviruses can activate *Myc* by similar mechanisms, e.g. the unrelated chicken syncytial virus (CSV: member of the reticuloendotheliosis virus (REV) family), and in mammals the T cell lymphomas caused by MuLV (Mo-MuLV and AKR-MuLV) and FeLV may involve activation of *Myc*.

Ranges and orientations of proviral insertion sites

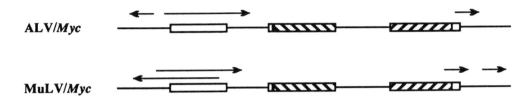

Insertion of ALV in chicken *Myc* and MuLV in rodent *Myc*. For the latter most insertions are within a 2 kb region upstream of exon 1 and in the opposite transcriptional orientation to *Myc*. As with ALV, however, some insertions have been detected within exon 1 and 3′ to the coding regions.

The overall effect of "promoter insertion" adjacent to *Myc* is that there is a 20- to 100-fold elevation in the concentration of *Myc* mRNA: occasional mutations occur in the coding domains, particularly in the vicinity of codon 60.

(2) CHROMOSOME TRANSLOCATION

Reciprocal translocation between the *Myc* locus and Ig gene sequences frequently occurs in Burkitt's lymphoma and murine plasmacytomas (Cory, 1986). This gives rise to increased expression of *Myc* in pre-B cells, it is presumed by the action of Ig elements (enhancers or the "Ig locus activation region" (LAR)) to which *Myc* becomes juxtaposed and/or by the mutation of promoters or the unmasking of cryptic promoter sites in the *Myc* gene (Croce, 1987). In many such rearrangements the first (non-coding) exon is lost from the gene: mutations may occur in exons 2 and 3 but are not typical. The other *Myc* allele is unchanged and not expressed. In general, overexpression of a *Myc* gene introduced into normal (but not transformed cells) suppresses expression of the endogenous *Myc* genes (Luscher and Eisenman, 1990). Thus endogenous MYC translation occurs in proliferating rat-1 cells (MYC protein concentration 600–700 molecules/cell) but is >90% suppressed when the MYC concentration is raised to ~5000 molecules/cell, the range reached ~2 h after quiescent cells are stimulated by serum. Repression requires *trans*-activating factors in addition to MYC, as indicated by the finding that *Myc* transcription in NIH 3T3 fibroblasts, which is not downregulated by MYC, is suppressed in somatic cell hybrids between NIH 3T3s and rat-1 (Penn *et al.*, 1990a). It appears that in the transformed cell phenotype *Myc* expression is suppressed and the translocated gene escapes the regulatory mechanism by its proximity to the Ig gene.

Translocations are generally believed to be caused by the aberrant activity of the VDJ recombinase, most breakpoint sites occurring in the IgH switch or VDJ join regions. Additional bases may be acquired during translocation (N regions – heterogeneous in length and sequence) due to the action of deoxynucleotidyl transferase (Desiderio *et al.*, 1984).

Chromosome translocations in human Burkitt's lymphoma

Burkitt's lymphoma (BL) is a tumour of B cell lineage in which translocations between chromosome 8 (*MYC*) and immunoglobulin (Ig) loci (chromosome 2, 14 or 22) cause an Ig gene to come to reside on the same chromosome as *MYC*. Almost all endemic (African form) BL tumours (eBL) contain Epstein–Barr virus (EBV) DNA whilst only ~25% of the sporadic (sBL) form do so, although >75% of individuals with sBL are EBV seropositive. The majority of sBL tumours but only a minority of eBL tumours secrete IgM. This appears to correlate with the locations of the chromosome 8 breakpoints which cause rearrangements of one *MYC* allele in most sBL, commonly occurring in the first intron, but lie upstream of the *MYC* locus in eBL (Pelicci *et al.*, 1986; Magrath, 1990). Thus translocations often cause mutation or truncation of exon 1, intron 1 or the 5′ flanking regions and loss of transcription elongation block. The evidence suggests that these effects are insufficient to cause the increase in *MYC* mRNA stability that occurs in BL. When exon 1 is retained, increased use of P1 occurs, which may be caused by the greatly decreased number of paused polymerases at the P2 promoter (Strobl *et al.*, 1993). Mutations may affect the p67 translation initiation site and thus change the proportion of p64 to p67 (Hann *et al.*, 1988). The DNAase I hypersensitive sites are retained in the translocated *MYC* allele but lost from the non-translocated allele.

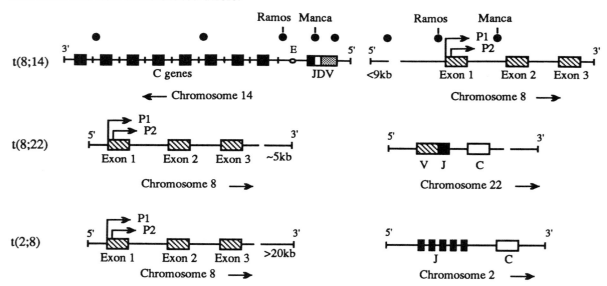

The black dots indicate breakpoints which may vary widely in position. Two specific examples are shown: Ramos, derived from an American Burkitt's lymphoma and Manca, a non-Hodgkin's lymphoma cell line. The breakpoints on chromosome 8 never disrupt the *MYC* protein coding regions and those on chromosomes 14, 22 and 2 never disrupt the constant regions of the Ig chains. Thus expression of a functional MYC protein is an invariable characteristic of BL cells.

t(8;14) is the most common translocation, involving the Ig$_H$ locus. Each family of Ig genes (κ and λ light chains and the heavy chains) consists of C, J and V gene clusters and, in the heavy chain, a cluster of D genes. The C genes are designated α, ε, γ2α, γ2β, γ1, γ3, δ and μ (Cμ adjacent to J). E represents the enhancer and the slashes between the C genes represent switch regions. Breakpoints are usually in the immediate 5′ non-transcribed region of *MYC* and translocation of *MYC*, generally to near the switch region of μ (Cμ), places *MYC* in a head-to-head configuration with the Ig genes. On the reciprocal chromosome the Ig$_H$ VJD region, often with the enhancer, is juxtaposed to the 5' end of *MYC*. In the BL67 cell line two promoters that give rise to antisense transcription of the μ gene also regulate activation of the translocated *MYC* gene (Apel *et al.*, 1992).

In the two translocations involving Igκ and Igλ, *MYC* remains on chromosome 8 and is joined at its 3' end by the Ig sequences facing the oncogene in a head-to-tail orientation. t(8;22) translocates the Vλ region to a breakpoint ~5 kb 3' to *MYC* exon 3 and t(2;8) translocates κ light chain locus to a breakpoint >20 kb 3' to *MYC* exon 3. These variant translocations occur equally in eBL and sBL. Cell lines bearing the 8;22 translocation tend to synthesize λ light chain whereas 2;8 variants synthesize κ light chain (Magrath, 1990), consistent with the hypothesis that translocation occurs during the period of differentiation in which Ig gene rearrangements take place.

The major chromosome translocation occurring in mouse plasmacytomas

Mouse plasmacytomas (MPCs) are a class of B cell tumours in which the *Myc* locus (chromosome 15) is translocated to chromosome 12 (Ig heavy chain) or, less often, the Igκ light chain (chromosome 6) is translocated to a region 3' of the *Myc* gene. As with Burkitt's lymphoma, rearrangements involving Ig$_H$ typically occur in the allelically excluded, α-switch region. The coding sequence of *Myc* is placed head-to-head with the Ig heavy chain gene. Deletions, duplications or insertions frequently occur near the breakpoint.

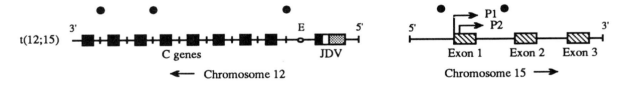

In the rarer translocation (6;15) the κ light chain locus (chromosome 6) is translocated to a breakpoint on chromosome 15 beyond a locus (*Pvt-1*) that is over 72 kb from the 3' end of *Myc*. A variant mouse plasmacytoma involves a 15;16 translocation and juxtaposes *Myc* head-to-tail with C3 in the λ light chain locus on chromosome 16 (Axelson *et al.*, 1991). Stable transcripts from the non-coding strand are produced in plasmacytomas using a promoter localized within intron 2 (Spicer and Sonenshein, 1992).

Some MPCs and some human cell lines appear to have acquired the same functional changes as are caused by the translocations described above via interstitial deletions (Wiener *et al.*, 1984; Ohno *et al.*, 1989). In Eμ-*Nmyc* transgenic mice treated with pristane and helper-free Ab-MuLV plasmacytomas develop as a result of the expression of *Nmyc* with no expression of *Myc* or endogenous *Nmyc* and without the normally associated translocations (Wang *et al.*, 1992). Most MPCs also express a putative oncogene, PC326, that is not expressed in normal plasma cells (Bergsagel *et al.*, 1992).

(3) GENE AMPLIFICATION

In cell lines *MYCN* is amplified from 5- to 600-fold and *MYCL* by up to 20-fold. In patients with neuroblastoma *MYCN* amplification to 10 copies correlates with a reduction in survival to 5% during a standard therapy course (Seeger *et al.*, 1985).

Effects of antisense oligodeoxynucleotide

Human T cells: Antisense *MYC* ODN (Weintraub, 1990) blocks entry into S phase (Heikkila *et al.*, 1987) and decreases the mitogen-stimulated increase in p34^{cdc2} mRNA (Furukawa *et al.*, 1990).

Burkitt's lymphoma cell lines: Antisense ODN directed against the cryptic promoter of the first intron inhibits proliferation of cell lines expressing abnormal transcripts (McManaway *et al.*, 1990).

Neuroectodermal cell lines: Inhibition of *MYCN* expression by an antisense ODN inhibits the spontaneous interconversion of phenotypes that often occurs in cell lines derived from pediatric neuroectoderm tumours (Whitesell *et al.*, 1991).

HL-60 leukaemia cells: Antisense *MYC* ODN decreases MYC protein by 50–80%: causes differentiation (Holt *et al.*, 1988).

Rat aortic smooth muscle cells: Antisense *Myc* ODN inhibits proliferation and migration *in vitro* (Biro *et al.*, 1993).

Mouse erythroleukaemia: Antisense *Myc* ODN inhibits progression to S phase; accelerates differentiation into mature erythroid precursors (Prochownik *et al.*, 1988).

F9 murine teratocarcinoma cells: Plasmids expressing antisense to *Myc* exon 1 or exons 2 and 3 (SV40 promoter-regulated) cause decrease in MYC protein and differentiation. Effects similar to those of retinoic acid. MYC downregulation necessary and sufficient for differentiation (Griep and Westphal, 1988).

Mouse embryo development: Inhibition of MYC protein synthesis by antisense *Myc* ODN severely attenuates blastocyst formation from two-cell embryos *in vitro* (Paria *et al.*, 1992).

Databank file names and accession numbers

	GENE	*EMBL*	*SWISSPROT*	*REFERENCES*
AMV_MC29	v-*myc*	Remh2mil V01173 Remc29 V01173 Remc29z V01174	MYC_AVIMC P01110	Alitalo *et al.*, 1983 Reddy *et al.*, 1983
AMV_CMII AMV_OK10 MH2	v-*myc* v-*myc* *gag–mil–myc*	Reacmmyc M15241 Reac2pol M11352 Remh2mil X00578 Rear01 X00534	MYC_AVIM2 P10395 MYC_AVIOK P12523 KMIL_AVIMH P00531	Walther *et al.*, 1986 Hayflick *et al.*, 1985 Galibert *et al.*, 1984 Sutrave *et al.*, 1984a Kan *et al.*, 1984
AMV_MH2E21 AMV_HBI	v-*myc* v-*myc*	ReaC2E21 M14008 ReaCMH01 M11784	MYC_AVIME P06647 MYC_AVIMD P06295	Patchinsky *et al.*, 1986 Smith *et al.*, 1985
Human	*MYC*	Hsmycc X00364 Hsmycl V00568 Hsmyce12 X00196	MYC_HUMAN P01106; P01107	Colby *et al.*, 1983 Saito *et al.*, 1983 Watt *et al.*, 1983 Bernard *et al.*, 1983 Rabbitts *et al.*, 1983 Gazin *et al.*, 1984
Human	*MYCL1*	Hsmyc3L M19720 Hslmycl X07262 Hslmyc2 X07263	MYCL_HUMAN P12524	Kaye *et al.*, 1988
Human	*MYCL2*	HsmycL2a J03069	MYCM_HUMAN P12525	Morton *et al.*, 1989

	GENE	*EMBL*	*SWISSPROT*	*REFERENCES*
Human	*MYCN*	Hsnmycla M13228 Hsnmyc2 X03294 Hsnmyc3a X03295 Hsnmyc01 M13241 Hsnmyc3 X02363 Hsnmyc Y00664	MYCN_HUMAN P04198	Slamon *et al.*, 1986 Stanton *et al.*, 1986 Kohl *et al.*, 1986 Ibson and Rabbitts, 1988 Michitsch and Melera, 1985
Human	*MAX*	Hsmax M64240		Blackwood and Eisenman, 1991
Human	Δ*MAX*	X60287		Makela *et al.*, 1992
Human	Δmax (3.5 kb mRNA)	X66867		Vastrik *et al.*, 1993
Mouse	*Myc*	Mmcmycl X01023 Mmb3 K00683	MYC_MOUSE P01108	Stanton *et al.*, 1984 Neuberger and Calabi, 1983
Mouse	*Lmyc*	MmcmycL X13945	MYCL_MOUSE P10166	Legouy *et al.*, 1987
Mouse	*Nmyc*	Mmnmyc X03919	MYCN_MOUSE P03966	DePinho *et al.*, 1986 Taya *et al.*, 1986
Rat	*Myc*	Rncmyc Y00396	MYC_RAT P09416	Hayashi *et al.*, 1987
Rat	*Bmyc*	Rnbmyca M21133 Rnbmyc5 X17455	MYCB_RAT P15063	Ingvarsson *et al.*, 1988 Asker *et al.*, 1989
Rat	*Smyc*			Sugiyama *et al.*, 1989
Chicken	*Myc*	Ggmyc J00889	MYC_CHICK P01109	Watson *et al.*, 1983 Shih *et al.*, 1984
Chicken	*Nmyc*	Ggnmyc D90071	MYCN_CHICK P18444	Sawai *et al.*, 1990
Feline	*Myc*	Fsmyccal M22726 Fsmycca2 M22727 Fsmycca3 M22728	MYC_FELCA P06877	Stewart *et al.*, 1986
Feline	*v-myc*	Fcftt M25762		Doggett *et al.*, 1989
FeLV	*v-myc*	Remyc M10973	MYC_FLV P06878	Braun *et al.*, 1985
Xenopus *laevis*	*myc* I	XlmycI X14806	MYC1_XENLA P06171	King *et al.*, 1986
Xenopus *laevis*	*myc* II	Xlmyc M14455 XlmycII X14807	MYC2_XENLA P15171	Vriz *et al.*, 1989
Trout	*Myc*			van Beneden *et al.*, 1986
Asterias *vulgaris*	pAv-*myc*	Avcmyc M80364		Walker *et al.*, 1992

Table 3.5.   *Cellular Myc mRNA expression*

Cell type	Agents	Comment
Proliferation		
Primary breast tumours	Tamoxifen	*MYC* and *HER2* mRNA decreased. *MYC* expression is stimulated by estrogen and downregulated by tamoxifen in estrogen-receptor-positive cells (Le Roy *et al.*, 1991)
Embryonic tissue (proliferating)		*Myc* and *Nmyc* expression generally high but patterns of distribution often distinct (Schmid *et al.*, 1989; Sawai *et al.*, 1990)
Partial hepatectomy		Transcription of *Myc*, *Fos* and the *Jun* family induced *in vivo* (Makino *et al.*, 1984)
Fibroblasts	Serum, PDGF, EGF, bombesin, A23187, TPA, UV light	*Myc* transcription maximal ~4 h after mitogenic stimulation of quiescent cells (i.e. significantly later than *Fos* and *Jun*)
Lymphocytes	ConA, PHA, anti-TCR antibody, Thy-1 (mice), LPS, A23187, TPA	Not all these agents cause PIP_2 hydrolysis and there is evidence that *Myc* expression, like *Fos*, does not depend on an increase in $[Ca^{2+}]_i$ (Kelly *et al.*, 1983; Moore *et al.*, 1986). The tenfold increase in the steady state concentration of mRNA is due to the relief of exon 1 elongation block (Schneider-Schaulies *et al.*, 1987). Downregulation of protein kinase C greatly reduces *Myc* expression without affecting PDGF-induced mitogenesis (Coughlin *et al.*, 1985)
Many cell types	Cycloheximide, actinomycin	Inhibition of protein synthesis causes superinduction of *Myc* transcription (see also **FOS**) but decreases *Lmyc* mRNA (Saksela, 1987). For *Myc*, this suggests that either short-lived proteins inhibit transcription and/or activate mRNA degradation or that inhibition of translation stabilizes the message (Wisdom and Lee, 1991; Bernstein *et al.*, 1992). Evidence for the latter has been found for β-tubulin and *Fos* (Wilson and Treisman, 1988)
Normal fibroblasts	Activated *Myc* genes (transfected pSV40–*Myc*)	Cells are non-tumorigenic but have increased sensitivity to growth factors, EGF alone causing DNA synthesis (Stern *et al.*, 1986)
Normal fibroblasts	Activated *Myc* genes (transfected pSV40–*Myc*)	*Myc* regulates the length of G_1, reducing G_1 from 6.5 to 4.6 h; *Myc* protein levels correlate with the rate of entry into S phase; S, G_2 and M are unaffected. When cells are deprived of growth factors and endogenously expressed *Myc* they continue to cycle for some time with increasing G_1 periods. Cells expressing *Myc* cease growth in the absence of growth factors and on re-stimulation with serum, enter S phase more rapidly and less synchronously than normal cells. Thus *Myc*-transformed cells may arrest at many points in G_1 or be reduced to a very slow rate of passage (Karn *et al.*, 1989)

Table 3.5. *Continued*

Cell type	Agents	Comment
Swiss 3T3 fibroblasts	Nuclear microinjection of *Myc* + co-mitogenic stimulation	Cells enter S phase (Kaczmarek *et al.*, 1985)
Mouse fibroblasts	Activated *Myc* (chimera of the binding domain of the human estrogen receptor and MYC C-terminus)	Cells re-enter the cycle and activate transcription of α-prothymosin that encodes a nuclear protein presumed to be involved in proliferation (Eilers *et al.*, 1991)
Human epidermal keratinocytes	EGF	Proliferation blocked by TGFβ$_1$ which downregulates *Myc*. This effect is prevented by SV40 T antigen, E1A or HPV-16 E7 but not when these proteins are mutated in their p105^{RB} binding domain (Pietenpol *et al.*, 1990)
Human epidermal keratinocytes	SV40, HPV-16 or HPV-18 transformation	Resistant to growth inhibition by TGFβ which does not suppress *MYC* mRNA levels in these transformed cells. Transient expression of p105^{RB} represses *MYC* promoter activity as effectively as TGFβ$_1$ and acts via the same TGFβ control element (TCE). The action of p105^{RB} on *MYC* transcription is mediated by a 106 kDa protein (Moses, 1992)
Lymphoma	Interferon	Expression downregulated: correlates with the anti-proliferative activity of IFN. 20-fold decrease in *Myc* mRNA level but no change in transcription rate (Dani *et al.*, 1985; Knight *et al.*, 1985)
Murine cell line (CTLL-2)	*Myb* expression vector	Expression of *Myb* strongly activates *Myc* transcription and CAT expression regulated by a *Myc* promoter (Evans *et al.*, 1990)
T cells	IL-2	*Myb* transcription correlates with the stimulation of proliferation by IL-2 and declines as the cells become insensitive to IL-2. *Myc* transcription is also activated by IL-2 (maximal by 4 h and sustained for up to 9 days). Antisense *Myc* or *Myb* blocks IL-2-stimulated DNA synthesis (Churilla *et al.*, 1989)
T helper cell clones	IL-1α	*Myb* (and *Myc*) transcription activated (Zubiaga *et al.*, 1991)
Myeloblastic leukaemia cell line (M1)	IL-6, leukaemia inhibitory factor (LIF)	Induce terminal differentiation: stimulate transient *Myc* transcription: rapidly (<12 h) suppress *Myb*. Sustained expression of *Myc* blocks terminal differentiation (Hoffman-Liebermann and Liebermann, 1991)
Human T cell leukaemia line (Jurkat)	TPA	TPA inhibits proliferation and induces expression of IL-2R and mRNA and terminal differentiation. TPA also reduces the high levels of *MYC*, *NRAS* and *BCL2* mRNAs in Jurkats and stimulates *FOS*, *JUN* and *EGR1* before IL-2R. It has no effect on *MYB*, *RAF1*, *LCK*, *FYN* or *FGR*. When *MYC* or *BCL2* expression is sustained (from plasmids), TPA still blocks growth and induces IL-2R expression (Makover *et al.*, 1991)

Table 3.5. *Continued*

Cell type	Agents	Comment
Mouse spleen	Regenerating *in vivo*	T cells have high *Myb* and *Myc* mRNA levels (Sihvola *et al.*, 1989)
Mouse T helper cell clones	Anti-CD3-antibody, IL-2	Activate *Myc* and *Myb* transcription (Bohjanen *et al.*, 1990)
Mouse pro-B cell line (BAF-B-3)	IL-2, EGF	IL-2 induces *Jun*, *Junb*, *Fos*, *Fra-1* and *Myc* transcription. With the exception of *Myc*, the stimulation of the EGFR activates the same pattern of transcription. Stimulation by EGF alone causes the cells to arrest in S phase of the cell cycle and progression to G$_2$/M requires ectopic expression of *Myc*. Thus in these cells expression of *Myc* is essential for mitosis (Shibuya *et al.*, 1992)
Mast cell line IL-3-dependent (MC)	*Myc* expression vector	*Myc* expression increases growth rate but cells remain IL-3-dependent (Hume *et al.*, 1988)
BALB-3T3	Polyoma mT	Transfected cells overexpressing mT are transformed and constitutively express *Myc* (and JE) but not *Fos* or *Jun* (Rameh and Armelin, 1991)
Human leukaemic cells (HL-60)	Electromagnetic radiation	Low-frequency fields (~60 Hz) stimulate *MYC*, β-actin and histone H2B transcription (Goodman *et al.*, 1989)
Differentiation		
NIH 3T3 fibroblasts	MyoD, myogenin	Sustained expression of MyoD or myogenin after transfection causes differentiation. Co-transfection and expression of *Myc* suppresses myogenesis independently of Id (Miner and Wold, 1991)
HL-60 leukaemia cells	DMSO, retinoic acid	*MYC* is amplified 20-fold in HL-60 cells. During the early stages of differentiation, a tenfold reduction in mRNA occurs due to a qualitative increase in the inhibition of transcriptional elongation at the 3′ end of exon 1. At later stages initiation is decreased (Siebenlist *et al.*, 1988)
Murine myeloid leukaemia cell line (WEHI-3B)	G-CSF and actinomycin D	Decrease in *Myc* (and *Myb*) transcription occurs only at a late stage of differentiation to macrophages. *Myc* decrease transient. *Fos* mRNA is increased (Gonda and Metcalf, 1984)
Murine erythroleukaemia cells (MELC DS19-sc9)	HMBA	*Myc* transiently downregulated during first 4 h; *Fos* mRNA is increased (Ramsay *et al.*, 1986)
Erythroleukaemic cells	DMSO, HMBA	Activation of differentiation correlates with a biphasic (down-then-up) modulation of transcription of *Myc* and *Myb*. Two H1 histone genes are induced, the expression of which is negatively regulated by *Myc* (Cheng and Skoultchi, 1989). Erythropoietin, which stimulates stem cell maturation to erythrocytes, increases *Myc* expression (Eilers *et al.*, 1991)

Table 3.5. *Continued*

Cell type	Agents	Comment
Rauscher-transformed cells (EM-SIII)	Erythropoietin	Rapid expression of *Myc* mRNA (~1 h) caused by erythropoietin blocked by staurosporine and other inhibitors of protein kinase C (Spangler *et al.*, 1991)
Erythroleukaemic cells	HMBA, Mo-MuLV LTRL–*Myc*	Transfection with *Myc* or *Lmyc* blocks HMBA-induced differentiation (Birrer *et al.*, 1989)
Rat pheochromocytoma cells (PC12)	NGF, SV40–*Myc*	Neuronal differentiation is blocked by expression of *Myc* and proliferation is stimulated (Maruyama *et al.*, 1987)
Human neuroblastoma	Retinoic acid, TPA	*MYCN* transcription decreases during differentiation (Hammerling *et al.*, 1989)
Murine embryonal carcinoma cells	Retinoic acid	Differentiation correlates with decrease in *Myc*, *Nmyc* and *Lmyc* expression (Ingvarsson *et al.*, 1989). *Nmyc* downregulation transient (Finklestein and Weinberg, 1988)
F9 murine teratocarcinoma cells	Interferon	20-fold decrease in *Myc* mRNA level but no change in transcription rate (Dony *et al.*, 1985)

Reviews

Alitalo, K. and Schwab, M. (1986). Oncogene amplification in tumor cells. Adv. Cancer Res., 47, 235–281.
Bister, K. and Jansen, H.W. (1986). Oncogenes in retroviruses and cells: biochemistry and molecular genetics. Adv. Cancer Res., 47, 99–188.
Cole, M.D. (1991). Myc meets its max. Cell, 65, 715–716.
Cory, S. (1986). Activation of cellular genes in hemopoietic cells by chromosome translocation. Adv. Cancer Res., 47, 189–234.
Croce, C.M. (1987). Role of chromosome translocations in human neoplasia. Cell, 49, 155–156.
DePinho, R.A., Schreiber-Agus, N. and Alt, F.W. (1991). *myc* family oncogenes in the development of normal and neoplastic cells. Adv. Cancer Res., 57, 1–46.
Hayman, M.J. (1983). Avian acute leukemia viruses. Curr. Top. Microbiol. Immunol., 103, 109–125.
Luscher, B. and Eisenman, R.N. (1990). New light on myc and myb. Part I. Myc. Genes Devel., 4, 2025–2035.
Magrath, I. (1990). The pathogenesis of Burkitt's lymphoma. Adv. Cancer Res., 55, 133–270.
Saksela, K. (1990). *myc* genes and their deregulation in lung cancer. J. Cell. Biochem., 42, 153–180.
Spencer, C.A. and Groudine, M. (1990). Control of c-myc regulation in normal and neoplastic cells. Adv. Cancer Res., 56, 1–48.
Varmus, H.E. (1984). The molecular genetics of cellular oncogenes. Annu. Rev. Genet., 18, 553–612.
Weintraub, H.M. (1990). Antisense RNA and DNA. Scientific American, Jan., pp. 34–40.
Williams, G.T. (1991). Programmed cell death: apoptosis and oncogenesis. Cell, 65, 1097–1098.

Papers

Adams, J.M., Harris, A.W., Pinkert, C.A., Corcoran, L.M., Alexander, W.S., Cory, S., Palmiter, R.D. and Brinster, R.L. (1985). The c-*myc* oncogene driven by immunoglobulin enhancers induces lymphoid malignancy in transgenic mice. Nature, 318, 533–538.
Adolph, S., Bartram, C.R. and Hameister, H. (1987). Mapping of the oncogenes *Myc*, *Sis* and *Int-1* to the distal part of mouse chromosome 15. Cytogenet. Cell Genet., 44, 65–68.

Aghib, D.F. and Bishop, M.J. (1991). A 3' truncation of *myc* caused by chromosomal translcoation in a human T-cell leukemia is tumorigenic when tested in established rat fibroblasts. Oncogene, 6, 2371–2375.

Akeson, R. and Bernards, R. (1990). N-*myc* down regulates neural cell adhesion molecule expression in rat neuroblastoma. Mol. Cell. Biol., 10, 2012–2016.

Alitalo, K., Bishop, J.M., Smith, D.H., Chen, E.Y., Colby, W.W. and Levinson, A.D. (1983). Nucleotide sequence of the v-*myc* oncogene of avian retrovirus MC29. Proc. Natl Acad. Sci. USA, 80, 100–104.

Alitalo, K., Schwab, M., Lin, C.C., Varmus, H.E. and Bishop, M.J. (1986). Homogenously staining chromosomal regions contain amplified copies of an abundantly expressed cellular oncogene (c-*myc*) in malignant neuroendocrine cells from a human colon carcinoma. Proc. Natl Acad. Sci. USA, 80, 1707–1711.

Alvarez, E., Northwood, I.C., Gonzalez, F.A., Latour, D.A., Seth, A., Abate, C., Curran, T. and Davis, R.J. (1991). Pro-Leu-Ser/Thr-Pro is a consensus primary sequence for substrate protein phosphorylation. J. Biol. Chem., 266, 15277–15285.

Amati, B., Dalton, S., Brooks, M.W., Littlewood, T.D.,. Evan, G.I. and Land, H. (1992). Transcriptional activation by the human c-myc oncoprotein in yeast requires interaction with max. Nature, 359, 423–426.

Apel, T.W., Mautner, J., Polack, A., Bornkamm, G.W. and Eick, D. (1992). Two antisense promoters in the immunoglobulin μ--switch region drive expression of c-*myc* in the Burkitt's lymphoma cell line BL67. Oncogene, 7, 1267–1271.

Asker C., Steinitz, M., Andersson, K., Sumegi, J., Klein, G., Ingvarsson, S. (1989). Nucleotide sequence of the rat B*myc* gene. Oncogene, 4, 1523–1527.

Askew, D.S., Ashmun, R.A., Simmons, B.C. and Cleveland, J.L. (1991). Constitutive c-*myc* expression in an IL-3-dependent myeloid cell line suppresses cell cycle arrest and accelerates apoptosis. Oncogene, 6, 1915–1922.

Axelson, H., Panda, C.K., Silva, S., Sugiyama, H., Wiener, F., Klein, G. and Sumegi, J. (1991). A new variant 15;16 translocation in mouse plasmacytoma leads to the juxtaposition of c-*myc* and immunoglobulin lambda. Oncogene, 6, 2263–2270.

Ayer, D.E., Kretzner, L. and Eisenman, R.N. (1993). Mad: a heterodimeric partner for max that antagonizes myc transcriptional activity. Cell, 72, 211–222.

Babiss, L.E. and Friedman, J.M. (1990). Regulation of N-*myc* gene expression: use of an adenovirus vector to demonstrate posttranscriptional control. Mol. Cell. Biol., 10, 6700–6708.

Baer, M.R., Augustinos, P. and Kinniburgh, A.J. (1992). Defective c-*myc* and c-*myb* RNA turnover in acute myeloid leukemia cells. Blood, 79, 1319–1326.

Barrett, J., Birrer, M.J., Kato, G.J., Dosaka-Akita, H. and Dang, C.V. (1992). Activation domains of L-myc and c-myc determine their transforming properties in rat embryo cells. Mol. Cell. Biol., 12, 3130–3137.

Bauters, C., de Groote, P., Adamantidis, M., Delcayre, C., Hamon, M., Lablanche, J.M., Bertrand, M.E., Dupuis, B. and Swynghedauw, B. (1992). Proto-oncogene expression in rabbit aorta after wall injury. First marker of the cellular process leading to restenosis after angioplasty? Eur. Heart J., 13, 556–559.

Beckman, H., Su, L.-K. and Kadesch. (1990). TFE3: a helix–loop–helix protein that activates transcription through the immunoglobulin enhancer mE3 motif. Genes Devel., 4, 167–179.

Benvenisty, N., Ornitz, D.M., Bennett, G.L., Sahagan, B.G., Kuo, A., Cardiff, R.D. and Leder, P. (1992a). Brain tumours and lymphomas in transgenic mice that carry HTLV-I LTR/c-*myc* and Ig/*tax* genes. Oncogene, 7, 2399–2405.

Benvenisty, N., Leder, A., Kuo, A., and Leder, P. (1992b). An embryonically expressed gene is a target for c-myc regulation via the c-myc-binding sequence. Genes Devel., 6, 2513–2523.

Berberich, S.J. and Cole, M.D. (1992). Casein kinase II inhibits the DNA-binding activity of max homodimers but not myc/max heterodimers. Genes Devel., 6, 166–176.

Bergsagel, P.L., Timblin, C.R., Eckhardt, L., Laskov, R. and Kuehl, W.M. (1992). Sequence and expression of a murine cDNA encoding PC326, a novel gene expressed in plasmacytomas but not in normal plasma cells. Oncogene, 7, 2059–2064.

Bernard, O., Cory, S., Gerndakis, S., Webb, E. and Adams, J.A. (1983). Sequence of the murine and human cellular *myc* oncogenes and two modes of *myc* transcription resulting from chromosome translocation in B-lymphoid tumours. EMBO J., 2, 2375–2383.

Bernards, R. (1991). N-*myc* disrupts protein kinase C-mediated signal transduction in neuroblastoma. EMBO J., 10, 1119–1125.

Bernards, R., Dessain, S.K. and Weinberg, R.A. (1986). N-*myc* amplification causes down-modulation of MHC class I antigen expression in neuroblastoma. Cell, 47, 667–674.

Bernstein, P.L., Herrick, D.J., Prokipcak, R.D. and Ross, J. (1992). Control of c-*myc* mRNA half-life in vitro by a protein capable of binding to a coding region stability determinant. Genes Devel., 6, 642–654.

Billaud, M., Isselbacher, K.J. and Bernards, R. (1993). A dominant-negative mutant of Max that inhibits sequence-specific DNA binding by Myc proteins. Proc. Natl Acad. Sci. USA, 90, 2739–2743.

Biro, S., Fu, Y.-M., Yu, Z.-X. and Epstein, S.E. (1993). Inhibitory effects of antisense oligodeoxynucleotides targeting c-*myc* mRNA on smooth muscle cell proliferation and migration. Proc. Natl Acad. Sci. USA, 90, 654–658.

Birrer, M.J., Raveh, L., Dosaka, H. and Segal, S. (1989). A transfected L-*myc* gene can substitute for c-*myc* in blocking murine erythroleukemia differentiation. Mol. Cell. Biol., 9, 2734–2737.

Blackwood, E.M. and Eisenman, R.N. (1991). Max: a helix-loop-helix zipper protein that forms a sequence-specific DNA-binding complex with myc. Science, 251, 1211–1217.

Blackwood, E.M., Luscher, B. and Eisenman, R.N. (1992). Myc and max associate in vivo. Genes Devel., 6, 71–80.

Bohjanen, P.R., Okajima, M. and Hodes, R.J. (1990). Differential regulation of interleukin 4 and interleukin 5 gene expression: a comparison of T-cell gene induction by anti-CD3 antibody or by exogenous lymphokines. Proc. Natl Acad. Sci. USA, 87, 5283–5287.

Bond, V.C. and Wold, B. (1993). Nucleolar localization of *myc* transcripts. Mol. Cell. Biol., 13, 3221–3230.

Bossone, S.A., Asselin, C., Patel, A.J. and Marcu, K.B. (1992). MAZ, a zinc finger protein, binds to c-*MYC* and *C2* gene sequences regulating transcriptional initiation and termination. Proc. Natl Acad. Sci. USA, 89, 7452–7456.

Braun M.J., Deininger, P.L. and Casey, J.W. (1985). Nucleotide sequence of a transduced *myc* gene from a defective feline leukemia provirus. J. Virol., 55, 177–183.

Campbell, G.R., Zimmerman, K., Blank, R.D., Alt, F.W. and D'Eustachio, P. (1989). Chromosome location of N-*myc* and L-*myc* genes in the mouse. Oncogene Res., 4, 47–54.

Carr, C.S. and Sharp, P.A. (1990). A helix–loop–helix protein related to the immunoglobulin E box-binding proteins. Mol. Cell. Biol., 10, 4384–4388.

Celano, P., Berchtold, C.M., Kizer, D.L., Weeraratna, A., Nelkin, B.D., Baylin, S.B. and Casero, R.A. (1992). Characterization of an endogenous RNA transcript with homology to the antisense strand of the human c-*myc* gene. J. Biol. Chem., 267, 15092–15096.

Chen, C., Biegalke, B.J., Eisenman, R.N. and Linial, M.L. (1989). FH3, a v-*myc* avian retrovirus with limited transforming ability. J. Virol., 63, 5092–5100.

Cheng, G. and Skoultchi, A.I. (1989). Rapid induction of polyadenylated H1 histone mRNA in mouse erythroleukemia cells is regulated by c-*myc*. Mol. Cell. Biol., 9, 2332–2340.

Churilla, A.M., Braciale, T.J. and Braciale, V.L. (1989). Regulation of T lymphocyte proliferation. Interleukin 2-mediated induction of c-myb gene expression is dependent on T lymphocyte activation state. J. Exp. Med., 170, 105–121.

Cogswell, J.P., Cogswell, P.C., Kuehl, W.M., Cuddihy, A.M., Bender, T.M., Engelke, U., Marcu, K.B. and Ting, J.P.-Y. (1993). Mechanism of c-*myc* regulation by c-myb in different cell lineages. Mol. Cell. Biol., 13, 2858–2869.

Colby, W.W., Chen, E.Y., Smith, D.H. and Levinson, A.D. (1983). Identification and nucleotide sequence of a human locus homologous to the v-*myc* oncogene of avian myelocytomatosis virus MC29. Nature, 301, 722–725.

Coll, J., Righi, M., de Taisne, C., Dissous, C., Gegonne, A. and Stehelin, D. (1983). Molecular cloning of the avian acute transforming retrovirus MH2 reveals a novel cell-derived sequence (v-*mil*) in addition to the *myc* oncogene. EMBO J., 2, 2189–2194.

Colledge, W.H., Gebhardt, A., Edge, M.D. and Bell, J.C. (1989). Analysis of A-MuLV transformed fibroblast lines for amplification of the c-*myc*, p53 and c-*fos* nuclear proto-oncogenes. Oncogene 4, 753–757.

Corcoran, L.M., Adams, J.M., Dunn, A.R. and Cory, S. (1984). Murine T lymphomas in which the cellular *myc* oncogene has been activated by retroviral insertion. Cell, 37, 113–122.

Coughlin, S.R., Lee, W.M.F., Williams, P.W., Giels, G.M. and Williams, L.T. (1985). c-*myc* gene expression is stimulated by agents that activate protein kinase C and does not account for the mitogenic effect of PDGF. Cell, 43, 243–251.

Crouch, D.H., Lang, C. and Gillespie, D.A.F. (1990). The leucine zipper domain of avian c-*myc* is required for transformation and autoregulation. Oncogene, 5, 683–689.

Cullen, B.R., Lomedico, P. and Ju, G. (1984). Transcriptional interference in avian retroviruses – implications for the promoter insertion model of leukaemogenesis. Nature, 307, 241–245.

Dahllof, B. (1990). Down-regulation of MHC class I antigens is not a general mechanism for the increased tumorigenicity caused by c-*myc* amplification. Oncogene, 5, 433–435.

Dang, C.V., McGuire, M., Buckmire, M. and Lee, W.M.F. (1989). Involvement of the "leucine zipper" region in the oligomerization and transforming activity of human c-*myc* protein. Nature, 337, 664–666.

Dani, C., Mechti, N., Piechaczyk, M., Lebleu, B., Jeanteur, P. and Blanchard, J.M. (1985). Increased rate of degradation of c-*myc* mRNA in interferon-treated Daudi cells. Proc. Natl Acad. Sci. USA, 82, 4896–4899.

Davis, L.J. and Halazonetis, T.D. (1993). Both the helix-loop-helix and the leucine zipper motifs of c-myc contribute to its dimerization specificity with max. Oncogene, 8, 125–132.

De Greve, J., Battey, J., Fedorko, J., Birrer, M., Evan, G., Kaye, F., Sausville, E. and Minna, J. (1988). The human L-myc gene encodes multiple nuclear phosphoproteins from alternatively processed mRNAs. Mol. Cell. Biol., 8, 4381–4388.

DePinho, R.A., Legouy, E., Feldman, L.B., Kohl, N.E., Yancopoulos, G.D. and Alt, F.W. (1986). Structure and expression of the murine N-myc gene. Proc. Natl Acad. Sci. USA, 83, 1827–1831.

DePinho, R.A., Hatton, K.S., Tesfaye, A., Yancopoulos, G.D. and Alt, F.W. (1987). The human myc gene family: structure and activity of L-myc and an L-myc pseudogene. Genes Devel., 1, 1311–1326.

Desiderio, S.V., Yancopoulos, G.D., Paskind, M., Thomas, E., Boss, M.A., Landau, N., Alt, F.W. and Baltimore, D. (1984). Insertion of N regions into heavy-chain genes is correlated with expression of terminal deoxytransferase in B cells. Nature, 311, 752–755.

Doggett, D.L., Drake, A.L., Hirsch, V., Rowe, M.E., Stallard, V. and Mullins, J.I. (1989). Structure, origin, and transforming activity of feline leukemia virus-myc recombinant provirus FTT. J. Virol. 63, 2108–2117.

Dolcetti, R., Rizzo, S., Viel, A., Maestro, R., De-Re, V., Feriotto, G. and Boiocchi, M. (1989). N-myc activation by proviral insertion in MCF 247-induced murine T-cell lymphomas. Oncogene, 4, 1009–1014.

Dony, C., Kessel, M. and Gruss, P. (1985). Posttranscriptional control of myc and p53 expression during differentiation of the embryonal carcinoma cell line F9. Nature, 317, 636–639.

Dosaka-Akita, H., Rosenberg, R.K., Minna, J.D. and Birrer, M.J. (1991). A complex pattern of translational initiation and phosphorylation in L-myc proteins. Oncogene, 6, 371–378.

Dotto, G.P., Gilman, M.Z., Maruyama, M. and Weinberg, R.A. (1986). c-myc and c-fos expression in differentiating mouse primary keratinocytes. EMBO J., 5, 2853–2857.

Downs, K.M., Martin, G.R. and Bishop, M.J. (1989). Contrasting patterns of myc and N-myc expression during gastrulation of the mouse embryo. Genes Devel., 3, 860–869.

Dufort, D., Drolet, M. and Nepveu, A. (1993). A protein binding site from the murine c-myc promoter contributes to transcriptional block. Oncogene, 8, 165–171.

Duyao, M.P., Kessler, D.J., Spicer, D.B., Bartholomew, C., Cleveland, J.L., Siekevitz, M. and Sonnenshein, G.E. (1992). Transactivation of the c-myc promoter by human T cell leukemia virus type 1 tax is mediated by NF-κB. J. Biol. Chem., 267, 16288–16291.

Eilers, M., Schirm, S. and Bishop, M.J. (1991). The MYC protein activates transcription of the α-prothymosin gene. EMBO J., 10, 133–141.

Escot, C., Simony-Lafontaine, J., Maudelonde, T., Puech, C., Pujol, H. and Rochefort, H. (1993). Potential value of increased MYC but not ERBB2 RNA levels as a marker of high-risk mastopathies. Oncogene, 8, 969–974.

Evan, G.I., Wyllie, A.H., Gilbert, C.S., Littlewood, T.D., Land, H., Brooks, M., Waters, C.M., Penn, L.Z. and Hancock, D.C. (1992). Induction of apoptosis in fibroblasts by c-myc protein. Cell, 69, 119–128.

Evans, J.L., Moore, T.L., Kuehl, W.M., Bender, T. and Ting, J.P. (1990). Functional analysis of c-Myb protein in T-lymphocytic cell lines shows that it trans-activates the c-myc promoter. Mol. Cell. Biol., 10, 5747–5752.

Ferre-D'Amare, A.R., Prendergast, G.C., Ziff, E.B. and Burley, S.K. (1993). Recognition by max of its cognate DNA through a dimeric b/HLH/Z domain. Nature, 363, 38–45.

Finklestein, R. and Weinberg, R.A. (1988). Differential regulation of N-myc and c-myc expression in F9 teratocarcinoma cells. Oncogene Res., 3, 287–292.

Forrest, D., Onions, D., Lees, G. and Neil, J.C. (1987). Altered structure and expression of c-myc in feline T-cell tumours. Virology, 158, 194–205.

Frykberg, L., Graf, T. and Vennstrom, B. (1987). The transforming activity of the chicken c-myc gene can be potentiated by mutations. Oncogene, 1, 415–421.

Furukawa, Y., Piwnica-Worms, H., Ernst, T.J., Kanakura, Y. and Griffin, J.D. (1990). cdc2 gene expression at the G_1 to S transition in human T lymphocytes. Science, 250, 805–808.

Galibert, F., de Dinechin, S.D., Righi, M. and Stehelin, D. (1984). The second oncogene mil of avian retrovirus MH2 is related to the src gene family. EMBO J. 3, 1333–1338.

Gazdar, A.F., Carney, D.N., Nau, M.M. and Minna, J.D. (1985). Characterization of variant subclasses of cell line derived from small cell lung cancer having distinctive biochemical, morphological and growth properties. Cancer Res., 45, 2924–2930.

Gazin, C., Dupont, S., de Dinechin, D., Hampe, A., Masson, J.M., Martin, P., Stehelin, D.and Galibert F. (1984). Nucleotide sequence of the human c-myc locus: provocative open reading frame within the first exon. EMBO J., 3, 383–387.

Gilladoga, A.D., Edelhoff, S., Blackwood, E.M., Eisenman, R.N. and Disteche, C.M. (1992). Mapping of

MAX to human chromosome 14 and mouse chromosome 12 by *in situ* hybridization. Oncogene, 7, 1249–1251.

Gillespie, D.A. and Eisenman, R.N. (1989). Detection of a myc-associated protein by chemical cross-linking. Mol. Cell. Biol., 9, 865–868.

Gonda, T.J. and Metcalf, D. (1984). Expression of *myb*, *myc* and *fos* proto-oncogenes during the differentiation of a murine myeloid leukemia. Nature, 310, 249–251.

Goodman, R., Wei, L.-X., Xu, J.-C. and Henderson, A. (1989). Exposure of human cells to low-frequency electromagnetic fields results in quantitative changes in transcripts. Biochim. Biophys. Acta, 1009, 216–220.

Goodrich, D.W. and Lee, W.-H. (1992). Abrogation by c-*myc* of G1 phase arrest induced by *RB* protein but not by p53. Nature, 360, 177–179.

Greenberg, R., Hawley, R. and Marcu, K.B. (1985). Acquisition of an intracisternal A-particle element by a translocated c-*myc* gene in a murine plasma cell tumor. Mol. Cell. Biol., 5, 3625–3628.

Gregor, P.D., Sawadogo, M. and Roeder, R.C. (1990). The adenovirus major late transcription factor USF is a member of the helix–loop–helix group of regulatory proteins and binds to DNA as a dimer. Genes Devel., 4, 1730–1740.

Griep, A.E. and Westphal, H. (1988). Antisense *myc* sequences induce differentiation of F9 cells. Proc. Natl Acad. Sci. USA, 85, 6806–6810.

Guerin, M., Barrois, M., Terrier, M.J., Spielmann, M. and Riou, G. (1988). Overexpression of either c-*myc* or c-*erb*B-2/*neu* proto-oncogenes in human breast carcinomas: correlation with poor prognosis. Oncogene Res., 3, 21–31.

Gupta, S., Seth, A. and Davis, R.J. (1993). Transactivation of gene expression by Myc is inhibited by mutation at the phosphorylation sites Thr-58 and Ser-62. Proc. Natl Acad. Sci. USA, 90, 3216–3220.

Gusse, M., Ghysdael, J., Evan, G., Soussi, T. and Mechali, M. (1989). Translocation of a store of maternal cytoplasmic c-*myc* protein into nuclei during early development. Mol. Cell. Biol., 9, 5395–5403.

Hamann, U., Wenzel., A., Frank, R. and Schwab, M. (1991). The MYCN protein of human neuroblastoma cells is phosphorylated by casein kinase II in the central region and at serine 367. Oncogene, 6, 1745–1751.

Hammerling, U., Bjelfman, C. and Pahlman, S. (1989). Different regulation of N- and c-*myc* expression during phorbol ester-induced maturation of human SH-SY5Y neuroblastoma cells. Oncogene, 2, 73–77.

Hann, S.R., King, M.W., Bentley, D.L., Anderson, C.W. and Eisenman, R.N. (1988). A non-AUG translational initiation in c-myc exon1 generates an N-terminally distinct protein whose synthesis is disrupted in Burkitt's lymphomas. Cell, 52, 185–195.

Hann, S.R., Sloan-Brown, K. and Spotts, G.D. (1992). Translational activation of the non-AUG-initiated c-*myc* 1 protein at high cell densities due to methionine deprivation. Genes Devel., 6, 1229–1240.

Haupt, Y., Alexander, W.S., Barri, G., Klinken, S.P. and Adams, J.M. (1991). Novel zinc finger gene implicated a *myc* collaborator by retrovirally accelerated lymphomagenesis in Eμ-*myc* transgenic mice. Cell, 65, 753–763.

Hayashi, K., Makino, R., Kawamura, H., Arisawa, A. and Yoneda, K. (1987). Characterization of rat c-*myc* and adjacent regions. Nucleic Acids Res., 15, 6419–6436.

Hayflick, J., Seeburg, P.H., Ohlsson, R., Pfeifer-Ohlsson, S., Watson, D., Papas, T. and Duesberg, P.H. (1985). Nucleotide sequence of two overlapping *myc*-related gene in avian carcinoma virus OK10 and their relation to the *myc* genes of other viruses and the cell. Proc. Natl Acad. Sci. USA, 82, 2718–2722.

Hayward, W.S., Neel, B.G. and Astrin, S.M. (1981). Activation of a cellular *onc* gene by promoter insertion in ALV-induced lymphoid leukosis. Nature, 290, 475–480.

Heaney, M.L., Pierce, J. and Parsons, J.T. (1986). Site-directed mutagenesis of the *gag-myc* gene of avian myelocytomatosis virus 29: biological activity and intracellular localization of structurally altered proteins. J. Virol., 60, 167–176.

Heikkila, R., Schwab, G., Wickstrom, E., Loke, S.L., Pluznik, D.H., Watt, R. and Neckers, L.M. (1987). A c-*myc* antisense oligodeoxynucleotide inhibits entry into S phase but not progress from G_0 to G_1. Nature, 328, 445–449.

Hiebert, S.W., Blake, M., Azizkhan, J. and Nevins, J.R. (1991). Role of E2F transcription factor in E1A-mediated trans activation of cellular genes. J. Virol., 65, 3547–3552.

Hiller, S., Breit, S., Wang, Z.-Q., Wagner, E.F. and Schwab, M. (1991). Localization of regulatory elements controlling human *MYCN* expression. Oncogene, 6, 969–977.

Hoffman-Liebermann, B. and Liebermann, D.A. (1991). Interleukin-6- and leukemia inhibitory factor-induced terminal differentiation of myeloid leukemia cells is blocked at an intermediate stage by constitutive c-*myc*. Mol. Cell. Biol., 11, 2375–2381.

Holt, J.T., Redner, R.L. and Nienhuis, A.W. (1988). An oligomer complementary to c-*myc* mRNA inhibits proliferation of HL-60 promyelocytic cells and induces differentiation. Mol. Cell. Biol., 8, 963–973.

Hu, Y.F., Luscher, B., Admon, A., Mermod, N. and Tjian, R. (1990). Transcription factor AP-4 contains multiple dimerization domains that regulate dimer specificity. Genes Devel., 4, 1741–1752.

Hume, C.R., Nocka, K.H., Sorrentino, V., Lee, J.S. and Fleissner, E.F. (1988). Constitutive c-*myc* expression enhances the response of murine mast cells to IL-3, but does not eliminate their requirement for growth factors. Oncogene, 2, 223–226.

Ibson, J.M. and Rabbitts, P.H. (1988). Sequence of a germ-line N-*myc* gene and amplification as a mechanism of activation. Oncogene, 2, 399–402.

Iguchi-Ariga, S.M.M., Okazaki, T., Itani, T., Ogata, M. Sato, Y. and Ariga, H. (1988). An initiation site of DNA replication with transcriptional enhancer activity present upstream of the c-*myc* gene. EMBO J., 7, 3135–3142.

Imagawa, M., Chiu, R. and Karin, M. (1987). Transcription factor AP-2 mediates induction by two different signal-transduction pathways: protein kinase C and cAMP. Cell, 51, 251–260.

Inghirami, G., Grignani, F., Sternas, L., Lombardi, L., Knowles, D.M. and Dalla-Favera, R. (1990). Down-regulation of LFA-1 adhesion receptor by the c-*myc* oncogene in human B lymphoblastoid cells. Science, 250, 682–686.

Ingvarsson, S., Asker, C., Axelson, H., Klein, G. and Sumegi, J. (1988). Structure and expression of B-*myc*, a new member of the *myc* gene family. Mol. Cell. Biol., 8, 3168–3174.

Ingvarsson, S., Sundaresan, S., Jin, P., Francke, U., Asker, C., Sumegi, J., Klein, G. and Sejersen T. (1989). Chromosome localization and expression pattern of Lmyc and Bmyc in murine embryonal carcinoma cells. Oncogene, 3, 679–685.

Jaffredo, T., Vandenbunder, B. and Dieterlen-Lievre, F. (1989). *In situ* study of c-*myc* protein expression during avian development. Development, 105, 679–695.

Jansen-Durr, P., Meichle, A., Steiner, P., Pagano, M., Finke, K., Botz, J., Wessbecher, J., Draetta, G. and Eilers, M. (1993). Differential modulation of cyclin gene expression by *MYC*. Proc. Natl Acad. Sci. USA, 90, 3685–3689.

Jin, P. and Ringertz, N.R. (1990). Cadmium induces transcription of proto-oncogenes c-*jun* and c-*myc* in rat L6 myoblasts. J. Biol. Chem., 265, 14061–14064.

Kaczmarek, L., Hyland, J.K., Watt, R., Rosenberg, M. and Baserga, R. (1985). Microinjected c-*myc* as a competence factor. Science, 228, 1313–1315.

Kaddurah-Daouk, R., Greene, J.M., Baldwin, A.S. and Kingston, R.E. (1987). Activation and repression of mammalian gene expression by the c-*myc* protein. Genes Devel., 1, 347–357.

Kakkis, E., Riggs, K.J., Gillespie, W. and Calame, K. (1989). A transcriptional repression of c-*myc*. Nature, 339, 718–721.

Kan, N.C., Flordellis, C.S., Garon, C.F., Duesberg, P.H. and Papas, T.S. (1983). Avian carcinoma virus MH2 contains a transformation-specific sequence, MHT, and shares the *myc* sequence with MC29, CMII and OK10 viruses. Proc. Natl Acad. Sci. USA, 80, 6566–6570.

Kan, N.C., Flordellis, C.S., Mark, G.E., Duesberg, P.H. and Papas, T.S. (1984). A common *onc* gene sequence transduced by avian carcinoma virus MH2 and by murine sarcoma virus 3611. Science, 223, 813–816.

Karn, J., Watson, J.V., Lowe, A.D., Green, S.M. and Vedeckis, W. (1989). Regulation of cell cycle duration by c-*myc* levels. Oncogene, 4, 773–787.

Kato, G.J., Barrett, J., Villa-Garcia, M. and Dang, C.V. (1990). An amino-terminal c-myc domain required for neoplastic transformation activates transcription. Mol. Cell. Biol., 10, 5914–5920.

Kato, G.J., Lee, W.M.F., Chen, L. and Dang, C.V. (1992). Max: functional domains and interaction with c-myc. Genes Devel., 6, 81–92.

Katzir, N., Rechavi, G., Cohen, J.B., Unger, T., Simoni, F., Segal, S., Cohen, D. and Givol, D. (1985). "Retroposon" insertion into the cellular oncogene c-*myc* in canine transmissible venereal tumor. Proc. Natl Acad. Sci. USA, 82, 1054–1058.

Kaye, F., Battey, J., Nau, M., Brooks, B., Seifter, E., de Greve, J., Birrer, M., Sausville, E. and Minna, J. (1988). Structure and expression of the human L-*myc* gene reveal a complex pattern of alternative mRNA splicing. Mol. Cell. Biol., 8, 186–195.

Kelly, K., Cochran, B.H., Stiles, C.D. and Leder, P. (1983). Cell-specific regulation of the c-myc gene by lymphocyte mitogens and platelet-derived growth factor. Cell, 35, 603–610.

Kerppola, T.K. and Kane, C.M. (1988). Intrinsic sites of transcription termination and pausing in the c-*myc* gene. Mol. Cell. Biol., 8, 4389–4394.

Kessler, D.J., Spicer, D.B., La Rosa, F.A. and Sonenshein, G.E. (1992). A novel NF-κB element within exon 1 of the murine c-*myc* gene. Oncogene, 7, 2447–2453.

King, M.W., Roberts, J.M. and Eisenman, R.N. (1986). Expression of the c-*myc* proto-oncogene during development of *Xenopus laevis*. Mol. Cell. Biol., 6, 4499–4508.

Knight, E., Anton, E.D., Fahey, D., Friedland, B.K. and Jonak, G.J. (1985). Interferon regulates c-*myc* gene expression in Daudi cells at the post-transcriptional level. Proc. Natl Acad. Sci. USA, 82, 1151–1154.

Kohl, N.E., Legouy, E., DePinho, R.A., Nisen, P.D., Smith, R.K., Gee, C.E. and Alt, F.W. (1986). Human N-*myc* is closely related in organization and nucleotide sequence to c-*myc*. Nature, 319, 73–77.

Koskinen, P.J., Sistonen, L., Evan, G., Morimoto, R. and Alitalo, K. (1991). Nuclear colocalization of cellular and viral *myc* proteins with HSP70 in *myc*-overexpressing cells. J. Virol., 65, 842–851.

Kretzner, L., Blackwood, E.M. and Eisenman, R.N. (1992). Myc and max proteins possess distinct transcriptional activities. Nature, 359, 426–429.

Krumm, A., Meulia, T., Brunvand, M. and Groudine, M. (1992). The block to transcriptional elongation within the human c-*myc* gene is determined in the promoter-proximal region. Genes Devel., 6, 2201–2213.

Krystal, G.W., Armstrong, B.C. and Battey, J.F. (1990). N-*myc* mRNA forms an RNA-RNA duplex with endogenous antisense transcripts. Mol. Cell. Biol., 10, 4180–4191.

Lang, J.C., Wilkie, N.M., Clark, A.M., Chudleigh, A., Talbot, A., Whitelaw, B. and Frame, M.C. (1991). Regulatory domains within the P0 promoter of human c-*myc*. Oncogene, 6, 2067–2075.

Le Roy, X., Escot, C., Brouillet, J.-P., Theillet, C., Maudelonde, T., Simony-Lafontaine, J., Pujol, H. and Rochefort, H. (1991). Decrease of c-*erb*B-2 and c-*myc* RNA levels in tamoxifen-treated breast cancer. Oncogene, 6, 431–437.

Legouy, E., DePinho, R., Zimmerman, K., Collum, R., Yancopoulos, G.D., Mitsock, L., Kriz, R. and Alt, F.W.; (1987). Structure and expression of the murine L-*myc* gene. EMBO J., 6, 3359–3366.

Lenardo, M., Rustgi, A.K., Schievella, A.R. and Bernards, R. (1989). Suppression of MHC class I gene expression by N-*myc* through enhancer inactivation. EMBO J., 8, 3351–3355.

Little, C.D., Nau, M.M., Carney, D.N., Gazdar, A.F. and Minna, J.D. (1983). Amplification and expression of the c-*myc* oncogene in human lung cancer cell lines. Nature, 306, 194–196.

Ludwig, S.R., Habera, L.F., Dellaporta, S.L. and Wessler, S.R. (1989). *Lc*, a member of the maize R gene family responsible for tissue-specific anthocyanin production, encodes a protein similar to transcriptional activators and contains the *myc*-homology region. Proc. Natl Acad. Sci. USA, 86, 7092–7096.

Luscher, B. and Eisenman, R.N. (1988). c-*myc* and c-*myb* protein degradation: effect of metabolic inhibitors and heat shock. Mol. Cell. Biol., 8, 2504–2512.

Luscher, B. and Eisenman, R.N. (1992). Mitosis-specific phosphorylation of the nuclear oncoproteins Myc and Myb. J. Cell. Biol., 118, 775–784.

Ma, A., Moroy, T., Collum, R., Weintraub, H., Alt, F.W. and Blackwell, T.K. (1993). DNA binding by N- and L-myc proteins. Oncogene, 8, 1093–1098.

McManaway, M.E., Neckers, L.M., Loke, S.L., Al-Nasser, A.A., Redner, R.L., Shiramizu, B.T., Goldschmidts, W.L., Huber, B.E., Bhatia, K. and Magrath, I.T. (1990). Tumour-specific inhibition of lymphoma growth by an antisense oligodeoxynucleotide. Lancet, 335, 808–811.

McWhinney, C. and Leffak, M. (1988). Episomal persistence of a plasmid containing human c-*myc* DNA. Cancer Cells, 6, 467–471.

Makela, T.P., Shiraishi, M., Borrello, M.G., Sekiya, T. and Alitalo, K. (1991). Rearrangement and co-amplification of L-*myc* and *rlf* in primary lung cancer. Oncogene, 7, 405–409.

Makela, T.P., Koskinen, P.J., Vastrik, I. and Alitalo, K. (1992). Alternative forms of max as enhancers or suppressors of myc-ras cotransformation. Science, 256, 373–377.

Makino, R., Hayashi, K. and Sugimura, T. (1984). c-*myc* transcription is induced in rat liver at a very early stage of regeneration or by cycloheximide treatment. Nature, 310, 697–698.

Makover, D., Cuddy, M., Yum, S., Bradley, K., Alpers, J., Sukhatme, V. and Reed, J.C. (1991). Phorbol ester-mediated inhibition of growth and regulation of proto-oncogene expression in the human T cell leukemia line JURKAT. Oncogene, 6, 455–460.

Mariani-Costantini, R., Escot, C., Theillet, C., Gentile, A., Merlo, G., Lidereau, R. and Callahan, R. (1988). *In situ* c-*myc* expression and genomic status of the c-*myc* locus in infiltrating ductal carcinomas of the breast. Cancer Res., 48, 199–205.

Maruyama, K., Schiavi, S.C., Huse, W., Johnson, G.L. and Ruley, H.E. (1987). *myc* and E1A oncogenes alter the responses of PC12 cells to nerve growth factor and block differentiation. Oncogene, 1, 361–367.

Michitsch, R.W. and Melera, P.W.; (1985). Nucleotide sequence of the 3′ exon of the human N-*myc* gene. Nucleic Acids Res., 13, 2545–2558.

Miner, J.H. and Wold, B.J. (1991). c-*myc* inhibition of myoD and myogenin-initiated myogenic differentiation. Mol. Cell. Biol., 11, 2842–2851.

Moberg, K.H., Logan, T.J., Tyndall, W.A. and Hall, D.J. (1992). Three distinct elements within the murine c-*myc* promoter are required for transcription. Oncogene, 7, 411–421.

Moens, C.B., Auerbach, A.B., Conlon, R.A., Joyner, A.L. and Rossant, J. (1992). A targeted mutation reveals a role for N-*myc* in branching morphogenesis in the embryonic mouse lung. Genes Devel., 6, 691–704.

Moore, J.P., Todd, J.A., Hesketh, T.R. and Metcalfe, J.C. (1986). c-*fos* and c-*myc* gene activation, ionic signals, and DNA synthesis in thymocytes. J. Biol. Chem., 261, 8158–8162.

Moore, J.P., Hancock, D.C., Littlewood, T.D. and Evan, G.I. (1987). A sensitive and quantitative enzyme-linked immunosorbence assay for the c-*myc* and N-*myc* oncoproteins. Oncogene Res., 2, 65–80.

Moroy, T., Verbeek, S., Ma, A., Achacoso, P., Berns, A. and Alt, F. (1991). Eμ N- and Eμ-L-*myc* cooperate with Eμ *pim*-1 to generate lymphoid tumors at high frequency in double-transgenic mice. Oncogene, 6, 1941–1948.

Morton, C.C., Nussenzweig, M.C., Sousa, R., Sorenson, G.D., Pettengill, O.S. and Shows, T.B. (1989). Mapping and characterization of an x-linked processed gene related to MYCL1. Genomics, 4, 367–375.

Moses, H.L. (1992). TGF-β regulation of epithelial cell proliferation. Mol. Reprod. Devel., 32, 179–184.

Mucenski, M.L., Gilbert, D.J., Taylor, B.A., Jenkins, N.A. and Copeland, N.G. (1987). Common sites of viral integration in lymphomas arising in AKXD recombinant inbred mouse strains. Oncogene Res., 2, 33–48.

Mukherjee, B., Morgenbesser, S.D. and DePinho, R.A. (1992). Myc family oncoproteins function through a common pathway to transform normal cells in culture: cross-interference by max and *trans*-acting dominant mutants. Genes Devel., 6, 1480–1492.

Nepveu, A. and Marcu, K.B. (1986). Intragenic pausing and anti-sense transcription within the murine c-*myc* locus. EMBO J., 5, 2859–2865.

Nepveu, A., Levine, A.A., Campisi, J., Greenberg, M.E., Ziff, E.B. and Marcu, K.B. (1987). Alternative modes of c-*myc* regulation in growth factor-stimulated and differentiating cells. Oncogene, 1, 243–250.

Neuberger, M.S. and Calabi, F. (1983). Reciprocal chromosome translocation between c-*myc* and immunoglobulin γ2b genes. Nature, 305, 240–243.

Ocadiz, R., Sauceda, R., Cruz, M., Graef, A.M. and Gariglio, P. (1987). High correlation between molecular alterations of the c-*myc* oncogene and carcinoma of the uterine cervix. Cancer Res., 47, 4173–4177.

O'Donnell, P.V., Fleissner, E., Lonial, H., Koehne, C.F. and Reicin, A. (1985). Early clonality and high-frequency proviral integration into the c-*myc* locus in AKR leukemias. J. Virol., 55, 500–503.

Ohno, H., Fukuhara, S., Doi, S., Amakawa, R., Horii, M., Akiyama, Y., Fukida, W., Hunjo, T., Sugiyama, T. and Uchino, H. (1989). Involvement of c-myc oncogene in lymphoma cell lines with no detectable chromosome rearrangement of band 8q24. Cancer Genet. Cytogenet., 40, 73–82.

Onclercq, R., Gilardi, P., Lavenu, A. and Cremisi, C. (1988). c-myc products trans-activate the adenovirus E4 genome in EL stem cells by using the same target sequence as E1A products. J. Virol., 62, 4533–4537.

Paria, B.C., Dey, S.K. and Andrews, G.K. (1992). Antisense c-*myc* effects on preimplantation mouse embryo development. Proc. Natl Acad. Sci. USA, 89, 10051–10055.

Parkes, J.L., Cardell, R.R., Hubbard, F.C., Hubbard, D., Meltzer, A. and Penn, A. (1991). Cultured human atherosclerotic plaque smooth muscle cells retain transforming potential and display enhanced expression of the *MYC* protooncogene. Am. J. Pathol., 138, 765–775.

Parkin, N.T. and Sonenberg, N. (1989). Identification of a protein that binds specifically to RNA from the first exon of c-*myc*. Oncogene 4, 815–822.

Patchinsky, T., Jansen, H.W., Blocker, H., Frank, R. and Bister, K. (1986). Structure and transforming function of transduced mutant alleles of the chicken c-*myc* gene. J. Virol., 59, 341–353.

Payne, G.S., Bishop, M.J. and Varmus, H.E. (1982). Multiple arrangements of viral DNA and an activated host oncogene in bursal lymphomas. Nature, 295, 209–214.

Pelicci, P.-G., Knowles, D.M., Magrath, I.M. and Dalla-Favera, R. (1986). Chromosomal breakpoints and structural alterations of the c-*myc* locus differ in endemic and sporadic forms of Burkitt lymphoma. Proc. Natl Acad. Sci. USA, 83, 2984–2988.

Penn, L.J.Z., Brooks, M.W., Laufer, E.M. and Land, H. (1990a). Negative autoregulation of c-*myc* transcription. EMBO J., 9, 1113–1121.

Penn, L.J.Z., Brooks, M.W., Laufer, E.M., Littlewood, T.D., Morgenstren, J., Evan, G.I., Lee, W.M.F. and Land, H. (1990b). Domains of human c-*myc* protein required for autosuppression and cooperation with *ras* oncogenes are overlapping. Mol. Cell. Biol., 10, 4961–4966.

Pfaff, S.L. and Duesberg, P.H. (1988). Two autonomous *myc* oncogenes in avian carcinoma virus OK10. J. Virol., 62, 3703–3709.

Pietenpol, J.A., Stein, R.W., Moran, E., Yaciuk, P., Schlegel, R., Lyons, R.M., Pittelkow, M.R., Munger, K., Howley, P.M. and Moses, H.L. (1990). TGF-β1 inhibition of c-*myc* transcription and growth in keratinocytes is abrogated by viral transforming proteins with pRB binding domains. Cell, 61, 777–785.

Pietenpol, J.A., Munger, K., Howley, P.M., Stein, R.W. and Moses, H.L. (1991). Factor-binding element in the human c-*myc* promoter involved in transcriptional regulation by transforming growth factor beta 1 and by the retinoblastoma gene product. Proc. Natl Acad. Sci. USA, 88, 10227–10231.

Plet, A., Tourkine, N., Mechti, N., Jeanteur, P. and Blanchard, J.-M. (1992). *In vivo* footprints between the murine c-*myc* P1 and P2 promoters. Oncogene, 7, 1847–1851.

Prendergast, G.C., Diamond, L.E., Dahl, D. and Cole, M.D. (1990). The c-*myc*-regulated gene *mrl* encodes plasminogen activator inhibitor 1. Mol. Cell. Biol., 10, 1265–1269.

Prendergast, G.C., Hopewell, R., Gorham, B.J. and Ziff, E.B. (1992). Biphasic effect of max on myc cotrans-formation activity and dependence on amino- and carboxy-terminal max functions. Genes Devel., 6, 2429–2439.

Prochownik, E.V., Kukowska, J. and Rodgers, C. (1988). c-*myc* antisense transcripts accelerate differen-tiation and inhibit G_1 progression in murine erythroleukemia cells. Mol. Cell. Biol., 8, 3683–3695.

Rabbitts, T.H., Hamlyn, P.H., Baer, R. (1983). Altered nucleotide sequences of a translocated c-*myc* gene in Burkitt lymphoma. Nature, 306, 760–765.

Rameh, L.E. and Armelin, M.C. (1991). T antigens' role in polyomavirus transformation: c-*myc* but not c-*fos* or c-*jun* expression is a target for middle T. Oncogene, 6, 1049–1056.

Ramsay, G., Graf, T. and Hayman, M.J. (1980). Mutants of avian myelocytomatosis virus with smaller *gag* gene-related proteins have an altered transforming ability. Nature, 288, 170–172.

Ramsay, R.G., Ikeda, K., Rifkind, R.A. and Marks, P.A. (1986). Changes in gene expression associated with induced differentiation of erythroleukemia: protooncogenes, globin genes, and cell division. Proc. Natl Acad. Sci. USA, 83, 6849–6853.

Rapp, U.R., Cleveland, J.L., Frederickson, T.N., Holmes, K.L., Morse, H.C., Jansen, H.W., Patchinsky, T. and Bister, K. (1985). Rapid induction of hemopoietic neoplasms in newborn mice by a *raf* (mil)/*myc* recombinant murine retrovirus. J. Virol., 55, 23–33.

Ray, R. and Miller, D.M. (1991). Cloning and characterization of a human c-*myc* promoter-binding protein. Mol. Cell. Biol., 11, 2154–2161.

Reddy, C.D., Dasgupta, P., Saikumar, P., Dudek, H., Rauscher, F.J. and Reddy, E.P. (1992). Mutational analysis of max: role of basic, helix-loop-helix/leucine zipper domains in DNA binding, dimerization and regulation of myc-mediated transcriptional activation. Oncogene, 7, 2085–2092.

Reddy, E.P., Reynolds, R.K., Watson, D.K., Schultz, R.A., Lautenberger, J. and Papas, T.S. (1983). Nucleotide sequence analysis of the proviral genome of avian myelocytomatosis virus (MC29). Proc. Natl Acad. Sci. USA, 80, 2500–2504.

Remmers, E.F., Yang, J.-Q. and Marcu, K.B. (1986). A negative transcriptional control element located upstream of the murine c-*myc* gene. EMBO J., 5, 899–904.

Resar, L.M.S., Dolde, C., Barrett, J.F. and Dang, C.V. (1993). B-myc inhibits neoplastic transformation and transcriptional activation by c-myc. Mol. Cell. Biol., 13, 1130–1136.

Roberts, S. and Bentley, D.L. (1992). Distinct modes of transcription read through or terminate at the c-*myc* attenuator. EMBO J., 11, 1085–1093.

Roberts, S., Purton, T. and Bentley, D.L. (1992). A protein binding site in the c-*myc* promoter functions as a terminator of RNA polymerase II transcription. Genes Devel., 6, 1562–1574.

Rogers, S., Wells, R. and Rechsteiner, M. (1986). Amino acid sequences common to rapidly degraded pro-teins: the PEST hypothesis. Science, 234, 364–368.

Rosenbaum, H., Webb, E., Adams, J.M., Cory, S. and Harris, A.W. (1989). N-*myc* transgene promotes B lymphoid proliferation, elicits lymphomas and reveals cross-regulation with c-*myc*. EMBO J., 8, 749–755.

Saito, H., Hayday, A.C., Wiman, K.G., Hayward, W.S., Tonegawa, S. (1983). Activation of the c-*myc* gene by translocation: a model for translational control. Proc. Natl Acad. Sci. USA, 80, 7476–7480.

Saksela, K. (1987). Expression of the L-*myc* gene is under positive control by short-lived proteins. Onco-gene, 1, 291–296.

Sawai, S., Kato, K., Wakamatsu, Y. and Kondoh, H. (1990). Organization and expression of the chicken N-*myc* gene. Mol. Cell. Biologist, 10, 2017–2026.

Sawai, S., Shimono, A., Hanaoka, K. and Kondoh, H. (1991). Embryonic lethality resulting from disruption of both N-*myc* allelesin mouse zygotes. New Biologist, 3, 861–869.

Schmid, P., Schulz, W.A. and Hameister, H. (1989). Dynamic expression of the *myc* protooncogene in midgestation mouse embryos. Science, 243, 226–229.

Schneider-Schaulies, J., Schimpl, A. and Wecker, E. (1987). Kinetics of cellular oncogene expression in mouse lymphocytes. II. Regulation of c-*fos* and c-*myc* gene expression. Eur. J. Immunol., 17, 713–718.

Schoenenberger, C.A., Andres, A.-C., Groner, B., van der Valk, M., LeMeur, M. and Gerlinger, P. (1988). Targeted c-*myc* gene expression in mammary glands of transgenic mice induces mammary tumours with constitutive milk protein gene transcription. EMBO J., 7, 169–175.

Schreiber-Agus, N., Torres, R., Horner, J., Lau, A., Jamrich, M. and DePinho, R.A. (1993a). Comparative analysis of the expression and oncogenic activities of *Xenopus* c-, N-, and L-*myc* homologs. Mol. Cell. Biol., 13, 2456–2468.

Schreiber-Agus, N., Horner, J., Torres, R., Chiu, F.-C. and DePinho, R.A. (1993b). Zebra fish *myc* family and *max* genes: differential expression and oncogenic activity throughout vertebrate evolution. Mol. Cell. Biol., 13, 2765–2775.

Schwab, M., Alitalio, K., Klempnauer, K.-H., Varmus, H.E., Bishop, M.J., Gilbert, F., Brodeur, G., Glodstein,

M. and Trent, J. (1983). Amplified DNA with limited homology to *myc* cellular oncogene is shared by human neuroblastoma cell lines and a neuroblastoma tumour. Nature, 305, 245–248.

Schweinfest, C.W., Fujiwara, S., Lau, L.F. and Pappas, T.S. (1988). c-*myc* can induce expression of G0/G1 transition genes. Mol. Cell. Biol., 8, 3080–3087.

Seeger, R.C., Brodeur, G.M., Sather, H., Dalton, A., Siegel, S.E., Wong, K.Y. and Hammond, D. (1985). Association of multiple copies of the N-*myc* oncogene with rapid progression of neuroblastomas. New. Engl. J. Med., 313, 1111–1116.

Selten, G., Cuypers, H.T., Zijlstra, M., Melief, C. and Berns, A. (1984). Involvement of c-*myc* in MuLV-induced T cell lymphomas in mice: frequency and mechanisms of activation. EMBO J., 3, 3215–3222.

Seth, A., Alvarez, E., Gupta, S. and Davis, R.J. (1991). A phosphorylation site located in the NH2-terminal domain of c-myc increases transactivation of gene expression. J. Biol. Chem., 266, 23521–23524.

Shaw, A.P., Poirier, V., Tyler, S., Mott, M., Berry, J. and Maitland, N.J. (1988). Expression of the N-*myc* oncogene in Wilms' tumour and related tissues. Oncogene, 3, 143–149.

Sheiness, D. and Bishop, M.J. (1979). DNA and RNA from infected vertebrate cells contain nucleotide sequences related to the putative transforming gene of avian myelocytomatosis virus. J. Virol., 31, 514–521.

Shi, Y., Glynn, J.M., Guilbert, L.J., Cotter, T.G., Bissonnette, R.P. and Green, D.R. (1992). Role for c-*myc* in activation-induced apoptotic cell death in T cell hybridomas. Science, 257, 212–214.

Shibuya, H., Yoneyama, M., Ninomiya-Tsuji, J., Matsumoto, K. and Taniguchi, T. (1992). IL-2 and EGF receptors stimulate the hematopoietic cell cycle via different signaling pathways: demonstration of a novel role for c-*myc*. Cell, 70, 57–67.

Shih, C.-K., Linial, M., Goodenow, M.M. and Hayward, W.S. (1984). Nucleotide sequence 5' of the chicken c-*myc* coding region: localization of a noncoding exon that is absent from *myc* transcripts in most avian leukemia virus-induced lymphomas. Proc. Natl Acad. Sci. USA, 81, 4697–4701.

Siebenlist, U., Henninghausen, L., Battey, J. and Leder, P. (1984). Chromatin structure and protein binding in the putative regulatory region of the c-*myc* gene in Burkitt lymphoma. Cell, 37, 381–391.

Siebenlist, U., Bressler, P. and Kelly, K. (1988). Two distinct mechanisms of transcriptional control operate on c-*myc* during differentiation of HL60 cells. Mol. Cell. Biol., 8, 867–874.

Sihvola, M., Sistonen, L., Alitalo, K. and Hurme, M. (1989). Mechanism of T cell proliferation in vivo: analysis of IL-2 receptor expression and activation of c-*myc* and c-*myb* oncogenes during lymphatic regeneration. Biochem. Biophys. Res. Commun., 160, 181–188.

Sinn, E., Muller, W., Pattengale, P.K., Tepler, I., Wallace, R. and Leder, P. (1987). Coexpression of MMTV/v-Ha-*ras* and MMTV/c-*myc* genes in transgenic mice: synergistic action of oncogenes in vivo. Cell, 49, 465–475.

Slamon, D.J., Boone, T.C., Seeger, R.C., Keith, D.E., Chazin, V., Lee, H.C. and Souza, L.M. (1986). Identification and characterization of the protein encoded by the human N-*myc* oncogene. Science, 232, 768–772.

Smith, D.R., Vennstrom, B., Hayman, M.J. and Enrietto, P.J. (1985). Nucleotide sequence of HBI, a novel recombinant MC29 derivative with altered pathogenic properties. J. Virol., 56, 969–977.

Spangler, R., Bailey, S.C. and Sytkowski, A.J. (1991). Erythropoietin increases c-*myc* mRNA by a protein kinase C-dependent pathway. J. Biol. Chem., 266, 681–684.

Spicer, D.B. and Sonenshein, G.E. (1992). An antisense promoter of the murine c-*myc* gene is localized within intron 2. Mol. Cell. Biol., 12, 1324–1329.

Stanton, L.W. and Bishop, M.J. (1987). Alternative processing of RNA transcribed from NMYC. Mol. Cell. Biol., 7, 4266–4272.

Stanton, L.W., Fahrlander, P.D., Tesser, P.M. and Marcu, K.B. (1984). Nucleotide sequence comparison of normal and translocated c-*myc* genes. Nature, 310, 423–425.

Stanton, L.W., Schwab, M. and Bishop, J.M. (1986). Nucleotide sequence of the human N-*myc* gene. Proc. Natl Acad. Sci. USA, 83, 1772–1776.

Stern, D.F., Roberts, A.B., Roche, N.S., Sporn, M.B. and Weinberg, R.A. (1986). Differential responsiveness of *myc*- and *ras*-transfected cells to growth factors: Selective stimulation of *myc*-transfected cells by epidermal growth factor. Mol. Cell. Biol., 6, 870–877.

Stewart, T.A., Bellve, A.R. and Leder, P. (1984). Transcription and promoter usage of the *myc* gene in normal somatic and spermatogenic cells. Science, 226, 707–710.

Stewart M.A., Forrest, D., McFarlane, R., Onions, D.E.,Wilkie, N. and Neil, J.C. (1986). Conservation of the c-myc coding sequence in transduced feline c-*myc* genes. Virology, 154, 121–134.

Strobl, L.J. and Eick, D. (1992). Hold back of RNA polymerase II at the transcription start site mediates down-regulation of c-*myc in vivo*. EMBO J., 11, 3307–3314.

Strobl, L.J., Kohlhuber, F., Mautner, J., Polack, A. and Eick, D. (1993). Absence of a paused transcription complex from the c-*myc* P$_2$ promoter of the translocation chromosome in Burkitt's lymphoma cells: implication for the c-*myc* P$_1$/P$_2$ promoter shift. Oncogene, 8, 1437–1447.

Sugiyama, A., Kume, A., Nemoto, K., Lee, S.Y., Asami, Y., Nemoto, F., Nishimura, S. and Kuchino, Y. (1989). Isolation and characterization of s-*myc*, a member of the rat *myc* gene family. Proc. Natl Acad. Sci. USA, 86, 9144–9148.

Sullivan, N.F., Willis, A.E., Moore, J.P. and Lindahl, T. (1989). High levels of the c-*myc* protein in cell lines of Bloom's syndrome origin. Oncogene, 4, 1509–1511.

Sutrave, P., Bonner, T.I., Rapp, U.R., Jansen, H.W. and Bister, K. (1984a). Nucleotide sequence of avian retroviral oncogene v-*mil*: homologue of murine retroviral oncogene v-*raf*. Nature, 309, 85–88.

Sutrave, P., Jansen, H.W., Bister, K. and Rapp, U.R. (1984b). The 3′-terminal region of avian carcinoma virus MH2 shares sequence elements with avian sarcoma viruses Y73 and SR-A. J. Virol., 52, 703–705.

Swift, R.A., Boerkoel, C., Ridgway, A., Fujita, D.J., Dodgson, J.B. and Kung, H.-J. (1987). B-lymphoma induction by reticuloendotheliosis virus: characterization of a mutated chicken syncytial virus provirus involved in c-*myc* activation. J. Virol., 61, 2084–2090.

Symonds, G., Hartshorn, A., Kennewell, A., O'Mara, M.-A., Bruskin, A. and Bishop, M.J. (1989). Transformation of murine myelomonocytic cells by *myc*: point mutations in v-*myc* contribute synergistically to transforming potential. Oncogene, 4, 285–294.

Taya, Y., Mizusawa, S. and Nishimura, S. (1986). Nucleotide sequence of the coding region of the mouse N-*myc* gene. EMBO J., 5, 1215–1219.

Tikhonenko, A.T. and Linial, M.L. (1992). *gag* as well as *myc* sequences contribute to the transforming phenotype of the avian retrovirus FH3. J. Virol., 66, 946–955.

Tikhonenko, A.T., Hartman, A.-R. and Linial, M.L. (1993). Overproduction of v-myc in the nucleus and its excess over max are not required for avian fibroblast transformation. Mol. Cell. Biol., 13, 3523–3631.

Tourkine, N., Mechti, N., Piechaczyk, M., Jeanteur, P. and Blanchard, J.-M. (1989). *In situ* and *in vitro* evidence for intragenic binding of nuclear factors at the murine c-*myc* locus. Oncogene, 4, 973–978.

Tsuda, H., Hirohashi, S., Shimosato, Y., Hirota, T., Tsugane, S., Yamamoto, H., Miyajima, N., Toyoshima, K., Yamamoto, T., Yokota, J., Yoshida, T., Sakamoto, H., Terada, M. and Sugimura, T. (1989). Correlation between long-term survival in breast cancer patients and amplification of two putative oncogene-coamplification units: hst-1/*int*-2 and c-*erb*B-2/*ear*-1. Cancer Res., 49, 3104–3108.

Ueno, K., Katoh, K. and Kondoh, H. (1988). Subnuclear localization and anti-transforming activity of N-*myc*:β-galactosidase fusion proteins. Mol. Cell. Biol., 8, 4529–4532.

van Antwerp, M.E., Chen, D.G., Chang, C. and Prochownik, E.V. (1992). A point mutation in the myoD basic domain imparts c-myc-like properties. Proc. Natl Acad. Sci. USA, 89, 9010–9014.

van Beneden, R.J., Watson, D.K., Chen, T.T., Lautenberger, J.A. and Papas, T.S. (1986). Cellular *myc* (c-*myc*) in fish (rainbow trout): its relationship to other vertebrate *myc* genes and to the transforming genes of the MC29 family of viruses. Proc. Natl Acad. Sci. USA, 83, 3698–3702.

van Lohuizen, M., Breuer, M. and Berns, A. (1989). N-*myc* is frequently activated by proviral insertion in MuLV-induced T cell lymphomas. EMBO J., 8, 133–136.

van Lohuizen, M., Verbeek, S., Scheijen, B., Wientjens, E., van der Gulden, H. and Berns, A. (1991). Identification of cooperating oncogene in Eμ-myc transgenic mice by provirus tagging. Cell, 65, 737–752.

van Straaten, J.P. and Rabbitts, T.H. (1987). The c-*myc* protein is associated with the nuclear matrix through specific metal interaction. Oncogene Res., 1, 221–228.

Van't Veer, L.J., Beijersbergen, R.L. and Bernards, R. (1993). N-*myc* suppresses major histocompatibility complex class I gene expression through down-regulation of the p50 subunit of NF-κB. EMBO J., 12, 195–200.

Vastrik, I., Koskinen, P.J., Alitalo, K. and Makela, T.P. (1993). Alternative mRNA forms and open reading frames of the *max* gene. Oncogene, 8, 503–507.

Verbeek, S., van Lohuizen, M., van der Valk, M., Domen, J., Kraal, G. and Berns, A. (1991). Mice bearing the Eμ-*myc* and Eμ-*pim*-1 transgenes develop pre-B-cell leukemia prenatally. Mol. Cell. Biol., 11, 1176–1179.

Versteeg, R., Kruse-Wolters, M., Plomp, A.C., van Leeuwen, A., Stam, N., Ploegh, H.L., Ruiter, D.J. and Schrier, P.I. (1989). Suppression of class I human histocompatibility leucocyte antigen by c-*myc* is locus specific. J. Exp. Med., 170, 621–635.

Vriz, S., Taylor, M. and Mechali, M. (1989). Differential expression of two *Xenopus* c-*myc* proto-oncogenes during development. EMBO J., 8, 4091–4097.

Vriz, S., Lemaitre, J.-M., Leibovici, M., Thierry, N. and Mechali, M. (1992). Comparative analysis of the intracellular localization of c-myc, c-fos, and replicative proteins during the cell cycle. Mol. Cell. Biol., 12, 3548–3555.

Wada, R.K., Seeger, R.C., Reynolds, C.P., Alloggiamento, T., Yamashiro, J.M., Ruland, C., Black, A.C. and

Rosenblatt, J.D. (1992). Cell type-specific expression and negative regulation by retinoic acid of the human N-*myc* promoter in neuroblastoma cells. Oncogene, 7, 711–717.

Walker, C.W., Boom, J.D.G. and Marsh, A.G. (1992). First non-vertebrate member of the *myc* gene family is seasonally expressed in invertebrate testis. Oncogene, 7, 2007–2012.

Walther, N., Jansen, H.W., Trachmann, C. and Bister, K. (1986). Nucleotide sequence of the CMII v-*myc* allele. Virology, 154, 219–223.

Wang, Y., Sugiyama, H., Axelson, H., Panda, C.K., Babonits, M., Ma, A., Steinberg, J.M., Alt, F.W., Klein, G. and Wiener, F. (1992). Functional homology between N-*myc* and c-*myc* in murine plasmacytomagenesis: plasmacytoma development in N-*myc* transgenic mice. Oncogene, 7, 1241–1247.

Wasson, J.C., Saylors, R.L., Zeltzer, P., Friedman, H.S., Bigner, S.H., Burger, P.C., Bigner, D.D., Look, A.T., Douglass, E.C. and Brodeur, G.M. (1990). Oncogene amplification in pediatric brain tumors. Cancer Res., 50, 2987–2990.

Waters, C.M., Littlewood, T.D., Hancock, D.C., Moore, J.P. and Evan, G.I. (1991). c-*myc* protein expression in untransformed fibroblasts. Oncogene, 6, 797–805.

Watson, D.K., Reddy, E.P., Duesberg, P.H. and Papas, T.S. (1983). Nucleotide sequence analysis of the chicken c-*myc* gene reveals homology and unique coding regions by comparison with the transforming gene of avian myelocytomatosis virus MC29, Δ*gag-myc*. Proc. Natl Acad. Sci. USA, 80, 2146–2150.

Watt, R., Stanton, L.W., Marcu, K.B., Gallo, R.C., Croce, C.M. and Rovera, G. (1983). Nucleotide sequence of cloned cDNA of human c-*myc* oncogene. Nature, 303, 725–728.

Wechsler, D.S. and Dang, C.V. (1992). Opposite orientations of DNA bending by c-myc and max. Proc. Natl Acad. Sci. USA, 89, 7635–7639.

Wenzel, A., Cziepluch, C., Hamann, U., Schurmann, J. and Schwab, M. (1991). The N-myc oncoprotein is associated in vivo with the phosphoprotein max (p20/22) in human neuroblastoma cells. EMBO J., 10, 3703–3712.

Whitesell, L., Rosolen, A. and Neckers, L.M. (1991). Episome-generated N-*myc* antisense RNA restricts the differentiation potential of primitive neuroectodermal cell lines. Mol. Cell. Biol., 11, 1360–1371.

Wiener, F., Ohno, S., Babonits, M., Sumegi, J., Wirschubsky, Z., Klein, G., Mushinski, J.F. and Potter, M. (1984). Hemizygous interstitial deletion of chromosome 15 (band D) in three translocation-negative murine plasmacytomas. Proc. Natl Acad. Sci. USA, 81, 1159–1163.

Wilson, T. and Treisman, R. (1988). Removal of poly(A) and consequent degradation of c-*fos* mRNA facilitated by 3′ AU-rich sequences. Nature, 336, 396–399.

Wisdom, R. and Lee, W. (1991). The protein-coding region of c-*myc* mRNA contains a sequence that specifies rapid mRNA turnover and induction by protein synthesis inhibitors. Genes Devel., 5, 232–243.

Wittig, B., Wolfl, S., Dorbic, T., Vahrson, W. and Rich, A. (1992). Transcription of human c-*myc* in permeabilized nuclei is associated with formation of Z-DNA in three discrete regions of the gene. EMBO J., 11, 4653–4663.

Yang, B.-S, Geddes, T.J., Pogulis, R.J., de-Crombrugghe, B. and Freytag, S.O. (1991). Transcriptional suppression of cellular gene expression by c-Myc. Mol. Cell. Biol., 11, 2291–2295.

Yokota, J., Wada, M., Yoshida, T., Noguchi, M., Terasaki, T., Shimosato, Y., Sugimura, T. and Terada, M. (1988). Heterogeneity of lung cancer cells with respect to the amplification and rearrangement of *myc* family genes. Oncogene, 2, 607–611.

Zajac-Kaye, M., Gelmann, E.P. and Levens, D. (1988). A point mutation in the c-*myc* locus of a Burkitt lymphoma abolishes binding of a nuclear protein. Science, 240, 1776–1780.

Zervos, A.S., Gyuris, J. and Brent, R. (1993). Mxi1, a protein that specifically interacts with max to bind myc-max recognition sites. Cell, 72, 223–232.

Zimmerman, K.A., Yancopoulos, G.D., Collum, R.G., Smith, R.K., Kohl, N.E., Denis, K.A., Nau, M.M., Witte, O.N., Toran-Allerand, D., Gee, C.E., Minna, J.D. and Alt, F.W. (1986). Differential expression of *myc* family genes during murine development. Nature, 319, 780–783.

Zubiaga, A.M., Munoz, E. and Huber, B.T. (1991). Production of IL-1a by activated Th type 2 cells. Its role as an autocrine growth factor. J. Immunol., 146, 3849–3856.

PDGFB/Sis

v-*sis* is the acutely transforming oncogene of simian sarcoma virus (SSV) isolated from woolly monkey sarcoma (Theilen *et al.*, 1971). Helper virus: simian sarcoma associated virus (SSAV), type C. *sis* is derived from the platelet-derived growth factor B chain gene (*Pdgfb*).

Related genes

The 3' untranslated regions of *Pdgfb* share sequence homology with the corresponding regions of human *IL2*, human β1-IFN, human and mouse β-NGF and proenkephalin (Ratner *et al.*, 1985). PDGFA is 60% similar to PDGFB.

Cross-species homology

PDGFB: 92% identity (human and cat); 89% (human and mouse). A non-coding region at the start of exon 7 that is deleted in v-*sis* is >92% conserved between human, mouse and cat *Pdgfb*. Loss of this region may increase v-*sis* mRNA stability (Bonthron *et al.*, 1991).

Transformation

MAN

PDGF and *PDGF* receptor genes are co-expressed in primary human astrocytomas (Maxwell *et al.*, 1990) and *PDGFB* transcription occurs in fibrosarcomas and glioblastomas. Expression is elevated in malignant mesothelioma cell lines but is barely detectable in normal mesothelial cells. The malignant cell line expresses primarily PDGFB receptors (and PDGFB) whereas the normal cells express only PDGFA receptors (Versnel *et al.*, 1991) and synthesize only PDGFA. This suggests that both types of cell may undergo autocrine stimulation, PDGF-AA acting via the α receptor and PDGF-BB via the B receptor (Heldin, 1992).

The *PDGFB* gene (22q13) is translocated to chromosome 9 in chronic myelogenous leukaemia (i.e. the reciprocal translocation to that undergone by *ABL*). There is no evidence that the translocated gene is transcribed, however, and *PDGFB* probably does not play a role in CML.

In a variety of sarcomas and astrocytomas cellular proliferation is promoted by autocrine PDGF stimulation (Fleming *et al.*, 1992).

ANIMALS

SSV induces fibrosarcomas and glioblastomas in monkeys (Wolfe *et al.*, 1972). In human WM9 melanoma cells expression of PDGF-BB promotes vascularization of the tumours that arise when the cells are injected into mice.

IN VITRO

SSV transforms rat kidney cells into a fibroblastic morphology unusual for cells infected by acute transforming viruses and also transforms fibroblasts. Suramin, a polyanionic drug used clinically for parasitic infections, disrupts PDGF ligand–receptor binding and induces reversion of fibroblasts transformed by v-*sis* (Fleming *et al.*, 1989).

Murine cell lines overexpressing v-*sis*/*Pdgfb* are highly tumorigenic: *in vitro* their growth is independent of the presence of PDGF and they show constitutively high expression of *Myc*, *Fos*, *Jun* and *Jund* but expression of other early response genes (*Fra-1*, *Fosb*, *Junb* and *Krox20*) is unaltered (Sonobe *et al.*, 1991), emphasizing the probable importance of *Myc*, *Fos*, *Jun* and *Jund* in the regulation of growth.

	PDGFB/Pdgfb	v-sis
Nucleotides (kb)		
Human	24	0.813 (*env–sis* fused ORF)
Mouse	~20	5.1 (SSV)
Chromosome		
Human	22q12.3–q13.1	
Mouse	15E	
Exons	7 (7th non-coding)	
Amino acids	241	220 (v-*sis*)
Mass (kDa)		
(predicted)	28	33
(expressed)	p26^{sis}	p28$^{v\text{-}sis}$ (forms p56 homodimer)
mRNA (kb)	2.7/4.2 (human)	
mRNA half-life (min)	40–100	

Protein location

v-*sis* (p28^{sis}) is detectable in SSV-transformed NRK cells (Devare *et al.*, 1983). It is synthesized on rough endoplasmic reticulum, glycosylated in the Golgi apparatus and retained at the cell surface by virtue of a hydrophilic membrane retention domain located at the C-terminus (LaRochelle *et al.*, 1991). Very little p28^{sis} is secreted from fibroblasts, whereas PDGF A chain is readily released.

Protein function

PDGF is released from the α granules of platelets during blood clotting but is also synthesized by many other types of cell (Heldin and Westermark, 1990). It is the major growth factor in human serum and *in vitro* it is a potent mitogen. PDGF is a disulfide-bonded dimer of two chains (A and B) that occurs in three forms (AA, BB and AB). PDGFB is generated by proteolytic cleavage of a precursor. All three forms of PDGF occur in both normal and transformed cells.

Structure of the simian sarcoma virus (SSV) genome

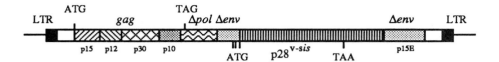

v-*sis* together with 5' (345 nucleotides) and 3' (305 nucleotides) segments of SSAV constitute the transforming gene (Robbins *et al.*, 1982). The entire SSAV *gag* gene is included in the SSV genome: there is a large 5' deletion from *pol* and the 3' end of *env* overlaps with the *pol* ORF such that the reading frame extends into v-*sis*. The ORF of v-*sis* initiates within the SSAV *env* gene.

Structure of the human *PDGFB* gene

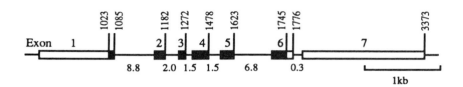

Black boxes: coding exons. The numbers between the exons are the intron sizes (kb). The nucleotides at the 3' ends of the exons are numbered and indicate that the size of the spliced mRNA is 3373 bp.

Structure of v-SIS and human PDGFB

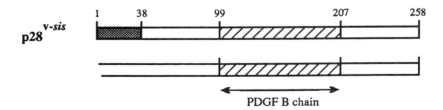

The initiation codon used in SSV is the normal one for the Mo-MuLV *env* gene product: the *env*-derived portion encodes a putative signal sequence (38 amino acids) but the transmembrane sequence present in the normal ENV protein has been deleted. v-*sis* encodes 220 amino acids. Residues 99–207 of v-SIS differ in only four positions from the 108 residues of PDGFB. The PDGFB precursor undergoes proteolytic cleavage to generate a final form in which the N- and C-termini correspond to amino acids 99 and 207 of v-SIS, respectively (Robbins *et al.*, 1983).

Sequences of p28$^{v\text{-}sis}$ and the precursors of human PDGFA and PDGFB and mouse PDGFB

```
v-SIS           (1)                                              MSPGSWKKLIILLSCV

Human PDGFA     (1)    -RTLAC-L-LG-G--AH-LA-EAE--R-VI-R-ARSQ-H-I-------EI-SVGSEDSL
Human PDGFB     (1)    MNRCWALFLSLCCYLRLVSAEGDPIPEELYEMLSDHSIRSFDDLQRLLHGDPGEEDGAE
Mouse PDGFB     (1)    --------P----------------------------------------R-SVD-----
v-SIS          (39)    FGGGGTSLQNKNPHQPMTLTWQ---------K---G------------Q--S-K-----

Human PDGFA    (60)    DTSLRAHGVHATKHVPEK-PLPIRRKRS-E- -VP-V-----VIY--P-SQV-P-S----
Human PDGFB    (60)    LDLNMTRSHSGGELESLARGRRSLGSLTIAEPAMIAECKTRTEVFEISRRLIDRTNANFL
Mouse PDGFB    (60)    -------A---V----SS---------AA----V----------Q---N---------
v-SIS          (77)    ------------------K------SV-------------------------------

Human PDGFA   (119)    I-------K--T----TSS-K-Q-SR-HH-S-K-A-V-Y-----KL-EVQ-R--E--E-A
Human PDGFB   (120)    VWPPCVEVQRCSGCCNNRNVQCRPTQVQLRPVQVRKIEIVRKKPIFKKATVTLEDHLACK
Mouse PDGFB   (120)    ---------------------AS---M------------------------------
v-SIS         (137)    ---------------------------------------------------------

Human PDGFA   (189)    -A-TSLNPDYREEDT-RPRESG-KRKRKRLKP- (211)
Human PDGFB   (180)    CETVAAARPVTRSPGGSQEQRAKTPQTRVTIRTVRVRRPPKGKHRKFKHTHDKTALKETLGA (241)
Mouse PDGFB   (180)    ---IVTP--------T-R--------A--------I----------------A------- (241)
v-SIS         (197)    --I-----A------T--------T-S----------------C-------------- (258)
```

Dashes indicate identity with PDGFB. Signal sequences are shown in underlined italics. The N-terminal 38 amino acids of v-SIS are encoded by the 5′ region of Mo-MuLV *env*. The region cleaved from the precursor (amino acids 82–190) to form PDGFB is underlined. This region corresponds to amino acids 99–207 of v-SIS.

Databank file names and accession numbers

	GENE	*EMBL*	*SWISSPROT*	*REFERENCES*
SSV	v-*sis*	RESSV1 V01201	TSIS_SMSAV P01128	Devare *et al.*, 1983
Human	*PDGFA* precursor	Hspdgfa1 M21571 Hspdgfar X03795 Hspdgfa X06374 Hspdga1 to Hspdga7, M20488 to M20494	PDGA_HUMAN P04085	Bonthron *et al.*, 1988 Rorsman *et al.*, 1988 Betsholtz *et al.*, 1986 Hoppe *et al.*, 1987 Tong *et al.*, 1987 Collins *et al.*, 1987
Human	*PDGFB* (*PDGF2* or *SIS*)	Hssispdg M12783 Hssis1 to Hssis4, K01913 to K01916 Hspdgfba M16288 Hspdgfb1 X03702	PDGB_HUMAN P01127	Rao *et al.*, 1986 Antoniades and Hunkapiller, 1983 Chiu *et al.*, 1984 Collins *et al.*, 1985 Josephs *et al.*, 1984 Ratner *et al.*, 1985 Waterfield *et al.*, 1983 Weich *et al.*, 1986
Human	*SIS* (v-*sis* homologous region)	Hscsis V00504		Josephs *et al.*, 1983

	GENE	EMBL	SWISSPROT	REFERENCES
Human	*SIS* (3′ flank)	Hscsisa M32009	P01127	Tong *et al.*, 1986
Human	*SIS* (clone pSM-1)	Hscsist X02744		Ratner *et al.*, 1985
Feline	*Sis* (exon 1)	Fssisg1 X06297		Van den Ouweland *et al.*, 1987
Cat	*Sis* 5′ region	Fssisg5 X03494		Van den Ouweland *et al.*, 1986
Mouse	*Sis* exon 1	Gbo:Muscsis01 M64844; M55394 Daily:Mmcsis01 M64844; M55394		Bonthron *et al.*, 1991
Human	*PDGFAR*	Hspdgf03 M21574 Hspdgf02 M22734	PGDS_HUMAN P16234	Matsui *et al.*, 1989 Claesson-Welsh *et al.*, 1989
Human	*PDGFBR*	Hspdgfra J03278 Hspdgfr M21616	PGDR_HUMAN P09619	Gronwald *et al.*, 1988 Claesson-Welsh *et al.*, 1988 Roberts *et al.*, 1988 Kazlauskas and Cooper, 1989
Mouse	*Pdgfa* (*PDGF-1*)	Mmpdgfa M29464	PDGA_MOUSE P20033	Mercola *et al.*, 1990
Mouse	*Pdgfbr*	Mmpdgfre X04367	PGDR_MOUSE P05622	Yarden *et al.*, 1986
Cat	*Pdgfb* (*PDGF-2*)	Fssismsg X05112	PDGB_FELCA P12919	van den Ouweland *et al.*, 1987
Pig	*Pdgfb* fragment		PDGB_PIG P20034	Stroobant and Waterfield, 1984
Xenopus laevis	*Pdgfa*	Xlpdgfa M23237 Xlpdgfaa M23238 Xlpdgfac X17545	PDGA_XENLA P13698	Mercola *et al.*, 1988 Bejcek *et al.*, 1990

Reviews

Heldin, C.-H. (1992). Structural and functional properties on platelet-derived growth factor. EMBO J., 11, 4251–4259.

Heldin, C.-H. and Westermark, B. (1990). Signal transduction by the receptors for platelet-derived growth factor. J. Cell Sci., 96, 193–196.

Papers

Aaronson, S.A., Igarashi, H., Rao, C.D., Finzi, E., Fleming, T.P., Segatto, O. and Robbins, K.C. (1986). Role of genes for normal growth factors in human malignancy. Int. Symp. Princess Takamatsu Cancer Res. Fund, 17, 95–108.

Antoniades, H.N. and Hunkapiller, M.W. (1983). Human platelet-derived growth factor (PDGF): amino-terminal amino acid sequence. Science, 220, 963–965.

Bejcek, B.E., Li, D.Y. and Deuel, T.F. (1990). Nucleotide sequence of a cDNA clone of *Xenopus* platelet-derived growth factor A-chain. Nucleic Acids Res., 18, 680.

Betsholtz, C., Johnsson, A., Heldin, C.-H., Westermark, B., Lind, P., Urdea, M.S., Eddy, R., Shows, T.B., Philpott, K., Mellor, A.L., Knott, T.J. and Scott, J. (1986). cDNA sequence and chromosomal localization of human platelet-derived growth factor A-chain and its expression in tumour cell lines. Nature, 320, 695–699.

Bonthron, D.T., Morton, C.C., Orkin, S.H. and Collins, T. (1988). Platelet-derived growth factor A chain: gene structure, chromosomal location, and basis for alternative mRNA splicing. Proc. Natl Acad. Sci. USA, 85, 1492–1496.

Bonthron, D.T., Sultan, P. and Collins, T. (1991). Structure of the murine c-*sis* proto-oncogene (*sis*, PDGF B) encoding the B chain of platelet-derived growth factor. Genomics, 10, 287–292.

Chiu, I.-M., Reddy, E.P., Givol, D., Robbins, K.C., Tronick, S.R. and Aaronson, S.A. (1984). Nucleotide sequence analysis identifies the human c-*sis* proto-oncogene as a structural gene for platelet-derived growth factor. Cell, 37, 123–129.

Claesson-Welsh, L., Eriksson, A., Moren, A., Severinsson, L., Ek, B., Ostman, A., Betsholtz, C. and Heldin, C.-H. (1988). cDNA cloning and expression of a human platelet-derived growth factor (PDGF) receptor specific for B-chain-containing PDGF molecules. Mol. Cell. Biol., 8, 3476–3486.

Claesson-Welsh, L., Eriksson, A., Westermark, B. and Heldin, C.-H. (1989). cDNA cloning and expression of the human A-type platelet-derived growth factor (PDGF) receptor establishes structural similarity to the B-type PDGF receptor. Proc. Natl Acad. Sci. USA, 86, 4917–4921.

Collins, T., Ginsburg, D., Boss, J.M., Orkin, S.H. and Pober, J.S. (1985). Cultured human endothelial cells express platelet-derived growth factor B chain: cDNA cloning and structural analysis. Nature, 316, 748–750.

Collins, T., Bonthron, D.T. and Orkin, S.H. (1987). Alternative RNA splicing affects function of encoded platelet-derived growth factor A chain. Nature, 328, 621–624.

Devare, S.G., Reddy, E.P., Law, J.D., Robbins, K.C. and Aaronson, S.A. (1983). Nucleotide sequence of the simian sarcoma virus genome: demonstration that its acquired cellular sequences encode the trans-forming gene product p28^{sis}. Proc. Natl Acad. Sci. USA, 80, 731–735.

Doolittle, R.F., Hunkapiller, M.W., Hood, L.E., Devare, S.G., Robbins, K.C., Aaronson, S.A. and Antoni-ades, H.N. (1983). Simian sarcoma virus onc gene, v-*sis*, is derived from the gene (or genes) encoding a platelet-derived growth factor. Science, 221, 275–277.

Fleming, T.P., Matsui, T., Molloy, C.J., Robbins, K.C. and Aaronson, S.A. (1992). Autocrine mechanism for v-*sis* transformation requires cell surface localization of internally activated growth factor receptors. Proc. Natl Acad. Sci. USA, 86, 8063–8067.

Fleming, T.P., Matsui, T., Heideran, M.A., Molloy, C.J., Artrip, J. and Aaronson, S.A. (1992). Demonstration of an activated platelet-derived growth factor autocrine pathway and its role in human tumor cell pro-liferation *in vitro*. Oncogene, 7, 1355–1359.

Gronwald, R.G., Grant, F.J., Haldeman, B.A., Hart, C.E., O'Hara, P.J., Hagen, F.S., Ross, R., Bowen-Pope, D.F., Murray, M.J. (1988). Cloning and expression of a cDNA coding for the human platelet-derived growth factor receptor: evidence for more than one receptor class. Proc. Natl Acad. Sci. USA, 85, 3435–3439.

Heldin, C.-H., Johnsson, A., Wennergren, S., Wernstedt, C., Betsholtz, C. and Westermark, B. (1986). A human osteosarcoma cell line secretes a growth factor structurally related to a homodimer of PDGF A-chains. Nature, 319, 511–514.

Hoppe, J., Schumacher, L., Eichner, W. and Weich, H.A. (1987). The long 3'-untranslated regions of the PDGF-A and -B mRNAs are only distantly related. FEBS Letts., 223, 243–246.

Johnsson, A., Betsholtz, C., Heldin, C.-H. and Westermark, B. (1986). The phenotypic characteristics of simian sarcoma virus-transformed human fibroblasts suggest that the v-*sis* gene product acts solely as a PDGF receptor agonist in cell transformation. EMBO J., 5, 1535–1541.

Josephs, S.F., Dalla Favera, R., Gelmann, E.P., Gallo, R.C., Wong-Staal, F. (1983). 5' viral and human cellu-lar sequences corresponding to the transforming gene of simian sarcoma virus. Science, 219, 503–505.

Josephs, S.F., Ratner, L., Clarke, M.F., Westin, E.H., Reitz, M.S. and Wong-Staal, F. (1984). Transforming potential of human c-*sis* nucleotide sequences encoding platelet-derived growth factor. Science, 225, 636–639.

Kazlauskas, A. and Cooper, J.A. (1989). Autophosphorylation of the PDGF receptor in the kinase insert region regulates interactions with cell proteins. Cell, 58, 1121–1133.

King, C.R., Giese, N.A., Robbins, K.C. and Aaronson, S.A. (1985). In vitro mutagenesis of the v-*sis* transforming gene defines functional domains of its growth factor-related product. Proc. Natl Acad. Sci. USA, 82, 5291–5299.

LaRochelle, W.J., May-Siroff, M., Robbins, K.C. and Aaronson, S.A. (1991). A novel mechanism regulating growth factor association with the cell surface: identification of a PDGF retention domain. Genes Devel., 5, 1191–1199.

Matsui, T., Heidaran, M., Miki, T., Popescu, N., La-Rochelle, W., Kraus, M., Pierce, J. and Aaronson, S. (1989). Isolation of a novel receptor cDNA establishes the existence of two PDGF receptor genes. Science, 243, 800–804.

Maxwell, M., Naber, S.P., Wolfe, H.J., Galanopoulos, T., Hedley-White, E.T., Black, P.McL. and Antoniades, H.N. (1990). Coexpression of platelet-derived growth factor (PDGF) and PDGF-receptor genes by primary human astrocytomas may contribute to their development and maintenance. J. Clin. Invest., 86, 131–140.

Mercola, M., Melton, D.A. and Stiles C.D. (1988). Platelet-derived growth factor A chain is maternally encoded in *Xenopus* embryos. Science, 241, 1223–1225.

Mercola, M., Wang, C.Y., Kelly, J., Brownlee, C., Jackson-Grusby, L., Stiles, C. and Bowen-Pope, D. (1990). Selective expression of PDGF A and its receptor during early mouse embryogenesis. Devel. Biol., 138, 114–122.

Rao, C.D., Igarashi, H., Chiu, I.M., Robbins, K.C. and Aaronson, S.A. (1986). Structure and sequence of the human c-*sis*/platelet-derived growth factor 2 (SIS/PDGF2) transcriptional unit. Proc. Natl Acad. Sci. USA, 83, 2392–2396.

Ratner, L., Josephs, S.F., Jarrett, R., Reitz, M.S. and Wong-Staal, F. (1985). Nucleotide sequence of transforming human c-*sis* cDNA clones with homology to platelet-derived growth factor. Nucleic Acids Res., 13, 5007–5018.

Robbins, K.C., Devare, S.G., Reddy, E.P. and Aaronson, S.A. (1982). *In vivo* identification of the transforming gene product of simian sarcoma virus. Science, 218, 1131–1133.

Robbins, K.C., Antoniades, H.N., Devare, S.G., Hunkapiller, M.W. and Aaronson, S.A. (1983). Structural and imunological similarities between simian sarcoma virus gene product(s) and human platelet-derived growth factor. Nature, 305, 605–608.

Roberts, W.M., Look, A.T., Roussel, M.F. and Sherr, C.J. (1988). Tandem linkage of human CSF-1 receptor (c-*fms*) and PDGF receptor genes. Cell, 55, 655–661.

Rorsman, F., Bywater, M., Knott, T.J., Scott, J. and Betsholtz, C. (1988). Structural characterization of the human platelet-derived growth factor A-chain cDNA and gene: alternative exon usage predicts two different precursor proteins. Mol. Cell. Biol., 8, 571–577.

Sonobe, M.H., Bravo, R. and Armelin, M.S. (1991). Imbalanced expression of cellular nuclear oncogenes caused by v-*sis*/PDGF-2. Oncogene, 6, 1531–1537.

Stroobant, P. and Waterfield, M.D. (1984). Purification and properties of porcine platelet-derived growth factor. EMBO J., 3, 2963–2967.

Theilen, G.P., Gould, D., Fowler, M. and Dungworth, D.L. (1971). C-type virus in tumor tissue of a woolly monkey (*Lagothrix* ssp.) with fibrosarcoma. J. Natl Cancer Inst., 47, 881–889.

Tong, B.D., Levine, S.E., Jaye, M., Ricca, G., Drohan, W., Maciag, T. and Deuel T.F. (1986). Isolation and sequencing of a cDNA clone homologous to the v-*sis* oncogene from human endothelial cells. Mol. Cell. Biol., 6, 3018–3022.

Tong, B.D., Auer, D.E., Jaye, M., Kaplow, J.M., Ricca, G., McConathy, E., Drohan, W. and Deuel, T.F. (1987). cDNA clones reveal differences between human glial and endothelial cell platelet-derived growth factor A-chains. Nature, 328, 619–621.

Van den Ouweland, A.M.W., Roebroek, A.J.M., Schalken, J.A., Claesen, C.A.A., Bloemers, H.P.J. and Van de Ven W.J.M. (1986). Structure and nucleotide sequence of the 5′ region of the human and feline c-*sis* proto-oncogenes. Nucleic Acids Res., 14, 765–778.

Van den Ouweland, A.M.W., Van Groningen, J.J.M., Schalken, J.A., Van Neck, H.W., Bloemers, P.J. and Van de Ven, W.J.M. (1987). Genetic organization of the c-*sis* transcription unit. Nucleic Acids Res.,15, 959–970.

Versnel, M.A., Claesson-Welsh, L., Hammacher, A., Bouts, M.J., van der Kwast, T.H., Eriksson, A., Willemsen, R., Weima, S.M., Hoogsteden, H.C., Hagemeijer, A. and Heldin, C.-H. (1991). Human malignant mesothelioma cell lines express PDGF β-receptors whereas cultured normal mesothelial cells express predominantly PDGF α-receptors. Oncogene, 6, 2005–2011.

Waterfield, M.D., Scrace, G.T., Whittle, N., Stroobant, P., Johnsson, A., Wasteson, A., Westermark, B. Heldin, C.-H., Huang, H.S. and Deuel, T.F. (1983). Platelet-derived growth factor is structurally related to the putative transforming protein p28^{sis} of simian sarcoma virus. Nature, 304, 35–39.

Weich, H.A., Sebald, W., Schairer, H.U. and Hoppe, J. (1986). The human osteosarcoma cell line U-2 OS expresses a 3.8 kilobase mRNA which codes for the sequence of the PDGF-B chain (published erratum appears in FEBS Letts., (1986) 201, 180). FEBS Letts., 198, 344–348.

Westermark, B., Johnsson, A., Paulsson, Y., Betsholtz, C., Heldin, C.H., Herlyn, M., Rodeck, U. and Koprowski, H. (1986). Human melanoma cell lines of primary and metastatic origin express the genes encoding the chains of platelet-derived growth factor (PDGF) and produce a PDGF-like growth factor. Proc. Natl Acad. Sci. USA, 83, 7197–7200.

Wolfe, L.G., Smith, R.K. and Deinhardt, F. (1972). Simian sarcoma virus, Type 1 (*Lagothrix*): focus assay and demonstration of nontransforming associated virus. J. Natl Cancer Inst., 48, 1905–1907.

Yarden, Y., Escobedo, J.A., Kuang, W.J., Yang-Feng, T.L., Daniel, T.O., Tremble, P.M., Chen, E.Y., Ando, M.E., Harkins, R.N., Francke, U., Fried, V.A., Ullrich, A. and Williams, L.T. (1986). Structure of the receptor for platelet-derived growth factor helps define a family of closely related growth factor receptors. Nature, 323, 226–232.

PIM

Pim-1 was first identified as a common *proviral integration* site in *M*uLV-induced murine T cell lymphomas (Cuypers *et al.*, 1986; Nagarajan *et al.*, 1986; Wirschubsky *et al.*, 1986; Hanecak *et al.*, 1988).

Related genes

Pim has extensive homology with the protein kinase gene family (van Beveren and Verma, 1986) and high homology with the γ subunit of phosphorylase kinase. PIM has C-terminal homology with ABL and N-terminal homology with MOS.

Cross-species homology

Human and mouse PIM1 are highly conserved: 94% identity overall; 98% for N-terminal 250 amino acids (Reeves *et al.*, 1990).

Transformation

MAN

Enhanced *PIM1* transcription occurs in some acute myeloid and lymphoid leukaemias (Nagarajan *et al.*, 1986; Amson *et al.*, 1989) although the 6;9 translocation is not the direct cause (von Lindern *et al.*, 1989). Thus, although the *PIM1* human chromosome site (6p21) is fragile, elevated PIM1 protein synthesis occurs in many human leukaemias by mechanisms other than translocation or amplification.

ANIMALS

Pim-1 and *Myc* are the most frequently occupied insertion sites in MuLV-induced tumours and both may be activated within the same cell lineage (Selten *et al.*, 1984; O'Donnell *et al.*, 1985). Activation of *Pim-1* also occurs in B cell lymphomas (Mucenski *et al.*, 1986, 1987) and in murine thymomas induced by NMU (Warren *et al.*, 1987).

IN VITRO

Pim-1 alone does not transform 3T3 fibroblasts but causes transformation in cooperation with *Myc* or *Ras*. *Pim-1* does not appear to be necessary for proliferation or differentiation of embryonic stem cells *in vitro* (te Riele *et al.*, 1990).

TRANSGENIC MICE

Pim-1 is the integration locus of Mo-MuLV in 35% of B cell lymphomas generated in Eμ–*myc* transgenic mice (van Lohuizen *et al.*, 1991). Transgenic animals overexpressing *Pim-1* in lymphoid cells show a low frequency of predisposition to lymphomagenesis but have a greatly increased susceptibility to tumour induction by MuLV or by *N*-ethyl-nitrosourea (Breuer *et al.*, 1991). It has been found that 78%, 22% and 44% of tumours overexpressing *Pim-1* also show activation of *Myc*, *Nmyc* and *Pal-1*, respectively (see **MYC**, page 316).

	PIM1/Pim-1
Nucleotides	~5 kb
Chromosome	
Human	6p21
Mouse	17 (Ark *et al.*, 1991)
Exons	6
mRNA (kb)	
Human	2.9
Mouse	2.8
	2.0–2.6 in some lymphomas with provirally activated *Pim-1* (Selten *et al.*, 1986)
mRNA half-life (min)	30
Amino acids	
Human, mouse	313
Mass (kDa)	
(predicted) (expressed)	35
Human	35 (Zakut-Houri *et al.*, 1987; Telerman *et al.*, 1988)
Mouse	34/44 (generated from two translational initiation codons, an ATG at the end of exon 1 and an in-frame CTG that extends the 5′ translated region of exon 1; Saris *et al.*, 1991)
Protein half-life	10 min (34 kDa); ~1 h (44 kDa) (Saris *et al.*, 1991)

Cellular location

Cytoplasmic.

Tissue location

Pim-1 is expressed at high concentrations in haematopoietic tissues, testis and ovaries and in embryonic stem cells (Amson *et al.*, 1989; Meeker *et al.*, 1990).

Transcripts shorter than the 2.8 kb mRNA occur in testis (Meijer *et al.*, 1987). A 2.4 kb *Pim-1* transcript is expressed in post-meiotic mouse spermatids (Sorrentino *et al.*, 1988) and a highly stable 2.3 kb mRNA in rat testes arises from the use of an alternative polyadenylation event that removes an A/U-rich regulatory element from the 3′ region (Wingett *et al.*, 1992).

Protein function

PIM1 is a serine/threonine protein kinase involved in early B and T cell lymphomagenesis (Dautry *et al.*, 1988). Expression is highly induced by IL-2, IL-3 or GM-CSF. In homozygous *Pim-1*-deleted mice bone marrow cell growth (colony formation) in response to IL-7 is inhibited (Berns *et al.*, 1992). However, complete inactivation of *Pim-1* loci in embryonic stem cells does not inhibit their differentiation (te Riele *et al.*, 1990). Physiological substrates have not been identified.

Proviral integration sites in murine *Pim-1*

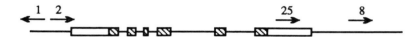

Hatched boxes: exon coding sequences (Cuypers *et al.*, 1984; Selten *et al.*, 1986). Arrows indicate regions of integration, orientation and number of proviruses detected.

Pim-1 does not have a TATAA sequence upstream from the putative transcription initiation site but has an eightfold repeat of a GC-rich motif (CCGCCC) that specifically binds SP-1 and the lymphoid-specific ATGCAAAT sequence.

Proviral activation of *Pim-1* involves elevated transcription by enhancer insertion and, usually, removal of 3′ untranslated (ATTT)$_5$ sequences that destabilize mRNAs. The protein coding domain is unaffected by insertions and the transforming effects of *Pim-1* are thus due to abnormally high expression of the gene. In most lymphomas the provirus is integrated within the *Pim-1* gene and has duplicated or triplicated enhancer regions within the LTRs. Integrations within the gene (in the 3′ untranslated region) or 3′ of the gene are all in the same transcriptional orientation as *Pim-1*. The concentration of *Pim-1* mRNA is higher in such tumours than when integration is outside the transcription unit: transcription is terminated at the polyadenylation signal in the 5′ LTR, generating truncated *Pim-1* transcripts lacking up to 1300 bases. Proviruses integrated upstream of *Pim-1* and in the same transcriptional orientation have intact 5′ and 3′ LTRs but major internal deletions. Such integrations do not provide a promoter for *Pim-1*, nor do they alter the transcript size: thus transcriptional enhancement appears to be the mechanism of activation for integrations outside coding regions of *Pim-1*.

Sequences of human and mouse PIM

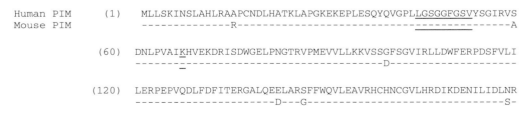

```
Human PIM   (180)   GELKLIDFGSGALLKDTVYTDFDGTRVYSPPEWIRYHRYHGRSAAVWSLGILLYDMVCGD
Mouse PIM           --I---------------------------------------------------------

            (240)   IPFEHDEEIIRGQVFFRQRVSSECQHLIRWCLALRPSDRPTFEEIQNHPWMQDVLLPQET
                    -----------------T---------K---S-------S----R------GD----AA

            (300)   AEIHLHSLSPGPSK (313)
                    S---------S-- (313)
```

Dashes indicate identity with human PIM. ATP binding sites underlined.

Databank file names and accession numbers

	GENE	EMBL	SWISSPROT	REFERENCES
Human	PIM1	Hspim1a M27903	KPIM_HUMAN	Reeves *et al.*, 1990
		Hspim1 M16750	P11309	Zakut-Houri *et al.*, 1987
		Hspim1e M54915		Domen *et al.*, 1987
Mouse	Pim-1	Mmpim1 P06803	KPIM_MOUSE P06803	Selten *et al.*, 1986

Papers

Amson, R., Sigaux, F., Przedborski, S., Flandrin, G., Givol, D. and Telerman, A. (1989). The human protoon-cogene product p33pim is expressed during fetal hematopoiesis and in diverse leukemias. Proc. Natl Acad. Sci. USA, 86, 8857–8861.

Ark, B., Gummere, G., Bennett, D. and Artzt, K. (1991). Mapping of the *pim*-1 oncogene in mouse t-haplotypes and its use to define the relative map positions of the *tcl* loci $t^0(t^6)$ and t^{w12} and the marker *tf* (*tufted*). Genomics, 10, 385–389.

Berns, A., Domen, J., van der Lugt, van Lohuizen, M., te Riele, H., Robanus Maandag, E., Saris, C., Laird, P., Clark, A. and Hooper, M. (1992). Effects of loss-of-function mutations in the *pim*-1 oncogene *in vitro* and *in vivo*. J. Cell. Chem., Suppl. 16F, 4.

Breuer, M., Wientjens, E., Verbeek, S., Slebos, R. and Berns, A. (1991). Carcinogen-induced lymphomagenesis in *pim*-1 transgenic mice: dose dependence and involvement of c-*myc* and *ras*. Cancer Res., 51, 958–963.

Cuypers, H.T., Selten, G., Quint, W., Zijlstra, M., Robanus-Maandag, E., Boelens, W., Van Wezenbeek, P., Melief, C. and Berns, A. (1984). Murine leukemia virus-induced T-cell lymphomagenesis: integration of proviruses in a distinct chromosomal region. Cell, 37, 141–150.

Cuypers, H.T., Selten, G., Berns, A and Geurts van Kessel, A.M.H. (1986). Assignment of the human homologue of *pim*-1, a mouse gene implicated in leukemogenesis, to the pter-q12 region of chromosome 6. Human Genet., 72, 262–265.

Dautry, F., Weil, D., Yu, J. and Dautry-Varsat, A. (1988). Regulation of pim and myb mRNA accumulation by interleukin 2 and interleukin 3 in murine hematopoietic cell lines. J. Biol. Chem., 263, 17615–17620.

Domen, J., Von Lindern, M., Hermans, A., Breuer, M., Grosveld, G. and Berns, A. (1987). Comparison of the human and mouse PIM-1 cDNAs: nucleotide sequence and immunological identification of the *in vitro* synthesized PIM-1 protein. Oncogene Res., 1, 103–112.

Hanecak, R., Pattengale, P.K. and Fan, H. (1988). Addition or substitution of simian virus 40 enhancer sequences into the Moloney murine leukemia virus (M-MuLV) long terminal repeat yields infectious M-MuLV with altered biological properties. J. Virol., 62, 2427–2436.

Meeker, T.C., Loeb, J., Ayres, M. and Sellers, W. (1990). The human *pim*-1 gene is selectively transcribed in different hemato-lymphoid cell lines in spite of a G+C rich housekeeping promoter. Mol. Cell. Biol., 10, 1680–1688.

Meijer, D., Hermans, A., von Lindern, M., van Agthoven, T., de Klein, A., Mackenbach, P., Grootegoed, A., Talarico, D., Della Valle, G. and Grosveld, G. (1987). Molecular characterization of the testes specific c-*abl* mRNA in mouse. EMBO J., 6, 4041–4048.

Mucenski, M.L., Taylor, B.A., Jenkins, N.A. and Copeland, N.G. (1986). AKXD recombinant inbred strains: models for studying the molecular genetic basis of murine lymphomas. Mol. Cell. Biol., 6, 4236–4243.

Mucenski, M.L., Gilbert, D.J., Taylor, B.A., Jenkins, N.A. and Copeland, N.G. (1987). Common sites of viral integration in lymphomas arising in AKXD recombinant inbred mouse strains. Oncogene Res., 2, 33–48.

Nadeau, J.H. and Phillips, S.J. (1987). The putative oncogene *pim*-1 in the mouse: its linkage and variation among t haplotypes. Genetics, 117, 533–541.

Nagarajan, L., Louie, E., Tsujimoto, Y., Ar-Rushdi, A., Huebner, K. and Croce, C.M. (1986). Localization of the human *pim* oncogene (*PIM*) to a region of chromosome 6 involved in translocations in acute leukemias. Proc. Natl Acad. Sci. USA, 83, 2556–2560.

O'Donnell, P.V., Fleissner, E., Lonial, H., Koehne, C.F. and Reicin, A. (1985). Early clonality and high-frequency proviral integration into the c-*myc* locus in AKR leukemias. J. Virol., 55, 500–503.

Reeves, R, Spies, G.A., Kiefer, M., Barr, P.J. and Power, M. (1990). Primary structure of the putative human oncogene, *pim*-1. Gene, 90, 303–307.

Saris, C.J.M., Domen, J. and Berns, A. (1991). The *pim*-1 oncogene encodes two related protein-serine/threonine kinases by alternative initiation at AUG and CUG. EMBO J., 10, 655–664.

Selten, G., Cuypers, H.T., Zijlstra, M., Melief, C. and Berns, A. (1984). Involvement of c-*myc* in MuLV-induced T cell lymphomas in mice: frequency and mechanisms of activation. EMBO J., 3, 3215–3222.

Selten, G., Cuypers, H.T., Boelens, W., Robanus-Maandag, E., Verbeek, J., Domen, J., van Beveren, C. and Berns, A. (1986). The primary structure of the putative oncogene *pim*-1 shows extensive homology with protein kinases. Cell, 46, 603–611.

Sorrentino, V., McKinney, M.D., Giorgi, M., Geremia, R. and Fleissner, E. (1988). Expression of cellular protooncogenes in the mouse male germ line: a distinctive 2.4-kilobase *pim*-1 transcript is expressed in haploid postmeiotic cells. Proc. Natl Acad. Sci. USA, 85, 2191–2195.

te Riele, H., Robanus Maandag, E., Clarke, A., Hooper, M. and Berns, A. (1990). Consecutive inactivation of both alleles of the *pim*-1 proto-oncogene by homologous recombination in embryonic stem cells. Nature, 348, 649–651.

Telerman, A., Amson, R., Zakut-Houri, R. and Givol, D. (1988). Identification of the human *pim*-1 gene product as a 33-kilodalton cytoplasmic protein with tyrosine kinase activity. Mol. Cell. Biol., 8, 1498–1503.

van Beveren, C. and Verma, I.M. (1986). Homology among oncogenes. Curr. Top. Microbiol., 123, 73–98.

van Lohuizen, M., Verbeek, S., Scheijen, B., Wientjens, E., van der Gulden, H. and Berns, A. (1991). Identification of cooperating oncogene in Eμ-*myc* transgenic mice by provirus tagging. Cell, 65, 737–752.

von Lindern, M., van Agthoven, T.M., Hagemeijer, A., Adriaansen, H. and Grosveld, G. (1989). The human *pim*-1 gene is not directly activated by the translocation (6;9) in acute nonlymphocytic leukemia. Oncogene, 4, 75–79.

Warren, W., Lawley, P.D., Gardner, E., Harris, G., Ball, J.K. and Cooper, C.S. (1987). Induction of thymomas by N-methyl-N-nitrosourea in AKR mice: interaction between the chemical carcinogen and endogenous murine leukaemia viruses. Carcinogenesis, 8, 163–172.

Wingett, D., Reeves, R. and Magnuson, N.S. (1992). Characterization of the testes-specific *pim*-1 transcript in rat. Nucleic Acids Res., 20, 3183–3189.

Wirschubsky, Z., Tsichlis, P., Klein, G. and Sumegi, J. (1986). Rearrangement of c-*myc*, *pim*-1 and *Mlvi*-1 and trisomy of chromosome 15 in MCF- and Moloney-MuLV-induced murine T-cell leukemias. Int. J. Cancer, 38, 739–745.

Zakut-Houri, R., Hazum, S., Givol, D. and Telerman, A. (1987). The cDNA sequence and gene analysis of the human *pim* oncogene. Gene, 54, 105–111.

v-*raf* is the oncogene of murine transforming retrovirus (MSV) 3611 (Rapp *et al.*, 1983a,b; Rapp, 1991). 3611-MSV arose after transforming gene rescue in culture with MuLV (Rapp and Todaro, 1978) followed by infection of a mouse treated with butylnitrosourea (BNU). This mouse developed histiocytic lymphoma and lung adenocarcinoma.

The avian (MH2) homologue of *Raf* is v-*mil* (or v-*mht*): it occurs in the Mill Hill 2 (MH2) virus isolated from a spontaneously arising ovarian tumour in chickens (Beard, 1980; Coll *et al.*, 1983; Jansen *et al.*, 1983, 1984; Kan *et al.*, 1983, 1984a; Sutrave *et al.*, 1984; see **MYC**, pages 314–325, for structure and properties of MH2).

RAF1, *RAFA1* and *RAFB1* (murine *Raf-1*, *Araf-1* and *Braf-1*) comprise the *Raf* family and encode serine/threonine kinases.

Related genes

RAF1, *RAFA1* and *RAFB1* (Huebner *et al.*, 1986; Huleihel *et al.*, 1986; Beck *et al.*, 1987; Grant and Chapman, 1991) and *RAFB1* (Ikawa *et al.*, 1988; Sithanandam *et al.*, 1990, 1992; Stephens *et al.*, 1992; Eychene *et al.*, 1992) belong to the *Src* superfamily of protein kinases (Hanks *et al.*, 1988). They have homology with the protein kinase C family in the N-terminal, cysteine-rich negative regulatory region in addition to the kinase domain.

RAF1P1 /*RAF2* (4pter) is a human pseudogene of *RAF1*. Where they share sequence homology it is 80% but there are numerous deletions and insertions in the pseudogene (Bonner *et al.*, 1985). *ARAF2* (7p14–q21) is a pseudogene of human *RAFA1* (Huebner *et al.*, 1986). *BRAF2* (7q33–36) is a pseudogene of human *RAFB1* (Sithanandam *et al.*, 1992). Xe-*raf* is a *Xenopus laevis* homologue of *Raf-1* (Le Guellec *et al.*, 1988).

PKS, a *RAF1*-related gene, is expressed in human fetal liver and shows elevated expression in peripheral blood mononuclear cells from individuals with angioimmunoblastic lymphadenopathy with dysproteinemia, in which auto-antibodies are produced following the stimulation of B cell proliferation (Mark *et al.*, 1986).

D-*raf-1* and D-*raf-2* are *Drosophila melanogaster* homologues of *RAFB1* and *RAF1* respectively (Mark *et al.*, 1987).

Elegans raf-1 is the *Caenorhabditis elegans Raf* family homologue (Georgi *et al.*, 1990).

Cross-species homology

Human *RAF1*: 87.7% (nucleotide)/99.2% (amino acid) with rat *Raf-1*; 87.6/98.8% with mouse *Raf-1*; 81.6/96.6% with chicken *Mil*; 75.7/92.6% with *Xenopus Raf*; 67.9/50.4% with *Drosophila Raf*.

Transformation

MAN

Oncogenic *RAF1* has been detected by NIH 3T3 fibroblast transfection with DNA from a primary stomach cancer (Shimizu *et al.*, 1985), laryngeal (Kasid *et al.*, 1987), lung and other carcinomas and sarcomas (Stanton and Cooper, 1987) and a glioblastoma cell line (Fukui *et al.*, 1985). High levels of *RAF1* expression occur in many small-cell lung cancers (SCLC) and derived cell lines (Graziano *et al.*, 1987). *RAF1* is also amplified in some non-small-cell lung cancers (Hajj *et al.*, 1990). The truncated versions of *RAF1* that have been isolated from tumours probably arose during transfection.

Deletions and translocations in the 3p25 region (*RAF1*) correlate with some human malignancies, including SCLC (Whang-Peng *et al.*, 1982), mixed salivary gland tumours (Mark *et al.*, 1980) and renal carcinoma (Zbar *et al.*, 1987).

ANIMALS

Tumorigenicity studies in mice as well as transformation in cell culture have been carried out with retroviral constructs containing *Raf* genes activated by truncation and/or mutation (Rapp *et al.*, 1983a,b, 1985b; Morse and Rapp, 1988; Fredrickson *et al.*, 1988; Klinken *et al.*, 1989; Troppmair *et al.*, 1989). Tumours arose most frequently in the haematopoietic lineages followed by pancreatic epithelium and connective tissues.

The oncogenically active v-*raf*, derived from mouse *Raf-1*, is capable of inducing a defined spectrum of tumours *in vivo*. Newborn mice inoculated intraperitoneally with the v-*raf*-expressing 3611-MSV develop fibrosarcomas, erythroblastosis and occasionally erythroleukaemia (Rapp *et al.*, 1988). Inoculation also results in foci of pancreatic acinar cells. Additionally, chickens infected with MH2 which expresses v-*myc* and the avian homologue of v-*raf*, v-*mil*, develop pancreatic carcinomas (Beard, 1980). The differences in tumour spectra induced by *Raf*- and *Myc*-expressing retroviruses suggest that the preferred *Myc* targets (lymphoid) differ from the preferred *Raf* targets (erythroid, fibroblast) in the rate limiting pathways through which their growth is normally controlled. Chemical induction (ENU) of lung adenocarcinomas and T cell lymphomas results in point mutated *Raf-1* in tumours without *Ras* mutations.

v-*raf* acts synergistically with v-*myc* to give rise to B cell tumours.

IN VITRO

Araf-1, *Braf-1* and *Raf-1* may be oncogenically activated *in vitro*. *Raf-1* preferentially transforms erythroid cells and also transforms fibroblasts and epithelial cells (Keski-Oja *et al.*, 1982). 3611-MSV-transformed fibroblasts release transforming growth factors (TGFs) with a corresponding decrease in the affinity of EGF for its receptor: other *Src* family oncogenes do likewise (e.g. *Fes*, *Abl*, *Mos*, and also v-*Kras*).

In IL-2- or IL-3-dependent cell lines 3611-MSV does not reduce growth factor dependence, although v-*myc* does so (Rapp *et al.*, 1985a).

In macrophages and B-lineage cells, v-*raf* alone does not transform but acts synergistically with v-*myc* (Blasi *et al.*, 1985). *Raf-1* does not activate *Myc* transcription.

NIH 3T3 cells are transformed by the activated *Raf* chimeric gene when its expression is directed by the RSV LTR (Ishikawa *et al.*, 1987a) and by microinjection of RAF from which the N-terminal (regulatory) domain has been removed (Smith *et al.*, 1990).

Raf and *Myc* act synergistically to transform cells of all haematopoietic lineages: their co-expression in lymphoid and erythroid cells induces differentiation to a myeloid form (Klinken, 1991).

Araf-1 transforms NIH 3T3 fibroblasts after incorporation into the genome of murine leukaemia virus and expression of the *gag–raf* gene product (Huleihel *et al.*, 1986).

	RAFA1/Araf-1	RAFB1/Braf-1	RAF1/Raf-1	v-raf
Nucleotides (kb)	11	?	>100	1.1 7.6 (3611-MSV)
Chromosome				
Human	Xp11.2	7q33–36	3p25	
Mouse	X	10	6	
Exons	16	?	17	
mRNA (kb)				
Human	2.6	2.6/4.5/10/13 (Storm et al., 1990)	3.4	6.9
Mouse	2.6/4.3	2.6/4.0	3.1	
Amino acids				
Human	606	766/651	648	323 (v-raf) 706 (gag–raf)
Mass (kDa)				
(predicted)	67.5	84/72.5	73	37 (v-raf)
(expressed)	pp68	pp73/pp95	70–74 (pp74–pp78)	gp90$^{gag-raf}$ p75$^{gag-raf}$

Cellular location

Cytosolic.

Tissue location

RAFA1/Araf-1: Predominantly urogenital tissues.
RAFB1/Braf-1: Cerebrum, testes.
RAF1/Raf-1: Ubiquitous (humans, mice).

In mouse testis *Raf-1, Araf* and *Braf* are differentially expressed during development, indicating specific regulatory roles in androgen production and/or spermatogenesis (Wadewitz et al., 1993).

Protein function

RAF genes encode serine/threonine protein kinases. RAF1 is positively regulated by serine/tyrosine phosphorylation. It has no autophosphorylating protein kinase activity (unlike Δgag–v-raf and Δgag–v-mil)(Schultz et al., 1988). The ubiquitous distribution of RAF1 suggests that it may have a basic regulatory function. In *Xenopus* RAF1 appears to mediate the developmental effects of basic fibroblast growth factor during mesoderm induction (MacNicol et al., 1993). In NIH 3T3 cells RAF1 undergoes rapid phosphorylation, mainly on serine and threonine, in response to PDGF, EGF, insulin, acidic FGF, CSF1 or TPA, and also in response to the oncoproteins of v-*fms*, v-*src*, v-*sis*, *Hras* or polyoma middle T antigen (Morrison et al., 1988; Baccarini *et al.*, 1990; Kovacina *et al.*, 1990; Blackshear *et al.*, 1990; App *et al.*, 1991). The RAF1 protein complexes with the activated PDGF β receptor (Morrison *et al.*, 1989). The activated enzyme is translocated to the perinuclear region and the nucleus. RAF1 is also activated by epithelial and lymphoid cell mitogens and is rapidly (15 min) tyrosine phosphorylated in response to IL-2 but not IL-4 in a T cell line (Turner *et al.*, 1991; Maslinski *et al.*, 1992) and by IL-3 or erythropoietin in murine myeloid cell lines (Carroll *et al.*, 1990, 1991) or by CD4 cross-linking (Thompson *et al.*, 1991). RAF1 is also activated via Thy-1 or the TCR in a protein kinase C-dependent manner (Siegel *et al.*, 1990) and by UV irradiation (Radler-Pohl *et al.*, 1993). RAF1 activates MAP kinase-kinase (MAPK-K) which in turn stimulates the mitogen-activated protein (MAP) kinases ERK1 and ERK2. MAPK-K, ERK1 and ERK2 are constitutively active in v-*raf*-transformed cells (Kyriakis *et al.*, 1992; Dent *et al.*, 1992; Howe *et al.*, 1992).

RAF oncoproteins *trans*-activate expression of genes driven by AP-1, ETS and NF-κB binding motifs (Wasylyk *et al.*, 1989; Bruder *et al.*, 1993; Bruder and Rapp, personal communication). The use of dominant inhibitory *Raf* mutants has demonstrated that RAF1 is required for AP-1/ETS-driven expression in response to serum or TPA stimulation and v-*Hras* expression. v-*Hras* appears to activate RAF1 through interactions with the cysteine-rich region located in the regulatory domain of RAF1 (Bruder *et al.*, 1992).

Transfection of a v-*raf* expression vector into NIH 3T3 cells induces transcription of the growth factor-regulated early response genes *Egr-1*, *Fos* and β-actin (Kaibuchi *et al.*, 1989; Jamal and Ziff, 1990; Qureshi *et al.*, 1991). Multiple *Fos* promoter elements are targets for the v-*raf*-mediated effect, including the dyad symmetry element (DSE), the octameric direct repeat (−76 to −97) and the region between nucleotides −99 and −225 (Rim *et al.*, 1992) and evidence from *Raf* revertant NIH 3T3 cell lines indicates that RAF1 kinase is essential for the activation of the AP-1 complex (Kolch *et al.*, 1993; see **FOS**).

Revertant cell lines that suppress transformation by *Kras* or *Hras* or BALB-MSV (v-*ras* carrying viruses) and by v-*fes* or v-*src* are transformed by v-*fms*, v-*mos* or v-*sis* and by 3611-MSV or *Araf*-MSV (Noda *et al.*, 1983; Rapp *et al.*, 1988). Furthermore, neither microinjection of anti-RAS antibody nor block of RAS activity by mutation (*Ras* revertant cells) affects growth in cells transformed by *Raf* or *Mos*. Thus *Raf* (and *Fms*, *Mos* and *Sis*) are the only oncogenes that appear to function independently of *Ras*. In NIH 3T3 cells expression of *Raf-1* antisense RNA inhibits proliferation, causes reversion of *Raf*-transformed cells and blocks transformation by *Kras* or *Hras* (Kolch *et al.*, 1991), indicating that RAF1 functions downstream of *Ras*. *Ras* and *Raf-1* cooperate to transform NIH 3T3 cells and dominant negative mutants of *Ras* inhibit the activation of RAF1 kinase in NIH 3T3 cells stimulated by serum or TPA and of both RAF-1 and BRAF-1 in NGF-stimulated PC-12 cells (Troppmair *et al.*, 1992), indicating that *Ras* may control the coupling of growth factor receptors and protein kinase C to cytosolic RAF kinases. This is consistent with the finding that N-terminally truncated, oncogenic RAF activates the MAP kinase ERK2 independently of $p21^{ras}$ function (Howe *et al.*, 1992) and that the kinase activity of RAF1 is enhanced as a result of direct phosphorylation by protein kinase C *in vitro* (Sozeri *et al.*, 1992).

The generalized scheme summarizes the above data, indicating that RAF1 kinase may be activated by a wide variety of receptors with intrinsic tyrosine kinase activity or by receptors that interact with tyrosine kinases (e.g. CD4). $p21^{ras}$ may mediate coupling to RAF1 of pathways that either require or are independent of protein kinase C. * Indicates activated form.

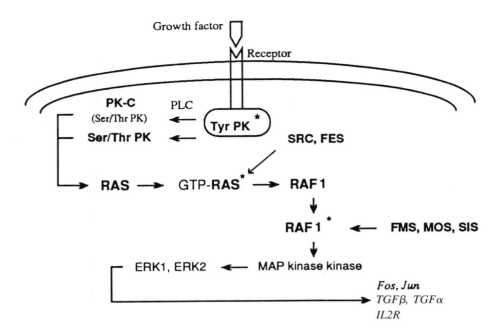

The human *RAF1* gene and the 3611-MSV genome

Human *RAF1*

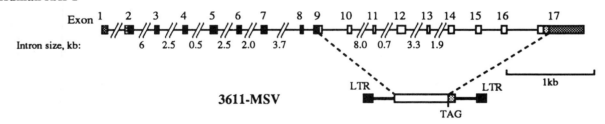

Open boxes: exons homologous to those in the mouse genome that are transduced in v-*raf*. The 3611-MSV genome has the structure 5′-*gag*(Δp15p12Δp30)–v-*raf*–Δ*pol*–*env*-3′. The C-terminal 172 amino acids of p30, all of p10^{gag} and p14 viral protease and 64 amino acids of *pol* N-terminus were deleted whereas the *env* gene is unchanged. The v-*raf* gene encodes amino acids 326–648 of the normal RAF-1 protein linked to *gag* sequences. Homologous recombination was involved in the acquisition of v-*raf*: the 5′ v-*raf* junction in 3611-MSV has 12 nucleotides identical to the 3′ end of mouse *Raf-1* exon 9 and differs from MuLV p30^{gag} by only one nucleotide. At the 3′ end, 8 nucleotides of v-*raf*, MuLV and mouse *Raf-1* exon 17 are identical. The homology between 3611-MSV and Mo-MuLV is the most extensive yet demonstrated for any retroviral/cell recombinant (Bonner *et al.*, 1985). The v-*mil* oncogene of the MH2 virus begins in exon 7 and encodes the last 380 amino acids of chicken *Mil* (*Raf*) with 19 amino acid substitutions and one deletion. In only one change (Asn522) do v-*mil* and v-*raf* differ from *Raf-1* but v-*mil* is identical to chicken *Raf* at this position. Thus none of the mutations appear critical for transformation.

Recombinant retroviruses containing v-*raf*–*mil* (J-1, J-2, J-3) have been constructed and the construct J-5 contains MC29 v-*myc* inserted in 3611-MSV *gag* with the elimination of v-*raf*.

Mo-MuLV LTR transfection into NIH 3T3 cells activates *Raf-1* by promoter insertion (Muller and Muller, 1984; Molders *et al.*, 1985), integrating into the fifth intron of *Raf-1*. The translation product is pp48, a cytosolic protein that, in contrast to p74^{raf}, is not myristylated or glycosylated but has Ser/Thr protein kinase activity *in vitro*.

The human *RAF1* promoter is located in an HTF-island and lacks TATA and CAAT boxes (Beck *et al.*, 1990). The 5' untranslated exon 1 is located at least 55 kb upstream of the body of the gene which spans 45 kb (Bonner *et al.*, 1985; Beck *et al.*, 1990). The last *RAF1* exon (17) contains 905 bp of 3' untranslated sequence. The large size of the gene may account for the relatively high frequency with which truncation-activated oncogenic versions of *RAF1* have been obtained.

Structure of RAF1

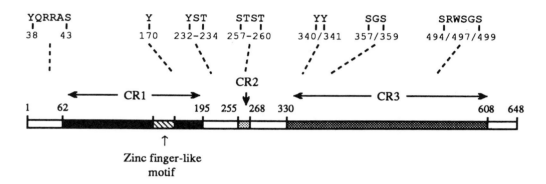

The N-terminal half of the protein comprises a regulatory domain that includes conserved region 1 (CR1) that contains a zinc finger-like motif and CR2 that is conserved in virtually all forms of RAF. The C-terminal region contains the kinase domain (CR3) that comprises the minimal transforming element (Heidecker *et al.*, 1990). Potential phosphorylation sites are shown above the figure. RAF1 is phosphorylated at multiple sites in the N-terminus that are deleted in the transforming protein. The major phosphorylation sites are Ser43, part of a consensus sequence for phosphorylation by protein kinase C (Kemp and Pearson, 1990), and Ser259. Deletion of residues 245–261 in CR2 causes oncogenic activation (Ishikawa *et al.*, 1988; Heidecker *et al.*, 1990) but mutation of Ser259 alone is not sufficient to activate transforming potential: the additional deletion of the region 283–309 activates weak transforming power but the complete removal of the N-terminal 303 residues (that includes nine serines) is required for maximal activity (McGrew *et al.*, 1992). Serines 357/359 are in the ATP binding domain and their phosphorylation may therefore exert a negative effect on RAF1 activity. Ser499 (replaced by Ala in RAFA1) may be a substrate for protein kinase C.

Sequences of human RAF1, human RAFA1, RAFB1, v-RAF and v-SRC proteins

Dashes indicate identity with human RAF1. Italics indicate the phorbol ester and diacylglycerol binding region. The consensus ATP binding site is underlined. Mutation of v-RAF Lys53 eliminates transforming capacity. Human RAFA1 is 60% homologous to RAF1 over 604 overlapping residues: including conservative exchanges, the homology is 89%. RAFB1 contains a second initiator codon (Met116), the use of which generates a 651 amino acid protein (Stephens *et al.*, 1992). Rat RAF1 differs from human RAF1 in 11 amino acids but has the same total number

```
RAFB1    (1)   MAALSGGGGGGADAGQALFNGDMEPEAGAGRPAASSAADPAIPEEVWNIKQMIKLTQEHI

RAF1     (1)                                     MEHIQGAWKTISNGFGFKDAVF
RAFB1   (61)   EALLDKFGGEHNPPSIYLEAYEEYTSKLDALQQREQQLL-SLGNGTDFSVSSSASM-T-T
                                                             ⟶ CR1
RAF1    (23)   DGSSCISPTIVQQFGYQRRASDDGKLTDPSKTSNTIRVFLPNKQRTVVNVRNGMSLHDCL
ARAF1    (1)             MEPPRGPPANGAE--RAVG-VK-Y---------T--D---VY-S-
RAFB1  (121)   SS--SSLSVLPSSLSVFQNPT-VARSNPK-PQKPIV-----------PA-C-VTVR-S-

RAF1    (83)   MKALKVRGLQPECCAVFRLLHEHKGKKARLDWNTDAASLIGEELQVDFLDHVPLTTHNFA
ARAF1   (46)   D--------NQD--V-Y--I...--R-TVTA-D-AI-P-D----I-EV-ED----M---V
RAFB1  (181)   K---MM---I------Y-I...QD-E-KPIG-D--ISW-T----H-EV-EN-------V
                                                          CR1  ⟵
RAF1   (143)   RKTFLKLAFCDICQKFLLNGFRCQTCGYKFHEHCSTKVPTMCVDWSNIRQLLLF......
ARAF1  (103)   ----FS-----F-L--FH-----------Q---S----V---M-TN--QFYH......
RAFB1  (238)   ----FT-----F-R-L-FQ-----------QR---E--L---NYDQLDL-FVSKFFEHH

RAF1   (197)   ....PNSTIGDSGVPALPSLTMRRMRESVSRMPVSSQHRYSTPHAFTFNTSSPSSEGSLS
ARAF1  (157)   ....SVQDLSG.-SRQHEAPSN-PLN-LLTPQGP-PRTQHCD-EH-P-....-APANAPL
RAFB1  (298)   PIPQEEASLAETALTSGS-PSAPASDSIGPQILT-PSPSK-I-IPQP-RPADEDHRNQFG
                              ⟶ CR2        ⟵
RAF1   (253)   QRQRSTSTPNVHMVSTTLPVDSRMIE      DAIRSHSESASPSALSSSPNNLSPTG
ARAF1  (208)   --I-------------A-M--NL-QLTGQSFST--AG-RGG-DGTPRG-P--ASV-SGR
RAFB1  (358)   --D--S-A----INTIEPVNIDDL-R........DQGFRGDGG--TTG--AT-PASL-GS
                                            ⟶ CR3
RAF1   (305)   WSQPK...TPVPAQRERAPVSGTQEKNKIRPRGQRDSSYYWEIEASEVMLSTRIGSGSFG
ARAF1  (268)   K-PHS...KSPAE----KSL..ADD-K-VKNL-Y-X-G----VPP---Q-LK---T----
RAFB1  (409)   LTNV-ALQKSPGP----KSS-SSEDR-RMKTL-R----DD---PDGQITVGQ--------
v-RAF    (1)                   -----------------KM-----------------
v-SRC  (243)                   VCPTSK-QT-GLAKDA-EIPRESLR-EAKL-Q-C--

RAF1   (362)   TVYKGKWHGDVAVKILKVVDPTPEQFQAFRNEVAVLRKTRHVNILLFMGYMTKDNLAIVT
ARAF1  (323)   --FR-R--------V---SQ--A-QA---K--MQ--------------F--RPGF--I-
RAFB1  (469)   -------------M-N-TA---Q-L---K---G---------------S--PQ-----
v-RAF   (37)   ----------------------L------------------------------------
v-SRC  (279)   E-WM-T-NDTTR-A-KTLK TGTMSPE--LQ-AQ-MK-L--EKLVQLYAVVSEEPIY--I

RAF1   (422)   QWCEGSSLYKHLHVQETKFQMF.QLIDIARQTAQGMDYLHAKNIIHRDMKSNNIFLHEGL
ARAF1  (383)   ---------H----AD-R-D-V.----V--------------------L--------
RAFB1  (529)   ---------H---II----E-I.K----------------S-----L--------D-
v-RAF   (97)   ---------------------.-------------------------------------
v-SRC  (338)   EYMSKG--LDF-KGEMG-YLRLPQ-V-M-A-I-S--A-VERM-YV---LRAA--LVG-NL

RAF1   (481)   TVKIGDFGLATVKSRWSGSQQVEQPTGSVLWMAPEVIRMQDNNPFSFQSDVYSYGIVLYE
ARAF1  (442)   -------------T----A-PL---S-------A-------P--Y-------A--V----
RAFB1  (588)   -------------------H-F--LS--I-----------K--Y-------AF------
v-RAF  (156)   -----------------------------------------------------------
v-SRC  (398)   VC-VA-----RLIED NEYTARQGAKFPIK-T---AALY...GR-TIK---W-F--L-T-

RAF1   (541)   LMT.GELPYSHINNRDQIIFMVGRGYASPDLSKLYKNCPKAMKRLVADCVKKVKEERPLF
ARAF1  (502)   ---.-S------GC------------L------ISS------R-LS--L-FQR-----
RAFB1  (648)   ---.-Q----N----------------L------VRS---------M-E-L--KRD-----
v-RAF  (216)   --A.-----A---------------------R--------I------------------
v-SRC  (455)   -TTK-RV--PGMV--E VLDQ-E---RM-CPP....E--ESLHD-MCQ-WR-DP----TF
               CR3  ⟵
RAF1   (600)   PQILSSIELLQHSLPKINRSASEPSLHRAA.HTEDINACTLTTSPRLPVF (648)
ARAF1  (561)   ----AT-----R-----E----------.T.QADELP--L-SAARLV- (606)
RAFB1  (707)   ----A-----AR-----H--------N--GFQ---FSLYA.CA--KT-IQAGGYGAFPVH (766)
v-RAF  (275)   --------------------P--------.------------------ (323)
v-SRC  (510)   .KY-QAQL-PACV-EVAE (526)
```

(648). pp79$^{\Delta gag\text{-}v\text{-}raf}$ contains 383 *gag* and 323 v-RAF residues and is *N*-myristylated (Beck *et al.*, 1987).

RAF proteins can be oncogenically activated by N-terminal fusion, truncation or point mutations (Ishikawa *et al.*, 1987a; Stanton and Cooper, 1987; Heidecker *et al.*, 1990). The generation of an activated oncoprotein by removal of the N-terminus of RAF1 indicates that myristylation and *gag* sequences are not essential for transformation (Schultz *et al.*, 1985). N-Terminally fused activated RAF1 (602 amino acids, 69 kDa) is identical from amino acid 232 to the C-terminus to the sequence of normal RAF1 from residue 278. The N-terminus of the activated fusion protein is comprised of 231 unrelated rat amino acids (TPR: see **MET**). Fusion occurs in the intron between exons 7 and 8. Activation by N-terminal deletion also occurs in the cellular transforming genes of *MET, RET, ROS* and *TRK* and in the viral oncogenes *abl, erbB, fgr* and *myb*.

Amino acid homologies (%) between conserved regions (CR1, CR2 and CR3) of human RAFA1, RAFB1 and RAF1

	CR1	CR2	CR3
RAFA1/RAFB1	71.1	61.5	75.7
RAFA1/RAF1	68.9	100.0	78.0
RAFB1/RAF1	64.4	61.5	79.1

Databank file names and accession numbers

	GENE	*EMBL*	*SWISSPROT*	*REFERENCES*
MSV-3611	v-*raf*	Revraf K01691	KRAF_MSV36 P00532	Kan *et al.*, 1984b
				Mark and Rapp, 1984
Human	*RAFA1*	Hsaraf1r X04790	KRAA_HUMAN P10398	Beck *et al.*, 1987
Human	*RAFB1*	Hsbraf3 M95712,	KRAB_HUMAN P15056	Ikawa *et al.*, 1988
		M95721,		Sithanandam *et al.*, 1990
		X54072		Eychene *et al.*, 1992
		Hsbrafa M21001		Stephens *et al.*, 1992
Human	*RAF1*	Hsrafr X03484	KRAF_HUMAN P04049	Bonner *et al.*, 1985, 1986
Mouse	*Araf*	Mmaraf M13071	KRAA_MOUSE P04627	Huleihel *et al.*, 1986
Rat	*Araf*	Rnaraf X06942	KRAA_RAT P14056	Ishikawa *et al.*, 1987b
Rat	*Raf*	Rnrafa M15427	KRAF_RAT P11345	Ishikawa *et al.*, 1987b
Drosophila	D-*raf-1/phl*	Dmraf1a M16598	KRAF_DROME P11346	Nishida *et al.*, 1988
		Dmrafpo X07181		Mark *et al.*, 1987
Xenopus laevis	*Raf*	Xlraf X12948	KRAF_XENLA P09560	Le Guellec *et al.*, 1988
				Le Guellec *et al.*, 1991

Reviews

Hanks, S.K., Quinn, A.M. and Hunter, T. (1988). The protein kinase family: conserved features and deduced phylogeny of the catalytic domains. Science, 241, 42–52.

Heidecker, G., Kolch, W., Morrison, D.K. and Rapp, U.R. (1992). The role of *Raf*-1 phosphorylation in signal transduction. Adv. Cancer Res., 58, 53–73.

Klinken, S.P. (1991). Transformation of hemopoietic cells by raf and myc oncogenes: a new perspective on lineage commitment. Cancer Cells, 3, 373–382.

Li, P., Wood, K., Mamon, H. and Roberts, T. (1991). raf-1: a kinase currently without a cause but not lacking in effects. Cell, 64, 479–482.

Morse, H.C. and Rapp, U.R. (1988). Tumorigenic activity of artificially activated oncogenes. In Klein, G. (ed.) Cellular Oncogene Activation: 335. Marcell Dekker, New York.

Rapp, U.R. (1991). Role of *raf*-1 serine/threonine protein kinase in growth factor signal transduction. Oncogene, 6, 495–500.

Rapp, U.R., Cleveland, J.L., Bonner, T.I. and Storm, S.M. (1988). The *raf* oncogene family. In Curran, T., Reddy, E.P. and Skalka, A. (eds) The Oncogene Handbook: 213–253. Elsevier, London.

Papers

App, H., Hazan, R., Zilberstein, A., Ullrich, A., Schlessinger, J. and Rapp, U.R. (1991). Epidermal growth factor (EGF) stimulates association and kinase activity of raf-1 with the EGF receptor. Mol. Cell. Biol., 11, 913–919.

Baccarini, M., Sabatini, D.M., App, H., Rapp, U.R. and Stanley, E.R. (1990). Colony stimulating factor-1 (CSF-1) stimulates temperature dependent phosphorylation and activation of the RAF-1 proto-oncogene product. EMBO J., 9, 3649–3657.

Beard, J.W. (1980). Biology of avian retroviruses. In Klein, G. (ed.) Viral Oncology: 79. Raven Press, New York.

Beck, T.W., Huleihel, M., Gunnell, M., Bonner, T.I. and Rapp, U.R. (1987). The complete coding sequence of the human A-*raf*-1 oncogene and transforming activity of a human A-*raf* carrying retrovirus. Nucleic Acids Res., 15, 595–609.

Beck, T.W., Brennscheidt, U., Sithanandam, G., Cleveland, J. and Rapp, U.R. (1990). Molecular organization of the human *raf*-1 promoter region. Mol. Cell. Biol., 10, 3325–3333.

Blackshear, P.J., Haupt, D.M., App, H. and Rapp, U.R. (1990). Insulin activates the raf-1 protein kinase. J. Biol. Chem., 265, 12131–12134.

Blasi, E., Mathieson, B., Varesio, L., Cleveland, J.L., Borchert, P.A. and Rapp, U.R. (1985). Selective immortalization of murine macrophages from fresh bone marrow by a *raf/myc* recombinant murine retrovirus. Nature, 318, 667–670.

Bonner, T.I., Kerby, S.B., Sutrave, P., Gunnell, M.A., Mark, G. and Rapp, U.R. (1985). Structure and biological activity of human homologs of the *raf/mil* oncogene. Mol. Cell. Biol., 5, 1400–1407.

Bonner, T.I., Oppermann, H., Seeburg, P., Kerby, S.B., Gunnell, M.A., Young, A..C. and Rapp, U.R. (1986). The complete coding sequence of the human *raf* oncogene and the corresponding structure of the c-*raf*-1 gene. Nucleic Acids Res., 14, 1009–1015.

Bruder, J.T., Heidecker, G. and Rapp, U.R. (1992). Serum-, TPA-, and *ras*-induced expression from Ap-1/Ets-driven promoters requires *raf*-1 kinase. Genes Devel., 6, 545–556.

Bruder, J.T., Tan, T.-H., Heidecker, G., Derse, D. and Rapp, U.R. (1993). *raf* transactivation of HIV-LTR-driven expression via the NF-κB binding sites. J. Virol., in press.

Carroll, M.P., Clark-Lewis, I., Rapp, U.R. and May, W.S. (1990). Interleukin-3 and granulocyte-macrophage colony-stimulating factor mediate rapid phosphorylation and activation of cytosolic c-*raf*. J. Biol. Chem., 265, 19812–19817.

Carroll, M.P., Spivak, J.L., McMahon, M., Weich, N., Rapp, U.R. and May, W.S. (1991). Erythropoietin induces raf-1 activation and raf-1 is required for erythropoietin-mediated proliferation. J. Biol. Chem., 266, 14964–14969.

Coll, J., Righi, M., de Taisne, C., Dissous, C., Gegonne, A. and Stehelin, D. (1983). Molecular cloning of the avian transforming retrovirus MH2 reveals a novel cell-derived sequence (v-*mil*) in addition to the *myc* oncogene. EMBO J., 2, 2189–2194.

Dent, P., Haser, W., Haystead, T.A.J., Vincent, L.A., Roberts, T.M. and Strugill, T.W. (1992). Activation of mitogen-activated protein kinase kinase by v-raf in NIH 3T3 cells and in vitro. Science, 257, 1404–1407.

Eychene, A., Barnier, J.V., Apiou, F., Dutrillaux, B. and Calothy, G. (1992). Chromosomal assignment of two human B-*raf*(Rmil) proto-oncogene loci: B-*raf*-1 encoding p94^{B}raf$^{\text{/Rmil}}$ and B-*raf*-2, a processed pseudogene. Oncogene, 7, 1657–1660.

Fredrickson, T.N., Hartley, J.W., Wolford, N.K., Resau, J.H., Rapp, U.R. and Morse, H.C. (1988). Histogenesis and clonality of pancreatic tumours induced by v-*myc* and v-*raf* oncogenes in NFS/N mice, Am. J. Pathol., 131, 444–451.

Fukui, M., Yamamoto, T., Kawai, S., Maruo, K. and Toyoshima, K. (1985). Detection of a *raf*-related and two other transforming DNA sequences in human tumors maintained in nude mice. Proc. Natl Acad. Sci. USA, 82, 5954–5958.

Georgi, L.L., Albert, P.S. and Riddle, D.L. (1990). *daf-1*, a C. elegans gene controlling dauer larva development, encodes a novel receptor protein kinase. Cell, 61, 635–645.

Grant, S.G. and Chapman, V.M. (1991). Detailed genetic mapping of the A-*raf* proto-oncogene on the mouse X chromosome. Oncogene, 6, 397–402.

Graziano, S.L., Cowan, B.Y., Carney, D.N., Bryke, C.R., Mitter, N.S., Johnson, B.E., Mark, G.E., Planas, A.T., Catino, J.J., Comis, R.L. and Poiesz, B.J. (1987). Small cell lung cancer line derived from a primary tumor with a characteristic deletion of 3p. Cancer Res., 48, 2148–2155.

Hajj, C., Akoum, R., Bradley, E., Paquin, F. and Ayoub, J. (1990). DNA alterations at proto-oncogene loci and their clinical significance in operable non-small cell lung cancer. Cancer, 66, 733–739.

Heidecker, G., Huleihel, M., Cleveland, J.L., Kolch, W., Beck, T.W., Lloyd, P., Pawson, T. and Raff, U.R. (1990). Mutational activation of c-*raf*-1 and definition of the minimal transforming sequence. Mol. Cell. Biol., 10, 2503–2512.

Howe, L.R., Leevers, S.J., Gomez, N., Nakielny, S., Cohen, P. and Marshall, C.J. (1992). Activation of the MAP kinase pathway by the protein kinase raf. Cell, 71, 335–342.

Huebner, K., Ar-Rushdi, A., Griffin, C.A., Isobe, M., Kozak, C., Emanuel, B.S., Nagarajan, L., Cleveland, J.L., Bonner, T.I., Goldsborough, M.D., Croce, C.M. and Rapp, U.R. (1986). Actively transcribed genes in the *raf* oncogene group, located on the X chromosome in mouse and human. Proc. Natl Acad. Sci. USA, 83, 3934–3938.

Huleihel, M, Goldsborough, M., Cleveland, J., Gunnell, M., Bonner, T. and Rapp, U.R. (1986). Characterization of murine A-*raf*, a new oncogene related to the v-*raf* oncogene. Mol. Cell. Biol., 6, 2655–2662.

Ikawa, S., Fukui, M., Ueyama, Y., Tamaoki, N., Yamamoto, T. and Toyoshima, K. (1988). B-*raf*, a new member of the *raf* family, is activated by DNA rearrangement. Mol. Cell. Biol., 8, 2651–2654.

Ishikawa, F., Takaku, F., Nagao, M. and Sugimura, T. (1987a). Rat c-*raf* oncogene activation by a rearrangement that produces a fused protein. Mol. Cell. Biol., 7, 1226–1232.

Ishikawa, F., Takaku, F., Nagao, M. and Sugimura, T. (1987b). The complete primary structure of the rat A-*raf* cDNA coding region: conservation of the putative regulatory regions present in rat c-*raf*. Oncogene Res., 1, 243–253.

Ishikawa, F., Sakai, R., Ochiai, M., Takaku, F., Sugimura, T. and Nagao, M. (1988). Identification of a transforming activity suppressing sequence in the c-*raf* oncogene. Oncogene, 3, 635–658.

Jamal, S. and Ziff, E., (1990). Transactivation of c-*fos* and β-actin genes by *raf* as a step in early response to transmembrane signals. Nature, 344, 463–466.

Jansen, H.W., Ruckert, B., Lurz, R. and Bister, K. (1983). Two unrelated cell-derived sequences in the genome of avian leukemia and carcinoma inducing retrovirus MH2. EMBO J., 2, 1969–1975.

Jansen, H.W., Lurz, R., Bister, K., Bonner, T.I., Mark, G.E. and Rapp, U.R. (1984). Homologous cell-derived oncogenes in avian carcinoma virus MH2 and murine sarcoma virus 3611. Nature, 307, 281–284.

Kaibuchi, K., Fukumoto, Y., Oku, N., Hori, Y., Yamamoto, T., Toyoshima, K. and Takai, Y. (1989). Activation of the serum response element and 12-O-tetradecanolyphorbol-13-acetate response element by the activated c-*raf*-1 protein in a manner independent of protein kinase C. J. Biol. Chem., 264, 20855–20858.

Kan, N.C., Flordellis, C.S., Garon, C.F., Duesberg, P.H. and Papas, T.S. (1983). Avian carcinoma virus MH2 contains a transformation-specific sequence, *mht*, and shares the *myc* sequence with MC29, CMII, and OK10 viruses. Proc. Natl Acad. Sci. USA, 80, 6566–6570.

Kan, N.C., Flordellis, C.S., Mark, G.E., Duesberg, P.H. and Papas, T.S. (1984a). A common *onc* gene sequence transduced by avian carcinoma virus MH2 and by murine sarcoma virus 3611. Science, 223, 813–816.

Kan, N.C., Flordellis, C.S., Mark, G.E., Duesberg, P.H., Papas, T.S. (1984b). Nucleotide sequence of avian carcinoma virus MH2: two potential onc genes, one related to avian virus MC29 and the other related to murine sarcoma virus 3611. Proc. Natl Acad. Sci. USA, 81, 3000–3004.

Kasid, U., Pfeifer, A., Weichselbaum, R.R., Dritschilo, A. and Mark, G.E. (1987). The *raf* oncogene is associated with a radiation-resistant human laryngeal cancer. Science, 237, 1039–1041.

Kemp, B.E. and Pearson, R.B. (1990). Protein kinse recognition sequence motifs. Trends Biol. Sci., 15, 342–346.

Keski-Oja, A., Rapp, U.R. and Vaheri, A. (1982). Transformation of MMC-E epithelial cells by acute 3611-MSV: inhibition of collagen synthesis and induction of novel polypeptides. J. Cell. Biochem., 20, 139–148.

Klinken, S.P., Rapp, U.R. and Morse, H.C. (1989). *raf/myc*-infected erythroid cells are restricted in their ability to terminally differentiate. J. Virol., 63, 1489–1492.

Kolch, W., Heidecker, G., Lloyd, P. and Rapp, U.R. (1991). *Raf*-1 protein kinase is requied for growth of induced NIH/3T3 cells. Nature, 349, 426–428.

Kolch, W., Heidecker, G., Troppmair, J., Yanagihara, K., Bassin, R.H. and Rapp, U.R. (1993). Raf revertant cells resist transformation by non-nuclear oncogenes and are deficient in the induction of early response genes by TPA and serum. Oncogene, 8, 361–370.

Kovacina, K.S., Yonezawa, K., Brautigan, D.L., Tonks, N.K., Rapp, U.R. and Roth, R.A. (1990). Insulin activates the kinase activity of the raf-1 proto-oncogene by increasing its serine phosphorylation. J. Biol. Chem., 265, 12115–12118.

Kyriakis, J.M., App, H., Zhang, X.-F., Banerjee, P., Brautigan, D.L., Rapp, U.R. and Avruch, J. (1992). Raf-1 activates MAP kinase-kinase. Nature, 358, 417–421.

Le Guellec, R., Le Guellec, K., Paris, J. and Philippe, M. (1988). Nucleotide sequence of *Xenopus* c-*raf* coding region. Nucleic Acids Res., 16, 10357.

Le Guellec, R., Couturier, A., Le Guellec, K., Paris, J., Le Fur, N. and Philippe, M. (1991). *Xenopus* c-*raf* proto-oncogene: cloning and expression during oogenesis and early development. Biol. Cell., 72, 39–45.

McGrew, B.R., Nichols, D.W., Stanton, V.P., Cai, H., Whorf, R.C., Patel, V., Cooper, G.M. and Laudano, A.P. (1992). Phosphorylation occurs in the amino terminus of the raf-1 protein. Oncogene, 7, 33–42.

MacNicol, A.M., Muslin, A.J. and Williams, L.T. (1993). Raf-1 kinase is essential for early Xenopus development and mediates the induction of mesoderm by FGF. Cell, 73, 571–583.

Mark, G.E. and Rapp, U.R. (1984). Primary structure of v-*raf*: relatedness to the *src* family of oncogenes. Science, 224, 285–289.

Mark, G.E., Seeley, T.W., Shows, T.B. and Mountz, J.D. (1986). *pks*, a *raf*-related sequence in humans. Proc. Natl Acad. Sci. USA, 83, 6312–6316.

Mark, G.E., MacIntyre, R.J., Digan, M.E., Ambrosio, L. and Perrimon, N. (1987). *Drosophila melanogaster* homologs of the *raf* oncogene. Mol. Cell. Biol., 7, 2134–2140.

Mark, J., Dahlenfors, Ekedahl, C. and Stenman, G. (1980). The mixed salivary gland tumor – a normally benign human neoplasm frequently showing specific chromosomal abnormalities. Cancer Genet. Cytogenet., 2, 231–241.

Maslinski, W., Remillard, B., Tsudo, M. and Strom, T.B. (1992). Interleukin-1 (IL-2) induces tyrosine kinase-dependent translocation of active raf-1 from the IL-2 receptor into the cytosol. J. Biol. Chem., 267, 15281–15284.

Molders, H., Defesche, J., Muller, D., Bonner, T.I., Rapp, U.R. and Muller, R. (1985). Integration of transfected LTR sequences into the c-*raf* proto-oncogene: activation by promoter insertion. EMBO J., 4, 693–698.

Morrison, D.K., Kaplan, D.R., Rapp, U.R. and Roberts, T.M. (1988). Signal transduction from membrane to cytosol: growth factors and membrane-bound oncogene products increase raf-1 phosphorylation and associated protein kinase activity. Proc. Natl Acad. Sci. USA, 85, 8855–8859.

Morrison, D.K., Kaplan, D.R., Escobedo, J.A., Rapp, U.R., Roberts, T.M. and Williams, L.T. (1989). Direct activation of the serine/threonine kinase activity of raf-1 through tyrosine phosphorylation by the PDGF β-receptor. Cell, 58, 649–657.

Muller, R. and Muller, D. (1984). Co-transfection of normal NIH/3T3 DNA and retroviral LTR sequences: a novel strategy for the detection of potential c-*onc* genes. EMBO J., 3, 1121–1127.

Nishida, Y., Hata, M., Ayaki, T., Ryo, H., Yamagata, M., Shimizu, K. and Nishizuka, Y. (1988). Proliferation of both somatic and germ cells is affected in the *Drosophila* mutants of *raf* proto-oncogene. EMBO J., 7, 775–781.

Noda, M., Selinger, Z., Scolnick, E.M. and Bassin, R.H. (1983). Flat revertants isolated from Kirsten sarcoma virus-transformed cells are resistant to the action of specific oncogene. Proc. Natl Acad. Sci. USA, 80, 5602–5606.

Qureshi, S.A., Rim, M., Bruder, J., Kolch, W., Rapp, U., Sukhatme, V.P. and Foster, D.A. (1991). An inhibitory mutant of c-*raf*-1 blocks v-*src*-induced activation of the *egr*-1 promoter. J. Biol. Chem., 266, 20594–20597.

Radler-Pohl, A., Sachsenmaier, C., Gebel, S., Auer, H.-P., Bruder, J.T., Rapp, U., Angel, P., Rahmsdorf, H.J. and Herrlich, P. (1993). UV-induced activation of AP-1 involves obligatory extranuclear steps including Raf-1 kinase. EMBO J., 12, 1005–1012.

Rapp, U.R. and Todaro, G.J. (1978). Generation of new mouse sarcoma viruses in cell culture. Science, 201, 821–824.

Rapp, U.R., Goldsborough, M.D., Mark, G.E., Bonner, T.I., Groffen, J., Reynolds, F.H. and Stephenson, J. (1983a). Structure and biological activity of v-*raf*, a unique oncogene transduced by a retrovirus. Proc. Natl Acad. Sci. USA, 80, 4218–4222.

Rapp, U.R., Reynolds, F.H. and Stephenson, J. (1983b). New mammalian transforming retrovirus: demonstration of a polyprotein gene product. J. Virol., 45, 914–924.

Rapp, U.R., Cleveland, J.L., Brightman, K., Scott, A. and Ihle, J.N. (1985a). Abrogation of IL-3 and IL-2 dependence by recombinant murine retroviruses expressing v-*myc* oncogenes. Nature, 317, 434–438.

Rapp, U.R., Cleveland, J.L., Fredrickson, T.N., Holmes, K.L., Morse, H.C., Jansen, H.W., Patchinsky, T. and Bister, K. (1985b). Rapid induction of hemopoietic neoplasms in newborn mice by a *raf(mil)/myc* recombinant murine retrovirus. J. Virol., 55, 23–33.

Rim, M., Qureshi, S.A., Gius, D., Nho, J., Sukhatme, V.P. and Foster, D.A. (1992). Evidence that activation of the egr-1 promoter by v-raf involves serum response elements. Oncogene, 7, 2065–2068.

Schultz, A.M., Copeland, T., Mark, G.E., Rapp, U.R. and Oroszlan, S. (1985). Detection of the myristylated *gag-raf* transforming protein with *raf*-specific antipeptide sera. Virology, 146, 78–89.

Schultz, A.M., Copeland, T.D., Oroszlan, S. and Rapp, U.R. (1988). Identification and characterization of c-*raf* phosphoproteins in transformed murine cells. Oncogene, 2, 187–193.

Shimizu, K., Nakatsu, Y., Sekiguchi, M., Hokamura, K., Tanaka, K., Terada, M. and Sugimura, T. (1985). Molecular cloning of an activated human oncogene, homologous to v-*raf*, from primary stomach cancer. Proc. Natl Acad. Sci. USA, 82, 5641–5645.

Siegel, J.N., Klausner, R.D., Rapp, U.R. and Samelson, L.E. (1990). T cell antigen receptor engagement stimulate c-*raf* phosphorylation and induces c-*raf*-associated kinase activation *via* a protein kinase C-dependent pathway. J. Biol. Chem., 265, 18472–18480.

Sithanandam, G., Kolch, W., Duh, F.M. and Rapp, U. (1990). Complete coding sequence of a human B-*raf* cDNA and detection of B-*raf* protein kinase with isozyme specific antibodies. Oncogene, 5, 1775–1780.

Sithanandam, G., Druck, T., Cannizzaro, L.A., Leuzzi, G., Huebner, K. and Rapp, U.R. (1992). B-*raf* and a B-*raf* pseudogene are located on 7q in man. Oncogene, 7, 795–799.

Smith, M.R., Heidecker, G., Rapp, U.R. and Kung, H.-F. (1990). Induction of transformation and DNA synthesis after microinjection of *raf* proteins. Mol. Cell. Biol., 10, 3828–3833.

Sozeri, O., Vollmer, K., Liyanage, M., Frith, D., Kour, G., Mark, G.E. and Stabel, S. (1992). Activation of the c-raf protein kinase by protein kinase C phosphorylation. Oncogene, 7, 2259–2262.

Stanton, V.P. and Cooper, G.M. (1987). Activation of human *raf* transforming genes by deletion of normal amino-terminal coding sequences. Mol. Cell. Biol., 7, 1171–1179.

Stephens, R.M., Sithanandam, G., Copeland, T.D., Kaplan, D.R., Rapp, U.R. and Morrison, D.K. (1992). 95-kilodalton B-raf serine/threonine kinase: identification of the protein and its major autophosphorylation site. Mol. Cell. Biol., 12, 3733–3742.

Storm, S.M., Cleveland, J.L. and Rapp, U. (1990). Expression of *raf* family proto-oncogenes in normal mouse tissues. Oncogene, 5, 345–351.

Sutrave, P., Bonner, T.I., Rapp, U.R., Jansen, H.W., Patschinsky, T. and Bister, K. (1984). Nucleotide sequence of avian retroviral oncogene v-*mil*: homologue of murine retroviral oncogene v-*raf*. Nature, 309, 85–88.

Thompson, P.A., Ledbetter, J.A., Rapp, U.R. and Bolen, J.B. (1991). The *raf-1* serine-threonine kinase is a substrate for the p56[lck] protein tyrosine kinase in human T-cells. Cell Growth Differ., 2, 609–617.

Troppmair, J., Potter, M., Wax, J.S. and Rapp, U.R. (1989). An altered v-*raf* is required in addition to v-*myc* in J3V1 virus for acceleration of murine plasmacytomagenesis. Proc. Natl Acad. Sci. USA, 86, 9941–9945.

Troppmair, J., Bruder, J.T., App, H., Cai, H., Liptak, L., Szeberenyi, J., Cooper, G.M. and Rapp, U.R. (1992). Ras controls coupling of growth factor receptors and protein kinase C in the membrane to *raf*-1 and B-*raf* protein serine kinases in the cytosol. Oncogene, 7, 1867–1873.

Turner, B., Rapp, U., App, H., Greene, M., Dobashi, K. and Reed, J. (1991). Interleukin 2 induces tyrosine phosphorylation and activation of p72–74 raf-1 kinase in a T-cell line. Proc. Natl Acad. Sci. USA, 88, 1227–1231.

Wadewitz, A.G., Winer, M.A. and Wolgemuth, D.J.. (1993). Developmental and cell lineage specificity of *raf* family gene expression in mouse testis. Oncogene, 8, 1055–1062.

Wasylyk, C., Wasylyk, B., Heidecker, G., Huleihel, M. and Rapp, U.R. (1989). Expression of *raf* oncogenes activates the PEA1 transcription factor motif. Mol. Cell. Biol., 9, 2247–2250.

Whang-Peng, J., Kao-Shan, C.S., Lee, E.C., Bunn, P.A., Carney, D.N., Gazdar, A.F. and Minna, J.D. (1982). Specific chromosome defects associated with human small-cell lung cancer; deletion 3p(14–23). Science, 215, 181–182.

Zbar, B., Brauch, H., Talmadge, C. and Linehan, M. (1987). Loss of alleles of loci on the short arm of chromosome 3 in renal cell carcinoma. Nature, 327, 721–724.

RAS

The *Ras* family form a group of closely related transforming genes that are evolutionarily the most highly conserved oncogenes known. There are three forms: *Hras* (the oncogene of Harvey murine sarcoma virus, Ha-MuSV), *Kras* (oncogene of Kirsten murine sarcoma virus, Ki-MuSV) and *Nras* (detected in tumours but not in retroviruses). Ha-MuSV and Ki-MuSV were first isolated by inoculating rats with the corresponding mouse leukaemia viruses (Mo-MuLV and Ki-MuLV): following the induction of leukaemia, plasma from these animals was injected into BALB/c mice which rapidly developed solid tumours (*rat* sarcomas) due to the effects of v-*ras*[H] or v-*ras*[K] (Harvey, 1964; Kirsten and Mayer, 1967; Harvey and East, 1971). BALB-MuSV, AF-1 and Rasheed-MuSV are additional murine sarcoma viruses that have acquired cellular *Ras* genes.

Murine sarcoma virus	Method of isolation	Acquired cellular gene
Ha-MuSV	Mo-MuLV passage in rats	*Hras-1* (rat)
Ki-MuSV	Ki-MuLV passage in rats	*Kras-2* (rat)
BALB-MuSV	Passage of cell-free extracts of spontaneous chloroleukaemia in mice	*Hras-1* (mouse)
AF-1	Friend-MuLV passage in mice	*Hras-1* (mouse)
Rasheed-MuSV	*In vitro* passage of rat leukaemia virus in rat fibroblasts	*Hras-1* (rat)

Related genes

The *RAS* superfamily comprises nearly 50 currently known *RAS*-related genes including *NRASL1*, *NRASL2* and *NRASL3*, *RRAS* (Lowe *et al.*, 1987), *RhoA*, *RhoB* and *RhoC* (Chardin *et al.*, 1988), *Rac-1* and *Rac-2* (ras-related *C3* botulinum toxin substrate; Moll *et al.*, 1991), *Ral* (Chardin *et al.*, 1986), *Rap-1A* (also called *Krev-1* or *Smg*-p21A) and *Rap-1B* (95% identical), *Rap-2* (Pizon *et al.*, 1988a,b; Beranger *et al.*, 1991b), the rat brain genes *Rab-1, 2, 3* and *4* (Touchot *et al.*, 1987), rat *BRL-Ras* (Bucci *et al.*, 1988), human *RAB2* (Tachibana *et al.*, 1988), yeast *YPT1* (Touchot *et al.*, 1987), human and mouse *MEL*, the *Drosophila* D-*ras* genes (Pizon *et al.*, 1988a), *let-60* (*C. elegans*; Han and Sternberg, 1990) and the plant *ara* gene (Matsui *et al.*, 1989).

The elongation factor EF-Tu in *E.coli* has four regions that are homologous with regions in the RAS family: most of the shared amino acids interact directly with GDP (Jurnak, 1985; see **Protein structure** below).

YEAST *RAS*

The yeast *Saccharomyces cerevisiae* has two *RAS* genes, *RAS1* and *RAS2* that encode G proteins with GTPase activity (see **Protein function** below), although they are larger than the RAS proteins of higher eukaryotes (309 and 322 amino acids, respectively). They show strong homology with human RAS proteins (90% up to position 86). The yeast proteins activate adenylate cyclase in a manner analogous to the action of G_s in mammalian plasma membranes, although it seems probable that there are additional regulatory proteins involved in yeast, with the *cdc*25 gene product regulating GTP binding to RAS and other proteins, including the 70 kDa cyclase-associated protein (CAP; Field *et al.*, 1990; Fedor-Chaiken *et al.*, 1990), that interact directly with adenylate cyclase. There is, however, no evidence that RAS proteins regulate adenylate cyclase in vertebrate cells, although they can substitute for RAS1 and RAS2 in yeast (Broach and Deschenes, 1990).

Recombinant data show that neither RAS1 nor RAS2 are necessary for viability but haploid cells require one *RAS* gene to germinate (a *RAS1/RAS2* double mutation is lethal). Mammalian *Ras* genes can substitute (50% of spores survive), hence there is functional conservation.

THE GTPase-ACTIVATING PROTEIN (GAP) FAMILY

Yeast RAS protein activity is inhibited by the *IRA* gene products of *S. cerevisiae* that stimulate GTPase activity. In yeast cells that depend upon the expression of transfected mammalian *Hras* for viability, the introduction of GAP protein complements the loss of the *IRA1* gene and inhibits growth caused by normal but not by oncogenic *Hras*^{Val12} (Tanaka *et al.*, 1989; Ballester *et al.*, 1989). Thus the *IRA1* and *IRA2* genes may code for a product with GAP-like activity (they share sequence homology with mammalian GAP) and deletions of either gene result in a phenotype similar to that caused by activating mutations in RAS, with high levels of RAS.GTP being constitutively expressed (Tanaka *et al.*, 1990).

NF1, the locus involved in hereditary neurofibromatosis (see **Tumour Suppressor Genes: NF1**), encodes a protein containing a region of 360 residues with 25% homology to the GAP catalytic domain (Xu *et al.*, 1990a, b). The homologous domain interacts with RAS proteins, stimulating the GTPase activity of yeast RAS2 and human HRAS but not that of oncogenic HRAS^{Val12} or RAS2^{Val19}. In *NF1*$^-$ cells RAS protein is predominantly in the GTP bound form and *NF1* may act as a dominant negative oncogene, its normal form decreasing p21^{ras} activity. However, the interaction with p21^{ras} is via the 32–40 amino acid effector domain and NF1 may therefore act downstream of p21^{ras} (See **Domains of RAS protein**, page 389).

Together with GAP, these proteins indicate the existence of a family providing a regulatory complement to the *Ras* family.

Cross-species homology

RAS N-termini are highly conserved (85 amino acids identical between NRAS and KRAS2 (human and mouse)). Residues 85–165: 85% homology between human RAS gene products. Residues 166–185: highly variable. CAAX C-terminus: absolutely conserved (see **Protein structure**).

Transformation

MAN

Activating mutations in *RAS* oncogenes have been detected in a wide variety of human tumours. The overall incidence of transforming *RAS* genes in human cancers is only between 10% and 15% but the variation extends from being rarely detectable in breast and stomach tumours through a 10% incidence in urinary tract tumours to a frequency as high as 95% in pancreatic carcinomas (Bos, 1988; Almoguera *et al.*, 1988). *HRAS* mutations have been detected in melanoma, and in bladder, lung and mammary carcinoma, *KRAS2* mutations in bladder, gall bladder and ovarian carcinoma and in neuroblastoma, rhabdomyosarcoma and acute lymphoblastic leukaemia (ALL) and *NRAS* mutations in lung carcinoma, teratocarcinoma, fibrosarcoma, melanoma, neuroblastoma, rhabdomyosarcoma, Burkitt's lymphoma, acute promyelocytic leukaemia, T cell leukaemia and chronic myelogenous leukaemia (CML). Individual *RAS* genes are commonly associated with specific tumours, for example, *KRAS2* with cancers of the lung (Rodenhuis and Slebos, 1992), colon or pancreas, *NRAS* with acute myeloblastic leukaemia (AML). However, there is no specificity in thyroid tumours and in thyroid adenomas and carcinomas mutations in all three genes (*HRAS, KRAS2* and *NRAS*) may occur within one tumour. Simultaneous mutations in *KRAS2* and *NRAS* have also been detected in multiple myeloma (Portier *et al.*, 1992). Even when these tumours are histologically identical, however, *RAS* expression is inconsistent. Although mutations in *RAS* occur only rarely in breast cancer, point mutations in *HRAS* or *KRAS2* have been detected in primary carcinomas and in some mammary tumour-derived cell lines (Kraus *et al.*, 1984; Rochlitz *et al.*, 1989).

These observations indicate the probable importance of *RAS* oncogenes in neoplasia although there is as yet no discernible pattern to the expression of activated *RAS* genes and they occur in benign as well as malignant tumours.

ANIMALS

Activated *Hras-1* caused by proviral insertion of myeloblastosis-associated virus has been detected in an avian nephroblastoma (Westaway *et al.*, 1986) and in a T lymphoma induced by murine leukaemia virus insertion (Ihle *et al.*, 1989). Proviral insertion of murine leukaemia virus has also been shown to cause activation of *Kras-2* (George *et al.*, 1986; Trusko *et al.*, 1989).

In model systems (tumours chemically or physically induced in rodents) the frequency of *Ras* mutations is usually ~70% (Barbacid, 1987). Thus in rats 86% of mammary tumours induced by a single dose of nitrosomethylurea (NMU) are caused by a point mutation of guanine to adenine in the second nucleotide in codon 12 (Gly12) of *Hras-1*. Dimethylbenzanthracene (DMBA) also activates *Hras-1* during the induction of mammary tumours in rats or mice and in cells transformed *in vitro*, creating an adenine to thymine transition in the second base of codon 61 (Nakazawa *et al.*, 1992). This mutation also occurs in chemically induced murine skin carcinomas, and mutations in the first two bases of codon 61 arise in both spontaneous and chemically induced hepatomas.

Nras or *Kras-2* may also be activated by chemical (e.g. NMU) or X-ray treatment (Sukumar *et al.*, 1986; Barbacid, 1987) and the alkylating carcinogen *N*-methyl-*N'*-nitro-*N*-nitrosoguanidine (MNNG) can activate *Kras-2* and/or *Hras-1* (Quintanilla *et al.*, 1986). Clonal cell populations derived from liver epithelial cells treated with MNNG that express one or both of these *Ras* genes have variable tumorigenicity when injected into rats. However, this treatment also gives rise to cell lines that are consistently highly tumorigenic, the *in vivo* action of which correlates with the co-expression of *Myc* and transforming growth factor α (TGFα) together with *Ras* (Lee *et al.*, 1991).

Chemical carcinogens are generally highly unstable (e.g. the half-life of NMU is 20 min), so their mutagenic activity must be expressed within a few hours of being administered, although the mammary carcinoma caused, for example, by NMU requires six months to appear. This indicates that in these chemically induced tumours direct mutagenesis of a *Ras* gene can play a critical role in the early stages of tumour development.

The subtlety of *Ras*-induced tumorigenesis is indicated by the finding that a single point mutation at Gly12 in chicken *Hras* generates a distinct pattern of tumours depending on whether the substituted amino acid is glutamine (predominantly lung and breast muscle tumours) or lysine (bone tumours; Givol *et al.*, 1992).

IN VITRO

The evidence from cellular studies of *Ras* is consistent with the pathology and epidemiology of spontaneously arising cancer in humans, suggesting that transformation is at least a two-stage process. Thus mutant *RAS* from human tumours only transforms transfected primary fibroblasts when supplemented with immortalizing oncogenes such as *Myc* (Land *et al.*, 1983), v-*myc*, *Nmyc* (Schwab *et al.*, 1985), adenovirus E1A (Ruley, 1983), mutant *P53* or polyoma large T antigen. E1B or polyoma middle T antigen can replace *Ras*. Normal fibroblasts are not transformed either by cellular or retroviral *Ras* oncogenes (Land *et al.*, 1983; Newbold and Overell, 1983; Ruley, 1983; Sager *et al.*, 1983). NIH 3T3 fibroblasts, however, can be transformed by overexpression of normal RAS proteins (Chang *et al.*, 1982; Pulciani *et al.*, 1985; Reynolds *et al.*, 1987b; Ricketts and Levinson, 1988), caused either by multiple copies of *Ras* genes or by linking low numbers of the genes to retroviral long terminal repeat (LTR) elements (DeFeo *et al.*, 1981; Chang *et al.*, 1982; McKay *et al.*, 1986; Doppler *et al.*, 1987). This indicates that the transforming function of proto-*Ras* genes depends on high expression due to heterologous promoters or enhancers and may be increased further by point mutations (Chakraborty *et al.*, 1991). These results suggest that NIH 3T3 fibroblasts are a partially transformed cell line, because other established cell lines (e.g. the rat embryo fibroblast line REF52), when transformed by *Hras*, arrest in G_2 or late S phase unless large T antigen is co-expressed, the role of large T antigen (or E1A) seemingly being to permit toleration by the cells of high concentrations of $p21^{ras}$ oncoprotein (Hirakawa and Ruley, 1988). Similarly, human bronchial epithelial cells (Yoakum *et al.*, 1985), epidermal keratinocytes (Rhim *et al.*, 1985), embryonic kidney cells (Pater and Pater, 1986) and fibroblasts (Namba *et al.*, 1986) are transformed by retroviral *ras* oncogenes but only when the cells have been immortalized by infection with DNA tumour viruses or other means.

Ras oncogenes efficiently transform erythroid (Hankins and Scolnick, 1981) and myeloid cells (Pierce and Aaronson, 1985) and murine mast cells (Rein *et al.*, 1985). In each of these types of cells the expression of *Ras* enhances growth without altering the differentiated phenotype. Thus, Harvey-MSV-transformed mast cells are immortalized but remain dependent on the continuous presence of interleukin-3 for survival. B lineage lymphoid cells can be stimulated by retroviral vectors expressing v-*Hras* to evolve into a clonal pre-B cell line. Double infection with v-*myc* and v-*Hras* increases the cell density *in vitro* and the cells become highly tumorigenic in animals (Schwartz *et al.*, 1986).

The patterns that have been established suggest that one oncogene may be needed for immortalization and another for transformation. However, massive overexpression of a single gene (e.g. v-*myc* or *Ras*) can probably override this distinction. It may be noted that the induction of *Hras* expression has been reported to cause the activation of both ornithine decarboxylase, *Fos*, *Jun* and *Junb* genes (Sistonen *et al.*, 1989) in NIH 3T3 cells. These are all early response genes, the expression of which correlates with activation of the mitogenic pathway and $p21^{ras}$ may stimulate at least some components of this pathway (see **RAS interactions in cell proliferation**, page 397).

The expression of oncogenic *Hras* can rapidly confer *in vivo* metastatic potential on benign rat mammary cells (Nicolson *et al.*, 1992). However, metastatic potential in these cells does not correlate with *Hras* copy number or the amount of RAS protein synthesized, and the expression of the putative metastasis-suppressor gene *NM23* is unchanged (see **Tumour Suppressor Genes: Metastasis**). These results are consistent with other findings, indicating that gene transfer to benign cells may affect the expression of genes encoding cell surface proteins and result in conversion to a metastatic phenotype.

The complexity of *Ras* is underlined by the isolation of cDNA encoding a 21 kDa protein with 50% homology to RAS (*Krev-1/Rap-1A*) from *Kras-2*-transformed NIH 3T3 cells that have reverted to a normal phenotype (Kitayama *et al.*, 1989). Thus *Krev-1* appears to be a *Ras*-related protein that suppresses the activity of v-*Kras-2*. Surprisingly, however, there is evidence that RAS and RAP1 proteins have different locations within the cell, RAS being associated with the plasma membrane and RAP1 with the Golgi apparatus (Beranger *et al.*, 1991a). Both proteins contain a CAAX box and the same "effector domain" (see below) but RAP1 lacks the upstream cysteine residues that undergo palmitoylation in RAS. RAP1 has a higher affinity for GAP than RAS and may also interact specifically with effector molecules (including GAP) by virtue of its different location to RAS. Rodent cells transformed by overexpression of the translation initiation factor eIF-4E have enhanced levels of GTP-bound p21^{ras} (see **Regulation of p21^{ras} by GAPs**, page 385) and reversion of the transformed phenotype occurs when GAP is overexpressed (Lazaris-Karatzas et al., 1992).

In a human lung cancer cell line with a homozygous *KRAS2* mutation, the introduction of a plasmid expressing a segment of *KRAS2* in an antisense orientation prevents translation of mutated *KRAS2*, inhibits cell growth and reduces the tumorigenicity of these cells in *nu/nu* mice (Mukhopadhyay et al., 1991). Anti-sense oligonucleotides directed against oncogenic human *HRAS* inhibit the growth of T24 bladder carcinoma cells but are without effect on the proliferation of the non-tumorigenic human mammary cell line HBL100 that carries two copies of the normal *HRAS* gene (Saison-Behmoaras et al., 1991). In mixed cell cultures photo-activated methyl-phosphonated antisense oligomers have been shown to inhibit selectively the synthesis of mutant p21^{ras} having only a point mutation at codon 61 (Chang et al., 1991).

TRANSGENIC ANIMALS

In transgenic mice expressing v-*Hras* under the control of an MMTV promoter, benign hyperplasia is induced in the Harderian lacrimal gland, i.e. the v-HRAS protein alone causes a non-neoplastic, proliferative effect in a tissue-specific manner. In other tissues (mammary, salivary and lymphoid), however, malignancies develop that appear to depend on additional factors. Co-expression of v-*Hras* and *Myc* causes a synergistic increase in the initiation of tumours, essentially all animals succumbing, with a marked increase in the incidence of B cell lymphomas (Sinn et al., 1987). Similar observations have been made using human *HRAS* under the control of murine whey acidic protein (Wap) promoter (Andres et al., 1987), indicating that the expression of the activated *HRAS* gene is not sufficient to transform differentiated cells *in vivo*. The overexpression of mouse *Nras* in the absence of somatic mutation has been shown to be tumorigenic in a variety of tissues (Mangues et al., 1992), whereas tumour development resulting from expression of human *HRAS* appears to be associated with somatic mutations in the majority of malignancies (Saitoh et al., 1990).

RAS AND DEVELOPMENT

Two *Ras* genes of *Dictyostelium*, Dd-*ras* and Dd-*rasG*, are differentially expressed, Dd-*rasG* protein being present only during vegetative growth whereas Dd-*ras* is maximally expressed during development after formation of the multicellular aggregate (Robbins et al., 1989). A third *Ras* gene, *RasB*, is expressed throughout *Dictyostelium* development (Daniel et al., 1993). An activated form of Dd-*ras* protein (Gly12 to Thr12) affects morphological differentiation, preventing aggregation. During multicellular development Dd-*ras* is located specifically in the prestalk region and appears to control spatial differentiation (Esch and Firtel, 1991).

	NRAS/Nras	HRAS/Hras	KRAS2/Kras-2
Nucleotides	The spliced junctions of all mammalian RAS genes correspond precisely but there is a wide variation between intron structures, giving rise to genes ranging from 4.5 kbp (*Hras-1*) to 50 kbp (*Kras-2*) in size. Of the three *Ras* genes thus far identified in the mammalian genome, *Hras-1* and *Kras-2* are so denoted to distinguish them from the pseudogenes *Hras-2* (*HRASP*; human Xpter-q26) and *Kras-1* (*KRAS1P*; human 6p12–p11). Murine *Kras-3* maps to chromosome 2 in close linkage with *Abl* and *Ltk* (Siracusa *et al.*, 1990) and an *Nras* pseudogene maps to chromosome 14 (Ryan *et al.*, 1984; Sakaguchi *et al.*, 1984)		
Chromosome			
Human	1p13	11p15.5	12p12.1
Mouse	3	7	6
Rat		1	4
Exons (coding)	4	4	4
mRNA (kb)			
Human	2.0/4.3	1.1–1.2	3.8/5.5
Amino acids	189	189	188/189 (Generated from two alternative fourth exons (*Kras-2* IVA and IVB): differ only in C-termini)
Mass (kDa)			
(expressed)	21	21	21

Cellular location

The three mammalian forms of RAS bind lipid tightly and are localized on the inner surface of the plasma membrane. They may function as homodimers or homotrimers (Santos *et al.*, 1988; Kikuchi *et al.*, 1988), in a manner similar to EF-Tu, SV40 large T antigen and *E. coli* CRP.

The concentration of RAS protein has been estimated as 6.8×10^4 molecules/cell in NIH 3T3 cells and 6.8×10^5 molecules/cell in v-*Hras*-transformed 3T3 cells (Hand *et al.*, 1987).

Tissue location

Ubiquitous.

Protein function

RAS-encoded proteins are membrane-bound GTPases. Normal p21^{ras} hydrolyses GTP at rates comparable with those reached by purified G proteins. Normal RAS proteins exist in an equilibrium between an active (GTP.p21^{ras}) and an inactive (p21^{ras}.GDP) state. The action of a variety of growth factors increases the cellular concentration of GTP.p21^{ras} and the conformational change induced by GTP binding activates p21^{ras}, enabling it to interact with target ("effector") molecule(s). The proto-oncogene forms are thought to be involved in the normal control of cell growth but any one of many single amino acid mutations can give rise to highly oncogenic proteins. The level of tyrosine phosphorylated proteins is elevated in *Ras*-transformed cells, indicating that RAS may cause transformation by cooperating with tyrosine kinases (Cuadrado, 1990).

The introduction of p21^{ras} oncoprotein into normal cells rapidly activates extracellular signal-related kinases (ERKs or MAP kinases) and p21^{ras} may mediate the activation of ERK2 by either insulin or PDGF (De Vries-Smits *et al.*, 1992). Oncogenic *Ras* also stimulates the activity of protein kinase C and the Na$^+$/H$^+$ exchange protein, phospholipid metabolism and in various types of cell has been reported to activate transcription of many genes, including ornithine decarboxylase, *Fos*, *Jun*, *Junb*, *Myc*, transin, p9Ka/42A, *TGFα* and *TGFβ* and to repress transcription of the *MyoD1*, *MyoH*, myogenin, PDGF receptor and fibronectin genes (see Tables 3.6 and 3.7 below).

Transformation by either *Kras* or *Hras* oncogenes of mouse mammary cells, rat intestinal epithelial cells, NIH 3T3 fibroblasts or NRK cells increases TGFα and TGFβ secretion. TGFα may function as an autocrine growth factor for *Ras*-transformed malignant cells although TGFα alone does not transform rat epithelial cells (Colletta *et al.*, 1991). Murine primary keratinocytes and papillomas in which v-*Hras* is expressed also have elevated expression of TGFα and TGFβ_1 (Glick *et al.*, 1991).

Transcriptional activation of *TGFβ* is regulated by a *Ras*-induced 120 kDa protein that binds to a TGACTCT upstream element (Owen and Ostrowski, 1990; Geiser *et al.*, 1991). TGFβs normally inhibit the growth of epithelial cells but this inhibitory action is lost in cells transformed by oncogenic *Ras* (Filmus *et al.*, 1992). The induction of this refractory behaviour is not caused by downregulation of TGFβ receptors from the cell surface but reflects the loss of regulation of p34^{cdc2} by TGFβ_1 (Longstreet *et al.*, 1992). Thus in *Ras*-transformed epithelial cells the phosphorylation state and kinase activity of p34^{cdc2} are not significantly decreased by TGFβ_1, in contrast to the changes in normal cells that correlate with TGFβ_1-induced inhibition of growth. Many transformed cells have high rates of secretion of TGFβ and in *Ras*-transformed fibroblasts this enhances the transcription of collagenase IV and procathepsin L and stimulates secretion of collagenolytic proteases (Samuel *et al.*, 1992). This suggests that the induction of TGFβ secretion may promote metastasis of transformed cells.

THE GTPASE CYCLE

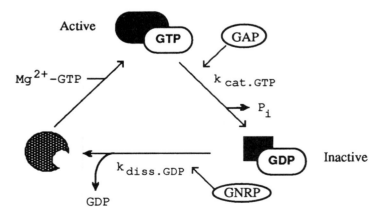

G proteins are "inactive" when bound to GDP; when this is released, the proteins assume a transient "empty" state: GTP then binds to convert the G protein to an "active" conformation that can allosterically stimulate target proteins. In many G proteins the intrinsic rate constants of GDP release ($k_{\text{diss.GDP}}$) and GTP hydrolysis ($k_{\text{cat.GTP}}$) are low (<0.03/min); these are increased by the actions of two classes of regulatory proteins: guanine nucleotide release proteins (GNRPs) that catalyse the release of bound GDP (Schweighoffer *et al.*, 1993) and GTPase activating proteins (GAPs) that increase the rate of hydrolysis of GTP (Bourne *et al.*, 1990).

REGULATION OF p21^{ras} BY GAPs

Most cells express two GAPs, type I p120^{GAP} and NF1–GAP, with similar activities. Type II GAP is an alternatively spliced form of type I GAP detected in placental trophoblasts (Trahey *et al.*, 1988). All RAS–GAPs contain an invariant Phe–Leu–Arg motif within the most conserved region of their catalytic domains: mutation of this motif can result in a protein defective in catalysis but not in binding to p21^{ras} (Brownbridge *et al.*, 1993). The C-terminal 40 kDa of p120^{GAP} acts catalytically on normal, but not transforming, RAS proteins to stimulate their relatively weak hydrolytic activity for bound GTP by 100-fold (Marshall *et al.*, 1989; McCormick, 1989). When p120^{GAP} or NF1–GAP proteins are tagged with RAS C-terminal motifs to target them to the plasma membrane, they suppress p21^{ras} function and inhibit fibroblast growth (Huang *et al.*, 1993). Nevertheless, there is evidence from microinjection studies that type I GAP, type II GAP and NF1–GAP have different activities (Al-Alawi *et al.*, 1993). The large increase in GTP.p21^{ras} that occurs in ligand-activated T cells or fibroblasts (see **Evidence for the function of *Ras*: Mitogenesis**) probably requires the inhibition of both p120^{GAP} and NF1–GAP during mitogenesis.

Purified p120^{GAP} itself does not possess nucleotide exchange activity but several proteins (p60, p100, p140$^{RAS-GRF}$) have been isolated from various tissues that markedly enhance the rate of guanine nucleotide exchange on p21^{ras} (Downward *et al.*, 1990a; West *et al.*, 1990; Wolfman and Macara, 1990; Kikuchi *et al.*, 1992). p140$^{RAS-GRF}$ has a region of sequence similarity to BCR and DBL (Shou *et al.*, 1992). The C-terminal domain of the *S. cerevisiae* Sdc25 gene product, which has GDP/GTP exchange activity for mammalian RAS proteins *in vitro*, promotes the formation of RAS–GTP in NIH 3T3 cells and renders them tumorigenic (Barlat *et al.*, 1993). The extent of RAS–GTP formation is directly proportional to *Ras* transforming potential. Mutations that reduce GTPase activity or increase guanine nucleotide exchange rates are complementary in promoting RAS–GTP formation (Patel *et al.*, 1992).

p120^{GAP} possesses SRC homology domains SH2 and SH3 through which it can associate with

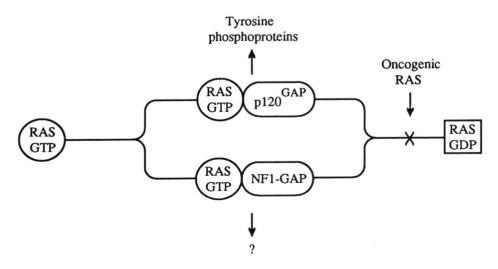

tyrosine phosphorylated proteins (Katan and Parker, 1988). The expression of GAP SH2/SH3 domains strongly induces expression from the *Fos* promoter in transfected cells (Medema *et al.*, 1992). The GAP SH2/SH3 domains do not activate p21^{ras} but this activity is required for full stimulation of transcription, suggesting that an additional signal(s) is generated by p21^{ras}. However, NF1–GAP does not contain the SH2/SH3 domains present in p120^{GAP}, indicating that different activated RAS complexes may have distinct cellular targets (McCormick, 1992).

The activity of p120^{GAP} is specifically inhibited by some lipids, the metabolism of which is altered during mitogenic stimulation (Tsai *et al.*, 1991). The most effective lipid inhibitors are phosphatidic acid, phosphatidylinositol phosphates and arachidonic acid and these bind to p120^{GAP} with high affinity in a Mg^{2+}-dependent interaction.

Structure of the Harvey sarcoma virus genome and the normal rat cellular homologue from which it is derived

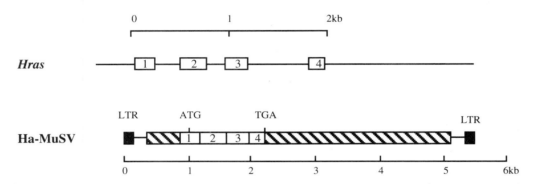

Open boxes: the four cellular exons. Black boxes and lines: LTRs and additional sequences derived from the helper virus. Hatched boxes: sequences derived from retrovirus-like rat 30S RNA. The viral genomes of Ha-MuSV (5.5 kb) and Ki-MuSV (6.5 kb) are similar: both are composed of three distinct types of nucleotide sequences: (1) sequences homologous to MuLV (0.2 kb at the 5′ end and the final 3′ 1 kb), (2) sequence homologous to rat retrovirus-like 30S RNA, located between the MuLV sequences, and (3) sequences derived from the host (rat) cell genome (1.05 kb in Ha-MuSV; 1.75 kb in Ki-MuSV), inserted towards the 5′ end of the 30S RNA. The 30S RNA is derived from a replication-defective, endogenous rat type C virus.

In the BALB-MuSV and NS.C58 MuSV-1 viruses mouse *Ras* has been transduced by a murine sarcoma virus replacing the 3′ end of *pol* and the 5′ end of the gp70 coding region of *env* (Reddy *et al.*, 1985; Fredrickson *et al.*, 1987). The sequence of the p21 protein of BALB-MuSV (v-*bas*) differs from that encoded by the human *HRAS* proto-oncogene only at positions 12 (lysine for glycine) and 143 (lysine for glutamate) and that of NS.C58 MuSV-1 differs from BALB-MuSV v-*bas* only at residues 12 (arginine) and 143 (glutamate).

Transcriptional regulation

The mammalian genes have an additional 5′ non-coding exon and mouse *Nras* contains two further non-coding exons (Paciucci and Pellicer, 1991). The promoter regions of *Ras* genes do not contain TATA or CAT boxes but have multiple GC boxes and utilize more than one transcription start site (Hoffman *et al.*, 1987). The human *NRAS* promoter contains sequences homologous to binding sites for CREB/ATF (consensus sequence: TGACGT^A/$_C$^{A}/$_G$), AP-1

(TGA$^G/_C$TCA), AP-2 (CCCCAGGC), MYB (C$^A/_C$GTT$^A/_G$), E4TF1 (GGAAGTG) and MLTF/MYC (CCACGTGA; Thorn *et al.*, 1991).

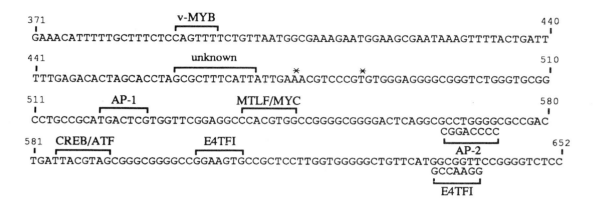

These sites reside within 439 bp comprising the 5' untranslated exon and adjacent 5' sequence that also contains Sp-1 sites that are, however, not protected in DNAase footprinting assays. An additional region is protected but has no homology to known consensus sequences. The base numbers refer to the 900 bp promoter region that has been sequenced (Hall and Brown, 1985).

A transcription unit (*Nras* upstream, *NRU* or upstream of *Nras*, *UNR*) encoding an ORF of 767 amino acids of no known function lies immediately upstream of *Nras* (Jeffers *et al.*, 1991; Nicolaiew *et al.*, 1991; Jacquemin-Sablon and Dautry, 1992). The last *NRU* polyadenylation signal is 150 nt from the *Nras* initiation sites (* in the above figure) so NRU may regulate *Nras* expression. *Kras* and murine *Nras* closely resemble human *NRAS* in their promoter regions (Paciucci and Pellicer, 1991). In murine *Nras* there is a site of premature transcription arrest in the first half of intron 1 (that separates the 5' non-coding exon and exon 1) and a positively acting region at the intron 1/exon 1 boundary that strongly enhances transcription from the *Nras* promoter (Jeffers and Pellicer, 1992).

☙ Protein structure ☙

Several different wild-type and oncogenic p21 complexes have been crystallized to provide the first atomic descriptions of proto-oncogenes and oncogenes (De Vos *et al.*, 1988; Pai *et al.*, 1989, 1990; Tong *et al.*, 1989, 1991a,b; Krengel *et al.*, 1990; Milburn *et al.*, 1990; Schlichting *et al.*, 1990; see Wittinghofer, 1992). p21 comprises a central, six-stranded β sheet and five helices, two of which (α2 and α3) lie below the plane defined by the β sheet. Of the ten loops in the protein, L1 contains Gly12 (the most frequent site of mutation in human tumours), L2 includes the residues believed to interact with the effector and L4 contains Gln61. The crystal structures are consistent with a transition state stabilization mechanism for GTP hydrolysis by p21^{ras} in which a complex is formed between the γ-phosphate of GTP and the Gln61 sidechain (Prive *et al.*, 1992). Substituents at position 61 are unable to stabilize the transition state, mutation of residue 59 from alanine to threonine disrupts the position of Gln61 and mutations at position 12 are assumed to interfere with the action of the Gln61 sidechain. Residues the mutation of which affects GAP/NF1 binding and activity (positions 12, 30–38, 59 and 61) occur in a localized region of the surface of GTP.p21 and GAP/NF1 may function by optimizing the position of Gln61.

Amino acid sequences of some RAS proteins.

```
                                  1        20         40         60         80        100
Human/rat HRAS       MTEYKLVVVGAGGVGKSALTIQLIQNHFVDEYDPTIEDSYRKQVVIDGETCLLDILDTAGQEEYSAMRDQYMRTGEGFLCVFAINNTKSFEDIHQYREQI
Chicken HRAS-1       ----------------------------------------------------------------------------------------------------
Human KRAS2A         ------------------------------------------------------------------------------------H---------------
Mouse KRAS-2A        ------------------------------------------------------------------------------------H---------------
Human KRAS2B         ------------------------------------------------------------------------------------H---------------
Mouse KRAS-2B        ------------------------------------------------------------------------------------H---------------
Human NRAS           ------------------------------------------------------------------------------S---A--NL-------------
Mouse NRAS           ------------------------------------------------------------------------------S---A--NL-------------
Drosophila Dras1     -----------------P----------------------------------RS-------------------L----SA----GT--------------
Drosophila Dras2/64B MQ-QT-------G------I--F-SY--TD--------------------------T-CN--DVPAK----------F--E---S----L-L-DHS--DE-PKFQR---
Dictiostelium DdRAS  ------I-G--------------I---------------------------------S-D-----------------------Q---YS-TSRS-YDE-ASF---
S.cerevisiae RAS1  MQGNKSTIR---I------G------------F-SY-------------------E-----------------------L-YSVTSRN--DELLS-YQ---
S.cerevisiae RAS2  MPLNKSNIR-------G------T-S--------------------------D-VSI---------------E---N---L-YS-TSKS-LDELMT-YQ---
S.pombe SPRAS      MRSTYLR--------D-------S--------------KCE----GA--V----------E---L-YN-TSRS--DE-STFYQ---

                                101       120        140        160        180
Human/rat HRAS1      KRVKDSDDVPMVLVGNKCDLAARTVESRQAQDLARSYGIPYIETSAKTRQGVEDAFYTLVREIRQHKLRKLNPPDESGPGCMSCK    CVLS (189)
Chicken HRAS-1       ----------------------------------------------------------------------------------N---    --I--
Human KRAS2A         ------E----------------------P-------T----------F------R-----YR-K-ISKEKTPGCVKIK-         --IIM
Mouse KRAS-2A        ------E----------------------PS--DTK---E-----F----------R-----YR-K-ISKEKTPGCVKIK-         --IM
Human KRAS2B         ------E----------------------PS--DTK-------F----D-----K--EKMSKDGKKKKKKSK T-               --IM
Mouse KRAS-2B        ------E----------------------PS--DTK---E---F----D-----K--EKMSKDGKKKKKKSR TR               --TVM
Human NRAS           ----------------------------PT--DTK--HE-K-----F----------YRMK---SS-DGTQ--GLP              --VM
Mouse NRAS           ----------------------------PT--DTK--HE-K-----F----------YR-K---SS-DGTQ---GSP             --M
Drosophila Dras1     -H--AEE---A-----SWN-NNE--REV-KQ-------------M--D-----KD-DN-GRRGRKMNKPNCRF-                --KML
Drosophila Dras2/64B L----R-EF--LM----KHQQQV-LEE--NTS-NLM----C---L-VN-DQ--HE---IV-KFQIAERPFIEQDYKKKGKR-        --C--M
Dictiostelium DdRAS  L---K-R--LI----A--DHERQV-VNEG-E--KDSLS FH-S---S-IN--E---S----KELKGDQSSGKAQKKKKQ           --LIL
S.cerevisiae RAS1    Q-----YI-V-V--L--ENERQV-YEDGLR--KQLNA-FL-----QAIN-DE---S-I-LV-DDGGKYNSMNRQLDNTNEIRD (111 aa)  --IIC
S.cerevisiae RAS2    L----T-Y--I-V--S--ENEKQV-Y-DGLNM-KQMNA-FL----QAIN-E-----A-LV-DEGGKYNKTLT-NDNSKQTSQ (114 aa)   --II-
S.pombe SPRAS        L--K-TF-V--A----E-ER-V--REGEQ--K-MHCL-V----L-LN--E---S---T-RYNKSEEKGFQNKQAVQIAQV (24 aa)      --IC
```

Dashes indicate residues identical to those of human/rat HRAS1. Regions with which nucleotides interact: 10–16, 57–62, 116–119, 143–145. "Effector domain": 32–40. CAAX box: 186–189. Murine sarcoma virus transforming HRAS differs from normal human HRAS by the substitutions G–K (at position 12) and E–K (143). Kirsten murine sarcoma virus KRAS differs from normal mouse KRAS2A by the substitutions G–S (at position 12), E–Q [37], A–T (59) and I–L (100).

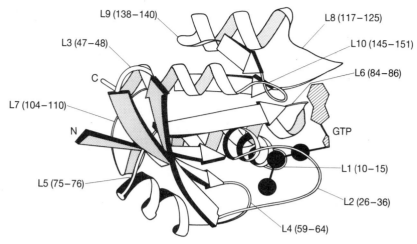

Domains of RAS proteins

(a) Evolutionary conservation

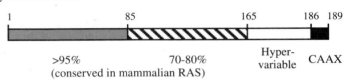

(b) Functional domains

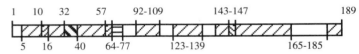

Five non-contiguous domains are essential for RAS transforming activity: residues 5–63, 77–92, 109–123, 139–165 and 186–189.

10–16, 57–62 and 116–119: Highly conserved nucleotide binding regions.

10–15 and 59–64: Two loops adjacent to the phosphate groups of the bound guanine nucleotide.

116–119 and 145–147: Form part of the pocket for the base. Substitution of Asn for Ser17 yields a dominant inhibitory protein: improper complexing of Mg^{2+} locks RAS in an inactive conformation (Farnsworth and Feig, 1991).

30 is apposed to the ribose sugar.

32–40: "Effector domain". Substitutions in this region reduce the biological effect of RAS proteins in both mammalian and yeast cells but do not affect GTP binding or hydrolysis (Sigal *et al.*, 1986). The inference from this is that the effector domain may be involved in the interaction of RAS proteins with cellular targets. Residues 32–40 are also essential for stimulation of GTPase activity by GAP.

61–65: Confer RAS–GAP sensitivity on RAS protein (Zhang *et al.*, 1991). The GTPase activity of RHO proteins, that do not have the normal RAS effector domain (Self *et al.*, 1993), is controlled by a different GAP protein (RHO–GAP, 29 kDa; Garrett *et al.*, 1989) and a GAP protein specific for KREV1/RAP1A has been isolated from HL-60 cells (Polakis *et al.*, 1991). RHO appears to play a role in maintaining cell shape by controlling actin polymerization, but it may be noted that about 30% of RHO in cells is bound to RAS. *RhoB* is an early response gene transiently induced in fibroblasts by v-*fps*, EGF or PDGF (Jahner and Hunter, 1991) and the overexpression of *Rho* renders NIH 3T3 cells tumorigenic (Perona *et al.*, 1993).

63–73: Recognized by monoclonal antibody Y13–259.

165–184: Highly divergent, function unknown. In v-RAS^H (identical to RAS^H except for two activating mutations, Arg12 and Thr59), most or all of these 20 residues can be deleted or duplicated without affecting activity (Willumsen *et al.*, 1985).

186–189: CAAX box: Cys186 essential for transforming activity. Mutations in v-*ras* that prevent membrane attachment of the protein destroy its transforming function.

White boxes: Dispensable domains (1–5, 63–77, 92–109, 123–139, 165–185).

Activating point mutations in naturally occurring *Ras* oncogenes: 12, 13, 59, 61.

Activating point mutations created by *in vitro* mutagenesis: 63, 116, 117, 119 and 146 (Barbacid, 1987; Reynolds *et al.*, 1987a; Sloan *et al.*, 1990).

Post-translational modification of RAS proteins

All RAS proteins are polyisoprenylated. HRAS, NRAS and KRAS proteins undergo two-step, post-translational modification. Step 1 involves the CAAX box (C = cysteine, A = aliphatic, X = non-aliphatic amino acid). Cys186 is alkylated by C_{15} farnesyl, the AAX amino acids are removed by proteolysis and methylesterification occurs at the α carboxyl of the new C-terminal Cys. The modified product (c-p21) is more hydrophobic than unmodified pro-p21 and associates weakly with cell membranes. In step 2 (p21^{Nras}, p21^{Hras} and p21$^{Kras(A)}$) palmitoylation of Cys residues in the hypervariable region (amino acids 165–185) increases the extent and avidity of membrane binding. Fatty acylation of Cys186 is reversible, the period of attachment being short compared to the lifetime of the protein itself (Magee *et al.*, 1987). Both modifications are necessary for plasma membrane localization (Hancock *et al.*, 1991a). p21$^{Kras(B)}$ lacks Cys in the hypervariable region and does not undergo the final palmitoylation step but has a polybasic region (six lysines at 175–180) essential for plasma membrane targeting (Hancock *et al.*, 1991b).

Phosphorylation

p21^{ras} is phosphorylated by protein kinases A or C on Ser177 in the hypervariable region linking the globular catalytic domain with the C-terminus (Saikumar *et al.*, 1988). The alternative fourth exons of the *Kras-2* gene give rise to two proteins, p21-IVA and p21-IVB, that differ only in their C-termini, p21-IVA being virtually identical to the C-terminus of v-*Kras*. In p21-IVB a serine residue at position 181 may be a target for phosphorylation. p21^{v-ras} of Ha- and Ki-MuSV are phosphorylated by autokinase activity at Thr59 but this residue is absent in p21^{ras}.

Oncogenic mutations

Mutations at the three residues critical for activating the oncogenic potential (Gly12, Ala59 and Gln61) inhibit GTP hydrolysis either by diminishing GTPase activity or (for Ala59) modulating the rate of nucleotide exchange. Any amino acid substitution at Gly12 (except Pro) causes transformation, correlating with α helix forming tendency (i.e. Gly and Pro are helix breakers). Gly12 lies within the loop that binds the β-phosphate and is enlarged in the oncoprotein forms, which may account for their reduced GTPase activity. Oncogenic mutations therefore enable the GTP.p21^{ras} complex to remain in an active form (analogous to the effect of hydrolysis-resistant GTP analogues or to cholera toxin on G proteins) that is presumed to stimulate a growth-promoting event. The Thr59 oncogenic mutation confers autophosphorylating activity on the protein: in p21^{ras}, this reaction is GTP specific.

In addition to the mutation at codon 12 in the *Hras* gene a second mutation (A to G in the fourth intron approximately 180 nucleotides 3' of the third coding exon) causes a tenfold increase in expression of p21^{ras} (Cohen and Levinson, 1988).

Evidence for the function of RAS

MITOGENESIS

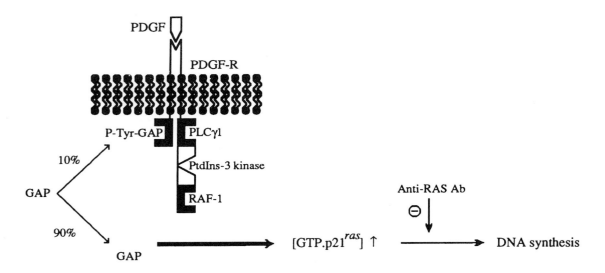

In fibroblasts the cellular concentration of active (GTP-bound) p21^{ras} is increased by PDGF, EGF or serum (Satoh *et al.*, 1990a,b) and, to a small extent by CSF1 which also causes strong phosphorylation on tyrosine residues of the GAP-associated p62 protein (Reedijk *et al.*, 1990). PDGF causes rapid tyrosine phosphorylation of ~10% of total cellular GAP through its association with the PDGFR (Molloy *et al.*, 1989; Kazlauskas *et al.*, 1990), together with PLC-γ, phosphatidylinositol 3-kinase and RAF1. Ligand-activated association of GAP with receptors may thus be a mechanism for switching on the mitogenic pathway. However, in CHO cells PDGF receptors mutated in the phosphatidylinositol 3-kinase binding sites (Tyr708, Tyr719) are unable to stimulate RAS whereas GAP-binding site mutants (Tyr739) do so, suggesting an important role for phosphatidylinositol 3-kinase or a protein binding to the same site in PDGF-stimulated RAS activation (Satoh *et al.*, 1993). In transfectants of a pro-B cell line, however, phosphatidylinositol 3-kinase, GAP or PLC-γ pathways can be eliminated without blocking RAS activation by PDGF. Furthermore, there is at present no evidence that the activated EGF receptor binds to directly to GAP *in vivo* even though it causes its phosphorylation and *in vitro* GAP SH2 domains associate with the activated receptors for EGF and PDGF (Kazlauskas *et al.*, 1990;

Moran *et al.*, 1990). Furthermore, although PDGF activates p21^{ras}, bombesin and insulin do not do so in normal fibroblasts, despite the fact that they form a potent co-mitogenic combination and bombesin activates all the other known responses stimulated by PDGF. In cells that overexpress high-affinity insulin receptors, however, insulin does activate p21^{ras} (Medema *et al.*, 1991) and in normal 3T3 fibroblasts anti-RAS antibody inhibits DNA synthesis stimulated by insulin with bombesin (Roden *et al.*, 1993).

Microinjection of anti-p21^{ras} antibody inhibits fibroblast mitogenesis in response to PDGF, EGF or serum (Mulcahy *et al.*, 1985), consistent with activation of p21^{ras} being essential for mitogenesis. In *Ras*-transformed cells, however, the activated PDGF receptor fails to undergo autophosphorylation (Rake *et al.*, 1991) or to associate with or to phosphorylate GAP even though the receptor tyrosine kinase activity is retained together with its capacity for binding to PLC-γ and phosphatidylinositol 3-kinase (Kaplan *et al.*, 1990).

Activated PDGF or EGF receptors that have undergone tyrosine phosphorylation associate with growth factor receptor-bound protein 2 (GRB2) via interaction with the SH2 domain of GRB2 (Lowenstein *et al.*, 1992; Gale *et al.*, 1993). The SH2 domain is also responsible for the interaction of GRB2 with the SRC tyrosine kinase substrate SHC. GRB2 is comprised of two SH3 domains flanking an SH2 domain and is the homologue of the *Drosophila E(sev)2b* gene product. GRB2 binds directly to murine SOS1, a mammalian homologue of *Drosophila* SOS (Rozakis-Adcock *et al.*, 1993). SOS1 is a guanine nucleotide exchange protein that activates RAS. Microinjection of HRAS together with GRB2 stimulates DNA synthesis in fibroblasts and expression of *Drosophila Sos* causes their transformation (Egan *et al.*, 1993). Thus GRB2 can bind tightly to SOS1 via its two SH3 domains and to tyrosine kinase substrates through its SH2 group. GRB2 also binds to the major insulin receptor substrate, IRS-1 (Skolnik *et al.*, 1993). Insulin also causes tyrosine phosphorylation of SHC which in turn then binds to GRB2. Thus GRB2 may be a component of an evolutionarily conserved pathway that couples growth factor receptors to the RAS signalling pathway.

In T lymphocytes anti-CD2 antibody or activation of the T cell receptor (TCR), either by monoclonal antibody or phytohaemagglutinin, increases the cellular concentration of GTP.p21^{ras} by tenfold (Downward *et al.*, 1990b; Graves *et al.*, 1991) and the direct activation of protein kinase C by TPA causes even greater increases. The effect of TPA appears to be due to inhibition of GAP activity, rather than an increase in the rate of nucleotide exchange. In LSTRA cells that overexpress p56^{lck} (by retroviral promoter insertion) GAP and the GAP-associated proteins p62 and p190 are tyrosine phosphorylated (Ellis *et al.*, 1991). In T cells activation of p21^{ras} is necessary but not sufficient to induce the expression of the growth factor interleukin-2 (IL-2). Thus activation of the IL-2 promoter in response to TPA or to stimulation of the TCR is inhibited by the expression of a dominant negative mutant of *RAS* (Rayter *et al.*, 1992).

In B lymphocytes cross-linking sIg causes co-capping of p21^{c-ras} (Graziadei *et al.*, 1990), a finding consistent with the observation that stimulation of the TCR activates p21^{ras}. This may reflect a role played by RAS proteins in receptor oligomerization, suggested by the involvement of RHO in actin filament rearrangement (Chardin *et al.*, 1989; Paterson *et al.*, 1990).

TRANSFORMATION BY OTHER ONCOGENES

Microinjection of anti-RAS antibodies transiently inhibits entry into S phase of NIH 3T3 cells transformed by *Src*, *Fes* or *Fms*, the products of which are membrane-associated tyrosine kinases (Smith *et al.*, 1986). In contrast, such antibodies have no effect on cells transformed by SV40 T antigen or by *Mos* or *Raf* (which encode cytoplasmic serine/threonine kinases). These observations suggest that *Fes*, *Fms* and *Src* may transform cells via a pathway involving *Ras* whereas *Raf* and *Mos* and the tumour suppressor genes *P53* and *RB1* that associate with T antigen activate pathways that converge downstream of *Ras*.

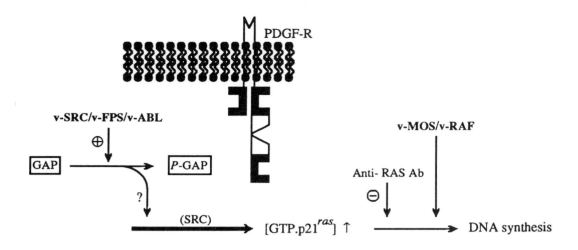

In addition to its activation by growth factors, GAP also undergoes rapid tyrosine phosphorylation in cells transformed by v-*src*, v-*fps* or v-*abl* (Ellis *et al.*, 1990) and it associates with pp62 and pp190 proteins that are themselves tyrosine phosphorylated in fibroblasts overexpressing the EGFR or *Src* (Chang *et al.*, 1993). *Src* (or *ErbB-2/Neu*) cause a 3- to 4-fold increase in the ratio of GTP.p21^{ras} to p21.GDP, similar to PDGF or EGF (Satoh *et al.*, 1990b). In p60^{v-src}-transformed rat-2 cells approximately equal proportions of GAP (~8% of the total) are complexed with p62 and localized at the plasma membrane and in the cytosol (Moran *et al.*, 1991). The majority of GAP forms a cytosolic complex with p190. EGF or expression of v-*src* also causes the formation of high molecular weight (300–500 kDa) complexes containing GAP. GAP–p190 complexes contain little phosphotyrosine but have high levels of phosphoserine and fourfold lower GTPase activity than monomeric GAP.

p190 contains N-terminal motifs that occur in all known GTPases and has C-terminal homology with BCR, *n*-chimerin and RHO–GAP, all of which possess GAP activity (Settleman *et al.*, 1992). The central 778 amino acids of p190 are 95% identical to those of GRF1, the transcriptional repressor of the human glucocorticoid receptor. p62 has significant sequence homology to the putative hnRNP protein GRP33 (Wong *et al.*, 1992). p190 is detectable in both the nucleus and its sequestration by GAP in the cytoplasm may represent a mechanism for modulating the expression of genes controlling cell growth. The putative action of p62 in the nucleus as a regulator of mRNA expression would similarly be susceptible to modulation as a result of complex formation with GAP.

EGG MATURATION

Microinjection of human RAS proteins induces maturation of *Xenopus* oocytes: this occurs with no change in cAMP levels (Birchmeier *et al.*, 1985) and independently of protein synthesis (Allende *et al.*, 1988) but may depend on the activation of protein kinase C (Chung *et al.*, 1992). The expression of oncogenic *Ras* in *Xenopus* oocytes activates MAP kinase: this precedes the activation of maturation promoting factor (MPF), the activation of S6 kinase and the induction of germinal vesicle breakdown (Hattori *et al.*, 1992). However, anti-RAS antibody inhibits maturation stimulated by progesterone but not by insulin (Korn *et al.*, 1987). Oncogenic RAS protein also exerts effects similar to those of cytostatic factor or MOS by causing unfertilized eggs to arrest in metaphase II of meiosis (Daar *et al.*, 1991).

Table 3.6. *Effects of oncogenic* Ras

Cell type/Method	Response	Comments
Fibroblasts/Microinjection of RAS	*Fos*	Induces *Fos* expression and DNA synthesis, evidently by activating SRF binding, because the responses are blocked by co-injection of antisense SRE oligonucleotide or antibodies to protein kinase C (Gauthier-Rouviere *et al.*, 1990), the latter result being consistent with other reports that protein kinase C activation is essential for *Ras*-induced proliferation
NIH 3T3/Transfected *Kras*$^{val-12}$	*Fos*	Expression of activated *Kras*^{val12} or stimulation by PDGF or TPA induces *Fos* transcription. Activation of *Fos* is inhibited by transfection of *Krev-1*. Activation of *Fos* transcription by expression of RAF1 kinase is unaffected by the co-expression of *Krev-1* (Sakoda *et al.*, 1992)
NIH 3T3 fibroblasts/Transfected *Hras*, v-*src* or v-*mos*	*Fos*	Activates *Fos* (Schonthal *et al.*, 1988)
NIH 3T3 fibroblasts/Transfected *Hras*	Osteopontin	*Ras*-transfection increases the secretion of osteopontin and the cells adhere strongly to osteopontin- or laminin-coated substrates (Chambers *et al.*, 1993)
HeLa cells/Transfection (*Ras* hsp70 promoter)	ODC, *Jun*	*Hras* stimulates transcription (Sistonen *et al.*, 1989). In HeLa H-TK$^-$ cells expression of oncogenic RAS disrupts the JUN/inhibitor complex, increasing *Jun* transcription (Baichwal *et al.*, 1991)
Fibroblasts/Anti-RAS antibody	*Fos*	Blocks serum-stimulated transcription (Stacey *et al.*, 1987)
Swiss 3T3 fibroblasts/Scrape loaded p21^{Hras}	*Myc*	Induces *Myc* transcription, maximal after 2 h (Lloyd *et al.*, 1989)
Murine myeloma cell line MPC11BU4, NIH 3T3 cells, F9 embryonal carcinoma cells/Transfected *Hras*	Polyoma virus	Oncogenic *Hras* activates the polyoma virus enhancer (Wasylyk *et al.*, 1987)
Rat-1 fibroblasts/Transfected Zn-inducible *Hras*	Transin, TGFα, TGFβ, PDGFR, fibronectin mRNAs	Causes morphological changes that are concurrent with the accumulation of 4–5 times the concentration of RAS protein that is present in normal cells. There is an accompanying increase in transin and TGFα mRNAs and a decrease in PDGFR and fibronectin transcripts. The expression of p29, a protein recognized by anti-RAS antibody, is also decreased (Godwin and Lieberman, 1990)
Normal rat kidney cells/Ki-MSV transformed	TGFα, TGFβ, Transin 2, p9Ka/42A	v-*Kras* activates transcription of TGFα, TGFβ, transin 2 and p9Ka/42A, an S100-related calcium binding protein (De Vouge and Mukherjee, 1992)
Rat epithelial cells/TGFβ_1 or TGFβ_2	GTP.p21^{ras}	TGFβ_1 or TGFβ_2 stimulate the formation of active GTP.p21^{ras}. A similar effect occurs in the CCL64 cell line that is highly sensitive to inhibition of proliferation by TGFβ (Mulder and Morris, 1992)

Table 3.6. *Continued*

Cell type/Method	Response	Comments
Fibroblasts/Microinjection of HRAS or v-HRAS	pH_i, Na^+/H^+ exchange	HRAS or v-HRAS proteins cause membrane ruffling and pinocytosis and, in HCO_3^--free medium, an increase in pH_i (Hagag *et al.*, 1987) – characteristics of the early stages of transformation. The effects of the cellular gene product are much shorter lived than those of the oncogene product (Bar-Sagi and Feramisco, 1986)
NIH 3T3 fibroblasts/MMTV-LTR-*Hras*, MMTV-LTR-v-*mos*	pH_i, Na^+/H^+ exchange, DNA synthesis	Activation of the Na^+/H^+ antiporter occurs after dexamethasone treatment (Doppler *et al.*, 1987; Maly *et al.*, 1989). *Hras* thus expressed in transfected cells appears to be able to activate the antiporter even in cells in which protein kinase C has been downregulated, which contrasts with the usual mechanism by which Na^+/H^+ exchange is thought to be stimulated. Expression of v-*mos* or *Hras* stimulates entry into S phase
NIH 3T3 and rat normal kidney fibroblasts/MMTV-LTR-*Nras*	$PtdIns(4,5)P_2$ hydrolysis	The evidence is conflicting: *Ras* has been reported to stimulate (Fleischman *et al.*, 1986; Wakelam *et al.*, 1986; Hancock *et al.*, 1988) and to have no effect on $PtdIns(4,5)P_2$ hydrolysis (Lacal *et al.*, 1987a; Seuwen *et al.*, 1988). It seems probable that *Ras*-expressing constructs transfected into 3T3 fibroblasts do not affect basal $PtdIns(4,5)P_2$ breakdown or inositol phosphate production but cause substantial enhancement of bombesin or bradykinin-induced breakdown and attenuation of the PDGF response (Parries *et al.*, 1987). This may reflect the increase in bradykin receptor expression that occurs in these transfected cells. Anti-phospholipase C-γ antibody blocks DNA synthesis in NIH 3T3s caused by microinjected oncogenic *ras* or PLC-γ. Anti-RAS antibody does not block PLC-γ-activated DNA synthesis, thus RAS protein is inferred to be an upstream regulator of PLC-γ activity that is necessary for DNA synthesis (Smith *et al.*, 1990). Oncogenic *Hras*, but not normal *Ras*, inhibits the immediate $[Ca^{2+}]_i$ response to serum (Maly *et al.*, 1988). This is not, however, due to release of Ca^{2+} by inositol phosphates which only accumulate over many hours in cells expressing *Ras*
NIH 3T3 fibroblasts/Bombesin	$PtdIns(4,5)P_2$ hydrolysis	Bombesin-PLC-γ coupling in NIH 3T3s is not pertussis toxin (PT) or cholera toxin (CT) sensitive. The enhanced phosphatidylinositol caused by $p21^{Nras}$ is the result of either a direct interaction or coupling by a PT/CT-insensitive G protein (Milligan *et al.*, 1989)
NIH 3T3/NRK/Transfected SV40-*Hras*, *Nras*, *Kras*	Diacylglycerol	DAG levels are elevated in *Ras*-transformed cells via breakdown of phosphatidylcholine not $PtdIns(4,5)P_2$. 80 kDa phosphorylation is increased, consistent with activation of protein kinase C: the latter may also be downregulated as TPA binding is reduced (Fleischman *et al.*, 1986; Lacal *et al.*, 1987a; Wolfman and Macara, 1987)

Table 3.6. *Continued*

Cell type/Method	Response	Comments
NIH 3T3/Transfected $Hras^{Asn17}$	DNA synthesis	The dominant inhibitory *Ras* mutant prevents cell proliferation induced by TPA or EGF and blocks EGF- or serum-stimulated hydrolysis of phosphatidylcholine. However, the mitogenic effect of phosphatidylcholine-specific phospholipase C is not inhibited by $Hras^{Asn17}$, suggesting that *Ras* signal transduction during mitogenesis involves phosphatidylcholine breakdown (Cai *et al.*, 1992)
Epithelial cell line/*Hras*-transformed	Phosphatidylinositol 3-kinase	In *Hras*-transformed epithelial cells p21^{ras} associates with phosphatidylinositol 3-kinase (Sjolander *et al.*, 1991). This indicates that phosphatidylinositol 3-kinase may be involved in *Ras*-mediated transformation but the importance of the products formed by phosphatidylinositol 3-kinase (PtdIns(4)P, PtdIns(4,5)P_2 and PtdIns(1,4,5)P_3) is unknown
NIH 3T3 fibroblasts/*Hras*, *Nras*, *Kras*	*Fos*	*Hras* but not *Nras* or *Kras* blocks *Fos* expression in response to TPA. In *TRK*- or *DBL*-transformed cells *Fos* induced normally by TPA (Carbone *et al.*, 1991)
NIH 3T3 fibroblasts/Transfection or retroviral infection with *ras*	cAMP	*Ras* expression may reduce adenylate cyclase activity in response to β agonists. However, most evidence indicates that *Ras* does not directly regulate PLC or PLA$_2$ (Yu *et al.*, 1988; Alonso *et al.*, 1988)
Scrape-loaded p21^{Hras}	Protein kinase C	Rapidly activated as assessed by phosphorylation of an 80 kDa Swiss 3T3 fibroblasts substrate (Morris *et al.*, 1989). Following the downregulation of protein kinase C, p21^{Hras} does not stimulate DNA synthesis in these cells (Lacal *et al.*, 1987b; Morris *et al.*, 1989) but the early 6–16 h) morphological changes associated with transformation together with the expression of *Myc* mRNA (2 h) are unaffected (Lloyd *et al.*, 1989). Protein synthesis is not required for the early changes (up to 6 h). The stimulation of protein kinase C activity precedes the detectable accumulation of diacylglycerol (DAG). In contrast to the source of DAG in ligand-activated cells (PtdIns(4,5)P_2), cells scrape-loaded with RAS release DAG from phosphatidylcholine (Price *et al.*, 1989)
3T3 and NRK fibroblasts/v-*Kras*	PDGFR autophosphorylation	PDGF-BB response blocked by v-*Kras*, indicating that KRAS can interact with the earliest stages of transmembrane signal transduction (Rake *et al.*, 1991)
In vitro/Normal or mutant *Nras* or *Hras*	Insulin receptor phosphorylation	Autophosphorylation of the receptor isolated from human placenta is inhibited (O'Brien *et al.*, 1987)
NIH 3T3 and rat fibroblasts/pMV7 retroviral ODC vector	Transformation	Sustained overexpression of ornithine decarboxylase (ODC) cooperates with activated *Hras* (Hibshoosh *et al.*, 1991)

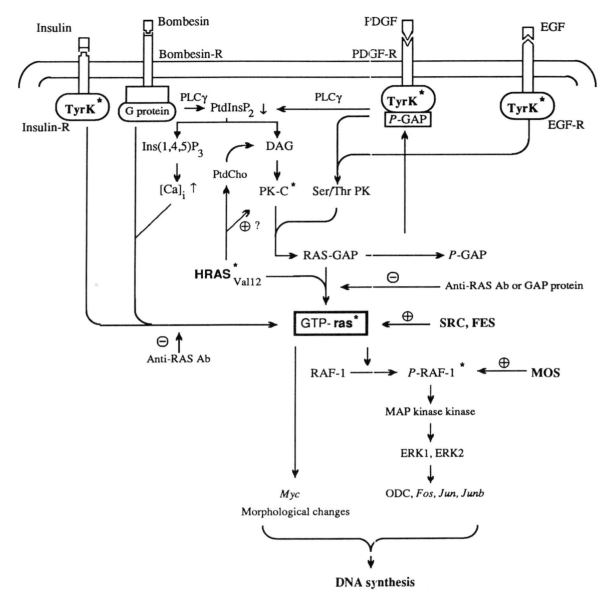

Bold type and asterisks indicate activated tyrosine kinase receptors. PLC: phospholipase C; PtdCho: phosphatidylcholine; PtdInsP2: phosphatidylinositol 4,5-bisphosphate; Ins(1,4,5)P_3: phosphatidylinositol 1,4,5-trisphosphate.

RAS interactions in cell proliferation

Insulin, together with any one of the other growth factors shown (bombesin, PDGF or EGF) forms a potent co-mitogenic combination. The receptors for insulin, PDGF and EGF each possess intrinsic tyrosine kinase activity and that for bombesin is a member of the guanine nucleotide binding protein-coupled receptor superfamily (Batty *et al.*, 1991). The activated forms of each of these receptors mediate different intracellular responses: bombesin or PDGF (AA, BB or AB) cause PtdIns(4,5)P_2 breakdown but only PDGF causes phosphorylated GAP (and also RAF1) to associate with its receptor. Neither insulin nor EGF causes PtdIns(4,5)P_2 breakdown in normal fibroblasts. EGF, PDGF or serum causes the activation of p21^{ras} (i.e. increases the p21^{ras}.GTP concentration) and the phosphorylation of GAP. Neither insulin nor bombesin activates RAS, although insulin has been shown to increase p21^{ras}.GTP levels in cells that overexpress high-affinity insulin receptors and to cause transient association of GAP with the insulin receptor (Pronk *et al.*, 1992). In Swiss 3T3 fibroblasts, microinjection of anti-RAS antibody inhibits DNA synthesis stimulated by PDGF or EGF (that are established as activating RAS) but also inhibits stimulation by insulin with bombesin. This suggests that RAS is involved in the insulin/bombesin-stimulated pathway, although increase in the concentration of activated RAS caused by these ligands in Swiss 3T3 cells has not been detected.

Oncogenic RAS (Val12) causes release of DAG: this originates from the hydrolysis of phosphatidylcholine rather than PtdIns(4,5)P_2 and precedes the activation of protein kinase C as assessed by p80 phosphorylation (Price *et al.*, 1989). Thus a direct interaction between HRAS and protein kinase C may occur.

The tyrosine kinase inhibitor genistein blocks the PDGF-induced expression of *Fos*, *Jun* and *Junb*: these genes are activated when genistein is removed and the cells progress to S phase without release of inositol 1,4,5-trisphosphate and increase in $[Ca^{2+}]_i$ caused by phospholipase C (Zwiller *et al.*, 1991).

PDGF, EGF, the activation of protein kinase C by TPA or the expression of *Hras* or the tyrosine kinase oncogenes *Src*, *Fes* or *Fms* causes the phosphorylation and activation of the cytoplasmic serine/threonine kinase RAF1 (Morrison *et al.*, 1988). v-SRC appears to activate protein kinase C (it causes p80 phosphorylation) and the induction of *TIS10* but not *Egr-1* transcription by activated v-*src* is dependent on protein kinase C (Qureshi *et al.*, 1991). The expression of activated *Raf* or *Mos* induces *Fos* transcription, and presumably the expression of other early genes that are activated before *Myc* by growth factors.

Microinjection of p21^{ras} stimulates *Fos* transcription but the constitutive expression of any of the members of the *Ras* family (*Hras*, *Nras*, *Kras*) inhibits *Fos* activation by growth factors. However, TPA activation of *Fos* is only inhibited by *Hras*, indicating that *Hras* differs functionally from *Nras* and *Kras*.

Microinjection of anti-RAS antibody blocks the effects of EGF or PDGF (the EGFR and PDGFR interact with GAP and increase the concentration of GTP.p21^{ras}) but it also inhibits the transcriptional activation pattern stimulated by bombesin or insulin, the receptors for which do not otherwise appear to interact with RAS.

Summary

The evidence indicates that, except for oncoproteins located in the cytosol, the stimulation of proliferation requires the activation of RAS. For some growth factors (PDGF, EGF) RAS has been shown to activated by the GTP binding assay. For others the evidence is less direct. In general, GAP appears to function as an upstream regulator of normal RAS, maintaining it in an inactive, GDP-bound state.

Consistent with this hypothesis is the finding that when transfected and expressed in 3T3 fibroblasts the *GAP* gene inhibits morphological transformation by normal *Hras* but not by v-*ras* (Zhang *et al.*, 1990). There is, however, evidence that GAP may be the target of RAS action. Thus mutant forms of RAS lacking effector function still associate with GAP but remain bound to GTP, although such complexes are not oncogenic (Krengel *et al.*, 1990; Adari *et al.*, 1988; Cales *et al.*, 1988). Furthermore, either RAS or GAP proteins inhibit the coupling of muscarinic receptors to atrial potassium channels (Yatani *et al.*, 1990) and antibodies directed against either block the action of the other. However, the transformation potential of a range of *Ras* mutants does not correlate with NF1-stimulated GTPase activity or with NF1 binding, suggest-

Table 3.7. Ras *and differentiation*

Cell type	Differentiation stimulus	Comments
Adrenal cells (PC12)	NGF, cAMP or oncogenic *Ras*	Each causes differentiation to chromaffin-like sympathetic neurons (Bar-Sagi and Feramisco, 1985; Noda *et al.*, 1985). NGF induces rapid accumulation of the GTP-bound form of p21^{ras} (Muroya *et al.*, 1992)
	Block by anti-RAS antibody	v-*Hras* expression elevates [cAMP] and [inositol phosphates], consistent with the finding that microinjection of anti-RAS antibody inhibits neurite formation induced by NGF but not be cAMP (Hagag *et al.*, 1986)
	Dominant inhibitory *Ras* (HRAS Asn17)	HRAS Asn17 blocks NGF-induced differentiation but does not inhibit inositol phosphates accumulation or increase in [Ca^{2+}]$_i$ (Szeberenyi *et al.*, 1992). Either NGF + db-cAMP or NGF + the Ca^{2+} ionophore ionomycin bypasses the HRAS Asn17 block to differentiation. Thus NGF-induced differentiation in PC12 cells appears to require both *Ras*-dependent and *Ras*-independent pathways
	Azatyrosine	Azatyrosine inhibits the differentiation of PC12 cells caused by microinjection of oncogenic RAS. It also causes *Ras* (or *Raf* or *Neu*)-transformed NIH 3T3 fibroblasts to revert to the normal phenotype (Fujita-Yoshigaki *et al.*, 1992)
	NGF	The activation of ERK1 and ERK2 kinases by NGF is inhibited by the expression of a dominant inhibitory *Ras* mutant, indicating that normal RAS acts upstream of an ERK activator (Robbins *et al.*, 1992)
Neuroectodermal (NF1$^-$)	RAS	Loss of *NF1* gene may lead to neurofibromatosis by removing a negative regulatory target of RAS (Basu *et al.*, 1992; DeClue *et al.*, 1992)
Murine embryonal carcinoma cells (F9)	Oncogenic *Ras* [*Hras*(Val12)]	Induces *Jun* transcription. *Jun* itself causes differentiation, i.e. JUN dimer binding to AP-1 is a sufficient trigger (Yamaguchi-Iwai *et al.*, 1990). *Hras* does not activate *Fos* in F9 cells
Rat thryoid cell line (TL)	v-*ras*	v-*ras* activates protein kinase C and induces de-differentiation in thyroid cells. The nuclear migration of the catalytic subunit of the cAMP-dependent protein kinase is inhibited, thereby regulating transcription factors that require phosphorylation by PKA for *trans*-activating capacity (Gallo *et al.*, 1992)

(*Continued on p. 400*)

ing that NF1–GAP does not function as a downstream effector of RAS (Marshall and Hettich, 1993).

There is evidence that in some types of cell dominant negative *Ras* mutants can inhibit the activation of ERK kinases. ERK kinases phosphorylate JUN and thereby modulate its activity as a transcription factor and it seems probable that RAS acts as an upstream regulator of this pathway.

Table 3.7. *Continued*

Cell type	Differentiation stimulus	Comments
Myoblasts	Block by *Hras*	Differentiation of myoblasts to myotubes is inhibited by the expression of *Ras* (Sternberg *et al.*, 1989). The mechanism involves inhibition of expression of the transcription factors for muscle-specific genes, MyoD1, MyoH and myogenin, and is similarly activated in *Fos*-transformed cells (Lassar *et al.*, 1989). Expression of a variety of other oncogenes (e.g. v-*src*, v-*fps*, v-*erbB*, v-*myc*, *Myc*, v-*erbA* and E1A) inhibits the differentiation of cells of several different lineages
C. elegans	*let-60*	*let-60* is 84% homologous to the first 164 amino acids of RAS and controls the vulval induction pathway (Han and Sternberg, 1990)
Drosophila melanogaster	*Ras-1*	Activation of *Ras* is required for signalling by the *sevenless* tyrosine protein kinase gene product. The *E(sev)2B* gene is required for signalling by sevenless and the product of this gene is a protein of the structure of SH3–SH2–SH3 that binds *in vitro* to sevenless and to son of sevenless (Sos), the latter being a putative guanine nucleotide exchange factor for p21^{ras1} (Simon *et al.*, 1993; Olivier *et al.*, 1993).

Substitution of His33 by Asp and Ser34 by Pro in the "effector domain" essentially blocks the transforming activity of oncogenic HRAS (Farnsworth *et al.*, 1991) but not that of normal HRAS when it is overexpressed. For both proteins, these mutations reduce the downstream coupling efficiency of RAS to adenylate cyclase in *S. cerevisiae* membranes and decrease GAP binding although the latter, of course, has no effect on the GTPase activity of the oncogenic form. Thus blockade of the GAP/effector binding domain preferentially inhibits the oncogenic form of RAS.

Databank file names and accession numbers

	GENE	*EMBL*	*SWISSPROT*	*REFERENCES*
Human	*NRAS*	Hsnrasr X02751 Hsnras1 to Hsnras4 (X00642 to X00645) Hsnrasn1 to Hsnrasn4 (L00040 to L00043) Hsrasnt1 M10055 Hsrasnt2 K03211	RASN_HUMAN P01111	Taparowsky *et al.*, 1983 Brown *et al.*, 1984 Yuasa *et al.*, 1984 Gambke *et al.*, 1985 Hall and Brown, 1985 Gambke *et al.*, 1985

	GENE	EMBL	SWISSPROT	REFERENCES
Human	NRU/UNR	Hsnru1 X68286		Jacquemin-Sablon and Dautry, 1992
Human	KRAS2/2A	Hsrask22 to Hsrask25 (L00045 to L00048) Hsckrasa K01519 Hsckrasb K01520 Hsckrasc X01669 Hsckrasd X02825 Hsrask1 K03209 Hsrask2 K03210	RASL_HUMAN P01118 RASK_HUMAN P01116	McGrath et al., 1983 Shimizu et al., 1983 Capon et al., 1983b McCoy et al., 1984 Nakano et al., 1984 Hirai et al., 1985 Yamamoto and Perucho, 1988
Human	HRAS1	Hsras1 V00574	RASH_HUMAN P01112	Capon et al., 1983a Reddy, 1983; Tabin et al., 1982 Sekiya et al., 1984
		X-ray crystallography		De Vos et al., 1988 Pai et al., 1989, 1990
Human	KRAS, exon 1	GB:Humkraspo M34904		Santos et al., 1984
Human	KRAS (promoter)	GB:Humkrasp X07918		Yamamoto and Perucho, 1988
Mouse	Nras	Mmnras1 to Mmnras4 (M12121 to M12124) Mmnrasr X13664	RASN_MOUSE P08556	Guerrero et al., 1985 Chang et al., 1987
MSV	Hras	GB: Msvras; Remsvras M10035	RASH_MSV P01113	Reddy et al., 1985
MSV	Hras	Rehmsv1 X00740	RASH_MSVHA P01115	Yasuda et al., 1984 Dhar et al., 1982
Mouse	Kras-2 (Kirsten MSV)	Rep21 J02228	RASK_MSVKI P01117	Tsuchida et al., 1982
Mouse	Kras-2B		RASL_MOUSE P08643; P04200	Guerrero et al., 1984 George et al., 1985
Mouse	Kras-2	Mmkiras1 to Mmkiras3 (X02452 to X02454) Mmkirasa X02455 Mmkirasb X02456 Mmrask K01927	RASK_MOUSE P04200 RASL_MOUSE P08643	George et al., 1985
Rat	Hras-1	Rnrash1c M13011	RASH_RAT P20171	Ruta et al., 1986
Rat	Hras (Rasheed SV)	Reras J02294	RASH_RRASV P01114	Rasheed et al., 1983
Rat	v-Hras	GB: Mshp21 J02207		Dhar et al., 1982

Reviews

Barbacid, M. (1987). *ras* genes. Annu. Rev. Biochem., 56, 779–827.

Bollag, G. and McCormick, F. (1991). Regulators and effectors of *ras* proteins. Annu. Rev. Cell Biol., 7, 601–632.

Bos, J.L. (1988). The *ras* gene family and human carcinogenesis. Mutat. Res., 195, 255–271.

Bourne, H.R., Sanders, D.A. and McCormick, F. (1990). The GTPase superfamily: a conserved switch for diverse cell functions. Nature, 348, 125–132.

Broach, J.R. and Deschenes, R.J. (1990). The function of *RAS* genes in *Saccharomyces cerevisiae*. Adv. Cancer Res., 54, 79–139.

Downward, J. (1992). Regulatory mechanisms for *ras* proteins. BioEssays, 14, 177–184.

Harvey, J.J. and East, J. (1971). The murine sarcoma virus (MSV). Int. Rev. Exp. Pathol., 10, 265–360.

Katan, M. and Parker, P.J. (1988). Oncogenes and cell control. Nature, 332, 203.

McCormick, F. (1989). ras GTPase activating protein: signal transmitter and signal terminator. Cell, 56, 5–8.

Santos, E. and Nebreda, A.R. (1989). Structural and functional properties of *ras* proteins. FASEB J., 3, 2151–2163.

Wittinghofer, F. (1992). Three-dimensional structure of p21$^{H\text{-}ras}$ and its implications. Seminars Cancer Biol., 3, 189–198.

Papers

Adari, H., Lowy, D.R., Willumsen, B.M., Der, C.J. and McCormick, F. (1988). Guanosine triphosphatase activity protein (GAP) interacts with the p21ras effector binding domain. Science, 240, 518–521.

Al-Alawi, N., Xu, G., White, R., Clark, R., McCormick, F. and Feramisco, J.R. (1993). Differential regulation of cellular activities by GTPase-activating protein and NF1. Mol. Cell. Biol., 13, 2497–2503.

Allende, C.A., Hinrichs, M.V., Santos, E. and Allende, J.E. (1988). Oncogenic *ras* protein induces meiotic maturation of amphibian oocytes in the presence of protein synthesis inhibitors. FEBS Letts., 234, 426–430.

Almoguera, C., Shibata, D., Forrester, K., Martin, J., Arnheim, N. and Perucho, M. (1988). Most human carcinomas of the exocrine pancreas contain mutant c-K-*ras* genes. Cell, 53, 549–554.

Alonso, T., Morgan, R.O., Marvizon, J.C., Zarbl, H. and Santos, E. (1988). Malignant transformation by *ras* and other oncogenes produces common alterations in inositol phospholipid signaling pathways. Proc. Natl Acad. Sci. USA, 85, 4271–4275

Andres, A.-C., Schonenberger, C.-A., Groner, B., Hennighausen, L., LeMeur, M. and Gerlinger, P. (1987). Ha-*ras* oncogene expression directed by a milk protein gene promoter: tissue specificity, hormonal regulation, and tumor induction in transgenic mice. Proc. Natl Acad. Sci. USA, 84, 1299–1303.

Baichwal, V.R., Park, A. and Tjian, R. (1991). v-src and EJ ras alleviate repression of c-jun by a cell-specific inhibitor. Nature, 352, 165–168.

Ballester, R., Michaeli, T., Ferguson, K., Xu, H.-P., McCormick, F. and Wigler, M. (1989). Genetic analysis of mammalian GAP expressed in yeast. Cell, 59, 681–686.

Barlat, I., Schweighoffer, F., Chevallier-Multon, M.C., Duchesne, M., Fath, I., Landais, D., Jacquet, M. and Tocque, B. (1993). The *Saccharomyces cerevisiae* gene product SDC25 C-domain functions as an oncoprotein in NIH 3T3 cells. Oncogene, 8, 215–218.

Bar-Sagi, D and Feramisco, J.R. (1985). Microinjection of the ras oncogene protein into PC12 cells induces morphological differentiation. Cell, 42, 841–848.

Bar-Sagi, D and Feramisco, J.R. (1986). Induction of membrane ruffling and fluid-phase pinocytosis in quiescent fibroblasts by *ras* proteins. Science, 233, 1061–1068.

Basu, T.N., Gutmann, D.H., Fletcher, J.A., Glover, T.W., Collins, F.S. and Downward, J. (1992). Aberrant regulation of *ras* proteins in malignant tumour cells from type 1 neurofibromatosis patients. Nature, 356, 713–715.

Batty, J.F., Way, J.M., Corday, M.H., Shapira, H., Kusano, K., Harkins, R., Wu, J.M., Slattery, T., Mann, E. and Feldman, R.I. (1991). Molecular cloning of the bombesin/gastrin-releasing peptide receptor from Swiss 3T3 cells. Proc. Natl Acad. Sci. USA, 88, 395–399.

Beranger, F., Goud, B., Tavitian, A. and de Gunzburg, J. (1991a). Association of the Ras-antagonistic Rap1/Krev-1 proteins with the Golgi complex. Proc. Natl Acad. Sci. USA, 88, 1606–1610.

Beranger, F., Tavitian, A. and de Gunzburg, J. (1991b). Post-translational processing and subcellular localization of the ras-related rap2 protein. Oncogene, 6, 1835–1842.

Birchmeier, C., Broek, D. and Wigler, M. (1985). *RAS* proteins can induce meiosis in *Xenopus* oocytes. Cell, 43, 615–621.

Brown, R., Marshall, C.J., Pennie, S.G. and Hall, A. (1984). Mechanism of activation of an N-ras gene in the human fibrosarcoma cell line HT1080. EMBO J., 3, 1321–1326.

Brownbridge, G.G., Lowe, P.N., Moore, K.J.M., Skinner, R.H. and Webb, M.R. (1993). Interaction of GTPase activating proteins (GAPs) with p21^{ras} measured by a novel fluorescence anisotropy method. J. Biol. Chem., 268, 10914–10919.

Bucci, C., Fruzio, R., Chiariotti, L., Brown, A.L., Rechler, M.M. and Bruni, C.B. (1988). A new member of the *ras* gene superfamily indeintified in a rat liver cell line. Nucleic Acids Res., 16, 9979–9986.

Cai, H., Erhardt, P., Szeberenyi, J., Diaz-Meco, M.T., Johansen, T., Moscat, J. and Cooper, G.M. (1992). Hydrolysis of phosphatidylcholine is stimulated by ras proteins during mitogenic signal transduction. Mol. Cell. Biol., 12, 5329–5335.

Cales, C., Hancock, J.F., Marshall, C.J. and Hall, A. (1988). The cytoplasmic protein GAP is implicated as the target for regulation by the *ras* gene product. Nature, 332, 548–551.

Capon, D.J., Chen, E.Y., Levinson, A.D., Seeburg, P.H. and Goeddel, D.V. (1983a). Complete nucleotide sequences of the T24 human bladder carcinoma oncogene and its normal homologue. Nature, 302, 33–37.

Capon, D.J., Seeburg, P.H., McGrath, J.P., Hayflick, J.S., Edman, U., Levinson, A.D. and Goeddel, D.V. (1983b). Activation of Ki-ras2 gene in human colon and lung carcinomas by two different point mutations. Nature, 304, 507–513.

Carbone, A., Gusella, G.L., Radzioch, D. and Varesio, L. (1991). Human Harvey-*ras* is biochemically different from Kirsten- or N-*ras*. Oncogene, 6, 731–737.

Chakraborty, A.K., Cichutek, K. and Duesberg, P.H. (1991). Transforming function of proto-*ras* genes depends on heterolgous promoters and is enhanced by specific point mutations. Proc. Natl Acad. Sci. USA, 88, 2217–2221.

Chambers, A.F., Hoth, C. and Prince, C.W. (1993). Adhesion of metastatic, *ras*-transformed NIH 3T3 cells to osteopontin, fibronectin, and laminin. Cancer Res., 53, 615–621.

Chang, E.H., Furth, M.E., Scolnick, E.M. and Lowy, D.R. (1982). Tumorigenic transformation of mammalian cells induced by a normal human gene homologous to the oncogene of Harvey murine sarcoma virus. Nature, 297, 479–483.

Chang, E.H., Miller, P.S., Cushman, C., Devadas, K., Pirollo, K.G., Ts'o, P.O.P. and Yu, Z.P. (1991). Antisense inhibition of ras p21 expression that is sensitive to a point mutation. Biochemistry, 30, 8283–8286.

Chang, H.Y., Guerrero, I., Lake, R., Pellicer, A. and D'Esutachio, P. (1987). Mouse Nras genes: organisation of the functional lcus and of a truncated cDNA-like pseudogene. Oncogene Res., 1, 29–136.

Chang, J.-H., Wilson, L.K., Moyers, J.S., Zhang, K. and Parsons, S.J. (1993). Increased levels of p21^{ras}-GTP and enhanced DNA synthesis accompany elevated tyrosyl phosphorylation of GAP-associated proteins, p190 and p62, in c-*src* overexpressors. Oncogene, 8, 959–967.

Chardin, P.C. and Tavitian, A. (1986). The *ral* gene: a new *ras* related gene isolated by the use of a synthetic probe. EMBO J., 5, 2203–2208.

Chardin, P.C., Madauce, P. and Tavitian, A. (1988). Coding sequence of human *rho* cDNAs clone 6 and clone 9. Nucleic Acids Res., 25, 2717.

Chardin, P., Boquet, P., Madaule, P., Popoff, M.R., Rubin, E.J. and Gill, D.M. (1989). The mammalian G protein *rhoC* is ADP-ribosylated by *Clostridium botulinum* exoenzyme C3 and affects actin microfilaments in Vero cells. EMBO J., 8, 1087–1092.

Chung, D.L., Brandt-Rauf, P.W., Weinstein, I.B., Nishimura, S., Yamaizumi, Z., Murphy, R.B. and Pincus, M.R. (1992). Evidence that the *ras* oncogene-encoded p21 protein induces oocyte maturation via activation of protein kinase C. Proc. Natl Acad. Sci. USA, 89, 1993–1996.

Cohen, J.B. and Levinson, A.D. (1988). A point mutation in the last intron responsible for increased expression and transforming activity of the c-Ha-*ras* oncogene. Nature, 334, 119–124.

Colletta, G., Cirafici, A.M., DiCarlo, A., Ciardiello, F., Salomon, D.S. and Vecchio, G. (1991). Constitutive expression of transforming growth factor α does not transform rat epithelial cells. Oncogene, 6, 583–587.

Cuadrado, A. (1990). Increased tyrosine phosphorylation in ras-transformed fibroblasts occurs prior to manifestation of the transformed phenotype. Biochem. Biophys. Res. Commun., 170, 526–532.

Daar, I., Nebreda, A.R., Yew, N., Sass, P., Paules, R., Santos, E., Wigler, M. and Vande Woude, G.F. (1991). The *ras* oncoprotein and M-phase activity. Science, 253, 74–76.

Daniel, J., Spiegelman, G.B. and Weeks, G. (1993). Characterization of a third *ras* gene, *rasB*, that is expressed throughout the growth and development of *Dictyostelium discoideum*. Oncogene, 8, 1041–1047.

DeClue, J.E., Papageorge, A.G., Fletcher, J.A., Diehl, S.R., Ratner, N., Vass, W.C. and Lowy, D.R. (1992).

Abnormal regulation of mammalian p21^{ras} contributes to malignant tumor growth in von Recklinghausen (type 1) neurofibromatosis. Cell, 69, 265–273.

DeFeo, D., Gonda, M.A., Young, H.A., Chang, E.H., Lowy, D.R., Scolnick, E.M. and Ellis, R.W. (1981). Analysis of two divergent rat genomic clones homologous to the transforming gene of Harvey murine sarcoma virus. Proc. Natl Acad. Sci. USA, 78, 3328–3332.

De Vos, A.M., Tong, L., Milburn, M.V., Matias, P.M., Jancarik, J., Noguchi, S., Nishimura, S., Miura, K., Ohtsuka, E. and Kim, S.-H. (1988). Three-dimensional structure of an oncogenic protein: catalytic domain of human c-H-*ras* p21. Science, 239, 888–893.

De Vouge, M.W. and Mukherjee, B.B. (1992). Transformation of normal rat kidney cells by v-K-*ras* enhances expression of transin 2 and an S-100-related calcium-binding protein. Oncogene, 7, 109–119.

De Vries-Smits, A.M.M., Burgering, B.M.T., Leevers, S.J., Marshall, C.J. and Bos, J.L. (1992). Involvement of p21^{ras} in activation of extracellular signal-regulated kinase 2. Nature, 357, 602–604.

Dhar, R., Ellis, R.W., Shih, T.Y., Oroszlan, S., Shapiro, B., Maizel, J., Lowy D. and Scolnick E.M. (1982). Nucleotide sequence of the p21 transforming protein of Harvey murine sarcoma virus. Science, 217, 934–937.

Doppler, W., Jaggi, R. and Groner, B. (1987). Induction of v-*mos* and activated Ha-*ras* oncogene expression in quiescent NIH 3T3 cells causes intracellular alkalinisation and cell-cycle progression. Gene, 54, 147–153.

Downward, J., Riehl, R., Wu, L. and Weinberg, R.A. (1990a). Identification of a nucleotide exchange-promoting activity for p21^{ras}. Proc. Natl Acad. Sci. USA, 87, 5998–6002.

Downward, J., Graves, J.D., Warne, P.H., Rayter, S. and Cantrell, D.A. (1990b). Stimulation of p21^{ras} upon T-cell activation. Nature, 346, 719–723.

Egan, S.E., Giddings, B.W., Brooks, M.W., Buday, L., Sizeland, A.M. and Weinberg, R.A. (1993). Association of Sos Ras exchange protein with Grb2 is implicated in tyrosine kinase signal transduction and transformation. Nature, 363, 45–51.

Ellis, C., Moran, M., McCormick, F. and Pawson, T. (1990). Phosphorylation of GAP and GAP-associated proteins by transforming and mitogenic tyrosine kinases. Nature, 343, 377–381.

Ellis, C., Liu, X., Anderson, D., Abraham, N., Veillette, A. and Pawson, T. (1991). Tyrosine phosphorylation of GAP and GAP-associated proteins in lymphoid and fibroblast cells expressing *lck*. Oncogene, 6, 895–901.

Esch, R.K. and Firtel, R.A. (1991). cAMP and cell sorting control the spatial expression of a developmentally essential cell-type-specific *ras* gene in *Dictyostelium*. Genes Devel., 5, 9–21.

Farnsworth, C.L. and Feig, L.A. (1991). Dominant inhibitory mutations in the Mg^{2+}-binding site of ras^H prevent its activation by GTP. Mol. Cell. Biol., 11, 4822–482.

Farnsworth, C.L., Marshall, M.S., Gibbs, J.B., Stacey, D.W. and Fieg, L.A. (1991). Preferential inhibition of the oncogenic form of ras^H by mutations in the GAP binding/"effector" domain. Cell, 64, 625–633.

Fedor-Chaiken, M., Deschenes, R.J. and Broach, J.R. (1990). *SRV2*, a gene required for RAS activation of adenylate cyclase in yeast. Cell, 61, 329–340.

Field, J., Vojtek, A., Ballester, R., Bolger, G. Colicelli, J., Ferguson, K., Gerst, J., Kataoka, T., Michaeli, T., Powers, S., Riggs, M., Rodgers, L., Wieland, I., Wheland, B. and Wigler, M. (1990). Cell, 61, 319–327.

Filmus, J., Zhao, J. and Buick, R.N. (1992). Overexpression of H-*ras* oncogene induces resistance to the growth-inhibitory action of transforming growth factor beta-1 (TGF-β1) and alters the number and type of TGF-β1 receptors in rat intestinal epithelial cell clones. Oncogene, 7, 521–526.

Fleischman, L.F., Chahwala, S.B. and Cantley, L. (1986). Cloning and characterisation of CAP, the S. cerevisiae gene encoding the 70kd adenylyl cyclase-associated protein. Science, 231, 407–410.

Fredrickson, T.N., O'Neill, R.R., Rutledge, R.A., Theodore, T.S., Martin, M.A., Ruscetti, S.K., Austin, J.B. and Hartley, J.W. (1987). Biologic and molecular characterization of two newly isolated *ras*-containing murine leukemia viruses. J. Virol., 61, 2109–2119.

Fujita-Yoshigaki, J., Yokoyama, S., Shindo-Okada, N. and Nishimura, S. (1992). Azatyrosine inhibits neurite outgrowth of PC12 cells induced by oncogenic ras. Oncogene, 7, 2019–2024.

Gale, N.W., Kaplan, S., Lowenstein, E.J., Schlessinger, J. and Bar-Sagi, D. (1993). Grb2 mediates the EGF-dependent activation of guanine nucleotide exchange on Ras. Nature, 363, 88–92.

Gallo, A., Benusiglio, E., Bonapace, I.M., Feliciello, A., Cassano, S., Garbi, C., Musti, A.M., Gottesman, M.E. and Avvedimento, E.V. (1992). v-ras and protein kinase C dedifferentiate thyroid cells by down-regulating nuclear cAMP-dependent protein kinase A. Genes Devel., 6, 1621–1630.

Gambke, C., Hall, A. and Moroni, C. (1985) Activation of an N-*ras* gene in acute myeloblastic leukemia through somatic mutation in the first exon. Proc. Natl Acad. Sci. USA, 82, 879–882.

Garrett, M.D., Self, A.J., van Oers, C. and Hall, A. (1989). Identification of distinct cytoplasmic targets for *ras*/R-*ras* and *rho* regulated proteins. J. Biol. Chem., 264, 10–13.

Gauthier-Rouviere, C., Fernandez, A. and Lamb, N.J.C. (1990). *ras*-induced c-*fos* expression and proliferation in living rat fibroblasts involves C-kinase activation and the serum response element pathway. EMBO J., 9, 171–180.

Geiser, A.G., Kim, S.-J., Roberts, A.B. and Sporn, M.B. (1991). Characterization of the mouse transforming growth factor-β1 promoter and activation by the Ha-*ras* oncogene. Mol. Cell. Biol., 11, 84–92.

George, D.L., Scott ,A.F., Trusko, S., Glick, B., Ford, E. and Dorney, D.J. (1985). Structure and expression of amplified cKi-*ras* gene sequences in Y1 mouse adrenal tumor cells. EMBO J., 4, 1199–1203.

George, D.L., Glick, B., Trusko, S. and Freeman, N. (1986). Enhanced c-Ki-*ras* expression associated with Friend virus integration in a bone marrow-derived mouse cell line. Proc. Natl Acad. Sci. USA, 83, 1651–1655.

Givol, I., Greenhouse, J.J., Hughes, S.H. and Ewert, D.L. (1992). Retroviruses that express different *ras* mutants cause different types of tumors in chickens. Oncogene, 7, 141–146.

Glick, A.B., Sporn, M.B. and Yuspa, S.H. (1991). Altered regulation of TGF-β1 and TGFα in primary keratinocytes and papillomas expressing v-Ha-*ras*. Mol. Carcinog., 4, 210–219.

Godwin, A.K. and Lieberman, M.W. (1990). Early and late responses to induction of *ras*T24 expression in Rat-1 cells. Oncogene, 5, 1231–1241.

Graves, J.D., Downward, J., Rayter, S., Warne, P., Tutt, A.L., Glennie, M. and Cantrell, D.A. (1991). CD2 antigen mediated activation of the guanine nucleotide binding proteins p21[ras] in human T lymphocytes. J. Immunol., 146, 3709–3712.

Graziadei, L., Riabowol, K. and Bar-Sagi, D. (1990). Co-capping of *ras* proteins with surface immunoglobulins in B lymphocytes. Nature, 347, 396–400.

Guerrero, I., Villasante, A., Corces, V. and Pellicer, A. (1984). Activation of a c-K-*ras* oncogene by somatic mutation in mouse lymphomas induced by gamma radiation. Science, 225, 1159–1162.

Guerrero, I., Villasante, A., Corces, V. and Pellicer, A. (1985). Loss of the normal N-*ras* allele in a mouse thymic lymphoma induced by a chemical carcinogen. Proc. Natl Acad. Sci. USA, 82, 7810–7814.

Hagag, N., Halegoua, S. and Viola, M. (1986). Inhibition of growth factor-induced differentiation of PC12 cells by microinjection of antibody to *ras* p21. Nature, 319, 680–682.

Hagag, N., Lacal, J.C., Graber, M., Aaronson, S. and Viola, M.V. (1987). Microinjection of *ras* p21 induces a rapid rise in intracellular pH. Mol. Cell. Biol., 7, 1984–1988.

Hall, A. and Brown, R. (1985). Human N-*ras*: cDNA cloning and gene structure. Nucleic Acids Res., 13, 5255–5268.

Han, M. and Sternberg, P.W. (1990). *let-60*, a gene that specifies cell fates during C.elegans vulval induction, encodes a *ras* proteins. Cell, 63, 921–931.

Hancock, J.F., Marshall, C.J., McKay, I.A., Gardner, S., Houslay, M.D., Hall, A. and Wakelam, M.J.O. (1988). Mutant but not normal p21 *ras* elevates inositol phospholipid breakdown in two different cell systems. Oncogene, 3, 187–193.

Hancock, J.F., Cadwallader, K. and Marshall, C.J. (1991a). Methylation and proteolysis are essential for efficient membrane binding of prenylated p21[K-ras(B)]. EMBO J., 10, 641–646.

Hancock, J.F., Cadwallader, K., Paterson, H. and Marshall, C.J. (1991b). A CAAX or a CAAL motif and a second signal are sufficient for plasma membrane targeting of *ras* proteins. EMBO J., 10, 4033–4039.

Hand, P.H., Vilasi, V., Caruso, A. and Schlom, J. (1987). Absolute values of *ras* p21 defined by direct binding liquid competition radioimmunoassays. Biochim. Biophys. Acta, 908, 131–142.

Hankins, W.D. and Scolnick, E.M. (1981). Harvey and Kirsten sarcoma viruses promote the growth and differentiation of erythroid precursor cells in vitro. Cell, 26, 91–97.

Harvey, J.J. (1964). An unidentified virus which causes the rapid production of tumours in mice. Nature, 204, 1104–1105.

Hattori, S., Fukuda, M., Yamashita, T., Nakamura, S., Gotoh, Y. and Nishida, E. (1992). Activation of mitogen-activated protein kinase and its activator by *ras* in intact cells and in a cell-free system. J. Biol. Chem., 267, 20346–20351.

Hibshoosh, H., Johnson, M. and Weinstein, I.B. (1991). Effects of overexpression of ornithine decarboxylase (ODC) on growth control and oncogene-induced cell transformation. Oncogene, 6, 739–743.

Hirai, H., Okabe, T., Anraku, Y., Fujisawa, M., Urabe, A. and Takaku, F. (1985). Activation of the c-K-*ras* oncogene in a human pancreas carcinoma. Biochem. Biophys. Res. Commun.,127, 68–174.

Hirakawa, T. and Ruley, H.E. (1988). Rescue of cells from *ras* oncogene-induced growth arrest by a second complementing, oncogene. Proc. Natl Acad. Sci. USA, 85, 1519–1523.

Hoffman, E.K., Trusko, S.P., Freeman, N. and George, D.L. (1987). Structural and functional characterization of the promoter region of the mouse c-Ki-*ras* gene. Mol. Cell. Biol., 7, 2592–2596.

Huang, D.C.S., Marshall, C.J. and Hancock, J.F. (1993). Plasma membrane-targeted *ras* GTPase-activating protein is a potent suppressor of p21[ras] function. Mol. Cell. Biol., 13, 2420–2431.

Ihle, J.N., Smith-White, B., Sisson, B., Parker, D., Blair, D.G., Schultz, A., Kozak, C., Lunsford, R.W., Askew, D., Weinstein, Y. and Isfort, R.J. (1989). Activation of the c-H-*ras* proto-oncogene by retrovirus insertion and chromosomal rearrangement in a Moloney leukemia virus-induced T-cell leukemia. J. Virol., 63, 2959–2966.

Jacquemin-Sablon, H. and Dautry, F. (1992). Organization of the unr/N-ras locus: characterization of the promoter region of the human unr gene. Nucleic Acids Res., 20, 6355–6361.

Jahner, D. and Hunter, T. (1991). The ras-related gene rhoB is an immediate-early gene inducible by v-fps, epidermal growth factor and platelet-derived growth factor in rat fibroblasts. Mol. Cell. Biol., 11, 3682–3690.

Jeffers, M. and Pellicer, A. (1992). Multiple elements regulate the expression of the murine N-ras gene. Oncogene, 7, 2115–2123.

Jeffers, M., Paciucci, R. and Pellicer, A. (1991). Characterization of unr; a gene closely linked to N-ras. Nucleic Acids Res., 18, 4891–4899.

Jurnak, F. (1985). Structure of the GDP domain of EF-Tu and location of the amino acids homologous to ras oncogene proteins. Science, 230, 32–36.

Kaplan, D.R., Morrison, D.K., Wong, G., McCormick, F. and Williams, L.T. (1990). PDGF β-receptor stimulates tyrosine phosphorylation of GAP and association of GAP with a signaling complex. Cell, 61, 125–133.

Kazlauskas, A., Ellis, C., Pawson, T. and Cooper, J.A. (1990). Binding of GAP to activated PDGF receptors. Science, 247, 1578–1581.

Kikuchi, A., Yamashita, T., Kawata, M., Yamamoto, K., Ikeda, K., Tanimoto, T. and Takai, Y. (1988). Purification and characterisation of a normal GTP-binding protein with a molecular weight of 24,000 from bovine brain membranes. J. Biol Chem., 263, 2897–2904.

Kikuchi, A., Kaibuchi, K., Hori, Y., Nonaka, H., Sakoda, T., Kawamura, M., Mizuno, T. and Takai, Y. (1992). Molecular cloning of the human cDNA for a stimulatory GDP/GTP exchange protein for c-Ki-ras p21 and smg p21. Oncogene, 7, 289–293.

Kirsten, W.H. and Mayer, C.A. (1967). Morphologic responses to a murine erythroblastosis virus. J. Natl Cancer Inst., 39, 311–335.

Kitayama, H., Sugimoto, Y., Matsuzaki, T., Ikawa, Y. and Noda, M. (1989). A ras-related gene with transformation suppressor activity. Cell, 56, 77–84.

Korn, L.J., Siebel, C.W., McCormick, F. and Roth, R.A. (1987). Ras p21 as a potential mediator of insulin action in Xenopus oocytes. Science, 236, 840–843.

Kraus, M.H., Yuasa, Y. and Aaronson, S.A. (1984). A position 12-activated H-ras oncogene in all HS578T mammary carcinosarcoma cells but not normal mammary cells of the same patient. Proc. Natl Acad. Sci. USA, 81, 5384–5388.

Krengel, U., Schlichting, I., Scherer, A., Schumann, R., Frech, M., John, J., Kabsch, W., Pai, E.F. and Wittinghofer, A. (1990). Three-dimensional structures of H-ras p21 mutants: molecular basis for their inability to function as signal switch molecules. Cell, 62, 539–548.

Lacal, J.C., Moscat, J. and Aaronson, S.A. (1987a). Novel source of 1,2-diacylglycerol elevated in cells transformed by Ha-ras oncogene. Nature, 330, 269–272.

Lacal, J.C., Fleming, T.P., Warren, B.S., Blumberg, P.M. and Aaronson, S.A. (1987b). Involvement of functional protein kinase C in the mitogenic response to the H-ras oncogene product. Mol. Cell. Biol., 7, 4146–4149.

Land, H., Parada, L.F. and Weinberg, R.A. (1983). Tumourigenic conversion of primary embryo fibroblasts requires at least two cooperating oncogenes. Nature, 304, 596–602.

Lassar, A.B., Thayer, M.J., Overell, R.W. and Weintraub, H. (1989). Transformation by activated ras or fos prevents myogenesis by inhibiting expression of MyoD. Cell, 58, 659–667.

Lazaris-Karatzas, A., Smith, M.R., Frederickson, R.M., Jaramillo, M.L., Liu, Y.-L., Kung, H.-F. and Sonenberg, N. (1992). Ras mediates translation inititation factor 4E-induced malignant transformation. Genes Devel., 6, 1631–1642.

Lee, L.W., Raymond, V.W., Tsao, M.-S., Lee, D.C., Earp, H.S. and Grisham, J.W. (1991). Clonal cosegregation of tumorigenicity with overexpression of c-myc and transforming growth factor α genes in chemically transformed rat liver epithelial cells. Cancer Res., 51, 5238–5244.

Lloyd, A.C., Paterson, H.F., Morris, J.D.H., Hall, A. and Marshall, C.J. (1989). p21[H-ras]-induced morphological transformation and increases in c-myc expression are independent of functional protein kinase C. EMBO J., 8, 1099–1104.

Longstreet, M., Miller, B. and Howe, P.H. (1992). Loss of transforming growth factor β1 (TGF-β1)-induced growth arrest and p34[cdc2] regulation in ras-transfected epithelial cells. Oncogene, 7, 1549–1556.

Lowe, D.G., Capon, D.J., Delwart, E., Sakaguchi, A.Y., Naylor, S.L. and Goeddel, D.V. (1987). Structure of the human and murine R-ras genes, novel genes closely related to ras proto-oncogenes. Cell, 48, 137–146.

Lowenstein, E.J., Daly, R.J., Batzer, A.G., Li, W., Margolis, B., Lammers, R., Ullrich, A., Skolnik, E.Y., Bar-

Sagi, D. and Schlessinger, J. (1992). The SH2 and SH3 domain-containing protein GRB2 links receptor tyrosine kinases to ras signaling. Cell, 70, 431–442.

McCormick, F. (1989). *ras* GTPase activity protein: signal transmitter and signal terminator. Cell, 56, 5–8.

McCormick, F. (1992). Coupling of ras p21 signalling and GTP hydrolysis by GTPase activating proteins. Phil. Trans. R. Soc. Lond. B, 336, 43–48.

McCoy, M.S., Bargmann, C.I. and Weinberg, R.A. (1984). Human colon carcinoma Ki-*ras*2 oncogene and its corresponding proto-oncogene. Mol. Cell. Biol., 4, 1577–1582.

McGrath, J.P., Capon, D.J., Smith, D.H., Chen, E.Y., Seeburg, P.H., Goeddel, D.V. and Levinson A.D. (1983). Structure and organization of the human Ki-*ras* proto-oncogene and a related processed pseudogene. Nature, 304, 501–506.

McKay, I.A., Marshall, C.J., Cales, C. and Hall, A. (1986). Transformation and stimulation of DNA synthesis in NIH 3T3 cells are a titratable function of normal p21^{N-ras} expression. EMBO J., 5, 2617–2621.

Magee, A.I., Gutierrez, L., McKay, I.A., Marshall, C.J. and Hall, A. (1987). Dynamic fatty acylation of p21^{N-ras}. EMBO J., 6, 3353–3357.

Maly, K., Doppler, W., Oberhuber, H., Meusburger, H., Hofmann, J., Jaggi, R. and Grunicke, H.H. (1988). Desensitization of the Ca^{2+}-mobilizing system to serum growth factors by Ha-*ras* and v-*mos*. Mol. Cell. Biol., 8, 4212–4216.

Maly, K., Uberall, F., Loferer, H., Doppler, W., Oberhuber, Groner, B. and Grunicke, H.H. (1989). Ha-*ras* activates the Na^+/H^+ antiporter by a protein kinase C-independent mechanism. J. Biol. Chem., 264, 11839–11842.

Mangues, R., Seidman, I., Gordon, J.W. and Pellicer, A. (1992). Overexpression of the N-*ras* proto-oncogene, not somatic mutational activation, associated with malignant tumors in transgenic mice. Oncogene, 7, 2073–2076.

Marshall, M.S. and Hettich, L.A. (1993). Characterization of ras effector mutant interactions with the NF1-GAP related domain. Oncogene, 8, 425–431.

Marshall, M.S., Hill, W.S., Ng, A.S., Vogel, V.S., Schaber, M.D., Scolnick, E.M., Dixon, R.A.F., Sigal, I.S. and Gibbs, J.B. (1989). A C-terminal domain of GAP is sufficient to stimulate *ras* p21 GTPase activity. EMBO J., 8, 1105–1110.

Matsui, M., Sasamoto, S., Kunieda, T., Nomura, N. and Ishizaki, R. (1989). Cloning of *ara*, a putative *Arabidopsis thaliana* gene homologous to the *ras*-related gene family. Gene, 76, 313–329.

Medema, R.H., Burgering, B.M.T. and Bos, J.L. (1991). Insulin-induced p21ras activation does not require protein kinase C, but a protein sensitive to phenylarsine oxide. J. Biol. Chem., 266, 21186–21189.

Medema, R.H., de Laat, W.L., Martin, G.A., McCormick, F. and Bos, J.L. (1992). GTPase-activating protein SH2-SH3 domains induce gene expression in a ras-dependent fashion. Mol. Cell. Biol., 12, 3425–3430.

Milburn, M.V., Tong, L., De Vos, A.M., Brunger, A., Yamaizumi, Z., Nishimura, S. and Kim, S.-H. (1990). Molecular switch for signal transduction: structural differences between active and inactive forms of protooncogenic *ras* proteins. Science, 247, 939–945.

Milligan, G., Davies, S.-A., Houslay, M.D. and Wakelam, M.J. (1989). Identification of the pertussis and cholera toxin substrates in normal and N-*ras* transformed NIH3T3 fibroblasts and an assessment of their involvement in bombesin-stimulation of inositol phospholipid metabolism. Oncogene, 4, 659–663.

Moll, J., Sansig, G., Fattori, E. and van der Putten, H. (1991). The murine *rac*1 gene: cDNA cloning, tissue distribution and regulated expression of *rac*1 mRNA by disassembly of actin microfilaments. Oncogene, 6, 863–866.

Molloy, C.J., Bottaro, D.P., Fleming, T.P., Marshall, M.S., Gibbs, J.B. and Aaronson, S.A. (1989). PDGF induction of tyrosine phosphorylation of GTPase activating protein. Nature, 342, 711–714.

Moran, M.F., Koch, C.A., Anderson, D.A., Ellis, C., England, L., Martin, G.S. and Pawson, T. (1990). src homology domains direct protein-protein interactions in signal transduction. Proc. Natl Acad. Sci. USA, 87, 8622–8626.

Moran, M.F., Polakis, P., McCormick, F., Pawson, T. and Ellis, C. (1991). Protein-tyrosine kinases regulate the phosphorylation, protein interactions, subcellular distribution and activity of p21^{ras} GTPase-activating protein. Mol. Cell. Biol., 11, 1804–1812.

Morris, J.D.H., Price, B., Lloyd, A.C., Self, A.J., Marshall, C.J. and Hall, A. (1989). Scrape-loading of Swiss 3T3 cells with *ras* protein rapidly activates protein kinase C in the absence of phosphoinositide hydrolysis. Oncogene, 4, 27–31.

Morrison, D.K., Kaplan, D.R., Rapp, U. and Roberts, T.M. (1988). Signal transduction from membrane to cytoplasm: growth factors and membrane-bound oncogene products increase *raf*-1 phosphorylation and associated protein kinase activity. Proc. Natl Acad. Sci. USA, 85, 8855–8859.

Mukhopadhyay, T., Tainsky, M., Cavender, A.C. and Roth, J.A. (1991). Specific inhibition of K-*ras* expression and tumorigenicity of lung cancer cells by antisense RNA. Cancer Res., 51, 1744–1748.

Mulcahy, L.S., Smith, M.R. and Stacey, D.W. (1985). Requirement for *ras* proto-oncogene function during serum-stimulated growth of NIH 3T3 cells. Nature, 313, 241–243.

Mulder, K.M. and Morris, S.L. (1992). Activation of p21^{ras} by transforming growth factor β in epithelial cells. J. Biol. Chem., 267, 5029–5031.

Muroya, K., Hattori, S. and Nakamura, S. (1992). Nerve growth factor induces rapid accumulation of the GTP-bound form of p21^{ras} in rat pheochromocytoma PC12 cells. Oncogene, 7, 277–281.

Nakano, H., Yamamoto, F., Neville, C., Evans, D., Mizuno, T. and Perucho, M. (1984). Isolation of transforming sequences of two human lung carcinomas: Structural and functional analysis of the activated c-K-*ras* oncogenes. Proc. Natl Acad. Sci. USA, 81, 71–75.

Nakazawa, H., Aguelon, A.-M. and Yamasaki, H. (1992). Identification and quantification of a carcinogen-induced molecular initiation event in cell transformation. Oncogene, 7, 2295–2301.

Namba, M., Nishitani, K., Fukushima, F., Kimoto, T. and Nose, K. (1986). Multistep process of neoplastic transformation of normal human fibroblasts by ^{60}CO gamma rays and Harvey sarcoma viruses. Int. J. Cancer, 37, 419–423.

Newbold, R.F. and Overell, R.W. (1983). Fibroblast immortality is a prerequisite for transformation by EJ c-Ha-*ras* oncogene. Nature, 304, 648–651.

Nicolaiew, N., Triqueneaux, G. and Dautry, F. (1991). Organization of the human *N-ras* locus: characterization of a gene located immediately upstream of *N-ras*. Oncogene, 6, 721–730.

Nicolson, G.L., Gallick, G.E., Spohn, W.H., Lembo, T.M. and Tainsky, M.A. (1992). Transfection of activated c-H-*ras*^{EJ}/pSV2neo or pSV2neo genes into rat mammary cells: rapid stimulation of clonal diversification of spontaneous metastatic and cell-surface properties. Oncogene, 7, 1127–1135.

Noda, M., Ko, M., Ogura, A., Liu, D.-G., Amano, T., Takano, T. and Ikawa, Y. (1985). Sarcoma viruses carrying *ras* oncogenes induce differentiation-associated properties in a neuronal cell line. Nature, 318, 73–75.

O'Brien, R.M., Siddle, K., Houslay, M.D. and Hall, A. (1987). Interaction of the human insulin receptor with the ras oncogene product p21. FEBS Letts., 217, 253–259.

Olivier, J.P., Raabe, T., Henkemeyer, M., Dickson, B., Mbamalu, G., Margolis, B., Schlessinger, J., Hafen, E. and Pawson, T. (1993). A Drosophila SH2-SH3 adaptor protein implicated in coupling the sevenless tyrosine kinase to an activator of Ras guanine nucleotide exchange, Sos. Cell, 73, 179–191.

Owen, R.D. and Ostrowski, M.C. (1990). Transcriptional activation of a conserved sequence element by *ras* requires a nuclear factor distinct from c-*fos* or c-*jun*. Proc. Natl Acad. Sci. USA, 87, 3866–3870.

Paciucci, R. and Pellicer, A. (1991). Dissection of the mouse N-*ras* gene upstream regulatory sequences and identification of the promoter and a negative regulatory element. Mol. Cell. Biol., 11, 1334–1343.

Pai, E.F., Kabsch, W., Krengel, U., Holmes, K.C., John, J. and Wittinghofer, A. (1989). Structure of the guanine nucleotide domain of the Ha-*ras* oncogene product p21 in the triphosphate conformation. Nature, 341, 209–214.

Pai, E.F., Krengel, U., Petsko, G.A., Goody, R.S., Kabsch, W. and Wittinghofer, A. (1990). Refined crystal structure of the triphosphate conformation of H-*ras* at 1.35A resolution: implications for the mechanism of GTP hydrolysis. EMBO J., 9, 2351–2359.

Parries, G.R., Hoebel, R. and Racker, E. (1987). Opposing effects of *ras* oncogene on growth factor-stimulated phosphoinositide hydrolysis: desensitization of platelet-derived growth factor and enhanced sensitivity to bradykinin. Proc. Natl Acad. Sci. USA, 84, 2648–2652.

Patel, G., MacDonald, M.J., Khosravi-Far, R., Hisaka, M.M. and Der, C.J. (1992). Alternate mechanisms of *ras* activation are complementary and favor formation of *ras*-GTP. Oncogene, 7, 283–288.

Pater, A. and Pater, M.M. (1986). Transformation of primary human embryonic kidney cells to anchorage independence by a combination of BK virus DNA and the Harvey-*ras* oncogene. J. Virol., 58, 680–683.

Paterson, H.F., Self, A.J., Garrett, M.D., Just, I., Aktories, K. and Hall, A. (1990). Microinjection of recombinant p21^{rho} induces rapid changes in cell morphology. J. Cell Biol., 111, 1001–1007.

Perona, R., Esteve, P., Jimenez, B., Ballestero, R.P., Cajal, S.R. and Lacal, J.C. (1993). Tumorigenic activity of *rho* genes from *Aplysia californica*. Oncogene, 8, 1285–1292.

Pierce, J.H. and Aaronson, S.A.(1985). Myeloid cell transformation by *ras*-containing murine sarcoma viruses. Mol. Cell. Biol., 5, 667–674.

Pizon, V., Chardin, P., Lerosey, I., Olofsson, B. and Tavitian, A. (1988a). Human cDNAs rap1 and rap2 homologous to the *Drosophila* gene DRAS3 encode proteins closely related to *ras* in the 'effector' region. Oncogene, 3, 201–204.

Pizon, V., Lerosey, I., Chardin, P. and Tavitian, A. (1988b). Nucleotide sequence of a human cDNA encoding a *ras*-related protein (*rap*1B). Nucleic Acids Res., 16, 7719.

Polakis, P.G., Rubinfeld, B., Evans, T. and McCormick, F. (1991). Purification of a plasma membrane-associated GTPase-activating protein specific for rap1/Krev-1 from HL60 cells. Proc. Natl Acad. Sci. USA, 88, 239–243.

Portier, M., Moles, J.-P., Mazars, G.-R., Jeanteur, P., Bataille, R., Klein, B. and Theillet, C. (1992). p53 and *RAS* gene mutations in multiple myeloma. Oncogene, 7, 2539–2543.

Price, B.D., Morris, J.D.H., Marshall, C.J. and Hall, A. (1989). Stimulation of phosphatidylcholine hydrolysis, diacylglycerol release, and arachidonic acid production by oncogenic ras is a consequence of protein kinase C activation. J. Biol. Chem., 264, 16638–16643.

Prive, G.G., Milburn, M.V., Tong, L., de Vos, A.M., Yamaizumi, Z., Nishimura, S. and Kim, S.-H. (1992). X-ray crystal structures of transforming p21 ras mutants suggest a transition-state stabilization mechanism for GTP hydrolysis. Proc. Natl Acad. Sci. USA, 89, 3649–3653.

Pronk, G.J., Medema, R.H., Burgering, B.M.T., Clark, R., McCormick, F. and Bos, J.L. (1992). Interaction between the p21ras GTPase activating protein and the insulin receptor. J. Biol. Chem., 267, 24058–24063.

Pulciani, S., Santos, E., Long, L.K., Sorrentino, V., Barbacid, M. (1985). ras gene amplification and malignant transformation. Mol. Cell. Biol., 5, 2836–2841.

Quintanilla, M., Brown, K., Ramsden, M. and Balmain, A. (1986). Carcinogen-specific mutation and amplification of Ha-*ras* during mouse skin carcinogenesis. Nature, 322, 78–80.

Qureshi, S.A., Joseph, C.K., Rim, M., Maroney, A. and Foster, D.A. (1991). v-*src* activates both protein kinase C-dependent and independent signaling pathway in murine fibroblasts. Oncogene, 6, 995–999.

Rake, J.B., Quinones, M.A. and Faller, D.V. (1991). Inhibition by platelet-derived growth factor-mediated signal transduction by transforming *ras*. J. Biol. Chem., 266, 5348–5352.

Rasheed, S., Norman, G.L. and Heidecker, G. (1983). Nucleotide sequence of the Rasheed rat sarcoma virus oncogene: New mutations. Science 221, 155–157.

Rayter, S.I., Woodrow, M., Lucas, S.C., Cantrell, D.A. and Downward, J. (1992). p21^{ras} mediates control of *IL-2* gene promoter function in T cell activation. EMBO J., 11, 4549–4556.

Reddy, E.P. (1983). Nucleotide sequence analysis of the T24 human bladder carcinoma oncogene. Science, 220, 1061–1063.

Reddy, E.P., Lipman, D., Andersen, P.R., Tronick, S.R. and Aaronson, S.A. (1985). Nucleotide sequence analysis of the BALB/c murine sarcoma virus transforming gene. J. Virol., 53, 984–987.

Reedijk, M., Liu, X. and Pawson, T. (1990). Interactions of phosphatidylinositol kinase, GTPase-activating protein (GAP), and GAP-associated proteins with the colony-stimulating factor 1 receptor. Mol. Cell. Biol., 10, 5601–5608.

Rein, A., Keller, J., Schultz, A.M., Holmes, K.L., Medicus, R. and Ihle, J.H. (1985). Infection of murine mast cells by Harvey sarcoma virus: immortalization without loss of requirement for interleukin-3. Mol. Cell. Biol., 5, 2257–2264.

Reynolds, S.H., Stowers, S., J., Patterson, R.M., Maronpot, R.R., Aaronson, S.A. and Anderson, M.W. (1987a). Activated oncogenes in B6C3F1 mouse liver tumors: implications for risk assessment. Science, 237, 1309–1316.

Reynolds, V.L., Lebovitz, R.M., Warren, S., Hawley, T.S., Godwin, A.K. and Lieberman, M.W. (1987b). Regulation of a metallothionein-*ras*T24 fusion gene by zinc results in graded alterations in cell morphology and growth. Oncogene, 1, 323–330.

Rhim, J.S., Jay, G., Arnstein, P., Price, F.M., Sanford, K.K. and Aaronson, S.A. (1985). Neoplastic transformation of human epidermal keratinocytes by AD12-SV40 and Kirsten sarcoma viruses. Science, 227, 1250–1252.

Ricketts, M.H. and Levinson, A.D. (1988). High-level exposure of c-H-*ras* fails to fully transform Rat-1 cells. Mol. Cell. Biol., 8, 1460–1468.

Robbins, S.M., Williams, J.G., Jermyn, K.A., Spiegelman, G.B. and Weeks, G. (1989). Growing and developing *Dictyostelium* cells express different *ras* genes. Proc. Natl Acad. Sci. USA, 86, 938–942.

Robbins, D.J., Cheng, M., Zhen, E., Vanderbilt, C.A., Feig, L.A. and Cobb, M.H. (1992). Evidence for a ras-dependent extracellular signal-regulated protein kinase (ERK) cascade. Proc. Natl Acad. Sci. USA, 89, 6924–6928.

Rochlitz, C.F., Scott, G.K., Dodson, J.M., Liu, E., Dollbaum, C., Smith, H.S. and Benz, C.C. (1989). Incidence of activating *ras* oncogene mutations associated with primary and metastatic human breast cancer. Cancer Res., 49, 357–360.

Roden, R.B.S., Cosulich, S.C., Hesketh, T.R. and Metcalfe, J.C. (1993). A common requirement for p21^{ras} function in the mitogenic signalling pathways of Swiss 3T3 fibroblasts. Cell Growth and Differentiation, in press.

Rodenhuis, S. and Slebos, R.J.C. (1992). Clinical significance of ras oncogene activation in human lung cancer. Cancer Res., 52, 2665s–2669s.

Rozakis-Adcock, M., Fernley, R., Wade, J., Pawson, T. and Bowtell, D. (1993). The SH2 and SH3 domains of mammalian Grb2 couple the EGF receptor to the Ras activator mSos1. Nature, 363, 83–88.

Ruley, H.E. (1983). Adenovirus early region 1A enables viral and cellular transforming genes to transform primary cells in culture. Nature, 304, 602–606.

Ruta, M., Wolford, R., Dhar, R., DeFeo-Jones, D., Ellis, R.W. and Scolnick, E.M. (1986). Nucleotide sequence of the two rat cellular ras-H genes. Mol. Cell. Biol., 6, 1706–1710.

Ryan, J., Hart, C.P. and Ruddle, F.H. (1984). Molecular cloning and chromosome assignment of murine N-ras. Nucleic Acids Res., 12, 6063–6072.

Sager, R., Tanaka, K., Lau, C.C., Ebina, Y. and Anisowicz, A. (1983). Resistance of human cells to tumorigenesis induced by cloned transforming genes. Proc. Natl Acad. Sci. USA, 87, 7601–7605.

Saikumar, P., Ulsh, L.S., Clanton, D.J., Huang, K.P. and Shih, T.Y. (1988). Novel phosphorylation of c-ras p21 by protein kinases. Oncogene Res., 3, 213–222.

Saison-Behmoaras, T., Tocque, B., Rey, I., Chassignol, M., Thuong, N.T. and Helene, C. (1991). Short modified antisense oligonucleotides directed against Ha-ras point mutation induce selective cleavage of the mRNA and inhibit T24 cells proliferation. EMBO J., 10, 1111–1118.

Saitoh, A., Kimura, M., Takahashi, R., Yokoyama, M., Nomura, T., Izawa, M., Sekiya, T., Nishimura, S. and Katsuki, M. (1990). Most tumors in transgenic mice with human c-Ha-ras gene contained somatically activated transgenes. Oncogene, 5, 1195–1200.

Sakaguchi, A.Y., Lalley, P.A., Zabel, B.U., Ellis, R., Skolnick, E. and Naylor, S.L. (1984). Mouse proto-oncogene assignments. Cytogenet. Cell Genet., 37, 573–574.

Sakoda, T., Kaibuchi, K., Kishi, K., Kishida, S., Doi, K., Hoshino, M., Hattori, S. and Takai, Y. (1992). smg/rap1/Krev-1 p21s inhibit the signal pathway to the c-fos promoter/enhancer from c-Ki-ras p21 but not from c-raf-1 kinase in NIH3T3 cells. Oncogene, 7, 1705–1711.

Samuel, S.K., Hurta, R.A.R., Kondaiah, P., Khalil, N., Turley, E.A., Wright, J.A. and Greenberg, A.H. (1992). Autocrine induction of tumor protease production and invasion by a metallothionein-regulated TGF-β_1 (Ser223, 225). EMBO J., 11, 1599–1605.

Santos, E., Martin-Zanca, D., Reddy, E.P., Pierotti, M.A., Della Porta, G. and Barbacid, M. (1984). Malignant activation of a K-ras oncogene in lung carcinoma but not in normal tissue of the same patient. Science, 223, 661–664.

Santos, E., Nebreda, A.R., Bryan, T. and Kempner, E.S. (1988). Oligomeric structure of p21ras proteins as determined by radiation inactivation. J. Biol. Chem., 263, 9853–9858.

Satoh, T., Endo, M., Nakafuku, M., Nakamura, S. and Kaziro, Y. (1990a). Platelet-derived growth factor stimulates formation of active $p21^{ras}$.GTP complex in Swiss mouse 3T3 cells. Proc. Natl Acad. Sci. USA, 87, 5993–5997.

Satoh, T., Endo, M., Nakafuku, M., Akiyama, T., Yamamoto, T. and Kaziro, Y. (1990b). Accumulation of $p21^{ras}$-GTP in response to stimulation with epidermal growth factor and oncogene products with tyrosine kinase activity. Proc. Natl Acad. Sci. USA, 87, 7926–7929.

Satoh, T., Fantl, W.J., Escobedo, J.A., Williams, L.T. and Kaziro, Y. (1993). Platelet-derived growth factor receptor mediates activation of Ras through different signaling pathways in different cell types. Mol. Cell. Biol., 13, 3706–3713.

Schlichting, I., Almo, S.C., Rapp, G., Wilson, K., Petratos, K., Lentfer, A., Wittinghofer, A., Kabsch, W., Pai, E.F., Petsko, G.A. and Goody, R.S. (1990). Time-resolved X-ray crystallographic study of the conformational change in Ha-ras p21 protein on GTP hydrolysis. Nature, 345, 309–315.

Schonthal, A., Herrlich, P., Rahmsdorf, H.J. and Ponta, H. (1988). Requirement for fos gene expression in the transient activation of collagenase by other oncogenes and phorbol ester. Cell, 54, 325–334.

Schwab, M., Varmus, H.E. and Bishop, J.M. (1985). Human N-myc gene contributes to neoplastic transformation of mouse cells in culture. Nature, 316, 160–162.

Schwartz, R.C., Stanton, L.W., Riley, S.C., Marcu, K.B. and Witte, O.N. (1986). Synergism of v-myc and v-Ha-ras in the in vitro neoplastic progression of murine lymphoid cells. Mol. Cell. Biol., 6, 3221–3231.

Schweighoffer, F., Faure, M., Fath, I., Chevallier-Multon, M.-C., Apiou, F., Dutrillaux, B., Sturani, E., Jacquet, M. and Tocque, B. (1993). Identification of a human guanine nucleotide-releasing factor (H-GRF55) specific for Ras proteins. Oncogene, 8, 1477–1485.

Self, A.J., Paterson, H. and Hall, A. (1993). Different structural organization of ras and rho effector domains. Oncogene, 8, 655–661.

Sefton, B.M. and Buss, J.E. (1987) The covalent modification of eukaryotic proteins with lipid. J.Cell Biol., 104, 1449–1453.

Sekiya, T., Fushimi, M., Hori, H., Hirohashi, S., Nishimura, S. and Sugimura, T. (1984). Molecular cloning and the total nucleotide sequence of the human c-Ha-ras-1 gene activated in a melanoma from a Japanese patient. Proc. Natl Acad. Sci. USA, 81, 4771–4775.

Settleman, J., Narasimhan, V., Foster, L.C. and Weinberg, R.A. (1992). Molecular cloning of cDNAs encoding the GAP-associated protein p190: implications for a signalling pathway from ras to the nucleus. Cell, 69, 539–549.

Seuwen, K., Lagarde, A., and Pouyssegur, J. (1988). Deregulation of hamster fibroblast proliferation by mutated *ras* oncogenes is not mediated by constant activation phosphoinositide-specific phospholipase C. EMBO J., 7, 161–168.

Shimizu, K., Birnbaum, D., Ruley, M.A., Fasano, O., Suard, Y., Edlund, L., Taparowsky, E., Goldfarb, M. and Wigler, M. (1983). Structure of the Ki-*ras* gene of the human lung carcinoma cell line calu-1. Nature, 304, 497–500.

Shou, C., Farnsworth, C.L., Neel, B.G. and Feig, L.A. (1992). Molecular cloning of cDNAs encoding a guanine-nucleotide-releasing factor for Ras p21. Nature, 358, 351–354.

Sigal, I.S., Gibbs, J.B., D'Alonzo, J.S. and Scolnick, E.M. (1986). Identification of effector residues and a neutralizing epitope of Ha-*ras*-encoded p21. Proc. Natl Acad. Sci. USA, 1986, 83, 4725–4729.

Simon, M.A., Dodson, G.S. and Rubin, G.M. (1993). An SH3-SH2-SH3 protein is required for p21^{Ras1} activation and binds to sevenless and Sos proteins in vitro. Cell, 73, 169–177.

Sinn, E., Muller, W., Pattengale, P., Tepler, I., Wallace, R. and Leder, P. (1987). Coexpression of MMTV/v-Ha-*ras* and MMTV/c-*myc* genes in transgenic mice: synergistic action of oncogenes *in vivo*. Cell, 49, 465–475.

Siracusa, L.D., Silan, C.M., Justice, M.J., Mercer, J.A., Bauskin, A.R., Ben-Neriah, Y., Duboule, D., Hastie, N.D., Copeland, N.G. and Jenkins, N.A. (1990). A molecular genetic linkage map of mouse chromosome 2. Genomics, 6, 491–504.

Sistonen, L., Holtta, E., Makela, T.P., Keski-Oja, J. and Alitalo, K. (1989). The cellular response to induction of the p21$^{c-Ha-ras}$ oncoprotein includes stimulation of *jun* gene expression. EMBO J., 8, 815–822.

Sjolander, A., Yamamoto, K., Huber, B.E. and Lapetina, E.G. (1991). Association of p21^{ras} with phosphatidylinositol 3-kinase. Proc. Natl Acad. Sci. USA, 88, 7908–7912.

Skolnik, E.Y., Lee, C.-H., Batzer, A., Vicentini, L.M., Zhou, M., Daly, R., Myers, M.J., Backer, J.M., Ullrich, A., White, M.F. and Schlessinger, J. (1993). The SH2/SH3 domain-containing protein GRB2 interacts with tyrosine-phosphorylated IRS1 and Shc: implications for insulin control of *ras* signalling. EMBO J., 12, 1929–1936.

Sloan, S.R., Newcomb, E.W. and Pellicer, A. (1990). Neutron radiation can activate K-*ras* via a point mutation in codon 146 and induces a different spectrum of *ras* mutations than does gamma radiation. Mol. Cell. Biol., 10, 405–408.

Smith, M.R., DeGudicibus, S.J. and Stacey, D.W. (1986). Requirement for c-*ras* proteins during viral oncogene transformation. Nature, 320, 540–543.

Smith, M.R., Liu, Y.-L., Kim, S., Rhee, S.F. and Kung, H.-F. (1990). Inhibition of serum- and ras-stimulated DNA synthesis by antibodies to phospholipase C. Science, 247, 1074–1077.

Stacey, D.W., Watson, T., Kung, H.F. and Curran, T. (1987). Microinjection of transforming *ras* protein induces c-*fos* expression. Mol. Cell. Biol., 7, 523–527.

Sternberg, E.A., Spizz, G., Perry, M.E. and Olson, E.N. (1989). A *ras*-dependent pathway abolishes activation of a muscle-specific enhancing system from the muscle creatine kinase gene. Mol. Cell. Biol., 9, 594–601.

Sukumar, S., Perantoni, A., Reed, C., Rice, J.M. and Wenk, M.L. (1986). Activated K-*ras* and N-*ras* oncogenes in primary renal mesenchymal tumors induced in F344 rats by methyl-(methoxymethyl)nitrosamine. Mol. Cell. Biol., 6, 2716–2720.

Szeberenyi, J., Erhardt, P., Cai, H. and Cooper, G.M. (1992). Role of ras in signal transduction from the nerve growth factor receptor: relationship to protein kinase C, calcium and cyclic AMP. Oncogene, 7, 2105–2113.

Tabin, C.J., Bradley, S.M., Bargmann, C.I., Weinberg, R.A., Papageorge, A.G., Scolnick, E.M., Dhar, R., Lowy, D.R. and Chang, E.H. (1982). Mechanism of activation of a human oncogene. Nature, 300, 143–149.

Tachibana, K., Umezana, A., Kato, S. and Takano, T. (1988). Nucleotide sequence of a new YPT1-related human cDNA which belongs to the *ras* gene superfamily. Nucleic Acids Res., 16, 10368.

Tanaka, K., Matsumoto, K. and Toh-E, A. (1989). *IRA1*, an inhibitory regulator of the RAS-cyclic AMP pathway in *Saccharomyces cerevisiae*. Mol. Cell. Biol., 9, 757–768.

Tanaka, K., Nakafuku, M., Satoh, T., Marschall, M.S., Gibbs, J.B., Matsumoto, K., Kaziro, Y. and Toh-e, A. (1990). S. cerevisiae genes *IRA1* and *IRA2* encode proteins that may be functionally equivalent to mammalian *ras* GTPase activity protein. Cell, 60, 803–807.

Taparowsky, E., Shimizu, K., Goldfarb, M., Wigler, M. (1983). Structure and activation of the human N-*ras* gene. Cell, 34, 581–586.

Thorn, J.T., Todd, A.V., Warrilow, D., Watt, F., Molloy, P.L. and Iland, H.J. (1991). Characterization of the human N-*ras* promoter region. Oncogene, 6, 1843–1850.

Tong, L., De Vos, A.M., Milburn, M.V., Jancarik, J., Noguchi, S., Nishimura, S., Miura, K., Ohtsuka, E.

and Kim, S.-H. (1989). Structural differences between a ras oncogene protein and the normal protein. Nature, 337, 90–93.

Tong, L., Milburn, M.V., De Vos, A.M. and Kim, S.-H. (1991a). Structure of ras protein. Science, 245, 244.

Tong, L., De Vos. A.M., Milburn, M.V. and Kim, S.-H. (1991b). Crystal structures at 2.2 resolution of the catalytic domains of normal and an oncogenic mutant complexed with GDP. J. Mol. Biol., 217, 503–516.

Touchot, N., Chardin, P. and Tavitian, A. (1987). Four additional members of the ras gene superfamily isolated by an oligomeric strategy: Molecular cloning of YPT-related cDNAs from a rat brain library. Proc. Natl Acad. Sci. USA, 84, 8210–8214.

Trahey, M., Wong, G., Halenbeck, R., Rubinfeld, B., Martin, G.A., Ladner, M., Long, C.M., Crosier, W.J., Watt, K., Koths, K. and McCormick, F. (1988). Molecular cloning of 2 types of GAP complementary DNA from human placenta. Science, 242, 1697–1700.

Trusko, S.P., Hoffman, E.H., and George, D.L. (1989). Transcriptional activation of cKi-ras proto-oncogene resulting from retroviral promoter insertion. Nucleic Acids Res., 17, 9259–9265.

Tsai, M.-H., Roudebush, M., Dobrowolski, S., Yu, C.-L., Gibbs, J.B. and Stacey, D.W. (1991). Ras GTPase-activating protein physically associates with mitogenically active phospholipids. Mol. Cell. Biol., 11, 2785–2793.

Tsuchida, N., Ryder, T. and Ohtsubo, E. (1982). Nucleotide sequence of the oncogene encoding the p21 transforming protein of kirsten murine sarcoma virus. Science 217, 937–939.

Wakelam, M.J.O., Davies, S.A., Houslay, M.D., McKay, I., Marshall, C.J. and Hall, A. (1986). Normal p21^{N-ras} couples bombesin and other growth factor responses to inositol phosphates production. Nature, 323, 173–176.

Wasylyk, C., Imler, J.L., Perez-Mutul, J. and Wasylyk, B. (1987). The c-Ha-ras oncogene and a tumor promoter activate the polyoma virus enhancer. Cell, 48, 525–534.

West, M., Kung, H.F. and Kamata, T. (1990). A novel membrane factor stimulates guanine nucleotide exchange reaction of ras proteins. FEBS Letts., 259, 245–248.

Westaway, D., Papkoff, J., Moscovici, C. and Varmus, H.E. (1986). Identification of a provirally activated c-Ha-ras oncogene in an avian nephroblastoma via a novel procedure: cDNA cloning of a chimaeric viral-host transcript. EMBO J., 5, 301–309.

Willumsen, B.M., Papageorge, A.G., Hubbert, N., Bekesi, E., Kung, H.-F. and Lowy, D.R. (1985). Transforming p21ras protein: flexibility in the major variable region binding the catalytic and membrane-anchoring domains. EMBO J., 4, 2893–2896.

Wolfman, A. and Macara, I.G. (1987). Elevated levels of diacylglycerol and decreased phorbol ester sensitivity in ras-transformed fibroblasts. Nature, 325, 359–361.

Wolfman, A. and Macara, I.G. (1990). A cytosolic protein catalyzes the release of GDP from p21^{ras}. Science, 248, 67–69.

Wong, G., Muller, O., Clark, R., Conroy, L., Moran, M.F., Polakis, P. and McCormick, F. (1992). Molecular cloning and nucleic acid binding properties of the GAP-associated tyrosine phosphoprotein p62. Cell, 69, 551–558.

Xu, G., O'Connell, P., Viskochil, D., Cawthon, R., Robertson, M., Culver, M., Dunn, D., Stevens, J., Gesteland, R., White, R. and Weiss, R. (1990a). The neurofibromatosis type 1 gene encodes a protein related to GAP. Cell, 62, 599–608.

Xu, G., Lin, B., Tanaka, K., Dunn, D., Wood, D., Gesteland, R., White, R., Weiss, R. and Tamanoi, F. (1990b). The catalytic domain of the neurofibromatosis type 1 gene product stimulates ras GTPase and complements ira mutants of S.cerevisiae. Cell, 63, 835–841.

Yamaguchi-Iwai, Y., Satake, M., Murakami, Y., Sakai, M., Muramatsu, M. and Ito, Y. (1990). Differentiation of F9 embryonal carcinoma cells induced by the c-jun and activated c-Ha-ras oncogenes. Proc. Natl Acad. Sci. USA, 87, 8670–8674.

Yamamoto, F. and Perucho, M. (1984). Activation of a human cK-ras oncogene. Nucleic Acids Res., 12, 8873–8885.

Yamamoto, F. and Perucho, M. (1988). Characterization of the human c-K-ras gene promoter. Oncogene Res., 3, 123–138.

Yasuda, S., Furuichi, M. and Soeda E. (1984). An altered DNA sequence encompassing the ras gene of Harvey murine sarcoma virus. Nucleic Acids Res., 12, 5583–5588.

Yatani, A., Okabe, K., Polakis, P., Halenbeck, R., McCormick, F. and Brown, A.M. (1990). ras p21 and GAP inhibit coupling of muscarinic receptors to atrial K$^+$ channels. Cell, 61, 769–776.

Yoakum, G.H., Lechner, J.F., Gabrielson, E.W., Korba, B.E., Malan-Shibley, L., Willey, J.C., Valerio, M.G., Shamsuddin, A.M., Trump, B.F. and Harris, C.C. (1985). Transformation of human bronchial epithelial cells transfected by Harvey ras oncogene. Science, 227, 1174–1179.

Yu, C.-L., Tsai, M.-H. and Stacey, D.W. (1988). Cellular ras activity and phospholipid metabolism. Cell, 52, 63–71.

Yuasa, Y., Gol, R.A., Chang, A., Chiu, I.-M., Reddy, E.P., Tronick, S.R. and Aaronson, S.A. (1984). Mechanism of activation of an N-*ras* oncogene of SW-1271 human lung carcinoma cells. Proc. Natl Acad. Sci. USA, 81, 3670–3674.

Zhang, K., DeClue, J.E., Vass, W.C., Papageorge, A.G., McCormick, F. and Lowy, D.R. (1990). Suppression of c-*ras* transformation by GTPase-activating protein. Nature, 346, 754–756.

Zhang, K., Papageorge, A.G., Martin, P., Vass, W.C., Olah, Z., Polakis, P.G., McCormick, F. and Lowy, D.R. (1991). Heterogeneous amino acids in ras and rap1A specifying sensitivity to GAP protein. Science, 254, 1630–1634.

Zwiller, J., Sassone-Corsi, P., Kakazu, K. and Boynton, A.L. (1991). Inhibition of PDGF-induced c-*jun* and c-*fos* expression by a tyrosine protein kinase inhibitor. Oncogene, 6, 219–221.

REL

v-*rel* is the oncogene of avian reticuloendotheliosis virus strain T (REV-T: Robinson and Twiehaus, 1974; Hoelzer *et al.*, 1979). Helper virus: REV-A: type C. REV-T was originally isolated from turkeys that had contracted lymphoid leukosis.

REL is a member of the nuclear factor κB (NF-κB) transcription factor family. Human *REL* encodes HIVEN86A, a κB site-binding transcription factor.

Related genes

v-REL is unrelated to any other known oncoprotein but is related to a number of cellular transcription factors, including KBF-1 and NF-κB. These proteins have an N-terminal conserved REL homology domain of ~300–350 amino acids that includes sequences important for DNA binding, dimerization and nuclear localization.

NF-κB is a transcription factor that consists of REL family proteins p50 and p65. p50 is synthesized as a precursor protein (p105) that is proteolytically cleaved to release the p50 DNA binding protein, comprised mainly of the REL homology domain. p65 is not processed and has a strong C-terminal transcription activation domain.

Human p49 (or p50B or *LYT-10*), like p50, is probably synthesized as a precursor (p100) that is processed to the mature DNA binding form (p49) by proteolysis. Both p49 and p50 contain C-terminal ankyrin-like repeats in their cleaved sequences that may function as inhibitory domains.

Murine REL-B (558 amino acids) has substantial regions of identity with REL (50%), murine NF-κB p50 (46%), human p49 (43%) and NF-κB p65 (52%). The C-terminal 180 residues of REL-B contain a transcriptional activation domain and REL-B/p50 heterodimers bind to κB sites with an affinity similar to that of p50 homodimers (Ryseck *et al.*, 1992). I-REL appears to be the human homologue of REL-B and I-REL may function as an inhibitor of REL proteins (Ruben *et al.*, 1992).

The *dorsal* gene product of *Drosophila melanogaster* binds to sequences related to NF-κB sites and is involved in establishment of dorsal–ventral polarity in fly blastoderm (Steward, 1987).

Cross-species homology

REL is highly conserved between species in the REL homology domain (human, chicken, mouse) but varies in the C-terminal half.

The N-terminus of REL-like proteins is highly conserved: for example, the N-terminal 296 amino acids of human REL are ~80% similar to the *Drosophila dorsal* gene product. The C-terminus diverges widely. The chicken and turkey (from which v-*rel* was transduced) *Rel* genes are highly conserved (REL 95% identical in sequence).

Xenopus laevis Xrel1: 72% identity with human REL within the ~300 amino acids of the N-terminal REL homology domain; probably the frog homologue of p65 (Kao and Hopwood, 1991).

Transformation

MAN

Rearrangement or amplification of the *REL* locus occurs in some lymphomas. A B cell lymphoma-associated chromosomal translocation, t(10;14)(q24;q32), translocates the immunoglobulin Cα₁ locus into that of *LYT10* (p49/p100): the fusion gene product includes the REL homology domain and binds κB sequences *in vitro* (Neri *et al.*, 1991). The chromosomal location (2p14–15; Mathew *et al.*, 1993) is associated with rearrangements in non-Hodgkin's lymphoma (Lu *et al.*, 1991).

A cell line derived from a diffuse large-cell lymphoma expresses a *REL* fusion mRNA (*NRG*, non-rel gene: Lu *et al.*, 1991).

ANIMALS

In REV-T infection v-REL causes acute neoplasia in birds that is rapidly fatal (Moore and Bose, 1989) and REV-A can cause an immunosuppressive runting disease. When injected into the wing web of young chickens, REV-T can cause sarcomas (Moore and Bose, 1988). The non-defective REVs (e.g. CSV or REV-A) can induce B cell lymphomas of long latency that are indistinguishable from those caused by ALV and arise from proviral insertion in the *Myc* locus. Tumours induced by REV-A are mainly IgM⁻: with a different helper virus (e.g. CSV) the target appears to change and most tumours are IgM⁺ (Barth and Humphries, 1987, 1988).

IN VITRO

v-*rel* only partially transforms CEFs (Moore and Bose, 1988; Morrison *et al.*, 1991). The expression of a v-REL/estrogen receptor fusion protein transforms chicken fibroblasts or bone marrow cells in the presence of estrogen which causes sequence-specific binding of the protein to DNA (Boehmelt *et al.*, 1992). v-*rel* primarily transforms lymphoid cells but may also transform erythroid and myeloid cells. Chicken spleen cells transformed *in vitro* by REV-T are tumorigenic on transplantation (Lewis *et al.*, 1981).

Alternative forms of REL (p50, p56, p58 and p62) occur in HP46 cells derived from an ALV-induced tumour. These are the result of promoter insertion causing de-regulation of the *Rel* locus (Kabrun *et al.*, 1990).

	REL/Rel	v-*rel*
Nucleotides (kb)	>24 (chicken, turkey)	1.4 (REV-T)
Chromosome		
Human	2p13–p12 (within the Igκ region)	
Mouse	11	
Exons	10	
mRNA (kb)		
Human	~12 (Abnormal 2.0–2.3 kb in lymphoma)	3
Chicken	2.6/4.0	
Mouse	2.5/7.5	
Amino acids		
Human	587	
Mouse	588	503
Chicken, turkey	598	

	REL/Rel	v-*rel*
Mass (kDa)		
(predicted)	p67	56
(expressed)	p68*rel*	pp59*v-rel*
Protein half-life (h)		4–10

Cellular location

p59*v-rel* is a nuclear protein in infected chick embryo fibroblasts (CEFs) (Gilmore and Temin, 1988). v-REL and REL are cytoplasmic in transformed avian and murine cells and exist in a complex with p68*rel*, p40 (I-κB), p115 and p124 (NF-κB p105) (Simek and Rice, 1988; Davis *et al.*, 1990, 1991; Capobianco *et al.*, 1992). In transformed lymphoid cells the majority of v-REL is complexed with p40, the minority with p115 and p124 and v-REL is 90% cytoplasmic, 10% nuclear. In the human lymphoblastoid cell line Jurkat, p40 is exclusively cytoplasmic and is not present in nuclear complexes of REL and NF-κB p105 (Neumann *et al.*, 1992).

REL/NF-κB proteins can translocate from cytoplasm to nucleus: for example, NF-κB after mitogenic stimulation and the *dorsal* protein in the *Drosophila* blastoderm during early development.

Tissue location

In humans high concentrations of *REL* mRNA occur in relatively mature lymphocytes (Lyt2+ and L3T4+ T cells and IgM+ B cells; Brownell *et al.*, 1987), consistent with REV-T (CSV) induction of B cell lymphomas. In chickens *Rel* mRNA is mainly in haematopoietic cells, particularly 4.0 kb mRNA (half-life ~2 h): the 2.6 kb transcript occurs in the ovary, not in muscle or brain (Moore and Bose, 1989).

Rel mRNA expression is depressed in immature thymocytes and may therefore play a role in lymphocyte differentiation, in contrast to the evidence for *Myb* and *Ets* (Brownell *et al.*, 1987).

Protein function

REL and v-REL are transcription factors that interact to form homo- or heterodimers and bind to NF-κB motifs (NGGNN$^A/_T$TTCC; Kamens and Brent, 1991; Kochel and Rice, 1992; Kunsch *et al.*, 1992). REL homodimers and heterodimers show distinct DNA-binding specificities and affinities for various κB motifs (Nakayama *et al.*, 1992). Human REL and NF-κB p105 protein synthesis is induced by the action of cytokines, mitogenic lectins, phorbol esters and viral gene products and both proteins are tyrosine kinase substrates (Neumann *et al.*, 1992).

The REL homodimer has a high affinity for interleukin-6 (IL-6) and interferon-β κB sites and binds to the interferon-γ intronic enhancer element that is not recognized by NF-κB (Sica *et al.*, 1992). The heterodimer of REL/NF-kB subunit p65 binds to the phorbol ester (TPA)-responsive sequence 5'-GGGAAAGTAC-3' in the 5' flanking region of the human urokinase gene (Hansen *et al.*, 1992).

v-REL is a sequence-specific DNA binding protein that can form heterodimers with NF-κB or its precursor p105 *in vitro* (Kieran *et al.*, 1990; Capobianco *et al.*, 1992). Immunoprecipitates of p59[v-rel] have an associated serine/threonine protein kinase activity (Rice *et al.*, 1986; Walro *et al.*, 1987).

In most cells v-REL represses gene expression from a number of promoters (Richardson and Gilmore, 1991; Ballard *et al.*, 1992; McDonnell *et al.*, 1992). When expressed in undifferentiated F9 cells v-REL acts as a κB-specific transcriptional activator rather than as a repressor (Walker *et al.*, 1992) and in chicken cells v-REL activates transcription of the MHC class I gene cluster and of high mobility group protein 14b (Boehmelt *et al.*, 1992). In rat fibroblasts v-REL also activates transcription but may have an anti-proliferative effect.

Human REL binds specifically to the HIV NF-κB motif and related enhancer elements found in the Igκ, class I MHC and IL-2 receptor genes (Muchardt *et al.*, 1992) and induction of REL synthesis correlates with expression of IL-2Rα expression at the cell surface (Tan *et al.*, 1992). REL can inhibit or activate expression of genes linked to mutant HIV LTRs containing intact NF-κB motifs and transfected into HeLa cells: activation occurs in the presence of low levels of endogenous κB binding activity and inhibition after TPA treatment of the cells which increases κB binding activity (McDonnell *et al.*, 1992). v-REL appears to compete with endogenous proteins of the *Rel* family, the expression and activity of which are cell specific. v-REL probably transforms cells by acting as a dominant negative version of REL (Gilmore, 1991).

v-*rel* downregulates *Myc* via NF-κB elements (see **MYC**) but an additional promoter site may also be involved.

KBF-1

The promoters of K^b and L^d class I MHC genes in the mouse include enhancer A which can potentiate the effect of an overlapping interferon response sequence. Enhancer A contains a 13 bp perfect palindrome recognized by a transcription-activating factor originally termed KBF1 (human κ binding factor). KBF-1 is an NF-κB p50 homodimer (Kieran *et al.*, 1990) that is induced as an early response gene (Bours *et al.*, 1990). The N-terminal 366 amino acids of p105 are highly related to REL and the C-terminal region of p105 is similar to sequences found in the *SW*14, *SW*16 and *cdc*10 gene products (essential for cell cycle progression of *S. cerevisiae* and *S. pombe*) and also in the human erythrocyte protein ankyrin.

NF-κB

The pleiotropic factor NF-κB occurs in an active form in the nucleus of mature B cells, differentiated monocytes and some T cell lines. It is generally inactive in the cytoplasm of other cells where it is complexed with I-κB (~37 kDa) which, when underphosphorylated, prevents translocation to the nucleus. I-κB is directly phosphorylated by protein kinase C. NF-κB binds to the Igκ enhancer and to the H-2K[b] palindrome. NF-κB has one 50 kDa DNA binding subunit identical to KBF-1 and one 65 kDa subunit via which I-κB operates. NF-κB p65 also has N-terminal (320 residues) sequence homology with REL and a C-terminal transcription activation domain (Nolan *et al.*, 1991). NF-κB p65 is a powerful *trans*-activating factor when transiently expressed in Jurkat T cells: its action is completely suppressed by v-REL.

A mutant of p50 that is unable to bind to DNA but can form homo- or heterodimers prevents transcriptional activation via the HIV LTR (that contains two potential NF-κB binding sites) or via the MHC class I H-2K[b] promoter (Logeat *et al.*, 1991).

NF-κB binding to the interferon-β promoter is activated by double-stranded RNA in intact cells (Visvanathan and Goodburn, 1989). This may be a consequence of the phosphorylation by the RNA-activated protein kinase (PKR) of one of the I-κB inhibitor proteins (see **Tumour Suppressor Genes: RNA-activated protein kinase**).

Structure of the REV-T genome

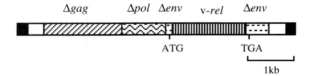

Integration of v-*rel* into REV-A causes deletion of a contiguous segment (the 3' end of *gag* and 5' end of *pol*) and v-*rel* replaces most of *env*. The *env* initiation codon is used and v-*rel* begins with the 12 N-terminal amino acids of *env*. The C-terminal 18 amino acids are also derived, out of frame, from *env*. The C-terminal 18 residues are not essential for transformation: the N-terminal *env*-encoded residues and the first 18 residues of exon 2 are essential (Sylla and Temin, 1986). REL contains 118 C-terminal amino acids not present in v-REL.

The promoter region of the normal chicken *Rel* gene is GC-rich, contains an NF-κB consensus binding sequence and lacks a TATA box. *In vitro* v-*rel* expression suppresses transcription from the *Rel* promoter by a mechanism that does not involve the NF-κB site (Capobianco and Gilmore, 1991).

Sequences of turkey REL, v-REL and human, mouse and chicken REL

```
Turkey REL   (1)        MA ----------------M-----------------------------
v-REL        (1)     MDFLTNLRFTEGISEPYIEIFEQPRQRGTRFRYKCEGRSAGSIPGEHSTDNNKTFPSIQ
Mouse REL    (1)        MASSGYN--V--I-------M----------------R-----R-Y--VD
Human REL    (1)        MASQLYN-----I-------M-----------------R-Y---N
Chicken REL  (1)        MA ----------------M-----------------------------

Turkey REL   (51)    ------------------------------D--------------R----------
v-REL        (60)    ILNYFGKVKIRTTLVTKNEPYKPHPHDLVGKGCRDGYYEAEFGPERQVLSFQNLGIQCVK
Mouse REL    (52)    -M--Y--G---I------D-----------D--P---------RP-F------R---
Human REL    (52)    -M--Y--G-V-I-------D------------------N--RP-F-----------
Chicken REL  (51)    ------------------------------D--------------R----------

Turkey REL   (111)   -------------------------------------------- ----------------
v-REL        (120)   KKDLKESISLRISKKINPFNVPEEQLHNIDEYDLNVVRLCFQA FLPDEHGNYTLALPPL
Mouse REL    (112)   --EV-GA-I----AG------G-Q--LD-EDC------ -VFMF-----D--F-T-V--I
Human REL    (112)   --EV--A-IT--KAG--------K--ND-EDC----------V --------L-T----V
Chicken REL  (111)   -------------------------------------------- ----------------

Turkey REL   (170)   ----------------- -----------------------------------------
v-REL        (179)   ISNPIYDNRAPNTAGLRI CRVNKNCGSVKGGDGIFLLCDKVQKDDIGVRFVLGNWEAKG
Mouse REL    (171)   V-------------E---LA---------R---E-------------E-----ND---R-
Human REL    (171)   V-------------E--- ---------R---E-------------E-----ND-----
Chicken REL  (170)   ----------------- ----------------------------------D------

Turkey REL   (229)   ------------------------------------------D--------------SY--
v-REL        (238)   SFSQADVHRQVAIVFRTPPFLGDITEPITVKMQLRRPSDQAVSEPVDFRTLPDEEDPSGN
Mouse REL    (231)   V--------------K---YCKA-L--V-----------E---SM---Y----K-AYA-
Human REL    (230)   I--------------K---YCKA----V-----------E---SM---Y----K-TY--
Chicken REL  (229)   -------------------R----------------D-------------K--Y--

Turkey REL   (289)   -----------L----------------------------I----------------
v-REL        (298)   KAKRQRSTLAWQKPIQDCGSAVTERPKAAPIPTVNPEGKL KKEPNMFSPTLMLPGLGTL
Mouse REL    (291)   -S-K-KT--IF--LL----H F--K-RT--LGSTGEGRF I---S-L--HGTV--EMPRS
Human REL    (290)   ---K-KT--LF--LC--H+VNFP---RPGLLGSIGEGRY F-----L--HDAVVREMPTG
Chicken REL  (289)   ---------AW--L--------------------------------------------
```

```
Turkey REL    (349)   A---------------------------------------- ----------M---N--------
v-REL         (357)   SSSQMYPACSQMPTQPAQLGPGKQDTLHSCWQQLYSP SPSASSLLSLHSHSSFTAEVP
Mouse REL     (349)   SGVPGQAEPYYSSCGSISSGL- HHPPAIPSVAHQPTS W-PVTHPT-HPVSTNTLSTFS
Human REL     (348)   V--  QAESYYPS-GPISSGLS HHASMAPL    PSSSWS-VAHPTPRSGNTNPLSSFS
Chicken REL   (349)   T-------P-----H------------P------F-S ---------M-P-N--------

Turkey REL    (408)   -------------HD---------D--------- -----------D-----------
v-REL         (415)   QPGAQGSSSLPAY  NPLNWPDGKNSSFYRNFGN THGMGAALVSAAGMQSVSSSSIVQG
Mouse REL     (407)   AGTLSSN-QGILP  FLEGPGVSDL-ASNSCLY- PDDLARMETPSMSPTDLY-I-D-NM
Human REL     (401)   TRTLPSN-QGIPP  FLRIPVGNDLNASNACIY-NADDIVGMEA-SMPSADLYGISDPNM
Chicken REL   (408)   -----------FHD---------D--------S -N-----M----D---A--N---HA

Turkey REL    (467)   -------A----N-ETNDMNCTSLNFEKYTGVLNMSNHRQQLHQVPATCPPVAAPGSTPF
v-REL         (472)   THQASATTASIMTMPRTPGEVPFLRQQVGYRS (503)
Mouse REL     (464)   LSTRPLSVMAPSTDGMGDTDNPRLVSINLENPSCNARLGPRDLRQLHQMSPASLSAGTSS
Human REL     (459)   LSNC-VNMMTTSSDSMGETDNPR-LSMNLENPSCNSVLDPRDLRQLHQMSSSSMSAGANS
Chicken REL   (467)   -------A---VN-ETNDMNCTS-NFEKYTGVLNVSNHRQQLHQAPAACPPVAAPGSTPF

Turkey REL    (527)   SSQPNVADTAVYSSFLDQEVLSDSRLSTNPLQNHQNSLTLTDNQFYDTDGVHTDELYQS
Mouse REL     (524)   SSVFVSQSDAFDRSNFSCVDNGLMNEPGLSDDANNPTFVQSSHYSVNTLQSEQLSDPFT
Human REL     (519)   NTTVFVSQSDAFEGSDFSCADNSMINESGPSNST NPNSHGFVQDSQYSGIGSMQNEQLS
Chicken REL   (527)   SSQPNLADTAVYNSFLDQEVISDSRLSTNPLQNHQNSLTLTDNQFYDTDGVHTDELYQS

Turkey REL    (586)   FQLDTNILQSYNH (598)
Mouse REL     (583)   YGFFKI (588)
Human REL     (578)   DSFPYEFFQV (587)
Chicken REL   (586)   FQLDTNILQSYNH (598)
```

Dashes indicate identity with v-REL. The two regions of underlined residues in v-REL are the *env* N- and C-termini derived from REV-A. + (position 308) Indicates an intron-derived insert (VETGFRHVDQDGLELLTSGDPPTLASQSAGIT) specific to human REL (Brownell *et al.*, 1989).

v-REL: 503 amino acids: rich in Pro/Ser (Pro-rich: 255–433). About 75% of the 45 serines in C-terminal half; 23 serines in 385–481.

Turkey: v-REL differs from REL (exons 0–7) in 14 amino acids (10 non-conservative) and there are three deletion sites in v-REL (that total five amino acids).

v-REL, REL, p50 and p65 protein domains

v-REL has lost two N-terminal amino acids and 118 C-terminal residues compared with REL (Wilhelmsen *et al.*, 1984; Capobianco *et al.*, 1990). Within the REL homology domain all REL proteins have a nuclear localization signal, although transformation of spleen cells appears independent of whether v-REL is nuclear or cytoplasmic (Gilmore and Temin, 1988). REL (and *dorsal*, see **Related genes**) contain C-terminal sequences, important for cytoplasmic retention and transcriptional activation, that are deleted in v-REL (Kamens *et al.*, 1990; Richardson and Gilmore, 1991). Small deletions of ~30 amino acids anywhere in the REL homology region of v-REL render the protein transformation defective, confer a principally cytosolic location in CEFs, and also inhibit association with p40 and κB site binding (Morrison *et al.*, 1992). p50 contains a unique ~40 amino acid insert in the REL domain. The p50 precursor is cleaved to release the REL domain, containing the DNA binding subunit, and a C-terminal region containing ~six ankyrin repeats that has I-κB activity (Ghosh *et al.*, 1990; Kieran *et al.*, 1990; Inoue *et al.*, 1992).

In the abnormal human *REL–NRG* gene product, the N-terminal 284 amino acids of REL are intact but the C-terminus is replaced by a 156 residue NRG sequence derived from a previously unknown gene (Lu *et al.*, 1991). This may promote transforming activity in a manner similar to the loss of the C-terminus in the generation of v-REL.

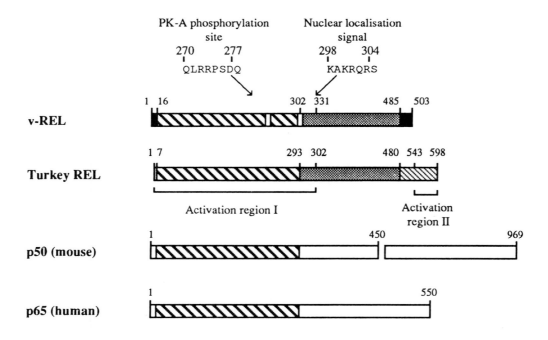

REL and v-REL are phosphorylated mainly on serine residues. The REL homology domain includes a conserved consensus sequence for cyclic AMP-dependent protein kinase phosphorylation (Arg–Arg–Pro–Ser). The insertion of two amino acids (Pro–Trp) within this sequence inhibits transformation of avian spleen cells and transcriptional repression by v-REL and, in chick embryo fibroblasts, changes the localization of REL from cytoplasmic to nuclear (Mosialos *et al.*, 1991). However, replacement of the serine phosphate acceptor with alanine does not affect the functions of v-REL, suggesting that phosphorylation is not crucial for the action of this domain (Mosialos *et al.*, 1991; Walker *et al.*, 1992; Mosialos and Gilmore, 1993).

Databank file names and accession numbers

	GENE	*EMBL*	*SWISSPROT*	*REFERENCES*
Chicken	*Rel*	Gdcrela M26381	TREL_CHICK P16236	Capobianco *et al.*, 1990
		Gsp68rel X52193		Hannink and Temin, 1989
				Kabrun *et al.*, 1990
Mouse	*Rel*	Mmcrelm X15842	TREL_MOUSE P15307	Grumont and Gerondakis, 1989
Turkey	*Rel*	Mgcrel0 to Mgcrel6a	TREL_MELGA P01125	Wilhelmsen *et al.*, 1984
		Mgcrel6b to Mgcrel7		
		X03508; X03616 to X03623		
		Mgrel1 K02447		

	GENE	EMBL	SWISSPROT	REFERENCES
Xenopus laevis	Xrel1	Xlrel M60785		Kao and Hopwood, 1991
AVIAN REV	p69^{v-rel}	Revtrel X02759	TREL_AVIRE P01126	Stephens *et al.*, 1983
				Wilhelmsen *et al.*, 1984

Reviews

Gilmore, T.D. (1990). NF-κB, KBF1, *dorsal* and *rel*ated matters. Cell, 62, 841–843.
Gilmore, T.D. (1991). Malignant transformation by mutant *rel* proteins. Trends Genet., 7, 318–322.
Gilmore, T.D. (1992). Role of *rel* family genes in normal and malignant lymphoid cell growth. Cancer Surveys, 15, 69–87.
Hannink, M. and Temin, H.M. (1991). Molecular mechanisms of transformation by the v-*rel* oncogene. Crit. Rev. Oncog., 2, 293–309.
Rushlow, C. and Warrior, R. (1992). The rel family of proteins BioEssays, 14, 89–95.

Papers

Ballard, D.W., Dixon, E.P., Peffer, N.J., Bogerd, H., Doerre, S., Stein, B. and Greene, W.C. (1992). The 65-kDa subunit of human NF-κB functions as a potent transcriptional activator and a target for v-rel-mediated repression. Proc. Natl Acad. Sci. USA, 89, 1875–1379.
Barth, C.F. and Humphries, E. (1987). A nonimmunosuppressive helper virus allows highly efficient induction of B cell lymphomas by reticuloendotheliosis virus strain T. J. Exp. Med., 167, 89–108.
Barth, C.F. and Humphries, E.H. (1988). Expression of v-*rel* induces mature B cell lines that reflect the diversity of avian immunoglobulin heavy- and light-chain rearrangements. Mol. Cell. Biol., 8, 5358–5368.
Boehmelt, G., Walker, A., Kabrun, N., Mellitzer, G., Beug, H., Zenke, M. and Enrietto, P.J. (1992). Hormone-regulated v-*rel* estrogen receptor fusion protein: reversible induction of cell transformation and cellular gene expression. EMBO J., 11, 4641–4652.
Bours, V., Villalobos, J., Burd, P.R., Kelly, K. and Siebenlist, U. (1990). Cloning of a mitogen-inducible gene encoding a κB DNA-binding protein with homology to the *rel* oncogene and to cell-cycle motifs. Nature, 348, 76–80.
Brownell, E., Mathieson, B., Young, H.A., Keller, J., Ihle, J.N. and Rice, N.R. (1987). Detection of c-*rel* related transcripts in mouse hematopoeitic tissues, fractionated lymphocyte populations and cell lines. Mol. Cell. Biol., 7, 1304–1309.
Brownell, E., Mittereder, N. and Rice, N.R. (1989). A human *rel* proto-oncogene cDNA containing an *Alu* fragment as a potential coding exon. Oncogene, 4, 935–942.
Bull, P., Morley, K.L., Hoekstra, M.F., Hunter, T. and Verma, I.M. (1990). The mouse c-*rel* protein has an N-terminal regulatory domain and a C-terminal transcriptional transactivation domain. Mol. Cell. Biol., 10, 5473–5485.
Capobianco, A.J. and Gilmore, T.D. (1991). Repression of the chicken c-*rel* promoter by vRel in chicken embryo fibroblasts is not mediated through a consensus NF-κB binding site. Oncogene, 6, 2203–2210.
Capobianco, A.J., Simmons, D.L. and Gilmore, T.D. (1990). Cloning and expression of a chicken c-*rel* cDNA: unlike p59^{v-rel}, p68^{c-rel} is a cytoplasmic protein in chicken embryo fibroblasts. Oncogene, 5, 257–265.
Capobianco, A.J., Chang, D., Mosialos, G. and Gilmore, T.D. (1992). p105, the NF-κB p50 precursor protein, is one of the cellular proteins complexed with the v-rel oncoprotein in transformed chicken spleen cells. J. Virol., 66, 3758–3767.
Davis, J.N., Bargmann, W. and Bose, H.R. (1990). Identification of protein complexes containing the c-rel proto-oncogene product in avian hematopoietic cells. Oncogene, 5, 1109–1115.
Davis, N., Ghosh, S., Simmons, D.L., Tempst, P., Liou, H.-C., Baltimore, D. and Bose, H.R. (1991). Rel-associated pp40: an inhibitor of the rel family of transcription factors. Science, 253, 1268–1271.

Ghosh, S., Gifford, A.M., Riviere, L.R., Tempst, P., Nolan, G.P. and Baltimore, D. (1990). Cloning of the p50 DNA binding subunit of NF-κB: homology to *rel* and *dorsal*. Cell, 62, 1019–1029.

Gilmore, T.D. and Temin, H.M. (1988). v-*rel* oncoproteins in the nucleus and in the cytoplasm transform chicken spleen cells. J. Virol., 62, 703–714.

Grumont, R.J. and Gerondakis, S. (1989). Structure of a mammalian c-*rel* protein deduced from the nucleotide sequence of murine cDNA clones. Oncogene Res., 4, 1–8.

Hannink, M. and Temin, H.M. (1989). Transactivation of gene expression by nuclear and cytoplasmic *rel* proteins. Mol. Cell. Biol., 9, 4323–4336.

Hansen, S.K., Nerlov, C., Zabel, U., Verde, P., Johnsen, M., Baeuerle, P.A. and Blasi, F. (1992). A novel complex between the p65 subunit of NF-kappa B and c-*rel* binds to a DNA element involved in the phorbol ester induction of the human urokinase gene. EMBO J., 11, 205–213.

Hoelzer, J.D., Franklin, R.B. and Bose, H.R. (1979). Transformation by reticuloendotheliosis virus: development of a focus assay and isolation of a nontransforming virus. Virology, 93, 20–30.

Inoue, J.-I., Kerr, L.D., Kakizuka, A. and Verma, I.M. (1992). IκBγ, a 70 kd protein identical to the C-terminal half of p110 NF-κB: a new member of the IκB family. Cell, 68, 1109–1120.

Kabrun, N., Bumstead, N., Hayman, M.J. and Enrietto, P.J. (1990). Characterization of a novel promoter insertion in the c-*rel* locus. Mol. Cell. Biol., 10, 4788–4794.

Kamens, J. and Brent, R. (1991). A yeast transcription assay defines distinct *rel* and *dorsal* DNA recognition sequences. New Biologist, 3, 1005–1013.

Kamens, J., Richardson, P., Mosialos, G., Brent, R. and Gilmore, T. (1990). Oncogenic transformation by vRel requires an amino-terminal activation domain. Mol. Cell Biologist, 10, 2840–2847.

Kao, K.R. and Hopwood, N.D. (1991). Expression of a mRNA related to c-*rel* and dorsal in early *Xenopus laevis* embryos. Proc. Natl Acad. Sci. USA, 88, 2697–2701.

Kieran, M., Blank, V., Logeat, R., Vandekerckhove, J., Lottspeich, F., LeBail, O., Urban, M., Kourilsky, P., Baeuerle, P.A. and Israel, A. (1990). The DNA binding subunit of NF-κB is identical to factor KBF1 and homologous to the *rel* oncogene product. Cell, 62, 1007–1018.

Kochel, T. and Rice, N.R. (1992). v-*rel* - and c-*rel* - protein complexes bind to the NF-κB site *in vitro*. Oncogene, 7, 567–572.

Kunsch, C., Ruben, S.M. and Rosen, C.A. (1992). Selection of optimal κB/rel DNA-binding motifs: interaction of both subunits of NF-κB with DNA is required for transcriptional activation. Mol. Cell. Biol., 12, 4412–4421.

Lewis, R.B., McClure, J., Rub, B., Niesel, D.W., Garry, R.F., Hoelzer, J.D., Nazerian, K. and Bose, H.R. (1981). Avian reticuloendotheliosis virus: identification of the hematopoietic target for transformation. Cell, 25, 421–431.

Logeat, F., Israel, N., Ten, R., Blank, V., Le Bail, O., Kourilsky, P. and Israel, A. (1991). Inhibition of transcription factors belonging to the rel/NF-κB family by a transdominant negative mutant. EMBO J., 10, 1827–1832.

Lu, D., Thompson, J.D., Gorski, G.K., Rice, N.R., Mayer, M.G. and Yunis, J.J. (1991). Alterations at the rel locus in human lymphoma. Oncogene, 6, 1235–1241.

McDonnell, P.C., Kumar, S., Rabson, A.B. and Gelinas, C. (1992). Transcriptional activity of *rel* family proteins. Oncogene, 7, 163–170.

Mathew, S., Murty, V.V.V.S., Dalla-Favera, R. and Chaganti, R.S.K. (1993). Chromosomal localization of genes encoding the transcription factors, c-*rel*, NF-κBp50, NF-κBp65, and *lyt*-10 by fluorescence *in situ* hybridization. Oncogene, 8, 191–193.

Moore, B.E. and Bose, H.R. (1988). Expression of the v-*rel* oncogene in reticuloendotheliosis virus-transformed fibroblasts. Virology, 162, 377–387.

Moore, B.E. and Bose, H.R. Jr. (1989). Expression of the c-*rel* and c-*myc* proto-oncogenes in avian tissues. Oncogene, 4, 845–852.

Morrison, L.E., Boehmelt, G., Beug, H. and Enrietto, P.J. (1991). Expression of v-*rel*-in a replication competent virus: transformation and biochemical characterization. Oncogene, 6, 1657–1666.

Morrison, L.E., Boehmelt, G. and Enrietto, P.J. (1992). Mutations in the *rel*-homology domain alter the biochemical properties of v-*rel* and render it transformation defective in chicken embryo fibroblasts. Oncogene, 7, 1137–1147.

Mosialos, G. and Gilmore, T.D. (1993). v-Rel and c-Rel are differentially affected by mutations at a consensus protein kinase recognition sequence. Oncogene, 8, 721–730.

Mosialos, G., Hamer, P., Capobianco, A.J., Laursen, R.A. and Gilmore, T.D. (1991). A protein kinase-A recognition sequence is structurally linked to transformation by p59^{v-rel} and cytoplasmic retention of p68^{c-rel}. Mol. Cell. Biol., 11, 5867–5877.

Muchardt, C., Seeler, J.S., Nirula, A., Shurland, D.L. and Gaynor, R.B. (1992). Regulation of human immunodeficiency virus enhancer function by PRDII-BF1 and c-*rel* gene products. J. Virol., 66, 244–250.

Nakayama, K., Shimizu, H., Mitomo, K., Watanabe, T., Okamoto, S. and Yamamoto, K. (1992). A lymphoid cell-specific nuclear factor containing c-REL-like proteins preferentially interacts with interleukin-6 kappa B-related motifs whose activities are repressed in lymphoid cells. Mol. Cell. Biol., 12, 1736–1746.

Neri, A., Chang, C.C., Lombardi, L., Salina, M., Corradini, P., Maiolo, A.T., Chaganti, R.S. and Dalla-Favera, R. (1991). B cell lymphoma-associated chromosomal translocation involves candidate oncogene *lyt*-10, homologous to NF-kappa B p50. Cell, 67, 1075–1087.

Neumann, M., Tsapos, K., Schleppler, J.A., Ross, J. and Franza, B.R. (1992). Identification of complex formation between two intracellular tyrosine kinase substrates: human c-rel and the p105 precursor of p50 NF-κB. Oncogene, 7, 2095–2104.

Nolan, G.P., Ghosh, S., Liou, H.-C., Tempst, P. and Baltimore, D. (1991). DNA binding and IκB inhibition of the cloned p65 subunit of NF-κB, a *rel*-related polypeptide. Cell, 64, 961–969.

Rice, N.R., Copeland, T.D., Simek, S., Oroszlan, S. and Gilden, R.V. (1986). Detection and characterization of the protein encoded by the v-*rel* oncogene. Virology, 149, 217–229.

Richardson, P.M. and Gilmore, T.D. (1991). vRel is an inactive member of the rel family of transcriptional activating proteins. J. Virol., 65, 3122–3130.

Robinson, F.R. and Twiehaus, M.J. (1974). Isolation of the avian reticuloendotheliosis virus (strain T). Avian Dis., 18, 278–288.

Ruben, S.M., Klement, J.F., Coleman, T.A., Maher, M., Chen, C.-H. and Rosen, C.A. (1992). I-rel: a novel *rel*-related protein that inhibits NF-κB transcriptional activity. Genes Devel., 6, 745–760.

Ryseck, R.-P., Bull, P., Takamiya, M., Bours, V, Siebenlist, U., Dobrzanski, P. and Bravo, R. (1992). relB, a new rel family transcription activator that can interact with p50-NF-κB. Mol. Cell. Biol., 12, 674–684.

Sica, A., Tan, T.H., Rice, N., Kretzschmar, M., Ghosh, P. and Young, H.A. (1992). The c-rel protooncogene product c-REL but not NF-kappa B binds to the intronic region of the human interferon-gamma gene at a site related to an interferon-stimulable response element. Proc. Natl Acad. Sci. USA, 89, 1740–1744.

Simek, S. and Rice, N.R. (1988). p59^{v-rel}, the transforming protein of reticuloendotheliosis virus, is complexed with at least four other proteins in transformed chicken lymphoid cells. J. Virol., 62, 4730–4736.

Stephens, R.M., Rice, N.R., Hiebsch, R.R., Bose, H.R. and Gilden, R.V. (1983). Nucleotide sequence of v-*rel*: the oncogene of reticuloendotheliosis virus. Proc. Natl Acad. Sci. USA, 80, 6229–6233.

Steward, R. (1987). *Dorsal*, an embryonic polarity gene in *Drosophila*, is homologous to the vertebrate proto-oncogene, c-*rel*. Science, 238, 692–694.

Sylla, B.S. and Temin, H.M. (1986). Activation of oncogenicity of the c-*rel* proto-oncogene. Mol. Cell. Biol., 6, 4709–4716.

Tan, T.-H., Huang, G.P., Sica, A., Ghosh, P., Young, H.A., Longo, D.L. and Rice, N.R. (1992). κB site-dependent activation of the interleukin-2 receptor α-chain gene promoter by human c-rel. Mol. Cell. Biol., 12, 4067–4075.

Visvanathan, K.V. and Goodburn, S. (1989). Double-stranded RNA activates binding of NF-κB to an inducible element in the human β-interferon promoter. EMBO J., 8, 1129–1138.

Walker, W.H., Stein, B., Ganchi, P.A., Hoffman, J.A., Kaufman, P.A., Ballard, D.W., Hannink, M. and Greene, W.C. (1992). The v-*rel* oncogene: insights into the mechanism of transcriptional activation, repression, and transformation. J. Virol., 66, 5018–5029.

Walro, D.S., Herzog, N.K., Zhang, J., Lim, M.Y. and Bose, H.R. (1987). The transforming protein of avian reticuloendotheliosis virus is a soluble cytoplasmic protein which is associated with a protein kinase activity. Virology, 160, 433–444.

Wilhelmsen, K.C., Eggleton, K. and Temin, H.M. (1984). Nucleic acid sequences of the oncogene v-*rel* in reticuloendotheliosis virus strain T and its cellular homolog, the proto-oncogene c-*rel*. J. Virol., 52, 172–182.

RET

RET is a human transforming gene with no homology with known viral oncogenes, originally detected by NIH 3T3 fibroblast transfection with DNA from a T cell lymphoma (Takahashi *et al.*, 1985).

Related genes

RET[TPC] and PTC (*p*apillary *t*hyroid *c*arcinoma) are identical. Human and mouse RET contain repeated sequence motifs in the extracellular domain that are homologous to regions in the Ca^{2+} binding sites of cadherins (Schneider, 1992; Iwamoto *et al.*, 1993). RET is related to mouse *Tek* receptor tyrosine kinase (see Table 2.5 Supplement).

Cross-species homology

RET: 84% homology (human and mouse) (Takahashi and Cooper, 1987; Iwamoto *et al.*, 1993).

Transformation

MAN

RET is probably the multiple endocrine neoplasia type 2A (MEN 2A) gene. Missense mutations in germline and/or tumour DNA have been detected in 20/23 unrelated MEN 2A patients (Mulligan *et al.*, 1993). *RET* may thus be the first gene detected in which dominantly acting point mutations initiate human hereditary neoplasia.

An activated form of *RET* (*RET/PTC1*) has been found with high frequency (11–33%) in papillary thyroid carcinomas (Fusco *et al.*, 1987; Grieco *et al.*, 1990; Jhiang *et al.*, 1992; Santoro *et al.*, 1992) and in the TPC-1 human papillary thyroid carcinoma cell line (Ishizaka *et al.*, 1990). There is one report of *RET/PTC1* activation in follicular adenomas and adenomatous goiters (Ishizaka *et al.*, 1991). A second type of *RET* oncogenic rearrangement, *RET/PTC2*, occurs with lower frequency in papillary thyroid carcinomas (Bongarzone *et al.*, 1993). *TRK* (*NTRK1*) is also activated with high frequency in papillary thyroid carcinomas (see **TRK**).

IN VITRO

Other activated forms of the *RET* proto-oncogene were generated *in vitro* during an NIH 3T3 transfection assay (Takahashi *et al.*, 1985; Koda, 1988).

TRANSGENIC ANIMALS

Mice carrying the metallothionein/*Ret* (MT/*Ret*) fusion gene develop melanosis and melanocytic tumours (Taniguchi *et al.*, 1992). In MMTV/*Ret* transgenic mice mammary and salivary gland adenocarcinomas develop in a stochastic manner (Iwamoto *et al.*, 1990).

	RET/Ret
Nucleotides (kb)	30
RET cDNA	4726 bp (including leader sequence and 5′ and 3′ untranslated regions) (Takahashi *et al.*, 1989)
RET/PTC1 cDNA	3642 bp (nucleotides 1–354 from the *D10S170* gene (formerly called *H4*) and nucleotides 355–3642 from *RET*)
RET/PTC2 cDNA	1867 bp (nucleotides 1–717 from the RIα subunit of cAMP-dependent protein kinase and 1150 nucleotides from *RET*)
RFP/RET cDNA	2486 bp (Takahashi and Cooper, 1987)
Chromosome	
Human	10q11.2
mRNA (kb)	
Human	2.3/1.4/0.9 (Mulligan *et al.*, 1991)
	3.9/4.5/6.0/7.0 (*RET*: neuroblastoma cells)
	3.3/4.2/6.0/7.6 (*RFP–RET*)
	1.8/2.8/4.5 (*PTC*)
Mouse	4.5/6.0
Amino acids	
Human	1072/1114
	(3′ alternative splicing creates 51 amino acids in the larger protein that are replaced by 9 unrelated residues in the smaller)
	478/520 (RET/PTC1)
	596/638 (RET/PTC2)
Mouse	1115
Mass (kDa)	
(predicted)	91 (RET)
	57–60 (RET/PTC1)
Human (expressed)	gp150/gp170
	(derived from a p120 precursor in neuroblastoma cells)

	RET/Ret
Human (expressed)	190 (monocytic leukaemia cell line: Takahashi *et al.*, 1991)
	pp96/pp100 (in *RET*-transformed cells)
	pp57$^{RET/TPC1}$
	p76$^{RET/PTC2}$/p81$^{RET/PTC2}$
	p64^{PTC1}
Mouse	gp140/gp160

Cellular location

RET is a plasma membrane receptor-like protein not phosphorylated on tyrosine. pp100 in transformed NIH 3T3 cells is predominantly in the membrane fraction; pp96 occurs in both membrane and cytosol fractions (Taniguchi *et al.*, 1991).

Tissue location

RET is expressed in a developmental stage-specific manner. It is undetectable or low in adult rat or mouse normal tissues but present in the rat placenta during the mid-term of gestation (Szentirmay *et al.*, 1990). It is expressed in neuroblastoma cells induced to differentiate by retinoic acid (Tahira *et al.*, 1991).

RET proto-oncogene is also expressed in human thyroid medullary carcinomas and pheochromocytomas and in a human thyroid medullary carcinoma cell line induced to differentiate by cAMP (Santoro *et al.*, 1990).

Protein function

RET encodes two forms of receptor tyrosine kinases. Ligand unknown. *RET* may be involved in neuronal differentiation (Takahashi and Cooper, 1987; Tahira *et al.*, 1991). p57$^{RET/TPC}$ is constitutively phosphorylated which may confer aberrant tyrosine kinase activity (Ishizaka *et al.*, 1992). The oncogenic forms of RET (p76$^{RET/PTC2}$/p81$^{RET/PTC2}$ and p64^{PTC1}) are constitutively phosphorylated on tyrosine, have autophosphorylation activity and are cytoplasmic (Ishizaka *et al.*, 1992; Lanzi *et al.*, 1992). p76$^{RET/PTC2}$ and p81$^{RET/PTC2}$ form homo- and heterodimers with each other (Bongarzone *et al.*, 1993).

The cell line derived from MT/*Ret* tumours (Mel-ret) causes rapid tumour formation and metastasis in nude mice and the tumours express a p85^{ret} protein that is highly tyrosine phosphorylated compared with the RET protein detected in primary, non-malignant melanocytic tumours (Taniguchi *et al.*, 1992).

Protein structure

The *RET* transforming gene isolated by Takahashi *et al.* (1985) had been activated *in vitro* during the transfection assay in a rearrangement that juxtaposed two unlinked human DNA segments, the *RET* proto-oncogene and the putative zinc finger-containing *RFP* gene (ret finger protein: Takahashi *et al.*, 1988b). A RET fusion protein of 435 amino acids has also been characterized after transfection of DNA from human stomach cancer into NIH 3T3 cells (Kunieda *et al.*, 1991).

RET/PTC1 is a different fusion protein of a 5' non-*RET* region (*D10S170*) and the kinase domain encoded by *RET*. These two 17 kb regions are normally ~25 kb apart (Sozzi *et al.*, 1991). The *PTC1* oncogene that results from the activation of proto-*RET* by recombination contains 520 amino acids: RET is truncated at amino acid 458 and its N-terminal region replaced by D10S170 (Grieco *et al.*, 1990). This is a somatic, tumour-specific event, in contrast to the recombination between *RET* and *RFP*. Alternative splicing of proto-*RET* gives rise to differing C-termini and corresponding *PTC* cDNAs have been isolated.

PTC/RET^TPC rearrangements occur at different sites in different tumours but the hybrid genes encode the same transcripts (Jhiang *et al.*, 1992).

A second rearrangement (RET/PTC2) has been detected in papillary thyroid carcinoma in which the C-terminal 360 amino acids of normal RET, including the tyrosine kinase domain, are fused with 236 residues of the RIα regulatory subunit of protein kinase A, creating a fusion protein of 596 amino acids (Lanzi *et al.*, 1992; Bongarzone *et al.*, 1993). Two isoforms having C-termini of 9 and 51 amino acid arise from the alternative splicing mechanism that generates two isoforms of the normal RET protein.

The point mutations that occur in MEN 2A affect Cys380 in 95% of cases (Mulligan *et al.*, 1993). In the remainder Cys364 is mutated. This suggests that the replacement of either of these residues may affect RET signal transduction, leading to the MEN 2A phenotype.

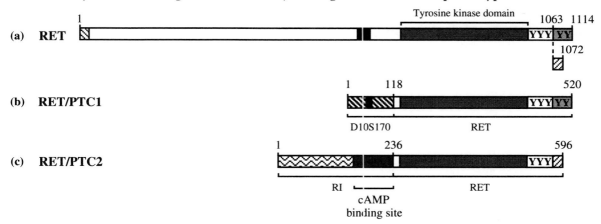

The promoter region of proto-*RET* contains a GC-rich region without a TATA box. Putative binding motifs for Sp-1, AP-2, epidermal growth factor receptor-specific transcription factor (ETF) and the transcription suppressor GC factor (GCF) occur in this repeated GC region (Itoh *et al.*, 1992).

Sequence of RET

```
RET    (1)   MVPFPVTVYDEDDSAPTFPAGVDTASAVVEFKRKEDTVVATLRVFDADVVPASGELVRRY
RET   (61)   TSTLLPGDTWAQQTFRVEHWPNETSVQANGSFVRATVHDYRLVLNRNLSISENRTMQLAV
RET  (121)   LVNDSDFQGPGAGVLLLHFNVSVLPVSLHLPSTYSLSVSRRARRFAQIGKVCVENCQAFS
RET  (181)   GINVQYKLHSSGANCSTLGVVTSAEDTSGILFVNDTKALRRPKCAELHYMVVATDQQTSR
RET  (241)   QAQAQLLVTVEGSYVAEEAGCPLSCAVSLRRLECEECGGLGSPTGRCEWRQGDGKGITRN
RET  (301)   FSTCSPSTKTCPDGHCDVVETQDINICPQDCLRGSIVGGHEPGEPRGIKAGYGTCNCFPE
             *          ***
RET  (361)   EEKCFCEPEDIQDPLCDELCRTVIAAAVLFSFVVSVLLSAFCIHCYHKFAHKPPISSAEM
```

```
RET  (421)  TFRRPAQAFPVSYSSSGARRPSLDSMENQVSVDAFKILEDPKWEFPRKNLVLGKTLGEGE
RET  (481)  FGKVVKATAFHLKGRAGYTTVAVKMLKENASPSELRDLLSEFNVLKQVNHPHVIKLYGAC
RET  (541)  SQDGPLLLIVEYAKYGSLRGFLRESRKVGPGYLGSGGSRNSSSLDHPDERALTMGDLISF
RET  (601)  AWQISQGMQYLAEMKLVHRDLAARNILVAEGRKMKISDFGLSRDVYEEDPYVKRSQGRIP
RET  (661)  VKWMAIESLFDHIYTTQSDVWSFGVLLWEIVTLGGNPYPGIPPERLFNLLKTGHRMERPD
RET  (721)  NCSEEMYRLMLQCWKQEPDKRPVFADISKDLEKMMVKRRDYLDLAASTPSDSLIYDDGLS
RET  (781)  EEETPLVDCNNAPLPRALPSTWIENKLYG*MSDPNWPGESPVPLTRADGTNTGFPRYPNDS*
RET  (841)  *VYANWMLSPSAAKLMDTFDS* (860)
```

Sequence of RFP

```
RFP    (1)  MASGSVAECLQQETTCPVCLQYFAEPMMLDCGHNICCACLARCWGTAETNVSCPQCRETF
RFP   (61)  PQRHMRPNRHLANVTQLVKQLRTERPSGPGGEMGVCEKHREPLKLYCEEDQMPICVVCDR
RFP  (121)  SREHRGHSVLPLEEAVEGFKEQIQNQLDHLKRVKDLKKRRRAQGEQARAELLSLTQMERE
RFP  (181)  KIVWEFEQLYHSLKEHEYRLLARLEELDLAIYNSINGAITQFSCNISHLSSLIAQLEEKQ
RFP  (241)  QQPTRELLQDIGDTLSRAERIRIPEPWITPPDLQEKIHIFAPKCLFLTESLKQFTEKMQS
RFP  (301)  DMEKIQELREAQLYSVDVTLDPDTAYPSLILSDNLRQVRYSYLQQDLPDNPERFNLFPCV
RFP  (361)  LGSPCFIAGRHYWEVEVGDKAKWTIGVCEDSVCRKGGVTSAPQNGFWAVSLWYGKEYWAL
RFP  (421)  TSPMTALPLRTPLQRVGIFLDYDAGEVSFYNVTERCHTFTFSHATFCGPVRPYFSLSYSG
RFP  (481)  GKSAAPLIICPMSGIDGFSGHVGNHGHSMETSP (513)
```

The chimeric gene product was generated *in vitro* by the fusion of the RET C-terminus to the first 315 amino acids of the 513 amino acid protein RFP (Takahashi *et al.*, 1988b). The N-terminus of RET and the N-terminus of RFP that replaces it in the chimeric protein are underlined. In the PTC1 fusion protein amino acids 1–458 of RET are replaced by D10S170 sequence.

The RET sequence is that encoded by one of the species of mRNA in the human monocytic leukaemia cell line THP-1 (Takahashi *et al.*, 1988a). It has been shown that 3.9, 4.5 and possibly 7.0 kb species encode a 1072 amino acid protein and a 6.0 kb and possibly a minor 4.6 kb form encode a 1114 amino acid protein (Tahira *et al.*, 1990). The italicized 51 C-terminal amino acids represent one isoform of RET. The alternative 9 amino acid terminus is shown in the RET/PTC2 sequence below.

*Indicates mutations detected in MEN 2A: Cys364 →Gly; Glu378–Leu379–Cys380 →Asp–Val–Arg or Cys380 →Gly, Tyr, Ser or Phe (Mulligan *et al.*, 1993).

Sequence of RET/PTC2

```
    (1)  MQSGSTAASQQARSLRQCQLYVEKHNIEALLKDSIVQLCTARPERPMAFLREYFERLEKE
   (61)  EAKQIQNLQKAGTRTDSREDEISPPPPNPVVKGRRRRGAISAEVYTEEDAASYVRKVIPK
  (121)  DYKTMAALAKAIEKNVLFSHLDDNERSDIFDAMFSVSFIAGETVIQQGDEGDNFYVIDQG
                                                        RIα/RET
  (181)  ETDVYVNNEWATSVGEGGSFGELALIYGTPRAATVKAKTNVKLWGIDRDSYRRILMEDPK
  (241)  WEFPRKNLVLGKTLGEGEFGKVVKATAFHLKGRAGYTTVAVKMLKENASPSELRDLLSEF
  (301)  NVLKQVNHPHVIKLYGACSQDGPLLLIVEYAKYGSLRGFLRESRKVGPGYLGSGGSRNSS
  (361)  SLDHPDERALTMGDLISFAWQISQGMQYLAEMKLVHRDLAARNILVAEGRKMKISDFGLS
  (421)  RDVYEEDPYVKRSQGRIPVKWMAIESLFDHIYTTQSDVWSFGVLLWEIVTLGGNPYPGIP
  (481)  PERLFNLLKTGHRMERPDNCSEEMYRLMLQCWKQEPDKRPVFADISKDLEKMMVKRRDYL
  (541)  DLAASTPSDSLIYDDGLSEEETPLVDCNNAPLPRALPSTWIENKLYG*RISHAFTRF* (596)
```

The underlined sequence is that of RIα and the RIα/RET fusion point (236/237), which is the same as in D10S170–RET, is shown. Italics: 9 amino acid form of C-terminus.

Databank file names and accession numbers

	GENE	*EMBL*	*SWISSPROT*	*REFERENCES*
Human	*RET*	Hstykret M16029	KRET_HUMAN P07949	Takahashi and Cooper, 1987
				Takahashi *et al.*, 1988a
Human	*RET/PTC2*	L03357		Bongarzone *et al.*, 1993
Mouse	*Ret*	Mmret X67812		Takahashi *et al.*, 1991
				Iwamoto *et al.*, 1993

Papers

Bongarzone, I., Monzini, N., Borrello, M.G., Carcano, C., Ferraresi, G., Arighi, E., Mondellini, P., Della Porta, G. and Pierotti, M.A. (1993). Molecular characterization of a thyroid tumor-specific transforming sequence formed by the fusion of *ret* tyrosine kinase and the regulatory subunit RIα of cyclic AMP-dependent protein kinase A. Mol. Cell. Biol., 13, 358–366.

Fusco, A., Grieco, M., Santoro, M., Berlingieri, M.T., Pilotti, S., Pierotti, M.A., Della Porta, G. and Vecchio, G. (1987). A new oncogene in human thyroid papillary carcinomas and their lymph-nodal metastases. Nature, 328, 170–172.

Grieco, M., Santoro, M., Berlingieri, M.T., Melillo, R.M., Donghi, R., Bongarzone, I., Pierotti, M.A., Della Porta, G., Fusco, A. and Vecchio, G. (1990). PTC is a novel rearranged form of the *ret* proto-oncogene and is frequently detected in vivo in human thyroid papillary carcinomas. Cell, 60, 557–563.

Ishizaka, Y., Ushijima, T., Sugimura, T. and Nagao, M. (1990). cDNA cloning and characterization of *ret* activated in a human papillary thyroid carcinoma cell line. Biochem. Biophys. Res. Commun., 168, 402–408.

Ishizaka, Y., Kobayashi, S., Ushijima, T., Hirohashi, S., Sugimura, T. and Nagao, M. (1991). Detection of *ret*^{TPC}/PTC transcripts in thyroid adenomas and adenomatous goiter by an RT-PCR method. Oncogene, 6, 1667–1672.

Ishizaka, Y., Shima, H., Sugimura, T. and Nagao, M. (1992). Detection of phosphorylated *ret*^{TPC} oncogene product in cytoplasm. Oncogene, 7, 1441–1444.

Itoh, F., Ishizaka, Y., Tahira, T., Yamamoto, M., Miya, A., Imai, K., Yachi, A., Takai, S., Sugimura, T. and Nagao, M. (1992). Identification and analysis of the *ret* proto-oncogene promoter region in neuroblastoma cell lines and medullary thyroid carcinomas from MEN2A patients. Oncogene, 7, 1201–1205.

Iwamoto, T., Takahashi, M., Ito, M., Hamaguchi, M., Isobe, K., Misawa, N., Asai, J., Yoshida, T. and Nakashima, I. (1990). Oncogenicity of the *ret* transforming gene in MMTV/*ret* transgenic mice. Oncogene, 5, 535–542.

Iwamoto, T., Taniguchi, M., Asai, N., Ohkusu, K., Nakashima, I. and Takahashi, M. (1993). cDNA cloning of mouse *ret* proto-oncogene and its sequence similarity to the cadherin family. Oncogene, 8, 1087–1091.

Jhiang, S.M., Caruso, D.R., Gilmore, E., Ishizaka, Y., Tahira, T., Nagao, M., Chiu, I.-M. and Mazzaferri, E.L. (1992). Detection of the PTC/*ret*^{TPC} oncogene in human thyroid cancers. Oncogene, 7, 1331–1337.

Koda, T. (1988). *Ret* gene from a human stomach cancer. Hokkaido J. Med. Sci., 63, 913–924.

Kunieda, T., Matsui, M., Nomura, N. and Ishizaki, R. (1991). Cloning of an activated human ret gene with a novel 5′ sequence fused by DNA rearrangement. Gene, 107, 323–328.

Lanzi, C., Borrello, M.G., Bongarzone, I., Migliazza, A., Fusco, A., Grieco, M., Santoro, M., Gambetta, R.A., Zunino, F., Della Porta, G. and Pierotti, M.A. (1992). Identification of the product of two oncogenic rearranged forms of the *RET* proto-oncogene in papillary thyroid carcinomas. Oncogene, 7, 2189–2194.

Mulligan, L.M., Gardner, E., Papi, L. and Ponder, B.A. (1991). A new polymorphism in the *ret* protooncogene (RET). Nucleic Acids Res., 19, 5795.

Mulligan, L., Kwok, J.B.J., Healey, C.S., Elsdon, M.J., Eng, C., Gardner, E., Love, D.R., Mole, S.E., Moore, J.K., Papi, L., Ponder, M.A., Telenius, H., Tunnacliffe, A. and Ponder, B.A.J. (1993). Germline mutations of the *RET* proto-oncogene in multiple endocrine neoplasia type 2A (MEN 2A). Nature, 363, 458–460.

Santoro, M., Rosati, R., Grieco, M., Berlingieri, M.T., D'Amato, G.L., de Franciscis, V. and Fusco, A. (1990).

The *ret* proto-oncogene is consistently expressed in human pheochromocytomas and thyroid medullary carcinomas. Oncogene, 5, 1595–1598.

Santoro, M., Carlomagno, F., Hay, I.D., Hermann, M.A., Grieco, M., Melillo, R., Pierotti, M.A., Bongarzone, I., Della Porta, G., Berger, N., Peix, J.L., Paulin, C., Fabien, N., Vecchio, G., Jenkins, R.B. and Fusco, A. (1992). Ret oncogene activation in human thyroid neoplasms is restricted to the papillary cancer subtype. J. Clin. Invest., 89, 1517–1522.

Schneider, R. (1992). The human protooncogene *ret*: a communicative cadherin? Trends Biochem. Sci., 17, 468–469.

Sozzi, G., Pierotti, M.A., Miozzo, M., Donghi, R., Radice, P., De Benedetti, V., Grieco, M., Santoro, M., Fusco, A., Vecchio, G., Mathew, C.G.P., Ponder, B.A.J., Spurr, N.K. and Della Porta, G. (1991). Refined localization to contiguous regions on chromosome 10q of the two genes (H4 and RET) that form the oncogenic sequence PTC. Oncogene, 6, 339–342.

Szentirmay, Z., Ishizaka, Y., Ohgaki, H., Tahira, T., Nagao, M. and Esumi, H. (1990). Demonstration by *in situ* hybridization of *ret* proto-oncogene mRNA in developing placenta during mid-term of rat gestation. Oncogene, 5, 701–705.

Tahira, T., Ishizaka, Y., Itoh, F., Nakayasu, M., Sugimura, T. and Nagao, M. (1990). Characterization of *ret* proto-oncogene mRNAs encoding two isoforms of the protein product in a human neuroblastoma cell line. Oncogene, 5, 97–102.

Tahira, T., Ishizaka, Y., Itoh, F., Nakayasu, M., Sugimura, T. and Nagao, M. (1991). Expression of the *ret* proto-oncogene in human neuroblastoma cell lines and its increase during neuronal differentiation induced by retinoic acid. Oncogene, 6, 2333–2338.

Takahashi, M. and Cooper, G.M. (1987). *ret* transforming gene encodes a fusion protein homologous to tyrosine kinases. Mol. Cell. Biol., 7, 1378–1385.

Takahashi, M., Ritz, J. and Cooper, M.G. (1985). Activation of a novel human transforming gene, *ret*, by DNA rearrangement. Cell, 42, 581–588.

Takahashi, M., Buma, Y., Iwamoto, T., Inaguma, Y., Ikeda, H. and Hiai, H. (1988a). Cloning and expression of the *ret* proto-oncogene encoding a tyrosine kinase with two potential transmembrane domains. Oncogene, 3, 571–578.

Takahashi, M., Inaguma, Y., Hiai, H. and Hirose, F. (1988b). Developmentally regulated expression of a human "finger"-containing gene encoded by the 5' half of the *ret* transforming gene. Mol. Cell. Biol., 8, 1853–1856.

Takahashi, M., Buma, Y. and Hiai, H. (1989). Isolation of *ret* proto-oncogene cDNA with an amino-terminal signal sequence. Oncogene, 4, 805–806.

Takahashi, M., Buma, Y. and Taniguchi, M. (1991). Identification of the *ret* proto-oncogene products in neuroblastoma and leukemia cells. Oncogene, 6, 297–301.

Taniguchi, M., Iwamoto, T., Hamaguchi, M., Matsuyama, M. and Takahashi, M. (1991). The *ret* oncogene products are membrane-bound glycoproteins phosphorylated on tyrosine residues *in vivo*. Biochem. Biophys. Res. Commun., 181, 416–422.

Taniguchi, M., Iwamoto, T., Nakashima, I., Nakayama, A., Ohbayashi, M., Matsuyama. M. and Takahashi, M. (1992). Establishment and characterization of a malignant melanocytic tumor cell line expressing the *ret* oncogene. Oncogene, 7, 1491–1496.

v-*ros* is the oncogene of the acutely transforming avian sarcoma virus UR2 (University of Rochester, Balduzzi *et al.*, 1981). Helper virus: UR2AV: host range: subgroup A. *ros* is so designated because it is unrelated to any other ASV gene (Wang *et al.*, 1982). Following transfection of cDNA derived from a human mammary carcinoma cell line (MCF-7) into NIH 3T3 cells and injection of these cells into nude mice, the *MCF3* gene was expressed in some of the tumours generated (Birchmeier *et al.*, 1986). *MCF3* is a 5' rearrangement of *Ros-1* that contains 99 N-terminal amino acids not present in v-*ros*.

Ros-1 encodes a receptor-type tyrosine kinase.

Related genes

Ros-1 is a member of the *Src* family (*Blk, Fes, Fgr, Fps, Fyn, Hck, Lck, Tkl, Yes*) and also has homology with receptor-type tyrosine kinases including the insulin and EGF receptors (61% and 45% in the kinase domain; Neckameyer and Wang, 1985).

Close similarity in overall structure and sequence exists between vertebrate ROS and *Drosophila sevenless* (Hafen *et al.*, 1987; Birchmeier *et al.*, 1990; Matsushime and Shibuya, 1990; Chen *et al.*, 1991).

MCF3 is probably the human homologue of chicken ROS but the identity is only 75% in the kinase domain, which is much lower than that for SRC (99%) or the EGFR (98%).

Cross-species homology

Human and chicken extracellular domains: 51% identity, 68% homology; intracellular kinase domains: 75% identity, 84% homology; none in the C-terminus. Human and rat kinase domains: 92% identity. Rat and chicken kinase domains: 75% identity (Matsushime and Shibuya, 1990).

Transformation

MAN

ROS1 expression is elevated in cell lines derived from human glioblastomas (Sharma *et al.*, 1989) but not in primary human glioblastomas (Wu and Chikaraishi, 1990).

ANIMALS

Injected UR2 induces tumours in chickens. UR2-transformed rat cells induce fatal fibrosarcomas on injection into rats (Neckameyer and Wang, 1985). *MCF3*-transformed NIH 3T3 cells form tumours in nude mice (Birchmeier *et al.*, 1986).

IN VITRO

Infected cells from chicken tumours transform chick embryo fibroblasts (CEFs) and infected CEFs transform rat-1 cell lines.

	ROS1/Ros-1	v-ros
Nucleotides		
Human	32 kb	
	(7041 coding nt)	1273
Chicken	11 kb	
	(6939 coding nt)	
Chromosome		
Human	6q21–q22	
Mouse	10	
Exons		
mRNA (kb)		
Human	8.5	3.3
Chicken	8.3	
Rat	1.9/2.4/6.9/8.2	
Amino acids		
Human	2347	552
Chicken	2313	
Rat	2317	
Mass (kDa)		
(predicted)		
Human	256	61
Chicken	252	
(expressed)	gp260	pp68$^{gag-ros}$

Cellular location

Plasma membrane.

Tissue location

Ros-1 mRNA expression in the mouse occurs transiently during the development of the kidney, intestine and lung and coincides with major morphogenetic and differentiation events (Sonnenberg *et al.*, 1991). Chicken *Ros-1* is significantly expressed in the kidney with low expression in the gonads, thymus, bursa and brain (Neckameyer *et al.*, 1986).

Rat *Ros-1* is expressed principally in the lung and kidney (8.2 kb mRNA), heart (6.9 kb) and testis (1.9 and 2.4 kb; Matsushime and Shibuya, 1990).

ROS1 is highly expressed in human glioblastoma cell lines as an 8.3 kb transcript or, in U-118 cells, as a 4.0 kb mRNA (Sharma *et al.*, 1989).

Protein function

Receptor-like tyrosine kinase with autophosphorylation capacity. p68$^{gag\text{-}ros}$ co-precipitates with phosphatidylinositol kinase and in UR2-transformed cells the levels of PtdIns(4)P, PtdIns(4,5)P_2 and PtdIns(1,4,5)P_3 are increased (Macara *et al.*, 1984). The pattern of phosphorylation of 26 proteins is altered in UR2-transformed fibroblasts in a manner similar to that seen in RSV-transformed cells (Maytin *et al.*, 1984).

The pattern of expression during the differentiation of normal tissues is unusual for a tyrosine kinase receptor and indicates a specific role for *Ros-1* during development (Sonnenberg *et al.*, 1991).

Structure of the UR2 genome and p68$^{gag\text{-}ros}$

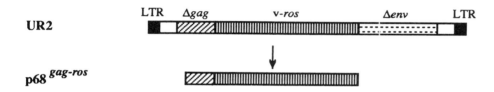

v-*ros* is inserted between p19^{gag} and gp37^{env} (*pol* deleted). The 5′ region of *Ros-1* is replaced by p19^{gag}. The chicken v-ROS sequence differs from ROS1 over the C-terminal 36 nucleotides. Chicken and human *Ros-1* contain an additional 5′ exon relative to v-*ros* with a potential *N*-linked glycosylation site. *Ros-1* contains further 5′ exons (Matsushime *et al.*, 1986). Thus v-ROS is a truncated version of ROS1 (cf. v-ERBB and the EGFR).

p68$^{gag\text{-}ros}$ comprises 150 p19^{gag} amino acids and 402 from ROS1. p19 and the transmembrane domain (28–29 hydrophobic residues) are essential for transformation.

The protein has a conserved ATP binding site and phosphate acceptor tyrosine residues but p68 has a six amino acid insert and three amino acid substitutions not found in other tyrosine protein kinases.

Human and chicken ROS

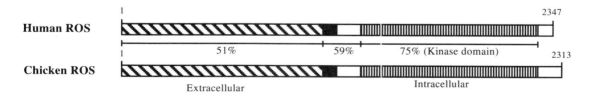

The percentage amino acid identity between the domains of the proteins is shown: the C-termini are completely divergent.

The genomic structure of *Ros-1* has only been incompletely characterized.

Structural similarity between rat ROS and the *Drosophila sev* gene product

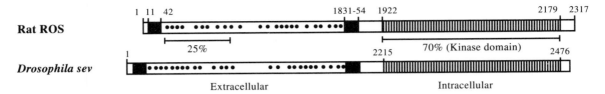

Percentages indicate amino acid homology. Dots: cysteine residues in the extracellular domains. Black boxes: hydrophobic regions (Matsushime and Shibuya, 1990).

Rat ROS1 is related to *Drosophila sev* protein and both have a unique 5–7 amino acid insert in the tyrosine kinase domain. They also contain a 20 residue hydrophobic sequence 50 amino acids downstream of the initiating Met residue and may form a loop structure from the plasma membrane.

Sequences of rat, human and chicken ROS1

```
Rat ROS1   (1)    MKRIRWLTPKPATFVVLGCVWISVAQGTILSSCLTSCVTNLGRQLDSGTRYNLSEACIQ
Human ROS1 (1)    --N-YC-I--LVN-AT---L----V-C-V-N---K-------Q---L--PH----P---

Rat        (60)   GCQFWNSIDQEKCALKCNDTYVTICERESCEVGCSNAEGSYEEEVLDNTELPTAPFASSI
Human      (60)   --H----V--KN-----        --------S---A------E-AD---------

Rat        (120)  GSNGVTLRWNPANISGVKYIIQWKYAQLPGSWAYTETVSKLSYMVEPLHPFTEYIFRVVW
Human      (111)  --HNM----KS--F-------------L---T--K---RP--V-K-----------

Rat        (180)  IFTAQLHLYSPPSPSYRTHPYGVPETAPFITNIESSSPDTVEVSWAPPYFPGGPILGYNL
Human      (171)  ------Q-------------H-------L-R-------------D--Q----------

Rat        (240)  RLISKTQKLDSGTQRTSFQFYSTLPNTTYRFSIAAVNEVGEGPEAESMITTPSPAVQEEE
Human      (231)  -----N----A---------------I------------------S---S-S---Q--

Rat        (300)  QWLFLSRKTSLRKRSLKYLVDEAHCLWSDAIRHNITGISVNTQQEVVYFSEGTIIWMKGA
Human      (291)  ----------------H--------RL---Y-------DVH-QI-------L--A-K-

Rat        (360)  ANMSDVSDLRIFYRGSALVSSISVDWLYQRMYFIMDNRVHVCDLKHCSNLEEITPFSIVA
Human      (351)  ---------------G-I----I-----------EL-C----EN---I-----P--S-

                         YVFYLLRDGIYRVHLPLPSVR
Rat        (420)  PQKVVVDSYNG DTKAVRIVESGTLKDFAVKPQSKRIIYFNGTMQVFMSTFLDGSAFHRV
                         YVFYLLRDGIYRADLPVPSGR
Human      (411)  ---I-A-----VCAE-------C------I---A-------D-A-----------S-LI

Rat        (479)  LPWVPLADVKSFACENNDFLITDGKAIFQQDSLSFNEFIVGCDLSHIEEFGFGNLVIFGS
Human      (491)  --RI-F-------------V----V-----A-------------------------

Rat        (539)  SVQSYPLPGHPQEVSVLFGSREALIQWKPPILAIGA          SPSAWQNWTY
Human      (551)  -S-LH----R---L------HQ--V-----A-----NVILISDIIELFELG---------

Rat        (585)  EVKVSSQDILETTQVFLNISRTVLNVPKLQSSTKYMVSVRASSPKGPGPWSEPSVGTTLV
Human      (611)  -----T--PP-V-HI-----G-M----E---AM--K--------R------------

Rat        (645)  PATEPPFIMAVKEDGLWSKPLSSFGPGEFLSSDVGNVSDMDWYNNSLYYSDTKGNVYVRP
Human      (671)  --S------------------N----------I-------------------D-F-WL

Rat        (705)  LNGMDISENYHISSIAGACALAFEWLGHFLYWAGKTYVIQRQSVLTGHTDIVTHVKLLVN
Human      (731)  ---T-------LP-----G-------------------------------------
```

```
Rat      (765)   DMAVDPVGGYLYWTTLYSVESTRLNGESSLVLQACPWLSGKKVIALTLDLSDGLLYWLVQ
Human    (891)   --V--S---------------------------T---F----------------------

Rat      (825)   DNQCIHLYTAVLRGWSGADATITEFAAWSTSEISQNALMYYSGRLFWINGFRIITAQEIG
Human    (851)   -S------------Q-TG-T--------------------------------T----

Rat      (985)   QRTSVSVSEPGKFNQFTIIQTSLKPLPGNFSSTPTVIPDSVQESSFRIEGHTSSFRILWN
Human    (911)   -K-----L--AR------------------F--K---------------NA---Q----

Rat      (945)   EPPAVDWGIVFYSVEFSAHSKFLAIEQQSLPVFTVEGLEPYALFNLSVTPYTYWGKGQKT
Human    (971)   G-------V--------------S--H-----------------------------P--

Rat      (1005)  SLSFRAPESVPSAPENPRIFILSLGRYTRKNEVVVEFRWNKPKHENGVLTKSEIFYHISK
Human    (1031)  ---L----T-------------PS-KCCN---------------------F----N--N

Rat      (1065)  QSGTNKSTEDWVSVSVTPPVMSFQLEAMSPGYIVSFQVRVFTSKGPGPFSDIVMSKTSEI
Human    (1091)  --I---TC---IA-N---S-------G--RCFIA----A--------YA-V-K-T----

Rat      (1125)  KPCPYLISLLGNKIEFLDMDQNQVVWTFSLEGAVSEVGYTADDEMGYFAQGDALFLLNLH
Human    (1151)  N-F-H--T------V-------------A-RVI-AVC----N----Y-E--S----H--

Rat      (1185)  NHSSSKLFQDVLASDIAVIAVDWIARHLYFALKASQDGTQIFDVDLEHKVKSPREVKICK
Human    (1211)  -R---E----S-VF--T--TI---S--------E--N-M-V---------Y------HN

Rat      (1245)  SHTAIISFSMYPLLSRLYWTEVSDLGYQMFYCNISSHTLHHVLQPKASNQ HGRRQCSCN
Human    (1271)  RNST-----V-------------NF------YS-I-----RI---T-T--QNK-N-----

Rat      (1304)  VTESELSGAMTVDTSDPDRPWIYFTKQQEIWAMDLEGCQCWKVIMVPA TPGKRIISLTV
Human    (1331)  ---F------AI---NLEK-L---A-A--------------R--T---MLA--TLV----

Rat      (1363)  DGEFIYWITTMKDDTEI YQAKKGSGAILSQVKAPRSKHILAYSSALQPFPDKAYLSVAS
Human    (1391)  --DL----I-A--S-Q-D------N---V-----L--R-------VM-------F--L--

Rat      (1422)  NMVEASILNATNTSLILKLPPVKTNLTWHGITTPTSTYLVYYMEAN RANSSDRKHNMLE
Human    (1451)  T --PT---------TIR--LA------Y---S--P------A-V-D-K----L-YRI--

Rat      (1581)  SQENVARIEGLQPFSTYVIQIAVKNYYSDPLEHLSLGKEIQGKTKSGVPGAVCHINATVL
Human    (1510)  F-DSI-L--D-------M---------------PP----W----N---E--QL--T--R

Rat      (1541)  SDTSLLVFWTESHKPNGPKELVRYQLVMSYLAPIPETPLRQDEFPSARLSLLVTKLSGGQ
Human    (1570)  -----IIS-R----------S-----AI-H--L---------S---NG--T----R----N

Rat      (1601)  QYVLKILACHSEEMWCTESHPVSVNMFDTPEKPSALVPENTSLLLDWKAPSNANLTRFWF
Human    (1630)  I----V---------------T-E--N-----YS--------QFN----L-V--I---V

Rat      (1661)  ELQKWKYSEFYHVKASCSQGPVYVCNIANLQPYTPYNIRVVVVYTTGENSSSIPESFKTK
Human    (1690)  -------N------T------A-----T------S--V------K-----T-L-------

Rat      (1721)  AGVPSKPGIPKLLEGSKNSIQWEKAEDNGNRLMYYTLEVRKSISNDSRDQSLRWTAVFNG
Human    (1750)  ----N----------------------------C-IT--I--I---T--NLQN-N---KMT---
Chicken  (1)                                      -QSG-TNKVKS- -VVVY----

Rat      (1781)  SCSSICTWRSKNLKGTFQFRAVASNAIGFGEYSEISEDITLVEDGFWITE*TSFILTIIVG*
Human    (1810)  ----V---K------I----V--A-NL------G---N-I--G-D---P----------
Chicken  (20)    --D-I----AE--E-T----AA---M--L----DT-KD-V-AK-TVTS-D*ITAIVAV-GA*

                                   ACH (1854)
Rat      (1841)  *IFLVAT VPL TFVWHRS*LKNHKATKEGLSVLNDNDCELAELRGLAAGVGLANACYAVHT
Human    (1870)  ----V- I-- ------R---Q-SA--VT--INE-K-------------------I--
Chicken  (80)    *VV-GL-I-I-FG*----Q-W-SR-P-ST-QI--VK------Q---M-ET---------VS-
```

```
Rat       (1899)  LPTQEEIESLPAFPREKLSLRLLLGSGAFGEVYEGTAVDILGRGSGEIKVAVKTLKKGST
Human     (1928)  --------N---------T-------------------V-----------------
Chicken    (140)  --S-A---S------D--N-HK--------------L---AD----SR-------R-A-
```

```
Rat       (1959)  DQEKIEFLKEAHLMSKFNHPNILKQLGVCLLSEPQYIILELMEGGDLLSYLRKARGTTLS
Human     (1988)  ----------------------------N----------------T------MA-FY
Chicken    (200)  ----S----V-------D--H---L-----------L-----------S---G--KQK-Q
```

```
Rat       (2019)  GPLLTLADLVELCVDISKGCVYLEQMHFIHRDLAARNCLVSVKDY TSPRVVKIGDFGLA
Human     (2048)  ------V---D-----------R-------------- ---I---------
Chicken    (260)  S-----T--L-I-L-VC-----K-R-------------E-Q-GSCS-V---------
```

```
Rat       (2078)  REIYKHDYYRKRGEGLLPVRWMAPENLMDGIFTSQSDVWSFGILVWEILTLGHQPYPAHS
Human     (2107)  -D-------------------------S-------T----------I------------
Chicken    (320)  ------------------------I--V--NL----A--V-V--T----Q----GL-
```

```
Rat       (2138)  NLDVLNYVQAGGRLEPPRNCPDDLWNLMFRCWAQEPDQRPTFYNIQDQLQLFRNVSLNNV
Human     (2167)  ---------T-----------------TQ-----------HR----------FF--SI
Chicken    (380)  -IE--HH-RS-----S-N-----IRD---R----D-HN----FY--HK--EI-HSP-CFS
```

```
Rat       (2198)  SHCGQAAPAGGVINKGFEGEDNEMATLNSDDTMPVALMETRNQEGLNYMVLATKCSQSED
Human     (2227)  YQ-RDE-NNS----ES-----GDVIC-----I---V----K-R----------E-G-G-E
Chicken    (440)  -FLG-KESVAGSSTKLLRVSLG-AVPTA-AQ-C-SVNVESQNGLGWKGP (488)
```

```
Rat       (2258)  RYEGPLGSKESGLHDLKKDERQP ADKDFCQQPQVAYGSPGHSEGLNYACLAHSGHGDVSE (2317)
Human     (2287)  KS------Q--ESCG-R-E-KE-H-------EK----CPS-KP--------T---Y--G-D (2347)
```

Italics: hydrophobic regions (11–42 and 1831–1854). Underlined: ATP binding site in the kinase domain. The sequence extending from above residue 431 of rat ROS1 is an insert present in the heart; the homologous human sequence is also shown as an insert but is numbered continuously. The sequence from above residue 1852 is a truncated form occurring in the rat lung.

Sequences of human ROS1, chicken ROS1 and the human insulin receptor

```
Human ROS1    (1790)  KSTSNNLQNQNLRWKMTFNGSCSSVCTWKSKNLKGIFQFRVVAANNLGFGEYSGISENI
Chicken ROS1     (1)  -QSG-TNKVKS- -VVVY----D-I----AE--E-T----AA---M--L----DT-KD-
```

```
Human ROS1    (1840)  ILVGDDFWIPETSFILTIIVGIFLVVT IPL TFVWHRRLKNQKSAKEGVTVLINEDKEL
Chicken ROS1     (59)  V-AK-TVTS-DITAIVAV-GAVV-GL-I-I-FG----Q-W-SR-P-ST-QI--VK-----
v-ROS            (1)  DTVTSPDITAIV*VIGAVVLGLTS************************************
```

```
Human Ins-R    (981)                        ---I--LRE--Q-S--M----N-R-
Human ROS1    (1907)  AELRGLAAGVGLANACYAIHTLPTQEEIENLPAFPREKLTLRLLLGSGAFGEVYEGTAVD
Chicken ROS    (119)  -Q---M-ET---------VS---S-A---S------D--N-HK--------------L-
v-ROS           (60)  ************************************************************
```

```
Human Ins-R   (1006)  -I K-EA-TR-----VNESASLR-R----N--SV-KG-TCHHVVRL---VSKGQ-TLVVM
Human ROS1    (1967)  ILGVGSGEIKVAVKTLKKGSTDQEKIEFLKEAHLMSKFNHPNILKQLGVCLLNEPQYIIL
Chicken ROS1   (179)  --AD----SR-------R-A-----S----V-------D--H---L-----------L--
v-ROS          (120)  *****************************E******************************
```

```
Human Ins-R   (1065)  ---AHGDLKSY-RS--PEAENNPGR-PPT-QEMIQMAAE-AD-MA--NAKK-V-------
Human ROS1    (2027)  ELME    GGDLLTYLRKARMATFYGPLLYLVDLVDLCVDISKGCVYLERMHFIHRDLAAR
Chicken ROS1   (239)  ----    -----S--G--KQK-QS---T-T--L-I-L-VC-----K-R---------
v-ROS          (180)  ****    ************************************I****I***********
```

```
Human Ins-R   (1125)  --M-AHDF    T-------MT---KN----G-K------------K--V---S-
Human ROS1    (2084)  NCLVSVKDY TSPRIVKIGDFGLARDIYKNDYYRKRGEGLLPVRWMAPESLMDGIFTTQS
Chicken ROS-1  (296)  -----E-Q-GSCS-V----------------------------------I--V--NL-
v-ROS          (237)  ****************************************************H*
```

```
Human Ins-R   (1179)   -N----VVL---TS-AE---QGL--EQ--KF-MD--Y-DQ-D---ERVTD--RM--WFN-
Human ROS1    (2143)   DVWSFGILIWEILTLGHQPYPAHSNLDVLNYVQTGGRLEPPRNCPDDLWNLMTQCWAQEP
Chicken ROS1  (356)    ---A--V-V--T----Q---GL--IE--HH-RS-----S-N-----IRD---R----D-
v-ROS         (297)    *********************************************************
```

```
Human Ins-R   (1239)   KM----LE-VNL-KDDLHPSFPEVSFFHS-E-KAPESE-LEMEFE-MENVPLDRSSHCQR
Human ROS1    (2203)   DQRPTFHRIQDQLQLFRNFFLNSIYKSRDEANNSGVINESFEGKFDSSEFSSFRCTVN (2347)
Chicken ROS1  (416)    HN----FY--HK--EI-HSP-CFS-FLG-KESVAGSSTKLLRVSLG-AVPTA-AQ-C-SV
v-ROS         (357)    ******************************PLRIQTAFFQPL (402)
```

```
Human Ins-R   (1299)   EEAGGRDGGSSLGFKRSYEEHIPYTTHMNGGKKNGRILTLPRSNPS (1343)
```

```
Chicken ROS1  (476)    NVESQNGLGWKGP (488)
```

Dashes indicate identity with human ROS1. * Indicates identity with chicken ROS. Common Tyr residues are in underlined bold type (corresponding to Ins-R residues 1110, 1146, 1150, 1151 and 1198).

Databank file names and accession numbers

	GENE	EMBL	SWISSPROT	REFERENCES
Human	ROS1	Humros1 M34353		Birchmeier et al., 1990
Chicken	Ros	Ggroscr X06770	KROS_CHICK P08941	Podell and Sefton, 1987
				Chen et al., 1991
Rat	Ros	Rncros1a M35104		Matsushime and Shibuya, 1990
		Rncros1b M35105		
Chicken	v-ros	ReacsUR2 M10455	KROS_AVISU P00529	Neckameyer and Wang, 1985
(ASVUR2)				

Papers

Balduzzi, P.C., Notter, M.F.D., Morgan, H.R. and Shibuya, M. (1981). Some biological properties of two new avian sarcoma viruses. J. Virol., 40, 268–275.

Birchmeier, C., Birnbaum, D., Waitches, G., Fasano, O. and Wigler, M. (1986). Characterization of an activated human c-ros gene. Mol. Cell. Biol., 6, 3109–3116.

Birchmeier, C., O'Neill, K., Riggs, M. and Wigler, M. (1990). Characterization of ROS1 cDNA from a human glioblastoma cell line. Proc. Natl Acad. Sci. USA, 87, 4799–4803.

Chen, J., Helier, D., Poon, B., Kang, L. and Wang, L.H. (1991). The proto-oncogene c-ros codes for a transmembrane tyrosine protein kinase sharing sequence and structural homology with sevenless protein of Drosophila melanogaster. Oncogene, 6, 257–264.

Hafen, E., Basler, K., Edstroem, J.-E. and Rubin, G.M. (1987). sevenless, a cell-specific homeotic transmembrane receptor with a tyrosine kinase domain. Science, 236, 55–63.

Macara, I.G., Marinetti, G.V. and Balduzzi, P.C. (1984). Transforming protein of avian sarcoma virus UR2 is associated with phosphatidylinositol kinase activity: possible role in tumorigenesis. Proc. Natl Acad. Sci. USA, 81, 2728–2732.

Matsushime, H. and Shibuya, M. (1990). Tissue-specific expression of rat c-ros-1 gene and partial structural similarity of its predicted products with sev protein of Drosophila melanogaster. J. Virol., 64, 2117–2125.

Matsushime, H., Wang, L.-H. and Shibuya, M. (1986). Human c-*ros*-1 gene homologous to the v-*ros* sequence of UR2 sarcoma virus encodes for a transmembrane receptor-like molecule. Mol. Cell. Biol., 6, 3000–3004.

Maytin, E.V., Balduzzi, P.C., Notter, M.F.D. and Young, D.A. (1984). Changes in the synthesis and phosphorylation of cellular proteins in chick fibroblasts transformed by two avian sarcoma viruses. J. Biol. Chem., 259, 12135–12143.

Neckameyer, W.S. and Wang, L.-H. (1985). Nucleotide sequence of avian sarcoma virus UR2 and comparison of its transforming gene with other members of the tyrosine protein kinase oncogene family. J. Virol., 53, 879–884.

Neckameyer, W.S., Shibuya, M., Hsu, M.-T. and Wang, L.-H. (1986). Proto-oncogene c-*ros* codes for a molecule with structural features common to those of growth factors receptors and displays tissue-specific and developmentally regulated expression. Mol. Cell. Biol., 6, 1478–1486.

Podell, S.B. and Sefton, B.M. (1987). Chicken proto-oncogene c-*ros* cDNA clones: identification of a c-*ros* RNA transcript and deduction of the amino acid sequence of the carboxyl terminus of the c-*ros* product. Oncogene, 2, 9–14.

Satoh, H., Yoshida, M.C., Matsushime, H., Shibuya, M. and Sasaki, M. (1987). Regional localization of the human c-*ros*-1 on 6q22 and *flt* on 13q12. Jpn J. Cancer Res., 78, 772–775.

Sharma, S., Birchmeier, C., Nikawa, J., O'Neill, K., Rodgers, L. and Wigler, M. (1989). Characterization of the *ros*1-gene products expressed in human glioblastoma cell lines. Oncogene Res., 5, 91–100.

Sonnenberg, E., Godecke, A., Walter, B., Bladt, F. and Birchmeier, C. (1991). Transient and locally restricted expression of the *ros 1* protooncogene during mouse development. EMBO J., 10, 3693–3702.

Wang, L.-H., Hanafusa, H., Notter, M.F.D. and Balduzzi, P.C. (1982). Genetic structure and transforming sequence of avian sarcoma virus UR2. J. Virol., 41, 833–841.

Wu, J.K. and Chikaraishi, D.M. (1990). Differential expression of *ros* oncogene in primary human astrocytomas and astrocytoma cell lines. Cancer Res., 50, 3032–3035.

SEA

v-*sea* is the oncogene of the acutely transforming virus AEV-S13 (Stubbs and Furth, 1935).

Related genes

Sea is a member of the tyrosine protein kinase family: it has strong homology with the insulin receptor family.

Cross-species homology

SEA: 72% homology with human MET within the tyrosine kinase domain.

Transformation

MAN

Expressed at low frequency (~1%) in breast carcinomas together with *BCL1*, *HSTF1* and *INT2* (Theillet *et al.*, 1990).

ANIMALS

Injection of AEV-S13 into young chickens causes sarcomas, erythroblastosis and anaemias (Stubbs and Furth, 1935). Fibroblasts transformed by v-*sea* are only weakly oncogenic when injected into chicks: cells expressing a retrovirus carrying both v-*sea* and v-*ski* are highly malignant (Larsen *et al.*, 1992).

IN VITRO

v-*sea* transforms fibroblasts and erythroblasts (Crowe and Hayman, 1991) but does not transform avian myeloid cells (Beug and Graf, 1989). It induces the synthesis of chicken myeloid growth factor (cMGF) and causes autocrine growth in myeloid cells transformed by v-*myb* or v-*myc* (Adkins *et al.*, 1984). The expression of v-*erbA* in v-*sea*-transformed erythroid cells represses the erythroid-specific genes carbonic anhydrase II (CAII), band III (the erythrocyte anion transporter) and δ-aminolevulinic acid synthase (Zenke *et al.*, 1990; Pain *et al.*, 1990). In contrast, the co-expression of v-*ski* and v-*sea* enhances the expression of CAII and β-globin, has little effect on band III and suppresses expression of histone H5, the latter being highly expressed in v-*erbA*/v-*sea*-transformed cells (Larsen *et al.*, 1992).

	SEA/Sea	v-*sea*
Nucleotides (kb)		8.5 (S13)
Chromosome		
Human	11q13	
Mouse .	19	

439

	SEA/Sea	v-*sea*
Exons		
mRNA (kb)		
Chicken	3.0/7.0	4.0
	4.2/5.0	
	(weakly expressed in fibroblasts)	
Amino acids		370 (v-SEA)
Mass (kDa)		
(predicted)		42 (v-SEA)
(expressed)		gp155$^{env\text{-}sea}$
		gp85^{env}/gp70$^{env\text{-}sea}$

Cellular location

Transmembrane.

Protein function

SEA is a growth factor receptor tyrosine protein kinase.

Gene structure of AEV-S13 and the *env* and v-*sea* products

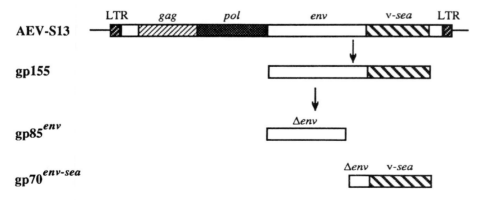

The *env* sequence is 96% homologous with that of the RAV2 strain of ALV. The ~1085 bp insert between *env* and the viral 3' non-coding region encodes the *sea* ORF. A single base deletion 14 bp upstream of the normal *env* termination codon permits read-through into the *sea* gene. The termination codon (TAG, nucleotides 1789–1791) lies within the 3' viral non-coding region; the 3' junction is at nucleotide 1776.

The S13 virus encodes normal *gag* and *gag–pol* proteins and an abnormal *env* glycoprotein (gp155) that is cleaved to gp85^{env} and gp70$^{env-sea}$. gp155$^{env-sea}$ retains the entire extracellular and transmembrane domains of *env*. Replacement of the entire *env* sequence by the myristylation target signal of pp60^{v-src} does not affect the capacity of *v-sea* to transform fibroblasts (Crowe and Hayman, 1991). The uncleaved but fully glycosylated gp155$^{env-sea}$ retains the capacity to transform chicken embryo fibroblasts (Crowe and Hayman, 1993).

Sequence of v-SEA

```
  (1)   ADSPGLARPHAHFASAGADAAGGGSPVLLLRTTSCCLEDLRPELLEEVKDILIPEERLI
 (60)   THRSRVIGRGHFGSVYHGTYMDPLLGNLHCAVKSLHRITDLEEVEEFLREGILMKGFHHP
(120)   QVLSLLGVCLPRHGLPLVVLPYMRHGDLRHFVRAQERSPTVKELIGFGLQVALGMEYLAQ
(180)   KKFVHRDLAARNCMLDETLTVKVADFGLARDVFGKEYYSIRQHRHAKLPVRWMALESLQT
(240)   QKFTTKSDVWSFGVLMWELLTRGASPYPEVDPYDMARYLLRGRRLPQPQPCPDTLYGVML
(300)   SCWAPTPEERPSFSGLVCELERVLASLEGEHYINMAVTYVNLESGPPFPPAPRGQLPDSE
(360)   DEEDEEEEVAE (370)
```

Databank file names and accession numbers

	GENE	EMBL	SWISSPROT	REFERENCES
AEV-S13	*env–sea*	Reac2tks M25158	KSEA_AVIET P23049	Smith *et al.*, 1989

Papers

Adkins, B., Leutz, A. and Graf, T. (1984). Autocrine growth induced by *src*-related oncogenes in transformed chicken myeloid cells. Cell, 39, 439–445.

Beug, H. and Graf, T. (1989). Co-operation between viral oncogenes in avian erythroid and myeloid leukemia. Eur. J. Clin. Invest., 19, 491–502.

Crowe, A.J. and Hayman, M.J. (1991). A myristylated form of the *sea* oncoprotein can transform chicken embryo fibroblasts. J. Virol., 65, 2533–2538.

Crowe, A.J. and Hayman, M.J. (1993). Post-translational modifications of the *env-sea* oncogene product: the role of proteolytic processing in transformation. Oncogene, 8, 181–189.

Larsen, J., Beug, H. and Hayman, M.J. (1992). The v-*ski* oncogene cooperates with the v-*sea* oncogene in erythroid transformation by blocking erythroid differentiation. Oncogene, 7, 1903–1911.

Pain, B., Melet, F., Jurdic, P. and Samurut, J. (1990). The carbonic anhydrase II gene, a gene regulated by thyroid hormone and erythropoietin, is repressed by the v-*erb*A oncogene in erythrocytic cells. New Biologist, 2, 284–294.

Smith, D.R., Vogt, P.K. and Hayman, M.J. (1989). The v-*sea* oncogene of avian erythroblastosis retrovirus S13: another member of the protein-tyrosine kinase gene family. Proc. Natl Acad. Sci. USA, 86, 5291–5295.

Stubbs, E.L. and Furth, J. (1935). The relation of leukosis to sarcoma of chickens. I. Sarcoma and erythroleukosis (Strain 13). J. Exp. Med., 61, 593–616.

Theillet, C., Adnane, J., Szepetowski, P., Simon, M.-P., Jeanteur, P., Birnbaum, D. and Gaudray, P. (1990). *BCL-1* participates in the 11q13 amplification found in breast cancer. Oncogene, 5, 147–149.

Zenke, M., Munoz, A., Sap, J., Vennstrom, B. and Beug, H. (1990). v-*erb*A oncogene activation entails the loss of hormone-dependent regulator activity of c-*erb*A. Cell, 61, 1035–1049.

SKI

v-*ski* is the common oncogene of Sloan–Kettering viruses (SKVs), a group of acutely transforming chicken retroviruses. First detected in chick embryo fibroblasts infected with an originally non-transforming ALV strain (Stavnezer *et al.*, 1981), from which three isolates (SKV770, SKV780, SKV790) were prepared.

Related genes

SNOA and *SNON* are produced by alternative splicing of the same gene (giving different C-termini) and are closely related to *SKI* (Nomura *et al.*, 1989). *SKI* and *SNO* show no marked sequence homology to other oncogenes. The homology between *SKI* and *SNO* lies in exon 1. SKI proteins contain an extensive C-terminal helical domain that has homology with the helical domains present in myosin, intermediate filaments and lamins (Sleeman and Laskey, 1993).

Cross-species homology

Thirteen cysteine residues are absolutely conserved among all known SKI/SNO proteins.

SKI: 73.4% identity (human and *Xenopus*); 90.6% conserved amino acids (Sleeman and Laskey, 1993).

Chicken SNON is six amino acids longer (690 residues) than human SNON; sequence identity: 75%.

Transformation

MAN

The chromosomal region 1q22–24, to which *SKI* maps, is a common site of breakage in carcinomas and haematopoietic tumours (Michael *et al.*, 1984; Atkin, 1986; Koduru *et al.*, 1987).

ANIMALS

In chickens injection of SKV CEFs causes non-metastasizing squamous cell carcinomas in 50% of animals (Stavnezer, 1988; Sutrave and Hughes, 1991). v-*ski* enhances the leukaemogenic potential of v-*sea* (Larsen *et al.*, 1992).

IN VITRO

v-*ski* or overexpressed *Ski* transforms chick embryo fibroblasts (CEFs) to flat, epithelioid cells with prominent nuclei and nucleoli, distinct from CEFs transformed by other avian retroviruses. These transformed cells grow more slowly than other retroviral transformants (Li *et al.*, 1986; Barkas *et al.*, 1986; Colmenares *et al.*, 1991b). v-*ski* or *Ski* also induce myogenic differentiation of quail embryo cells (Colmenares and Stavnezer, 1989; Colmenares *et al.*, 1991a). The differentiation of v-*sea*-transformed erythroid cells into erythrocytes is blocked by the expression of v-*ski* (Larsen *et al.*, 1992). This effect of v-*ski* is similar to that of v-*erbA* but is associated with different effects on gene expression (see **SEA**).

Chicken *SnoN* expression at high levels causes transformation of chick embryo fibroblasts and muscle differentiation of quail embryo cells (Boyer *et al.*, 1993).

TRANSGENIC ANIMALS

Transgenic mice expressing a region of chicken *Ski* have distinctive muscle growth caused by selective hypertrophy of fast skeletal muscle fibres (Sutrave *et al.*, 1990b, 1992).

	SKI/Ski	v-*ski*
Nucleotides	>70 kb (chicken)	3.0–8.9 kb (SKV-derived genomes)
		1305 bp (v-*ski*)
Chromosome		
Human	1q22–q24	
Mouse	4	
Exons	At least 8	
	(chicken cDNAs containing 7 exons or lacking exons 2 or 6 have been isolated (Sutrave and Hughes, 1989).	
	Equivalent human cDNA lacks exon 2 (Nomura *et al.*, 1989)	
mRNA (kb)	5.6, 8.0 (homologous to v-*ski*)	
	Alternative splicing generates multiple mRNAs in chicken (Li *et al.*, 1986; Sutrave and Hughes, 1989)	
Amino acids		
Human	728 (SKI)	437
Chicken	448/510/750	
	415 (SNOA); 684 (SNON)	
Mass (kDa)		
(predicted)	p80^{ski}	p49$^{v\text{-}ski}$
	p46^{SNOA}; p77^{SNON}	
(expressed)	p90 (7 exons)	P125$^{\Delta gag\text{-}ski}$; P110$^{\Delta gag\text{-}ski\text{-}pol}$; P45$^{\Delta gag\text{-}ski}$
	(3 chicken SKI proteins: p50 (lacking exon 7), p60 (lacking exon 6), p90 (Sutrave *et al.*, 1990a))	(P110 contains p19$^{\Delta gag}$, *ski*, p27^{gag} and *pol*)
Protein half-life (min)		
Chicken	45 (p60)/130 (p90)	

Cellular location

Nuclear (Barkas *et al.*, 1986).

Tissue location

Detectable at low levels in all chicken and quail tissues (Stavnezer, 1988). Maximal in sternal and vertebral cartilage (20 copies per cell): minimal in liver and kidney (2 copies per cell).

Xenopus Ski RNA accumulates in developing oocytes: following fertilization, the level declines during the mid-blastula transition. In *Xenopus* adult tissues *Ski* expression is high in the lungs and ovaries (Sleeman and Laskey, 1993).

Protein function

Unknown. v-*ski* induces MyoD and myogenin expression and myogenesis in non-muscle cells (Colmenares *et al.*, 1991a). These genes are also induced by a transformation-defective v-*ski* mutant that does not induce myotube formation. However, in *Ski* transgenic mice the levels of MyoD and myogenin are not affected (Sutrave *et al.*, 1992). The effect of wild-type v-*ski* is the opposite to that of v-*jun* which inhibits myogenic differentiation.

The combination of v-*ski* and v-*sea* is highly malignant, indicating that v-*ski* can cooperate with a tyrosine kinase oncogene, as occurs with v-*erbA* and v-*erbB* (Larsen *et al.*, 1992).

The C-terminal helical domain, deleted in v-SKI, may permit the formation of homodimers or interaction with other proteins. Phosphorylation in the C-terminal region of the normal *Ski* gene product may release the protein to function via its N-terminus as a regulator of transcription (Sleeman and Laskey, 1993).

SKV770-derived proviral genomes and their translation products

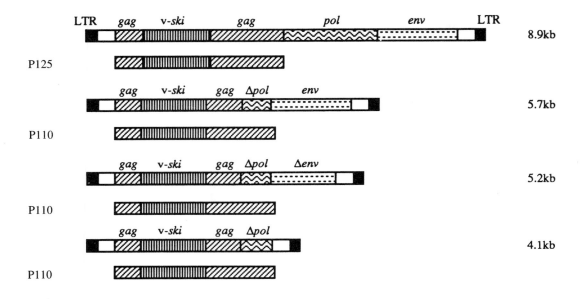

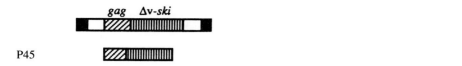

gag Δv-*ski*

P45

3.0kb

(Adapted from Stavnezer, E. (1988). In Curran, T., Reddy, E.P. and Skalka, A. (eds) The Oncogene Handbook. Elsevier, Amsterdam.)

The maps represent the sites of insertion of *ski* into the 7.6 kb tdB77 genome (Stavnezer *et al.*, 1986). The 8.9, 5.7, 5.2, 4.1 and 3.0 kb genomes are represented above; 4.2, 4.6 and 7.2 kb genomes have also been isolated. Each SKV genome has identical 5' regions but different 3' deletions. The prototype SKV genome (SKV775.7, 5.7 kb) has a deletion of 3.2 kb (3' half of *gag* and 5' 80% of *pol*); the p19^{Δgag} generated is in phase with v-*ski*. The smallest genome, SKV773.0, has a deletion of at least 150 bp from the 3' end of *ski*. The 8.9 kb genome is comprised of the entire tdB77 genome and the 1.3 kb *ski* gene.

Partial structure of the chicken *Ski* gene

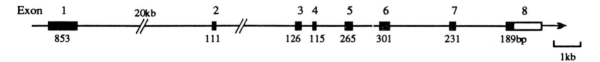

Exon 1   20kb   2   3 4   5   6   7   8

853   111   126 115   265   301   231   189bp   1kb

Black boxes: coding exons. Exons 1 and 2 are separated by at least 20 kb. The region between exons 2 and 3 has not been fully mapped. The open box indicates the untranslated region of exon 8 and the arrow indicates the the 3' end has not been defined (Grimes *et al.*, 1992).

Sequences of human SKI and v-SKI

```
Human SKI  (1)    MEAAAGGRGCFQPHPGLQKTLEQFHLSSMSSLGGPAAFSARWAQEAYKKESAKEAGAAA
v-SKI      (1)    -------------------------M---DNG-DPAEPV

Human SKI  (60)   VPAPVPAATEPPPVLHLPAIQPPPPVLPGPFFMPSDRSTERCETVLEGETISCFVVGGEK
v-SKI      (37)   LHL- -            ----- -M-----------------I--------------

Human SKI  (120)  RLCLPQILNSVLRDFSLQQINAVCDELHIYCSRCTADQLEILKVMGILPFSAPSCGLITK
v-SKI      (82)   --------------------S-----------------------------------

Human SKI  (180)  TDAERLCNALLYGGAYPPPCKKELAASLALGLELSERSVRVYHECFGKCKGLLVPELYSS
v-SKI      (142)  --------------T--------F  -STIE---T-K-FK----------------N

Human SKI  (240)  PSAACIQCLDCRLMYPPHKFVVHSHKALENRTCHWGFDSANWRAYILLSQDYTGKEEQAR
v-SKI      (200)  -------------------------S------------------S-----------K--

Human SKI  (300)  LGRCLDDVKEKFDYGNKYKRRVPRVSSEPPASIRPKTDDTSSQSPAPSEKDKPSSWLRTL
v-SKI      (260)  --QL--EM------N-----KA--NRES-RVQL-RNKMFKTMLWDPAGGSAVLQRQPDGN

Human SKI  (360)  AGSSNKSLGCVHPRQRLSAFRPWSPAVSASEKELSPHLPALIRDSFYSYKSFETAVAPNV
v-SKI      (320)  EVPSDPPASKKTKIDD SASQ  ---  ST---  KQSSRLRSL-SS-N--IGCVHPRQR
```

```
Human SKI (420) ALAPPAQQKVVSSPPCAAAVSRAPEPLATCTQPRKRKLTVDTPGAPETLAPVAAPEEDKD
v-SKI     (373) LS-FRPWSPA--ANEKELSTHLPALIRDSSFYSY-SFENAVA-NVALAPPAQQKVVSNPP
                                                                      ⟶1
Human SKI (480) SEAEVEVESREEFTSSLSSLSSPSFTSSSSAKDLGSPGARALPSAVPDAAAPADAPSGLE
v-SKI     (433) CATVV (437)
                           ⟵⟶2                        ⟵⟶3
Human SKI (540) AELEHLRQALEGGLDTKEAKEKFLHEVVKMRVKQEEKLSAALQAKRSLHQELEFLRVAKK
                     ⟵⟶4                    ⟵⟶           ⟵⟶
Human SKI (600) EKLREATEAKRNLRKEIERLRAENEKKMKEANESRLRLKRELEQARQARVCDKGCEAGRL
                           ⟵
Human SKI (660) RAKYSAQIEDLQVKLQHAEADREQLRADLLREREAREHLEKVVKELQEQLWPRARPEAAG

Human SKI (720) SEGAAELEP (728)
```

Dashes indicate identity with SKI. The numbered arrows indicate the four major contiguous 25-mer repeated elements defined by the regular position of five hydrophobic, one acidic and two basic residues. Two other partially homologous regions are also indicated by arrows (Sleeman and Laskey, 1993).

Databank file names and accession numbers

	GENE	EMBL	SWISSPROT	REFERENCES
Human	*SKI*	Hsskir X15218	SKI_HUMAN P12755	Nomura *et al.*, 1989
Human	*SNOA*	Hssnoar X15217	SNOA_HUMAN P12756	
Human	*SNON*	Hssnonr X15219	SNOB_HUMAN P12757	Nomura *et al.*, 1989
Chicken	*Ski* (exon 1)	Ggcski1 M28491		Stavnezer *et al.*, 1989
Chicken	Ski	Gdcski3 X62159		Grimes *et al.*, 1992
Chicken	Ski	Ggcski M28517		Sutrave and Hughes, 1989
	(cDNA)			
Xenopus	Ski	Xlskica X68683		Sleeman and Laskey, 1993
AEV	v-*ski*	Ggvski M28490	SKI_AVIES P17863	Stavnezer *et al.*, 1989
(strain Sloan–Kettering)				

Reviews

Stavnezer, E. (1988). The *ski* oncogene. In Curran, T., Reddy, E.P. and Skalka, A. (eds) The Oncogene Handbook: 393–401. Elsevier, London.
Sutrave, P. and Hughes, S.H. (1991). The *ski* oncogene. Oncogene, 6, 353–356.

Papers

Atkin, N.B. (1986). Chromosome 1 aberrations in cancer. Cancer Genet. Cytogenet., 21, 279–285.
Barkas, A.E., Brodeur, D. and Stavnezer, E. (1986). Polyproteins containing a domain encoded by the v-*ski* oncogene are located in the nuclei of SKV-transformed cells. Virology, 151, 131–138.

Boyer, P.L., Colmenares, C., Stavnezer, E. and Hughes, S. (1993). Sequence and biological activity of chicken *sno*N cDNA clones. Oncogene, 8, 457–466.

Colmenares, C. and Stavnezer, E. (1989). The *ski* oncogene induces muscle differentiation in quail embryo cells. Cell, 59, 293–303.

Colmenares, C., Teumer, J.K. and Stavnezer, E. (1991). Transformation-defective v-*ski* induces myoD and myogenin expression but not myotube formation. Mol. Cell. Biol., 11, 1167–1170.

Colmenares, C., Sutrave, P., Hughes, S.H. and Stavnezer, E. (1991). Activation of c-*ski* oncogene by over-expression. J. Virol., 65, 4929–4935.

Grimes, H.L., Szente, B.E. and Goodenow, M.M. (1992). c-*ski* cDNAs are encoded by eight exons, six of which are closely linked within the chicken genome. Nucleic Acids Res., 20, 1511–1516.

Koduru, P.R.K., Filippa, D.A., Richardson, M.E., Jhanwar, S.C., Chaganti, S.R., Koziner, B., Clarkson, B.D., Lieberman, P.H. and Chaganti, R.S.K. (1987). Cytogenetic and histologic correlations in malignant lymphoma. Blood, 69, 97–102.

Larsen, J., Beug, H. and Hayman, M.J. (1992). The v-*ski* oncogene cooperates with the v-*sea* oncogene in erythroid transformation by blocking erythroid differentiation. Oncogene, 7, 1903–1911.

Li, Y., Turck, C.M., Teumer, J.K. and Stavnezer, E. (1986). Unique sequence, *ski*, in Sloan-Kettering avian retroviruses with prioperties of a new cell-derived oncogene. J. Virol., 57, 1065–1072.

Michael, P.M., Levin, M.D. and Garson, O.M. (1984). Translocation 1;19 - a new cytogenetic abnormality in acute lymphocytic leukemia. Cancer Genet. Cytogenet., 12, 333–341.

Nomura, N., Sasamoto, S., Ishii, S., Matsui, M. and Ishizaki, R. (1989). Isolation of human cDNA clones of *ski* and the *ski*-related gene, *sno*. Nucleic Acids Res., 17, 5489–5500.

Sleeman, J.P. and Laskey, R.A. (1993). *Xenopus* c-*ski* contains a novel coiled-coil protein domain, and is maternally expressed during development. Oncogene, 8, 67–77.

Stavnezer, E., Gerhard, D.S., Binari, R.C. and Balazs, I. (1981). Generation of transforming viruses in cultures of chicken fibroblasts infected with an avian leukosis virus. J. Virol., 39, 920–934.

Stavnezer, E. Barkas, A.E., Brennan, L.A., Brodeur, D. and Li, Y. (1986). Transforming Sloan-Kettering viruses generated from the cloned v-*ski* oncogene by *in vitro* and *in vivo* recombinations. J. Virol., 57, 1073–1083.

Stavnezer, E., Brodeur, D. and Brennan, L.A. (1989). The v-*ski* oncogene encodes a truncated set of c-*ski* coding exons with limited sequence and structural relatedness to v-*myc*. Mol. Cell. Biol., 9, 4038–4045.

Sutrave, P. and Hughes, S.H. (1989). Isolation and characterization of three distinct cDNAs for the chicken c-*ski* gene. Mol. Cell. Biol., 9, 4046–4051.

Sutrave, P., Copeland, T.D., Showalter, S.D. and Hughes, S.H. (1990a). Characterization of chicken c-*ski* oncogene products expressed by retrovirus vectors. Mol. Cell. Biol., 10, 3137–3144.

Sutrave, P., Hughes, S.H., Kelly, A.M. and Hughes, S.H. (1990b). *ski* can cause selective growth of skeletal muscle in transgenic mice. Genes Devel., 4, 1462–1473.

Sutrave, P., Leferovich, J., Kelly, A.M. and Hughes, S.H. (1992). c-*ski* expression can increase the skeletal musculature of transgenic mice. In Kelly, A.M. and Blau, H.M. (eds) Neuromuscular Development and Disease, Molecular and Cellular Biology: vol. 2, 107–114. Raven Press, New York.

v-*src* is the the transforming gene of Rous *sarc*oma virus (RSV) that infects chickens (Jove and Hanafusa, 1987). *Src* (originally *sarc*), is the prototype of the SRC family of membrane-associated protein tyrosine kinases.

Related genes

Protein tyrosine kinases may have been required for the evolution of multicellular organisms and *Src*-like genes have been found in all vertebrates that have been examined, including man (Anderson *et al.*, 1985; Parker *et al.*, 1985; Tanaka *et al.*, 1987) and *Xenopus laevis* (*Src, Src-2*; Steele, 1985; Steele *et al.*, 1989; Ghosn *et al.*, 1992) and in *Drosophila melanogaster* (D-*src28c*, D-*src64* and D*ash* (homologous to *Abl*); Hoffmann *et al.*, 1983; Simon *et al.*, 1985; Wadsworth *et al.*, 1985; Gregory *et al.*, 1987) and in simple metazoan organisms including *Hydra attenuata* (Bosch *et al.*, 1989) and *Spongilla lacustris* (*srk1–4*; Ottilie *et al.*, 1992).

In vertebrates eight genes of the *Src* family have been identified (*Src, Blk, Fgr* (*Src-2*), *Fyn, Hck, Lck/Tkl, Lyn, Yes*) of which *Src, Fgr* and *Yes* have viral homologues (Bolen *et al.*, 1991). There is a high degree of similarity within the family: all the proteins contain glycine 2 that becomes myristylated and contributes to membrane anchoring of the proteins; all share sequences throughout the SRC homology domains 1 (the tyrosine kinase catalytic region), 2 and 3 (SH1, SH2, SH3) and all have the capacity to be regulated by phosphorylation of a common C-terminal tyrosine residue. The major differences reside in the N-terminal 80 amino acids distal to Gly2.

All known tyrosine kinases possess conserved domains of 260 amino acids. A superfamily of kinases arises from the presence of eleven major sub-domains conserved between all known kinase catalytic units (Hanks *et al.*, 1988): thus, cAMP- and cGMP-dependent protein kinases have two regions of homology with p60^{src} (250 out of 520 residues: see Fig. 2.1, page 73).

Proteins having homology with the kinase and regulatory domains of p60^{src}

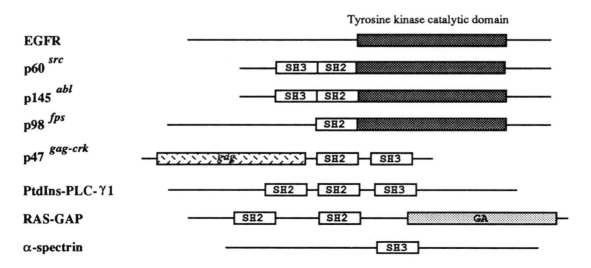

SH = sequence homology domain; GA = GTPase activating region of RAS–GAP.

The SH3 domain (~50 amino acids) and SH2 domain (~110 amino acids immediately N-terminal to the kinase domain), located N-terminally with respect to the tyrosine kinase region of members of the SRC family, are strongly homologous to regions in the ABL/ARG family of non-receptor tyrosine kinases (Pawson and Gish, 1992). The FPS/FES family contains a similarly located SH2 domain. An SH2 domain occurs in the growth factor receptor coupling protein SHC (Pelicci *et al.*, 1992) and in v-AKT and two SH2 regions are present in the PTP1 and PTP2 tyrosine phosphatases (Plutzky *et al.*, 1992; Freeman *et al.*, 1992) and in RAS–GAP (Vogel *et al.*, 1988; Trahey *et al.*, 1988; McCormick, 1989) and SYK (Ohta *et al.*, 1992). SH2 and SH3 domains occur in the tyrosine kinases TEC, ATK and ITK (Mano *et al.*, 1990, 1993; Vetrie *et al.*, 1993; Siliciano *et al.*, 1992), in the CT10 avian sarcoma virus-encoded hybrid protein p47$^{gag-crk}$ (Stahl *et al.*, 1988), in the human melanoma NCK protein (Lehmann *et al.*, 1990) and in ISGF3α, the transcription factor that regulates interferon-responsive genes (Fu, 1992; Schindler *et al.*, 1992). Phospholipase C-γ1 contains a duplicated SH2 region and an SH3 region transposed with respect to SRC (Stahl *et al.*, 1988) and phosphatidylinositol 3-kinase (p85α and p85β) also contains one SH3 and two SH2 domains (Escobedo *et al.*, 1991; Booker *et al.*, 1992). ASH (abundant SRC homology) protein (Matuoka *et al.*, 1992), *C. elegans Sem-5* (Clark *et al.*, 1992) and growth factor receptor-bound protein 2 (GRB2; Lowenstein *et al.*, 1992) contain one SH2 and two SH3 domains and other GRBs containing SH2 domains have been identified (Margolis *et al.*, 1992). Regions of strong homology to SH3 occur in the yeast actin binding protein ABP1p, myosin-I (Drubin *et al.*, 1990), tensin (Davis *et al.*, 1991) and α-spectrin (Lehto *et al.*, 1988; Musacchio *et al.*, 1992). TYK2 (see **Glossary**, Tyrosine kinases) contains an SH2-like domain preceding two tandem kinase domains.

Cross-species homology

Src is highly conserved: exons 3–12 are 98% conserved and exon 2 is 71% conserved between human and chicken genes. The three *Drosophila* SRC proteins are between 51% and 54% identical to human SRC in their kinase domains (Simon *et al.*, 1983; Gregory *et al.*, 1987).

Transformation

MAN

SRC protein kinase activity is enhanced in human colon cancers (Cartwright *et al.*, 1990; Garcia *et al.*, 1991) and skin tumours (Barnekow *et al.*, 1987). SRC expression and kinase activity are increased in some human neuroblastoma-derived cells lines, some of which also express pp60^{src+} (see **Tissue location,** below; Yang and Walter, 1988; Veillette *et al.*, 1989).

ANIMALS

The original RSV strain is tumorigenic in only a few strains of chicken: later variants are tumorigenic in a range of avian species. Injection of RSV causes fibrocytic and histiocytic sarcomas, particularly in young, immunologically immature birds. In young chickens cloned v-*src* DNA is also tumorigenic (Fung *et al.*, 1983).

IN VITRO

Infection with RSV transforms many types of cell including myoblasts, chondroblasts, retinal melanoblasts, iris epithelial cells and neuroblasts (Fiszman and Fuchs, 1975; Pacifici *et al.*, 1977; Boettiger *et al.*, 1977; Ephrussi and Temin, 1960; Keane *et al.*, 1984). Antisense oligodeoxynucleotide directed against the LTRs of RSV blocks viral production in infected chick embryo fibroblasts (Zamencik and Stephenson, 1978).

Expression of pp60$^{v\text{-}src}$ is sufficient to initiate and maintain cellular transformation of chicken or mammalian fibroblasts. p60^{src} is non-transforming, even when expressed at high levels (Iba *et al.*, 1984; Parker *et al.*, 1984; Shalloway *et al.*, 1984). Co-transfection of NIH 3T3 cells with *Src* and either E1A, v-*myc*, *Myc* or the 5' half of polyoma large T antigen does cause transformation. v-*src* has also been shown to cause differentiation in PC12 rat pheochromocytoma cells, indicating the probable multifunctional nature of the protein.

TRANSGENIC ANIMALS

Mice homozygous for a null mutation in *Src* have impaired osteoclast function, are deficient in bone remodelling and develop osteopetrosis (Soriano *et al.*, 1991; Lowe *et al.*, 1993).

	SRC/Src	v-*src*
Nucleotides (kb)	19.5 (human); 7 (chicken)	7–9
Chromosome		
Human	20q13.3	
Mouse	2	
Exons	12 (1 non-coding)	
mRNA (kb)		
Human	5.0	
Chicken	3.0/4.0	
Amino acids		
Human	536	526 (Prague, Schmidt–
Chicken	533	Ruppin)
Mouse	541 (SRC⁺)	
Xenopus	532	
Mass (kDa)		
(expressed)	pp60^{src}	pp60$^{v\text{-}src}$
Protein half-life (h)	20–24	2–7

Cellular location

Plasma membrane associated. (Krueger *et al.*, 1983; Resh and Erikson, 1985; Nigg *et al.*, 1986; Ferrell *et al.*, 1990). Nuclear in differentiating keratinocytes (Zhao *et al.*, 1992). Targeting of v-SRC to adhesion plaques is sufficient to transform chicken embryo fibroblasts (Liebl and Martin, 1992).

Tissue location

pp60^{src} is expressed in most avian and mammalian cells although it is barely detectable in lymphocytes. The highest concentrations of protein and tyrosine kinase activity occur in neuronal tissues (Brugge *et al.*, 1987) and in platelets where pp60^{src} comprises 0.2–0.4% of total protein (Golden *et al.*, 1986) and in which pp60^{src} kinase activity and the total phosphotyrosine content is rapidly increased following thrombin stimulation (Golden and Brugge, 1989; Wong *et al.*, 1992). *Src* is expressed in myeloid leukaemia cells at all stages of differentiation (Willman *et al.*, 1987). The tyrosine kinase activity of pp60^{src} but not its expression is increased in differentiating HL-60 cells (Barnekow and Gessler, 1986) and keratinocytes (Zhao *et al.*, 1992).

An alternative splicing mechanism occurs in normal avian and rodent neurons and in some human neuroblastomas that yields a variant (p60^{src+}) with six additional amino acids (Arg–Lys–Val–Asp–Val–Arg). This arises from the presence of an 18 nucleotide exon (the NI exon) between *Src* exons 3 and 4 (Martinez *et al.*, 1987; Levy *et al.*, 1987; Wiestler and Walter, 1988). A second neuronal exon (NII) between exons 3 and 4 has been isolated from human adult and fetal brain (Pyper and Bolen, 1990). Exon NII contains 33 nucleotides encoding 11 amino acids (Gln–Thr–Trp–Phe–Thr–Phe–Arg–Trp–Leu–Gln–Arg). The NII exon is utilized primarily in conjunction with the NI exon to encode products with 17 additional amino acids. Splicing between the NI and NII exons alters the sixth amino acid encoded by the NI exon from an arginine to a serine residue, producing a new potential phosphorylation site. The expression of *Src* RNA containing both NI and NII exons is similar in fetal and adult brain but that of non-neuronal *Src* and *Src* RNA containing only the NI exon is significantly higher in fetal brain tissues. Neuron-specific splicing is regulated by a positive acting RNA sequence residing in the intron between exon NI and exon 4 (Black, 1992).

The predominant form of *Src* in chicken tissues is expressed as a 4 kb mRNA. In adult skeletal muscle alternative splicing generates a 3 kb form (*Sur: src* upstream region) encoding a membrane-associated protein (p24) that lacks the tyrosine kinase domain of pp60^{src} (Dorai and Wang, 1990). p24^{sur} is developmentally regulated and is inversely expressed with respect to pp60^{src}.

Protein function

Both v-SRC and SRC are membrane-associated phosphoproteins with tyrosine-specific kinase activity but that of v-SRC greatly exceeds that of SRC. SRC activity is normally inhibited *in vivo* by nearly stoichiometric phosphorylation of Tyr527. The activation of SRC correlates with the phosphorylation on tyrosine residues of a wide range of substrates, many of which are similarly phosphorylated during the mitogenesis of normal cells and in transformed cells. pp60^{src} phosphorylates p34^{cdc2} *in vitro* and in fibroblasts p60^{src} is itself phosphorylated during mitosis (see **SRC and the cell cycle**, page 462). However, in intact cells essential targets of SRC involved in regulating cell proliferation have not been identified (see **SRC substrates**, page 466).

The existence of neuron-specific forms of SRC, their increased protein kinase activity and altered substrate specificity suggests that they are involved in neuronal differentiation and the maintenance of mature neuronal cell function (Cartwright *et al.*, 1987b; Sudol *et al.*, 1988; Maness *et al.*, 1988; Flynn *et al.*, 1992). However, disruption of the *Src* gene in mice does not appear to cause abnormalities in the brain or in platelets but rather to indicate that *Src* is essential for bone formation (Soriano *et al.*, 1991).

In the rat basophilic leukaemia cell line RBL-2H3 the kinase activity of SRC is increased after cellular stimulation via the high affinity IgE receptor (Eiseman and Bolen, 1992). However, p56^{lyn} but not SRC immunoprecipitates with the receptor and may therefore be responsible for the tyrosine phosphorylation of the activated receptor. The activation of other members of the SRC family (e.g. pp62^{yes} and pp60^{fyn}) by transmembrane signalling receptors occurs in a number of cell lines (Eiseman and Bolen, 1990; see **YES**).

Overexpression of *Src* in mouse fibroblasts increases by threefold the accumulation of cAMP in response to β-adrenergic agonists (Bushman *et al.*, 1990).

The SH2 domain contained in SRC family kinases and a number of other proteins regulates protein interactions (Heldin, 1991). Phosphatidylinositol 3-kinase, which possesses two SH2 domains, immunoprecipiates with SRC in cells transformed by polyoma virus and also associates with oncogenic tyrosine kinases including v-SRC, suggesting that SRC is involved in the modulation of phosphatidylinositol metabolism that occurs in transformed cells (see **SRC and phosphatidylinositol metabolism** and **Association between SRC and polyoma virus middle T antigen**, pages 463 and 464). Proteins encoded by the *Shc* gene (p46^{shc}, p56^{shc} and p66^{shc}) that transform NIH 3T3 fibroblasts when overexpressed are highly tyrosine phosphorylated in rat-2 cells transformed by v-*src* or v-*fps* (McGlade *et al.*, 1992). Tyrosine phosphorylated SHC proteins form complexes with the *Grb-2/Sem-5* gene product and, as *Shc* overexpression causes *Ras*-dependent neurite outgrowth in PC12 cells, the SHC–GRB2/SEM5 complex may couple tyrosine kinases to the *Ras* signalling pathway (Rozakis-Adcock *et al.*, 1992). In cells transformed by v-*src* the mouse phosphotyrosine phosphatase SYP that is a variant of the the mouse homologue of PTP1D is constitutively phosphorylated on tyrosine (Feng *et al.*, 1993). The tyrosine phosphorylation of human PTP1D correlates with enhancement of its catalytic activity (Vogel *et al.*, 1993).

v-SRC induces sustained transcription of the *Egr-1*, *Junb*, *TIS10* and *CEF-4/9E3* genes that are transiently activated by exposure of fibroblasts to serum (Dehbi *et al.*, 1992; Apel *et al.*, 1992). Induction of *TIS10* but not of *Egr-1* is dependent on protein kinase C, consistent with the evidence that v-SRC activates promoters under the control of either TPA response elements (TREs) or serum response elements (SREs). The activation of SRE-mediated gene expression appears to be regulated by RAF1 kinase and both SRE- and TRE-mediated expression are dependent on *Hras* (Qureshi *et al.*, 1992b). v-SRC does not activate *Fos* transcription and the sustained expression of *Egr-1* may be due to the absence of the transcriptional repression that FOS normally exerts on the *Egr-1* gene (Qureshi *et al.*, 1992a). Transformation of fibroblasts by v-SRC also activates S6 kinase II, although it is not a substrate for v-SRC *in vitro* (Sweet *et al.*, 1990; Chung *et al.*, 1991). Activation of S6 kinase II also occurs when quiescent cells are stimulated by serum or TPA and may arise from phosphorylation by p42 mitogen-activated kinase. In the embryonic avian neuroretina the QR1 gene is transcriptionally downregulated by v-SRC (Pierani *et al.*, 1993).

Transformation by v-*src* causes a two- to fivefold increase in glucose transport and in the level of immunoprecipitable glucose transporter protein. The human glucose transport protein expressed in chicken fibroblasts transformed by a temperature-sensitive *Src* mutant (tsNY68) is also stablilized against turnover at the permissive temperature (White and Weber, 1990).

Structures of avian leukosis virus (ALV) and RSV genomes

A variety of mutations have given rise to a number of strains of RSV (e.g. Schmidt–Ruppin, Prague) in which the insertion of the *src* oncogene does not affect the three retroviral genes *gag*, *pol* and *env*. Such viruses are thus able to replicate normally, in contrast to all other known, rapidly transforming retroviruses (and some RSV strains, e.g. the Bryan high-titre RSV) which are replication defective and require the presence of another virus for reproduction.

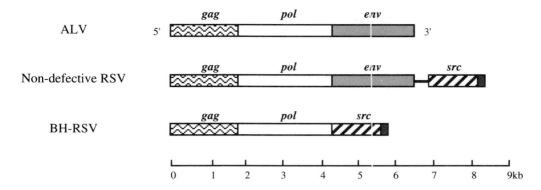

RSV: Rous sarcoma virus; BH-RSV: Bryan high-titre strain of RSV.

Structure of *Src* and v-*src* genomic DNA

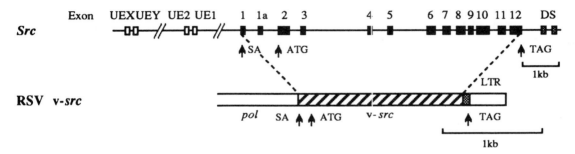

The numbered boxes denote the 12 exons of *Src*; SA, splice acceptor site; ATG, initiation codon; TAG, termination codon; DS downstream sequences (see below).

In addition to exons 1–12, four 5' exons (UE1, UE2, UEX, UEY) are present in chicken *Src* (Dorai *et al.*, 1991). These are spliced to exons 1 and 2 or to exon 1a that maps in the region formerly defined as intron 1. All of the mRNAs generated by the differential splicing of these exons and by the use of distinct initiation sites have the potential to encode pp60^{src} as their 5' exons are all eventually joined to exon 2. Translation of all v-*src* sequences begins at an ATG codon derived from exon 2 of *Src*.

Organization of the 5' exons of *Src* mRNAs

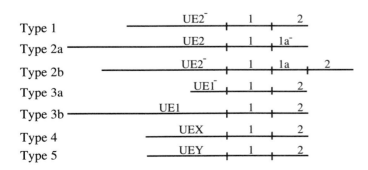

Seven cDNA clones of the 5′ ends of mRNAs are shown (Dorai *et al.*, 1991). UE1⁻ and UE2⁻ represent truncated forms of the upstream exons and in one form (type 2a) exon 1a is truncated (1a⁻).

Origin of the 3′ end of v-*src*

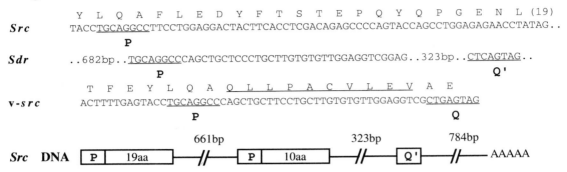

```
                        Y   L   Q   A   F   L   E   D   Y   F   T   S   T   E   P   Q   Y   Q   P   G   E   N   L  (19)
Src        TACCTGCAGGCCTTCCTGGAGGACTACTTCACCTCGACAGAGCCCCAGTACCAGCCTGGAGAGAACCTATAG..
                   P

Sdr        ..682bp..TGCAGGCCCAGCTGCTCCCTGCTTGTGTGTTGGAGGTCGGAG..323bp..CTCAGTAG..
                     P                                                              Q'

                        T   F   E   Y   L   Q   A   Q   L   L   P   A   C   V   L   E   V   A   E
v-src      ACTTTTGAGTACCTGCAGGCCCAGCTGCTTCCTGCTTGTGTGTTGGAGGTCGCTGAGTAG
                        P                                               Q
```

```
                         661bp             323bp      784bp
Src  DNA  [ P |   19aa   ] —//— [ P |  10aa  ] —//— [ Q' ] —//—— AAAAA
```

The 19 C-terminal amino acids of SRC are indicated. An ORF of 217 amino acids commences 105 nucleotides 3′ of the pp60^{src} termination codon (*Sdr*: src downstream region). This region contains the 39 bp sequence that comprises the 3′ end of v-*src*. The 10 amino acids of SDR that are acquired at the C-terminus of v-*src* are underlined. The nucleotide sequence P (underlined) is present 57 bases upstream and 661 bases downstream from the *Src* termination codon and immediately preceding the 10 amino acid sequence of v-*src*. The sequence Q that encodes the last two amino acids and the stop codon of v-*src* is also present 323 bp downstream from the 10 amino acid sequence of *Sdr* (Q′)(Dorai *et al.*, 1991).

Sequences of chicken SRC, v-SRC and SDR proteins

```
Chicken SRC            (1)    MGSSKSKPKDPSQRRRSLEPPDSTHHGGFPASQTPNKTAAPDTHRTPSRSFGTVATEPK
v-SRC (Prague C)       (1)    ---------------H------------------DE-----A--N-------------
v-SRC (Schmidt-Ruppin) (1)    ----------------------------------------------------------

Chicken SRC           (60)    LFGGFNTSDTVTSPQRAGALAGGVTTFVALYDYESRTETDLSFKKGERLQIVNNTEGDWW
v-SRC (PC)            (60)    --W------------------------------------W------------------
v-SRC (SR)            (60)    ---D-----------------------------------WI---------------N--

Chicken SRC          (120)    LAHSLTTGQTGYIPSNYVAPSDSIQAEEWYFGKITRRESERLLLNPENPRGTFLVRESET
v-SRC (PC)           (120)    --------------------------------------------------------K---
v-SRC (SR)           (120)    ----V-----------------------------------------------------

Chicken SRC          (180)    TKGAYCLSVSDFDNAKGLNVKHYKIRKLDSGGFYITSRTQFSSLQQLVAYYSKHADGLCH
v-SRC (PC)           (180)    A---------------P-------Y--Y-----------G------------------
v-SRC (SR)           (180)    ----------------------------------------------------------

Chicken SRC          (240)    RLTNVCPTSKPQTQGLAKDAWEIPRESLRLEVKLGQGCFGEVWMGTWNGTTRVAIKTLKP
v-SRC (PC)           (240)    --A------------------------------A---------------D---------
v-SRC (SR)           (240)    ----------------------------------------------------------

Chicken SRC          (300)    GNMSPEAFLQEAQVMKKLRHEKLVQLYAVVSEEPIYIVTEYMSKGSLLDFLKGEMGKYLR
v-SRC (PC)           (300)    -T--------------------------------------------------------
v-SRC (SR)           (300)    -T----------------K-----------------I---------------------

Chicken SRC          (360)    LPQLVDMAAQIASGMAYVERMNYVHRDLRAANILVGENLVCKVADFGLARLIEDNEYTAR
v-SRC (PC)           (360)    ----------------------------------------------------------
v-SRC (SR)           (360)    ----------------------------------------------------------
```

```
Chicken SRC     (420)   QGAKFPIKWTAPEAALYGRFTIKSDVWSFGILLTELTTKGRVPYPGMVNREVLDQVERGY
v-SRC (PC)      (420)   ------------------------------------------------------------
v-SRC (SR)      (420)   -------------------------------------------------G-G----R-----
                                                                         *
Chicken SRC     (480)   RMPCPPECPESLHDLMCQCWRKDPEERPTFEYLQAFLEDYFTSTEPQYQPGENL (533)
v-SRC (PC)      (480)   -------------------------K----Q-LPACVLEVAE (526)
v-SRC (SR)      (480)   ---------------S----R------------Q-LPACVLEVAE (526)


SDR      (1)   MVRCRVLHRSLKLCWATLNEVARGAPALPQRSWGSGWQMEQQDCSCTATAFRTLFSQQPEKLGDSPLPPQTHCP
        (75)   TPPAPPFLNQHKFLHPFTPHFALVCPRPFAETFGDAEGTALDRMQLESRPWDAPWRLMVSLLRHRVLGPGLSVL
       (149)   GNYLSFSAAFVHRSVSSHHPPPLLPSLIREHGATASRLQAQLLFACVLEVGVIHAQPGAAAAPIEHPCT (217)
```

Dashes indicate residues identical to SRC. The chicken SRC sequence is that of Takeya and Hanafusa (1983: Acc. P00523) except for the presence of Lys at position 501 (Dorai *et al.*, 1991). *Indicates Tyr527.

Unique domain: 8–84; SH3: 85–136 (underlined); SH2: 137–248; catalytic: 249–514; regulatory: 515–533. The ATP binding domain (273–281 and 295) is in italics. The SDR ORF commences 105 nucleotides downstream from the *Src* termination codon. The 10 amino acids acquired by v-SRC are underlined.

Sequences of SRC family proteins

```
SRC     (1)    MG  SNKS K P KDASQRRRSLEPAENVHGAGGGAFPASQTPSKPASADGHRGP SAA
FGR     (1)    --CVFC-KLEPVATAKEDAGLEGDFRSYGAADHYGPD-TKAR-ASSFAH IPNYSNFSS
FYN     (1)    --CVQC-DKEATKLTEERDGSLNQSSGYR   YGTD-TPQHYPSFGVTSIPYNNFHA
LCK     (1)    --CGCSS            H-EDDWMENIDVCENCHY-IVPL
YES     (1)    --CIKS-EN-S-AIKYRPENTPEPVSTS-SHY-AEPTTV-PC--SS-KGTAVNFSSLSM
BLK     (1)    --LL-  - -RQVSEKGKGWSPVKIRTQDKAPPPLPPLVVFNHLA-PSPN
HCK     (1)    --  -M-- -FLQVGGNTFSKTETSASPHCPV YVPD-T-TIKPG-NSHNSN
LYN     (1)    --CIKS-GKDSLSD-GVDLKTQPVRNTERTIY


SRC     (54)   F APAAAEPKLFGGFNSSDTVTSPQRAGPLAGGVT TFVALYDYESRTETDLSFKKGERLQ
FGR     (59)   Q         AINPGFLD-GTIR-VSGIG--L-I------A---D--T-T---KFH
FYN     (56)   A  GGQGLTVFG-VNS-SH-G-LRTRG  GTG--L-------A---D----H---KF-
LCK     (31)   D GKGTLLIRNGSEVRDPLVTYEGSNPPASPLQDNLVI--HS--PSHDG--G-E---QLR
YES     (60)   TPFGGSSGVTPF--AS--FS-VPSSYPAG-T----I--------A--TE--------F-
BLK     (48)                  QDPDEEERFV---F--AAVNDR--QVL---K--
HCK     (49)               TPGIREAGSEDIIV------AIHHE----Q--DQMV
LYN     (33)   VRDPTSNKQQRPVPESQLLPGQRFQTKDPEEQGDIV----P-DGIHPD--------KMK
TKL     (1)                PLVSYEGAMSPPCSPLQDKLV-------PTHDG--GL-Q--KLR


SRC     (113)  IVNNTEGDWWLAHSLSTGQTGYIPSNYVAPSDSIQAEEWYFGKITRRESERLLLNAENPR
FGR     (106)  -L--------E-R---S-K-C--------V------------G-KDA--Q--SPG--Q
FYN     (111)  -L-SS-----E-R--T--E----------V------------IG-KDA--Q--SFG---
LCK     (90)   -LEQS -E--K-Q--T---E-F--F-F--KAN-LEP-P-F-KNLS-KDA--Q--APG-TH
YES     (118)  -I--------E-R-IA--KN----------A----------MG-KDA------PG-Q-
BLK     (81)   VLRS- ------R--V--RE--V---F----VETLEV-K-F-RT-S-KDA--Q--APM-KA
HCK     (86)   VLEES -E--K----A-RKE-------RV--LET---F-KG-S-KDA--Q--APG-ML
LYN     (90)   -LEEH-E--K-K--L-KKE-F-------KLNTLET---F-KD---KDA--Q--APG-SA
TKL     (45)   -LEES-E--R-Q--T---E-L--H-F--MVN-LEP-P-PPLNLS-KNA-AR--ASG-TH


SRC     (173)  GTFLVRESETTKGAYCLSVSDFDNAKGLNVKHYKIRKLDSGGFYITSRTQFNSLQQLVAY
FGR     (166)  -A--I----------S--IR-W-QTR-DH----------M--Y---T-V----V-E--QH
FYN     (171)  ----I---------S--IR-W-DM--DH----------N--Y---T-A--ET----QH
LCK     (149)  -S--I-----S-A-SFS---R---QNQ-EV-------N--N-----SP-IT-PG-HE--RH
YES     (178)  -I------------S--IR-W-EIR-D----------N--Y---T-A--DT--K--KH
BLK     (140)  -S--I----SN---FS---K-IT TQ-EV-------S--N--Y--SP-IT-PT--A--QH
HCK     (145)  -S-MI-D------S-S---R-Y-PRQ-DT-------T--N-----SP-ST-ST--E--DH
LYN     (151)  -A--I------L--SFS---R---PVH-DVI------S--N--Y--SP-IT-PCISDMIKH
TKL     (104)  -S--I-----S--S-S---R-----N-ET-------AM-A--Y--SP-VT-S--HE--E-
```

```
SRC   (233)  YSKHADGLCHRLTTVCPTSKPQTQGLA    KDAWEIPRESLRLEVKLGQGCFGEVWMGTW
FGR   (226)  -MEVN----NL-IAP-TIM----L---    ------S-S-IT--RR--T----D--L---
FYN   (231)  --ER-A---C--VVP-HKGM-RLTD-SVKT--V--------Q-IKR--N-Q---------
LCK   (209)  -TNAS----T--SRP-Q-Q---KPWWE    -E--V---T-K-VER--A-Q------YY
YES   (238)  -TE-------K------V---------    --------------------------
BLK   (199)  ---KG----QK--LP-VNLA-KNLWA     Q-E----Q--K-VR---S-Q------YY
HCK   (199)  -K-GN----QK-SVP-MS----KPWE     -----------K--K---A-Q-----ATY
LYN   (205)  -Q-Q-----R--EKA-ISP---KPWD     ----------IK-VKR--A-Q-------YY
TKL   (156)  --SSS----T--GKP-R-Q---KPWWQ    -E--V-----K-VE---A-Q-------FY


SRC   (290)  NGTTRVAIKTLKPGTMSPEAFLQEAQVMKKLRHEKLVQLYAVVSEE  PIYIVTEYMSKGS
FGR   (283)  --S-K--V----------K---E------L---D------------  -------F-CH--
FYN   (291)  --N-K-------------S--E------K-D---------_       --------N---
LCK   (265)  --H-K--V-S--Q-S---D--A--NL--Q-Q-QR--R-----TQ-   ----I----EN--
YES   (295)  ----K----------M---------IMK----D---P--------   -------F-----
BLK   (255)  KNNMK-------E---------G--N---T-Q--R--R-----TR-  ---------AR-C
HCK   (261)  -KH-K--V--M---S--V----A--N---T-Q-DK--K-H---TK-  ----I--F-A---
LYN   (267)  -NS-K--V---------VQ---E--NL--T-Q-DK--R-----TR-E----I----A---
TKL   (213)  --H-K----N--Q-S---S---A--NL--N-Q-PR--R-----TK-  ----I----E---


SRC   (349)  LLDFLKGETGKYLRLPQLVDMAAQIASGMAYVERMNYVHRDLRAANILVGENLVCKVADF
FGR   (342)  ------NPE-QD------------VAE----M-----I-------------R-A--I---
FYN   (350)  ------DGE-RA-K--N-------VAA----I-----I-----S------NG-I--I---
LCK   (324)  -V----TPS-IK-TINK-L-------E---FI-ER--I-----------SDT-S--I---
YES   (356)  ------EGD----K----------D----I-----I--------------I---
BLK   (314)  ------TDE-SR-S--R-I--S--VAE----SI---------S-T-C--I---
HCK   (320)  ------SDE-SKQP--K-I-FS----E---FI-QR--I-----------SAS----I---
LYN   (327)  ------SDE-GKVL--K-I-FS----E----I--K--I--------V--S-S-M--I---
TKL   (272)  -V----TSE-IK-SINK-L-------E---FI-AK--I-----------S-A-C--I---


SRC   (409)  GLARLIEDNEYTARQGAKFPIKWTAPEAALYGRFTIKSDVWSFGILLTELTTKGRVPYPG
FGR   (402)  ------K-D--NPC--S------------F------------------I----I----
FYN   (410)  ------------------------------------------------V--------
LCK   (384)  -------------E-----------IN--T---------------IV-H--I----
YES   (416)  ---------------------------------------------Q---V--------
BLK   (374)  ----  -I-S----QE-----------IHF-V----A------V--MVIV-Y-------
HCK   (380)  ----V---------E-----------INF-S-------------M-IV-Y--I----
LYN   (387)  ----V---------E-----------INF-C-------------Y-IV-Y-KI----
TKL   (332)  -------------E-----------IN--T---------------IV-Y--I----


SRC   (469)  MVNREVLDQVERGYRMPCPPECPESLHD  LMCQCWRKEPEERPTFEYLQAFLEDYFTSTEPQYQPGENL  (536)
FGR   (462)  -NK----E---Q--H-----G--A--YE  A-EQT--LD-----------S-------A-------DQT  (529)
FYN   (470)  -N-----E----------QD--I---E   --IH--K-D-----------S-------A-----------  (537)
LCK   (444)  -T-P--IQNL------VR-DN---E-YQ  --RL--KER--D----D--RSV---F--A--G----QP  (509)
YES   (476)  ----------------QG------E     --NL--K-D-D-------I-S---------A----------  (543)
BLK   (433)  -S-P--IRSL-H-------ET--PE-YNDIITE---GR--------F--SV---FY-A--G--ELQP  (499)
HCK   (440)  -S-P--IRAL-------R-EN---E-YN  I-MR--KNR---------I-SV-D-FY-A--S---QQP  (505)
LYN   (447)  RT-AD-MTALSQ-----RVEN--DE-Y-  I-KM--KEKA------D---SV-D-FY-A--G---QQP  (512)
TKL   (392)  -T-P--IQNL------Q-DN--QE-YE   --M---KEQ---------MKSV---F--A--G---QQP  (457)
```

The sequences are of human SRC, FGR, FYN, HCK, LYN and YES, mouse BLK and LCK and its chicken homologue TKL. Dashes indicate sequence identity with SRC. Italics: SH3 domain (88–139). Underlined: SH2 domain (140–251) and the ATP binding region (276–284 and 298). The SRC family consensus ATP binding site is Gly–X–Gly–X–X–Gly–Glu–X–Trp–X–Gly–X–X–X–X–X–X–X–Val–Ala–X–Lys–X–Leu–Lys–X (Hanks *et al.*, 1988).

DOMAINS OF SRC

Residues 1–7: myristylation domain.
Residues 8–87: unique domain.
Residues 88–139: SH3 domain.
Residues 140–251: SH2 domain.
Residues 252–517: catalytic domain.
Residues 518–536: regulatory domain.

PERCENTAGE SEQUENCE IDENTITY WITH SRC IN DOMAINS OF THE SRC FAMILY PROTEINS

	Myristylation and unique domains	SH2 and SH3 domains	Catalytic domain
YES	22	74	89
FYN	20	67	81
FGR	11	57	78
LCK	4	50	67
HCK	17	56	69
LYN	11	52	66
BLK	18	53	67

Structures of SRC and v-SRC

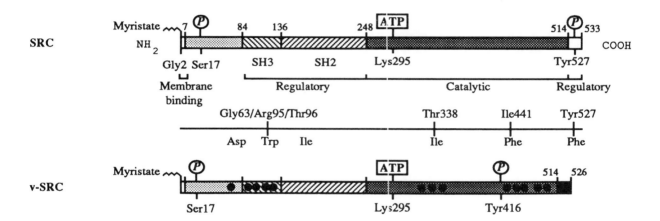

Dots indicate point mutations scattered through v-SRC in Schmidt–Ruppin strains of RSV. The C-terminal regions (of 12 amino acids of v-SRC and 19 in SRC) are unrelated in sequence.

SRC can be converted to a transforming protein by various amino acid substitutions (Kato *et al.*, 1986; Levy *et al.*, 1986), by replacement or truncation of the C-terminus (Reynolds *et al.*, 1987; Yaciuk *et al.*, 1988) or by dephosphorylation of Tyr527 (Courtneidge, 1985). The critical mutations that confer transforming activity are shown in the centre of the above figure (Hunter, 1987; see below). For a summary of mutational effects on SRC see Parsons and Weber (1989).

Functions of SRC domains

MYRISTYLATION DOMAIN

The seven N-terminal amino acids of SRC are necessary and sufficient for myristylation at Gly2 and this domain is presumed to form a recognition sequence for *N*-myristyl transferase (Kaplan *et al.*, 1988; Towler and Gordon, 1988). The N-terminal 14 amino acids of v-SRC are required for stable association with the plasma membrane (Kaplan *et al.*, 1990), which is potentially mediated via a 32 kDa N-terminal SRC receptor protein (Resh and Ling, 1990; Resh, 1990) and is essential for transformation. Substitution of Gly2 by Ala (p60$^{2A/527F}$) yields an activated, soluble tyrosine kinase that is transformation defective (Buss *et al.*, 1986). However, myristylation is neither necessary nor sufficient for membrane attachment of p60^{src}. Some non-myristylated forms of the protein associate with membranes and some myristylated cytoplasmic forms have been detected (Stoker *et al.*, 1986). For example, two isolates of recovered avian sarcoma viruses (rASVs), strains rASV157 and rASV1702, encode mutant proteins (62.5 kDa and 56 kDa respectively) that are not myristylated (Garber and Hanafusa, 1987). The N-terminus of rASV157 has 30 *env* amino acids attached to Ser6: rASV1702 has 45 *env* amino acids attached to Ala76, thus preventing their myristylation and tight binding to the plasma membrane. Neither rASV157 nor rASV1702 are tumorigenic but they cause morphological changes through their specific association with adhesion plaques.

In addition to the extreme N-terminal region, amino acids 38–111 mediate attachment to the plasma membrane and to perinuclear membranes and residues 204–259 primarily mediate association with perinuclear membranes (Kaplan *et al.*, 1990).

Ser12 and Ser17 are phosphorylated by protein kinase C and cAMP-dependent protein kinase, respectively (Patschinsky *et al.*, 1986). However, mutation of these residues does not affect transformation by v-*src* (Cross and Hanafusa, 1983; Parsons and Weber, 1989; Yaciuk *et al.*, 1989) and the significance of their phosphorylation state is unclear.

UNIQUE DOMAIN

The region of significant sequence variability between non-membrane receptor tyrosine kinases includes Ser48 that is phosphorylated by protein kinase C. However, deletions or insertions within this region have little effect on transformation potential (Raymond and Parsons, 1987; DeClue and Martin, 1989).

SH2 AND SH3 DOMAINS

(a)

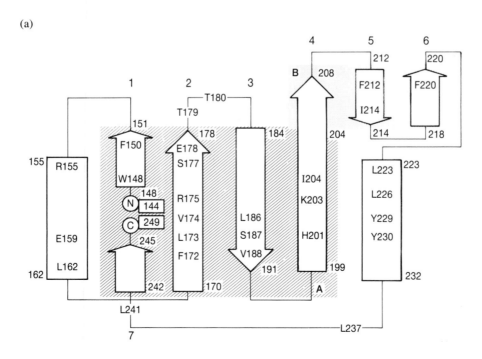

(b)

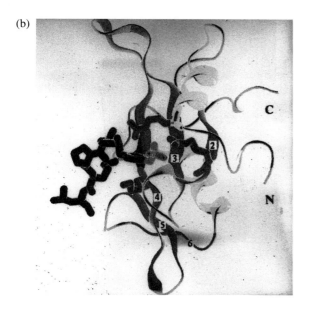

(c)

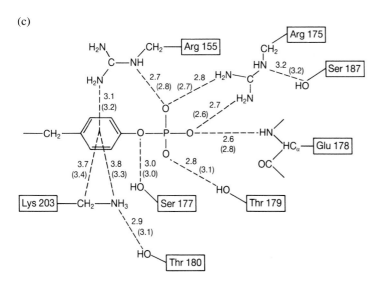

The v-SRC SH2 domain contains a central anti-parallel β sheet flanked by two α helices (Waksman *et al.*, 1992, 1993). The central β sheet may be divided into two connected sheets. (Adapted from Waksman *et al.* (1992). Crystal structure of the phosphotyrosine recognition domain SH2 of v-*src* complexed with tyrosine-phosphorylated peptides. Nature, 358, 646–653.)

(a) The strands of the β sheets are represented as arrows, the α helices as rectangles and the conserved or functionally important amino acids are numbered. Peptide binding is mediated by the sheet, intervening loops and one of the helices.

(b) The ribbon diagram represents the SH2 domain complexed with a peptide comprised of residues 751–755 of the human PDGF receptor (peptide in **WHITE**).

(c) This figure represents the phosphotyrosine binding site, showing distances between non-hydrogen atoms and from the centre of the ring for the PDGFR peptide and, in brackets, for a peptide comprised of residues 1174–1178 of the human EGF receptor. The sequence specificity of the peptide binding sites of SH2 domains have been determined for two groups of domains: SRC, FYN, LCK, FGR, ABL, CRK and NCK (pTyr–hydrophilic–hydrophilic–Ile/Pro) and p85, phospholipase C-γ and SHPTP2 (pTyr–hydrophobic–X–hydrophobic). Individual members of these groups select unique sequences except for the SRC subfamily SRC, FYN, LCK and FGR that are specific for pTyr–Glu–Glu–Ile (Songyang *et al.*, 1993).

(d)

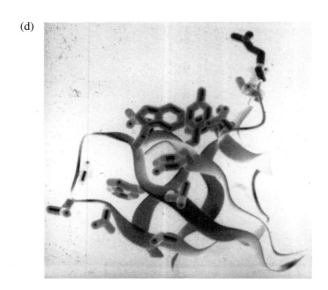

The SRC SH3 domain contains two short three-stranded anti-parallel β sheets (Yu *et al.*, 1992). The first of these (residues 107–111, 118–124 and 129–132) has a strong right-handed twist and the second (residues 85–92, 99–102 and 137–140) is packed at approximately right angles to the first. There is also a type II β turn (103–106) and a 3_{10} helix (133–137). The ligand binding site, defined using peptides with sequences occurring in the protein 3BP-1 that binds to SH3 domains of SRC and ABL *in vitro* (Cicchetti *et al.*, 1992), is a slightly curved, hydrophobic depression on the surface lined with the sidechains of aromatic amino acids. The loop containing Asn113 and Thr114 is the site of the insertions present in neuronal forms of SRC (see **Tissue location**). (Adapted from Yu *et al.* (1992). Solution structure of the SH3 domain of src and identification of its ligand binding site. Science, 258, 1665–1668.)

The importance of the SH2 region for transformation has been shown by the use of deletion mutants that are either transformation defective, partially transforming or temperature sensitive. Deletion of amino acids 15–169 or 149–169 attenuate but do not abolish transformation (Kitamura and Yoshida, 1983; Nemeth *et al.*, 1989) and deletion of 202–255 or 169–225 gives rise to temperature-sensitive variants (Bryant and Parsons, 1982; Raymond and Parsons, 1987). Point mutations of highly conserved residues in SRC (Arg95, Trp148, Arg155, Gly170) activate transforming potential (Kato *et al.*, 1986; O'Brien *et al.*, 1990).

The SH2 and SH3 domains also regulate substrate specificity in a host-dependent manner. Thus, insertions after 225 and 227 or deletion of 149–174 or 77–225 abolish transformation in rat-2 cells but in chick embryo fibroblasts complete removal of both the SH2 and SH3 domains does not inhibit kinase activity or transformation capacity (DeClue and Martin, 1989; Liebl *et al.*, 1992). When Phe172 is eliminated from SH2 the kinase activity of the v-*src* mutant is indistinguishable from that of wild-type v-*src* in chicken cells but significantly reduced in rat cells (Verderame *et al.*, 1989). Comparison of the effects of substitution and deletion mutants on chick embryo and mouse NIH 3T3 fibroblasts has defined 11 mutants that are host-dependent for transformation (Hirai and Varmus, 1990).

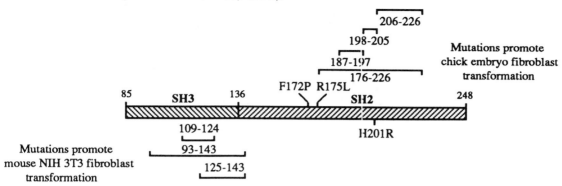

The substitution of Arg for His201 in the SH2 domain and the deletions Δ93–143, Δ109–124 or Δ125–143 cause preferential transformation of mouse fibroblasts (Hirai and Varmus, 1990). Although these mutants transform only one type of host cell, they do so with efficiencies similar to that of the Src^{Y527F} mutation. Thus species-specific differences in proteins interacting with these regions may regulate transformation efficiency. The region from residues 155 to 177 within SH2 also appears to influence the stability of SRC, mutations in this domain reducing the half-life of the protein and inhibiting transformation (Wang and Parsons, 1989). In general, the transforming capacity correlates with *in vitro* tyrosine kinase activity which depends on the type of host cell.

SH2 domains bind directly to tyrosine phosphorylated proteins. Thus the SH2 domains of v-SRC, v-CRK and RAS–GAP bind directly to the tyrosine phosphorylated protein p62 and p130 in rat-2 cells and the SH2 domains of RAS–GAP and v-CRK bind to the GAP-associated protein p190 (Koch *et al.*, 1992; Liebl *et al.*, 1992; see **RAS**). The corresponding domain of ABL binds to tyrosine phosphorylated cellular proteins with high affinity (Mayer *et al.*, 1991).

p47$^{gag-crk}$ immunoprecipitates with tyrosine phosphorylated proteins, including v-SRC but association with the latter is prevented if autophosphorylation of Tyr416 is blocked (Matsuda *et al.*, 1990). Mutational studies indicate that the SH2 domain of p47$^{gag-crk}$ binds specifically to tyrosine phosphorylated regions of peptides. SH2 domains also mediate the interaction of this diverse group of proteins with other phosphotyrosine ligands including the EGFR and a 62 kDa protein (Moran *et al.*, 1990) and the phosphorylation of p62 by v-SRC or v-FPS (which correlates with transformation) is dependent on their SH2 domains.

Two mutations in the SH2 domain of SRC (Arg for Trp148 or Ile for Gly170) increase phosphatidylinositol 3-kinase association and transformation without dephosphorylation of Tyr527 or phosphorylation of Tyr416 (O'Brien *et al.*, 1990).

SRC contains potential tyrosine phosphorylation sites in the N-terminal region (residues 90, 92, 131, 136 and 149): the phosphorylation of each of these amino acids does not directly affect kinase activity although, as the total kinase activity is dependent on the overall phosphorylation state of this region, it presumably influences the structure of SRC (Espino *et al.*, 1990).

CATALYTIC DOMAIN

This region shares sequence homology with other tyrosine kinases and contains the consensus sequence Gly–X–Gly–X–X–Gly (274–279 in chicken SRC) present in many nucleotide binding proteins. Mutations of Lys295 or in the vicinity of the consensus sequence block kinase activity and transformation (Kamps and Sefton, 1986; DeClue and Martin, 1989). Mutations in the highly conserved sequence Ala–Pro–Glu (430–432) also inhibit kinase activity and transformation (Bryant and Parsons, 1984). The transforming potential of p60^{src} is activated by point mutations at Thr338, Glu378 or Ile441 (Kato *et al.*, 1986; Levy *et al.*, 1986) and by mutations at positions 517, 518 or 523 that truncate the protein (Reynolds *et al.*, 1987; Yaciuk *et al.*, 1988).

The site of pp60^{src} *trans*-phosphorylation, Tyr416 is highly conserved in tyrosine kinases (although it is not present in the uncharacterized cellular kinase, designated *Csk* (*c*Src *k*inase)) and is the major phosphorylation site in v-SRC (Tyr527 is deleted). All transforming p60^{src} mutants have increased kinase activity that correlates with Tyr416 *trans*-phosphorylation: in such mutants the extent of Tyr527 phosphorylation (see below) varies from low to high (Jove *et al.*, 1989; Sato *et al.*, 1989). Mutation of Tyr416 suppresses tumorigenic activity of mutant forms of SRC but overexpression of the gene product that has reduced kinase activity can still transform cells *in vitro* (Cross and Hanafusa, 1983). The effect on the phosphorylation of target substrates varies with different mutants, however, and does not correlate with total tyrosine kinase activity (Ferracini and Brugge, 1990).

REGULATORY DOMAIN

In normal cells Tyr527 of SRC is phosphorylated to almost stoichiometric levels which inhibits its tyrosine kinase activity (Courtneidge, 1985; Cooper *et al.*, 1986). The substitution of Tyr527 in SRC by Phe produces an oncogenic mutant (*Src*^{Y527F}) that has high kinase activity throughout the cell cycle (Cartwright *et al.*, 1987a; Kmiecik and Shalloway, 1987; Piwnica-Worms *et al.*, 1987; Reynolds *et al.*, 1987). Treatment with phosphatase or an antibody directed against the C-terminal region of pp60^{src} generates a kinase activity comparable to that of v-SRC (Cooper and King, 1986). Phosphorylation of Tyr527 probably occurs by an intermolecular mechanism (Cooper and MacAuley, 1988) and both *in vitro* and in yeast has been shown to be caused by *Csk* rather than by autophosphorylation (Okada and Nakagawa, 1989; Nada *et al.*, 1991; Okada *et al.*, 1991). However, kinases other than CSK also phosphorylate Tyr527 in intact fibroblasts (MacAuley *et al.*, 1993). The phosphorylation of Tyr527, and hence the activity of SRC, is little affected by the nature of adjacent residues but depends critically on the spacing between Tyr527 and the kinase domain, deletions or insertions of as few as two amino acids at residue 518 stimulating the kinase and activating transforming potential (MacAuley and Cooper, 1990; Cobb *et al.*, 1991).

SRC and the cell cycle

The serine/threonine protein kinase p34^{cdc2} is the major regulator of progression through the eukaryotic cell cycle. Entry into M phase is controlled by the activation of p34^{cdc2} caused by its dephosphorylation and association with cyclin (see **Tumour Suppressor Genes**). p34^{cdc2} can be phosphorylated on tyrosine by SRC *in vitro* but whether this occurs *in vivo* is controversial. The major site of p34^{cdc2} phosphorylation *in vivo*, Tyr15, is also phosphorylated *in vitro* by an *Src*-related kinase (p67) that is distinct from SRC and other previously detected tyrosine kinases and that associates tightly with the cyclin B–p34^{cdc2} complex (Ferris *et al.*, 1991; Cheng *et al.*, 1991).

The stimulation of quiescent fibroblasts by PDGF causes the rapid phosphorylation and activation (within 10 min) of a small proportion of SRC and the stoichiometry of SRC association with the PDGFR suggests that activation during the G_0–G_1 transition may result from the formation of this complex (Gould and Hunter, 1988; Kypta *et al.*, 1990). SRC is also phosphorylated during mitosis, principally on Ser12, following stimulation by serum, PDGF, FGF, vasopressin, prostaglandin $F_{2\alpha}$ or phorbol ester. Of these agents, only PDGF causes an increase (4- to 7-fold) in the kinase activity of immune complexes of SRC. This correlates with the phosphorylation of multiple N-terminal serine and tyrosine residues, in addition to Ser12 (Ralston and Bishop, 1985; Gould and Hunter, 1988; Kypta *et al.*, 1990). Phosphorylation is due to the activity of p34^{cdc2} (i.e. p34 co-purifies and phosphorylates *in vitro*), and occurs on Thr34, Thr46 and Ser72 in chicken SRC (Chackalaparampil and Shalloway, 1988; Morgan *et al.*, 1989; Shenoy *et al.*, 1989). The equivalent conserved residue in human SRC is Thr37. This region is generally not highly conserved but the phosphorylated residues all occur in a conserved consensus sequence (basic/polar–S/T–PX–basic). p34^{cdc2} itself contains the consensus sequence, as do the retinoblastoma and chicken and human MYC proteins. The phosphorylation of Thr34, Thr46 and Ser72 is not sufficient for mitotic activation of SRC, which appears to be directly caused by the partial dephosphorylation of Tyr527 (Shenoy *et al.*, 1992). The N-terminal phosphorylations by p34^{cdc2} may, therefore, sensitize Tyr527 of SRC to phosphatase action or desensitize it to a kinase. In rat embryo fibroblasts the overexpression of protein tyrosine phosphatase PTPα causes sustained activation of SRC and dephosphorylation of Tyr527 with concomitant cell transformation and tumorigenesis (Zheng *et al.*, 1992). Thus the phosphatase PTPα may regulate cell proliferation and is oncogenic when overexpressed. SRC can promiscuously phosphorylate many non-physiological substrates but p34^{cdc2} (MPF) does not – apart from histone H1 and MAP-2. Thus it appears that the major regulator of the mammalian cell cycle, p34^{cdc2}, may activate SRC. However, it has not been shown to activate SRC kinase *in vitro*, in contrast to what happens at mitosis *in vivo*. The role of SRC is unknown but it may be noted that the cytoskeletal alterations that occur at mitosis and are associated with chromosome condensation, mitotic spindle assembly and nuclear envelope breakdown resemble those induced by v-SRC-activated transformation.

SRC and phosphatidylinositol metabolism

v-SRC causes multiple alterations in the metabolism of phosphatidylinositol and its derivatives. It stimulates PtdIns(4,5)P_2 hydrolysis and the accumulation of inositoltrisphosphate and inositolbisphosphate in chick embryo fibroblasts (Chiarugi *et al.*, 1987; Martins *et al.*, 1989), enhances by 6- to 8-fold the activity of inositol(1,4,5)P_3 3-kinase in rat-1 fibroblasts (Johnson *et al.*, 1989) and activates phosphatidylinositol 3-kinase (PI 3-kinase) in chick embryo fibroblasts (Fukui *et al.*, 1991a) and in the murine haematopoietic cell line 32D (Ruggiero *et al.*, 1991).

PI 3-kinase (formerly type I kinase) phosphorylates the D-3 position of inositol phospholipids: PI 4-kinase (type II) phosphorylates the D-4 position (Whitman *et al.*, 1988). Both kinases are present in normal and transformed fibroblasts and are activated in thrombin-stimulated platelets (Grondin *et al.*, 1991). PI 3-kinase utilizes phosphatidylinositol, PtdIns(4)P and PtdIns(4,5)P_2 as substrates and the concentrations of the products (PtdIns(3)P, PtdIns(3,4)P_2 and PtdIns(3,4,5)P_3) are increased in response to PDGF, CSF1 or insulin (Auger *et al.*, 1989). PI 3-kinase co-precipitates with v-SRC, with the products of the *fyn* and *yes* oncogenes and with the receptors for PDGF, CSF1, insulin or EGF, and its activity in anti-phosphotyrosine immunoprecipitates increases 50-fold after PDGF stimulation. Bovine brain PI 3-kinase contains two related proteins, p85α and β (both contain one SH3 and two SH2 regions), and p110. p85α and p85β are substrates for receptor tyrosine kinases and appear to restrict the binding specificity of the PI 3-kinase complex (Otsu *et al.*, 1991). p110 is the catalytic component (Hiles *et al.*, 1992).

The SH3 domain of SRC is important for complex formation with PI 3-kinase. A point mutation in SH3 (Lys106 to Glu) and other mutations in this region give rise to partially transforming mutants that have a decreased affinity for PI 3-kinase (Wages *et al.*, 1992). In cells transformed by v-SRC, v-*yes* or v-*fps* the enhancement of PI 3-kinase activity correlates with the accumulation of PtdIns(3)P, PtdIns(3,4)P_2 and PtdIns(3,4,5)P_3 (Fukui *et al.*, 1991a) and the inositol phosphate response to serum, although not that to PDGF or thrombin, is doubled (Gray and Macara 1989). This suggests the existence of serum factor(s) that can couple to SRC.

In rat-1 fibroblasts transformed by v-SRC there is a sixfold increase in the concentration of D-inositol $(1,4,5,6)P_4$ (Mattingly *et al.*, 1991). Substantial inositol $(1,3,4)P_3$ 6-kinase activity is present in both normal and transformed cells and the specific production of inositol $(1,4,5,6)P_4$ that occurs in the latter may result from the activation of PI 3-kinase (Johnson *et al.*, 1989) generating inositol $(1,3,4,5)P_4$ and the production of inositol $(1,3,4,5,6)P_5$ as an intermediate.

The significance of these effects on phosphatidylinositol metabolism by v-*src* is unknown although their probable importance is emphasized by the partial reversal of v-*src* transformation that occurs after the microinjection of antibody directed against PtdIns$(4,5)P_2$ (Fukami *et al.*, 1988). The stimulus-induced hydrolysis of PtdIns$(4,5)P_2$ that produces the second messengers inositol $(1,4,5)P_3$ and diacylglycerol is a ubiquitous cellular signalling system (Berridge and Irvine, 1989) but, with the exception of inositol $(1,4,5)P_3$, the function of inositol polyphosphates is also unknown.

Association between SRC and polyomavirus middle T antigen

pp60^{src}, pp59^{fyn} and pp60^{yes} form stable 1:1 complexes with polyoma middle T antigen (58 kDa; see **DNA Tumour Viruses**). Only a small proportion of SRC associates with middle T antigen in polyoma-transformed cells (Courtneidge and Smith, 1983) but the interaction augments many fold the tyrosine kinase activity of SRC and is necessary but not sufficient for transformation by polyoma virus. Activation of SRC is partly caused by the enzyme being locked in a conformation that prevents its being negatively regulated by Tyr527 phosphorylation (Courtneidge, 1985; Bolen *et al.*, 1984; Cartwright *et al.*, 1985) but it also undergoes tyrosine phosphorylation in the N-terminal domain (Yonemoto *et al.*, 1985). The essential region for middle T antigen binding is from Asp518 to Pro525 (Cheng *et al.*, 1988).

In contrast to the transient increase in SRC kinase activity that occurs during mitosis in normal cells, cells expressing middle T antigen maintain high kinase activity throughout the cell cycle (Kaech *et al.*, 1991). The importance of SRC in polyomavirus transformation has been indicated by studies with antisense RNA to the *Src* message (Amini *et al.*, 1986). In polyoma-transformed cells transfected with a recombinant plasmid containing the mouse metallothionein I promoter upstream of the *Src* gene in an antisense orientation, the activation of transcription of RNA complementary to *Src* by the addition of Cd^{2+} causes a significant decrease in growth rate, focus formation and tumorigenicity of the cells.

Complexes between tyrosine kinases and middle T antigen also associate with PI 3-kinase (p85 and p110) and PI 3-kinase is present in immunoprecipitates of all transforming and some non-transforming middle T antigen mutants (Courtneidge and Heber, 1987; Pallas *et al.*, 1988; Cohen *et al.*, 1990). Cells in which middle T antigen associates with PI 3-kinase have increased concentrations of PtdIns$(3,4)P_2$ and PtdIns$(3,4,5)P_3$ and accumulate inositol $(3,4)P_2$ (Ulug *et al.*, 1990). However, activation of SRC by association with middle T antigen is not sufficient to activate PI 3-kinase and middle T antigen lacking its major phosphorylation site does not bind PI 3-kinase, although it complexes with and activates SRC (Talmage *et al.*, 1989). Inositol $(3,4)P_2$ is derived from inositol $(1,3,4,5)P_4$ and the increased synthesis of these metabolites may occur in all cells in which PI 3-kinase is activated.

In rat cell lines in which the expression of middle T antigen is regulatable, the synthesis of levels of middle T antigen sufficient to cause transformation correlates with the expression of high PI 3-kinase activity (Marcellus *et al.*, 1991). This suggests that, although other independent signals may be necessary for transformation, for example, activation of protein kinase C, the stimulation of PI 3-kinase is also essential.

The strategy of viruses modulating the activity of normal cellular gene products is not confined to polyomavirus: other examples include SV40 large T antigen/p53 and adenovirus E1B/p53 and E1B/p105^{RB}. This affects either catalytic activity (as in SRC) or stability (e.g. p53, see **Tumour Suppressor Genes**).

Models for the regulation of SRC tyrosine kinase activity

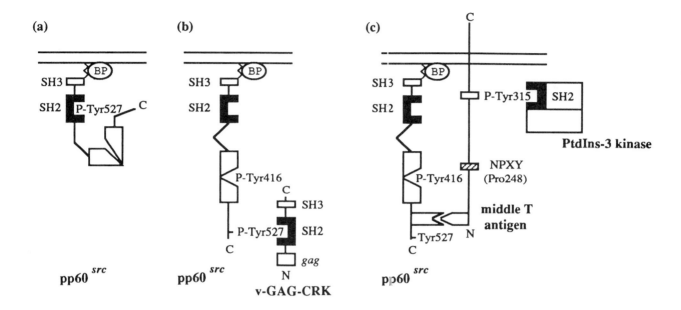

(Adapted from Cantley *et al.* (1991). Oncogenes and signal transduction. Cell, 64, 281–302.)

(a) Representation of SRC in normal, unstimulated cells in which Tyr527 is phosphorylated and its interaction with the SH2 domain results in very low kinase activity (Liu *et al.*, 1993). SRC binds *in vitro* to a peptide comprised of the 13 amino acids surrounding Tyr527 when the peptide is phosphorylated on tyrosine and the SH2 domain of SRC is intact (Roussel *et al.*, 1991). BP: binding protein.

(b) Possible interaction of v-GAG–CRK (the hybrid protein encoded by the avian sarcoma virus CT10, see **Proteins having homology with the kinase and regulatory domains of SRC** (above) and **CRK**) with phosphotyrosine527, causing activation of SRC.

(c) Interaction of polyoma middle T antigen with the region adjacent to Tyr527, thereby preventing phosphorylation of that residue and activating the kinase. The major site of tyrosine phosphorylation in middle T antigen (Tyr315) may provide a binding site for the SH2 domain of the 85 kDa subunit of PI 3-kinase (Talmage *et al.*, 1989). In cells transformed by v-*src*, tyrosine phosphorylation of p85 may provide a recognition site for the SH2 domain of v-SRC. The sequence NPXY in middle T antigen is identical to the coated vesicle localization signal of the low density lipoprotein receptor: a mutated middle T antigen (Pro248 to Leu) forms complexes with SRC, is tyrosine phosphorylated and binds to PI 3-kinase but is non-transforming (Drucker *et al.*, 1990). This suggests that middle T antigen may require to be endocytosed to cause transformation. The SH2 domain of v-SRC appears to bind to the inhibitor protein that regulates the transcriptional activity of JUN (see ***JUN***).

SRC substrates

The only known function of pp60^{src} is as a tyrosine kinase and it is generally believed that the loss of anchorage dependence and growth control, together with the changes in metabolite transport and the organization of the cytoskeleton that occur in v-*src*-transformed cells derive from the phosphorylation of specific target proteins (Kellie *et al.*, 1991). SRC phosphorylation, for example of integrins, may also be a component of signalling mechanisms in normal cells.

Tyrosine phosphorylation accounts for only 0.03% of the phosphorylated amino acids in unstimulated (chick embryo) fibroblasts. This is increased by tenfold in cells transformed by v-*src*, v-*yes* and v-*fps*, but by much less for v-*ros* and v-*erbB*, despite the fact that there is a common set of proteins in chick embryo fibroblasts that undergoes tyrosine-specific phosphorylation in response to the products of each of these oncogenes (Kamps and Sefton, 1988). Approximately 20 substrates that are tyrosine phosphorylated in response to v-*src* or activated *Src* have been identified, as summarized below. However, cells expressing high levels of SRC show little evidence of transformation and the stoichiometry of phosphorylation generally low (<1%). Many of the proteins of known function seem unlikely determinants of transformation, for example, the glycolytic proteins that undergo tyrosine phosphorylation (lactate dehydrogenase, enolase and phosphoglycerate mutase; Cooper *et al.*, 1983b) are not major regulatory enzymes, and it seems probable that substrates critical for transformation remain to be discovered.

p42: This is an M-phase-specific serine/threonine kinase (Cooper and Hunter, 1981; Cooper *et al.*, 1983a; Rossomando *et al.*, 1989; Ferrell and Martin, 1990), phosphorylated on tyrosine residues by maturation-promoting factor (MPF) *in vivo* and in cell free systems and also in fibroblasts transformed by v-*src*, which cause much greater phosphorylation of serine and threonine than of tyrosine residues. p42 phosphorylates a ribosomal S6 kinase and microtubule-associated protein MAP-2. In general, phosphorylation of p42 correlates well with cell transformation and mitogenesis: it is, however, a poor *in vitro* substrate for SRC and may not therefore be a primary target.

p50: p50 binds to newly synthesized v-SRC, together with the p90 heat shock protein but the phosphorylation of p50 does not correlate with transformation (Brugge, 1986).

p75: In murine fibroblasts the phosphotyrosine content of p75 is cooperatively increased by *Src* overexpression and EGF. p75 co-localizes with SRC at the plasma membrane and in the perinuclear region (Maa *et al.*, 1992).

p80/85: The product of the *EMS1* gene that is frequently co-amplified and overexpressed in human breast cancer and squamous cell carcinomas of the head and neck that maps to chromosome 11q13 in proximity to the *PRAD1*/cyclin D1 gene (see **BCL**). EMS1 is 85% homologous to a chicken protein that is a substrate for oncogenic SRC (Schuuring *et al.*, 1993; Wu *et al.*, 1991). In carcinoma cells EMS1 is present at cell–substrate contact sites and may therefore be involved in metastasis.

p110 and p130: These form stable complexes with activated SRC (Kanner *et al.*, 1991). p110 and p130 are substrates for serine/threonine and tyrosine kinases and there is some correlation between their phosphorylation state and cell transformation. The SH3 domain of SRC mediates association with p110 and the formation of the ternary complex requires SH2.

p120: Tyrosine phosphorylation of p120 correlates with transformation and also occurs in NIH 3T3 cells in response to PDGF, CSF1 or EGF (Downing and Reynolds, 1991). p120 is not phosphorylated by the expression of non-myristylated SRC (Reynolds *et al.*, 1989b). p120 contains four copies of an imperfect repeat that occurs in human plakoglobulin and *Xenopus laevis* β-catenin (see **Tumour Suppressor Genes: Cadherins**) and in the *Drosophila armadillo* segment polarity protein (Reynolds *et al.*, 1992).

gp130: This is highly phosphorylated in cells transformed by v-SRC, Fujinami sarcoma virus or Y73 (Hamaguchi *et al.*, 1990). This glycoprotein is distinct from the fibronectin receptor and the use of temperature-sensitive mutants indicates that its phosphorylation correlates with morphological transformation.

CD3-ζ: Normal lymphocytes express very low levels of SRC. When v-SRC is constitutively expressed in murine T cell hybridomas CD3-ζ is phosphorylated on tyrosine residues (O'Shea *et al.*, 1991). However, although these cells also spontaneously secrete low levels of IL-2, the amount of IL-2 released, the level of tyrosine phosphorylation and the range of phosphorylated substrates is increased when the cells are challenged with antigen, indicating that the expression of v-SRC in these cells is much less effective as a stimulus than the physiologically coupled protein kinase(s).

Clathrin and calmodulin: Phosphorylated on tyrosine residues in v-SRC-transformed cells (Fukami *et al.*, 1986).

Connexin43 (cx43): Activation of v-SRC causes tyrosine phosphorylation of the major gap junction protein cx43 that correlates with inhibition of intercellular communication via gap junctions (Crow *et al.*, 1992).

G proteins: The α subunits of several heterotrimeric G proteins are phosphorylated on tyrosine residues *in vitro* (Hausdorff *et al.*, 1992). This increases the rate of receptor-stimulated GTP hydrolysis by $G_{\alpha s}$ subunits.

NCK: This 47 kDa SH2/SH3 domain protein is phosphorylated on tyrosine in v-*src*-transformed NIH 3T3 fibroblasts (Meisenhelder and Hunter, 1992).

Platelet fibrinogen receptor (gpIIb/gpIIIa): Both subunits of the isolated receptor are phosphorylated by purified SRC although only gpIIIa is a substrate in platelet plasma membrane preparations (Findik *et al.*, 1990; Elmore *et al.*, 1990).

RAS–GAP: RAS–GAP associates stably in an interaction dependent on the SH2 domain of SRC with SRC proteins of low kinase activity but poorly with activated SRC (e.g. lacking Tyr527; Brott *et al.*, 1991b). GAP immunoprecipitates with SRC but is tyrosine phosphorylated only in complexes with v-SRC from transformed cells (Brott *et al.*, 1991a) indicating a link between tyrosine kinase and *Ras* signalling pathways. Overexpression of GAP or (more effectively) of the C-terminus of GAP inhibits transformation and causes reversion of NIH 3T3 cells transformed by *Src*, *Src*^{Y527F} or v-*src* (DeClue *et al.*, 1991). In *src*-transformed cells or after EGF stimulation of normal cells, tyrosine and serine phosphorylated GAP stably associates with tyrosine phosphorylated p62/64 and p190 (Bouton *et al.*, 1991). A minor fraction of GAP associates with 15–25% of the total pp62/64: the majority forms a cytosolic, predominantly serine phosphorylated complex with p190 (Moran *et al.*, 1991). These various complexes are potential regulators or targets of p21^{ras} (see **RAS**).

Synaptophysin: Synaptophysin (p38) is a substrate for SRC in neuronal tissues (Cheng and Sahyoun, 1988; Matten *et al.*, 1990; Barnekow *et al.*, 1990). It is a major component of the synaptic vesicle membrane and its phosphorylation by SRC may be part of the mechanism of synaptic vesicle exocytosis in neuroendocrine cells.

Cytoskeletal proteins: The cytoskeletal changes correlated with transformation include a reduction in microfilament bundles, redistribution of the actin-associated proteins α-actinin, vinculin and talin, and loss of the extracellular matrix protein fibronectin. In cells infected with the temperature-sensitive mutant LA29 (Ala for Pro507), SRC undergoes rapid and reversible cytoskeletal binding on switching from the permissive to the non-permissive temperature (Welham and Wyke, 1988) that is prevented by deletion of amino acids 149–169 in the SH2 domain (Fukui *et al.*, 1991b). Vinculin, talin and the fibronectin receptor (a member of the integrin family) occur in adhesion plaques that are disrupted by the expression of v-SRC (Rohrschneider and Reynolds, 1985; Nigg *et al.*, 1986). However, use of a considerable number of morphological mutants of RSV has shown that well-developed adhesion plaques can exist that contain high concentrations of enzymatically active v-SRC (Kellie *et al.*, 1986; Stoker *et al.*, 1986).

Annexin II (p36, calpactin I or lipocortin II): This is a major Ca^{2+} binding protein of unknown function that is highly conserved (mammalian, avian and *Xenopus* proteins are >80% identical; Izant and Bryson, 1991), is induced in v-*src*-transformed rat cells (Ozaki and Sakiyama, 1993) and is phosphorylated when *Src* is expressed (Radke *et al.*, 1980). It is associated with the inner face of the plasma membrane and binds to cytoskeletal elements including actin and fodrin. Annexin II synthesis is modulated during differentiation and passage through the cell cycle (Keutzer and Hirschorn, 1990; Schlaepfer and Haigler, 1990) but does not occur in all cells. In rodent tissues there is high expression in the lung, intestine and thymus, intermediate expression in the spleen, lymph nodes and testis and none in brain and muscle. Annexin II is phosphorylated by all cytosolic tyrosine kinases and phosphorylation of Tyr23 by SRC decreases its *in vitro* affinity for actin (Glenney, 1985). The significance of this is unknown but observations with non-myristylated mutants (Buss *et al.*, 1986) and temperature-sensitive mutants of SRC that phosphorylate p36 at restrictive temperatures (Kamps *et al.*, 1986; Stoker *et al.*, 1986) indicate that phosphorylation of p36 does not correlate with transformation.

α-fodrin, α- and β-tubulin and the microtubule-associated proteins MAP2 and TAU: These are phosphorylated *in vitro* by v-SRC (Akiyama *et al.*, 1986) and tubulin is phosphorylated by SRC in neuronal tissues (Cheng and Sahyoun, 1988; Matten *et al.*, 1990).

Integrin: Integrin is a transmembrane receptor for fibronectin (complex of 120, 140 and 160 kDa polypeptides). The two smaller subunits are phosphorylated on tyrosine in response to transformation by RSV (Hirst *et al.*, 1986) and there is evidence that tyrosine phosphorylation of the receptor correlates with loss of surface fibronectin in rounded cells (Horvath *et al.*, 1990) and decreased affinity for talin (Tapley *et al.*, 1989). Immunolabelling studies of the three-dimensional structure of adhesion plaques in cells undergoing transformation suggests that v-*src*-mediated phosphorylation does not affect the interaction of actin with the plasma membrane (Nermut *et al.*, 1991).

v-SRC expressed by the ASV variant 2234.3 has high tyrosine kinase activity and is co-localized with the integrin receptor but causes little increase in receptor phosphorylation or disruption of adhesion plaques (Horvath *et al.*, 1990). v-*src* transformation blocks myogenic differentiation of primary embryonic myoblasts, in part by causing phosphorylation of integrin α and β chains (Aneskievich *et al.*, 1991). There appears to be a good correlation between the phosphotyrosine content of integrin and morphological change.

p125^{FAK}: This protein undergoes a large increase in tyrosine phosphorylation when activated *Src* (*Src*^{Y527F}) is expressed in NIH 3T3 fibroblasts (Guan and Shalloway, 1992). p125 is itself a tyrosine kinase but the sequences flanking the catalytic domain do not have significant homology with other kinases (Schaller *et al.*, 1992). p125 co-localizes with components of focal adhesion plaques, including tensin, vinculin and talin and has thus been designated p125^{FAK} (*focal adhesion kinase*: see **Tumour Suppressor Genes: Integrins**).

Paxillin: This is an adhesion plaque protein (68 kDa) that binds to the rod domain of vinculin and is ~20-fold more highly phosphorylated on tyrosine residues in v-SRC-transformed cells than either vinculin or talin (Turner *et al.*, 1990). Paxillin is one of the major tyrosine kinase substrates during embryonic development (Turner, 1991).

Talin: Talin is an adhesion plaque protein (215 kDa) tyrosine phosphorylated in RSV-transformed cells but also phosphorylated in other cells which lack any of the morphological features of the transformed phenotype (Pasquale *et al.*, 1986; DeClue and Martin, 1989). Intercellular junctions, at which both talin and vinculin are localized, are major sites of protein tyrosine kinase activity in both normal and transformed cells (Volberg *et al.*, 1991).

Vinculin: This is an adhesion plaque protein (130 kDa) that undergoes a 20-fold increase in tyrosine phosphorylation in RSV-transformed cells (Sefton *et al.*, 1981, 1982) that could account for the disruption of actin bundles. However, not all tyrosine kinase oncogenes induce phosphorylation of vinculin (e.g. *Ros* does not). At most only about 1–2% of the vinculin in transformed cells is tyrosine phosphorylated and so it is difficult to see how this would cause gross morphological changes. The lack of correlation between vinculin phosphorylation and transformation extends to cells infected with an RSV variant that encodes a truncated but fully active tyrosine kinase (that phosphorylates vinculin) but is nevertheless transformation defective (Felice *et al.*, 1990).

Databank file names and accession numbers

	GENE	*EMBL*	*SWISSPROT*	*REFERENCES*
RSV	v-*src*	GB: Alrgsrca M11753		Nishizawa *et al.*, 1985
RSV (Prague C)	v-*src*	Rersv6 V01197	KSRC_RSVP P00526	Schwartz *et al.*, 1983 Neil *et al.*, 1981
RSV (Schmidt–Ruppin)	v-*src*	Rsvsrc X13745 Reasv5 V01169	KSRC_RSVSR P00524	Barnier *et al.*, 1989 Czernilofsky *et al.*, 1983 Takeya and Hanafusa, 1983 Neil *et al.*, 1981
ASV (PR2257)	v-*src*	Realrs04 M21526	KSRC_AVIS2 P15054	Geryk *et al.*, 1989
ASV (RASV1441)	v-*src*	EReensr K00928	KSRC_AVISR P00525	Takeya *et al.*, 1982 Neil *et al.*, 1981
ASV-S1	v-*src*		KSRC_AVISS P14084	
ASV-S2	v-*src*		KSRC_AVIST P14085	Ikawa *et al.*, 1986
ASV (rASV157)	v-*src*	GB: Acsmuta M1517rASV1702 GB: Acsmutb M15172		Garber and Hanafusa 1987
GR-FeSV	v-*fgr*/*src-2*	Refesv X00255	KFGR_FSVGR P00544	Naharro *et al.*, 1984
Human	*SRC1*	Hssrcex3 to Hssrcex5 (M16243 to M16245) Hssrc101 to Hssrc107 (K03212 to K03218) Hssrce7 to Hssrce12 (X03995 to X04000)	KSRC_HUMAN P12931	Anderson *et al.*, 1985 Tanaka *et al.*, 1987 Parker *et al.*, 1985
Human	*SLK*	GB: Humslk M14676		Kawakami *et al.*, 1986
Human	*FGR*/*SRC2*	GB: Humsrc2b K03219 Hsfgr2 to Hsfgr7 (M12719 to M12724)	KFGR_HUMAN P09769	Parker *et al.*, 1985 Katamine *et al.*, 1988 Nishizawa *et al.*, 1986 Inoue *et al.*, 1987

	GENE	EMBL	SWISSPROT	REFERENCES
Human	*NCK*	Hsnck X17576	NCK_HUMAN P16333	Lehmann *et al.*, 1990
Human	*SHC*	Hsshc X68148		Pelicci *et al.*, 1992
Chicken	*Src*	Ggcsrc V00402GB	KSRC_CHICK P00523	Takeya and Hanafusa, 1983
		Chksrc J00844		Kamps *et al.*, 1984
				Gould *et al.*, 1985
				Smart *et al.*, 1981
				Cooper *et al.*, 1986
Mouse	*Scr+*	GB: Mussrcpp6 M17031	KSRN_MOUSE P05480	Martinez *et al.*, 1987
		Mmsrcpp6 M17031		
Drosophila	*Src*	Dmsrcc M11917	KSR1_DROME P00528	Simon *et al.*, 1985
		Dmdsrc K01043		Hoffmann *et al.*, 1983
Drosophila	*Src-2*	Dmsrc28c M16599	KSR2_DROME P08630; P11361	Gregory *et al.*, 1987
		Dmsrc4 X02305		Wadsworth *et al.*, 1985
Xenopus laevis	*Src*	Xlsrca M24704	KSR1_XENLA P13115	Steele *et al.*, 1989
Xenopus laevis	*src-2*	Xlsrc M23422	KSR2_XENLA P13116	Steele *et al.*, 1989
		Xlsrc2 M30858		Steele, 1985
Hydra attenuata Src-related		Hastk M25245	KSTK_HYDAT P17713	Bosch *et al.*, 1989

Reviews

Berridge, M.J. and Irvine, R.F. (1989). Inositol phosphates and cell signalling. Nature, 341, 197–205.

Bolen, J.B., Thompson, P.A., Eiseman, E. and Horak, I.D. (1991). Expression and interactions of the *Src* family of tyrosine protein kinases in T lymphocytes. Adv. Cancer Res., 57, 103–149.

Brickell, P.M. (1991). The c-*src* family of protein-tyrosine kinases. Int. J. Exp. Pathol., 72, 97–108.

Cantley, L.C., Auger, K.R., Carpenter, C., Duckworth, B., Graziani, A., Kapeller, R. and Soltoff, S. (1991). Oncogene and signal transduction. Cell, 64, 281–302.

Eiseman, E. and Bolen, J.B. (1990). *src*-related tyrosine protein kinases as signaling components in hematopoietic cells. Cancer Cells 2, 303–310.

Hanks, S.K., Quinn, A.M. and Hunter, T. (1988). The protein kinase family: conserved features and deduced phylogeny of the catalytic domains. Science, 241, 42–52.

Heldin, C.-H. (1991). SH2 domains: elements that control protein interactions during signal transduction. Trends Biochem. Sci., 16, 450–452.

Hunter, T. (1987). A tail of two *src*'s: mutatis mutandis. Cell, 49, 1–4.

Jove, R. and Hanafusa, H. (1987). Cell transformation by the viral *src* oncogene. Ann. Rev. Cell Biol., 3, 31–56.

Kellie, S., Horvath, A.R. and Elmore, M.A. (1991). Cytoskeletal targets for oncogenic tyrosine kinases. J. Cell Sci., 99 (Pt 2), 207–211.

McCormick, F. (1989). *ras* GTPase activating protein: signal transmitter and signal terminator. Cell, 56, 5–8.

Parsons, J.T. and Weber, M.J. (1989). Genetics of *src*: structure and functional organization of a protein tyrosine kinase. Curr. Top. Microbiol. Immunol., 147, 80–127.

Pawson, T. and Gish, G.D. (1992). SH2 and SH3 domains: from structure to function. Cell, 71, 359–362.

Resh, M.D. (1990). Membrane interactions of pp60$^{v\text{-}src}$: a model for myristylated tyrosine protein kinases. Oncogene, 5, 1437–1444.

Towler, D.A. and Gordon, J.I. (1988). The biology and enzymology of eukaryotic protein acylation. Annu. Rev. Biochem., 57, 69–99.

Papers

Akiyama, T., Kadowaki, T., Nishida, E., Kadooka, T., Ogawara, H., Fukami, Y., Sakai, H., Takaku, F. and Kasuga, M. (1986). Substrate specificities of tyrosine-specific protein kinases toward cytoskeletal proteins *in vitro*. J. Biol. Chem., 261, 14797–14803.

Amini, S., DeSeau, V., Reddy, S., Shalloway, D. and Bolen, J.B. (1986). Regulation of pp60$^{c\text{-}src}$ synthesis by inducible RNA complementary to c-*src* mRNA in polyomavirus-transformed rat cells. Mol. Cell. Biol., 6, 2305–2316.

Anderson, S.K., Gibbs, C.P., Tanaka, A., Kung, H.-J. and Fujita, D.J. (1985). Human cellular *src* gene: nucleotide sequence and derived amino acid sequence of the region coding for the carboxy-terminal two-thirds of pp60$^{c\text{-}src}$. Mol. Cell. Biol., 5, 1112–1129.

Aneskievich, B.J., Haimovich, B. and Boettiger, D. (1991). Phosphorylation of integrin in differentiating ts-Rous sarcoma virus-transformed myogenic cells. Oncogene, 6, 1381–1390.

Apel, I., Yu, C.-L., Wang, T., Dobry, C., van Antwerp, M.E., Jove, R. and Prochownik, E.V. (1992). Regulation of the *jun*B gene by v-*src*. Mol. Cell. Biol., 12, 3356–3364.

Auger, K.R., Serunian, L.A., Soltoff, S.P., Libby, P. and Cantley, L. (1989). PDGF-dependent tyrosine phosphorylation stimulates production of novel polyphosphoinositides in intact cells. Cell, 57, 167–175.

Barnekow, A. and Gessler, M. (1986). Activation of the pp60$^{c\text{-}src}$ kinase during differentiation of monomyelocytic cells *in vitro*. EMBO J., 5, 701–705.

Barnekow, A., Paul, E. and Schartl, M. (1987). Expression of the c-src protein in human skin tumors. Cancer Res., 47, 235–240.

Barnekow, A., Jahn, R. and Schartl, M. (1990). Synaptophysin: a substrate for the protein tyrosine kinase pp60c-src in intact synaptic vesicles. Oncogene, 5, 1019–1024.

Barnier, J.V., Dezelee, P., Marx, M. and Calothy, G. (1989). Nucleotide sequence of the *src* gene of the Schmidt-Ruppin strain of Rous sarcoma virus type E. Nucleic Acids Res., 17, 1252.

Black, D.L. (1992). Activation of c-*src* neuron-specific splicing by an unusual RNA element in vivo and in vitro. Cell, 69, 795–807.

Boettiger, D., Roby, K., Brumbaugh, J., Briehl, J. and Holtzer, H. (1977). Transformation of chicken embryo retinal melanoblasts by a temperature-sensitive mutant of Rous sarcoma virus. Cell, 11, 881–890.

Bolen, J.B., Thiele, C.J., Israel, M.A., Yonemoto, W., Lipsich, L.A. and Brugge, J.S. (1984). Enhancement of cellular *src* gene product associated tyrosyl kinase activity following polyoma virus infection and transformation. Cell, 38, 767–777.

Booker, G.W., Breeze, A.L., Downing, A.K., Panayotou, G., Gout, I., Waterfield, M.D. and Campbell, I.D. (1992). Structure of an SH2 domain of the p85α subunit of phosphatidylinositol-3-OH kinase. Nature, 358, 684–687.

Bosch, T.C.G., Unger, T.F., Fisher, D.A. and Steele, R.E. (1989). Structure and expression of *STK*, a src-related gene in the simple metazoan *Hydra attenuata*. Mol. Cell. Biol., 9, 4141–4151.

Bouton, A.H., Kanner, S.B., Vines, R.R., Wang, H.-C.R., Gibbs, J.B. and Parsons, J.T. (1991). Transformation by pp60^{src} or stimulation of cells with epidermal growth factor induces the stable association of tyrosine-phosphorylated cellular proteins with GTPase-activating protein. Mol. Cell. Biol., 11, 945–953.

Brott, B.K., Decker, S., Shafer, J., Gibbs, J.B. and Jove, R. (1991a). GTPase-activating protein interactions with the viral and cellular src kinases. Proc. Natl Acad. Sci. USA, 88, 755–759.

Brott, B.K., Decker, S., O'Brien, M.C. and Jove, R. (1991b). Molecular features of the viral and cellular src kinases involved in interactions with the GTPase-activating protein. Mol. Cell. Biol., 11, 5059–5067.

Brugge, J. S. (1986). Interaction of the Rous sarcoma virus protein pp60^{src} with the cellular proteins pp50 and pp90. Curr. Top. Microbiol. Immunol., 123, 1–22.

Brugge, J., Cotton, P., Lustig, A., Yonemoto, W., Lipsich, L., Coussens, P., Barrett, J.N., Nonner, D. and Keane, R.W. (1987). Characterization of the altered form of the c-*src* gene product in neuronal cells. Genes Devel., 1, 287–296.

Bryant, D. and Parsons, J.T. (1982). Site-directed mutagenesis of the *src* gene of Rous sarcoma virus: construction and characterization of a deletion mutant temperature sensitive for transformation. J. Virol., 44, 683–691.

Bryant, D. and Parsons, J.T. (1984). Amino acid alterations within a highly conserved region of the Rous sarcoma virus *src* gene product pp60^{src} inactivate tyrosine kinase activity. Mol. Cell. Biol., 4, 862–866.

Bushman, W.A., Wilson, L.K., Luttrell, D.K., Moyers, J.S. and Parsons, S.J. (1990). Overexpression of c-src enhances β-adrenergic-induced cAMP accumulation. Proc. Natl Acad. Sci. USA., 87, 7462–7466.

Buss, J.E., Kamps, M.P., Gould, K. and Sefton, B.M. (1986). The absence of myristic acid decreases membrane binding of p60^{src} but does not affect tyrosine protein kinase activity. J. Virol., 58, 468–474.

Cartwright, C.A., Hutchinson, M.A. and Eckhart, W. (1985). Structural and functional modification of pp60^{c-src} associated with polyoma middle tumor antigen from infected or transformed cells. Mol. Cell. Biol., 5, 2647–2652.

Cartwright, C.A., Eckhart, W., Simon, S. and Kaplan, P.L. (1987a). Cell transformation by pp60^{c-src} mutated in the carboxy-terminal regulatory domain. Cell, 49, 83–91.

Cartwright, C.A., Simantov, R., Kaplan, P.L., Hunter, T. and Eckhart, W. (1987b). Alterations in pp60^{c-src} accompany differentiation of neurons from rat embryo striatum. Mol. Cell. Biol., 7, 1830–1840.

Cartwright, C.A., Meisler, A.I. and Eckhart, W. (1990). Activation of the pp60^{c-src} protein kinase is an early event in colonic carcinogenesis. Proc. Natl Acad. Sci. USA, 87, 558–562.

Chackalaparampil, I. and Shalloway, D. (1988). Altered phosphorylation and activation of pp60^{c-src} during fibroblast mitosis. Cell, 52, 801–810.

Cheng, H.-C., Litwin, C.M., Hwang, D.M. and Wang, J.H. (1991). Structural basis of specific and efficient phosphorylation of peptides derived from p34^{cdc2} by a pp60^{src}-related protein tyrosine kinase. J. Biol. Chem., 266, 17919–17925.

Cheng, N. and Sahyoun, N. (1988). The growth cone cytoskeleton. Glycoprotein association, calmodulin binding, and tyrosine/serine phosphorylation of tubulin. J. Biol. Chem., 263, 3935–3942.

Cheng, S.H., Piwnica-Worms, H., Harvey, R.W., Roberts, T.M. and Smith, A.E. (1988). The carboxy terminus of pp60^{c-src} is a regulatory domain and is involved in complex formation with the middle-T antigen of polyomaviruses. Mol. Cell. Biol., 8, 1736–1747.

Cheng, S.H., Espino, P.C., Marshall, J., Harvey, R. and Smith, A.E. (1990). Stoichiometry of cellular and viral components in the polyomavirus middle-T antigen-tyrosine kinase complex. Mol. Cell. Biol., 10, 5569–5574.

Chiarugi, V., Porciatti, F., Pasquali, F., Magnelli, L., Giannelli, S. and Ruggiero, M. (1987). Polyphosphoinositide metabolism is rapidly stimulated by activation of a temperature-sensitive mutant of Rous sarcoma virus in rat fibroblasts. Oncogene, 2, 37–40.

Chung, J., Chen, R.-Y. and Blenis, J. (1991). Coordinate regulation of pp90^{rsk} and a distinct protein-serine/threonine kinase activity that phosphorylates recombinant pp90^{rsk} in vitro. Mol. Cell. Biol., 11, 1868–1874.

Cicchetti, P., Mayer, B.J., Thiel, G. and Baltimore, D. (1992). Identification of a protein that binds to the SH3 region of Abl and is similar to Bcr and GAP-rho. Science, 257, 803–806.

Clark, S.G., Stern, M.J. and Horvitz, H.R. (1992). *C. elegans* cell-signalling gene *sem*-5 encodes a protein with SH2 and SH3 domains. Nature, 356, 340–344.

Cobb, B.S., Payne, D.M., Reynolds, A.B. and Parsons, J.T. (1991). Regulation of the oncogenic activity of the cellular *src* protein requires the correct spacing between the kinase domain and the C-terminal phosphorylated tyrosine (Tyr-527). Mol. Cell. Biol., 11, 5832–5838.

Cohen, B., Liu, Y., Druker, B., Roberts, T.M. and Schaffhausen, B.S. (1990). Characterization of pp85, a target of oncogenes and growth factor receptors. Mol. Cell. Biol., 10, 2909–2915.

Cooper, J.A. and Hunter, T. (1981). Changes in protein phosphorylation in Rous sarcoma virus-transformed chicken embryo cells. Mol. Cell. Biol., 1, 165–178.

Cooper, J.A. and King, C.S. (1986). Dephosphorylation or antibody binding to the carboxy terminus stimulates pp60^{c-src}. Mol. Cell. Biol., 6, 4467–4477.

Cooper, J.A. and MacAuley, A. (1988). Potential positive and negative autoregulation of p60^{c-src} by intermolecular autophosphorylation. Proc. Natl Acad. Sci. USA, 85, 4232–4236.

Cooper, J.A., Nakamura, K.D., Hunter, T. and Weber, M.J. (1983a). Phosphotyrosine-containing proteins and expression of transformation parameters in cells infected with partial transformation mutants of Rous sarcoma virus. J. Virol., 46, 15–28.

Cooper, J.A., Reiss, N.A., Schwartz, R.J. and Hunter, T. (1983b). Three glycolytic enzymes are phosphorylated at tyrosine in cells transformed by Rous sarcoma virus. Nature, 302, 218–223.

Cooper, J.A., Gould, K.L., Cartwright, C.A. and Hunter, T. (1986). Tyr^{527} is phosphorylated in pp60^{c-src}: implications for regulation. Science, 231, 1431–1434.

Courtneidge, S.A. (1985). Activation of the pp60^{src} kinase by middle T antigen binding or by dephosphorylation. EMBO J., 4, 1471–1477.

Courtneidge, S.A. and Heber, A. (1987). An 81kd protein complexed with middle T antigen and pp60^{c-src}: a possible phosphatidylinositol kinase. Cell, 50, 1031–1037.

Courtneidge, S.A. and Smith, A.E. (1983). Polyoma virus transforming protein associates with the product of the c-*src* cellular gene. Nature, 303, 435–439.

Cross, F.R. and Hanafusa, H. (1983). Local mutagenesis of Rous sarcoma virus: the major sites of tyrosine and serine phosphorylation of p60*src* are dispensable for transformation. Cell, 34, 597–607.

Cross, F.R., Garber, E.A. and Hanafusa, H. (1985). N-terminal deletions in Rous sarcoma virus p60*src*: effects on tyrosine kinase and biological activities and on recombination in tissue culture with the cellular *src* gene. Mol. Cell. Biol., 5, 2789–2795.

Crow, D.S., Kurata, W.E. and Lau, A.F. (1992). Phosphorylation of connexin43 in cells containing mutant *src* oncogenes. Oncogene, 7, 999–1003.

Czernilofsky, A.P., Levinson, A.D., Varmus, H.E., Bishop, J.M., Tischer, E. and Goodman, H. (1983). Corrections to the nucleotide sequence of the *src* gene of Rous sarcoma virus. Nature, 301, 736–738.

Davis, S., Lu, M.L., Lo, S.H., Lin, S., Butler, J.A., Druker, B.J., Roberts, T.M., An, Q. and Chen, L.B. (1991). Presence of an SH2 domain in the actin-binding protein tensin. Science, 252, 712–715.

DeClue, J.E. and Martin, G.S. (1989). Linker insertion-deletion mutagenesis of the v-*src* gene: isolation of host- and temperature-dependent mutants. J. Virol., 63, 542–554.

DeClue, J.E., Sadowski, I., Martin, G.S. and Pawson, T. (1987). A conserved domain regulates interactions of the v-*fps* protein-tyrosine kinase with the host cell. Proc. Natl Acad. Sci. USA, 84, 9064–9068.

DeClue, J.E., Zhang, K., Redford, P., Vass, W.C. and Lowy, D.R. (1991). Suppression of *src* transformation by overexpression of full-length GTPase-activating protein (GAP) or of the GAP C terminus. Mol. Cell. Biol., 11, 2819–2825.

Dehbi, M., Mbiguino, A., Beauchemin, M., Chatelain, G. and Bedard, P.-A. (1992). Transcriptional activation of the CEF-4/9E3 cytokine gene by pp60*v-src*. Mol. Cell. Biol., 12, 1490–1499.

Dorai, T. and Wang, L.-H. (1990). An alternative non-tyrosine protein kinase product of the c-*src* gene in chicken skeletal muscle. Mol. Cell. Biol., 10, 4068–4079.

Dorai, T., Levy, J.B., Kang, L., Brugge, J.S. and Wang, L.-H. (1991). Analysis of cDNAs of the proto-oncogene c-*src*: heterogeneity in 5' exons and possible mechanism for the genesis of the 3' end of v-*src*. Mol. Cell. Biol., 11, 4165–4176.

Downing, J.R. and Reynolds, A.B. (1991). PDGF, CSF-1, and EGF induce tyrosine phosphorylation of p120, a pp60*src* transformation-associated substrate. Oncogene, 6, 607–613.

Drubin, D.G., Mulholland, J., Zhu, Z. and Botstein, D. (1990). Homology of a yeast actin-binding protein to signal transduction proteins and myosin-I. Nature, 343, 288–290.

Druker, B.J., Ling, L.E., Cohen, B., Roberts, T.M. and Schaffhausen, B.S. (1990). A completely transformation-defective point mutant of polyomavirus middle t antigen which retains full associated phosphatidylinositol kinase activity. J. Virol., 64, 4454–4461.

Eiseman, E. and Bolen, J.B. (1992). Engagement of the high-affinity IgE receptor activates *src* protein-related tyrosine kinases. Nature, 355, 78–80.

Elmore, M.A., Anand, R., Horvath, A.R. and Kellie, S. (1990). Tyrosine-specific phosphorylation of gpIIIa in platelet membranes. FEBS Letts., 269, 283–287.

Ephrussi, B. and Temin, H.M. (1960). Infection of chick iris epithelium with Rous sarcoma virus in vitro. Virology, 11, 547–552.

Escobedo, J.A., Navankasattusas, S., Kavanaugh, W.M., Milfay, D., Fried, V.A. and Williams, L.T. (1991). cDNA cloning of a novel 85 kd protein that has SH2 domains and regulates binding of PI3-kinase to the PDGF β-receptor. Cell, 65, 75–82.

Espino, P.C., Harvey, R., Schweickhardt, R.L., White, G.A., Smith, A.E., and Cheng, S.H. (1990). The amino-terminal region of pp60c-*src* has a modulatory role and contains multiple sites of tyrosine phosphorylation. Oncogene, 5, 283–293.

Felice, G., Horvath, A.R. and Kellie, S. (1990). Tyrosine kinase activities and neoplastic transformation. Biochem. Soc. Trans., 18, 69–72.

Feng, G.-S., Hui, C.-C. and Pawson, T. (1993). SH2-containing phosphotyrosine phosphatase as a target of protein-tyrosine kinases. Science, 259, 1607–1611.

Ferracini, R. and Brugge, J. (1990). Analysis of mutant forms of the c-*src* gene product containing a phenylalanine substitution for tyrosine 416. Oncogene Res., 5, 205–219.

Ferrell, J.E. and Martin, G.S. (1990). Identification of a 42-kilodalton phosphotyrosyl protein as a serine (threonine) protein kinase by renaturation. Mol. Cell. Biol., 10, 3020–3026.

Ferrell, J.E., Noble, J.A., Martin, G.S., Jacques, Y.V. and Bainton, D.F. (1990). Intracellular localization of pp60c-*src* in human platelets. Oncogene, 5, 1033–1036.

Ferris, D.K., White, G.A., Kelvin, D.J., Copeland, T.D., Li, C.C. and Longo, D.L. (1991). p34*cdc2* is physically associated with and phosphorylated by a *cdc2*-specific tyrosine kinase. Cell Growth Differ., 2, 343–349.

Findik, D., Reuter, C. and Presek, P. (1990). Platelet membrane glycoproteins IIb and IIIa are substrates of purified pp60c-*src* protein tyrosine kinase. FEBS Letts. March 12, 262(1), 1–4.

Fiszman, M.Y. and Fuchs, P. (1975). Temperature-sensitive expression of differentiation in transformed myoblasts. Nature, 254, 429–431.

Flynn, D.C., Schaller, M.D. and Parsons, J.T. (1992). Tyrosine phosphorylation of a 120 000 dalton membrane-associated protein by the neural form of pp60$^{c\text{-}src}$, pp60$^{c\text{-}src+}$. Oncogene, 7, 579–583.

Freeman, R.M., Plutzky, J. and Neel, B.G. (1992). Identification of a human src homology 2-containing protein-tyrosine-phosphatase: a putative homolog of *Drosophila* corkscrew. Proc. Natl Acad. Sci. USA, 89, 11239–11243.

Fu, X.-Y. (1992). A transcription factor with SH2 and SH3 domains is directly activated by an interferon α-induced cytoplasmic protein tyrosine kinase(s). Cell, 70, 323–335.

Fukami, Y., Nakamura, T., Nakayama, A. and Karehisa, T. (1986). Phosphorylation of tyrosine residues of calmodulin in Rous sarcoma virus-transformed cells. Proc. Natl Acad. Sci. USA, 83, 4190–4193.

Fukami, K., Matsuoka, K., Nakanishi, O., Yamakawa, A., Kawai, S. and Takenawa, T. (1988). Antibody to phosphatidylinositol 4,5-bisphosphate inhibits oncogene-induced mitogenesis. Proc. Natl Acad. Sci. USA, 85, 9057–9061.

Fukui, Y., Saltiel, A.R. and Hanafusa, H. (1991a). Phosphatidylinositol-3 kinase is activated in v-src, v-yes and v-fps transformed chicken embryo fibroblasts. Oncogene, 6, 407–411.

Fukui, Y., O'Brien, M.C. and Hanafusa, H. (1991b). Deletions in the SH2 domain of p60$^{v\text{-}src}$ prevent association with the detergent-insoluble cellular matrix. Mol. Cell. Biol., 11, 1207–1213.

Fung, Y.-K., Crittenden, L.B., Fadly, A.M. and Kung, H.-J. (1983). Tumor induction by direct injection of cloned v-src DNA into chickens. Proc. Natl Acad. Sci. USA, 80, 353–357.

Garber, E.A. and Hanafusa, H. (1987). NH2-terminal sequences of two src proteins that cause aberrant transformation. Proc. Natl Acad. Sci. USA, 84, 80–84.

Garcia, R., Parikh, N.U., Saya, H. and Gallick, G.E. (1991). Effect of herbimycin A on growth and pp60$^{c\text{-}src}$ activity in human colon tumor cell lines. Oncogene, 6, 1983–1989.

Geryk, J., Dezelee, P., Barnier, J.V., Svoboda, J., Nehyba, J., Karakoz, I., Rynditch, A.V., Yatsula, B.A. and Calothy, G. (1989). Transduction of the cellular src gene and 3′ adjacent sequences in avian sarcoma virus PR2257. J. Virol., 63, 481–492.

Ghosn, C.R., Ral., B.B.A., Winokur, S.T., Unger, T.F. Steele, R.E. (1992). Structural organization of a src gene from *Xenopus laevis*. Oncogene, 7, 2345–2350.

Glenney, J.R. (1985). Phosphorylation of p36 in vitro with pp60^{src}. FEBS Letts., 192, 79–82.

Golden, A. and Brugge, J. S. (1989). Thrombin treatment induces rapid changes in tyrosine phosphorylation in platelets. Proc. Natl Acad. Sci. USA, 86, 901–905.

Golden, A., Nemeth, S.P. and Brugge, J. S. (1986). Blood platelets express high levels of the pp60$^{c\text{-}src}$-specific tyrosine kinase activity. Proc. Natl Acad. Sci. USA, 83, 852–856.

Gould, K. and Hunter, T. (1988). Platelet-derived growth factor induces multisite phosphorylation of pp60$^{c\text{-}src}$ and increases its protein-tyrosine kinase activity. Mol. Cell. Biol., 8, 3345–3356.

Gould, K.L., Woodgett, J.R., Cooper, J.A., Buss, J.E., Shalloway, D. and Hunter, T. (1985). Protein kinase C phosphorylates pp60^{src} at a novel site. Cell, 42, 849–857.

Gray, G.M. and Macara, I.G. (1989). Serum-stimulated phosphatidylinositol turnover is enhanced in 3T3 cells with active pp60v-src. Oncogene, 4, 1213–1217.

Gregory, R.J., Kammermeyer, K.L., Vincent, W.S. and Wadsworth, S.G. (1987). Primary sequence and developmental expression of a novel *Drosophila melanogaster* src gene. Mol. Cell. Biol., 7, 2119–2127.

Grondin, P., Plantavid, M., Sultan, C., Breton, M., Mauco, G. and Chap, H. (1991). Interaction of pp60$^{c\text{-}src}$, phospholipase C, inositol-lipid, and diacyglycerol kinases with the cytoskeletons of thrombin-stimulated platelets. J. Biol. Chem., 266, 15705–15709.

Guan, J.-L. and Shalloway, D. (1992). Regulation of focal adhesion-associated protein tyrosine kinase by both cellular adhesion and oncogenic transformation. Nature, 358, 690–692.

Hamaguchi, M., Matsuda, M. and Hanafusa, H. (1990). A glycoprotein in the plasma membrane matrix as a major potential substrate of p60$^{v\text{-}src}$. Mol. Cell. Biol., 10, 830–836.

Hausdorff, W.P., Pitcher, J.A., Luttrell, D.K., Linder, M.E., Kurose, H., Parsons, S.J., Caron, M.G. and Lefkowitz, R.J. (1992). Tyrosine phosphorylation of G protein α subunits by pp60$^{c\text{-}src}$. Proc. Natl Acad. Sci. USA, 89, 5720–5724.

Hiles, I.D., Otsu, M., Volinia, S., Fry, M.J., Gout, I., Dhand, R., Panayotou, G., Ruiz-Larrea, F., Thompson, A., Totty, N.F., Hsuan, J.J., Courtneidge, S.A., Parker, P.J. and Waterfield, M.D. (1992). Phosphatidylinositol 3-kinase: structure and expression of the 110 kd catalytic subunit. Cell, 70, 419–429.

Hirai, H. and Varmus, H. (1990). Mutations in src homology regions 2 and 3 of activated chicken c-src that result in preferential transformation of mouse or chicken cells. Proc. Natl Acad. Sci. USA, 87, 8592–8596.

Hirst, R., Horwitz, A., Buck, C. and Rohrschneider, L. (1986). Phosphorylation of the fibronectin receptor complex in cells transformed by oncogenes that encode tyrosine kinases. Proc. Natl Acad. Sci. USA, 83, 6470–6474.

Hoffmann, F.M., Fresco, L.D., Hoffman-Falk, H., Shilo, B.Z. (1983). Nucleotide sequences of the Drosophila *src* and *abl* homologs: conservation and variability in the *src* family oncogenes. Cell, 35, 393–401.

Horvath, A.R., Elmore, M.A. and Kellie, S. (1990). Differential tyrosine-specific phosphorylation of integrin in Rous sarcoma virus transformed cells with differing transformed phenotypes. Oncogene, 5, 1349–1357.

Iba, H., Takeya, T., Cross, F.R., Hanafusa, T. and Hanafusa, H. (1984). Rous sarcoma virus variants that carry the cellular *src* gene instead of the viral *src* gene cannot transform chicken embryo fibroblasts. Proc. Natl Acad. Sci. USA, 81, 4424–4428.

Ikawa, S., Hagino-Yamagishi, K., Kawai, S., Yamamoto, T. and Toyoshima, K. (1986). Activation of the cellular *src* gene by transducing retrovirus. Mol. Cell. Biol., 6, 2420–2428.

Inoue, K., Ikawa, S., Semba, K., Sukegawa, J., Yamamoto, T. and Toyoshima, K. (1987). Isolation and sequencing of cDNA clones homologous to the v-*fgr* oncogene from a human B lymphoma line, IL-9. Oncogene, 1, 301–304.

Izant, J.G. and Bryson, L.J. (1991). *Xenopus* annexin II (calpactin I) heavy chain has a distinct amino terminus. J. Biol. Chem., 266, 18560–18566.

Johnson, R.M., Wasilenko, W.J., Mattingly, R.R., Weber, M.J. and Garrison, J.C. (1989). Fibroblasts transformed with v-*src* show enhanced formation of an inositol tetrakisphosphate. Science, 246, 121–124.

Jove, R., Hanafusa, T., Hamaguchi, M. and Hanafusa, H. (1989). *In vivo* phosphorylation states and kinase activities of transforming p60$^{c\text{-}src}$ mutants. Oncogene Res., 5, 49–60.

Kaech, S., Covic, L., Wyss, A. and Ballmer-Hofer, K. (1991). Association of p60$^{c\text{-}src}$ with polyoma virus middle-T antigen abrogating mitosis-specific activation. Nature, 350, 431–433.

Kamps, M.P. and Sefton, B.M. (1986). Neither arginine nor histidine can carry out the function of lysine-295 in the ATP-binding site of p60^{src}. Mol. Cell. Biol., 6, 751–757.

Kamps, M.P. and Sefton, B.M. (1988). Identification of multiple novel polypeptide substrates of the v-*src*, v-*yes*, v-*fps*, v-*ros*, and v-*erb*-B oncogenic tyrosine protein kinases utilizing antisera against phosphotyrosine. Oncogene, 2, 305–315.

Kamps, M.P., Taylor, S.S. and Sefton, B.M. (1984). Direct evidence that oncogenic tyrosine kinases and cyclic AMP-dependent protein kinase have homologous ATP-binding sites. Nature, 310, 589–592.

Kamps, M.P., Buss, J.E. and Sefton, B.M. (1986). Rous sarcoma virus transforming protein lacking myristic acid phosphorylates known polypeptide substrates without inducing transformation. Cell, 45, 105–112.

Kanner, S.B., Reynolds, A.B., Wang, H.-C.R., Vines, R.R. and Parsons, J.T. (1991). The SH2 and SH3 domains of pp60^{src} direct stable association with tyrosine phosphorylated proteins p130 and p110. EMBO J., 10, 1689–1698.

Kaplan, J.M., Mardon, G., Bishop, J.M. and Varmus, H.E. (1988). The first seven amino acids encoded by the v-*src* oncogene act as a myristylation signal: lysine 7 is a critical determinant. Mol. Cell. Biol., 8, 2435–2441.

Kaplan, J.M., Varmus, H.E. and Bishop, J.M. (1990). The *src* protein contains multiple domains for specific attachment to membranes. Mol. Cell. Biol., 10, 1000–1009.

Katamine, S., Notario, V., Rao, C.D., Miki, T., Cheah, M.S.C., Tronick, S.R. and Robbins, K.C. (1988). Primary structure of the human fgr proto-oncogene product p55$^{c\text{-}fgr}$. Mol. Cell. Biol., 8, 259–266.

Kato, J.-Y., Takeya, T., Grandori, C., Iba, H., Levy, J.B. and Hanafusa, H. (1986). Amino acid substitutions sufficient to convert the nontransforming p60$^{c\text{-}src}$ protein to a transforming protein. Mol. Cell. Biol., 6, 4155–4160.

Kawakami, T., Pennington, C.Y. and Robbins, K.C. (1986). Isolation and oncogenic potential of a novel human *src*-like gene. Mol. Cell. Biol., 6, 4195–4201.

Keane, R.W., Lipsich, L.A. and Brugge, J.S. (1984). Differentiation and transformation of neural plate cells. Devel. Biol., 103, 38–52.

Kellie, S., Patel, B., Wigglesworth, N.M., Mitchell, A., Critchley, D.R. and Wyke, J.A. (1986). The use of Rous sarcoma virus transformation mutants with differing tyrosine kinase activities to study the relationships between vinculin phosphorylation, pp60$^{v\text{-}src}$ location and adhesion plaque integrity. Exp. Cell Res., 165, 216–228.

Keutzer, J.C. and Hirschorn, R.R. (1990). The growth regulated gene 1B6 is identified as the heavy chain of calpactin I. Exp. Cell Res., 188, 153–159.

Kitamura, N. and Yoshida, M. (1983). Small deletion in *src* of Rous sarcoma virus modifying transformation phenotypes: identification of 207-nucleotide deletion and its smaller product with protein kinase activity. J. Virol., 46, 985–992.

Kmiecik, T.E. and Shalloway, D. (1987). Activation and suppression of pp60$^{c\text{-}src}$ transforming ability by mutation of its primary sites of tyrosine phosphorylation. Cell, 49, 65–73.

Koch, C.A., Moran, M.F., Anderson, D., Liu, X., Mbamalu, G. and Pawson, T. (1992). Multiple SH2-mediated interactions in v-*src*-transformed cells. Mol. Cell. Biol., 12, 1366–1374.

Krueger, J.G., Garber, E.A. and Goldberg, A.R. (1983). Subcellular localization of pp60^{src} in RSV-transformed cells. Curr. Top. Microbiol. Immunol., 107, 51–124.

Kypta, R.M., Goldberg, Y., Ulug, E.T. and Courtneidge, S.A. (1990). Association between the PDGF receptor and members of the *src* family of tyrosine kinases. Cell, 62, 481–492.

Lehmann J.M., Riethmueller G., Johnson J.P. (1990). *Nck*, a melanoma cDNA encoding a cytoplasmic protein consisting of the *src* homology units SH2 and SH3. Nucleic Acids Res., 18, 1048.

Lehto, V.-P., Wasenius, V.-M., Salven, P. and Saraste, M. (1988). Transforming and membrane proteins. Nature, 334, 388.

Levy, J.B., Iba, H. and Hanafusa, H. (1986). Activation of the transforming potential of p60^{c-src} by a single amino acid change. Proc. Natl Acad. Sci. USA, 83, 4228–4232.

Levy, J.B., Dorai, T., Wang, L.-H. and Brugge, J.S. (1987). The structurally distinct form of pp60^{c-src} detected in neuronal cells is encoded by a unique c-*src* mRNA. Mol. Cell. Biol., 7, 4142–4145.

Liebl, E.C. and Martin, G.S. (1992). Intracellular targeting of pp60^{src} expression: localization of v-*src* to adhesion plaques is sufficient to transform chicken embryo fibroblasts. Oncogene, 7, 2417–2428.

Liebl, E.C., England, L.J., DeClue, J.E. and Martin, G.S. (1992). Host range mutants of v-*src*: alterations in kinase activity and substrate interactions. J. Virol., 66, 4315–4324.

Liu, X., Brodeur, S.R., Gish, G., Songyang, Z., Cantley, L.C., Laudano, A.P. and Pawson, T. (1993). Regulation of c-Src tyrosine kinase activity by the Src SH2 domain. Oncogene, 8, 1119–1126.

Lowenstein, E.J., Daly, R.J., Batzer, A.G., Li, W., Margolis, B., Lammers, R., Ullrich, A., Skolnik, E.Y., Bar-Sagi, D. and Schlessinger, J. (1992). The SH2 and SH3 domain-containing protein GRB2 links receptor tyrosine kinases to ras signaling. Cell, 70, 431–442.

Lowe, C., Yoneda, T., Boyce, B.F., Chen, H., Mundy, G.R. and Soriano, P. (1993). Osteopetrosis in Src-deficient mice is due to an autonomous defect of osteoclasts. Proc. Natl Acad. Sci. USA, 90, 4485–4489.

Maa, M.-C., Wilson, L.K., Moyers, J.S., Vines, R.R., Parsons, J.T. and Parsons, S.J. (1992). Identification and characterization of a cytoskeleton-associated, epidermal growth factor sensitive pp60^{c-src} substrate. Oncogene, 7, 2429–2438.

MacAuley, A. and Cooper, J.A. (1990). Acidic residues at the carboxyl terminus of p60^{c-src} are required for regulation of tyrosine kinase activity and transformation. New Biologist, 2, 828–840.

MacAuley, A., Okada, M., Nada, S., Nakagawa, H. and Cooper, J.A. (1993). Phosphorylation of src mutants at Tyr 527 in fibroblasts does not correlate with *in vitro* phosphorylation by CSK. Oncogene, 8, 117–124.

McGlade, J., Cheng, A., Pelicci, G., Pelicci, P.G. and Pawson, T. (1992). Shc proteins are phosphorylated and regulated by the v-src and v-fps protein-tyrosine kinases. Proc. Natl Acad. Sci. USA, 89, 8869–8873.

Maness, P.F., Aubry, M., Shores, C.G., Frame, L. and Pfenninger, K.H. (1988). c-*src* gene product in developing rat brain is enriched in nerve growth cone membranes. Proc. Natl Acad. Sci. USA, 85, 5001–5005.

Mano, H., Ishikawa, F., Nishida, J., Hirai, H. and Takaku, F. (1990). A novel protein-tyrosine kinase, *tec*, is preferentially expressed in liver. Oncogene, 5, 1781–1786.

Mano, H., Mano, K., Tang, B., Koehler, M., Yi, T., Gilbert, D.J., Jenkins, N.A., Copeland, N.G. and Ihle, J.N. (1993). Expression of a novel form of *tec* kinase in hematopoietic cells and mapping of the gene to chromosome 5 near *kit*. Oncogene, 8, 417–424.

Marcellus, R., Whitfield, J.F. and Raptis, L. (1991). Polyoma virus middle tumor antigen stimulates membrane-associated protein kinase C at lower levels than required for phosphatidylinositol kinase activation and neoplastic transformation. Oncogene, 6, 1037–1040.

Margolis, B., Silvennoinen, O., Comoglio, F., Roonprapunt, C., Skolnik, E., Ullrich, A. and Schlessinger, J. (1992). High-efficiency expression/cloning of epidermal growth factor-receptor-binding proteins with src homology 2 domains. Proc. Natl Acad. Sci. USA, 89, 8894–8898.

Martinez, R., Mathey-Prevot, B., Bernards, A. and Baltimore, D. (1987). Neuronal pp60^{c-src} contains a six-amino acid insertion relative to its non-neuronal counterpart. Science, 237, 411–415.

Martins, T. J., Sugimoto, Y. and Erikson, R.L. (1989). Dissociation of inositol trisphosphate from diacylglycerol production in Rous sarcoma virus-transformed fibroblasts. J. Cell Biol., 108, 683–691.

Matsuda, M., Meyer, B.J., Fukui, Y. and Hanafusa, H. (1990). Binding of transforming protein p47$^{gag-crk}$ to a broad range of phosphotyrosine-containing proteins. Science, 248, 1537–1539.

Matten, W.T., Aubry, M., West, J. and Maness, P.F. (1990). Tubulin is phosphorylated at tyrosine by pp60^{c-src} in nerve growth cones. J. Cell Biol., 111, 1959–1970.

Mattingly, R.R., Stephens, L.R., Irvine, R.F. and Garrison, J.C. (1991). Effects of transformation with the v-*src* oncogene on inositol phosphate metabolism in rat-1 fibroblasts. J. Biol. Chem., 266, 15144–15153.

Matuoka, K., Shibata, M., Yamakawa, A. and Takenawa, T. (1992). Cloning of ASH, a ubiquitous protein composed of one src homology region (SH) 2 and two SH3 domains, from human and rat cDNA libraries. Proc. Natl Acad. Sci. USA, 89, 9015–9019.

Mayer, B.J., Jackson, P.K. and Baltimore, D. (1991). The non-catalytic *src* homology region 2 segment of *abl* tyrosine kinase binds to tyrosine-phosphorylated cellular proteins with high affinity. Proc. Natl Acad. Sci. USA, 88, 627–631.

Meisenhelder, J. and Hunter, T. (1992). The SH2/SH3 domain-containing protein nck is recognized by certain anti-phospholipase C-γ1 monoclonal antibodies, and its phosphorylation on tyrosine is stimulated by platelet-derived growth factor and epidermal growth factor treatment. Mol. Cell. Biol., 12, 5843–5856.

Moran, M.F., Koch, C.A., Anderson, D., Ellis, C., England, L., Martin, G.S. and Pawson, T. (1990). Src homology domains direct protein-protein interactions in signal transduction. Proc. Natl Acad. Sci. USA, 87, 8622–8626.

Moran, M.F., Polakis, P., McCormick, F., Pawson, T. and Ellis, C. (1991). Protein-tyrosine kinases regulate the phosphorylation, protein interactions, subcellular distribution, and activity of p21^{ras} GTPase-activating protein. Mol. Cell. Biol., 11, 1804–1812.

Morgan, D.O., Kaplan, J.M., Bishop, M.J. and Varmus, H.E. (1989). Mitosis-specific phosphorylation of p60^{c-src} by p34^{cdc2}-associated protein kinase. Cell, 57, 775–786.

Musacchio, A., Noble, M., Pauptit, R., Wierenga, R. and Saraste, M. (1992). Crystal structure of a src-homology 3 (SH3) domain. Nature, 359, 851–855.

Nada, S., Okada, M., MacAuley, A., Cooper, J.A. and Nakagawa, H. (1991). Cloning of a complementary DNA for a protein-tyrosine kinase that specifically phosphorylates a negative regulatory site of p60^{c-src}. Nature, 351, 69–72.

Naharro, G., Robbins, K.C. and Reddy, E.P. (1984). Gene product of v-*fgr onc*: hybrid protein containing a portion of actin and a tyrosine-specific protein kinase. Science, 223, 63–66.

Neil, J.C., Ghysdael, J., Vogt, P.K. and Smart, J.E. (1981). Homologous tyrosine phosphorylation sites in transformation-specific gene products of distinct avian sarcoma viruses. Nature, 291, 675–677.

Nemeth, S.P., Fox, L.G., DeMarco, M. and Brugge, J.S. (1989). Deletions within the amino-terminal half of the c-*src* gene product that alter the functional activity of the protein. Mol. Cell. Biol., 9, 1109–1119.

Nermut, M.V., Eason, P., Hirst, E.M. and Kellie, S. (1991). Cell/substratum adhesions in RSV-transformed rat fibroblasts. Exp. Cell Res., 193, 382–397.

Nigg, E.A., Sefton, B.A., Hunter, T., Walter, G. and Singer, S.J. (1986). Immunofluorescent localisation of the transforming protein of Rous sarcoma virus with antibodies against a synthetic *src* peptide. Proc. Natl Acad. Sci. USA, 79, 5322–5366.

Nishizawa, M., Mayer, B.J., Takeya, T., Yamamoto, T., Toyoshima, K., Hanafusa, H. and Kawai, S. (1985). Two independent mutations are required for temperature-sensitive cell transformation by a Rous sarcoma virus temperature-sensitive mutant. J. Virol. 56, 743–749.

Nishizawa, M., Semba, K., Yoshida, M.C., Yamamoto, T., Sasaki, M. and Toyoshima, K. (1986). Structure, expression and chromosomal location of the human c-*fgr* gene. Mol. Cell. Biol., 6, 511–517.

O'Brien, M.C., Fukui, Y. and Hanafusa, H. (1990). Activation of the proto-oncogene p60^{c-src} by point mutations in the SH2 domain. Mol. Cell. Biol., 10, 2855–2862.

Ohta, S., Taniguchi, T., Asahi, M., Kato, Y., Nakagawara, G. and Yamamura, H. (1992). Protein-tyrosine kinase p72^{syk} is activated by wheat germ agglutinin in platelets. Biochem. Biophys. Res. Commun., 185, 1128–1132.

O'Shea, J.J., Ashwell, J.D., Bailey, T.L., Cross, S.L., Samelson, L.E. and Klausner, R.D. (1991). Expression of v-*src* in a murine T-cell hybridoma results in constitutive T-cell receptor phosphorylation and interleukin 2 production. Proc. Natl Acad. Sci. USA, 88, 1741–1745.

Okada, M. and Nakagawa, H. (1989). A protein tyrosine kinase involved in regulation of pp60^{c-src} function. J. Biol. Chem., 264, 20886–20893.

Okada, M., Nada, S., Yamanashi, Y., Yamamoto, T. and Nakagawa, H. (1991). CSK: a protein-tyrosine kinase involved in regulation of *src* family kinases. J. Biol. Chem., 266, 24249–24252.

Otsu, M., Hiles, I., Gout, I., Fry, M.J., Ruiz-Larrea, F., Panayotou, G., Thompson, A., Dhand, R., Hsuan, J., Totty, N., Smith, A.D., Morgan, S.J., Courtneidge, S.A., Parker, P.J. and Waterfield, M.D. (1991). Characteriation of two 85 kd proteins that associate with receptor tyrosine kinases, middle-T/pp60^{c-src} complexes, and pI3-kinase. Cell, 65, 91–104.

Ottilie, S., Raulf, F., Barnekow, A., Hannig, G. and Schartl, M. (1992). Multiple *src*-related kinase genes, *srk*1–4, in the fresh water sponge *Spongilla lacustris*. Oncogene, 7, 1625–1630.

Ozaki, T. and Sakiyama, S. (1993). Molecular cloning of rat calpactin I heavy-chain cDNA whose expression is induced in v-*src*-transformed rat culture cell lines. Oncogene, 8, 1707–1710.

Pacifici, M., Boettiger, D., Roby, K. and Holtzer, H. (1977). Transformation of chondroblasts by Rous sarcoma virus and synthesis of the sulfated proteoglycan matrix. Cell, 11, 891–899.

Pallas, D.C., Cherington, V., Morgan, W., DeAnda, J., Kaplan, D., Schaffhausen, B. and Roberts, T.M. (1988). Cellular proteins that associate with the middle and small T antigens of polyomavirus. J. Virol., 62, 3934–3940.

Parker, R.C., Varmus, H.E. and Bishop, J.M. (1984). Expression of v-*src* and chicken c-*src* in rat cells demonstrates qualitative differences between pp60^{v-src} and pp60^{c-src}. Cell, 37, 131–139.

Parker, R.C., Mardon, G., Lebo, R.V., Varmus, H.E. and Bishop, J.M. (1985). Isolation of duplicated human c-*src* genes located on chromosomes 1 and 20. Mol. Cell. Biol., 5, 831–838.

Pasquale, E.B., Maher, P.A. and Singer, S.J. (1986). Talin is phosphorylated on tyrosine in chicken embryo fibroblasts transformed by Rous sarcoma virus. Proc. Natl Acad. Sci. USA, 83, 5507–5511.

Patschinsky, T., Hunter, T. and Sefton, B.M. (1986). Phosphorylation of the transforming protein of Rous sarcoma virus: direct demonstration of phosphorylation of serine 17 and identification of an additional site of tyrosine phosphorylation in p60^{v-src} of Prague Rous sarcoma virus. J. Virol., 59, 73–81.

Pelicci, G., Lanfrancone, L., Grignani, F., McGlade, J., Cavallo, F., Forni, G., Nicoletti, I., Grignani, F., Pawson, T. and Pelicci, P.G. (1992). A novel transforming protein (SHC) with an SH2 domain is implicated in mitogenic signal transduction. Cell, 70, 93–104.

Pierani, A., Pouponnot, C. and Calothy, G. (1993). Transcriptional downregulation of the retina-specific QR1 gene by pp60^{v-src} and identification of a novel v-*src*-responsive unit. Mol. Cell. Biol., 13, 3401–3414.

Piwnica-Worms, H., Saunders, K.B., Roberts, T.M., Smith, A.E. and Cheng, S.H. (1987). Tyrosine phosphorylation regulates the biochemical and biological properties of pp60^{c-src}. Cell, 49, 75–82.

Plutzky, J., Neel, B.G. and Rosenberg, R.D. (1992). Isolation of a src homology 2-containing tyrosine phosphatase. Proc. Natl Acad. Sci. USA, 89, 1123–1127.

Potts, W.M., Reynolds, A.B., Lansing, T.J. and Parsons, J.T. (1988). Activation of pp60^{c-src} transforming potential by mutations altering the structure of an amino terminal domain containing residues 90–95. Oncogene Res., 3, 343–355.

Pyper, J.M. and Bolen, J.B. (1990). Identification of a novel neuronal C-*SRC* exon expressed in human brain. Mol. Cell. Biol., 10, 2035–2040.

Qureshi, S.A., Rim, M., Alexandropoulos, K., Berg, K., Sukhatme, V. and Foster, D.A. (1992a). Sustained induction of *egr*-1 by v-*src* correlates with a lack of fos-mediated repression of the *egr*-1 promoter. Oncogene, 7, 121–125.

Qureshi, S.A., Alexandropoulos, K., Rim, M., Joseph, C.K., Bruder, J.T., Rapp, U.R. and Foster, D.A. (1992b). Evidence that Ha-ras mediates two distinguishable intracellular signals activated by v-src. J. Biol. Chem., 267, 17635–17639.

Radke, K., Gilmore, T. and Martin, G.S. (1980). Transformation by Rous sarcoma virus: a cellular substrate for transformation-specific protein phosphorylation contains phosphotyrosine. Cell, 21, 821–828.

Ralston, R. and Bishop, M.J. (1985). The product of the proto-oncogene c-*src* is modified during the cellular response to platelet-derived growth factor. Proc. Natl Acad. Sci. USA, 82, 7845–7849.

Raymond, V.W. and Parsons, J.T. (1987). Identification of an amino terminal domain required for the transforming activity of the Rous sarcoma virus *src* protein. Virology, 160, 400–410.

Resh, M.D. and Erikson, R.L. (1985). Highly specific antibody to Rous sarcoma virus *src* gene product recognizes a novel population of pp60^{v-src} and pp60^{c-src} molecules. J. Cell Biol., 100, 409–417.

Resh, M.D. and Ling, H.-P. (1990). Identification of a 32K plasma membrane protein that binds to the myristylated amino-terminal sequence of p60^{v-src}. Nature, 346, 84–86.

Reynolds, A.B., Vila, J., Lansing, T.J., Potts, W.M., Weber, M.J. and Parsons, J.T. (1987). Activation of the oncogenic potential of the avian cellular *src* protein by specific structural alteration of the carboxy terminus. EMBO J., 6, 2359–2364.

Reynolds, A.B., Roesel, D.J., Kanner, S.B.. and Parsons, J.T. (1989a). Transformation-specific tyrosine phosphorylation of a novel cellular protein in chicken cells expressing oncogenic variants of the avian cellular *src* gene. Mol. Cell. Biol., 9, 629–638.

Reynolds, A.B., Kanner, S.B., Wang, H.C. and Parsons, J.T. (1989b). Stable association of activated pp60^{src} with two tyrosine-phosphorylated cellular proteins. Mol. Cell. Biol., 9, 3951–3958.

Reynolds, A.B., Herbert, L., Cleveland, J.L., Berg, S.T. and Gaut, J.R. (1992). p120, a novel substrate of protein tyrosine kinase receptors and of p60^{v-src}, is related to cadherin-binding factors β-catenin, plakoglobulin and *armadillo*. Oncogene, 7, 2439–2445.

Rohrschneider, L. and Reynolds, S. (1985). Regulation of cellular morphology by Rous sarcoma virus *src* gene: analysis of fusiform mutants. Mol. Cell. Biol., 5, 3097–3107.

Rossomando, A.J., Payne, D.M., Weber, M.J and Sturgill, T.W. (1989). Evidence that pp42, a major tyrosine kinase target protein, is a mitogen-activated serine/threonine protein kinase. Proc. Natl Acad. Sci. USA, 86, 6940–6943.

Roussel, R.R., Brodeur, S.R., Shalloway, D. and Laudano, A.P. (1991). Selective binding of activated pp60^{c-src}

by an immobilized synthetic phosphopeptide modeled on the carboxyl terminus of pp60^{c-src}. Proc. Natl Acad. Sci. USA, 88, 10696–10700.

Rozakis-Adcock, M., McGlade, J., Mbamalu, G., Pelicci, G., Daly, R., Li, W., Batzer, A., Thomas, S., Brugge, J., Pelicci, P.G., Schlessinger, J. and Pawson, T. (1992). Association of the shc and grb2/sem-5 SH2-containing proteins is implicated in activation of the ras pathway by tyrosine kinases. Nature, 360, 689–692.

Ruggiero, M., Wang, L.M. and Pierce, J.H. (1991). Mitogenic signal transduction in normal and transformed 32D hematopoietic cells. FEBS Letts., 291, 203–207.

Sato, M., Kato, J. and Takeya, T. (1989). Characterization of partially activated p60^{c-src} in chicken embryo fibroblasts. J. Virol., 63, 683–688.

Schaller, M.D., Borgman, C.A., Cobb, B.S., Vines, R.R., Reynolds, A.B. and Parsons, J.T. (1992). pp125^{FAK}, a structurally distinctive protein-tyrosine kinase associated with focal adhesions. Proc. Natl Acad. Sci. USA, 89, 5192–5196.

Schindler, C., Shuai, K., Prezioso, V.R. and Darnell, J.E. (1992). Interferon-dependent tyrosine kinase phosphorylation of a latent cytoplasmic transcription factor. Science, 257, 809–813.

Schlaepfer, D.D. and Haigler, H.T. (1990). Expression of annexins as a function of cellular growth state. J. Cell Biol., 111, 229–238.

Schuuring, E., Verhoeven, E., Litvinov, S. and Michalides, R.J.A M. (1993). The product of the *EMS1* gene, amplified and overexpressed in human carcinomas, is homologous to a v-*src* substrate and is located in cell-substratum contact sites. Mol. Cell. Biol., 13, 2891–2898.

Schwartz, D.E., Tizard, R. and Gilbert, W. (1983). Nucleotide sequence of Rous sarcoma virus. Cell, 32, 853–869.

Sefton, B.M., Hunter, T., Ball, E.H. and Singer, S.J. (1981). Vinculin: a cytoskeletal target of the transforming protein of Rous sarcoma virus. Cell, 24, 165–174.

Sefton, B.M., Hunter, T., Nigg, E.A., Singer, S.J. and Walker, G. (1982). Cytoskeletal targets for viral transforming proteins with tyrosine protein kinase activity. Cold Spring Harbor Symp. Quant. Biol., 46, 939–951.

Shalloway, D., Coussens, P.M. and Yaciuk, P. (1984). Overexpression of the c-*src* protein does not induce transformation of NIH 3T3 cells. Proc. Natl Acad. Sci. USA, 81, 7071–7075.

Shenoy, S., Choi, J.-K., Bagrodia, S., Copeland, T.D., Maller, J.L. and Shalloway, D. (1989). Purified maturation promoting factor phosphorylates pp60^{c-src} at the sites phosphorylated during fibroblast mitosis. Cell, 57, 763–774.

Shenoy, S., Chackalaparampil, I., Bagrodia, S., Lin, P.-H. and Shalloway, D. (1992). Role of p34^{cdc2}-mediated phosphorylations in two-step activation of pp60^{c-src} during mitosis. Proc. Natl Acad. Sci. USA, 89, 7237–7241.

Siliciano, J., Morrow, T.A. and Desiderio, S.V. (1992). *itk*, a T-cell-specific tyrosine kinase gene inducible by interleukin 2. Proc. Natl Acad. Sci. USA, 89, 11194–11198.

Simon, M.A., Kornberg, T.B. and Bishop, J.M. (1983). Three loci related to the *src* oncogene and tyrosine-specific protein kinase activity in *Drosophila*. Nature, 302, 837–839.

Simon, M.A., Drees, B., Kornberg, T. and Bishop, J.M. (1985). The nucleotide sequence and the tissue-specific expression of *Drosophila* c-*src*. Cell, 42, 831–840.

Smart, J.E., Oppermann, H., Czernilofsky, A.P., Purchio, A.F., Erikson, R.L. and Bishop, J.M. (1981). Characterization of sites for tyrosine phosphorylation in the transforming protein of Rous sarcoma virus (pp60^{v-src}) and its normal cellular homologue (pp60^{c-src}). Proc. Natl Acad. Sci. USA, 78, 6013–6017.

Songyang, Z., Shoelson, S.E., Chaudhuri, M., Gish, G., Pawson, T., Haser, W.G., King, F., Roberts, T., Ratnofsky, S., Lechleider, R.J., Neel, B.G., Birge, R.B., Fajardo, J.E., Chou, M.M., Hanafusa, H., Schaffhausen, B. and Cantley, L. (1993). SH2 domains recognize specific phosphopeptide sequences. Cell, 72, 767–778.

Soriano, P., Montgomery, C., Geske, R. and Bradley, A. (1991). Targeted disruption of the *src* proto-oncogene leads to osteoporosis in mice. Cell, 64, 693–702.

Stahl, M.L., Ferenz, C.R., Kelleher, K.L., Kriz, R.W. and Knopf, J.L. (1988). Sequence similarity of phospholipase C with the non-catalytic region of *src*. Nature, 332, 269–272.

Steele, R.E. (1985). Two divergent cellular *src* genes are expressed in *Xenopus laevis*. Nucleic Acids Res., 13, 1747–1761.

Steele, R.E., Unger, T.F., Mardis, M.J. and Fero, J.B. (1989). The two *Xenopus laevis* SRC genes are co-expressed and each produces functional pp60^{src}. J. Biol. Chem., 264, 10649–10653.

Stoker, A.W., Kellie, S. and Wyke, J.A. (1986). Intracellular localization and processing of pp60^{v-src} proteins expressed by two distinct temperature-sensitive mutants of Rous sarcoma virus. J. Virol., 58, 876–883.

Sudol, M., Alvarez-Buylla, A. and Hanafusa, H. (1988). Differential developmental expression of cellular *yes* and cellular *src* proteins in cerebellum. Oncogene Res, 2, 345–355.

Sweet, L.J., Alcorta, D.A., Jones, S.W., Erikson, E. and Erikson, R.L. (1990). Identification of mitogen-responsive ribosomal protein S6 kinase pp90^{rsk}, a homolog of *Xenopus* S6 kinase II, in chicken embryo fibroblasts. Mol. Cell. Biol., 10, 2413–2417.

Takeya, T. and Hanafusa, H. (1983). Structure and sequence of the cellular gene homologous to the RSV *src* gene and the mechanism for generating the transforming virus. Cell, 32, 881–890 (and correction: Cell, 34, 319, 1983).

Takeya, T., Feldman, R.A. and Hanafusa, H. (1982). DNA sequence of the viral and cellular src gene of chickens. J. Virol., 44, 1–11.

Talmage, D.A., Freund, R., Young, A.T., Dahl, J., Dawe, C.J. and Benjamin, T.L. (1989). Phosphorylation of middle T by pp60$^{c\text{-}src}$: a switch for binding of phosphatidylinositol 3-kinase and optimal tumorigenesis. Cell, 59, 55–65.

Tanaka, A., Gibbs, C.P., Arthur, R.R., Anderson, S.K., Kung, H.-J. and Fujita, D.J. (1987). DNA sequence encoding the amino-terminal region of the human c-*src* protein: implications of sequence divergence among *src*-type kinase oncogenes. Mol. Cell. Biol., 7, 1978–1983.

Tapley, P., Horwitz, A., Buck, C., Duggan, K. and Rohrschneider, L. (1989). Integrins isolated from Rous sarcoma virus-transformed chicken embryo fibroblasts. Oncogene, 4, 325–333.

Trahey, M., Wong, G., Halenbeck, R., Rubinfeld, B., Martin, G.A., Ladner, M., Long, C.M., Crosier, W.J., Watt, K., Koths, K. and McCormick, F. (1988). Molecular cloning of two types of GAP complementary DNA from human placenta. Science, 242, 1697–1700.

Turner, C.E. (1991). Paxillin is a major phosphotyrosine-containing protein during embryonic development. J. Cell Biol., 115, 201–207.

Turner, C.E., Glenney, J.R. and Burridge, K. (1990). Paxillin: a new vinculin-binding protein present in focal adhesions. J. Cell Biol., 111, 1059–1068.

Ulug, E.T., Hawkins, P.T., Hanley, M.R. and Courtneidge, S.A. (1990). Phosphatidylinositol metabolism in cells transformed by polyomavirus middle T antigen. J. Virol., 64, 3895–3904.

Veillette, A., O'Shaughnessy, J., Horak, I.D., Israel, M.A., Yee, D., Rosen, N., Fujita, D.J., Kung, H.-J., Biedler, J.L. and Bolen, J.B. (1989). Coordinate alteration of pp60$^{c\text{-}src}$ abundance and c-*src* RNA expression in human neuroblastoma variants. Oncogene, 4, 421–427.

Verderame, M.F., Kaplan, J.M. and Varmus, H.E. (1989). A mutation in v-*src* that removes a single conserved residue in the SH2 domain of pp60$^{v\text{-}src}$ restricts transformation in a host-dependent manner. J. Virol., 63, 338–348.

Vetrie, D., Vorechovsky, I., Sideras, P., Holland, J., Davies, A., Flinter, F., Hammarstrom, L., Kinnon, C., Levinsky, R., Bobrow, M., Smith, C.I.E. and Bentley, D.R. (1993). The gene involved in X-linked agammaglobulinaemia is a member of the *src* family of protein-tyrosine kinases. Nature, 361, 226–233.

Vogel, U.S., Dixon, R.A.F., Schaber, M.D., Diehl, R.E., Marshall, M.S., Scolnick, E.M., Sigal, I.S. and Gobbs, J.R. (1988). Cloning of bovine GAP and its interaction with oncogenic *ras* p21. Nature, 335, 90–93.

Vogel, W., Lammers, R., Huang, J. and Ullrich, A. (1993). Activation of a phosphotyrosine phosphatase by tyrosine phosphorylation. Science, 259, 1611–1614.

Volberg, T., Geiger, B., Dror, R. and Zick, Y. (1991). Modulation of intercellular adherens-type junctions and tyrosine phosphorylation of their components in RSV-transformed cultured chick lens cells. Cell. Regul., 2, 105–120.

Wadsworth, S.C., Madhavan, K. and Bilodeau-Wentworth, D. (1985). Maternal inheritance of transcripts from three *Drosophila src*-related genes. Nucleic Acids Res., 13, 2153–2170.

Wages, D.S., Keefer, J., Rall, T.B. and Weber, M.J. (1992). Mutations in the SH3 domain of the *src* oncogene which decrease association of phosphatidylinositol 3'-kinase activity with pp60$^{v\text{-}src}$ and alter cellular morphology. J. Virol., 66, 1866–1874.

Waksman, G., Kominos, D., Robertson, S.C., Pant, N., Baltimore, D., Birge, R.B., Cowburn, D., Hanafusa, H., Mayer, B.J., Overduin, M., Resh, M.D., Rios, C.B., Silverman, L. and Kuriyan, J. (1992). Crystal structure of the phosphotyrosine recognition domain SH2 of v-*src* complexed with tyrosine-phosphorylated peptides. Nature, 358, 646–653.

Waksman, G., Shoelson, S.E., Pant, N., Cowburn, D. and Kuriyan, J. (1993). Binding of a high affinity phosphotyrosyl peptide to the Src SH2 domain: crystal structures of the complexed and peptide-free forms. Cell, 72, 779–790.

Wang, H.-C.R. and Parsons, J.T. (1989). Deletions and insertions within an amino-terminal domain of pp60$^{v\text{-}src}$ inactivate transformation and modulate membrane stability. J. Virol., 63, 291–302.

Welham, M.J. and Wyke, J.A. (1988). A single point mutation has pleiotropic effects on pp60$^{v\text{-}src}$ function. J. Virol., 62, 1898–1906.

Wendler, P.A. and Boschelli, F. (1989). Src homology 2 domain deletion mutants of p60$^{v\text{-}src}$ do not phosphorylate cellular proteins of 120–150 kDa. Oncogene, 4, 231–236.

White, M.K. and Weber, M.J. (1990). The *src* oncogene can regulate a human glucose transporter expressed in chicken embryo fibroblasts. Mol. Cell. Biol., 10, 1301–1306.

Whitman, M., downes, C.P., Keeler, M., Keller, T. and Cantley. L. (1988). Type I phosphatidylinositol kinase makes a novel inositol phospholipid, phosphatidylinositol-3–phosphate. Nature, 332, 644–646.

Wiestler, O.D. and Walter, G. (1988). Developmental expression of two forms of pp60$^{c\text{-}src}$ in mouse brain. Mol. Cell. Biol., 8, 502–504.

Willman, C.L., Stewart, C.C., Griffith, J.K., Stewart, S.J. and Tomasi, T.B. (1987). Differential expression and regulation of c-*src* and c-*fgr* protooncogenes in myelomonocytic cells. Proc. Natl Acad. Sci. USA, 84, 14480–14484.

Wong, S., Reynolds, A.B. and Papkoff, J. (1992). Platelet activation leads to increased c-*src* kinase activity and association of c-*src* with an 85-kDa tyrosine phosphoprotein. Oncogene, 7, 2407–2415.

Wu, H., Reynolds, A.B., Kanner, S.B., Vines, R.R. and Parsons, J.T. (1991). Identification and characterization of a novel cytoskeleton-associated pp60^{src} substrate. Mol. Cell. Biol., 11, 5113–5124.

Wyke, J.A. and Stoker, A.W. (1987). Genetic analysis of the form and function of the viral *src* oncogene product. Biochim. Biophys. Acta, 907, 47–69.

Yaciuk, P., Cannella, M.T. and Shalloway, D. (1988). Comparison of the effects of carboxyl terminal truncation and point mutations on pp60$^{c\text{-}src}$ activities. Oncogene Res., 3, 207–212.

Yaciuk, P., Choi, J.-K. and Shalloway, D. (1989). Mutation of amino acids in pp60$^{c\text{-}src}$ that are phosphorylated by protein kinases C and A. Mol. Cell. Biol., 9, 2453–2463.

Yang, X. and Walter, G. (1988). Specific kinase activity and phosphorylation state of pp60$^{c\text{-}src}$ from neuroblastomas and fibroblasts. Oncogene, 3, 237–244.

Yonemoto, W., Jarvis-Morar, M., Brugge, J.S., Bolen, J.B. and Israel, M.A. (1985). Tyrosine phosphorylation within the amino-terminal domain of pp60$^{c\text{-}src}$ molecules associated with polyoma middle-sized tumor antigen. Proc. Natl Acad. Sci. USA, 82, 4568–4572.

Yu, H., Rosen, M.K., Shin, T.B., Seidel-Dugan, C., Brugge, J.S. and Schreiber, S.L. (1992). Solution structure of the SH3 domain of src and identification of its ligand binding site. Science, 258, 1665–1668.

Zamencik, P.C. and Stephenson, M.L. (1978). Inhibition of Rous sarcoma virus replication and cell transformation by a specific oligodeoxynucleotide. Proc. Natl Acad. Sci. USA, 75, 280–284.

Zhao, Y., Sudol, M., Hanafusa, H. and Krueger, J. (1992). Increased tyrosine kinase activity of c-src during calcium-induced keratinocyte differentiation. Proc. Natl Acad. Sci. USA, 89, 8298–8302.

Zheng, X.M., Wang, Y. and Pallen, C.J. (1992). Cell transformation and activation of pp60$^{c\text{-}src}$ by overexpression of a protein tyrosine phosphatase. Nature, 359, 336–339.

TAL1

TAL1 (also called SCL (stem cell leukaemia) or TCL5) was identified in a chromosome trans-location in a stem cell leukaemia (Begley et al., 1989a).

Cross-species homology

TAL1: 94% identity (human and mouse); 68% identity (human and chicken; Goodwin et al., 1992).

Transformation

In 3% of T cell acute lymphoblastic leukaemias (T-ALLs) the translocation (1;14)(p32;q11) transposes TAL1 into the T cell receptor δ gene.

	TAL1/Tal-1
Nucleotides (kb)	16
Chromosome	
Human	1p32
Exons	6
mRNA	Type A (exons 1a–4–5/6); type B (exons 1b–2–3–4–5/6)
	~3.0/4.7 kb
	Alternative splicing can link exon 1a to 2 or 1b to 4 or utilize an alternative intron to split exons 5 and 6
Amino acids	
Human	331
Mouse	329
Chicken	311
Mass (kDa)	
(predicted)	34
(expressed)	22/42

Tissue location

TAL1 is expressed in developing brain, normal bone marrow and mast cells, mast cell lines, leukaemic T cell, megakaryocytic and erythroleukaemic cell lines (Green et al., 1992), but not in normal T cells. *TAL1* is thus expressed in cells of the same three lineages as the haematopoietic transcription factor *Gata-1*. In non-haematopoietic murine tissues *Tal-1* is only expressed in adult and developing brain, in which *Gata-1* has not been detected.

Protein function

TAL1 is a transcription factor. It forms heterodimers with E12 or E47 that bind to the E box (CANNTG) eukaryotic enhancer element, as does MyoD (Hsu *et al.*, 1991). *Tal-1* expression is necessary for erythroid cell differentiation and is regulated by the erythroid transcription factor GATA1 (Aplan *et al.*, 1992). In the early myeloid cell line 416B, *Gata-1* but not *Tal-1* induces differentiation into megakaryocytes (Visvader *et al.*, 1992). *Tal-1* may be involved in neural differentiation (Green *et al.*, 1992).

The transposition of *TAL1* into the T cell receptor δ gene in the T-ALL translocation (1;14)(p32;q11) results in elevated expression of *TAL1* mRNA in the leukaemic cells. In 25% of T-ALL there is a 90 kb deletion (*tal*^d or *tal*^{d1}) upstream from one allele of the *TAL1* locus, probably due to aberrant Ig recombinase activity (Aplan *et al.*, 1990; Brown *et al.*, 1990). A second specific deletion (*tal*^{d2}) occurs in 6% of T-ALLs. The t(1;14) translocations and both *tal*^d deletions disrupt the 5′ end of the *TAL1* gene so that its expression is controlled by the regulatory elements of the TCRδ or *SIL* genes that are both normally expressed in T cell ontogeny (Bernard *et al.*, 1991).

Protein structure

Helix–loop–helix protein.

Sequences of human, mouse and chicken TAL1

```
Human    (1)   MT ERPPSEAAR SDPQLEGR DA AEAS        MAPPH  QVLLNGVAKETSR        AAAAEP
Mouse    (1)   -- --------- -------Q -- ---R        -----  ------------        --P---
Chicken  (1)   --MD---APPPPS---RDAR-H-PE-D-TSEPDSSRGG-E--AEP-L----A---AG-PSPGPP---VP

Human    (50)  PVIELGARGGPGGGPAGGGGAARDLKGRDAATAEARHRVPTTELCRPPGPAPAPAPASVTAELPGDGRMV
Mouse    (50)  --------S-A-----S------------VA----L------------------AP---------
Chicken  (70)  ----VR---SL        ---S-E--G  --MQ-A-GA-P--            A--AACEA---

Human    (120) QLSPPALAAPAAPGRALLYSLSQPLASLGSGFFGEPDAFPMFTTNNRVKRRPSPYEMEITDGPHTKVVRR
Mouse    (120) ----------G-------------------------------N----------------S--------__
Chicken  (114) -------PLQ P----M--N-G---GTI---------S-S-YGS- ---------------------

Human    (190) IFTNSRERWRQQNVNGAFAELRKLIPTHPPDKKLSKNEILRLAMKYINFLAKLLNDQEEEGTQRAKTGKD
Mouse    (190) --------------------------------------------------------------P ---
Chicken  (172) -------------------------------------------------------------N--G-VN--

Human    (260) PVVGAGGGGGGGGGAPPDDLLQDVLSPNSSCGSSLDGAASPDSYTEE   PAPKHTARSLHPAMLPAADGAGPR (331)
Mouse    (249) --------A--- I--E-------------------------       -T----S------L---------- (329)
Chicken  (242) SGIVQ        E-----M------------------F---HDTLDS-- --N--H-I--VEGS-Q - (311)
```

The helix–loop–helix and upstream hydrophilic region is underlined.

Databank file names and accession numbers

	GENE	EMBL	SWISSPROT	REFERENCES
Human	TAL1	Hsscl M29038 Hsscll-3 M61103–M61105 Hssc14–7 M63572; M63576; M63584; M63589	SCL_HUMAN P17542	Aplan et al., 1990 Begley et al., 1989b
Chicken	Tal-1	Gdasclpro X63371	SCL_CHICK P24899	Goodwin et al., 1992
Mouse	Tal-1	Mmscl M59764	SCL_MOUSE P22091	Begley et al., 1991

Papers

Aplan, P.D., Begley, C.G., Bertness, V., Nussmeier, M., Ezquerra, A., Coligan, J. and Kirsch, I.R. (1990). The SCL gene is formed from a transcriptionally complex locus. Mol. Cell. Biol., 10, 6426–6435.

Aplan, P.D., Nakahara, K., Orkin, S.H. and Kirsch, I.R. (1992). The SCL gene product: a positive regulator of erythroid differentiation. EMBO J., 11, 4073–4081.

Begley, C.G., Aplan, P.D., Davey, M.P., Nakahara, K., Tchorz, K., Kurtzberg, J., Hershfield, M., Haynes, B.F., Cohen, D.I., Waldmann, T.A. and Kirsch, I.R. (1989a). Chromosomal translocation in a human leukemic stem-cell line disrupts the T-cell antigen receptor δ-chain diversity region and results in a previously unreported fusion transcript. Proc. Natl Acad. Sci. USA, 86, 2031–2035.

Begley, C.G., Aplan, P.D., Denning, S.M., Haynes, B.F., Waldmann, T.A. and Kirsch, I.R. (1989b). The gene SCL is expressed during early hematopoiesis and encodes a differentiation-related DNA-binding motif. Proc. Natl Acad. Sci. USA, 86, 10128–10132.

Begley, C.G., Visvader, J., Green, A.R., Aplan, P.D., Metcalf, D., Kirsch, I.R. and Gough, N.M. (1991). Molecular cloning and chromosomal localization of the murine homolog of the human helix–loop–helix gene SCL. Proc. Natl Acad. Sci. USA, 88, 869–873.

Bernard, O., Lecointe, N., Jonveaux, P., Souyri, M., Mauchauffe, M., Berger, R., Larsen, C.J. and Mathieu-Mahul, D. (1991). Two site-specific deletions and t(1;14) translocation restricted to human T-cell acute leukemias disrupt the 5′ part of the TAL1 gene. Oncogene, 6, 1477–1488.

Brown, L., Cheng, J.-T., Chen, Q., Siciliano, M.J., Crist, W., Buchanan, G. and Baer, R. (1990). Site-specific recombination of the TAL1 gene is a common occurrence in human T cell leukemia. EMBO J., 9, 3343–3351.

Goodwin, G., MacGregor, A., Zhu, J. and Crompton, M.R. (1992). Molecular cloning of the chicken SCL cDNA. Nucleic Acids Res., 20, 368.

Green, A.R., Lints, T., Visvader, J., Harvey, R. and Begley, C.G. (1992). SCL is coexpressed with GATA-1 in hemopoietic cells but is also expressed in developing brain. Oncogene, 7, 653–660.

Hsu, H.-L., Cheng, J.-T. and Baer, R. (1991). Enhancer-binding activity of the TAL1 oncoprotein in association with the E47/E12 helix–loop–helix proteins. Mol. Cell. Biol., 11, 3037–3042.

Visvader, J.E., Elefanty, A.G., Strasser, A. and Adams, J.M. (1992). GATA-1 but not SCL induces megakaryocytic differentiation in an early myeloid line. EMBO J., 11, 4557–4564.

THR/ErbA, EGFR/ErbB-1, HER2/Neu, HER3 and HER4

v-*erbB* is the oncogene of the avian *erythroblastosis virus* (AEV), strain AEV-H. Strain AEV-ES4 carries the v-*erbA* and v-*erbB* oncogenes (Rothe Meyer and Engelbreth-Holm, 1933).

ErbA-1 encodes thyroid hormone receptor α (human *THRA1*) and *ErbA-2* encodes thyroid hormone receptor β (human *THRB*), both of which are receptors for triiodothyronine (T_3).

EGFR (*ErbB-1*) encodes the receptor for epidermal growth factor.

HER2 (human)/*ErbB-2* are homologues of rat *Neu*, closely related to but distinct from *ErbB-1*/*EGFR*. *Neu* was first identified by transfection with DNA from *neuroglioblastomas* that had arisen in rats exposed *in utero* to ethylnitrosourea (Shih *et al.*, 1981). *HER2* was identified by screening genomic and cDNA libraries (Semba *et al.*, 1985; King *et al.*, 1985; Coussens *et al.*, 1985).

HER3/*ErbB-3* and *HER4*/*ErbB-4* are additional members of the *EGFR* family, distinct from *ErbB-1* and *ErbB-2*.

Related genes

THRA1 and *THRB* are members of a superfamily numbering nearly 30 that includes the receptors for steroids, retinoic acid and vitamin D_3 (Giguere *et al.*, 1987; Arriza *et al.*, 1987). The subfamily of thyroid hormone receptors (THRs) and retinoic acid receptors (RARs) comprises three RARs (α, β and γ), three retinoid X receptors (RXR-α, β, γ), two THRs (α and β) and several "orphan receptors" for which ligands have yet to be identified.

EAR2 (erbA-related/*ERBAL2*: chromosome 19) and *EAR3* (*ERBAL3*: chromosome 5) are human *THRA1*-related genes encoding DNA binding proteins (Miyajima *et al.*, 1988). *EAR3* (or chicken ovalbumin upstream promoter, COUP) binds to the ovalbumin promoter and, in conjunction with another protein (S300-II), stimulates transcriptional initiation (Wang *et al.*, 1989). It is closely similar to *Drosophila seven-up*.

In *Drosophila*, DER is homologous in the extracellular (41%) and kinase domains (55%) to human EGFR (Livneh *et al.*, 1985; Wadsworth *et al.*, 1985).

In *Xiphophorus maculatus*, *Xmrk*, a melanoma-inducing gene, encodes a receptor tyrosine kinase closely related to the EGFR (Adam *et al.*, 1991).

There is extensive genetic linkage conservation between the *Erb* genes in the human and murine genomes and *Erbb*, *Csfgm*, *Evi-2*, *Erba*, *Myla* and *Hox-2* map to the same region of mouse chromosome 11 (Buchberg *et al.*, 1989).

Cross-species homology

THRA1 and THRB: >91% identity (man, chicken and rat). Human EGFR: 75%, 97% and 65% identity with the chicken ERBB1 in the extracellular, tyrosine kinase and C-terminal (227 amino acid) regions, respectively. HER2 and NEU: 80% identity (humans and rats).

Transformation

MAN

THRA1/*THRB*: In colon carcinomas expression of the larger transcript (6 kb) of *THRB* is suppressed; expression of *THRA1* and *THRA2* is unaffected (Markowitz *et al.*, 1989).

EGFR: *EGFR* is amplified by up to 50-fold in some primary tumours (squamous cell carcinomas and glioblastomas) and derived cell lines (Liberman *et al.*, 1985; Yamamoto *et al.*, 1986b; Lacroix *et al.*, 1989; Gullick, 1991), in ~20% of bladder tumours (Proctor *et al.*, 1991) and in cell lines derived from a human bladder carcinoma (A431; Lin *et al.*, 1984; Ullrich *et al.*, 1984) and a human gastric cancer (Fukushige *et al.*, 1986). Amplification also occurs in ~20% of primary breast tumours where it is strongly associated with early recurrence and death in lymph node-positive patients (Tsuda *et al.*, 1989; Zhou *et al.*, 1989; Thor *et al.*, 1989; Horak *et al.*, 1991; Borg *et al.*, 1991; Paterson *et al.*, 1991). In breast tumours *EGFR* expression correlates with that of *P53* but is inversely correlated with *MYB* amplification.

Although elevated transcription of *EGFR* correlates with the absence of steroid hormone receptors, it is reduced by tamoxifen, presumably acting via targets other than the estrogen receptor (Le Roy *et al.*, 1991). *EGFR* is infrequently amplified in pediatric gliomas (Wasson *et al.*, 1990). Monoclonal antibody directed against EGFR has been used for radioimaging in patients with squamous cell carcinoma of the lung (Divgi *et al.*, 1991).

HER2: Unlike the rat *Neu* oncogene, *HER2* does not have an activated mutant form. However, it is overexpressed with high frequency in human adenocarcinomas of the breast, stomach and ovary, in bladder carcinomas (Slamon *et al.*, 1987; Yokota *et al.*, 1988; Wright *et al.*, 1990) and in 20–36% of breast and ovarian cancers (Guerin *et al.*, 1988; Slamon *et al.*, 1989). In some breast cancer cell lines *HER2* is overexpressed but not amplified (Kraus *et al.*, 1987). In lymph-node-positive patients there is a strong correlation between *HER2* amplification and poor prognosis although the expression of *HER2* does not appear to promote metastasis (Rio *et al.*, 1987; Ro *et al.*, 1989; Slamon *et al.*, 1989; Berchuck *et al.*, 1990). It has been found that 12.5% of breast cancers overexpress both *HER2* and *MYC* and this co-expression correlates with the worst prognosis. *HER2* overexpression is also an indicator of high risk of recurrence in node-negative patients (Paterson *et al.*, 1991). Co-amplification of *HER2* and topoisomerase IIα has also been detected in some primary breast cancers (Smith *et al.*, 1993).

HER2 overexpression or amplification has also been correlated with poor prognosis in endometrial cancer (Borst *et al.*, 1990; Berchuck *et al.*, 1991), adenocarcinoma of the lung (Kern *et al.*, 1990) and in gastric cancer (Yonemura *et al.*, 1991). Amplified or overexpressed *HER2* has also been detected in colon cancer (Tal *et al.*, 1988; D'Emilia *et al.*, 1989), salivary gland adenocarcinoma (Riviere *et al.*, 1991), squamous cell carcinoma of the lung (Kern *et al.*, 1990), thyroid tumours (Aasland *et al.*, 1988) and in a malignant lymphoma (Imamura *et al.*, 1990).

HER3: This is expressed in carcinomas and, with low frequency, in sarcomas. It is not detectable in cell lines derived from haematopoietic tumours. It is overexpressed in a subset of mammary tumour-derived cell lines (Kraus *et al.*, 1989).

ANIMALS

v-*erbA* alone is not tumorigenic but cooperates with v-*ets* to cause avian erythroleukaemia (Metz and Graf, 1992). v-*erbB* is the transduced gene in avian retroviruses (e.g. avian leukosis virus) that causes rapid induction of erythroblastosis and (after intramuscular injection of the virus) sarcomas. Inoculation of cells or plasmids expressing non-mutated *erbB* causes renal neoplasia in chickens (Taglienti-Sian *et al.*, 1993).

The RAV-1 retrovirus that does not carry an oncogene induces clonal erythroleukaemia in some strains of chicken; this is due to the activation of the *ErbB* gene by proviral insertion. The resulting transcript suffers a deletion of the ligand binding domain (Beug *et al.*, 1986).

Cells derived from human epidermoid lung tumours are tumorigenic in nude mice but transfected cells expressing *RARB* are markedly less tumorigenic, indicating a possible tumour suppressor gene function for *RARB* (Houle *et al.*, 1993).

The expression of oncogenic NEU in mouse mammary epithelium can cause frank ductal carcinoma but may also induce epithelial abnormalities resembling those of human sclerosing adenosis and atypical hyperplasia that may be precursors of ductal carcinoma (Bradbury *et al.*, 1993).

IN VITRO

v-*erbA* cooperates with v-*erbB* and related sarcoma-inducing oncogenes (and with *Hras*) to block erythroid cell differentiation (into erythrocytes) and promote transformation. The capacity of v-*erbA* to block differentiation correlates with transcriptional arrest of erythrocyte-specific genes (see **Protein function**; Zenke *et al.*, 1988). v-*erbA* alone can transform erythrocytic progenitor cells, although by itself it does not cause tumours. v-*erbB* alone stimulates proliferation of erythrocyte progenitor cells but does not completely block their differentiation. v-*erbB* alone transforms chick embryo fibroblasts (CEFs) whereas v-*erbA* only stimulates CEF growth *in vitro* but enhances the tumorigenicity of v-*erbB*-transformed CEFs (Zenke *et al.*, 1990). v-*erbB* transformation of cells causes phosphorylation on tyrosine residues of fibronectin receptor proteins (Hirst *et al.*, 1986). v-*erbA* is a thyroid hormone and retinoic acid receptor antagonist and the corresponding protein does not bind thyroid hormones (Sap *et al.*, 1986; Sande *et al.*, 1993).

EGFR and NEU differ quantitatively and qualitatively in their effects: NEU is a 100-fold better transforming agent than EGFR in NIH 3T3 cells (DiFiore *et al.*, 1987b; Hudziak *et al.*, 1987; Riedel *et al.*, 1988) but in an interleukin-3-dependent myeloid precursor line expression of the EGFR induces ligand-independent proliferation whereas NEU is without effect. Differences depend strongly on the N-terminal region of the tyrosine kinase domains (EGFR residues 660–667; Segatto *et al.*, 1991).

The DNA from tumours (neuro- and glio-blastomas) induced in BDIX rats by ethylnitrosourea transforms NIH 3T3 cells due to the action of NEU. The transformed cells induce tumours in mice (Padhy *et al.*, 1982). Expression of the normal *Neu* cDNA does not usually cause transformation; however, massive overexpression caused by driving the gene with the Mo-MuLV LTR can transform NIH 3T3 cells (DiFiore *et al.*, 1987a).

Overexpression of either human *HER2* or rat *Neu* transforms NIH 3T3 fibroblasts and *Neu*-induced transformation can occur independently of the EGF receptor (Chazin *et al.*, 1992). Transformation of NIH 3T3 fibroblasts by oncogenic *Neu* causes the cells to exhibit metastatic properties both *in vitro* and *in vivo* (Yu and Hung, 1991). *Neu*-transformed NIH 3T3 cells revert to the normal phenotype on treatment with azatyrosine (Fujita-Yoshigaki *et al.*, 1992). Adenovirus E1A protein binds to the element (G)TGG$^A/_T$$^A/_T$$^A/_T$(G) in the *Neu* promoter (human −296 to −289; mouse −268 to −261) and suppresses *Neu*-induced metastasis of NIH 3T3 cells (Yu *et al.*, 1992). p105^{RB} suppresses *Neu* transformation by binding to the *cis*-acting element GTTGGAGGGGTGGGGGGGCGAGCC (mouse −258 to −235). The GGTGGGGGGG sequence (GTG element) is also the target for *Neu*-mediated autorepression of transcription (Zhao and Hung, 1992). *Myc* reverses the transformed morphology of NIH 3T3 cells induced by *Neu*, MYC protein binding to a 140 bp element (−312 to −173) of the *Neu* promoter (Suen and Hung, 1991). The sequence AAGATAAAACC (mouse −439 to −429) binds a *trans*-acting factor (RVF: *EcoRV* Factor on the *Neu* promoter) required for maximal transcription (Yan and Hung, 1991; White and Hung, 1992).

Monoclonal antibodies directed against p185^{HER2} specifically inhibit the proliferation of human breast carcinoma cells (Carter *et al.*, 1992).

TRANSGENIC ANIMALS

Transgenic mice carrying an activated *Neu* oncogene develop mammary adenocarcinomas and, occasionally, other tumours. Polyclonal (Muller *et al.*, 1988) or monoclonal (Bouchard *et al.*,

1989) mammary tumours develop in these animals depending on whether the MMTV LTR is adjacent to *Neu* cDNA or whether the two are separated by 600 bp, the latter construct presumably encoding an elongated NEU protein.

	THRA1/ErbA-1	*THRB/ErbA-2*	*v-erbA*
Nucleotides (kb)	27	60	
Chromosome			
Human	17q11.2–q12	3p24.1–p22	
Mouse	11		
Rat	10	15	
mRNA (kb)			
Human	2.7/5.2 (alternative splicing generates α-1 and α-2 receptors)	2.0/6.2	
Chicken	3.0/4.5/6.8	7.0	5.4
Exons			
Human	10	>7	
Chicken	8		
Amino acids			
Human	410 (α-1); 490 (α-2)	461	639 (*gag–erbA*)
Chicken	408	369	
Mass (kDa)			
(predicted)	47 (α-1); 55 (α-2)	52 42 (chicken)	72
(expressed)	48;58	52;55	p75$^{gag–erbA}$

Cellular location

Nuclei of normal and transformed cells.

Tissue location

THRA1 is ubiquitous. *THRB* is restricted: chicken *THRB/ErbA-2* is substantially expressed in brain, lung, kidney, eye and yolk sac, but undetectable in haematopoietic tissues (Forrest *et al.*, 1990). In chick brain ontogenesis *THRA1/ErbA-1* is expressed from the early embryonic stages; *THRB/ErbA-2* is rapidly induced after embryonic day 19 (Forrest *et al.*, 1991).

Protein function

v-ERBA suppresses transcription of avian erythrocyte anion transport (band III), carbonic anhydrase II and β-globin genes. v-ERBA is phosphorylated on Ser16/17 by protein kinase A or protein kinase C. Mutation of Ser16/17 to block phosphorylation releases the block of v-*erbB*- or v-*sea*-induced differentiation normally exerted by v-*erbA* and also allows band II and carbonic anhydrase II expression. v-*erbA* affects transformed erythroblasts in two ways: (i) it increases the pH range within which the cells will grow and (ii) it blocks the differentiation of erythroblasts into erythrocytes. The potent repressor function of v-ERBA requires the formation of heterodimeric complexes with retinoid X receptor (RXR-α) and C-terminal mutations in v-ERBA that abolish heterodimer formation also block v-ERBA repressor function (Hermann *et al.*, 1993). Despite being a constitutive repressor in animal cells, v-ERBA is a hormone-activated transcriptional activator in yeast. The functional domains of the protein required for activation of gene expression in yeast and for transformation of avian cells are closely similar (Smit-McBride and Privalsky, 1993).

THRA1 and THRB are transcription factors possessing zinc finger domains. Human THRA1 and THRB are the high-affinity receptors (k_d = 0.2 nM) for T_3 (Sap *et al.*, 1986; Weinberger *et al.*, 1986). THRA1 binds to the palindromic response element TCAGGTCATGACCTGA, repressing its activity as a promoter; T_3 binding to THRA1 activates transcription (Damm *et al.*, 1989). A second functional form of human THRB (*THRB2/ErbA-2*) exists.

Structure of viral genomes and major translation products

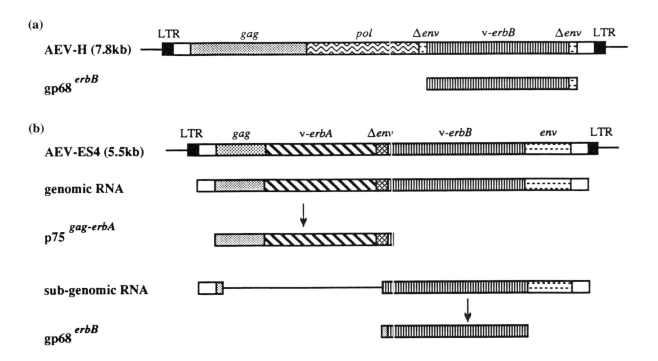

(a) The AEV-H genome carries genes encoding active *gag* proteins and reverse transcriptase (*pol*) as well as the oncogene *erbB* that is closely related to a portion of *EGFR* (see below) (Yamamoto *et al.*, 1983). *pol* and *erbB* are joined by a 66 nucleotide sequence of intronic ErbB. The four C-terminal amino acids of p68*erbB* are encoded by *env* but in a different reading frame to that used to translate the *env* product. In other strains of ALV that have transduced *ErbB*, the size of the captured 5' *ErbB* intron sequence and the site of the 3' junction differ from AEV-H. In most strains the 3′ junction is in the untranslated region of the *ErbB* gene, the C-terminal domain of *ErbB* remaining intact (Raines *et al.*, 1988).

(b) In the AEV-ES4 viral genome most of the multiple introns have been lost. The two *Erb* genes are inserted between *gag* and *env* and are separated by an *ErbB* intron sequence (nucleotides 1181–1370). The C-terminal four amino acids and the termination codon of P75$^{gag\text{-}erbA}$ are encoded by the 5′ region of the *ErbB* intron sequence (191 nucleotides). The 11 preceding P75$^{gag\text{-}erbA}$ amino acids are encoded by nucleotides 1151–1183 that are derived from *env*. Nucleotide 1371 of v-*erbB* corresponds to the beginning of homology with *EGFR* (Henry *et al.*, 1985). The *erb* genes are independently expressed and remain colinear with the coding domains of their cellular progenitors. P75$^{gag\text{-}erbA}$ is translated from 5.4 kb genomic RNA; p68^{erbB} from 3.5 kb spliced, subgenomic RNA containing AUG and six codons of *gag* that are spliced onto the codons of v-*erbB*.

v-ERBB is almost identical to the transmembrane and cytoplasmic domains of the EGFR (it has lost all but 61 amino acids of the extracellular domain). In the AEV-ES4 and AEV-H strains the C-terminal terminal autophosphorylation site is also deleted: they lack 73 and 34 amino acids, respectively, compared to the normal receptor. It is assumed that this confers constitutive activity on the protein, although it possesses only weak tyrosine kinase activity *in vitro*. Deletion of the E domain of v-ERBB (corresponding to residues 961–1102 of chicken EGFR) abolishes the capacity of AEV-H to transform erythroid cells without substantially affecting fibroblast transformation. The deletion of a negative regulatory region within the E domain (residues 1031–1055) enhances erythroid cell transformation (Lee *et al.*, 1993). Only 5–20% of v-ERBB is plasma membrane-associated, presumably due to the deletion of the signal sequence. In most of the other strains of ALV that have transduced *ErbB*, however, the C-terminal region remains intact, the 3′ junction being in the untranslated region (Raines *et al.*, 1988).

Transduced *erbB* was identified in derivatives of ALV (Graf and Beug, 1978). When ALV induces erythroblastosis, the proviral insertion sites are within the *ErbB* locus but upstream of the sequences represented in v-*erbB*. This is an example of promoter insertion: the provirus is in the same transcriptional orientation as *ErbB* and transcripts are initiated in the 5′ LTR and continue through the 3′ LTR into the *ErbB* sequence. RNA splicing removes most of the intervening sequences and links a viral splice donor to a splice acceptor site at the point in *ErbB* where homology with v-*erbB* begins (Nilsen *et al.*, 1985). This causes N-terminal truncation of the *ErbB* gene and the presence of the 5′ LTR causes enhanced transcription. Viral insertion occasionally introduces C-terminal deletions as well as N-terminal truncations; this confers the capacity for isolates of such viruses to transform fibroblasts as well as erythroid cells *in vitro* (Gamett *et al.*, 1986).

v-*erbB* carried by the ES4 or R strains of ASV induces erythroleukaemia and fibrosarcomas, whereas *ErbB* activated by proviral insertion induces only leukaemia. The critical mutations introduced into the transduced gene that are responsible for activating sarcomagenic potential are Arg263 to His, Ile384 to Ser and deletion of the C-terminal regulatory domain (residues 494–514). The Arg263 mutation increases kinase and autophosphorylation activity (Shu *et al.*, 1991).

The virus AEV-5005 contains a complete *ErbB* C-terminal domain whereas AAV-5005 has a deletion of 59 amino acids between positions 993 and 1051 of the chicken EGFR (Robinson *et al.*, 1992). Expression of either of these *erbB* genes causes erythroblastosis but the deletion in AAV-5005 confers the potential to induce angiosarcoma.

Structure of the human *THRA1* gene

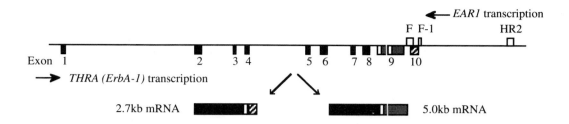

Boxes below the line represent *THRA1* (*ErbA-1*) exons 1–10: open boxes above the line represent the exons of the *THRA*-related *EAR1* gene (F: final, F–1: adjacent to final, HR2: homologue of rat exon 2) that is transcribed in the reverse direction (Miyajima *et al.*, 1989). An alternative splice site in *THRA1* exon 9 generates a 2.7 kb mRNA (THRA2, 490 amino acids: exons 1–8, the first 128 nucleotides of exon 9 and exon 10): the 5.0 kb mRNA (THRA1, 410 amino acids) contains sequences from exons 1 to 9. The initiation codon is in exon 2 (Laudet *et al.*, 1991). The product of the 5.0 kb transcript, human THRA1, binds T_3 and activates transcription of target genes. Human THRA2 does not bind T_3 and has been proposed to act as a dominant negative regulator of thyroid hormone receptors.

The human *THRA* promoter lacks TATA elements but is very GC-rich and contains many Sp-1 sites as well as hormone-responsive elements (Laudet *et al.*, 1993).

The intron–exon organization of the human and chicken *THRA/ErbA-1* genes is highly conserved within the DNA binding region. The intron–exon organization of human *THRB1* closely resembles that of chicken *THRA/ErbA-1*, although the sequences encoded differ (see below).

Sequences of chicken THRA/ERBA and v-ERBA proteins

```
Chicken THRA        (1)   MEQKPSTLDPLSEPEDTRWLDGKRKRKSSQCLVKSSMSGYIPSYLDKDEQCVVCGDKAT
v-ERBA (gag-erbA)         ------------------------------C---------------

                   (60)   GYHYRCITCEGCKGFFRRTIQKNLHPTYSCKYDGCCVIDKITRNQCQLCRFKKCISVGMA
                   (46)   -------------S---------------T-----------------------------

                  (120)   MDLVLDDSKRVAKRKLIEENRERRRKEEMIKSLQHRPSPSAEEWELIHVVTEAHRSTNAQ
                  (104)   ----------------------------------------------------------

                  (180)   GSHWKQKRKFLPEDIGQSPMASMPDGDKVDLEAFSEFTKIITPAITRVVDFAKKLPMFSE
                  (164)   ------R----L-----------L----------------------------N-----

                  (240)   LPCEDQIILLKGCCMEIMSLRAAVRYDPESETLTLSGEMAVKREQLKNGGLGVVSDAIFD
                  (224)   ----------------------------------------------------------

                  (300)   LGKSLSAFNLDDTEVALLQAVLLMSSDRTGLICVDKIEKCQETYLLAFEHYINYRKHNIP
                  (286)   ---------------------------------------------S------------

                  (360)   HFWPKLLMKVTDLRMIGACHASRFLHMKVECFTELFPPLFLEVFEDQEV   (408)
                  (346)   ---S------A-------Y---------------S-          QEV   (385)
```

The 12 N-terminal amino acids of THRA1 are deleted in v-ERBA. There are 13 single substitutions and a C-terminal deletion in v-ERBA. Dashes indicate identical residues.

Sequences of human THRA and THRB proteins

```
                                      K                    P
Human THRA1    (1)   MEQKPSKVECGSDPEENSARSPDGKRKRKNGQCSLKTSMSGYIPSYLDKDEQCVVCGDK
Human THRA2          ----------------------------------------------------------
Human THRB1          MTPNSMTENGLTAWDKPKHCPDREHDWKLVGMSEACLHRKSHSERRSTLKNEQSSPHLI

Human THRA1   (60)   ATGYHYRCITCEGCKGFFRRTIQKNLHPTYSCKYDSCCVIDKITRNQCQLCRFKKCIAVG
                     ----------------------------------------------------------
                     QTTWTSSIFHLDHDDVNDQSVSSAQTFQTEEKKCKGYIPSYLDKDELCVVCGDKATGYHY

                                                                 V
Human THRA1  (120)   MAMDLVLDDSKRVAKRKLIEQNRERRRKEEMIRSLQQRPEPTPEEWDLIHIATEAHRSTN
                     ----------------------------------------------------------
                     RCITCEGCKGFFRRTIQKNLHPSYSCKYEGKCVIDKVTRNQCQECRFKKCIYVGMATDLV

Human THRA1  (181)   AQGSHWKQRRKFLPDDIGQSPIVSMPDGDKVDLEAFSEFTKIITPAITRVVDFAKKLPMF
                     ----------------------------------------------------------
                     LDDSKRLAKRKLIEENREKRRREELQKSIGHKPEPTDEEWELIKTVTEAHVATNAQGSHW

                                                          T   K
Human THRA1  (240)   SELPCEDQIILLKGCCMEIMSLRAAVRYDPESDTLTLSGEMAVKREQLKNGGLGVVSDAI
                     ----------------------------------------------------------
                     KQKRKFLPEDIGQAPIVNAPEGGKVDLEAFSHFTKIITPAITRVVDFAKKLPMFCELPCE

Human THRA1  (300)   FELGKSLSAFNLDDTEVALLQAVLLMSTDRSGLLCVDKIEKSQEAYLLAFEHYVNHRKHN
                     ----------------------------------------------------------
                     DQIILLKGCCMEIMSLRAAVRYDPESETLTLNGEMAVTRGQLKNGGLGVVSDAIFDLGMS

Human THRA1  (360)   IPHFWPKLLMKVTDLRMIGACHASRFLHMKVECPTELFPPLFLEVFEDQEV(410)
Human THRA2          ----------EREVQSSILYKGAAAEGRPGGSLGVHPEGQQLLGMHVVQGPQVRQLEQQ
Human THRB1          LSSFNLDDTEVALLQAVLLMSSDRPGLACVERIEKYQDSFLLAFEHYINYRKHHVTHFWP

Human THRA2  (420)   LGEAGSLQGPVLQHQSPKSPQQRLLELLHRSGILHARAVCGEDDSSEADSPSSSEEEPEV
Human THRB1          KLLMKVTDLRMIGACHASRFLHMKVECPTELFPPLF451LEVFED(461)

Human THRA2  (480)   CEDLAGNAASP(490)
```

Human THRA1 and THRA2 are identical up to amino acid 370 (codon 43 in exon 9); the sequence of THRA2 is continued as the lower line from that position. Underlined amino acids differ from those of v-ERBA. Rat THRA1 is identical to human THRA1 but for the five substitutions shown above the human sequence (positions 17, 34, 171, 281 and 285).

Relationship between rat THRB, chicken THRA and THRB and v-ERBA proteins (see figure on p. 493)

The percentage figures indicate sequence homology within the DNA binding and hormone binding regions. P75$^{v\text{-}gag\text{-}erbA}$ is a highly mutated version of 385 ERBA amino acids of chicken THRA. v-ERBA has acquired two point mutations in the DNA binding domain and 11 others in the hormone binding domain (shown as dots), a 9 amino acid C-terminal deletion in the hormone binding domain and an N-terminal third (254 amino acids) encoded by *gag*. These changes result in the loss of triiodothyronine binding capacity (though the hormone binding region is retained) but the retention of sequence-specific DNA binding. v-ERBA acts as a constitutive repressor of T_3-regulated genes.

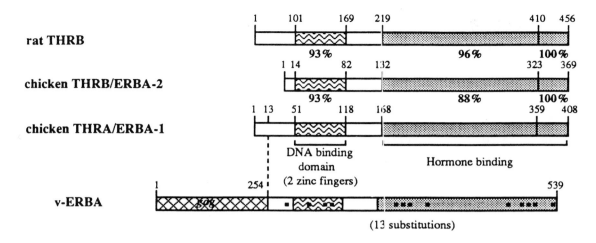

Comparison of sequences in the putative second zinc binding finger of THRA and THRB

```
Human/rat THRA    (75)   GFFRRTIQKNLHPTYSCKYDSCCVIDKITRNQCQLCRFKKCIAVGM
Chicken THRA      (75)   GFFRRTIQKNLHPTYSCKYDGCCVIDKITRNQCQLCRFKKCISVGM
                                          *         *        *          *
Chicken THRB      (37)   GFFRRTIQKNLHPTYSCKYEGCCVIDKVTRNQCQECRFKKCIFVGM
Rat THRB         (124)   GFFRRTIQKSLHPSYSCKYEGCCIIDKVTRNQCQECRFKKCIYVGM
Human THRB       (124)   GFFRRTIQKNLHPSYSCKYEGCCVIDKVTRNQCQECRFKKCIYVGM
```

Bold letters show the conserved Cys residues. * Indicates differences between chicken THRA and THRB. The underlined Lys (K) in chicken THRA is the only amino acid in this region that is mutated in v-ERBA (where it is changed to Thr).

	EGFR/ErbB-1	HER2/ErbB-2/Neu	HER3/ErbB-3	HER4/ErbB-4	v-erbB
Nucleotides (kb)					
Human	110				
Chromosome					
Human	7p13–p12	17q21–q22	12q13		
Mouse	11	11			
Rat	14	10			
Exons	26				
mRNA (kb)					
Human	5.8/10.5	4.8/5.8/10.5 2.3 (*HER2 ECD*)	6.2	~6.0/>15	
Chicken	2.6/5.8/8.6/12.0				3.5
mRNA half-life (h)		7			
Amino acids	1186 (human, chicken) (signal sequences:	1255 (human)	1323	1308 (19)	604 (25)

493

	EGFR/ErbB-1	HER2/ErbB-2/Neu	HER3/ErbB-3	HER4/ErbB-4	v-erbB
	human 24; chicken: 30)	1260 (rat)			
Mass (kDa)					
(predicted)	134 139 (rat)	138 (human)	146	144	62
(expressed)	gp170	gp185 100 (HER2 ECD)	gp 160	gp180	68/74

Cellular location

Plasma membrane glycoproteins. HER2 ECD is a perinuclear cytoplasmic protein. In chickens the 2.6 kb *ErbB* mRNA encodes a truncated, secreted 70 kDa receptor that binds TGFα (Flickinger *et al.*, 1992).

Tissue location

EGFR: Human *EGFR* is widely distributed, except in haematopoietic tissues, and is amplified in epidermal and glial malignancies. *EGFR* is expressed, however, in chicken erythrocytic progenitor cells and is responsible for mitogenic stimulation by TGFα (Pain *et al.*, 1991). Most cells express between 2×10^4 and 2×10^5 receptors. *EGFR* is overexpressed by 20 to 50-fold in the A431 cell line derived from a human epidermoid carcinoma of the vulva (2×10^6 receptors/cell).

HER2: The pattern of expression is closely similar to that of *EGFR* (Coussens *et al.*, 1985; Semba *et al.*, 1985), although high levels of *HER2* mRNA occur in melanocytes in which *EGFR* is undetectable. It is present in fetal epithelial cells but only at low levels post-natally. The overexpression of *HER2* in tumour cell lines reflects increased synthesis rather than stabilization of the mRNA (Pasleau *et al.*, 1993).

HER2 ECD is an alternatively processed form of *HER2* produced in some human breast carcinoma cell lines (Scott *et al.*, 1993). The 5′ 2.1 kb of *HER2 ECD* is identical to that of *HER2* and diverges 61 nucleotides before the transmembrane region.

HER3: The pattern of expression is closely similar to that of *HER2* although *HER3* is undetectable in fetal or adult skin fibroblasts. It is transcribed in term placenta, the respiratory and urinary tracts, stomach, lung, kidney and brain but not in skeletal muscle or lymphoid cells (Prigent *et al.*, 1992). It is expressed in normal fetal liver, kidney and brain but not in the heart. It is overexpressed in tumour cell lines derived from mammary carcinomas (Kraus *et al.*, 1989).

HER4: Maximum expression in brain, heart and kidney but also expressed in parathyroid, cerebellum, pituitary, spleen, testis and breast with lower levels detectable in thymus, lung, salivary gland and pancreas. It is also expressed in a variety of mammary adenocarcinoma and neuroblastoma cell lines (Plowman *et al.*, 1993).

Protein function

EGFR

EGFR is the receptor for epidermal growth factor (EGF), heparin-binding EGF-like factor (HB-EGF; Higashiyama *et al.*, 1991), transforming growth factor α (TGFα; Marquardt *et al.*, 1984), amphiregulin (Johnson *et al.*, 1993) and vaccinia virus growth factor (Stroobant *et al.*, 1985). The stoichiometry of EGF:EGFR binding is 1:1. The chicken receptor binds human TGFα with 100 times the affinity of human EGF (k_d 10^{-9}–10^{-10}M, approximately the same as that of human EGF for the human EGFR). EGF binding increases receptor–receptor affinity, activating the cytoplasmic tyrosine kinase domain of EGFR by dimerization and transphosphorylation: the ligand–receptor complex undergoes receptor-mediated endocytosis. A mutated form of EGFR that lacks intrinsic tyrosine kinase activity retains the capacity to activate MAP kinase and may do so via an EGFR-associated kinase (Selva *et al.*, 1993). Mutation of the tyrosine autophosphorylation sites does not inhibit EGF-stimulated [^{3}H]-thymidine incorporation in NIH 3T3 cells, suggesting that the interaction of SH2 domain proteins with the receptor may not be essential for DNA synthesis (Decker, 1993).

EGFR activation causes transient membrane hyperpolarization and increases the intracellular free concentration of Ca^{2+}. In A431 cells the EGFR activates a membrane-potential-independent Ca^{2+} channel and the resulting Ca^{2+} influx in turn activates Ca^{2+}-dependent K^+ channels causing membrane hyperpolarization. The activation of these Ca^{2+} channels is mimicked by leukotriene C_4, suggesting that the EGFR stimulates phospholipase A2 and 5-lipoxygenase-mediated leukotriene C_4 production (Peppelenbosch *et al.*, 1992).

EGF acts synergistically with insulin to stimulate DNA synthesis and cell proliferation in fibroblasts. One effect of EGF in these cells is to activate p21^{ras}. The activated EGFR phosphorylates GTPase-activating protein (GAP) at Tyr460 immediately C-terminal to the second GAP SH2 domain (Liu and Pawson, 1991), which may cause the modulation of p21^{ras} activity and also regulate other protein–protein interactions. The EGFR also associates with phosphatidylinositol 3-kinase and phospholipase Cγ. The SH2 domains of phospholipase Cγ mediate binding which also requires the EGF-stimulated phosphorylation of the EGFR (Zhu *et al.*, 1992).

The EGFR also phosphorylates pp81 (Krieg and Hunter, 1992), lipocortins (or calpactins, pp34–39) and pp42 in intact cells and calmodulin *in vitro* (Jose *et al.*, 1992). In A431 cells EGF inhibits proliferation and this also correlates with an increase in cellular phosphotyrosine content (Gill and Lazar, 1981). HB-EGF is a fibroblast, keratinocyte and smooth muscle cell mitogen (Higashiyama *et al.*, 1991).

HER2

Receptor-like tyrosine kinase activated by NEU differentiation factor (NDF: 44 kDa; Wen *et al.*, 1992), the heregulins and glial growth factors that are all alternatively spliced products of the same gene (Marchionni *et al.*, 1993). NDF stimulates tyrosine phosphorylation of HER2 and the differentiation of human breast cancer cells *in vitro* (Peles *et al.*, 1992). The expression of NDF is activated by *Ras*. The NDF precursor is a transmembrane protein with an extracellular EGF-like domain and an immunoglobulin homology domain and contains both *O*- and *N*-linked sugars. The extracellular region is proteolytically released from COS-7 cells in a form that activates p185^{neu}.

NEU has also been shown to bind to a 30 kDa glycoprotein secreted from human breast cancer cells and a 25 kDa peptide secreted by activated macrophages (Tarakhovsky *et al.*, 1991). NEU protein-specific activating factor (NAF) isolated from medium conditioned by the human T cell line ATL-2 increases the tyrosine kinase activity of p185 and causes its dimerization and internalization (Dobashi *et al.*, 1991).

TPA stimulates serine/threonine phosphorylation of normal and oncogenic NEU and inhibits the tyrosine kinase activity of oncogenic NEU: thus, like the EGFR, oncogenic NEU may be negatively regulated by protein kinase C (Cao *et al.*, 1991).

In cells that co-express EGFR and p185^{neu}, EGF or TGFα causes the formation of highly tyrosine phosphorylated heterodimers with enhanced protein kinase activity (Qian *et al.*, 1992).

The truncated version of HER2, HER2 ECD, suppresses the growth-inhibitory effects of antibodies directed against HER2 (Scott *et al.*, 1993).

HER3

This is the third member of the EGFR family. Ligand unknown. Although HER3 has a tyrosine kinase domain that is highly homologous to those of EGFR and HER2, the C-terminal domain and a 29 amino acid region C-terminal to the ATP binding domain diverge markedly. These regions may confer functional specificity.

HER4

The intrinsic tyrosine kinase activity of HER4 is specifically stimulated by a heparin-binding growth factor that has no direct effect on EGFR, HER2 or HER3 (Plowman *et al.*, 1993). This growth factor causes phenotypic differentiation of a human mammary tumour cell line.

Structure of the human *EGFR* gene

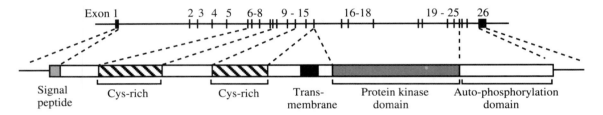

Exon 1 comprises a 5′ untranslated region and the sequence encoding the first 29 amino acids of the EGFR, including the signal peptide. The remainder of the 26 exons encode the ligand binding domain including two cysteine-rich regions, the transmembrane region, the tyrosine kinase domain, the autophosphorylation region and the 3′ untranslated region. The *EGFR* gene promoter is rich in GC regions but lacks a TATA box (Ishii *et al.*, 1985).

Sequences of the chicken (CEF) and human EGF receptors and avian v-ERBB

```
CEF    (-30)  MGVRSPLSASGPRGAAVLVLLLLGVALCSAVEEKKVCQGTNNKLTQLGHVEDHFTSLQRMYNNCEVVLS
EGFR   (-24)       MRP--TA---L-A--AALCPASR-L---------S-------TF----L-----F-------G

CEF     (40)  NLEITYVEHNRDLTFLKTIQEVAGYVLIALNMVDVIPLENLQIIRGNVLYDNSFALAVLSNYHMNKTQGL
EGFR    (40)  -------QR-Y--S-----------------T-ER-----------MY-E--Y--------DA--- --

CEF    (110)  RELPMKRLSEILNGGVKISNNPKLCNMDTVLWNDIIDTSRKPLTVLDFASNLSSCPKCHPNCTEDHCWGA
EGFR   (109)  K----RN-Q---H-A-RF----A---VESIQ-R--VSSDFLSNMSM--QNH-G--Q--D-S-PNGS----

CEF    (180)  GEQNCQTLTKVICAQQCSGRCRGKVPSDCCHNQCAAGCTGPRESDCLACRKFRDDATCKDTCPPLVLYNP
EGFR   (179)  --E---K---I------------S-------------------V------E---------M----

CEF    (250)  TTYQMDVNPEGKYSFGATCVRECPHNYVVTDHGSCVRSCNTDTYEVEENGVRKCKKCDGLCSKVCNGIGI
EGFR   (249)  ------------------KK--R-----------A-GA-S--M--D-------E-P-R-------

CEF    (320)  GELKGILSINATNIDSFKNCTKINGDVSILPVAFLGDAFTKTLPLDPKKLDVFRTVKEISGFLLIQAWPD
EGFR   (319)  --F-DS--------KH-----S-S--LH------R--S--H-P----QE--ILK-----T--------E
```

```
CEF     (390)   NATDLYAFENLEIIRGRTKQHGQYSLAVVNLKIQSLGLRSLKEISDGDIAIMKNKNLCYADTMNWRSLFA
EGFR    (389)   -R---H----------------F-----S-N-T------------VI-SG-------N-I--KK--G

CEF     (460)   TQSQKTKIIQNRNKNDCTADRHVCDPLCSDVGCWGPGPFHCFSCRFFSRQKECVKQCNILQGEPREFERD
EGFR    (459)   -SG------S--GE-S-K-TGQ--HA---PE-----E-RD-V---NV--GR---DK--L-E------VEN

CEF     (530)   SKCLPCHSECLVQNSTAYNTTCSGPGPDHCMKCAHFIDGPHCVKACPAGVLGENDTLVWKYADANAVCQL
EGFR    (529)   -E-IQ--P---P-   -M-I--T-R---N-IQ---Y---……----T-----M---N---------GH--H-
v-ERBB  (1)                     -------------------------------R----------

CEF     (600)   CHPNCTRGCKGPGLEGCP NGSKTPS IAAGVVGGLLCLVVVGLGIGLYLRRRHIVRKRTLRRLLQERELV
EGFR    (596)   ------Y--T--------T--P-I---- T-M--A--L-L--A-----FM--------------------
v-ERBB  (41)    -----------------  -----------------------------------------------------
                                          # #  #                             £
CEF     (669)   EPLTPSGEAPNQAHLRILKETEFKKVKVLGSGAFGTVYKGLWIPEGEKVKIPVAIKELREATSPKANKEI
EGFR    (666)   ------------L----------I---------------------------------------------
v-ERBB  (110)   ---------------------------------I-----------------------------------

CEF     (739)   LDEAYVMASVDNPHVCRLLGICLTSTVQLITQLMPYGCLLDYIREHKDNIGSQYLLNWCVQIAKGMNYLE
EGFR    (736)   --------------------------------F------V----------------------------
v-ERBB  (180)   -------------------------------------------------------------------

CEF     (809)   ERRLVHRDLAARNVLVKTPQHVKITDFGLAKLLGADEKEYHAEGGKVPIKWMALESILHRIYTHQSDVWS
EGFR    (806)   D----------------------------------E--------------------------------
v-ERBB  (250)   -------------------------------------------------------------------

CEF     (879)   YGVTVWELMTFGSKPYDGIPASEISSVLEKGERLPQPPICTIDVYMIMVKCWMIDADSRPKFRELIAEFS
EGFR    (876)   -----------------------I------------------------------------------I---
v-ERBB  (320)   -------------------------------------------------------------------

CEF     (949)   KMARDPPRYLVIQGDERMHLPSPTDSKFYRTLMEEEDMEDIVDADEYLVPHQGFFNSPSTSRTPLLSSLS
EGFR    (946)   ------Q----------------------N---A--D----D-V-------I-Q----S--------
v-ERBB  (390)   -------------------------------------------------------------------
                                                                             +
CEF     (1019)  ATSNNSATNCIDRNG QGHPVREDSFVQRYSSDPTGNFLEESIDDGFLPAPEYVNQLMPKKPSTAMVQNQ
EGFR    (1016)  ------TVA------L-SC-IK----L---------ALT-D----T---V---I--SV--R-AGS ---P
v-ERBB  (460)   ---------------
                  +                                                            +
CEF     (1088)  IYNNISLTAISKLPMDSRYQNSHSTAVDNPEYLNTNQSPLAKTVFESSPYWIQSGNHQINLDNPDYQQDF
EGFR    (1085)  V-H-QP-NPAP  SR-PH--DP-----G-------V-PTCVNST-D-PAH-A-K-S---S---------
v-ERBB  (529)   -------------------------------------------------------------------
                  +
CEF     (1158)  FPNETKPNGLLKVPAAENPEYLRVAAPKSEYIEASA(1194)
EGFR    (1153)  F-K-A----IF-GST---A------PQS--F-G-- (1186)
v-ERBB  (599)   L-TSCS (604)
```

Dashes indicate identity with the CEF sequence. Italicized and underlined: signal peptides. Italics: transmembrane regions. # Indicates conserved ATP binding site residues (human EGFR: 695–700 and 721). + Indicates major tyrosine autophosphorylation sites in human EGFR (1068, 1086, 1148 and 1173). The E domain of v-ERBB (see **Structure of viral genomes and major translation products**, page 489) corresponds to residues 961–1102 of CER.

Structures of the v-ERBB oncoprotein, EGFR, HER2, HER3 and HER4

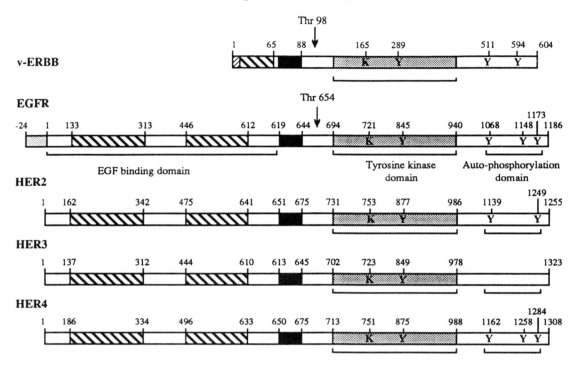

Hatched boxes: extracellular cysteine-rich domains. Black boxes: transmembrane domains. Shaded boxes: tyrosine protein kinase domains. Dotted box: 24 amino acid signal sequence that is proteolytically cleaved from the EGFR. The *gag*-encoded (6 amino acids) of v-ERBB (lightly hatched box) also encodes a (putative, cleaved) signal sequence. In v-ERBB the receptor binding domain is lost and the C-terminus truncated.

EGFR

The extracellular domain contains 51 cysteines in two clusters and 12 potential sites for *N*-linked glycosylation. Similar cysteine-rich regions occur in the receptors for insulin, insulin-like growth factor (IGF-I), nerve growth factor (NGF) and low-density lipoprotein (LDL). The cytoplasmic region (13 amino acids) adjacent to the membrane is a basic "stop transfer" sequence. Thr654 in the centre of this region is phosphorylated by protein kinase C: this decreases the affinity of EGF binding. In the tyrosine kinase domain, residues 695–700 (Gly–X–Gly–X–X–Gly) recognize the C-2 and N-1 atoms on the adenine moiety of ATP and Lys721 forms a salt bridge with an oxygen atom on the β phosphate. The three C-terminal tyrosines of EGFR are phosphorylated on EGF activation and positively regulate the kinase and transforming activity (Helin *et al.*, 1991). The EGF receptor, when expressed in *src*-transformed rat fibroblasts, is constitutively phosphorylated, as is PLC-γ (Wasilenko *et al.*, 1991): the EGFR site is probably Tyr845, rather than the major sites (Tyr1173, 1148, 1068).

EGFR mutants lacking most of the cytoplasmic domain form heterodimers with wild-type receptors when co-expressed. The heterodimers do not undergo tyrosine autophosphorylation in response to EGF. EGFR mutants defective in kinase activity also interact with normal receptors and block EGF-stimulated cell proliferation (Redemann *et al.*, 1992). Substitution of Thr for Arg662 in the juxtamembrane region does not affect the ligand binding properties of EGFR but confers the mitogenic characteristics of gp185^{HER2} (DiFiore *et al.*, 1992). Thus, the EGFR^{Thr662} mutant protein conveys potent mitogenic signals to NIH 3T3 cells, as does gp185^{HER2}, indicating that the point mutation strongly affects cytoplasmic signalling.

HER2

HER2 is ~80% homologous to EGFR but does not bind EGF. The sequence divergence is greatest in the N-terminal region of the tyrosine kinase domains (Schechter *et al.*, 1984). HER2 and EGFR both encode transmembrane proteins with two repeats of an extracellular, cysteine-rich domain (the 50 Cys residues are identically positioned) and an intracellular tyrosine kinase domain. Potential sites for *N*-linked glycosylation are not conserved. Mutation of the ATP binding site (Lys753) blocks transforming activity.

The dominant transforming *Neu* oncogene isolated from rat neuroblastoma DNA was oncogenically activated by a single point mutation (Val664 to Glu: A to T mutation at nucleotide 2012) in the transmembrane domain. Substitution of Gln is almost as effective as Glu; Lys, His, Gly or Tyr do not activate. The adjacent residues Ala661, Val663 and Gly665 are also essential for transforming activity (Cao *et al.*, 1992). The Glu664 mutation confers high-affinity ligand binding on the receptor (Ben-Levy *et al.*, 1992) and enhances tyrosine kinase activity and autophosphorylation of Tyr1248 (the major autophosphorylation site). Mutation of Tyr1248 to Phe lowers tyrosine kinase and transforming activities. Thus Tyr1248 negatively regulates transformation, the effect being blocked by phosphorylation (Akiyama *et al.*, 1991). However, complete removal of 230 C-terminal amino acids enhances transformation.

About 90% of non-transforming sequences contain a sharp bend at positions 664/665, whereas a similar proportion of transforming sequences are α-helical (Brandt-Rauf *et al.*, 1990). In the human breast carcinoma cell line SK-BR-3 there is evidence that the extracellular domain (p105 or p130) is released from the cell surface into the medium (Zabrecky *et al.*, 1991; Lin and Clinton, 1991), as also occurs with CSF, IL-2 and EGFR.

Oncogenic activation of *Neu* (by point mutation, overexpression or by truncation of non-catalytic sequences) results in its constitutive phosphorylation and in the tyrosine phosphorylation of PtdIns(4,5)P_2-specific phospholipase Cγ, which is permanently associated with activated NEU (Peles *et al.*, 1991).

HER3

HER3 is ~44% identical in amino acid sequence to EGFR and HER2 in the extracellular domain and ~60% identical in the tyrosine kinase domain. The tyrosine kinase domain homology with EPH, MET, FMS and the insulin receptor is ~30%. The extracellular domain contains 50 cysteines, 47 of which occur in two clusters, that have a similar distribution to those in EGFR and HER2.

HER4

HER4 has all the structural features of the EGFR family of receptor tyrosine kinases. The extracellular 625 residues includes two cysteine-rich regions (186–334 and 496–633) and domains II–IV (186–649) that are between 56% and 67% identical to the corresponding regions of HER3 and 43–51% and 34–46% identical to EGFR and HER2. The 50 conserved extracellular cysteines of EGFR, HER2 and HER3 are also conserved in HER4 except for the fourth cysteine in domain IV. The transmembrane 37 amino acids are 73% identical with those of EGFR and the 276 catalytic domain is 79%, 77% and 63% identical to those of EGFR, HER2 and HER3, respectively. In the C-terminus homology is much lower (19% (EGFR), 27% (HER2), respectively) but the major tyrosine autophosphorylation sites of EGFR (1068, 1086, 1148 and 1173) are conserved (1058, 1162, 1188 and 1284).

Sequence homology between the protein kinase domains of HER2 and some viral oncogenes

Viral oncogene:	*erbB*	*src*	*abl*	*yes*	*fgr*	*ros*	*fps*	*mil*	*fms*	*mos/rel*
% homology:	82	43	42	42	41	38	37	28	27	<25

Sequences of human EGFR, HER2, HER3 and HER4

```
EGFR  (-24)  MRPSGTAGAALLALLAALCPAS  RALEEKKVCQGTSNKLTQLGTFEDHFLSLQRMFNNCEVVLGNLEITYVQRNYD
HER2   (1)   M   ELAALCRWG--LA-LPPGAA     STQ--T--DMK-RLPASP-THLDM-RHLYQG-Q--Q----LVLLPT-AS
HER3  (-19)  M-ANDAL   QV-*--FS-ARG-EV   GN*QA--P--L-G-SVT-DA-NQYQT-YK**ER----M-----**TGH-*-
HER4   (1)   MK-A     TG-*VWVSL-VA-*TVQPSD*QS--A--E---SS-SDL-QQYRA-*KY*E-----M------SIEH-R-

EGFR  (52)   LSFLKTIQEVAGYVLIALNTVERIPLENLQIIRGNMYYENSYALAVLSN        YDANKT GLKELPMRNLQE
HER2  (71)   ----QD-Q--Q----I-H-QVRQV--QR-RIV--TQLFEDNY-LA-LD-GDPLNNTTPVTGASPGG-RE-QLRS---
HER3  (55)   ----*W-R--T----V-M-EFSTL--P--*V*--**V-DGKF-IF-ML-        -NT-*SHA-*Q-R*TQ---
HER4  (74)   ----RSVR--T----V---QFRYL-----R----TKL--DR----IFL-       -RKDGNF--Q--GLK--T-

EGFR  (119)  ILHGAVRFSNNPALCNVESIQWRDIVSSDFLSNMSMDFQNHLGSCQKCDPSCPNGSCWGAGEENCQKLTKIICAQQC
HER2  (148)  --K-G-LIQR-PQ--YQDT-L-K--FHKNNQLALTLIDT-RSRA-HP-SPM-KGSR---ESS-D--S--R-V--GG-
HER3  (123)  --S-*-Y*EK-DK--HM**-D-----RDRDAEIVVK-  - G*--P*-HEV-K -*---P-*-*--T---T---P--
HER4  (142)  --N-GVYVDQNKF--YADT-H-Q---RNPWP--LTLVST-GSSG-GR-HK--T -R---PT-NH--T--RTV--E--

EGFR  (196)  SGRCRGKSPSDCCHNQCAAGCTGPRESDCLVCRKFRDEATCKDTCPPLMLYNPTTYQMDVNPEGKYSFGATCVKKCP
HER2  (225)  A R-K-PL-TD---EQ--A--T--KHS--LA-LH-NHSGI-ELH--ALVT--TD-FESMP--EGR-TF-AS--TA--
HER3  (196)  N-H-F-*N-NQ---DE--G--S--QDT--F*--*-*-**A-VPR--QPLV--KL-F-LE*--HT--QY-GV--AS--
HER4  (218)  D---Y-PYV-----RE--G--S--KDT--FA-MN-N-SGA-VTQ--QTFV-----F-LEH-FNA--TY--F-----

EGFR  (273)  RNYVVTDHGSCVRACGADSYEME EDGVRKCKKCEGPCRKVCNGIGIGEFKDSLSINATNIKHFKNCTSISGDLHIL
HER2  (301)  Y-YLST-VG--TLV-PLHNQ-VTAED-TQR-EK-SKP-ARV-Y-L-MEHLREVRAVTSA--QE-AG-KK-F-S-AF-
HER3  (273)  H-F-- -QT------*P-KM-*D KN-LKM-*P-G-L-P-A-E-T- SGSRFQT*D*S---DG-V---*-L-N-D*-
HER4  (295)  H-F-- -SS------PSSKM-V- -N-IKM-P-TDI-P-A-D---T-SLMSAQTVDSS--DK-I---K-N-N-IFL

EGFR  (349)  PVAFRGDSFTHTPPLDPQELDILKTVKEITGFLLIQAWPENRTDLHAFENLEIIRGRTKQHGQFSL AVVSLNITSL
HER2  (378)  PESFD--PASNTAP-Q-EQ-QVFE-LE----Y-Y-SA--DSLPDLSV-Q--QV-R--ILHNGAY-- TLQG-GISW-
HER3  (346)  ITGLN--*WHKI-A---*K-N**R--R----*-N--S---PHMHNF**-S--TT-G--S*Y*RG---LIMKN--V---
HER4  (370)  VTGIH--PYNAIEAI--EK-NVFR--R------N--S--P-M--FSV-S--VT-G--VLYS-LSL- ILKQQG----

EGFR  (425)  GLRSLKEISDGDVIISGNKNLCYANTINWKKLFGTS GQKTKIIISNRGENSCKATGQVCHALCSPEGCWGPEPRDCV
HER2  (454)  -L---R-LGS-LAL-HH-TH--FVHTVP-DQLFRNP HQALLHTA--PEDE-VGE-LA-HQ--ARRALL-SG-TQ-V
HER3  (423)  -F-------A-RIY--A-RQ---H*SL--T-VL*-PTEER*D-KH--*RRD-V-*-K--DP---SG-----*-G*-L
HER4  (446)  QFQ------A-NIY-TD-S----YH----TT--S-I N-RIV-RD--KAEN-T-E-M--NH---SD-----G-DQ-L

EGFR  (501)  SCRNVSRGRECVDKCNLLEGEPREFVENSECIQCHPEC LPQAMNITCTGRGPDNCIQCAHYIDGPHCVKTCPAGV
HER2  (530)  N-SQFL--QE--EE-RV-Q-L---YVNARH-LP-----Q -QN-SV--F-PEA-Q-VA---YK-P-F--AR--S--
HER3  (500)  ----Y---GV--TH--F-N------AHEA--FS-----*PM GGTA--N-S-S-T-A----FR------SS--H--
HER4  (522)  ---RFS---I-IES-N-YD--F---ENG-I-VE-D-Q-EKMEDGL L--H-P-----TK-S-FK---N--EK--D-L

EGFR  (576)  MGENNTL VWKYADAGHVCHLCHPNCTYGCTGPGLEGCP        TNGPKIPS *IATGMVGALLLLLVVALGIG*
HER2  (605)  KPDLSYMPIW-FP-EEGA-QP-PI---HS-VDLDDKG-P        AEQRASP *LTSIVSAVVG ILLVVVLGVVFG*
HER3  (575)  L-AKG **Y--*-VQNE-R*--E---Q--K--E-QD-L        *GQTLVLI-KTHLTM-LTVIAG-**IFMM --GT*
HER4  (598)  Q-A-S F IF----PDRE--P------Q--N--TSHD-IYYPWTGHSTLPQHAR *T-L--A-VI-G-FI-VI-G-TFA*
                                                              #  #   #
EGFR  (642)  *LFM*RRRHIV RKRTLRRLLQERELVEPLTPSGEAPNQALLRILKETEFKKIKVLGSGAFGTVYKGLWIPEGEKVKIP
HER2  (673)  *ILI*KRRQQKIR-YTM--L-QET-LV---T--GAMP-QAQM--L----LR-V-------------I---D--NV---
HER3  (644)  *FLYW*-GRRIQN--A*--Y-ERG-SI---D-- -KA-KV-A--F----**-L------V----H--V------SI---
HER4  (673)  *VYV*--KS-K K--A---F- -T----------T-----Q--------L-RV-------------I-V----T----
               #
```

```
EGFR   (718)   VAIKELREATSPKANKEILDEAYVMASVDNPHVCRLLGICLTSTVQLITQLMPFGCLLDYVREHKDNIGSQYLLNWC
HER2   (750)   ----V---N----------------G-GS-Y-S-------------V-----Y-----H---NRGRL---D-----
HER3   (720)   -C--*IEDKSGRQSFQAVT-HMLAIG-L-HA-IV----L-PG-SL--*--YL*L-S---*--Q-**A*-P-L----G
HER4   (748)   ----I-N-T-G----V-FM---LI---M-HP-LV----V--GP-I--V-----H----E--H---------L-----

EGFR   (795)   VQIAKGMMYLEDRRLVHRDLAARNVLVKTPQHVKITDFGLAKLLGAEEKEYHAEGGKVPIKWMALESILHRIYTHQS
HER2   (827)   M------S----V----------------S-N---------R--DI--T----D---V---------R-RF----
HER3   (797)   V------Y---EHGM---N-------L-*-SQ-QVA---V-D--PPDD-QLLYSEA-T----------HFGK-----
HER4   (825)   ----------E-------------*-*---------*--EGD----N-*---M--------C-HY-K*----

EGFR   (872)   DVWSYGVTVWELMTFGSKPYDGIPASEISSILEKGERLPQPPICTIDVYMIMVKCWMIDADSRPKFRELIIEFSKMA
HER2   (904)   ---------------A--------R--PDL------------------------SEC--R----VS---R--
HER3   (874)   ---------------*E--A-LRLA-V***-------A--Q--------V--------ENI--T-K--AN--T*--
HER4   (902)   --------I-------G-------T*--***---------------V------------K--AA---*--

EGFR   (949)   RDPQRYLVIQGDERMHL PSPTDSNFYRALMDEEDMDDVVDADEYLIPQQGFFSSPS  TSR
HER2   (981)   -----FV---NED LGP A--L--T----S-LEDD--G-L---E---V------CPDPAPGAGGMVHHRHRSSSTRSG
HER3   (951)   ---P-----KR*SGP*IA-G-EPHGLTNKKL--VELEPEL-L-LD-EAEEDNLATTTLGSALSLPVGTLNRPRGSQS
HER4   (979)   -----------D--K- ---N--K-FQN-L----LE-MM--E---V-- A-NIP-PIY---ARIDSNRSEIGHSPP

EGFR   (1008)                               TPLLSSLSATSN  NSTVACIDRNGLQSCPIKEDSFLQRY
HER2   (1056)  GGDL            TL    GLEPSEEEAPRS--AP-EG-G-DVFDGDLGMGAAK----L-THDP-P----
HER3   (1028)  LLSPSSGYMPMNQGNLGESCQESAVS*SSERCPRPVSLHPM*RGCLASESSEGHVTGSEAELQEKVSMCRSRSRS-S
HER4   (1054)  PAYTPMSGNQFVYRDGGFAAEQGVSVPYRAPTSTI*EA-V*  Q*--AEI**DSCCNGTLRKPVAPHVQ---ST---
                                             +                        +
EGFR   (1046)  SSDPTGALTEDSI     DDTFL    PVPEYINQS    VPKRPAGSV   QNPVYHNQPLNPAPS    RD
HER2   (1113)  -E---VP-PS      ET-GYVAPLTCS-Q---V--PDVRFQP-SP-E-PLPAARPAGATLERPKTLSPGKNGVVK
HER3   (1105)  PRPRGDSAYHSQRHSLLTPV-PLS*PGLEEEDVNGYVMPDTH-LKGT*SSREGTLSSVGLSSVLGTEEEDEDEEYEYM
HER4   (1129)  -A---*FA*-R-PRGELDEE**MT*MRDK-KQ--L-PVEEN*F-SR-KN-DLQALD--E---ASNG-PKAEDEYVNE
                                                         +
EGFR   (1099)  PHYQDPHSTAVGNPEYLNT   VQPTCVNSTFDSPA   HWAQKGSHQISLDNPDYQQDFFPKEA KPNGIFKGS
HER2   (1183)  DVF  AFGG--E-----TPQGGAA-QPHPPPAF---FDNLYY-D-DPPERGAPPST        ---T
HER3   (1182)  NRRRRHSPPHPPR-SS-EEL*YEYMDVGSDLSA-LGSTQSCFLHPVPIMPT*GTT--EDYEYMNRQRDGGGPGGDYA
HER4   (1206)  -L-LNTFANTL-KA---K    NNILSM*EKAKK-***PD*-NHSL*PRST-QH---L-EYST-YFY-Q--RIRPI
                       +
EGFR   (1167)   TAENAEYLRVAPQSSEFIGA (1186)
HER2   (1241)  P----P---GLDVPV (1255)
HER3   (1259)  AMGAC*ASEQGYEEMRAFQGPGHQAPHVHYARLKTLRSLEATDSAFDNPDYWHSRLFPKANAQRT (1323)
HER4   (1278)  V---*---SEFSLKPGTVLPPPPYRHRNTVV (1308)
```

Dashes indicate identity with EGFR. Underlined regions: signal sequences. Italicized and underlined regions: transmembrane domains. # Indicates conserved ATP binding site residues (EGFR: 795–800 and 821). + Indicates major tyrosine autophosporylation sites in EGFR (1068, 1086, 1148 and 1173). There is no significant homology within the C-terminal 353 amino acids of HER3.

Databank file names and accession numbers

	GENE	EMBL	SWISSPROT	REFERENCES
AEV-ES4	erbA(gag–erbA–erbB)	Reaeverb Y00044	ERBA_AVIER P03373	Damm et al., 1987, 1989 Debuire et al., 1984
AEV	v-erbB	Reerbbh K01216 Reacbver M13179	KERB_AVIER P00535 KER2_CHICK P11273	Yamamoto et al., 1983 Choi et al., 1986 Scotting et al., 1987
Human	THRA1 THRA2	Hscerbar X55005 Hsthra2a J03239 Hserbt1 Y00479	THA1_HUMAN P21205 THA2_HUMAN P10827	Nakai et al., 1988 Pfahl and Benbrook, 1989 Miyajima et al., 1989 Laudet et al., 1991

	GENE	EMBL	SWISSPROT	REFERENCES
Human	THRB	Hserbar X04707	THB_HUMAN P10828	Weinberger *et al.*, 1986 Sakurai *et al.*, 1990
Human	EGFR	Hsegfpre X00588 Hsegfr K02047 Hsegfrcp K01885 Hsegfr1 X06370 Hsegfr01 M38425	EGFR_HUMAN P00533	Ullrich *et al.*, 1984 Lin *et al.*, 1984 Simmen *et al.*, 1984 Haley *et al.*, 1987 Mroczkowski *et al.*, 1984 Margolis *et al.*, 1989
Human	HER2		ERB2_HUMAN P04626	Semba *et al.*, 1985 Yamamoto *et al.*, 1986a
Human	HER3	Hsegfrbb M29366	ERB3_HUMAN P21860	Kruas *et al.*, 1989 Plowman *et al.*, 1990
Human	HER4	L07868		Plowman *et al.*, 1993
Human	EAR2	Hsear2 X12794	EAR2_HUMAN P10588	Miyajima *et al.*, 1988
Human	EAR3	Hsear3 X12795	COTF_HUMAN P10589	Miyajima *et al.*, 1988
Chicken	THRα	Ggcerbar Y00987	THA_CHICK P04625	Sap *et al.*, 1986
Chicken	THRβ	Ggthrb X17504	THB_CHICK P18112	Forrest *et al.*, 1990
Chicken	EGFR	Ggegfr M20386	EGFR_CHICK P13387	Lax *et al.*, 1988
Chicken	gag–env–erbB	Ggerbbf M10066	KER1_CHICK P00534	Nilsen *et al.*, 1985
Rat	Neu	Rnneur X03362	NEU_RAT P06494	Bargmann *et al.*, 1986

Reviews

Carpenter, G. (1987). Receptors for epidermal growth factor and other polypeptide mitogens. Annu. Rev. Biochem., 56, 881–914.

Graf, T. and Beng, H. (1978). Avian leukemia viruses: interaction with their target cells in vivo and in vitro. Biochim. Biophys. Acta, 516, 269–299.

Gullick, W.J. (1991). Prevalence of aberrant expression of the epidermal growth factor receptor in human cancers. Brit. Med. Bull., 47, 87–98.

Laurence, D.J.R. and Gusterson, B.A. (1990). The epidermal growth factor: a review of structural and functional relationships in the normal organism and in cancer cells. Tumor Biol., 11, 229–261.

Papers

Aasland, R., Lillehaug, J.R., Male, R., Josendal, O., Varhaug, J.E. and Kleppe, K. (1988). Expression of oncogenes in thyroid tumours: coexpression of c-*erb*B2/*neu* and c-*erb*B. Brit. J. Cancer, 57, 358–363.

Adam, D., Maueler, W. and Schartl, M. (1991). Transcriptional activation of the melanoma inducing *Xmrk* oncogene in *Xiphophorus*. Oncogene 6, 73–80.

Akiyama, T., Matsuda, S., Namba, Y., Saito, T., Toyoshima, K. and Yamamoto, T. (1991). The transforming potential of the c-*erb*B-2 protein is regulated by its autophosphorylation at the carboxyl-terminal domain. Mol. Cell. Biol., 11, 833–842.

Arriza, J.L., Weinberger, C., Cerelli, G., Galser, T.M., Handelin, B.L., Houseman, D.E. and Evans, R.M. (1987). Cloning of human mineralocorticoid receptor complementary DNA: structural and functional kinship with the glucocorticoid receptor. Science, 237, 268–275.

Bargmann, C.I., Hung, M.-C. and Weinberg, R.A. (1986). The *neu* oncogene encodes an epidermal growth factor receptor-related protein. Nature, 319, 226–230.

Ben-Levy, R., Peles, E., Goldman-Michael, R. and Yarden, Y. (1992). An oncogenic point mutation confers high affinity ligand binding to the *neu* receptor. J. Biol. Chem., 267, 17304–17313.

Berchuck, A., Kamel, A., Whitaker, R., Kerns, B., Olt, G., Kinney, R., Soper, J.T., Dodge, R., Clarke-Pearson, D.L., Marks, P., McKenzie, S., Yin, S. and Bast, R.C. (1990). Over expression of HER2/*neu* is associated with poor survival in advanced epithelial ovarian cancer. Cancer Res., 50, 4087–4091.

Berchuck, A., Rodriguez, G., Kinney, R.B., Soper, J.T., Dodge, R.K., Clarke-Pearson, D.L. and Bast, R.C. (1991). Overexpression of HER2/neu in endometrial cancer is associated with advanced stage disease. Am. J. Obstet. Gynecol., 164, 15–21.

Beug, H., Hayman, M.J., Raines, M.B., Kung, H.J. and Vennstrom, B. (1986). RAV-1 induced erythroleukemic cells exhibit a weakly transformed phenotype in vitro and release c-erbB containing virus unable to transform fibroblasts. J. Virol., 57, 1127–1138.

Borg, A., Baldetorp, B., Ferno, M., Killander, D., Olsson, H. and Sigurdsson, H. (1991). ERBB2 amplification in breast cancer with a high rate of proliferation. Oncogene, 6, 137–143.

Borst, M.P., Baker, V.V., Dixon, D., Hatch, K.D., Shingleton, H.M. and Miller, D.M. (1990). Oncogene alterations in endometrial carcinoma. Gynecol. Oncol., 38, 364–366.

Bouchard, L., Lamarre, L., Tremblay, P.J. and Jolicoeur, P. (1989). Stochastic appearance of mammary tumors in transgenic mice carrying the MMTV/c-neu oncogene. Cell, 57, 931–936.

Bradbury, J.M., Arno, J. and Edwards, P.A.W. (1993). Induction of epithelial abnormalities that resemble human breast lesions by the expression of the neu/erbB-2 oncogene in reconstituted mouse mammary gland. Oncogene, 8, 1551–1558.

Brandt-Rauf, P.W., Rackovsky, S. and Pincus, M.R. (1990). Correlation of the structure of the transmembrane domain of the neu oncogene-encoded p185 protein with its function. Proc. Natl Acad. Sci. USA, 87, 8660–8664.

Buchberg, A.M., Brownell, E., Nagata, S., Jenkins, N.A. and Copeland, N.G. (1989). A comprehensive genetic map of murine chromosome 11 reveals extensive linkage conservation between mouse and human. Genetics, 122, 153–161.

Cao, H., Decker, S. and Stern, D.F. (1991). TPA inhibits the tyrosine kinase activity of the neu protein in vivo and in vitro. Oncogene, 6, 705–711.

Cao, H., Bangalore, L., Bormann, B.J. and Stern, D.F. (1992). A subdomain in the transmembrane domain is necessary for p185^{neu*} activation. EMBO J., 11, 923–932.

Carter, P., Presta, L., Gorman, C.M., Ridgway, J.B.B., Henner, D., Wong, W.L.T., Rowland, A.M., Kotts, C., Carver, M.E. and Shepard, H.M. (1992). Humanization of an anti-p185^{HER2} antibody for human cancer therapy. Proc. Natl Acad. Sci. USA, 89, 4285–4289.

Chazin, V.R., Kaleko, M., Miller, A.D. and Slamon, D.J. (1992). Transformation mediated by the human HER2 gene independent of the epidermal growth factor receptor. Oncogene, 7, 1859–1866.

Choi, O.-R., Trainor, C., Graf, T., Beug, H. and Engel, J.D. (1986). A single amino acid substitution in v-erbB confers a thermolabile phenotype to ts167 avian erythroblastosis virus-transformed erythroid cells. Mol. Cell. Biol., 6, 1751–1759.

Coussens, L., Yang-Feng, T.L., Liao, Y.-C., Chen, E., Gray, A., McGrath, J., Seeburg, P.H., Libermann, T.A., Schlessinger, J., Francke, U., Levinson, A. and Ullrich, A. (1985). Tyrosine kinase receptor with extensive homology to epidermal growth factor receptor shares chromosomal location with neu oncogene. Science, 230, 1132–1139.

D'Emilia, J., Bulovas, K., D'Ercole, K., Wolf, B., Steele, G. and Summerhayes, I.C. (1989). Expression of the c-erbB-2 gene product (p185) at different stages of neoplastic progression in the colon. Oncogene, 4, 1233–1239.

Damm, K., Beug, H., Graf, T. and Vennstrom, B. (1987). A single point mutation in erbA restores the erythroid transforming potential of a mutant avian erythroblastosis virus (AEV) defective in both erbA and erbB oncogenes. EMBO J., 6, 375–382.

Damm, K., Thompson, C.C., Evans, R.M. (1989). Protein encoded by v-erbA functions as a thyroid-hormone receptor antagonist. Nature, 339, 593–597.

Debuire, B., Henry, C., Benaissa, M., Biserte, G., Claverie, J.M., Saule, S., Martin, P. and Stehelin, D. (1984). Sequencing the erbA gene of avian erythroblastosis virus reveals a new type of oncogene. Science, 224, 1456–1459.

Decker, S.J. (1993). Transmembrane signaling by epidermal growth factor receptors lacking autophosphorylation sites. J. Biol. Chem., 268, 9176–9179.

DiFiore, P.P., Pierce, J., Kraus, M.H., Segatto, O., King, C.R. and Aaronson, S.A. (1987a). erbB-2 is a potent oncogene when overexpressed in NIH/3T3 cells. Science, 237, 178–182.

DiFiore, P.P., Pierce, J.H., Fleming, T.P., Hazen, R., Ullrich, A., King, C.R., Schlessinger, and Aaronson, S.A. (1987b). Overexpression of the human EGF receptor confers an EGF-dependent transformation phenotype to NIH 3T3 cells. Cell, 51, 1063–1070.

DiFiore, P.P., Helin, K., Kraus, M.H., Pierce, J.H., Artrip, J., Segatto, O. and Bottaro, D.P. (1992). A single amino acid substitution is sufficient to modify the mitogenic properties of the epidermal growth factor receptor to resemble that of gp185^{erbB-2}. EMBO J., 11, 3927–3933.

Divgi, C.R., Welt, S., Kris, M., Real, F.X., Yeh, S.D.J., Gralla, R., Merchant, B., Schweighart, S., Unger, M., Larson, S.M. and Mendelsohn, J. (1991). Phase I and imaging trial of indium 111-labeled anti-epidermal growth factor receptor monoclonal antibody 225 in patients with squamous cell lung carcinomas. J. Natl Cancer Inst., 83, 97–104.

Dobashi, K., Davis, J.G., Mikami, Y., Freeman, J.K., Hamuro, J. and Greene, M.I. (1991). Characterization of a neu/c-erbB-2 protein-specific activating factor. Proc. Natl Acad. Sci. USA, 88, 8582–8586.

Flickinger, T.W., Maihle, N.J. and Kung, H.-J. (1992). An alternatively processed mRNA from the avian c-*erb*B gene encodes a soluble, truncated form of the receptor that can block ligand-dependent transformation. Mol. Cell. Biol., 12, 883–893.

Forrest, D., Sjoberg, M. and Vennstrom, B. (1990). Contrasting developmental and tissue-specific expression of α and β thyroid hormone receptor genes. EMBO J., 9, 1519–1528.

Forrest, D., Hallbook, F., Persson, H. and Vennstrom, B. (1991). Distinct functions for thyroid hormone receptors α and β in brain development indicated by differential expression of receptor genes. EMBO J., 10, 269–275.

Fujita-Yoshigaki, J., Yokoyama, S. Shindo-Okada, N. and Nishimura, S. (1992). Azatyrosine inhibits neurite outgrowth pf PC12 cells induced by oncogenic *ras*. Oncogene, 7, 2019–2024.

Fukushige, S.-I., Matsubara, K.-I., Yoshida, M., Sasaki, M., Suzuki, T., Semba, K., Toyoshima, K. and Yamamoto, T. (1986). Localization of a novel v-*erb*B-related gene, c-*erb*B-2, on human chromosome 17 and its amplification in a gastric cancer cell line. Mol. Cell. Biol., 6, 955–958.

Gamett, D.C., Tracy, S.E. and Robinson, H.L. (1986). Differences in sequences encoding the carboxyl-terminal domain of the epidermal growth factor receptor correlate with differences in the disease potential of viral *erb*B genes. Proc. Natl Acad. Sci. USA, 83, 6053–6057.

Giguere, V., Ong, E.S., Prudimar, S. and Evans, R.M. (1987). Identification of a receptor for the morphogen retinoic acid. Nature, 330, 624–629.

Gill, G.N. and Lazar, C.S. (1981). Increased phosphotyrosine content and inhibition of proliferation in EGF-treated A431 cells. Nature, 293, 305–307.

Guerin, M., Barrois, M., Terrier, M.J., Spielmann, M. and Riou, G. (1988). Overexpression of either c-*myc* or c-*erb*B-2/*neu* proto-oncogenes in human breast carcinomas: correlation with poor prognosis. Oncogene Res., 3, 21–31.

Haley, J., Whittle, N., Bennett, P., Kinchington, D., Ullrich, A. and Waterfield, M. (1987). The human EGF receptor gene: structure of the 110 kb locus and identification of sequences regulating its transcription. Oncogene Res., 1, 375–396.

Helin, K., Velu, T., Martin, P., Vass, W.C., Allevato, G., Lowy, D.R. and Beguinot, L. (1991). The biological activity of the human epidermal growth factor receptor is positively regulated by its C-terminal tyrosines. Oncogene, 6, 825–832.

Henry, C., Coquillaud, M., Saule, S., Stehelin, D. and Debuire, B. (1985). The four C-terminal amino acids of the v-*erb*A polypeptide are encoded by an intronic sequence of the v-*erb*B oncogene. Virology, 140, 179–182.

Hermann, T., Hoffmann, B., Piedrafita, F.J., Zhang, X. and Pfahl, M. (1993). V-erbA requires auxiliary proteins for dominant negative activity. Oncogene, 8, 55–65.

Higashiyama, S., Abraham, J.A., Miller, J., Fiddes, J.C. and Klagsbrun, M. (1991). A heparin-binding growth factor secreted by macrophage-like cells that is related to EGF. Science, 251, 936–939.

Hirst, R., Horwitz, A., Buck, C. and Rohrschneider, L. (1986). Phosphorylation of the fibronectin receptor complex in cells transformed by oncogenes that encode tyrosine kinases. Proc. Natl Acad. Sci. USA, 83, 6470–6474.

Horak, E., Smith, K., Bromley, L., LeJeune, S., Greenall, M., Lane, D. and Harris, A.L. (1991). Mutant p53, EGF receptor and c-*erb*B-2 expression in human breast cancer. Oncogene, 6, 2277–2284.

Houle, B., Rochette-Egly, C. and Bradley, W.E.C. (1993). Tumor-suppressive effects of the retinoic receptor β in human epidermoid lung cancer cells. Proc. Natl Acad. Sci. USA, 90, 985–989.

Hudziak, R.M., Schlessinger, J. and Ullrich, A. (1987). Increased expression of the putative growth factor receptor p185[HER2] causes transformation and tumorigenesis of NIH 3T3 cells. Proc. Natl Acad. Sci. USA, 84, 7159–7163.

Imamura, N., Miyazawa, T., Mtasiwa, D. and Kuramoto, A. (1990). Co-expression of N-*ras* p21 and c-*erb*B-2 (*neu*) oncogene products by common ALL antigen-positive aggressive diffuse lymphoma. Lancet, 336, 825–826.

Ishii, S., Xu, Y.-H., Stratton, R.H., Roe, B.A., Merlono, G.T. and Pastan, I. (1985). Characterization and sequence of the promoter region of the human epidermal growth factor receptor gene. Proc. Natl Acad. Sci. USA, 82, 4920–4924.

Johnson, G.R., Kannan, B., Shoyab, M. and Stromberg, K. (1993). Amphiregulin induces tyrosine phosphorylation of the epidermal growth factor receptor and p185[erbB2]. J. Biol. Chem., 268, 2924–2931.

Jose, E.S., Benguria, A., Geller, P. and Villalobo, A. (1992). Calmodulin inhibits the epidermal growth factor receptor tyrosine kinase. J. Biol. Chem., 267, 15237–15245.

Kern, J.A., Schwartz, D.A., Nordberg, J.E., Weiner, D.B., Greene, M.I., Torney, L. and Robinson, R.A. (1990). p185^{neu} expression in human lung adenocarcinomas predicts shortened survival. Cancer Res., 50, 5184–5191.

King, C.R., Kraus, M.H. and Aaronson, S.A. (1985). Amplification of a novel v-*erb*B-related gene in a human mammary carcinoma. Science, 229, 974–976.

Kraus, M.H., Popescu, N.C., Amsbaugh, S. and King, C.R. (1987). Overexpression of the EGF receptor-related proto-oncogene *erb*B-2 in human mammary tumor cell lines by different molecular mechanisms. EMBO J., 6, 605–610.

Kraus, M.H., Issing, W., Miki, T., Popescu, N.C. and Aaronson, S.A. (1989). Isolation and characterization of *ERBB3*, a third member of the *ERBB*/epidermal growth factor receptor family: evidence for over-expression in a subset of human mammary tumors. Proc. Natl Acad. Sci. USA, 86, 9193–9197.

Krieg, J. and Hunter, T. (1992). Identification of the two major epidermal growth factor-induced tyrosine phosphorylation sites in the microvillar core protein ezrin. J. Biol. Chem., 267, 19258–19265.

Lacroix, H., Iglehart, J.D., Skinner, M.A. and Kraus, M.H. (1989). Overexpression of *erb*B-2 or EGF receptor proteins present in early stage mammary carcinoma is detected simultaneously in matched primary tumors and regional metastases. Oncogene, 4, 145–151.

Laudet, V., Begue, A., Henry, C., Joubel, A., Martin, P., Stehelin, D. and Saule, S. (1991). Genomic organis-ation of the human thyroid hormone receptor a (c-*erb*A-1) gene. Nucleic Acids Res. 19, 1105–1112.

Laudet, V., Vanacker, J.M., Adelmant, G., Begue, A. and Stehelin, D. (1993). Characterization of a func-tional promoter for the human thyroid hormone receptor alpha (c-*erb*A-1) gene. Oncogene, 8, 975–982.

Lax, I., Johnson, A., Howk, R., Sap, J., Bellot, F., Winkler, M., Ullrich, A., Vennstrom, B., Schlessinger, J. and Givol, D. (1988). Chicken epidermal growth factor (EGF) receptor: cDNA cloning, expression in mouse cells, and differential binding of EGF and transforming growth factor alpha. Mol. Cell. Biol., 8, 1970–1978.

Lee, E.B., Beug, H. and Hayman, M.J. (1993). Mutational analysis of the role of the carboxy-terminal region of the v-*erb*B protein in erythroid cell transformation. Oncogene, 8, 1317–1327.

Le Roy, X., Escot, C., Brouillet, J.-P., Theillet, C., Maudelonde, T., Simony-Lafontaine, J., Pujol, H. and Rochefort, H. (1991). Decrease of c-*erb*B-2 and c-*myc* RNA levels in tamoxifen-treated breast cancer. Oncogene, 6, 431–437.

Liberman, T.A., Nusbaum, H.R., Razon, N., Kris, R., Lax, I., Soreq, H., Whittle, N., Waterfield, M.D., Ullrich, A. and Schlessinger, J. (1985). Amplification, enhanced expression and possible rearrangement of EGF receptor gene in primary human brain tumours of glial origin. Nature, 313, 144–147.

Lin, C.R., Chen, W.S., Kruiger, W., Stolarsky, L.S., Weber, W., Evans, R.M., Verma, I.M., Gill, G.N. and Rosenfeld, M.G. (1984). Expression cloning of human EGF receptor complementary DNA: gene amplifi-cation and three relatd messenger RNA products in A431 cells. Science, 224, 843–848.

Lin, Y.J. and Clinton, G.M. (1991). A soluble protein related to the HER2 proto-oncogene product is released from human breast carcinoma cells. Oncogene, 6, 639–643.

Liu, X. and Pawson, T. (1991). The epidermal growth factor receptor phosphorylates GTPase-activating protein (GAP) at Tyr-460, adjacent to the GAP SH2 domains. Mol. Cell. Biol., 11, 2511–2516.

Livneh, E., Glazer, L., Segal, D., Schlessinger, J. and Shilo, B.-Z. (1985). The *Drosophila* EGF receptor gene homolog: conservation of both hormone binding and kinase domains. Cell, 40, 599–607.

Marchionni, M.A., Goodearl, A.D.J., Chen, M.S., Bermingham-McDonogh, O., Kirk, C., Hendricks, M., Danehy, F., Misumi, D., Sudhalter, J., Kobayashi, K., Wroblewski, D., Lynch, C., Baldassare, M., Hiles, I., Davis, J.B., Hsuan, J.J., Totty, N.F., Otsu, M., McBurney, R.N., Waterfield, M.D., Stroobant, P. and Gwynne, D. (1993). Glial growth factors are alternatively spliced erbB2 ligands expressed in the nervous system. Nature, 362, 312–318.

Margolis, B.L., Lax, I., Kris, R., Dombalagian, M., Honegger, A.M., Howk, R., Givol, D., Ullrich, A. and Schlessinger, J. (1989). All autophosphorylation sites of epidermal growth factor (EGF) receptor and HER2/neu are located in their carboxyl-terminal tails. J. Biol. Chem., 264, 10667–10671.

Markowitz, S., Haut, M., Stellato, T., Gerbic, C. and Molkentin, K. (1989). Expression of the erbA-β class of thyroid hormone receptors is selectively lost in human colon carcinoma. J. Clin. Invest., 84, 1683–1687.

Marquardt, H., Hunkapiller, M.W., Hood, L.E. and Todaro, G.J. (1984). Rat transforming growth factor type 1: structure and relationship to epidermal growth factor. Science, 223, 1079–1082.

Metz, T. and Graf, T. (1992). The nuclear oncogenes v-*erb*A and v-*ets* cooperate in the induction of avian erythroleukemia. Oncogene, 7, 597–605.

Miyajima, N., Kadowaki, Y., Fukushige, S., Shimizu, S., Semba, K., Yamanashi, Y., Matsubara, K., Toyo-shima, K. and Yamamoto T. (1988). Identification of two novel members of erbA superfamily by molecu-lar cloning: the gene products of the two are highly related to each other. Nucleic Acids Res., 16, 11057–11074.

Miyajima, N., Horiuchi, R., Shibuya, Y., Fukushige, S.-I., Matsubara, K.-I., Toyoshima, K. and Yamamoto,

T. (1989). Two *erbA* homologs encoding proteins with different T_3 binding capacities are transcribed from opposite DNA strands of the same genetic locus. Cell, 57, 31–39.

Mroczkowski, B., Mosig, G. and Cohen, S. (1984). ATP-stimulated interaction between epidermal growth factor receptor and supercoiled DNA. Nature, 309, 270–273.

Muller, W.J., Sinn, E., Pattengale, P.K., Wallace, R. and Leder, P. (1988). Single-step induction of mammary adenocarcinoma in transgenic mice bearing the activated c-*neu* oncogene. Cell, 54, 105–115.

Nakai, A., Seino, S., Sakurai, A., Szilak, I., Bell, G.I. and DeGroot, L.J. (1988). Characterization of a thyroid hormone receptor expressed in human kidney and other tissues. Proc. Natl Acad. Sci. USA, 85, 2781–2785.

Nilsen, T.W., Maroney, P.A., Goodwin, R.G., Rottman, F.M., Crittenden, L.B., Raines, M.A. and Kung, H.-J. (1985). c-*erbB* activation in ALV-induced erythroblastosis: novel RNA processing and promoter insertion result in expression of an amino-truncated EGF receptor. Cell, 41, 719–726.

Padhy, L.C., Shih, C., Cowing, D., Finklestein, R. and Weinberg, R.A. (1982). Identification of a phosphoprotein specifically induced by the transforming DNA of rat neuroblastomas. Cell, 28, 865–871.

Pain, B., Woods, C.M., Saez, J., Flickinger, T., Raines, M., Peyrol, S., Moscovici, C., Moscovici, M.G., Kung, H.-J., Jurdic, P., Lazarides, E. and Samarut, J. (1991). EGFR as a hemopoietic growth factor receptor: the c-*erbB* product is present in chicken erythrocytic progenitors and controls their self-renewal. Cell, 65, 37–46.

Pasleau, F., Grooteclaes, M. and Gol-Winkler, R. (1993). Expression of the c-*erbB2* gene in the BT474 human mammary tumor cell line: measurement of c-*erbB2* mRNA half-life. Oncogene, 8, 849–854.

Paterson, M.C., Dietrich, K.D., Danyluk, J., Paterson, A.H., Lees, A.W., Jamil, N., Hanson, J., Jenkins, H., Krause, B.E., McBlain, W.A., Slamon, D.J. and Fourney, R.M. (1991). Correlation between c-*erbB*-2 amplification and risk of recurrent disease in node-negative breast cancer. Cancer Res., 51, 556–567.

Peles, E., Levy, R.B., Or, E., Ullrich, A. and Yarden, Y. (1991). Oncogenic forms of the *neu*/HER2 tyrosine kinase are permanently coupled to phospholipase Cγ. EMBO J., 10, 2077–2086.

Peles, E., Bacus, S.S., Koski, R.A., Lu, H.S., Wen, D., Ogden, S.G., Levy, R.B. and Yarden, Y. (1992). Isolation of the neu/HER2 stimulating ligand: a 44 kd glycoprotein that induces differentiation of mammary tumor cells. Cell, 69, 205–216.

Peppelenbosch, M.P., Tertoolen, L.G.J., den Hertog, J. and de Laat, S.W. (1992). Epidermal growth factor activates calcium channels by phospholipase A_2/5-lipoxygenase-mediated leukotriene C_4 production. Cell, 69, 295–303.

Pfahl, M. and Benbrook, D. (1987). Nucleotide sequence of cDNA encoding a novel human thyroid hormone receptor. Nucleic Acids Res., 15, 9613.

Plowman, G.D., Whitney, G.S., Neubauer, M.G., Green, J.M., McDonald, V.L., Todaro, G.J. and Shoyab, M. (1990). Molecular cloning and expression of an additional epidermal growth factor receptor-related gene. Proc. Natl Acad. Sci. USA, 87, 4905–4909.

Plowman, G.D., Culouscou, J.-M., Whitney, G.S., Green, J.M., Carlton, G.W., Foy, L., Neubauer, M.G. and Shoyab, M. (1993). Ligand-specific activation of HER4/p180[erbB4], a fourth member of the epidermal growth factor receptor family. Proc. Natl Acad. Sci. USA, 90, 1746–1750.

Prigent, S.A., Lemoine, N.R., Hughes, C.M., Plowman, G.D., Selden, C. and Gullick, W.J. (1992). Expression of the c-*erbB*-3 protein in normal human adult and fetal tissues. Oncogene, 7, 1273–1278.

Proctor, A.J., Coombs, L.M., Cairns, J.P. and Knowles, M.A. (1991). Amplification at chromosome 11q13 in transitional cell tumours of the bladder. Oncogene, 6, 789–795.

Qian, X., Decker, S.J. and Greene, M.I. (1992). p185[c-neu] and epidermal growth factor receptor associate into a structure composed of activated kinases. Proc. Natl Acad. Sci. USA, 89, 1330–1334.

Raines, M.A., Maihle, N.J., Moscovici, C., Crittenden, L. and Kung, H.-J. (1988). Mechanism of c-*erbB* transduction: newly released transducing viruses retain poly(A) tracts of *erbB* transcripts and encode C-terminally intact *erbB* proteins. J. Virol., 62, 2437–2443.

Redemann, N., Holzmann, B., von Ruden, T., Wagner, E.F., Schlessinger, J. and Ullrich, A. (1992). Anti-oncogenic activity of signalling-defective epidermal growth factor receptor mutants. Mol. Cell. Biol., 12, 491–498.

Riedel, H., Massoglia, S., Schlessinger, J. and Ullrich, A. (1988). Ligand activation of overexpressed epidermal growth factor receptors transforms NIH 3T3 mouse fibroblasts. Proc. Natl Acad. Sci. USA, 85, 1477–1481.

Rio, M.C., Bellocq, J.P., Gairard, B., Rasmussen, U.B., Krust, A., Koehl, C., Calderoli, H., Schiff, V., Renaud, R. and Chambon, P. (1987). Specific expression of the pS2 gene in subclasses of breast cancers in comparison with expression of the estrogen and progesterone receptors and the oncogene *ERBB2*. Proc. Natl Acad. Sci. USA, 84, 9243–9247.

Riviere, A., Becker, J. and Loning, T. (1991). Comparative investigation of c-*erbB2*/*neu* expression in head and neck tumors and mammary cancer. Cancer, 67, 2142–2149.

Ro, J., El-Naggar, A., Ro, J.Y., Blick, M., Frye, D., Fraschini, G., Fritsche, H. and Hortobagyi, G. (1989). c-*erb*B-2 amplification in node-negative human breast cancer. Cancer Res., 49, 6941–6944.

Robinson, H.L., Tracy, S.E., Nair, N., Taglienti-Sian, C. and Gamett, D.C. (1992). Characterization of an angiosarcoma-inducing mutation in the *erb*B oncogene. Oncogene, 7, 2025–2030.

Rothe Meyer, A. and Engelbreth-Holm, J. (1933). Experimentelle studien uber die beziehungen zwischen hunerleukose und sarkom an der hand eines stammes von ubertragbarer leukose-sarkom-kombination. Acta Pathol. Microbiol. Scand., 10, 380–427.

Sager, R. (1989). Tumor suppressor genes: the puzzle and the promise. Science, 246, 1406–1412.

Sakurai, A., Nakai, A. and DeGroot, L.J. (1990). Structural analysis of human thyroid hormone receptor β gene. Mol. Cell. Endocrinol., 71, 83–91.

Sande, S., Sharif, M., Chen, H. and Privalsky, M. (1993). v-*erb*A acts on retinoic acid receptors in immature avian erythroid cells. J. Virol., 67, 1067–1074.

Sap, J., Munoz, A., Damm, K., Goldberg, Y., Ghysdael, J., Leutz, A., Beug, H. and Vennstrom, B. (1986). The c-*erb*A protein is a high-affinity receptor for thyroid hormone. Nature, 324, 635–640.

Schechter, A.L., Stern, D.F., Vaidyanathan, L., Decker, S.J., Drebin, J.A., Greene, M.I. and Weinberg, R.A. (1984). The *neu* oncogene: an *erb*B-related gene encoding a 185,000-M$_r$ tumor antigen. Nature, 312, 513–516.

Scott, G.K., Robles, R., Park, J.W., Montgomery, P.A., Daniel, J., Holmes, W.E., Lee, J., Keller, G.A., Li, W.-L., Fendly, B.M., Wood, W.I., Shepard, H.M. and Benz, C.C. (1993). A truncated intracellular HER2/*neu* receptor produced by alternative RNA processing affects growth of human carcinoma cells. Mol. Cell. Biol., 13, 2247–2257.

Scotting, P., Vennstrom, B., Jansen, M., Graf, T., Beug, H. and Hayman, M.J. (1987). Common site of mutation in the *erb*B gene of avian eryhtroblastosis virus mutants that are temperature sensitive for transformation. Oncogene Res., 1, 265–278.

Segatto, O., Lonardo, F., Wexler, D., Fazioloi, F., Pierce, J.H., Bottaro, D.P., White, M.F. and Di Fiore, P.P. (1991). The juxtamembrane regions of the epidermal growth factor receptor and gp185^{erbB-2} determine the specificity of signal transduction. Mol. Cell. Biol., 11, 3191–3202.

Selva, E., Raden, D.L. and Davis, R.J. (1993). Mitogen-activated protein kinase stimulation by a tyrosine kinase-negative epidermal growth factor receptor. J. Biol. Chem., 268, 2250–2254.

Semba, K., Kamata, N., Toyoshima, K. and Yamamoto, T. (1985). A v-*erb*B-related protooncogene, c-*erb*B-2, is distinct from the c-*erb*B-1/epidermal growth factor-receptor gene and is amplified in a human salivary gland adenocarcinoma. Proc. Natl Acad. Sci. USA, 82, 6497–6501.

Shih, C., Padhy, L.C., Murray, M. and Weinberg, R.A. (1981). Transforming genes of carcinomas and neuroblastomas introduced into mouse fibroblasts. Nature, 290, 261–264.

Shu, H.-K.G., Pelley, R.J. and Kung, H.-J. (1991). Dissecting the activating mutations in v-*erb*B of avian erythroblastosis virus strain R. J. Virol., 65, 6177–6180.

Simmen, F.A., Gope, M.L., Schulz, T.Z., Wright, D.A., Carpenter, G. and O'Malley, B.W. (1984). Isolation of an evolutionarily conserved epidermal growth factor receptor cDNA from human A431 carcinoma cells. Biochem. Biophys. Res. Commun., 124, 125–132.

Slamon, D.J., Clark, G.M., Wong, S.G., Levin, W.J., Ullrich, A. and McGuire, W.L. (1987). Human breast cancer: correlation of relapse and survival with amplification of the HER2/*neu* oncogene. Science, 235, 177–182.

Slamon, D.J., Godolphin, W., Jones, L.A., Holt, J.A., Wong, S.G., Keith, D.E., Levin, W.J., Stuart, S.G., Udove, J., Ullrich, A. and Press, M.F. (1989). Studies of the HER2/*neu* proto-oncogene in human breast and ovarian cancer. Science, 244, 707–712.

Smit-McBride, Z. and Privalsky, M.L. (1993). Functional domains of the v-*erb*A protein necessary for oncogenesis are required for transcriptional activation in *Saccharomyces cerevisiae*. Oncogene, 8, 1465–1475.

Smith, K., Houlbrook, S., Greenall, M., Carmichael, J. and Harris, A.L. (1993). Topoisomerase IIα co-amplification with *erb*B2 in human primary breast cancer and breast cancer cell lines: relationship to *m*-AMSA and mitoxantrone sensitivity. Oncogene, 8, 933–938.

Stroobant, P., Rice, A.P., Gullick, W.J., Cheng, D.J., Kerr, I.M. and Waterfield, M.D. (1985). Purification and characterization of vaccinia virus growth factor. Cell, 42, 383–393.

Suen, T.-C. and Hung, M.-C. (1991). c-*myc* reverses *neu*-induced transformed morphology by transcriptional repression. Mol. Cell. Biol., 11, 354–362.

Taglienti-Sian, C.A., Banner, B., Davis, R.J. and Robinson, H.L. (1993). Induction of renal adenocarcinoma by a nonmutated *erb*B oncogene. J. Virol., 67, 1132–1136.

Tal, M., Wetzler, M., Josefberg, Z., Deutch, A., Gutman, M., Assaf, D., Kris, R., Shiloh, Y., Givol, D. and Schlessinger, J. (1988). Sporadic amplification of the HER2/neu proto-oncogene in adenocarcinomas of various tissues. Cancer Res., 48, 1517–1520.

Tarakhovsky, A., Zaichuk, T., Prassolov, V. and Butenko, Z.A. (1991). A 25 kDa polypeptide is the ligand for p185neu and is secreted by activated macrophages. Oncogene, 6, 2187–2196.

Thor, A.D., Schwartz, L.H., Koerner, F.C., Edgerton, S.M., Skates, S.J., Yin, S., McKenzie, S.J., Panicali, D.L., Marks, P.J., Fingert, H.J. and Wood, W.C. (1989). Analysis of c-*erb*B-2 expression in breast carcinomas with clinical follow-up. Cancer Res., 49, 7147–7152.

Tsuda, H., Hirohashi, S., Shimosato, Y., Hirota, T., Tsugane, S., Yamamoto, H., Miyajima, N., Toyoshima, K., Yamamoto, T., Yokota, J., Yoshida, T., Sakamoto, H., Terada, M. and Sugimura, T. (1989). Correlation between long-term survival in breast cancer patients and amplification of two putative oncogene-coamplification units: *hst*-1/*int*-2 and c-*erb*B-2/*ear*-1. Cancer Res., 49, 3104–3108.

Ullrich, A., Coussens, L., Hayflick, J.S., Dull, T.J., Gray, A., Tam, A.W., Lee, J., Yarden, Y., Liberman, T.A., Schlessinger, J., Downward, J., Mayes, E.L.V., Whittle, N., Waterfield, M.D. and Seeburg, P.H. (1984). Human epidermal growth factor receptor cDNA sequence and aberrant expression of the amplified gene in A431 epidermoid carcinoma cells. Nature, 309, 418–425.

Wadsworth, S.C., Vincent, W.S. and Bilodeau-Wentworth, D. (1985). A *Drosophila* genomic sequence with homology to human epidermal growth factor receptor. Nature, 314, 178–180.

Wang, L.-H., Tsai, S.Y., Cook, R.G., Beattie, W.G., Tsai, M.-J. and O'Malley, B.W. (1989). COUP transcription factor is a member of the steroid receptor family. Nature, 340, 163–166.

Wasilenko, W.J., Payne, D.M., Fitzgerald, D.L. and Weber, M.J. (1991). Phosphorylation and activation of epidermal growth factor receptors in cells transformed by the *src* oncogene. Mol. Cell. Biol., 11, 309–321.

Wasson, J.C., Saylors, R.L., Zeltzer, P., Friedman, H.S., Bigner, S.H., Burger, P.C., Bigner, D.D., Look, A.T., Douglass, E.C. and Brodeur, G.M. (1990). Oncogene amplification in pediatric brain tumors. Cancer Res., 50, 2987–2990.

Weinberger, C., Thompson, C.C., Ong, E.S., Lebo, R., Gruol, D.J. and Evans, R.M. (1986). The c-*erb*A gene encodes a thyroid hormone receptor. Nature, 324, 641–646.

Wen, D., Peles, E., Cupples, R., Suggs, S.V., Bacus, S.S., Luo, Y., Trail, G., Hu, S., Silbiger, S.M., Levy, R.B., Koski, R.A., Lu, H.S. and Yarden, Y. (1992). Neu differentiation factor: a transmembrane glycoprotein containing an EGF domain and an immunoglobulin homology unit. Cell, 69, 559–572.

White, M.R.-A. and Hung, M.-C. (1992). Cloning and characterization of the mouse *neu* promoter. Oncogene, 7, 677–683.

Wright, C., Mellon, K., Neal, D.E., Johnston, P., Corbett, I.P. and Horne, C.H.W. (1990). Expression of c-*erb*B-2 protein product in bladder cancer. Brit. J. Cancer, 62, 764–765.

Yamamoto, T., Nishida, T., Miyajima, N., Kawai, S., Ooi, T. and Toyoshima, K. (1983). The *erb*B gene of avian erythroblastosis virus is a member of the *src* gene family. Cell, 35, 71–78.

Yamamoto, T., Ikawa, S., Akiyama, T., Semba, K., Nomura, N., Miyajima, N., Saito, T. and Toyoshima, K. (1986a). Similarity of protein encoded by the human c-*erb*B-2 gene to epidermal growth factor receptor. Nature, 319, 230–234.

Yamamoto, T., Kamata, N., Kawano, H., Shimizu, S., Kuroki, T., Toyoshima, R., Rikimaru, K., Nomura, N., Ishizaki, R., Pastan, I., Gamou, S. and Shimizu, N. (1986b). High incidence of amplification of the EGF receptor gene in human squamous carcinoma cell lines. Cancer Res., 46, 414–416.

Yan, D.-H. and Hung, M.-C. (1991). Identification and characterization of a novel enhancer for the rat n*eu* promoter. Mol. Cell. Biol., 11, 1875–1882.

Yang-Feng, T.L., Schechter, A.L., Weinberg, R.W. and Francke, U. (1988). Oncogene from rat neuro/glioblastomas (human gene symbol *NGL*) is located on the proximal long arm of human chromosome 17 and *EGFR* is confirmed at 7p13–q11.2. Cytogen. Cell Genet., 40, 784.

Yokota, J., Yamamoto, T., Miyajima, N., Toyoshima, K., Nomura, N., Sakamoto, H. Yoshida, T., Terada, M. and Sugimura, T. (1988). Genetic alterations of the c-*erb*B-2 oncogene occur frequently in tubular adenocarcinoma of the stomach and are often accompanied by amplification of the v-*erb*A homologue. Oncogene, 2, 283–287.

Yonemura, Y., Ninomiya, I., Yamaguchi, A., Fushida, S., Kimura, H., Ohoyama, S., Miyazaki, I., Endou, Y., Tanaka, M. and Sasaki, T. (1991). Evaluation of immunoreactivity for *erb*B-2 protein as a marker of poor short term prognosis in gastric cancer. Cancer Res., 51, 1034–1038.

Yu, D. and Hung, M.-C. (1991). Expression of activated rat *neu* oncogene is sufficient to induce experimental metastasis in 3T3 cells. Oncogene, 6, 1991–1996.

Yu, D., Hamada, J., Zhang, H., Nicolson, G.L. and Hung, M.-C. (1992). Mechanisms of c-*erb*B2/*neu* oncogene-induced metastasis and repression of metastatic properties by adenovirus 5 E1A gene products. Oncogene, 7, 2263–2270.

Zabrecky, J.R., Lam, T., McKenzie, S.J. and Carney, W. (1991). The extracellular domain of p185/*neu* is released from the surface of human breast carcinoma cells, SK-BR-3. J. Biol. Chem., 266, 1716–1720.

Zenke, M., Kahn, P., Disela, C., Vennstrom, B., Leutz, A., Keegan, K., Hayman, M.J., Choi, H.R., Yew, N.,

Engel, J.D. and Beug, H. (1988). v-*erb*A specifically suppresses transcription of the avian erythrocyte anion transporter (Band 3) gene. Cell, 52, 107–119.

Zenke, M., Munoz, A., Sap, J., Vennstrom, B. and Beug, H. (1990). v-*erb*A oncogene activation entails the loss of hormone-dependent regulator activity of c-*erb*A. Cell, 61, 1035–1049.

Zhao, X.-Y. and Hung, M.-C. (1992). Negative autoregulation of the *neu* gene is mediated by a novel enhancer. Mol. Cell. Biol., 12, 2739–2748.

Zhou, D.-J., Ahuja, H. and Cline, M.J. (1989). Proto-oncogene abnormalities in human breast cancer: c-ERBB-2 amplification does not correlate with recurrence of disease. Oncogene, 4, 105–108.

Zhu, G., Decker, S.J. and Saltiel, A.R. (1992). Direct analysis of the binding of src-homology 2 domains of phospholipase C to the activated epidermal growth factor receptor. Proc. Natl Acad. Sci. USA, 89, 9559–9563.

TRK

TRK (tropomyosin-receptor-*k*inase, originally designated *onc*D) is a human transforming gene having no homology with known viral oncogenes. It was originally detected by NIH 3T3 fibroblast transfection with genomic DNA from a colon carcinoma (Pulciani *et al.*, 1982; Martin-Zanca *et al.*, 1986). Additional *TRK* oncogenes have been isolated from thyroid tumours and over 40 *TRK* oncogenes have been generated *in vitro* (Barbacid, 1993).

Normal *TRK* alleles (*TRK* (or *TRKA*), *TRKB* and *TRKC*) encode tyrosine kinase receptors for the nerve growth factor (NGF) family of neurotrophins.

Related genes

TRK genes encode a distinct subfamily of tyrosine kinase receptors. The N-terminal, extracellular regions of TRK proteins contain three leucine-rich motifs (LRMs) flanked by conserved cysteine residues, a characteristic of the LRM superfamily that includes human platelet von Willebrand factor receptor, ribonuclease/angiogenin inhibitor, cell adhesion proteins and extracellular matrix proteins (Schneider and Schweiger, 1991). The extracellular domains also contain two C_2 Ig-like loops similar to those present in neural cell adhesion molecules and in the receptors for fibroblast growth factors (see **HSTF1/Hst-1**), PDGF and CSF1, in KIT and in *Drosophila* D-*trk* (Pulido *et al.*, 1992). The 3' TRK sequence is >50% homologous to receptor tyrosine kinase domains (EGFR, insulin-R, SRC family).

The human putative tyrosine kinase receptors ROR1 and ROR2 share homology with TRK in the kinase domain, ROR1 being 47% identical in sequence to TRK in this region (Masiakowski and Carroll, 1992).

A muscle-specific receptor in *Torpedo californica* contains a TRK-related kinase domain but has a kringle domain close to the transmembrane region (Jennings *et al.*, 1993).

Cross-species homology

TRK (human), TRKB (mouse) and TRKC (pig): 67% overall amino acid homology. TRK and TRKB: overall identity 38%; 88% protein sequence homology in kinase domains: ~40% homology in extracellular, ligand binding domains. TRK and TRKC kinase domains are 87% homologous (76% identical); TRKB and TRKC kinase domains are 88% homologous (83% identical).

Twelve extracellular cysteine residues are conserved in all known TRK proteins.

Drosophila D-*trk* and the mammalian *Trk* gene products are 42–48% homologous in the extracellular domains and 60–63% homologous in the kinase domains.

Transformation

MAN

Transforming *TRK* (*NTRK1*) alleles are found in human colon carcinomas and with high frequency in thyroid papillary carcinomas (Martin-Zanca *et al.*, 1986; Bongarzone *et al.*, 1989). *TRK* maps to a region of chromosome 1 that includes breakpoints associated with some cancers and also the TGFβ and poly(ADP-ribose)-polymerase genes. *TRK* expression is high in most stage I, II, and IV-S neuroblastomas but undetectable in most advanced tumours and appears to correlate inversely with amplification of *MYCN* (Nakagawara *et al.*, 1992).

The colon carcinoma *TRK* oncogene encodes a hybrid protein in which the N-terminal portion of non-muscle tropomyosin is fused to the transmembrane and cytoplasmic domains of TRK. The 5' region shares 90% homology with horse platelet tropomyosin and >96% homology with a cloned, human, non-muscle tropomyosin pseudogene.

Some *TRK* oncogenes detected in thyroid tumours encode TRK oncoprotein sequences identical to that of the colon carcinoma protein but others have different sequences replacing the TRK ligand binding domain, including those derived from the *TPR* locus (see **TRK oncoproteins**, page 515).

IN VITRO

NIH 3T3 fibroblasts are transformed by NGF, the ligand for TRKA (Cordon-Cardo *et al.*, 1991), or by co-transfection of plasmids expressing *TrkB* and brain-derived neurotropic factor (BDNF) or neurotropin-3 (NT-3; Klein *et al.*, 1991b) or by co-expression of *TrkC* and NT-3 (Lamballe *et al.*, 1991). The human oncogene *TRK-T1* transforms NIH 3T3 cells (Greco *et al.*, 1992).

	TRK/Trk	*TRKB/TrkB*	*TRKC/TrkC*
Nucleotides (kb)	20	>100	
Chromosome			
Human	1q23–1q24 (*NTRK1*) (Morris *et al.*, 1991)	1q23–q31 (*NTRK2*)	1q23–q31 (*NTRK3*)
Mouse	3	13	
mRNA (kb)			
Human	3.2		
Mouse	3.0	2.0–9.0 (>6)	
Rat		0.7–9.0 (>8)	
Pig			4.7/6.1
Amino acids			
Human	790 619 (TRK1) 439 (TRK2)		
Mouse, rat		821 (gp145^{trkB})	
Mouse, pig			825 (gp145^{trkC}) 839 (gp145^{trkC}K1) 850 (gp145^{trkC}K2)
Mass (kDa)			
(predicted)	87 70 (TRK1)/49 (TRK2)	95	90
(expressed)	gp140^{trk} 70^{trk} (tropomyosin-TRK) 55 (TRK-T1)	gp95^{trkB}/gp145^{trkB}	gp145^{trkC} gp145^{trkC}K1 gp145^{trkC}K2

Cellular location

Plasma membrane.

Tissue location

Trk and *TrkB* are primarily expressed in the nervous system (Barbacid *et al.*, 1991). In the mouse the earliest developmental stage at which *Trk* mRNA is detectable coincides with the onset of neurogenesis. The pattern of *Trk* expression is highly specific, being confined to a subpopulation of neural crest-derived sensory neurons in the peripheral nervous system (Martin-Zanca *et al.*, 1990).

TrkB is widely expressed in both the central nervous system and the peripheral nervous system (Klein *et al.*, 1990a,b). gp145^{trkB} mRNA (5.5 and 9.0 kb) occurs in the mouse cerebral cortex and the pyramidal cell layer of the hippocampus. Murine gp95^{trkB} mRNA (2.5 and 8.2 kb) is expressed in the ependymal linings of the cerebral ventricles and the choroid plexus; this non-catalytic receptor may not be expressed in neurons. *TrkB* mRNA is also found in non-neuronal cells (glia, Schwann cells) and in the adult mouse low expression occurs in lung and muscle (2.0, 2.5 and 8.2 kb), in ovaries (2.5 and 8.2 kb) and in testes (2.5 and 2.8 kb). In rats *TrkB* is detectable in spleen, testes and submaxillary gland, as well as in brain (Middlemas *et al.*, 1991).

TrkC is widely expressed in both the central nervous system and the peripheral nervous system. *TrkC* mRNA occurs in the cerebral cortex, the dentate gyrus, the pyramidal cell layer of the hippocampus and in specific regions of the cerebellum (Lamballe *et al.*, 1991). The arterial walls and the gut lining also express *TrkC* but not *TrkB* (Barbacid, 1993).

In the rat forebrain *Trk* and low-affinity NGFR (LNGFR) mRNAs are co-localized in the medial septal nucleus and the nucleus of Broca's diagonal band, whereas *TrkB* is widely distributed (Vazquez and Ebendal, 1991).

Protein function

TRK genes encode transmembrane tyrosine kinases that are receptors for NGF, BNDF, NT-3, NT-4 or NT-5 and probably mediate specific cell adhesion events during neuronal cell development. Some of the multiple *TrkB* transcripts encode receptors from which the tyrosine kinase domain has been truncated. The *TrkC* locus may also encode truncated, non-catalytic receptors. TRK tyrosine kinase activity is specifically inhibited by the alkaloid-like compound K252a (Tapley *et al.*, 1992; Ohmichi *et al.*, 1992a; Berg *et al.*, 1992).

gp140^{trkA}

gp140^{trkA} is a high-affinity (k_d ~30 pM) receptor for NGF (Klein *et al.*, 1991a; Berkemeier *et al.*, 1991; Kaplan *et al.*, 1991a). There is controversial evidence indicating that high-affinity binding by NGF requires the co-expression of a distinct, low-affinity (k_d ~1 nM) receptor, gp75^{LNGFR} (Hempstead *et al.*, 1991). However, there is only limited co-expression of gp140^{trkA} and gp75^{LNGFR} in the CNS (Barbacid, 1993). Furthermore, the ectopic expression of gp140^{trkA} in NIH 3T3 fibroblasts that do not normally express either type of receptor confers high-affinity NGF binding that is unaffected by the co-expression of gp75^{LNGFR} (Klein *et al.*, 1991a). Targeted mutation of gp75^{LNGFR} in mice indicates that this neurotrophin receptor is involved in the development of sensory neurons (Lee *et al.*, 1992). The nine N-terminal amino acids of NGF are essential for interaction with the receptor (Kahle *et al.*, 1992).

NGF binding stimulates the tyrosine kinase activity and rapid tyrosine phosphorylation of p140^{trkA} (Kaplan *et al.*, 1991b). The activation of chimeric receptors comprised of the EGFR extracellular ligand binding domain and TRK transmembrane and intracellular sequences promotes association of phosphorylated PLC-γ, RAS–GTP and the non-catalytic subunit of phosphatidylinositol 3-kinase, p85, with TRK (Obermeier *et al.*, 1993). TRK Tyr785 is a major site of interaction with PLC-γ. In PC12 cells the activation of gp140^{trkA} by NGF stimulates RAF1 and mitogen-activated protein (MAP) kinases and results in differentiation into neuronal-type cells (Ohmichi *et al.*, 1992b). In transfected NIH 3T3 fibroblasts expressing gp140^{trkA} NGF causes *Fos* transcription, DNA synthesis and morphological transformation (Cordon-Cardo *et al.*, 1991) and in *Xenopus* oocytes expressing gp140^{trkA} NGF induces meiotic maturation (Nebreda *et al.*, 1991). In both PC12 and NIH 3T3 cells there is evidence that NT-3 is a weak agonist of the gp140^{trkA} receptor (Cordon-Cardo *et al.*, 1991) but it remains to be established whether this observation has significance for the *in vivo* effects of NT-3. Isoforms of gp140^{trkA} that may represent post-translational modification and dimerization have been detected in PC12 cells (Hartman *et al.*, 1992).

gp145^{trkB}

gp145^{trkB} is a receptor for BDNF, NT-3 and *Xenopus* NT-4 (Klein *et al.*, 1991b; Soppet *et al.*, 1991; Squinto *et al.*, 1991; Klein *et al.*, 1992). When expressed in NIH 3T3 fibroblasts gp145^{trkB} is rapidly phosphorylated on tyrosine residues in response to BDNF or NT-3 but in neither 3T3 cells nor hippocampal cells does gp145^{trkB} bind NGF (Soppet *et al.*, 1991). *TrkB* mediates the survival and proliferation of NIH 3T3 cells in response to BDNF in the absence of p75^{LNGFR} expression (Glass *et al.* 1991) and the co-expression of gp145^{trkB} and either BDNF or XNT-4 transforms these cells (Klein *et al.*, 1991b, 1992). BDNF, NT-3 or XNT-4 induce PC12 cells expressing gp145^{trkB} to differentiate (Klein *et al.*, 1992; Squinto *et al.*, 1991). However, NT-3 is at least tenfold less potent than BDNF in promoting survival or differentiation of cells expressing gp145^{trkB} and may not therefore be a physiological ligand for this receptor.

NT-5, which is closely related to XNT-4, also activates both p140^{trkA} and gp145^{trkB} (Berkemeier *et al.*, 1991).

gp95^{trkB}

The function of gp95^{trkB} is unknown but the differential pattern of expression with respect to gp145^{trkB} (see **Tissue location**) suggests that this non-catalytic form may transport gp145^{trkB} ligands within or to the brain.

gp145^{trkC}

This protein is a high-affinity (k_d ~26 pM) NT-3 receptor, but it does not bind BDNF, NT-4 or NGF (Lamballe *et al.*, 1991). When expressed in NIH 3T3 fibroblasts gp145^{trkC} is rapidly phosphorylated on tyrosine residues in response to NT-3 but not to other neurotrophins and the co-expression of gp145^{trkC} and NT-3 transforms these cells. gp145^{trkC}K1 contains an insert of 14 amino acids in the sequence of gp145^{trkC} (see **Protein structure** below). When expressed in NIH 3T3 cells gp145^{trkC}K1 also undergoes rapid tyrosine phosphorylation in response to NT-3 (Barbacid, 1993).

Protein structure

THE TRK FAMILY OF NEUROTROPHIN RECEPTORS

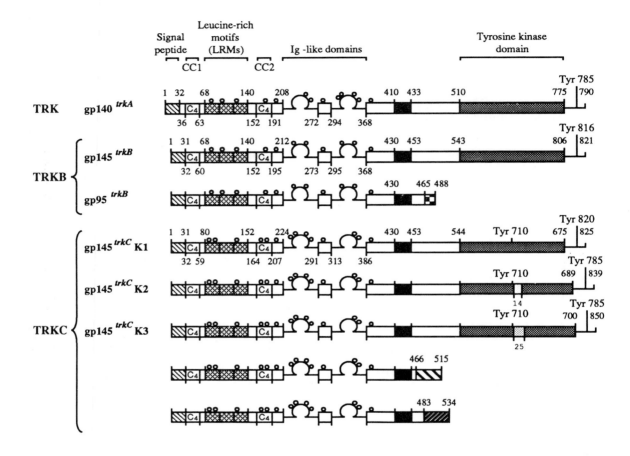

(Adapted from Barbacid, M. (1993). The Trk family of neurotrophin receptors: molecular characterization and oncogenic activation in human tumors. In Molecular Genetics of Nervous System Tumors: 123–135. Wiley-Liss, New York.)

The N-terminal region of the extracellular domains contains a signal peptide, two cysteine clusters (C_4) each including four of the 12 cysteine residues conserved in all known TRK proteins, three tandem repeats of a 24 amino acid leucine-rich motif (LRM: consensus sequence L–X–X–L–X–y–X–X–N– –X–L–X–X–y–X–X– – –X–X–y–X–X–X–X–X, where X is any amino acid and y is hydrophobic) and two C_2 Ig-like domains. Homologous features occur in the *Drosophila toll* gene product that mediates cell adhesion. Black boxes indicate transmembrane regions and circles ($\circ$) denote conserved potential *N*-glycosylation sites (Schneider and Schweiger, 1991).

gp145[trkB] and gp95[trkB] have identical extracellular and transmembrane domains (465 amino acids): gp95[trkB] lacks a tyrosine kinase domain, possessing only 23 cytoplasmic amino acids, the C-terminal 11 of which are unique to gp95[trkB]. The range of mRNAs detected in rat and mouse brain suggests the existence of other truncated receptors (Middlemas *et al.*, 1991) and the two major RNA species (2.0 and 8.0 kb) may encode a protein identical to gp95[trkB] in its C-terminus but having a different N-terminus (Klein *et al.*, 1990a). Five putative TRKC receptors have been identified: gp145*trkC*K1 is identical to gp145*trkC* except for the insertion of 14 amino acids two residues after Tyr598, the putative autophosphorylation site. gp145*trkC*K2 has a 25 amino acid insertion at the same point. Two putative non-catalytic isoforms have also been identified that correspond in structure to gp95*trkB* but have 49 and 51 amino acid cytoplasmic domains. In one of these isoforms the point of divergence from gp145*trkC* is identical to that of gp95*trkB* from gp145*trkB*. In the other isoform the novel cytoplasmic region is attached 30 amino acids beyond the C-terminus of the transmembrane region (Barbacid, 1993).

TRK ONCOPROTEINS

The *TRK* oncogene first isolated from a colon carcinoma was generated by rearrangement of the first seven coding exons of a non-muscle tropomyosin gene and a tyrosine kinase (Martin-Zanca *et al.*, 1986). Tropomyosin has 27 residues deleted at the C-terminus and the N-terminal 360 amino acids of TRK are truncated but the transmembrane region and the tyrosine kinase domain are unmodified ((b) below). Thus activation of *TRK* to an oncogene is the result of fusion of the tropomyosin sequences. The non-muscle isoform of tropomyosin involved in the activation of *TRK* maps to 1q31, suggesting that the generation of the hybrid transforming gene may be caused by an intra-chromosomal rearrangement of the long arm of chromosome 1 (Radice *et al.*, 1991).

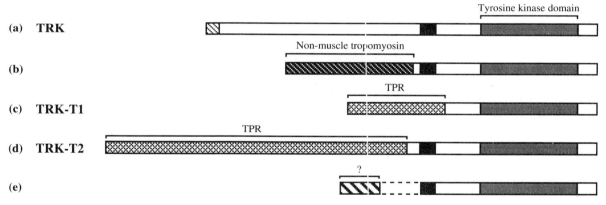

(Adapted from Barbacid, M. (1993). The Trk family of neurotrophin receptors: molecular characterization and oncogenic activation in human tumors. In Molecular Genetics of Nervous System Tumors: 123–135. Wiley-Liss, New York).

The tropomyosin-activated *TRK* oncogene has also been isolated from human thyroid papillary carcinomas but chimeric *TRK* oncogenes have also been isolated from these tumours that contain different activating sequences (Bongarzone *et al.*, 1989). Thyroid *TRK* oncogenes activated by fusion with sequences other than those of tropomyosin have been designated *TRK-T* (Greco *et al.*, 1992). *TRK-T1* contains 598 bp of the *TPR* gene (see **MET**) fused 5' to 1148 bp of *TRK* proto-oncogene. The 2.2 kb mRNA encodes a 503 amino acid protein (55 kDa) containing 192 TPR and 310 TRK residues ((c) above). *TRK-T2* contains additional *TPR* sequences ((d) above) and a third *TPR/TRK* oncogene has also been detected. A further isolate contains uncharacterized sequences ((e) above).

TRK ONCOPROTEINS ACTIVATED *IN VITRO*

Activation of *TRK* can also occur by recombination *in vitro* and over 40 such *TRK* oncogenes have been detected (Kozma *et al.*, 1988; Oskam *et al.*, 1988). The products of these *TRK* oncogenes retain the parental tyrosine kinase activity and have an intact C-terminus. However, the

N-termini acquired may generate non-glycosylated cytoplasmic molecules or transmembrane glycoproteins.

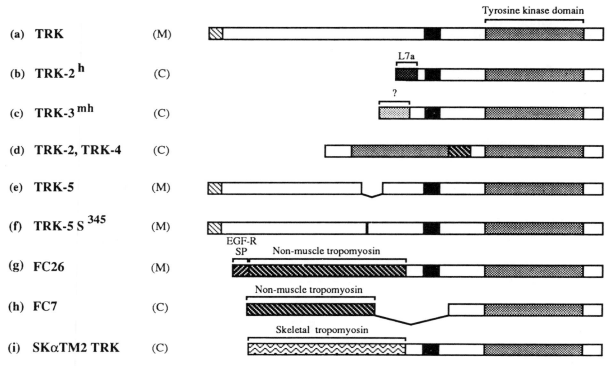

(Adapted from Barbacid, M. (1993). The Trk family of neurotrophin receptors: molecular characterization and oncogenic activation in human tumors. In Molecular Genetics of Nervous System Tumors: 123–135. Wiley-Liss, New York).

The figure shows the structures of a number of TRK oncoproteins generated *in vitro*. Transfection of either human genomic DNA or the TRK kinase domain into fibroblasts (Kozma *et al.*, 1988) generated the chimeric proteins TRK-2[h] in which the N-terminus is derived from the human ribosomal protein L7a (b) and TRK-3[mh] containing a mouse 5' sequence (c). TRK-2 and TRK-4 (d) comprise head-to-tail arrangements of tyrosine kinase domains and TRK-5 (e) is identical to gp140[trkA] save for a 51 amino acid deletion in the second Ig-like domain. A transforming *TRK* gene (TRK-5 S[345], (f)) has also been generated by substituting the conserved cysteine residue that is removed in the TRK-5 deletion with serine (Coulier *et al.*, 1990). Other fusions conferring transforming capacity involve the EGF receptor signal peptide (EGFR SP) and tropomyosin ((g) and (h)) and skeletal muscle tropomyosin (i).

Chimeric proteins that have lost the signal peptide are converted from a membrane (M) to a cytosolic (C) location.

Sequences of human TRK, mouse TRKB and rat TRKB and pig TRKC

```
                                    →  CC1
Human TRK   (1) MLRGGRRGOLGWHSWAAGPGSLLAWLIL ASAGAAPCPDAC CPHGSSGLRCTR  DGALD
Mouse TRKB  (1) -SPWL  KWH-PAMARLWGLC-IVLGFWR--  LA--TS-K-SSAR  IW--EPSP-IVA
Rat TRKB    (1) ****P  ************************  ****M * ****TT************
Pig TRKC    (1) -DVSL  CPAKCSFWRIF-LGSVW-DYVGSVLA--AN-V-SKTE  IN-R-PD--N-
```

```
                      CC1 ←                              →       LRM-1        ←→ LRM-2
Human TRK    (58)  SLHHLPG                     AENLTELYIENQQHLQHLELRDLRGLGELRNLTIVKSG
Mouse TRKB   (55)  FPRLE-NSVD                  P--I--IL-A--KR-HIINED-VEAYVG-------D--
Rat TRKB     (55)  ********I*                  ***********************K********
Pig TRKC     (54)  FPLLEGQDSGNSNGNASINITDISR-I-SIH-E-WRG-HT-NAV-MELYTG-QK---KN--
                          LRM-2     ←→       LRM-3          ←              → CC-2
Human TRK   (103)  LRFVAPDAFHFTPRLSRLNLSFNALESLSWKTVQGLSLQELVLSGNPLHCSCALRWLQRVE
Mouse TRKB  (103)  -K---YK--LKNSN-RHI-FTR-K-T---RRHFRH-D-SD-I-T---FT---DIM--KTLQ
Rat TRKB    (103)  *************************G*********
Pig TRKC    (115)  --SIQ-R--AKN-H-RYI---S-R-TT---QLF-T---R--R-EQ-FFN---DI--M-LWQ
                                   CC-2      ←                       → Ig-like I
Human TRK   (164)  EEGLGGVPEQKLQC  HGQGPLAHMPNASCGVPTLKVQVPNASVDVGDDVLLRCQVEGR
Mouse TRKB  (164)  - TKSSPDT-D-Y-LNESSKNM---NLQIPN--L-SARLAA--LT-EE-KS-T-S-S-G-D
Rat TRKB    (164)  * ********************T***********************I*******
Pig TRKC    (176)  -Q-EAKLNS-S-Y-ISADGS-L--FR-NISQ-DL-EIS-SHV-LT-RE--NAVVT-NGS-S
                                                              Ig-like I    ←
Human TRK   (221)  GLEQAGWILTELEQS   ATKVMSGGLPSLGLTLANVTSDLNRKNLTCWAENDVGRAEVSV
Mouse TRKB  (224)  P-PTLY-DVGN-VS   KHMNET-HTQG--RI-  -IS--DSG-QIS-V---L--EDQD--
Rat TRKB    (224)  **************   ***************   **********************
Pig TRKC    (237)  P-PDVD--V-G-QSINTHQ-NLNWTNVHAIN---V----ED-GFT---I---V--MSNAS-
                          →  Ig-like II
Human TRK   (279)  QVNVSFPASVQLHTAVEM HHWSIPESVDGQPAPSLRWLFNGSVLNETSFIFTEFLEPAAN
Mouse TRKB  (280)  NLT-H-APTITFLESPTSD---C---T-R-N-K-A-Q-FY--AI---SKY-C-KIHVT -
Rat TRKB    (280)  *******************************************t*********** *
Pig TRKC    (298)  ALT-HY-PR-VSLEEP-LRLEHC-EFV-R-N-P-T-H--H--QP-R-SKITHVEYYQEG
                                         Ig-like II  ←
Human TRK   (339)  ETVRHGCLRLNQPTHVNNGNYTLLAANPFGQASASIMAAFMDNP  FEFNPEDP
Mouse TRKB  (339)  H-EY----Q-DN---M---D---M-K-EY-KDERQ-S-H--GR-GVDY-T--NY-EVLYED
Rat TRKB    (339)  ****************************************H*****************
Pig TRKC    (357)  E-SE---LF-K---Y-------NRQE-L-T-NQT-NGH-LKE-       F-EST DN
                          ++
Human TRK   (391)     IPDTNSTSGD   PVEKKDET PFGVSVAVGLAVFACLFLSTLLLVLNKCGRRN
Mouse TRKB  (400)  WTTPTD-G--TNK-N-IPSTD-ADQSNREHLS-YAVVVIASVVG-CLLVM-L-L -LA-HS
Rat TRKB    (400)  *********************************T***************** ******
Pig TRKC    (407)  FVSFYEVSPT     PPITVTHKPEEDT----I-----A--VL-VV-FIMI--Y---S
Human TRK   (441)  KFGINRPA VLAPEDGLAMSLHFMTLGGSSLSPTEG KGSGLQG      HIIENPQYF
Mouse TRKB  (460)  ---MKG--S-ISND-DS-SP--HISN-SNTP-SS--GPDAVIIGMTKIPV-------GITN
Rat TRKB    (460)  ***********************************************************
Pig TRKC    (461)  ---MKG-VA-ISG-EDS-SP--HDQPWHHHTLI-GRRA-HSVI-MTRIPV-------RQGH
                                   →  Tyrosine kinase domain
Human TRK   (492)       SDACVHHIKRRDIVLKWELGEGAFGKVFLAECHNLLPEQDKMLVAVKALKEASESAR
Mouse TRKB  (521)  SQLKP-TF-Q----HN----R--------------Y--C-----I-----T--D--DN--
Rat TRKB    (521)  ***********************************************************
Pig TRKC    (522)  NCHKP-TY-Q----------R--------------Y--S-TKV-------A--DPTLA--
Human TRK   (549)  QDFQREAELLTMLQHQHIVRFFGVCTEGRPLLMVFEYMRHGDLNRFLRSHGPDAKLLAGGE
Mouse TRKB  (581)  K--H-------N---E---K-Y---V--D--I------K-----K---A-----V-M---N
Rat TRKB    (581)  ***********************************************************
Pig TRKC    (583)  K----------N---E---K-Y---GD-D--I------K-----K---A-----MI-VD-Q
Human TRK   (610)  D VAPGPLGLGQLLAVASQVAAGMVYLAGLHFVHRDLATRNCLVGQGLVVKIGDFGMSRDI
Mouse TRKB  (643)  PP  TE-TQS-M-HI-Q-I--------SQ---------------EN-L----------V
Rat TRKB    (643)  ** ***********************************************************
Pig TRKC    (644)  PRQ-K-E---S-M-HI---ICS------SQ---------------AN-L----------V
Human TRK   (670)  YSTDYYRVGGRTMLPIRWMPPESILYRKFTTESDVWSFGVVLWEIFTYGKQPWYQLSNTEA
Mouse TRKB  (701)  ----------H-------------M-----------L-----------------N-V
Rat TRKB    (701)  ***********************************************************
Pig TRKC    (705)  ----------H-------------M--------------I-----------F------V
```

517

```
                                        Tyrosine kinase domain  ⟵
Human TRK  (731)  IDCITQGRELERPRACPPEVYAIMRGCWQREPQQRHSIKDVHARLQALAQAPPVYLDVLG  (790)
Mouse TRKB (762)  -E------V-Q---T--Q---EL-L-------HT-KN--SI-TL--N--K-S-----I--  (821)
Rat TRKB   (762)  ***********************************************NI***********  (821)
Pig TRKC   (766)  -E------V-----V--K---DV-L----------LN--EIYKI-H--GK-T-I---I--  (825)
```

Dashes indicate identity of mouse TRKB and pig TRKC with human TRK. * Indicates identity of rat TRKB with mouse TRKB. The transmembrane regions are in italics. Human TRK tyrosine kinase domain: residues 510–775. The TRK kinase domain is unique in containing a threonine residue instead of Ala647 (TRKB Thr678, TRKC Thr682), tryptophan instead of Tyr722 (TRKB Trp753, TRKC Trp757) and histidine instead of Pro766 (TRKB Lys797, TRKC Leu801). There is 37% identity between the extracellular domains and 75% identity within the kinase domains. ++ Indicates the breakpoint between residues 393 and 394 generated in the human tropomyosin/*TRK* oncogene. The 266 residue TRKA tyrosine kinase domain is 25% identical in sequence to that of SRC (Martin-Zanca *et al.*, 1986, 1989).

Sequences of human TRK-1[h] and human TRK-2[h]

```
Human TRK-1ʰ  (1)    MAGITTIEAVKRKIQVLQQQADDAEERAERLQREVEGERRAREQAEAEVASLNRRIQLV
Human TRK-1ʰ  (60)   EEELDRAQERLATALQKLEEAEKAADESERGMKVIENRALKDEEKMELQEIQLEEAKHIA
Human TRK-1ʰ  (120)  EEADRKYEEVARKLVIIEGDLERTEERAELAESRCREMDEQIRLMDQNLKCLSAAEEKYS

Human TRK-1ʰ  (180)  QKEDKYEEEIKILTDKLKEAETRAEFAERSVAKLEKTIDDLEDTNSTSGDPVEKKDETPF
Human TRK-2ʰ  (1)    MPKGKKAKG-KVAPAPAVVKKQEAKKVVNPLFEKRPKNFGI----------------

Human TRK-1ʰ  (240)  GVSVAVGLAVFACLFLSTLLLVLNKCGRRNKFGINRPAVLAPEDGLAMSLHFMTLGGSSL
Human TRK-2ʰ  (60)   --------------------------------------------------------

Human TRK-1ʰ  (300)  SPTEGKGSGLQGHIIENPQYFSDACVHHIKRRDIVLKWELGEGAFGKVFLAECHNLLPEQ
Human TRK-2ʰ  (120)  --------------------------------------------------------

Human TRK-1ʰ  (360)  DKMLVAVKALKEASESARQDFQREAELLTMLQHQHIVRFFGVCTEGRPLLMVFEYMRHGD
Human TRK-2ʰ  (180)  --------------------------------------------------------

Human TRK-1ʰ  (420)  LNRFLRSHGPDAKLLAGGEDVAPGPLGLGQLLAVASQVAAGMVYLAGLHFVHRDLATRNC
Human TRK-2ʰ  (240)  --------------------------------------------------------

Human TRK-1ʰ  (480)  LVGQGLVVKIGDFGMSRDIYSTDYYRVGGRTMLPIRWMPPESILYRKFTTESDVWSFGVV
Human TRK-2ʰ  (300)  --------------------------------------------------------

Human TRK-1ʰ  (540)  LWEIFTYGKQPWYQLSNTEAIDCITQGRELERPRACPPEVYAIMRGCWHGEPQQRHSIKD
Human TRK-2ʰ  (360)  --------------------------------------------------------

Human TRK-1ʰ  (600)  VHARLQALAQAPPVYLDVLG  (619)
Human TRK-2ʰ  (420)  -------------------  (439)
```

The transmembrane region is underlined. The ATP binding site is in bold type and underlined.

In TRK-1[h] amino acids 1–221 are non-muscle tropomyosin: 222–619 is the kinase domain. The chimeric oncogene *TRK-2[h]* was generated *in vitro* by transfection of DNA from the human breast carcinoma cell line MDA-MB231. Amino acids 42–439 of TRK-2[h] are identical to 222–619 of TRK-1[h]; the N-terminal 41 amino acids of TRK-2[h] are derived from human ribosomal protein 7a (Ziemiecki *et al.*, 1990). The 5′ region of *TRK-2[h]* is homologous to C5 RNA, the transcription of which is increased by UV irradiation or other DNA-damaging treatment (Ben-Ishai *et al.*, 1990). Thus the chimeric oncogene may have enhanced responsiveness to carcinogens.

The tyrosine kinase product of the *TRK* oncogene, p70^{rk}, is autophosphorylated *in vitro* on tyrosine and phosphorylated on serine, threonine and tyrosine in *TRK*-transformed cells. Its activity is abolished by mutation of Lys367. Mutation of Tyr503 and Tyr504, the putative auto-phosphorylation sites, greatly reduces the tyrosine kinase activity and transforming potential of the protein (Mitra, 1991).

Databank file names and accession numbers

	GENE	EMBL	SWISSPROT	REFERENCES
Human	*TRK*	Hstrkpoa M23102	TRKA_HUMAN P04629	Martin-Zanca *et al.*, 1986, 1989
Human	*TRK-2*[h]	Hstrk2H X06704	TRK2_HUMAN P08119	Kozma *et al.*, 1988
	TRK-1[h]	Hstrkr X03541	TRK1_HUMAN P04629	Martin-Zanca *et al.*, 1986 Kozma *et al.*, 1988
Mouse	*TrkB*	Mstrkb X17647	TRKB_MOUSE P15209	Klein *et al.*, 1989
Pig	*TrkC*	Sstrkc M80800	TRKC_PIG P24786	Lamballe *et al.*, 1991
Rat	*Trk*	Rrtrkprec M85214		Meakin *et al.*, 1992
Rat	*TrkB*	RntrkB1 M55291		Middlemas *et al.*, 1991
Drosophila	*D-trk*	Dmdtrk X63453		Pulido *et al.*, 1992

Reviews

Barbacid, M. (1993). The Trk family of neurotrophin receptors: molecular characterization and oncogenic activation in human tumors. In Molecular Genetics of Nervous System Tumors: 123–135. Wiley-Liss, New York.

Barbacid, M., Lamballe, F., Pulido, D. and Klein, R. (1991). The *trk* family of tyrosine protein kinase receptors. Biochim. Biophys. Acta, 1072, 115–127.

Papers

Ben-Ishai, R., Scharf, R., Sharon, R. and Kapten, I. (1990). A human cellular sequence implicated in *trk* oncogene activation is DNA damage inducible. Proc. Natl Acad. Sci. USA, 87, 6039–6043.

Berg, M.M., Sternberg, D.W., Parada, L.F. and Chao, M.V. (1992). K-252a inhibits nerve growth factor-induced *trk* proto-oncogene tyrosine phosphorylation and kinase activity. J. Biol. Chem., 267, 13–16.

Berkemeier, L.R., Winslow, J.W., Kaplan, D.R., Nikolics, K., Goeddel, D.V. and Rosenthal, A. (1991). Neur-otrophin-5: a novel neurotrophic factor that activates *trk* and *trk*B. Neuron, 7, 857–866.

Bongarzone, I., Pierotti, M.A., Monzini, N., Mondellini, P., Manenti, G., Donghi, R., Pilotti, S., Grieco, M., Santoro, M., Fusco, A., Vecchio, G. and Della Porta, G. (1989). High frequency of activation of tyrosine kinase oncogenes in human papilloma thyroid carcinoma. Oncogene, 4, 1457–1462.

Cordon-Cardo, C., Tapley, P., Jing, S., Nanduri, V., O'Rourke, E., Lamballe, F., Kovary, K., Klein, R., Jones, K.R., Reichardt, L. and Barbacid, M. (1991). The *trk* tyrosine protein kinase mediates the mitogenic properties of nerve growth factor and neurotropin-3. Cell, 66, 173–183.

Coulier, F., Kumar, R., Ernst, M., Klein, R., Martin-Zanca, D. and Barbacid, M. (1990). Human *trk* onco-genes activated by point mutation, in-frame deletion and duplication of the tyrosine kinase domain. Mol. Cell. Biol., 10, 4202–4210.

Glass, D.J., Nye, S.H., Hantzopoulos, P., Macchi, M.J., Squinto, S.P., Goldfarb, M. and Yancopoulos, G.D. (1991). trkB mediates BDNF/NT-3-dependent survival and proliferation in fibroblasts lacking the low affinity NGF receptor. Cell, 66, 405–413.

Greco, A., Pierotti, M.A., Bongarzone, I., Pagliardini, S., Lanzi, C. and Della Porta, G. (1992). *TRK*-T1 is a novel oncogene formed by the fusion of *TPR* and *TRK* genes in human papillary thyroid carcinomas. Oncogene, 7, 237–242.

Hartman, D.S., McCOrmack, M., Schubenel, R. and Hertel, C. (1992). Multiple trkA proteins in PC12 cells bind NGF with a slow association rate. J. Biol. Chem., 267, 24516–24522.

Hempstead, B.L., Kaplan, D., Martin-Zanca, D., Parada, L.F. and Chao, M. (1991). High affinity NGF binding requires co-expression of the *trk* proto-onocgene product and the low affinity NGF receptor. Nature, 350, 678–683.

Jennings, C.G.B., Dyer, S.M. and Burden, S.J. (1993). Muscle-specific *trk*-related receptor with a kringle domain defines a distinct class of receptor tyrosine kinases. Proc. Natl Acad. Sci. USA, 90, 2895–2899.

Kahle, P., Burton, L.E., Schmelzer, C.H. and Hertel, C. (1992). The amino terminus of nerve growth factor is involved in the interaction with the receptor tyrosine kinase p140^{trkA}. J. Biol. Chem., 267, 22707–22710.

Kaplan, D.R., Hempstead, B.L., Martin-Zanca, D., Chao, M.V. and Parada, L.F. (1991a). The *trk* proto-oncogene product: a signal transducing receptor for nerve growth factor. Science, 252, 554–558.

Kaplan, D.R., Martin-Zanca, D. and Parada, L.F. (1991b). Tyrosine phosphorylation and tyrosine kinase activity of the trk proto-oncogene product induced by NGF. Nature, 350, 158–160.

Klein, R., Parada, L.F., Coulier, F. and Barbacid, M. (1989). *trk*B, a novel tyrosine protein kinase expressed during mouse neural development. EMBO J., 8, 3701–3709.

Klein, R., Conway, D., Parada, L.F. and Barbacid, M. (1990a). The *trk*B tyrosine protein kinase gene codes for a second neurogenic receptor that lacks the catalytic kinase domain. Cell, 61, 647–656.

Klein, R., Martin-Zanca, D., Barbacid, M. and Parada, L.F. (1990b). Expression of the tyrosine kinase receptor gene *trk*B is confined to the murine embryonic and adult nervous system. Development, 109, 845–850.

Klein, R., Jing, S., Nanduri, V., O'Rourke, E. and Barbacid, M. (1991a). The *trk* proto-oncogene encodes a receptor for nerve growth factor. Cell, 65, 189–197.

Klein, R., Nanduri, V., Jing, S., Lamballe, F., Tapley, P., Bryant, S., Cordon-Cardo, C., Jones, K.R., Reichardt, L. and Barbacid, M. (1991b). The *trk*B tyrosine protein kinase is a receptor for brain-derived neurotropic factor and neurotropin-3. Cell, 66, 395–403.

Klein, R., Lamballe, F., Bryant, S. and Barbacid, M. (1992). The *trk*B tyrosine protein kinase is a receptor for neurotrophin-4. Neuron, 8, 947–956.

Kozma, S.C., Redmond, S.M.S., Saurer, S.M., Groner, B. and Hynes, N.E. (1988). Activation of the receptor kinase domain of the *trk* oncogene by recombination with two different cellular sequences. EMBO J. 7, 147–154.

Lamballe, F., Klein, R. and Barbacid, M. (1991). *trk*C, a new member of the *trk* family of tyrosine protein kinases, is a receptor for neurotropin-3. Cell, 66, 967–979.

Lee, K.-F., Li, E., Huber, J., Landis, S.C., Sharpe, A.H., Chao, M.V. and Jaenisch, R. (1992). Targeted mutation of the gene encoding the low affinity NGF receptor p75 leads to deficits in the peripheral sensory nervous system. Cell, 69, 737–749.

Martin-Zanca, D., Hughes, S.H. and Barbacid, M. (1986). A human oncogene formed by the fusion of truncated tropomyosin and protein tyrosine kinase sequences. Nature, 319, 743–748.

Martin-Zanca, D., Oskam, R., Mitra, G., Copeland, T. and Barbacid, M. (1989). Molecular and biochemical characterization of the human *trk* proto-oncogene. Mol. Cell. Biol., 9, 24–33.

Martin-Zanca, D., Barbacid, M. and Parada, L.F. (1990). Expression of the *trk* proto-oncogene is restricted to the sensory cranial and spinal ganglia of neural crest origin in mouse development. Genes Devel., 4, 683–694.

Masiakowski, P. and Carroll, R.D. (1992). A novel family of cell surface receptors with tyrosine kinase-like domain. J. Biol. Chem., 267, 26181–26190.

Meakin, S.O., Suter, U., Drinkwater, C.C., Welcher, A.A. and Shooter, E.M. (1992). The rat *trk* proto-oncogene product exhibits properties characteristic of the slow nerve growth factor receptor. Proc. Natl Acad. Sci. USA, 89, 2374–2378.

Middlemas, D.S., Lindberg, R.A. and Hunter, T. (1991). *trk*B, a neural receptor protein-tyrosine kinase: evidence for a full-length and two truncated receptors. Mol. Cell. Biol., 11, 143–153.

Mitra, G. (1991). Mutational analysis of conserved residues in the tyrosine kinase domain of the human *trk* oncogene. Oncogene, 6, 2237–2241.

Mitra, G., Martin-Zanca, D. and Barbacid, M. (1987). Identification and biochemical characterization of p70*trk*, the gene product of the human *TRK* oncogene. Proc. Natl Acad. Sci. USA, 84, 6707–6711.

Morris, C.M., Hao, Q.L., Heisterkamp, N., Fitzgerald, P.H. and Groffen, J. (1991). Localization of the TRK proto-oncogene to human chromosome bands 1q23–1q24. Oncogene, 6, 1093–1095.

Nakagawara, A., Arima, M., Azar, C.G., Scavarda, N.J. and Brodeur, G.M. (1992). Inverse relationship between *trk* expression and N-*myc* amplification in human neuroblastomas. Cancer Res., 1364–1368.

Nebreda, A.R., Martin-Zanca, D., Kaplan, D.R., Parada, L.F. and Santos, E. (1991). Induction by NGF of meiotic maturation of *Xenopus* oocytes expressing the *trk* proto-oncogene product. Science, 252, 558–561.

Obermeier, A., Halfter, H., Wiesmuller, K.-H., Jung, G., Schlessinger, J. and Ullrich, A. (1993). Tyrosine 785 is a major determinant of Trk-substrate interaction. EMBO J., 12, 933–941.

Ohmichi, M., Decker, S.J., Pang, L. and Saltiel, A.R. (1992a). Inhibition of the cellular actions of nerve growth factor by staurosporine and K252A results from the attenuation of the activity of the *trk* tyrosine kinase. Biochemistry, 31, 4034–4039.

Ohmichi, M., Pang, L., Decker, S.J. and Saltiel, A.R. (1992b). Nerve growth factor stimulates the activities of the *raf*-1 and the mitogen-activated protein kinases via the *trk* protooncogene. J. Biol. Chem., 267, 14604–14610.

Oskam, R., Coulier, F., Ernst, M., Martin-Zanca, D. and Barbacid, M. (1988). Frequent generation of oncogenes by *in vitro* recombination of *TRK* protooncogene sequences. Proc. Natl Acad. Sci. USA, 85, 2964–2968.

Pulciani, S., Santos, S., Lauver, A.V., Long, L.K., Aaronson, S.A. and Barbacid, M. (1982). Oncogenes in solid human tumors. Nature, 300, 579.

Pulido, D., Campuzano, S., Koda, T., Modolell, J. and Barbacid, M. (1992). D*trk*, a Drosophila gene related to the *trk* family of neurotrophin receptors, encodes a novel class of neural cell adhesion molecule. EMBO J., 11, 391–404.

Radice, P., Sozzi, G., Miozzo, M., De Benedetti, V., Cariani, T., Bongarzone, I., Spurr, N.K., Pierotti, M.A. and Della Porta, G. (1991). The human tropomyosin gene involved in the generation of the *TRK* oncogene maps to chromosome 1q31. Oncogene, 6, 2145–2148.

Schneider, R. and Schweiger, M. (1991). A novel modular mosaic of cell adhesion motifs in the extracellular domains of the neurogenic *trk* and *trkB* tyrosine kinase receptors. Oncogene, 6, 1807–1811.

Soppet, D., Escandon, E., Maragos, J., Middlemas, D.S., Reid, S.W., Blair, J., Burton, L.E., Stanton, B.R., Kaplan, D.R., Hunter, T., Nikolics, K. and Parada, L.F. (1991). The neurotrophic factors brain-derived neurotrophic factors and neurotrophin-3 are ligands for the *trk*B tyrosine kinase receptor. Cell, 65, 895–903.

Squinto, S.P., Stitt, T.N., Aldrich, T.H., Davis, S., Bianco, S.M., Radziejewski, C., Glass, D.J., Masiakowski, P., Furth, M.E., Valenzuela, D.M., DiStefano, P.S. and Yancopoulos, G.D. (1991). *trk*B encodes a functional receptor for brain-derived neurotrophic factor and neurotrophin-3 but not nerve growth factor. Cell, 65, 886–893.

Tapley, P., Lamballe, F. and Barbacid, M. (1992). K252a is a selective inhibitor of the tyrosine protein kinase activity of the *trk* family of oncogenes and neurotrophin receptors. Oncogene, 7, 371–382.

Vazquez, M.E. and Ebendal, T. (1991). Messenger RNAs for *trk* and the low-affinity NGF receptor in rat basal forebrain. Neuroreport, 2, 593–596.

Ziemiecki, A., Muller, R.G., Fu, X.-C., Hynes, N, E. and Kozma, S. (1990). Oncogenic activation of the human *trk* proto-oncogene by recombination with the ribosomal large subunit protein L7a. EMBO J., 9, 191–196.

Tumour Suppressor Genes

...istence of what are now variously known as tumour suppressor genes, recessive onco-genes, anti-oncogenes or growth suppressor genes was originally inferred from the finding that when tumorigenic and non-tumorigenic cells were fused in culture the resulting hybrids were generally non-tumorigenic. When such hybrid cells do give rise to tumours in animals, this usually involves the loss of a specific chromosome derived from the non-tumorigenic cell. In many spontaneously arising tumours, individual chromosomes or specific regions of a chromosome are lost or deleted.

These observations suggest the existence of a substantial class of tumour suppressor genes, the normal function of which is to govern cell proliferation, and indicate that when non-tumorigenic hybrids are formed from two different tumorigenic cells genetic complementation may be occurring. The two best understood tumour suppressor genes are the retinoblastoma (*RB1*) gene and *TP53*: the properties of these and of other emerging potential tumour suppressor genes are summarized below. *RB1* provides the classical model for a recessive tumour suppressor gene in that both paternal and maternal copies of the gene must be inactivated for the tumour to develop. For *TP53* and some other tumour suppressor genes, mutation at one allele may be sufficient to give rise to the altered cell phenotype.

Table 3.8. *Human tumour suppressor genes* (Genes detected by loss of heterozygosity, molecular probing, cell hybridization or chromosome transfer)

Chromosome	Cancer
1p	Melanoma (Bale *et al.*, 1989) Multiple endocrine neoplasia (MEN) type 2 Neuroblastoma (Bader *et al.*, 1991) Medullary thyroid carcinoma Pheochromocytoma (Ponder, 1988) Ductal breast carcinoma (Genuardi *et al.*, 1989)
1q	Breast carcinoma (Chen *et al.*, 1989)
3p	Lung cancer (Takahashi *et al.*, 1989; Yokota *et al.*, 1987) Renal cell carcinoma (Kovacs *et al.*, 1988) Cervical carcinoma (Yokota *et al.*, 1989) von Hippel–Lindau disease (Tory *et al.*, 1989)
5q	Familial adenomatous polyposis (Bodmer *et al.*, 1987) Sporadic colorectal cancer (Solomon *et al.*, 1987)
9q	Bladder carcinoma (Fearon *et al.*, 1985; Tsai *et al.*, 1990)
10q	Astrocytoma (Fujimoto *et al.*, 1989) MEN type 2 (Mathew *et al.*, 1987; Simpson *et al.*, 1987)
11p	Wilms' tumour (Francke *et al.*, 1979) Lung carcinoma (Shiraishi *et al.*, 1987) Breast carcinoma (Theillet *et al.*, 1987) Rhabdomyosarcoma Hepatoblastoma Transitional bladder carcinoma (Ponder, 1988)
11q	MEN type 1 (Larsson *et al.*, 1988; Ponder, 1988) Cervical carcinoma (Srivatsan *et al.*, 1991; Koi *et al.*, 1989; Saxon *et al.*, 1986)

Table 3.8. *Continued*

Chromosome	Cancer
13q	Retinoblastoma (Knudson, 1985) Osteosarcoma (Toguchida *et al.*, 1988) Lung cancer (Takahashi *et al.*, 1989) Breast cancer (Lee *et al.*, 1988) Stomach cancer (Ponder, 1988)
17p	Astrocytoma (James *et al.*, 1989) Lung cancer (Takahashi *et al.*, 1989) Colorectal carcinoma (Baker *et al.*, 1989) Breast cancer (Mackay *et al.*, 1988) Osteosarcoma (Toguchida *et al.*, 1988)
17q	NF-1 (Viskochil *et al.*, 1990; Wallace *et al.*, 1990; Cawthon *et al.*, 1990) Ovarian cancer (Eccles *et al.*, 1992) Breast cancer (Smith *et al.*, 1992)
18q	Colorectal carcinoma (Fearon and Vogelstein, 1990)
22q	Acoustic neuroma (Seizinger *et al.*, 1987) NF-2 (Rouleau *et al.*, 1987) Meningioma Pheochromocytoma (Ponder, 1988)

Papers

Bader, S.A., Fasching, C., Brodeur, G.M. and Stanbridge, E.J. (1991). Dissociation of suppression of tumorigenicity and differentiation *in vitro* effected by transfer of single human chromosomes into human neuroblastoma cells. Cell Growth Differ., 2, 245–255.

Baker, S.J., Fearon, E.R., Nigro, J.M., Hamilton, S.R., Preisinger, A.C., Jessup, J.M., van Tuinen, P., Ledbetter, D.H., Barker, D.F., Nakamura, Y., White, R. and Vogelstein, B. (1989). Chromosome 17 deletion and p53 mutations in colorectal carcinomas. Science, 244, 217–221.

Bale, S.J., Dracopoli, N.C., Tucker, M.A., Clark, W.H., Fraser, M.C., Stanger, B.Z., Green, P., Donis-Keller, H., Housman, D.E. and Greene, M.H. (1989). Mapping the gene for hereditary cutaneous malignant melanoma-dysplasia nevus to chromosome 1p. New Engl. J. Med., 320, 1367–1372.

Bodmer, W.F., Bailey, C.J., Bodmer, J., Bussey, H.J.R., Ellis, A., Gorman, P., Lucibello, F.C., Murday, V.A., Rider, S.H., Scambler, P., Sheer, D., Solomon, E. and Spurr, N.K. (1987). Localization of the gene for familial adenomatous polyposis on chromosome 5. Nature, 328, 614–616.

Cawthon, R.M., Weiss, R., Xu, G., Viskochil, D., Culver, M., Stevens, J., Robertson, M., Dunn, D., Gesteland, R., O'Connell, P. and White, R. (1990). A major segment of the neurofibromatosis type 1 gene: cDNA sequence, genomic structure, and point mutations. Cell, 62, 193–201.

Chen, L.-C., Dollbaum, C. and Smith, H.S. (1989). Loss of heterozygosity on chromosome 1q in human breast cancer. Proc. Natl Acad. Sci. USA, 86, 7204–7207.

Eccles, D.M., Russell, S.E.H., Haites, N.E., Atkinson, R., Bell, D.W., Gruber, L., Hickey, I., Kelly, K., Kitchener, H., Leonard, R., Lessells, A., Lowry, S., Miller, I., Milner, B. and Steel, M. (1992). Early loss of heterozygosity on 17q in ovarian cancer. Oncogene, 7, 2069–2072.

Fearon, E.R. and Vogelstein, B. (1990). A genetic model for colorectal tumorigenesis. Cell, 61, 759–767.

Fearon, E.R., Feinberg, A.P., Hamilton, S.H. and Vogelstein, B. (1985). Loss of genes on the short arm of chromosome 11 in bladder cancer. Nature, 318, 377–380.

Francke, U., Holmes, L.B., Atkins, L. and Riccardi, V.M. (1979). Aniridia-Wilms' tumor association: evidence for specific deletion of 11p13. Cytogenet. Cell Genet., 24, 185–192.

Fujimoto, M., Fults, D.W., Thomas, G.A., Nakamura, Y., Heilbrun, M.P., White, R., Story, J.L., Naylor, S.L., Kagan-Hallet, K.S. and Sheridan, P.J. (1989). Loss of heterozygosity on chromosome 10 in human glioblastoma multiforme. Genomics, 4, 210–214.

Genuardi, M., Tsihira, H., Anderson, D.E. and Saunders, G.F. (1989). Distal deletion of chromosome 1p in ductal carcinoma of the breast. Am. J. Hum. Genet., 45, 73.

James, C.D., Carlbom, E., Nordenskjold, M., Collins, P.V. and Cavenee, W.K. (1989). Mitotic recombination of chromosome 17 in astrocytomas. Proc. Natl Acad, Sci. USA, 86, 2858–2862.

Knudson, A.G. (1985). Hereditary cancer, oncogenes, and antioncogenes. Cancer Res., 45, 1437–1443.

Koi, M., Morita, H., Yamada, H., Satoh, H., Barrett, J.C. and Oshimura, M. (1989). Normal human chromosome 11 suppresses tumorigenicity of human cervical tumor cell line SiHa. Mol. Carcinog., 2, 12–21.

Kovacs, G., Erlandsson, R., Boldog, F., Ingvarsson, S., Muller-Brechlin, R., Klein, G. and Sumegi, J. (1988). Consistent chromosome 3p deletion and loss of heterozygosity in renal cell carcinoma. Proc. Natl Acad. Sci. USA, 85, 1571–1575.

Larsson, C., Skogseid, B., Oberg, K., Nakamura, Y. and Nordenskjold, M. (1988). Multiple endocrine neoplasmia type 1 gene maps to chromosome 11 and is lost in insulinoma. Nature, 332, 85–87.

Lee, E.Y.-H.P., To, H., Shew, J.-Y., Bookstein, R., Scully, P. and Lee, W.-H. (1988). Inactivation of the retinoblastoma susceptibility gene in human breast cancers. Science, 241, 218–221.

Mackay, J., Elder, P.A., Steel, C.M., Forest, A.P.M. and Evans, H.J. (1988). Allele loss on short arm of chromosome 17 in breast cancers. Lancet, ii, 1384–1385.

Mathew, C.G.P., Smith, B.A., Thorpe, K., Wong, Z., Royle, N.J., Jeffreys, A.J. and Ponder, B.A.J. (1987). Deletion of genes on chromosome 1 in endocrine neoplasia. Nature, 328, 524–526.

Ponder, B.A.J. (1988). Gene losses in human tumours. Nature, 335, 400–402.

Rouleau, G.A., Wertelecki, W., Haines, J.L., Hobb, W.J., Trofatter, J.A., Seizinger, B.R., Martuza, R.L., Superneau, D.W., Conneally, D.M. and Gusella, J.F. (1987). Genetic linkage of bilateral acoustic neurofibromatosis to a DNA marker on chromosome 22. Nature, 329, 246–248.

Saxon, P.J., Srivatsan, E.S. and Stanbridge, E.J. (1986). Introduction of human chromosome 11 via microcell transfer controls tumorigenic expression of HeLa cells. EMBO J., 5, 3461–3466.

Seizinger, B.R., Rouleau, G., Ozelius, L.J., Lane, A.H., George-Hislop, S.P., Huson, S., Gusella, J.F. and Martuza, R.L. (1987). Common pathogenetic mechanism for three tumor types in bilateral acoustic neurofibromatosis. Science, 236, 317–319.

Shiraishi, M., Morinaga, S., Noguchi, M., Shimosato, Y. and Sekiya, T. (1987). Loss of genes on the short arm of chromosome 11 in human lung carcinomas. Jpn J. Cancer Res., 78, 1302–1308.

Simpson, N.E., Kidd, K.K., Goodfellow, P.J., McDonald, H., Myers, S., Kidd, J.R., Jackson, C.E., Duncan, A.M.V., Farrer, L.A., Brasch, K., Castiglione, C., Genel, M., Gertner, J., Greenberg, C.R., Gusella, J.F., Holden, J.J. and White, B.N. (1987). Assignment of multiple endocrine neoplasia type 2A to chromosome 10 by linkage. Nature, 328, 528–530.

Smith, S.A., Easton, D.F., Evans, D.G.R. and Ponder, B.A.J. (1992). Allele losses in the region 17q12–21 in familial breast and ovarian cancer involve the wild-type chromosome. Nature Genetics, 2, 128–131.

Solomon, E., Voss, R., Hall, V., Bodmer, W.F., Jass, J.R., Jeffreys, A.J., Lucibello, F.C., Patel, I. and Rider, S.H. (1987). Chromosome 5 allele loss in human colorectal carcinomas. Nature, 328, 616–619.

Srivatsan, E.S., Misra, B.C., Venugopalan, M., Wilczynski, S.P. (1991). Loss of heterozygosity for alleles on chromosome II in cervical carcinoma. Am. J. Hum. Genet., 49, 868–877.

Takahashi, T., Nau, M.M., Chiba, I., Birrer, M.J., Rosenberg, R.K., Vincour, M., Levitt, M., Pass, H., Gazdar, A.F. and Minna, J.D. (1989). p53: a frequent target for genetic abnormalities in lung cancer. Science, 246, 491–594.

Theillet, C., Lidereau, R., Escot, C., Hutzell, P., Brunet, M., Gest, J., Schlom, J. and Callahan, R. (1987). Loss of a c-H-ras-1 allele and aggressive human primary breast carcinomas. Cancer Res., 46, 4776–4781.

Toguchida, J., Ishizaki, K., Sasaki, M.S., Ikenaga, M., Sugimoto, M., Kotoura, Y. and Yamamuro, T. (1988). Chromosomal reorganization for the expression of recessive mutation of retinoblastoma susceptibility gene in the development of osteosarcoma. Cancer Res., 48, 3939–3943.

Tory, K., Brauch, H., Linehan, M., Barba, D., Oldfield, E., Filling-Katz, M., Seizinger, B., Nakamura, Y., White, R., Marshall, F.F., Lerman, M.I. and Zbar, B. (1989). Specific genetic change in tumors associated with von Hippel-Lindau disease. J. Natl Cancer Inst., 81, 1097–1101.

Tsai, Y.C., Nichols, P.W., Hiti, A.L., Williams, Z., Skinner, D.G. and Jones, P.A. (1990). Allelic losses of chromosomes 9, 11, and 17 in human bladder cancer. Cancer Res., 50, 44–47.

Viskochil, D., Buchberg, A.M., Xu, G., Cawthon, R.M., Stevens, J., Wolff, R.K., Culver, M., Carey, J.C., Copeland, N.G., Jenkins, N.A., White, R. and O'Connell, P. (1990). Deletions and a translocation interrupt a cloned gene at the neurofibromatosis type 1 locus. Cell, 62, 187–192.

Wallace, M.R., Marchuk, D.A., Andersen, L.B., Letcher, R., Odeh, H.M., Saulino, A.M., Fountain, J.W., Brereton, A., Nicholson, J., Mitchell, A.L., Brownstein, B.H. and Collins, F.S. (1990). Type 1 neurofibromatosis gene: identification of a large transcript disrupted in three NF1 patients. Science, 249, 181–186.

Weston, A., Willey, J.C., Modali, R., Sugimura, H., McDowell, E.M., Resau, J., Light, B., Haugen, A., Mann, D.L., Trump, B.F. and Harris, C.C. (1989). Differential DNA sequence deletions from chromosomes 3, 11, 13 and 17 in squamous-cell carcinoma, large-cell carcinoma, and adenocarcinoma of the human lung. Proc. Natl Acad, Sci. USA, 86, 5099–5103.

Yokota, J., Wada, M., Shimosato, Y., Terada, M. and Sugimura, T. (1987). Loss of heterozygosity on chromosomes 3, 13, and 17 in small-cell carcinoma and on chromosome 3 in adenocarcinoma of the lung. Proc. Natl Acad, Sci. USA, 84, 9252–9256.

Yokota, J., Tsukada, Y., Nakajima, T., Gotoh, M., Shimosato, Y., Mori, N., Tsunokawa, Y., Sugimura, T. and Terada, M. (1989). Loss of heterozygosity on the short arm of chromosome 3 in carcinoma of the uterine cervix. Cancer Res., 46, 3598–3601.

Retinoblastoma (*RB*)

Related genes

The protein encoded by the *RB1* (*RB*) gene, p105^{RB}, has homology with a 564 amino acid region in the cellular protein p107 that binds independently to T antigen or E1A (Ewen *et al.*, 1991).

Cross-species homology

The human and mouse proteins are 91% identical in sequence.

Transformation

MAN

Retinoblastoma is a rare hereditary disease, occurring in 1 child in 20 000, that affects the precursors of retina cells that normally become cones. In 60% of the cases the condition is termed sporadic, when there is no family history of the disease and a single tumour occurs in one eye; in the remaining 40% of cases (familial or germinal retinoblastoma) tumours are bilateral and more than one independently derived tumour is frequently present (Knudson, 1971). The disease is caused by the loss of both copies of the gene by inactivating mutations resulting in null alleles. Knudson pointed out that familial retinoblastoma might occur because one of the alleles was mutated at conception with the other undergoing somatic mutation. In sporadic retinoblastoma both mutations must occur somatically within one cell to give rise to a tumour clone. The gene, located on the long arm of chromosome 13, is defective in all retinoblastomas and in a number of other cancers: inactive *RB* alleles are very common in small-cell lung carcinoma, and they occur in ~30% of bladder carcinomas, in 25% of cell lines derived from human breast carcinomas (Horowitz *et al.*, 1990; Friend *et al.*, 1987; Weichselbaum *et al.*, 1988) and in 20% of pancreatic carcinomas (Ruggeri *et al.*, 1992). Individuals with inherited retinoblastoma are also susceptible to malignant tumours in mesenchymal tissues, often osteosarcomas or soft tissue sarcomas.

TRANSGENIC ANIMALS

Mice carrying a homozygous mutation in the retinoblastoma gene die before the 16th day of gestation (Lee *et al.*, 1992; Jacks *et al.*, 1992). The major defects are manifested in the haematopoietic system, in which the number of immature, nucleated erythrocytes is increased, and in the central nervous system, with ectopic mitoses and death of neuronal cells. The expression in transgenic mice of T antigen, which binds to p105^{RB} (see **Protein function** below), in the retina causes hereditable ocular tumours apparently identical to those of retinoblastoma (Windle *et al.*, 1990).

	RB/Rb-1
Nucleotides (kb)	180
Chromosome	
Human	13q14.2
Mouse	14
Rat	15
Exons	27
mRNA (kb)	
Human	4.7
Mouse	2.8 (adult testes)/4.7 in most normal tissues
mRNA half-life (h)	2 (quiescent cells)
	3.5 (stimulated monocytes)
	6 (stimulated T cells)
Amino acids	
Human	928
Mouse	921
Mass (kDa)	
(predicted)	
Human	106
Mouse	105
(expressed)	
Human	pp105
Mouse	pp104–110
Protein half-life (h)	4–6 (fibroblasts; monkey kidney cells; Chen *et al.*, 1989; Xu *et al.*, 1989)
	>10 (human cell lines; Mihara *et al.*, 1989)

Cellular location

Nuclear. RB^+ and RB^- tumours are distinguishable by protein staining (Xu *et al.*, 1991). Hypophosphorylated forms are more tightly associated with the nucleus than hyperphosphorylated species (Mittnacht and Weinberg, 1991). Some mutant forms are cytoplasmic (Shew *et al.*, 1990).

Tissue location

In normal cells $p105^{RB}$ is undetectable by immunohistochemistry (Xu *et al.*, 1991). It is detectable by immunofluorescence in a variety of normal and tumour-derived cell lines (Bartek *et al.*, 1992). Low or undetectable expression in 30% of acute myelogenous leukaemia (AML) patients is caused by abnormal regulation rather than by defects in the gene (Zhang *et al.*, 1993).

Protein function

p105^{RB} binds to double-stranded DNA in a non-sequence-specific manner. It immunoprecipitates with the E1A protein of human adenovirus (Whyte *et al.*, 1988), SV40 large T antigen, the E7 oncoprotein of human papillomavirus 16 (HPV-16) and cyclins D1, D3, B1 and C (Dowdy *et al.*, 1993; Ewen *et al.*, 1993). These proteins show sequence homology only over the small putative p105^{RB}-binding region (see **DNA Tumour Viruses: EBV**). Each of the viral gene products can immortalize primary cells *in vitro*, transform embryonic cells when co-expressed with *Ras* and act as transcriptional regulators of viral and host cell genes. The p105^{RB} binding regions of T antigen and E1A are the domains essential for immortalization of primary cells *in vitro*. Mutations in T antigen or E1A that block p105^{RB} binding also inhibit transforming power, suggesting that the prevention of normal p105^{RB} function is a crucial common step in cell transformation by these viruses. HPV-16 E7 inhibits DNA binding by p105^{RB} (Stirdivant *et al.*, 1992a). Ser31 and Ser32 of E7 are phosphorylated by casein kinase II and this appears to be necessary for transformation but not for p105^{RB} binding.

T antigen forms a complex with DNA polymerase α that stimulates the activity of the enzyme. *In vitro*, p105^{RB} inhibits this stimulation, suggesting that p105^{RB} competes with DNA polymerase α in binding to T antigen (Savoysky *et al.*, 1993).

p105^{RB} acts through a motif (the retinoblastoma control element, RCE) to repress *MYC* transcription in human keratinocytes (see **MYC**), to repress *FOS* transcription, to enhance transcription of insulin-like growth factor II and to regulate either positively or negatively the expression of *TGFβ$_1$* depending on cell type (see **FOS**). The transcription factor Sp-1 also interacts with the RCE and p105^{RB} enhances the *trans*-activating capacity of Sp-1 (Udvadia *et al.*, 1993). p105^{RB} also negatively regulates expression of p34^{CDC2} (Dalton, 1992).

The neoplastic phenotype of retinoblastoma, osteosarcoma or human prostate carcinoma cells carrying inactivated *RB* genes can be suppressed by transfection of a cloned *RB* gene (Huang *et al.*, 1988; Bookstein *et al.*, 1990b). p105^{RB} suppresses transformation and metastasis induced in fibroblasts by *Neu*. Studies with transgenic mice (see above) indicate that *RB* is essential for normal mouse development but not for cell proliferation and differentiation in the early stages of organogenesis.

At least ten cellular proteins have been detected that bind to p105^{RB} in a manner similar to T antigen, E1A and E7. The distinct human genes encoding retinoblastoma binding proteins RBP1 (Otterson *et al.*, 1993) and RBP2 have no homology to other known human proteins but contain the p105^{RB} binding motif conserved between large T antigen, E1A and E7 (Defeo-Jones *et al.*, 1991). Human RBAP46 competes with T antigen for binding to p105^{RB} (Huang *et al.*, 1991). Underphosphorylated p105^{RB} also associates with the ubiquitous transcription factor E2F and the complex is dissociated by E1A, SV40 T antigen or HPV E7 (Chellappan *et al.*, 1991, 1992; Hamel *et al.*, 1992; Pagano *et al.*, 1992). The p105^{RB}–E2F complex occurs in G$_1$ in human primary cells and tumour cell lines and functions as a transcriptional repressor in the presence of an additional factor, RBP60 (Weintraub *et al.*, 1992; Ray *et al.*, 1992). One target of the p105^{RB}–E2F complex is the *CDC2* promoter which includes E2F binding sites (Dalton, 1992). As the cells enter S phase, a second E2F complex forms containing the p105^{RB}-related protein p107 and cyclin A (Shirodkar *et al.*, 1992). p107 has been shown to inhibit E2F-dependent transcription in a co-transfection assay (Schwarz *et al.*, 1993). The human proteins RBAP1 and RBAP2 also bind to unphosphorylated p105^{RB} (Helin *et al.*, 1992; Kaelin *et al.*, 1992). RBAP1 is an E2F-like protein that binds specifically to E2F recognition sequences. The RCE, discussed earlier, is a variant of the consensus Sp-1 binding site and it is possible that p105^{RB} regulation of promoter activity is mediated by complex interactions between Sp-1, E2F and E2F-related proteins and p105^{RB} (Kim *et al.*, 1992). p105^{RB} also interacts with the transcription factor DRTF1 that recognizes the same motif in the adenovirus E2A promoter as E2F (TTTTCGCGCAATT) and complexes containing p105^{RB} bind to related motifs with high affinity (Ouellette *et al.*, 1992). The transcription factor PU.1 binds directly to the "pocket" domain of p105^{RB} and to a related sequence in the transcription factor TFIID (Hagemeier *et al.*, 1993). p105^{RB} also contains a region of sequence similarity to TFIIB and these two domains may be involved in the activity of p105^{RB} as a transcription factor.

The catalytic subunit of the type 1 protein phosphatase PP-1α2 binds to the same region of p105^{RB} as T antigen (Durfee *et al.*, 1993). The complex forms during M phase and exists well into the G$_1$ phase of the next cycle, the period in which p105^{RB} is active, and cell cycle progression may be promoted by the opposing action of cdk/cyclin complexes that phosphorylate and inactivate p105^{RB} (see below).

MYC and MYCN proteins bind to p105^{RB} via their N-termini and HPV E7 competes for binding with MYC (Rustgi *et al.*, 1991). Antisense *MYC* oligonucleotides or overexpression of p105^{RB} inhibit the G$_1$ to S phase transition (see below), suggesting that the direct interaction between MYC and p105^{RB} regulates cell proliferation.

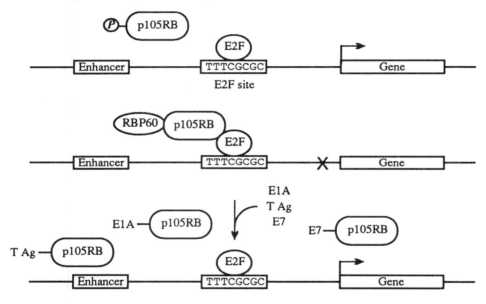

E2F was originally identified as activating the adenovirus E2 promoter via TTTCGCGC sequences. Similar sequence motifs in the promoters of the *MYC*, *MYCN*, *MYB*, *CDC2* and EGF receptor genes appear to be important for regulation of their transcription.

Phase-specific phosphorylation of p105^{RB} in HeLa cells

Mitogenically activated lymphocytes have enhanced levels of phosphorylated p105^{RB} (Chen *et al.*, 1989; Terada *et al.*, 1991) and when proliferation is inhibited by interferon-α these cells accumulate in G$_1$ and contain mainly hypophosphorylated p105^{RB} protein (Burke *et al.*, 1992). Hypoxic stress also induces hypophosphorylation of p105^{RB} and cell cycle arrest (Ludlow *et al.*, 1993a). The induction of differentiation in several human leukaemia cell lines also leads to underphosphorylation of p105^{RB} (Chen *et al.*, 1989). In the human osteosarcoma-derived line Saos-2 high expression of p105^{RB}, which remains unphosphorylated, blocks passage through G$_1$ but not the G$_1$ to S phase transition (Goodrich *et al.*, 1991). However, when human cyclin A or cyclin E is co-transfected, p105^{RB} is hyperphosphorylated, migrates to the nucleus and the

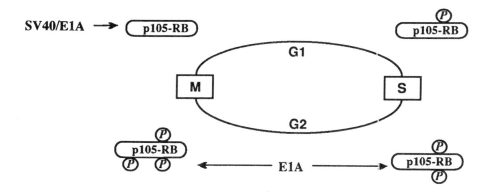

cells revert to the transformed phenotype (Hinds *et al.*, 1992). Cell cycle arrest in G_1 by p105^{RB} is inhibited by microinjection of MYC, with which p105^{RB} physically associates *in vitro* (Goodrich and Lee, 1992). HeLa cells synthesize p105^{RB} throughout the cell cycle but the protein is only detectably phosphorylated during S, G_2 and M phases (Buchkovich *et al.*, 1989; DeCaprio *et al.*, 1989). In chronic myelogenous leukaemia (CML) cells, however, p105^{RB} is phosphorylated early in G_1 and hyperphosphorylated by the time the cells enter S phase (Zhang *et al.*, 1992). Phosphorylation of p105^{RB} is probably due to the activity of p33^{CDK2}/p58^{cyclinA} or p34^{CDC2}/p58$^{cyclin\ A}$ (Lin *et al.*, 1991) with which p105^{RB} associates (Hu *et al.*, 1992; Williams *et al.*, 1992), and which also phosphorylate p53 (see *P53*). p105^{RB} is phosphorylated *in vitro* by p33^{CDK2} (Akiyama *et al.*, 1992). The period of the cycle in which p105^{RB} is hypophosphorylated (G_1) coincides with that when p34^{CDC2} transcription is minimal. Okadaic acid, an inhibitor of type 1 and type 2A protein phosphatases, inhibits p105^{RB} phosphorylation and thus causes cell cycle arrest, possibly by inhibiting the expression of the p105^{RB} kinases (Schonthal and Feramisco, 1993). Microinjection of type 1 and type 2A protein phosphatases also inhibits progression to S phase, presumably by direct dephosphorylation of p105^{RB} protein (Alberts *et al.*, 1993). The late mitotic dephosphorylation of p105^{RB} correlates with an increase in cellular phosphatase activity (Ludlow *et al.*, 1993b).

Phosphorylated p105^{RB} may activate transcription of thymidine kinase (Dou *et al.*, 1992). This suggests that in normal cells the phosphorylation of p105^{RB} is necessary for transition of the G_1/S boundary and that this is functionally equivalent to the inhibition of activity caused by binding to oncoproteins in virally infected cells. SV40 T antigen will only bind to the unphosphorylated (or underphosphorylated) form of p105^{RB}. E1A proteins, however, appear to be less specific in that they bind to p105^{RB} throughout the cell cycle. It is not known whether p105^{RB} binds directly to DNA although it can regulate *FOS*, *MYC* and *TGFβ₁* transcription, attach to DNA cellulose columns and contains a putative metal binding site, in common with known transcription factors (Lee *et al.*, 1987b). In contrast to these observations, however, human embryonic lung fibroblasts are stimulated to a high rate of mitosis by the complete inhibition of p105^{RB} synthesis in the presence of antisense oligonucleotide (Strauss *et al.*, 1992).

Senescence

Depletion of p105^{RB} by the use of an antisense oligomer in fibroblasts that are about to senesce extends the lifespan of the cells (Hara *et al.*, 1991), an effect potentiated by co-treatment with antisense *P53* oligomer. SV40-immortalized fibroblasts become senescent when expression of T antigen is inhibited (Shay *et al.*, 1991). Senescent hamster embryo cells express only unphosphorylated p105^{RB} (Futreal and Barrett, 1991) which inhibits proliferation.

Gene structure

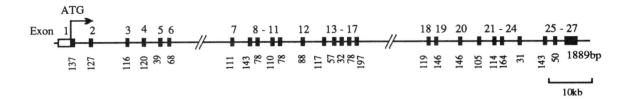

Black boxes: exons. Numbers below boxes indicate exon size in base pairs (T'Ang *et al.*, 1989).

The region extending 600 bases upstream from the initiation codon (ATG, exon 1) includes potential AP-1 and ATF (CREB family) binding sites and three Sp-1 sites to which RBF1 (distinct from Sp-1) binds. Major deletions in the gene occur in 15–40% of retinoblastomas. More subtle effects are presumed to occur in all other cases, including (1) hypermethylation in the 5′ region of the gene which inhibits binding of ATF-like and RBF1 transcription factors (Ohtani-Fujita *et al.*, 1993), (2) point mutations in the ATF and Sp-1 sites (G to T at −189 and G to A at −198) that are known to cause hereditary retinoblastoma (Sakai *et al.*, 1991), (3) a point mutation that results in the loss of exon 21 and inactivation of the protein, (4) Cys706 to Phe706 mutation in a small-cell lung carcinoma line resulting in an underphosphorylated protein that does not bind to SV40 T antigen or E1A (Kaye *et al.*, 1990) but retains the capacity to bind MYC and MYCL proteins (Kratzke *et al.*, 1992), and (5) loss of 103 nucleotides in the promoter preventing expression of *RB* in human prostate tumours (Bookstein *et al.*, 1990a).

Structure of human p105^{RB}

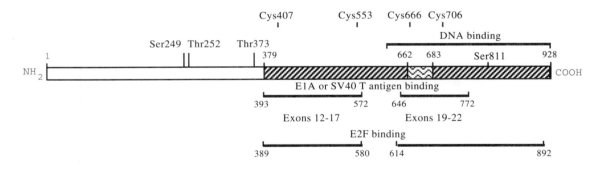

The major phosphorylation sites and the leucine zipper motif (662–683) are shown. The E1A and SV40 T antigen binding regions overlap sites of naturally occurring mutations, notably in exon 21 (bladder carcinoma and small-cell lung carcinoma) and these regions also mediate E2F binding (Qian *et al.*, 1992; Hiebert, 1993). The minimal region necessary for growth suppression by p105^{RB} is from 379 to 928 (Qin *et al.*, 1992). Of the eight cysteine residues in the "binding pocket" (393–772), the four at positions 407, 553, 666 and 706 contribute to the binding of E7 protein (Stirdivant *et al*, 1992b). The pocket contains domain A (393–573) and domain B (645–772) that include residues 399–564 and 658–816 which have regions of similarity to TFIID and TFIIB, respectively (Hagemeier *et al.*, 1993).

Interactions between p105*RB*, p53 and the oncoproteins of SV40, adenovirus and human papilloma virus

A. SV40

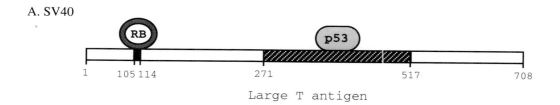

Large T antigen

B. Adenovirus type 5

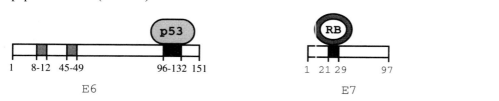

E1A (26kDa)   E1B (55kDa)

C. Human papilloma virus (HPV 16)

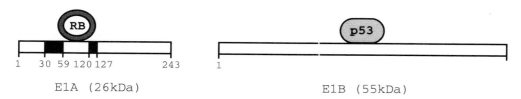

E6   E7

Sequences of human and mouse p105*RB*

```
Human RB        MPPKTPRKTAATAAAAAAEPPAPPPPPPPEEDPEQDSGPEDLPLVRLEFEETEEPDFTA
Mouse RB        MPPKAPR    R-------P------R-D--A------E---A------I---E-I-
       (60)     LCQKLKIPDHVRERAWLTWEKVSSVDGVLGGYIQKKKELWGICIFIAAVDLDEMSFTFTE
       (54)     ------V-------------------I-E----------------------P-----

      (120)     LQKNIEISVHKFFNLLKEIDTSTKVDNAMSRLLKKYDVLFALFSKLERTCELIYLTQPSS
      (114)     ---S--T--Y---D--------------------N--C--Y----------------

      (180)     SISTEINSALVLKVSWITFLLAKGEVLQMEDDLVISFQLMLCVLDYFIKLSPPMLLKEPY
      (174)     AL------M----I------------------------V-----F---A--R---

      (240)     KTAVIPINGSPRTPRRGQNRSARIAKQLENDTRIIEVLCKEHECNIDEVKNVYFKNFIPF
      (234)     ---A---------------------------------------------------

      (300)     MNSLGLVTSNGLPEVENLSKRYEEIYLKNKDLDARLFLDHDKTLQTDSIDSFETQRTPRK
      (294)     I----I-S--------S-------V----------------P------E-----

      (360)     SNLDEEVNVIPPHTPVRTVMNTIQQLMMILNSASDQPSENLISYFNNCTVNPKESILKRV
      (354)     N-P---A--VT------------------V-------------------N-----

      (420)     KDIGYIFKEKFAKAVGQGCVEIGSQRYKLGVRLYYRVMESMLKSEEERLSIQNFSKLLND
      (414)     --V-H-------N-------D-GV------------------------------
```

```
(480)  NIFHMSLLACALEVVMATYSRSTSQNLDSGTDLSFPWILNVLNLKAFDFYKVIESFIKAE
(474)  ----------------------L-H-----------------------------V-

(540)  GNLTREMIKHLERCEHRIMESLAWLSDSPLFDLIKQSKDREGPTDHLESACPLNLPLQNN
(534)  A-------------------------------------G--- -N--P----S----G-

(600)  HTAADMYLSPVRSPKKKGSTTRVNSTANAETQATSAFQTQKPLKSTSLSLFYKKVYRLAY
(593)  ---------------L-----RT-------A--T----A---H----------A----------

(660)  LRLNTLCERLLSEHPELEHIIWTLFQHTLQNEYELMRDRHLDQIMMCSMYGICKVKNIDL
(653)  --------A-----D-------------------------------

(720)  KFKIIVTAYKDLPHAVQETFKRVLIKEEEYDSIIVFYNSVFMQRLKTNILQYASTRPPTL
(713)  --------------A---------R---F-----------------------

(780)  SPIPHIPRSPYKFPSSPLRIPGGNIYISPLKSPYKISEGLPTPTKMTPRSRILVSIGESF
(773)  -----------------S-----------------------------------

(840)  GTSEKFQKINQMVCNSDRVLKRSAEGSNPPKPLKKLRFDIEGSDEADGSKHLPGESKFQQ
(833)  -----------------------G-------NV------A----------A------

(900)  KLAEMTSTRTRMQKQKMNDSMDTSNKEEK (928)
(893)  --------------R--E-K-V------ (921)
```

Leucine zipper motifs are shown in bold and underlined. Potential serine/threonine phosphorylation sites conserved between human and mouse are underlined: these comprise seven of the most stringent consensus sequence for p34^{CDC2} phosphorylation (basic/polar–Ser/Thr–Pro–X–basic (human: Thr252, Thr356, Thr373, Ser612, Ser788, Ser795, Ser811)), three sites in which Leu, Ile and Pro replace the first consensus residue (Ser608, Ser807, Thr821) and five groups of Ser/Thr–Pro (Ser230, Ser249, Ser567, Ser780, Thr826).

Databank file names and accession numbers

	GENE	*EMBL*	*SWISSPROT*	*REFERENCES*
Human	*RB1*	Hsrbs M15400 Harbsa M28419 Hsrb1ra M33647 Hsrb1g X16439	RB_HUMAN P06400	Lee *et al.*, 1987a,b Friend *et al.*, 1987 T'ang *et al.*, 1989
Mouse	*Rb-1*	Mmpp105r	RB_MOUSE P13405	Bernards *et al.*, 1989
Human	*RBAP1*	M26391 M96577		Helin *et al.*, 1992 Kaelin *et al.*, 1992

Reviews

Cooper, J.A. and Whyte, P. (1989). RB and the cell cycle: entrance or exit? Cell, 58, 1009–1011.
Green, M.R. (1989). When the products of oncogenes and anti-oncogenes meet. Cell, 56, 1–3.
Klein, G. (1987). The approaching era of the tumor suppressor genes. Science, 238, 1539–1545.
Levine, A.J. (1990). Tumor suppressor genes. BioEssays. 12, 60–66.
Schwab, M. (1989). Genetic principles of tumor suppression. Biochim. Biophys. Acta, 989, 49–64.
Weinberg, R.A. (1991). Tumor suppressor genes. Science, 254, 1138–1146.

Papers

Akiyama, T., Ohuchi, T., Sumida, S., Matsumoto, K. and Toyoshima, K. (1992). Phosphorylation of the retinoblastoma protein by cdk2. Proc. Natl Acad. Sci. USA, 89, 7900–7904.

Alberts, A.S., Thorburn, A.M., Shenolikar, S., Mumby, M.C. and Feramisco, J.R. (1993). Regulation of cell cycle progression and nuclear affinity of the retinoblastoma protein by protein phosphatases. Proc. Natl Acad. Sci. USA, 90, 388–392.

Bartek, J., Vojtesek, B., Grand, R.J.A., Gallimore, P.H. and Lane, D.P. (1992). Cellular localization and T antigen binding of the retinoblastoma protein. Oncogene, 7, 101–108.

Bernards R., Schackleford G.M., Gerber M.R., Horowitz J.M., Friend S.H., Schartl M., Bogenman E., Rapaport J., McGee T., Dryja T., Weinberg R.A. (1989). Structure and expression of the murine retinoblastoma gene and characterization of its encoded protein. Proc. Natl Acad. Sci. USA, 86, 6474–6478.

Bookstein, R., Rio, P., Madreperla, S.A., Hong, F., Allred, C., Grizzle, W.E. and Lee, W.-H. (1990a). Promoter deletion and loss of retinoblastoma gene expression in human prostate carcinoma. Proc. Natl Acad. Sci. USA, 87, 7762–7766.

Bookstein, R., Shew, J.-Y., Chen, P.-L., Scully, P. and Lee, W.-H. (1990b). Suppression of tumorigenicity of human prostate carcinoma cells by replacing a mutated *RB* gene. Science, 247, 712–715.

Buchkovich, K., Duffy, L.A. and Harlow, E. (1989). The retinoblastoma protein is phosphorylated during specific phases of the cell cycle. Cell, 58, 1097–1105.

Burke, L.C., Bybee, A. and Thomas, N.S.B. (1992). The retinoblastoma protein is partially phosphorylated during early G_1 in cycling cells but not in G_1 cells arrested with α-interferon. Oncogene, 7, 783–788.

Chellappan, S.P., Hiebert, S., Mudryj, M., Horowitz, J.M. and Nevins, J.R. (1991). The E2F transcription factor is a cellular target for the RB protein. Cell, 65, 1053–1061.

Chellappan, S.P., Kraus, V.B., Kroger, B., Munger, K., Howley, P.M., Phelps, W.C. and Nevins, J.R. (1992). Adenovirus E1A, simian virus 40 tumor antigen, and human papillomavirus E7 protein share the capacity to disrupt the interaction between transcription factor E2F and the retinoblastoma gene product. Proc. Natl Acad. Sci. USA, 89, 4549–4553.

Chen, P.-L., Scully, P., Shew, J.-Y., Wang, J.Y.J. and Lee, W.-H. (1989). Phosphorylation of the retinoblastoma gene product is modulated during the cell cycle and cellular differentiation. Cell, 58, 1193–1198.

Dalton, S. (1992). Cell cycle regulation of the human *cdc2* gene. EMBO J., 11, 1797–1804.

DeCaprio, J.A., Ludlow, J.W., Lynch, D., Furukawa, Y., Griffin, J., Piwnica-Worms, H. and Huang, C.M. (1989). The product of the retinoblastoma susceptibility gene has properties of a cell cycle regulatory element. Cell, 58, 1085–1095.

Defeo-Jones, D., Huang, P.S., Jones, R.E., Haskell, K.M., Vuocolo, G.A., Hanobik, M.G., Huber, H.E. and Oliff, A. (1991). Cloning of cDNAs for cellular proteins that bind to the retinoblastoma gene product. Nature, 352, 251–254.

Dou, Q.-P., Markell, P.J. and Pardee, A.B. (1992). Thymidine kinase transcription is regulated at G_1/S phase by a complex that contains retinoblastoma-like protein and a cdc2 kinase. Proc. Natl Acad. Sci. USA, 89, 3256–3260.

Dowdy, S.F., Hinds, P.W., Louie, K., Reed, S.I., Arnold, A. and Weinberg, R.A. (1993). Physical interaction of the retinoblastoma protein with human D cyclins. Cell, 73, 499–511.

Durfee, T., Becerer, K., Chen, P.-L., Yeh, S.-H., Yang, Y., Kilburn, A.E., Lee, W.-H. and Elledge, S.J. (1993). The retinoblastoma protein associates with the protein phosphatase type 1 catalytic subunit. Genes Devel., 7, 555–569.

Dyson, N., Buchkovich, K., Whyte, P. and Harlow, E. (1989). The cellular 107K protein that binds to adenovirus E1A also associates with the large T antigens of SV40 and JC virus. Cell, 58, 249–255.

Ewen, M.E., Ludlow, J.W., Marsilio, E., DeCaprio, J.A., Millikan, R.C., Cheng, S.H., Paucha, E. and Livingston, D.M. (1989). An N-terminal transformation-governing sequence of SV40 large T antigen contributes to the binding of both $p110^{Rb}$ and a second cellular protein, p120. Cell, 58, 257–267.

Ewen, M.E., Xing, Y., Lawrence, J.B. and Livingston, D.M. (1991). Molecular cloning, chromosomal mapping, and expression of the cDNA for p107, a retinoblastoma gene product-related protein. Cell, 66, 1155–1164.

Ewen, M.E., Sluss, H.K., Sherr, C.J., Matsushime, H., Kato, J. and Livingston, D.M. (1993). Functional interactions of the retinoblastoma protein with mammalian D-type cyclins. Cell, 73, 487–497.

Friend, S.H., Horowitz, J.M., Berger, M.R., Wang, X.-F., Bogenmann, E., Li, F.P. and Weinberg, R.A. (1987). Deletions of a DNA sequence in retinoblastoma and mesenchymal tumors: Organization of the sequence and its encoded protein. Proc. Natl Acad. Sci. USA, 84, 9059–9063.

Futreal, P.A. and Barrett, J.C. (1991). Failure of senescent cells to phosphorylate the RB protein. Oncogene, 6, 1109–1113.

Goodrich, D.W. and Lee, W.-H. (1992). Abrogation by c-*myc* of G_1 phase arrest induced by *RB* protein but not by p53. Nature, 360, 177–179.

Goodrich, D.W., Wang, N.P., Qian, Y.-W., Lee, E.Y.-H.P. and Lee, W.-H. (1991). The retinoblastoma gene product regulates progression through the G1 phase of the cell cycle. Cell, 67, 293–302.

Hagemeier, C., Bannister, A., Cook, A. and Kouzarides, T. (1993). The activation domain of transcription factor PU.1 binds the retinoblastoma (RB) protein and the transcription factor TFIID *in vitro*: RB shows sequence similarity to TFIID and TFIIB. Proc. Natl Acad. Sci. USA, 90, 1580–1584.

Hamel, P.A., Gill, R.M., Phillips, R.A. and Gallie, B.L. (1992). Transcriptional repression of the E2-containing promoters EIIaE, c-*myc*, and *RB1* by the product of the *RB1* gene. Mol. Cell. Biol., 12, 3431–3438.

Hara, E., Tsurui, H., Shinozaki, A., Nakada, S. and Oda, K. (1991). Cooperative effect of antisense-Rb and antisense-p53 oligomers on the extension of life span in human diploid fibroblasts, TIG-1. Biochem. Biophys. Res. Commun., 179, 528–534.

Helin, K., Lees, J.A., Vidal, M., Dyson, N., Harlow, E. and Fattaey, A. (1992). A cDNA encoding a pRB-binding protein with properties of the transcription factor E2F. Cell, 70, 337–350.

Hiebert, S.W. (1993). Regions of the retinoblastoma gene product required for its interaction with the E2F transcription factor are necessary for E2 promoter repression and pRb-mediated growth suppression. Mol. Cell. Biol., 13, 3384–3391.

Hinds, P.W., Mittnacht, S., Dulic, V., Arnold, A., Reed, S.I. and Weinberg, R.A. (1992). Regulation of retinoblastoma protein functions by ectopic expression of human cyclins. Cell, 70, 993–1006.

Horowitz, J.M., Park, H.-H., Bogenmann, E., Cheng, J.-C., Yandell, D.W., Kaye, F.J., Minna, J.D., Dryja, T.P. and Weinberg, R.A. (1990). Frequent inactivation of the retinoblastoma anti-oncogene is restricted to a subset of human tumor cells. Proc. Natl Acad. Sci. USA, 87, 2775–2779.

Horowitz, J.M., Yandell, D.W., Park, S.-H., Canning, S., Whyte, P., Buchkovich, K., Harlow, E., Weinberg, R.A. and Dryja, T.P. (1989). Point mutational inactivation of the retinoblastoma antioncogene. Science, 243, 937–940.

Hu, Q., Lees, J.A., Buchkovitch, K.J. and Harlow, E. (1992). The retinoblastoma protein physically associates with the human cdc2 kinase. Mol. Cell. Biol., 12, 971–980.

Huang, H.-J.S., Yee, J.K., Shew, J.-Y., Chen, P.-L., Bookstein, R., Friedmann, T., Lee, E.Y.-H.P. and Lee, W.-H. (1988). Suppression of the neoplastic phenotype by replacement of the RB gene in human cancer cells. Science, 242, 1563–1566.

Huang, S., Lee, W.-H. and Lee, E.Y.-H.P. (1991). A cellular protein that competes with SV40 T antigen for binding to the retinoblastoma gene product. Nature, 350, 160–162.

Jacks, T., Fazeli, A., Schmitt, E.M., Bronson, R.T., Goodell, M.A. and Weinberg, R.A. (1992). Effects of an *Rb* mutation in the mouse. Nature, 359, 295–300.

Kaelin, W.G., Krek, W., Sellers, W.R., DeCaprio, J.A., Ajchenbaum, F., Fuchs, C.S., Chittenden, T., Li, Y., Farnham, P.J., Blanar, M.A., Livingston, D.M. and Flemington, E.K. (1992). Expression cloning of a cDNA encoding a retinoblastoma-binding protein with E2F-like properties. Cell, 70, 351–364.

Kaye, F.J., Kratzke, R.A., Gerster, J.L. and Horowitz, J.M. (1990). A single amino acid substitution results in a retinoblastoma protein defective in phosphorylation and oncoprotein binding. Proc. Natl Acad. Sci. USA, 87, 6922–6926.

Kim, S.-J., Onwuta, U.S., Lee, Y.I., Li, R., Botchan, M.R. and Robbins, P.D. (1992). The retinoblastoma gene product regulates Sp1-mediated transcription. Mol. Cell. Biol., 12, 2455–2463.

Knudson, A.G. (1971). Mutation and cancer - statistical study of retinoblastoma. Proc. Natl Acad. Sci. USA, 68, 820–823.

Kratzke, R.A., Otterson, G.A., Lin, A.Y., Shimizu, E., Alexandrova, N., Zajac-Kaye, M., Horowitz, J.M and Kaye, F.J. (1992). Functional analysis at the Cys[706] residue of the retinoblastoma protein. J. Biol. Chem., 267, 25998–26003.

Lee W.-H., Bookstein R., Hong F., Young L.J., Shew J.-Y., Lee E.Y.-H.P. (1987a). Human retinoblastoma susceptibility gene: Cloning, identification, and sequence. Science 235, 1394–1399.

Lee W.-H., Shew J.-Y., Hong F.D., Sery T.W., Donoso L.A., Young L.J., Bookstein R., Lee E.Y.-H.P. (1987b). The retinoblastoma susceptibility gene encodes a nuclear phosphoprotein associated with DNA binding activity. Nature 329, 642–645.

Lee, E.Y.-H.P., Chang, C.-Y., Hu, N., Wang, Y.-C.J., Lai, C.-C., Herrup, K., Lee, W.-H. and Bradley, A. (1992). Mice deficient for Rb are nonviable and show defects in neurogenesis and haematopoiesis. Nature, 359, 288–294.

Lin, B.T.-Y., Gruenwald, S., Morla, A.O., Lee, W.-H. and Wang, J.Y.J. (1991). Retinoblastoma cancer suppressor gene product is a substrate of the cell cycle regulator cdc2 kinase. EMBO J., 10, 857–864.

Ludlow, J.W., Howell, R.L. and Smith, H.C. (1993a). Hypoxic stress induces reversible hypophosphorylation of pRB and reduction in cyclin A abundance independent of cell cycle progression. Oncogene, 8, 331–339.

Ludlow, J.W., Glendening, C.L., Livingston, D.M. and DeCaprio, J.A. (1993b). Specific enzymatic dephosphorylation of the retinoblastoma protein. Mol. Cell. Biol., 13, 367–372.

Mihara, K., Cao, X.-R., Yen, A., Chandler, S., Driscoll, B., Murphree, A.L., T'Ang, A. and Fung, Y.-K.T. (1989). Cell cycle-dependent regulation of phosphorylation of the human retinoblastoma gene product. Science, 246, 1300–1303.

Mittnacht, S. and Weinberg, R.A. (1991). G1/S phosphorylation of the retinoblastoma protein is associated with an altered affinity for the nuclear compartment. Cell, 65, 381–393.

Ohtani-Fujita, N., Fujita, T., Aoike, A., Osifchin, N.E., Robbins, P.D. and Sakai, T. (1993). CpG methylation inactivates the promoter activity of the human retinoblastoma tumor-suppressor gene. Oncogene, 8, 1063–1067.

Otterson, G.A., Kratzke, R.A., Lin, A.Y., Johnston, P.G. and Kaye, F.J. (1993). Alternative splicing of the *RBP1* gene clusters in an internal exon that encodes potential phosphorylation sites. Oncogene, 8, 949–957.

Ouellette, M.M., Chen, J., Wright, W.E. and Shay, J.W. (1992). Complexes containing the retinoblastoma gene product recognize different DNA motifs related to the E2F binding site. Oncogene, 7, 1075–1081.

Pagano, M., Durst, M., Joswig, S., Draetta, G. and Jansen-Durr, P. (1992). Binding of the human E2F transcription factor to the retinoblastoma protein but not to cyclin A is abolished in HPV-16-immortalized cells. Oncogene, 7, 1681–1686.

Qian, Y., Luckey, C., Horton, L., Esser, M. and Templeton, D.J. (1992). Biological function of the retinoblastoma protein requires distinct domains for hyperphosphorylation and transcription factor binding. Mol. Cell. Biol., 12, 5363–5372.

Qin, X.-Q., Chittenden, T., Livingston, D.M. and Kaelin, W.G. (1992). Identification of a growth suppression domain within the retinoblastoma gene product. Genes Devel., 6, 953–964.

Ray, S.K., Arroyo, M., Bagchi, S. and Raychaudhuri, P. (1992). Identification of a 60-kilodalton Rb-binding protein, RBP60, that allows the Rb-E2F complex to bind DNA. Mol. Cell. Biol., 12, 4327–4333.

Ruggeri, B., Zhang, S.-Y., Caamano, J., DiRado, M., Flynn, S.D. and Klein-Szanto, A.J.P. (1992). Human pancreatic carcinomas and cell lines reveal frequent and multiple alterations in the p53 and Rb-1 tumor-suppressor genes. Oncogene, 7, 1503–1511.

Rustgi, A.K., Dyson, N. and Bernards, R. (1991). Amino-terminal domains of c-*myc* and N-*myc* proteins mediate binding to the retinoblastoma gene product. Nature, 352, 541–544.

Sakai, T., Ohtani, N., McGee, T.L., Robbins, P.D. and Dryja, T. (1991). Oncogenic germ-line mutations in Sp1 and ATF sites in the human retinoblastoma gene. Nature, 353, 83–86.

Savoysky, E., Suzuki, M., Simbulan, C., Tamai, K., Ohuchi, T., Akiyama, T. and Yoshida, S. (1993). Immunoprecipitated Rb protein inhibits SV40 T antigen-dependent stimulation of DNA polymerase α. Oncogene, 8, 319–325.

Schonthal, A. and Feramisco, J.R. (1993). Inhibition of histone H1 kinase expression, retinoblastoma protein phosphorylation, and cell proliferation by the phosphatase inhibitor okadaic acid. Oncogene, 8, 433–441.

Schwarz, J.K., Devoto, S.H., Smith, E.J., Chellappan, S.P., Jakoi, L. and Nevins, J.R. (1993). Interactions of the p107 and Rb proteins with E2F during the cell proliferation cycle. EMBO J., 12, 1013–1020.

Shay, J.W., Pereira-Smith, O.M. and Wright, W.E. (1991). A role for both RB and p53 in the regulation of human cellular senescence. Exp. Cell Res., 196, 33–39.

Shew, J.-Y., Lin, B.T.-Y., Chen, P.-L., Tseng, B.Y., Yang-Feng, T.L. and Lee, W.-H. (1990). C-terminal truncation of the retinoblastoma gene product leads to functional inactivation. Proc. Natl Acad. Sci. USA, 87, 6–10.

Shirodkar, S., Ewen, M., DeCaprio, J.A., Morgan, J., Livingston, D.M. and Chittenden, T. (1992). The transcription factor E2F interacts with the retinoblastoma product and a p107-cyclin A complex in a cell cycle-regulated manner. Cell, 68, 157–166.

Stirdivant, S.M., Huber, H.E., Patrick, D.R., Defeo-Jones, D., McAvoy, E.M., Garsky, V.M., Oliff, A. and Heimbrook, D.C. (1992a). Human papillomavirus type 16 E7 protein inhibits DNA binding by the retinoblastoma gene product. Mol. Cell. Biol., 12, 1905–1914.

Stirdivant, S.M., Ahern, J.D., Oliff, A. and Heimbrook, D.C. (1992b). Retinoblastoma protein binding properties are dependent on 4 cysteine residues in the protein binding pocket. J. Biol. Chem., 267, 14846–14851.

Strauss, M., Hering, S., Lieber, A., Herrmann, G., Griffin, B.E. and Arnold, W. (1992). Stimulation of cell division and fibroblast focus formation by antisense repression of retinoblastoma protein synthesis. Oncogene, 7, 769–773.

T'Ang, A., Wu, K.-J., Hashimoto, T., Liu, W.-Y., Takahashi, R., Shi, X.-H., Mihara, K., Zhang, F.-H., Chen, Y.Y., Du, C., Qian, J., Lin, Y.-G., Murphree, A.L., Qiu, W.-R., Thompson, T., Benedict, W.F. and Fung, Y.-K.T. (1989). Genomic organization of the human retinoblastoma gene. Oncogene, 4, 401–407.

Terada, N., Lucas, J.J. and Gelfand, E.W. (1991). Differential regulation of the tumor suppressor molecules, retinoblastoma susceptibility gene product (Rb) and p53, during cell cycle progression of normal human T cells. J. Immunol., 147, 698–704.

Udvadia, A.J., Rogers, K.T., Higgins, P.D.R., Murata, Y., Martin, K.H., Humphrey, P.A. and Horowitz, J.M.

(1993). Sp-1 binds promoter elements regulated by the RB protein and Sp-1 mediated transcription is stimulated by RB coexpression. Proc. Natl Acad. Sci. USA, 90, 3265–3269.

Weichselbaum, R.R., Beckett, M. and Diamond, A. (1988). Some retinoblastomas, osteosarcomas, and soft tissue sarcomas may share a common etiology. Proc. Natl Acad. Sci. USA, 85, 2106–2109.

Weintraub, S.J., Prater, C.A. and Dean, D.C. (1992). Retinoblastoma protein switches the E2F site from positive to negative element. Nature, 358, 259–261.

Whyte, P., Buchkovich, K.J., Horowitz, J.M., Friend, S.H., Raybuck, M., Weinberg, R.A. and Harlow, E. (1988). Association between an oncogene and an anti-oncogene: the adenovirus E1A proteins bind to the retinoblastoma gene product. Nature, 334, 124–129.

Williams, R.T., Carbonaro-Hall, D.A. and Hall, F.L. (1992). Co-purification of $p34^{cdc2}/p58^{cyclin\ A}$ proline-directed protein kinase and the retinoblastoma tumor susceptibility gene product: interaction of an oncogenic serine/threonine protein kinase with a tumor-suppressor protein. Oncogene, 7, 423–432.

Windle, J.J., Albert, D.M., O'Brien, J.M., Marcus, D.M., Disteche, C.M., Bernards, R. and Mellon, P.L. (1990). Retinoblastoma in transgenic mice. Nature, 343, 665–669.

Xu, H.-J., Hu, S.-X., Hashimoto, T., Takahashi, R. and Benedict, W.F. (1989). The retinoblastoma susceptibility gene product: a characteristic pattern in normal cells and abnormal expression in malignant cells. Oncogene, 4, 807–812.

Xu, H.-J., Hu, S.-X. and Benedict, W.F. (1991). Lack of nuclear RB protein staining in G0/middle G1 cells: correlation to changes in total RB protein level. Oncogene, 6, 1139–1146.

Zhang, W., Drach, J., Andreeff, M. and Deisseroth, A. (1993). Growth factor-induced changes in the expression of the retinoblastoma gene in acute myelogenous leukemia cells. Blood, in press.

Zhang, W., Hittelman, W., Van, N., Andreeff, M. and Deisseroth, A. (1992). The phosphorylation of retinoblastoma gene product in human myeloid leukemia cells during the cell cycle. Biochem. Biophys. Res. Commun., 184, 212–216.

P53

Chromosome 17p is frequently lost in human cancers and in most tumours that have been examined point mutations have occurred in one allele of the *TP53* (tumour protein 53)/*P53* gene (Bartek *et al.*, 1991). In Li–Fraumeni syndrome the mutated gene is transmitted in the germ line and this autosomal dominant syndrome is characterized by the occurrence of a variety of mesenchymal and epithelial neoplasms at multiple sites (Srivastava *et al.*, 1990).

Cross-species homology

High degree of homology in 5 domains (human, chicken, mouse, rat, *Xenopus*; Harlow *et al.*, 1985; Soussi *et al.*, 1987; Zakut-Houri *et al.*, 1983, 1985). P53: 76% identity (human and mouse).

Transformation

MAN (see Table 3.9)

Mutations in *P53* and in *RAS* occur in 74% and 35% respectively of cell lines derived from non-small-cell lung cancers (Mitsudomi *et al.*, 1992). These appear to be independent mutations that exert differing effects but, in those lines in which both *P53* and *RAS* are abnormal, the *P53* mutations tend to occur in exon 8, suggesting that this region may encode a domain that interacts with RAS. Mutations in *P53* occur with low frequency in AML but the normal protein is overexpressed in the peripheral blood cells of 75% of patients (Zhang *et al.*, 1992).

Table 3.9. *Incidence of P53 mutations*

Cancer	Percentage of samples in which *P53* mutations occur	References
Acute myeloblastic leukaemia (AML)	6	Zhang and Deisseroth, 1993
Brain tumours	~10	Mashiyama *et al.*, 1991
Breast cancer	53–86	Horak *et al.*, 1991; Varley *et al.*, 1991
Burkitt's lymphoma cell lines	60	Wiman *et al.*, 1991
Colorectal cancer	50	Rodrigues *et al.*, 1990
Epithelial skin (basal cell) carcinomas	48	Moles *et al.*, 1993
Oesophageal cancers	50	Bennett *et al.*, 1991
Gastric carcinoma	57	Martin *et al.*, 1992
HBV-positive hepatoma	18	Hosono *et al.*, 1993
Lung tumours:		
Small-cell carcinoma	44–73	Iggo *et tal.*, 1990; Takahashi *et al.*, 1991
Non-small-cell carcinoma	45	Takahashi *et al.*, 1991
Adenocarcinoma	57	Iggo *et al.*, 1990
Squamous cell carcinomas	34–82	Gusterson *et al.*, 1991; Iggo *et al.*, 1990
Carcinoid	0	Iggo *et al.*, 1990
Malignant astrocytomas	~30	Mashiyama *et al.*, 1991
Melanomas (primary)	97	Akslen and Morkve, 1992
Multiple myeloma	20	Portier *et al.*, 1992
Neuroblastoma cell lines	80	Davidoff *et al.*, 1992
Osteosarcoma cell lines	90	Diller *et al.*, 1990
Osteosarcomas	41	Mulligan *et al.*, 1990
Ovarian carcinomas	44	Milner *et al.*, 1993
Pancreatic carcinomas	40	Ruggeri *et al.*, 1992
Rhabdomyosarcomas	45	Mulligan *et al.*, 1990
Squamous cell carcinoma of the larynx	60	Maestro *et al.*, 1992
Thyroid carcinomas	50	Dongi *et al.*, 1992

ANIMALS

Disruption of *P53* by proviral insertion of murine leukaemia viruses has been detected in erythroid and lymphoid tumours (Munroe *et al.*, 1990).

IN VITRO

Mutant (but not wild-type) *P53* plus *Ras* causes transformation of primary rat embryo fibroblasts (Finlay *et al.*, 1989) and mutant *P53*, like E1A, can immortalize cells. In transfected primary fibroblasts expression of wild-type *P53* inhibits the ability of mutant *P53* plus *Ras* (or E1A plus *Ras*) to cause transformation. The transfection of some breast carcinoma, osteosarcoma, colorectal carcinoma and glioblastoma cell lines that carry mutations in *P53* with a wild-type *P53* gene suppresses growth (Baker *et al.*, 1990; Diller *et al.*, 1990; Mercer *et al.*, 1990). The tumorigenicity of breast carcinoma cell lines that harbour mutations in both *P53* and *RB* genes is reduced by the expression of wild-type forms of either *P53* or *RB* (Wang *et al.*, 1993). These *in vitro* findings are consistent with the occurrence of *trans*-dominant mutations in *P53*, as are those from analysis of a number of animal and human tumours. However, the growth of some other breast carcinoma cell lines is not prevented by wild-type *P53* (Casey *et al.*, 1991). This is consistent with the fact that a significant proportion of such tumours do not appear to involve mutations in *P53* but may reflect a dominant negative effect being exerted by mutant *P53*.

TRANSGENIC ANIMALS

Mice homozygous for the null allele develop normally but are predisposed to spontaneous tumour formation at an early age (Donehower *et al.*, 1992). 74% of homozygote animals develop neoplasms within 6 months, most commonly malignant lymphomas and sarcomas. This frequency greatly exceeds that observed in mice carrying a mutant *P53* transgene (20%). Tumour development in *P53*-deficient mice is sporadic, indicating that additional genetic or epigenetic events are required.

	P53
Nucleotides (kb)	12.5
Chromosome	
Human	17p13.1
Mouse	11
Exons	
Human, mouse	11 (1st exon non-coding)
Rat	10
mRNA (kb)	
Human	2.5
Mouse	2.0
	P53 mRNA is detectable in all mammalian cells: levels are low in normal cells (Rogel *et al.*, 1985) but high in early embryonic development (Louis *et al.*, 1988)
mRNA half-life (h)	>12
Amino acids	
Human	393
Mouse	390
Mass (kDa)	
(predicted)	
Human	43.5
Mouse	43.5
(expressed)	
Human	pp53
Mouse	pp53 (high proline content may cause the anomalous electrophoretic behaviour seen also in a number of other nuclear oncoproteins (SV40 large T, adenovirus E1A, FOS and MYC) that share structural properties)
Protein half-life	5–20 min (normal cells) 4–20 h (transformed cells)

Cellular location

Normally nuclear but detectable at the plasma membrane during mitosis in normal and transformed cells (Milner and Cook, 1986; Shaulsky *et al.*, 1990). The conformational phenotype (see below) may determine its location (Zerrahn *et al.*, 1992).

Tissue location

Ubiquitous. In most transformed and tumour cells the concentration of p53 is increased 5- to 100-fold (Hassapoglidou *et al.*, 1993) over the minute concentration in normal cells (~1000 molecules/cell), principally due to the half-life of the mutant forms (4 h) compared with that of the wild-type (20 min). Normal p53 is undetectable by immunofluorescent staining: thus positive staining indicates the presence of mutant protein (detected in 40% of human mammary carcinomas and 30% of colon cancers). High concentrations of p53 protein are transiently expressed in human epidermis and superficial dermal fibroblasts following mild ultraviolet irradiation (Hall *et al.*, 1993).

Protein function

p53 binds to a DNA consensus sequence, the p53 response element, comprised of two copies of 5'-PuPuPuC(^{A}/$_T$)(^{T}/$_A$)GPyPy-3' separated by 0–13 bp (Kern *et al.*, 1991; El-Deiry *et al.*, 1992). Wild-type p53 has weak sequence-specific DNA binding activity that is strongly enhanced by factors acting on its C-terminal regulatory domain. These factors include casein kinase II, monoclonal antibody binding, *E. coli* dnaK or deletion of the C-terminus (Hupp *et al.*, 1992). Sequences to which wild-type p53 specifically binds occur in the human ribosomal gene cluster (RGC), the mouse muscle creatine kinase gene (*MCK*) and SV40, binding affinity being slightly lower for the latter site (Bargonetti *et al.*, 1992). p53 also interacts with CCAAT binding factor (CBF) to repress transcription from the heat shock protein 70 (hsp70) promoter (Agoff *et al.*, 1993). Point mutations in *P53* generally abolish sequence-specific DNA binding although the Trp248 mutant that occurs in Li–Fraumeni syndrome binds with almost undiminished affinity to RGC DNA.

p53 contains a powerful transcription activation domain (Fields and Jang, 1990; Raycroft *et al.*, 1990) and fusion proteins of GAL4 and the N-terminal 160 amino acids of p53 have transcription-activating capacity (O'Rourke *et al.*, 1990). Transcriptional activation by these fusion proteins is prevented by mutant p53 proteins or by adenovirus E1B and inhibition of *trans* activation by p53 correlates with transformation of primary cells by E1B in cooperation with E1A (Yew and Berk, 1992). SV40 T antigen and HPV-16 E6 protein also inhibit *trans* activation by wild-type p53 (Mietz *et al.*, 1992). The first 42 amino acids of p53 comprise the minimum region sufficient for *trans*-activating function in GAL4 fusion proteins (Unger *et al.*, 1992). In constructs containing a reporter gene downstream of the p53 DNA binding sequence and a minimal promoter, wild-type p53 activates transcription *in vitro* in both yeast and human cells and transcription is suppressed by dominant negative p53 mutants (Farmer *et al.*, 1992; Kern *et al.*, 1992; Scharer and Iggo, 1992). The 59 amino acids between residues 302 and 360 of mouse p53 constitute a minimum transforming domain that will oligomerize with wild-type p53 and inhibit sequence-specific DNA binding (Shaulian *et al.*, 1992).

Wild-type p53 activates transcription of genes with a p53 response element but it can suppress transcription of a variety of genes that lack a p53 response element, including human IL-6, *Fos*, *Jun* or β-actin genes and the porcine MHC class I gene (Santhanam *et al.*, 1991; Ginsberg *et al.*,

1991). In glioblastoma cells the expression of wild-type p53 represses transcription of proliferating cell nuclear antigen (PCNA), DNA polymerase α and *Mybb*, but not of *Fos*, *Jun*, *Junb* or *Myc*, consistent with its causing growth arrest at the G_1/S transition of the cell cycle (Mercer *et al.*, 1991; Lin *et al.*, 1992). Wild-type but not mutant p53 binds to human TATA-binding protein and *in vitro* this inhibits transcription from minimal promoters (Seto *et al.*, 1992; Mack *et al.*, 1993). The region of p53 that interacts with TBP lies in the activation domain between residues 20 and 57: residues 93 to 160 are responsible for *trans* repression (Liu *et al.*, 1993). p53 also binds to a *cis*-acting element (GGAAGTGA) in the *RB* promoter: as this element overlaps the basal transcription unit of the *RB* promoter, p53 may repress *RB* transcription (Shiio *et al.*, 1992). A similar sequence is present in the SV40 enhancer/promoter (GGAACTGG) to which p53 may bind specifically to repress transcription (Jackson *et al.*, 1993).

p53 binds via its acidic activation domain (residues 20–42) to the 95 kDa product of the murine double minute 2 (*Mdm-2*) gene in intact cells and *in vitro* the formation of this complex inhibits p53-mediated *trans* activation (Momand *et al.*, 1992; Oliner *et al.*, 1993). The expression of *Mdm-2* is itself induced by p53 which may serve to autoregulate p53 activity in normal cells (Barak and Oren, 1992; Barak *et al.*, 1993). *MDM2* is amplified in 36% of human sarcomas analysed and the overexpression of this gene may enable p53-regulated growth control to be overridden in these tumours (Oliner *et al.*, 1992).

p53 was first discovered as a component of immunoprecipitates of SV40 large T antigen. In cells transformed by SV40 or adenovirus and in tumours induced by these viruses, p53 is found in an oligomeric complex with SV40 large T antigen (at a site between residues 271 and 517; this region contains the ATPase-helicase activity and is distinct from that to which p105^{RB} binds) or with adenovirus type 5 E1B 58 kDa protein. Both E1A and E1B proteins are necessary for adenoviral transformation of primary cells: the former binds p105^{RB} and the latter p53. Transformation by T antigen alone may arise because the single protein encompasses binding sites for both p105^{RB} and p53. T antigen inhibits transcriptional activation by p53 *in vitro* (Farmer *et al.*, 1992). p53/T antigen complexes also contain β-tubulin (Maxwell *et al.*, 1991).

Although the sites of interaction are distinct, the mechanisms by which DNA tumour viruses inactivate p105^{RB} and p53 to cause transformation and tumorigenesis are highly conserved. Other nuclear phosphoproteins have been shown to bind to the large T antigens of SV40 and JC virus (Dyson *et al.*, 1989), and to E1A, indicating the presence of a family of normal proteins the regulatory functions of which can be modulated by DNA viruses. p53 forms complexes with at least three proteins in growth-arrested cells. p53 also forms stable homo-oligomers that principally result from the α helix (334–356) and basic regions (363–386) of the C-terminus (Milner *et al.*, 1991; Sturzbecher *et al.*, 1992; Friedman *et al.*, 1993; Iwabuchi *et al.*, 1993). *In vitro*, p53 also binds to protein kinase C and S100b (Baudier *et al.*, 1992).

p53 AND THE CELL GROWTH CYCLE

One role of p53 may be in regulating the normal cell growth cycle by activating transcription of genes that cause arrest in G_1 when the genome is damaged (Lane, 1992). This hypothesis was prompted by the observations that γ-irradiation of cells or treatment with actinomycin D to inhibit DNA synthesis induces an increase in the level of p53 protein that correlates with arrest in G_1 and nuclear accumulation of p53 (Kastan *et al.*, 1991) and also by the evidence from transgenic mouse studies indicating that p53 is not essential for cell growth control during early development. In normal cells ionizing radiation increases the concentration of p53 and transgenic studies indicate that p53 is essential for the apoptotic response to radiation or to the topoisomerase 2 inhibitor etoposide but not for the response to other DNA damaging agents such as glucocorticoids (Clarke *et al.*, 1993; Lowe *et al.*, 1993). The *GADD* (*G*rowth *A*rrest on *D*NA *D*amage) genes are induced in a wide variety of mammalian cells by DNA-damaging agents

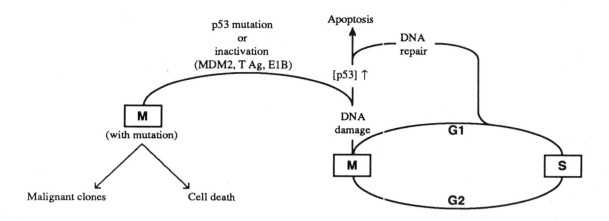

or other causes of growth arrest (Kastan *et al.*, 1992) and p53 induces *GADD45* transcription by a mechanism in which wild-type but not mutant p53 binds to a DNA motif that is an almost perfect consensus p53 binding sequence. Cells from patients with ataxia telangietasia, a human autosomal recessive disorder characterized by hypersensitivity to ionizing radiation and a markedly enhanced susceptibility to cancer, lack the normal ionizing radiation-induced increase in p53 protein. Thus p53 may function via *GADD45* to inhibit progression to S phase. The accumulation of p53 may merely inhibit the cell cycle until damaged DNA has been repaired or, if sustained, cause the activation of programmed cell death. The latter mechanism is consistent with the finding that expression of wild-type p53 (or p105^{RB}) can mediate apoptosis in the absence of appropriate differentiation or proliferation signals. Thus, murine leukaemia cells or human colon tumour-derived cells that normally do not express p53 enter apoptosis when wild-type *P53* is expressed from a transfected vector (Yonish-Rouach *et al.*, 1991; Shaw *et al.*, 1992), as do Burkitt's lymphoma cells that carry mutant P53 (Ramqvist *et al.*, 1993). Commitment to cell death coincides with the appearance of fragmented DNA (Ryan *et al.*, 1993). The inactivation of p53 may thus permit replication of damaged DNA and promote the development of malignant cell clones, as occurs with high frequency in *P53* null mice and in patients with Li–Fraumeni syndrome.

p53 does, however, appear to be essential for normal proliferation in that antisense mRNA or anti-p53 antibody blocks entry into S phase (Shohat *et al.*, 1987; Mercer *et al.*, 1984). Cells expressing wild-type p53 arrest in G$_1$ when uridine synthesis is inhibited by *N*-(phosphonacetyl)-L-aspartate (PALA) and do not show the gene amplification characteristic of transformed cells. However, cells that have lost both *P53* alleles are insensitive to inhibitors of cell cycle progression and have a high frequency of gene amplification (Livingstone *et al.*, 1992; Yin *et al.*, 1992).

When 3T3 cells are stimulated by TPA or serum there is a 10- to 20-fold rise in *P53* mRNA within 6 h. Transcription of p34^{CDC2}, a critical regulator of mammalian cell cycle progression, also increases in serum-stimulated fibroblasts, reaching a maximum after 18 h, shortly before S phase. p53 is phosphorylated by p34^{CDC2} when the latter is complexed with either p60 (cyclin A) or cyclin B (Sturzbecher *et al.*, 1990; Bischoff *et al.*, 1990). These two active forms of p34 occur in late G$_1$ and M phases of the cell cycle, respectively, and the fact that, in addition to p53, p105^{RB} and SV40 T antigen are substrates, suggests that either suppressing the action of these proteins or redirecting their activity is a crucial requirement for both DNA synthesis and mitosis to occur. Both T antigen and p53 are phosphorylated by p34^{CDC2} at sites adjacent to the nuclear targeting signal, T antigen on Thr124 (nuclear signal: residues 126–133) and p53 on Ser315 (nuclear signal: SSSPQPKKKP, residues 313–322 (Marshak *et al.*, 1991). p34^{CDC2} complexes preferentially with wild-type (suppressor) p53 but p53–p34^{CDC2} complexes are undetectable during mitosis (Milner *et al.*, 1990). This suggests that p53–p34^{CDC2} interaction is critical for progression through the early phases of the cell cycle and p53 (and T antigen in infected cells) may be prevented from entering the nucleus when p34 is active. Serine phosphorylation of p53 is increased in transformed cells by comparison with normal cells: serines 4, 6 and 9 are phosphorylated by casein kinase I (Milne *et al.*, 1992a) and phosphorylation of Ser389 by casein kinase II (Meek *et al.*, 1990; Herrmann *et al.*, 1991; Filhol *et al.*, 1992) may activate the antiproliferative capacity of p53 (Milne *et al.*, 1992b). The capacity of wild-type p53 to inhibit transformation by *Ras* and either E1A or mutant *P53* is dependent on the nuclear localization signal in p53 (Shaulsky *et al.*, 1991). The co-transforming activity of mutant *P53* also requires the nuclear targeting signal, confirming that p53 must enter the nucleus to manifest activity. p53 and T antigen are dephosphorylated at specific sites by protein phosphatase 2A; the dephosphorylation is blocked by SV40 small t antigen (Scheidtmann *et al.*, 1991).

A mutant form of p53 derived from a human tumour blocks the growth of yeast cells and its inhibitory effects are reversed by the co-expression of p34^{CDC2} (Wagner *et al.*, 1991). Other mutant forms of p53 do not affect yeast cell growth, consistent with the evidence that there are functional subclasses of mutants, but the rescue from growth arrest by p34^{CDC2} indicates a functional interaction with p53.

Structure of the mouse *P53* gene

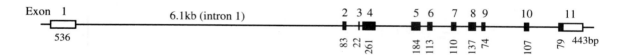

Open boxes: non-coding exons. Black boxes: coding exons. Numbers below boxes indicate exon size in base pairs (Bienz *et al.*, 1984). The *P53* promoter lacks a TATA sequence but contains a helix–loop–helix consensus binding sequence (Ronen *et al.*, 1991) either downstream of the transcription initiation site (+70 to +75, mouse) or upstream (−29 to −34, human). In the murine promoter this element is required for full promoter activity and it contains the sequence CACGTG which is the recognition site for the transcription factors MYC, USF and TFE3 (Reisman and Rotter, 1993). The region between +22 and +67 are involved in *trans* activation of the *P53* promoter by p53 itself (Deffie *et al.*, 1993). Two G nucleotides at intron 4 positions 33 and 44 bind a protein that is necessary for transformation by p53 (Beenken *et al.*, 1991). Intron 4 is essential for *P53* expression in transgenic mice (Lozano and Levine, 1991). Differentiating mouse erythroleukaemia cells accumulate antisense RNA to the first intron that may be involved in the downregulation of *P53* mRNA (Khochbin and Lawrence, 1989).

Sequences of human and mouse p53

```
Human p53    (1)    MEEPQSDPSVEPPLSQETFSDLWKLL PENNVLSPLPS QAMDDLMLSPDDIEQWFTEDPG
Mouse p53    (1)    MTA---S---I-L-L--------G-----P--DI    ---PHC----L-PQ- V-EF- -  -

            (60)    PDEAPRMPEAAPPVAPAPAAPTPAAPAPAPSWPLSSSVPSQKTYQGSYGFRLGFLHSGTA
            (57)    -S--L-VSG-PAAQD-VTET-G-V-----TP-----F---------N---H----Q----

            (120)   KSVTCTYSPALNKMFCQLAKTCPVQLWVDSTPPPGTRVRAMAIYKQSQHMTEVVRRCPHH
            (117)   ---M-----P---L-------------SA---A-S--------K-------------
```

```
(180)  ERCSDSDGLAPPQHLIRVEGNLRVEYLDDRNTFRHSVVVPYEPPEVGSDCTTIHYNYMCN
(177)  -----G---------------YP---E--Q-------------A--EY----K----

(240)  SSCMGGMNRRPILTIITLEDSSGNLLGRNSFEVRVCACPGRDRRTEEENLRKKGEPHHEL
(237)  -------------------------D-------------------F---EVLCP--

(300)  PPGSTKRALPNNTSSSPQPKKKPLDGEYFTLQIRGRERFEMFRELNEALELKDAQAGKEP
(297)  ----A-----TC--A--PQ-----------K----K----------------H-TE-S

(360)  GGSRAHSSHLKSKKGQSTSRHKKLMFKTEGPDSD (393)
(357)  -D------Y--T-----------T-V-KV----- (390)
```

Protein structure

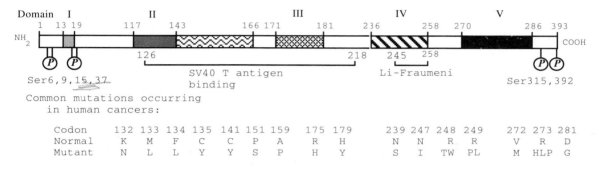

Common mutations occurring in human cancers:

Codon	132	133	134	135	141	151	159	175	179	239	247	248	249	272	273	281
Normal	K	M	F	C	C	P	A	R	H	N	N	R	R	V	R	D
Mutant	N	L	L	Y	Y	S	P	H	Y	S	I	TW	PL	M	HLP	G

The N-terminal domain (residues 1–75 in human p53) is very acidic and this highly charged region is predicted to form an α helix. The central region (residues 75–150) is a proline-rich, hydrophobic region and the C-terminus (residues 319–393 (276–390 in the mouse)) is a basic DNA binding domain containing helix–coil–helix motifs. The T antigen binding region mapped by mutagenesis is shown (Ruppert and Stillman, 1993) although, as these mutant proteins have altered tertiary structure, the precise T antigen binding site remains undefined. The "hot-spot" in exon 7 for Li–Fraumeni germ line mutations is indicated; some Li–Fraumeni families have also been identified with *P53* mutations outside exon 7 (Prosser *et al.*, 1992). The serine residues indicated are major phosphorylation sites (see below and Wang and Eckhart, 1992). Serines 15 and 37 are phosphorylated *in vitro* by the nuclear serine/threonine proteins kinase DNA-PK that requires double-stranded DNA for activity (Lees-Miller *et al.*, 1992) and mutation of Ser15 reduces the capacity of p53 to block cell cycle progression (Fiscella *et al.*, 1993). Both wild-type and mutant murine p53 are linked to 5.8S rRNA at Ser389 (Samad and Carroll, 1991; Fontoura *et al.*, 1992). This residue (human Ser392) is also the target for casein kinase II (Hupp *et al.*, 1992). Two putative Zn^{2+} binding domains ($Cys135-X_5-Cys141-X_{34}-Cys176-X_2-His179$ and $Cys238-X_3-Cys242-X_{32}-Cys275-X_1-Cys277$) may form a bridge between conserved domains II and III and IV and V, providing an explanation of how mutations scattered over more than 150 residues may have a common effect on tertiary structure (Hainaut and Milner, 1993).

Mutations in *P53*

A large number of *P53* mutations lead to a single substitution of a nucleic acid base pair (Hollstein *et al.*, 1991) but ~10% of human cancers are characterized by deletions or insertions in this gene (Jego *et al.*, 1993). Mutations are mainly clustered in four domains highly conserved among vertebrates involving exons 5–10 (amino acids 120–290). The resultant mutant proteins fail to bind monoclonal antibody PAb246 (which recognizes an epitope between amino acids 88 and 109 of wild-type p53), bind to DNA or to SV40 T antigen with much reduced affinity, but bind with high affinity to the hsp70 protein via the C-terminal 28 amino acids of p53 (Hainaut and Milner, 1992). In cells transformed by *Ras* with *P53*, mutant p53 protein occurs in a trimeric complex with the heat shock protein and wild-type p53. Mutations producing an abnormal protein that inhibits the function of its normal allelic gene product by formation of mutant/wild-type protein complexes are called *trans*-dominant mutations.

Codons 144–166 lie outside the evolutionarily conserved domains but include frequent sites of mutation in non-small-cell lung cancer. Eight of these p53 mutants isolated from human lung carcinomas react with a monoclonal antibody (PAb240) that is normally non-reactive with wild-type p53. Size fractionation indicates that the quaternary structure adopted by these mutant proteins is similar to that of wild-type p53, with the exception of p53-Tyr135 (Medcalf *et al.*, 1992). Three of the mutants (247, 248 and 273 (Arg to Leu)) have conformations that are temperature-sensitive: they bind PAb1620 (that recognizes wild-type p53) at 30°C but not at 37°C. In hepatocellular carcinomas there is a mutational hot-spot involving G to C or T transversions in codon 249 (Hsu *et al.*, 1991; Bressac *et al.*, 1991) and the *in vitro* growth of hepatocellular carcinoma cells that contain integrated hepatitis B virus sequences is inhibited by exogenous wild-type p53 (Puisieux *et al.*, 1993). Tobacco smoke can cause G to C mutations in lung cancer (Chiba *et al.*, 1990) and a point mutation in intron 5 has been detected in a colorectal tumour that deletes amino acids 172–186 and generates a protein derived from truncation of exon 7 (Ishioka *et al.*, 1991). A germ line mutation in intron 5 has also been detected (Felix *et al.* 1993). Normal and epidermal carcinoma cells express an alternatively spliced RNA at ~30% of the level of the normal transcript that contains an additional 96 bases derived from intron 10 (Arai *et al.*, 1986; Han and Kulesz-Martin, 1992).

In glioblastoma cells wild-type p53 is more highly phosphorylated than the mutant protein and the change in phosphorylation state correlates with the loss of a specific epitope at the C-terminus (Ullrich *et al.*, 1992). However, a murine temperature-sensitive *P53* gene product has been described that appears not to undergo a change in phosphorylation state on switching between the oncogenic and tumour suppressor forms (Picksley *et al.*, 1992).

Mutations in p53 may (1) be of the dominant negative type when the protein overrides the action of the suppressor wild-type p53 or (2) result in the loss of suppressor function or (3) result in a protein that functions as a tumour promoter (Milner, 1991). The selectivity of binding of two monoclonal antibodies to p53 indicates the existence of two conformational forms that correspond to suppressor and promoter activities. The switch from suppressor to promoter conformation occurs transiently in serum-stimulated fibroblasts (Milner and Watson, 1990), a finding consistent with the inhibition of proliferation by microinjected monoclonal antibody against p53. Evidence from antibody binding studies indicates that wild-type p53 assumes a "mutant-like" conformation when it binds to DNA, undergoing conformational changes at both its N- and C-termini (Halazonetis *et al.*, 1993). The equivalent permanent conformational change would account for the action of the temperature-sensitive mouse mutant p53 that carries a substitution from alanine to valine at position 135 (Michalovitz *et al.*, 1990; Milner and Medcalf, 1990). p53-Val135 cooperates with *Ras* to transform rat embryo fibroblasts at 37.5°C but represses transformation by microinjected RAS at 32.5°C, as does wild-type p53. Some p53 mutants form complexes with wild-type p53 within which the wild-type protein is driven to adopt the mutant tertiary structure (Milner and Medcalf, 1991). This conformational effect may account for the dominant negative effect of some mutants whereas others, for example those occurring in Li–Fraumeni syndrome, fail to have this dominant effect on the tertiary structure of the wild-type protein and are therefore recessive in nature.

p53 protein synthesized by normal human bone marrow blast cells and by resting or activated peripheral lymphocytes is recognized by the monoclonal antibody PAb240 that is usually specific for the mutant protein (Rivas *et al.*, 1992). Thus normal human haematopoietic cells may express p53 in an activated conformation. p53 protein from a high proportion (86%) of samples of AML cells is precipitated by PAb240, although the frequency of mutations in AML is only 6% (Zhang *et al.*, 1992). The half-life of the non-mutated protein from these cells is 2–5 h, approximately that observed in proliferating lymphocytes, whilst the half-life of the mutant forms (>10 h) is similar to that in other transformed cells. Thus the characteristics of AML, abnormal proliferation and inhibition of differentiation, are correlated in the majority of cases with enhanced expression of normal p53 having an altered conformation.

HPV-mediated degradation of p53

Cervical carcinomas expressing HPV DNA sequences normally co-express wild-type p53 mRNA, mutant p53 being present in the absence of HPV DNA (Crook *et al.*, 1991a), although p53 mutations do occur in some HPV-associated cancers (Crook and Vousden, 1992) and mutant p53 can convert HPV-immortalized cells to a more transformed state (Chen *et al.*, 1993). p53 binds to the HPV E6 protein (see above) in a process dependent on an additional cellular factor (E6-associated protein, E6-AP; Huibregtse *et al.*,1993) and this interaction targets the suppressor form of p53 for ubiquitin-mediated degradation (Scheffner *et al.*, 1990). The E6 proteins of both benign and oncogenic HPVs associate *in vitro* with p53 but only oncogenic HPVs direct p53 degradation (Crook *et al.*, 1991b). p53 binds to the C-terminus of HPVs (amino acids 106–115 of HPV-16 E6) but the binding site that is specific for degradation is in the N-terminus (residues 8–12 and 45–49) and is conserved in oncogenic HPVs. The expression of E6 in keratinocyte cell lines decreases the stability of p53 by between 2- and 4-fold and also prevents the inhibition by p53 of transcription from various TATA-containing promoters (Hubbert *et al.*, 1992; Lechner *et al.*, 1992; Band *et al.*, 1993) and abolishes the arrest in G_1 that normally occurs following DNA damage (Kessis *et al.*, 1993).

Databank file names and accession numbers

	GENE	*EMBL*	*SWISSPROT*	*REFERENCES*
Human	*TP53*	Hsp53t K03199 Hsp53r X01405 Hsp53 X02469	P53_HUMAN P04637	Harlow *et al.*, 1985 Zakut-Houri *et al.*, 1985 Harris *et al.*, 1986 Buchman *et al.*, 1988 Matlashewski *et al.*, 1984 Addison *et al.*, 1990 Rodrigues *et al.*, 1990 Malkin *et al.*, 1990 Hsu *et al.*, 1991
	intron 10 promoter	M13874 Hsp53a J04238		Han and Kulesz-Martin, 1992 Tuck and Crawford, 1989

	GENE	EMBL	SWISSPROT	REFERENCES
Mouse	P53	Mmant02 to Mmant11 (X00876 to X00885) Mmp53a to Mmp53c (M13872 to M13874) Mmp53r X01237 Mmp53 X00741	P53_MOUSE P02340	Zakut-Houri *et al.*, 1983 Bienz *et al.*, 1984 Jenkins *et al.*, 1984 Samad *et al.*, 1986 Meek *et al.*, 1990
Rat	P53	Rnp53 X13058 L07781	P53_RAT P10361	Soussi *et al.*, 1988a Hulla and Schneider, 1993
Chicken	P53	Ggp53 X13057	P53_CHICK P10360	Soussi *et al.*, 1988b
Green monkey	P53	Cap53 X16384	P53_CERAE P13481	Rigaudy and Eckhart, 1989
Xenopus laevis	P53	Xlp53r X05191	P53_XENLA P07193	Soussi *et al.*, 1987

Reviews

Fearon, E.R. and Vogelstein, B. (1990). A genetic model for colorectal tumorigenesis. Cell, 61, 759–767.

Hollstein, M., Sidransky, D., Vogelstein, B. and Harris, C.C. (1991). p53 mutations in human cancers. Science, 253, 49–53.

Lane, D.P. (1992). p53, guardian of the genome. Nature, 358, 15–16.

Levine, A.J., Momand, J. and Finlay, C.A. (1991). The p53 tumour suppressor gene. Nature, 351, 453–456.

Milner, J. (1991). A conformational hypothesis for the suppressor and promoter functions of *p53* in cell growth control and in cancer. Proc. R. Soc. Lond. B, 245, 139–145.

Oren, M. (1985). The p53 cellular tumor antigen: gene structure, expression and protein properties. Biochim. Biophys. Acta, 823, 67–78.

Vogelstein, B. and Kinzler, K.W. (1992). p53 function and dysfunction. Cell, 70, 523–526.

Papers

Addison, C., Jenkins, J.R. and Sturzbecher, H.-W. (1990). The p53 nuclear localisation signal is structurally linked to a p34[cdc2] kinase motif. Oncogene, 5, 423–426.

Agoff, S.N., Hou, J., Linzer, D.I.H. and Wu, B. (1993). Regulation of the human hsp70 promoter by p53. Science, 259, 84–87.

Akslen, L.A. and Morkve, O. (1992). Expression of p53 protein in cutaneous melanoma. Int. J. Cancer, 52, 13–16.

Arai, N., Nomura D., Yokota K., Wolf D., Brill E., Shohat O., Rotter V. (1986). Immunologically distinct p53 molecules generated by alternative splicing. Mol. Cell. Biol., 6, 3232–3239.

Baker, S.J., Markowitz, S., Fearon, E.R., Willson, J.K.V. and Vogelstein, B. (1990). Suppression of human colorectal carcinoma cell growth by wild-type p53. Science 249, 912–915.

Band, V., Dalal, S., Delmolino, L. and Androphy, E.J. (1993). Enhanced degradation of p53 protein in HPV-6 and HPV-1 E6-immortalized human mammary epithelial cells. EMBO J., 12, 1847–1852.

Barak, Y. and Oren, M. (1992). Enhanced binding of a 95 kDa protein to p53 in cells undergoing p53-mediated growth arrest. EMBO J., 11, 2115–2121.

Barak, Y., Juven, T., Haffner, R. and Oren, M. (1993). *mdm2* expression is induced by wild type p53 activity. EMBO J., 12, 461–468.

Bargonetti, J., Reynisdottir, I., Friedman, P.N. and Prives, C. (1992). Site-specific binding of wild-type p53 to cellular DNA is inhibited by SV40 T antigen and mutant p53. Genes Devel., 6, 1886–1898.

Bartek, J., Bartkova, J., Vojtesek, B., Staskova, Z., Lukas, J., Rejthar, A., Kovarik, J., Midgley, C.A., Gannon,

J.V. and Lane, D.P. (1991). Aberrant expression of the p53 oncoprotein is a common feature of a wide spectrum of human malignancies. Oncogene, 6, 1699–1703.

Baudier, J., Delphin, C., Grunwald, D., Khochbin, S. and Lawrence, J.J. (1992). Characterization of the tumor suppressor protein p53 as a protein kinase C substrate and a S100b-binding protein. Proc. Natl Acad. Sci. USA, 89, 11627–11631.

Beenken, S.W., Karsenty, G., Raycroft, L. and Lozano, G. (1991). An intron binding protein is required for transformation ability of p53. Nucleic Acids Res., 19, 4747–4752.

Bennett, W.P., Hollstein, M.C., He, A., Zhu, S.M., Resau, J.H., Trump, B.F., Metcalf, R.A., Welsh, J.A., Midgley, C., Lane, D.P. and Harris, C.C. (1991). Archival analysis of p53 genetic and protein alterations in Chinese esophageal cancer. Oncogene, 6, 1779–1784.

Bienz, B., Zakut-Houri, R., Givol, D. and Oren, M. (1984). Analysis of the gene coding for the murine cellular tumour antigen p53. EMBO J., 3, 2179–2183.

Bischoff, J.R., Friedman, P.N., Marshak, D.R., Prives, C. and Beach, D. (1990). Human p53 is phosphorylated by p60-cdc2 and cyclin B-cdc2. Proc. Natl Acad. Sci. USA, 87, 4766–4770.

Bressac, B., Kew, M., Wands, J. and Ozturk, M. (1991). Selective G to T mutations of p53 gene in hepatocellular carcinoma from southern Africa. Nature, 350, 429–431.

Buchman, V.L., Chumakov, P.M., Ninkina, N.N., Samarina, O.P. and Georgiev, G.P. (1988). A variation in the structure of the protein-coding region of the human p53 gene. Gene, 70, 245–252.

Casey, G., Lo-Hsueh, M., Lopez, M.E., Vogelstein, B. and Stanbridge, E.J. (1991). Growth suppression of human breast cancer cells by the introduction of a wild-type p53 gene. Oncogene, 6, 1791–1797.

Chen, T.-M., Chen, C.-A., Hsieh, C.-Y., Chang, D.-Y., Chen, Y.-H. and Defendi, V. (1993). The state of p53 in primary human cervical carcinomas and its effects in human papillomavirus-immortalized human cervical cells. Oncogene, 8, 1511–1518.

Chiba, I., Takahashi, T., Nau, M.M., D'Amico, D., Curiel, D.T., Mitsudomi, T., Buchhagen, D.L., Carbone, D., Piantadosi, S., Koga, H., Reissman, P.T., Slamon, D.J., Holmes, E.C. and Minna, J.D. (1990). Mutations in the p53 gene are frequent in primary, resected non-small cell lung cancer. Oncogene, 5, 1603–1610.

Clarke, A.R., Purdie, C.A., Harrison, D.J., Morris, R.G., Bird, C.C., Hooper, M.L. and Wyllie, A.H. (1993). Thymocyte apoptosis induced by p53-dependent and independent pathways. Nature, 362, 849–852.

Crook, T. and Vousden, K.H. (1992). Properties of p53 mutations detected in primary and secondary cervical cancers suggest mechanisms of metastasis and involvement of environmental carcinogens. EMBO J., 11, 3935–3940.

Crook, T., Wrede, D. and Vousden, K.H. (1991a). p53 point mutation in HPV negative human cervical carcinoma cell lines. Oncogene, 6, 873–875.

Crook, T., Tidy, J.A. and Vousden, K.H. (1991b). Degradation of p53 can be targeted by HPV E6 sequences distinct from those required for p53 binding and trans-activation. Cell, 67, 547–556.

Davidoff, A.M., Pence, J.C., Shorter, N.A., Iglehart, J.D. and Marks, J.R. (1992). Expression of p53 in human neuroblastoma- and neuroepithelioma-derived cell lines. Oncogene, 7, 127–133.

Deffie, A., Wu, H., Reinke, V. and Lozano, G. (1993). The tumor suppressor p53 regulates its own transcription. Mol. Cell. Biol., 13, 3415–3423.

Diller, L., Kassel, J., Nelson, C.E., Gryka, M.A., Litwak, G., Gebhardt, M., Bressac, B., Ozturk, M., Baker, S.J., Vogelstein, B. and Friend, S.H. (1990). p53 functions as a cell cycle control protein in osteosarcoma. Mol. Cell. Biol., 10, 5772–5781.

Donehower, L.A., Harvey, M., Slagle, B.L., McArthur, M.J., Montgomery, C.A., Butel, J.S. and Bradley, A. (1992). Mice deficient for p53 are developmentally normal but susceptible to spontaneous tumours. Nature, 356, 215–221.

Dongi, R., Longoni, A., Michieli, P., Della Porta, G. and Pierotti, M.A. (1992). Analysis of p53 mutations in human thyroid carcinoma. In Lemoine, N. and Epenetos, A. (eds) Mutant Oncogenes: 187–192. Chapman and Hall, London.

Dyson, N., Buchkovich, K., Whyte, P. and Harlow, E. (1989). The cellular 107K protein that binds to adenovirus E1A also associates with the large T antigens of SV40 and JC virus. Cell, 58, 249–255.

El-Deiry, W.S., Kern, S.E., Pietenpol, J.A., Kinzler, K.W. and Vogelstein, B. (1992). Definition of a consensus binding site for p53. Nature Genetics, 1, 45–49.

Farmer, G., Bargonetti, J., Zhu, H., Friedman, P., Prywes, R. and Prives, C. (1992). Wild-type p53 activates transcription in vitro. Nature, 358, 83–86.

Felix, C.A., Strauss, E.A., D'Amico, D., Tsokos, M., Winter, S., Mitsudomi, T., Nau, M.M., Brown, D.L., Leahey, A.M., Horowitz, M.E., Poplack, D.G., Costin, D. and Minna, J.D. (1993). A novel germline p53 splicing mutation in a pediatric patient with a second malignant neoplasm. Oncogene, 8, 1203–1210.

Fields, S. and Jang, S.K. (1990). Presence of a potent transcription activating sequence in the p53 protein. Science, 249, 1046–1049.

Filhol, O., Baudier, J., Delphin, C., Loue-Mackenbach, P., Chambaz, E.M. and Cochet, C. (1992). Casein kinase II and the tumor suppressor protein P53 associate in a molecular complex that is negatively regulated upon p53 phosphorylation. J. Biol. Chem., 267, 20577–20583.

Finlay, C., Hinds, P.W. and Levine, A.J. (1989). The p53 proto-oncogene can act as a suppressor of transformation. Cell, 57, 1083–1093.

Fiscella, M., Ullrich, S.J., Zambrano, N., Shields, M.T., Lin, D., Lees-Miller, S.P., Anderson, C.W., Mercer, W.E. and Appella, E. (1993). Mutation of the serine 15 phosphorylation site of human p53 reduces the ability of p53 to inhibit cell cycle progression. Oncogene, 8, 1519–1528.

Fontoura, B.M.A., Sorokina, E.A., David, E. and Carroll, R.B. (1992). p53 is covalently linked to 5.8S rRNA. Mol. Cell. Biol., 12, 5145–5151.

Fritsche, M., Haessler, C. and Brandner, G. (1993). Induction of nuclear accumulation of the tumor-suppressor protein p53 by DNA-damaging agents. Oncogene, 8, 307–318.

Ginsberg, D., Mechta, F., Yaniv, M. and Oren, M. (1991). Wild-type p53 can down-modulate the activity of various promoters. Proc. Natl Acad. Sci. USA, 88, 9979–9983.

Gusterson, B.A., Anbazhagan, R., Warren, W., Midgely, C., Lane, D.P., O'Hare, M., Stamps, A., Carter, R. and Jayatilake, H. (1991) Expression of p53 in premalignant and malignant squamous epithelium. Oncogene, 6, 1785–1789.

Hainaut, P. and Milner, J. (1992). Interaction of heat-shock protein 70 with p53 translated *in vitro*: evidence for interaction with dimeric p53 and for a role in the regulation of p53 conformation. EMBO J., 11, 3513–3520.

Hainaut, P. and Milner, J. (1993). A structural role for metal ions in the "wild-type" conformation of the tumour suppressor protein p53. Cancer Res., 53, 1739–1742.

Halazonetis, T., Davis, L.J. and Kandil, A.N. (1993). Wild-type p53 adopts a 'mutant'-like conformation when bound to DNA. EMBO J., 12, 1021–1028.

Hall, P.A., McKee, P.H., Menage, H.du P., Dover, R. and Lane, D.P. (1993). High levels of p53 protein in UV-irradiated normal human skin. Oncogene, 8, 203–207.

Han, K.-A. and Kulesz-Martin, M.F. (1992). Alternatively spliced p53 RNA in transformed and normal cells of different tissue types. Nucleic Acids Res., 20, 1979–1981.

Harlow, E., Williamson, N.M., Ralston, R., Helfman, D.M. and Adams, T.E. (1985). Molecular cloning and in vitro expression of a cDNA clone for human cellular tumor antigen p53. Mol. Cell. Biol., 5, 1601–1610.

Harris, N., Brill, E., Shohat, O., Prokocimer, M., Wolf, D., Arai, N. and Rotter, V. (1986). Molecular basis for heterogeneity of the human p53 protein. Mol. Cell. Biol., 6, 4650–4656.

Hassapoglidou, S., Diamandis, E.P. and Sutherland, D.J.A. (1993). Quantification of p53 protein in tumor cell lines, breast tissue extracts and serum with time-resolved immunofluorometry. Oncogene, 8, 1501–1509.

Herrmann, C.P., Kraiss, S. and Montenarh, M. (1991). Association of casein kinase II with immunopurified p53. Oncogene, 6, 877–884.

Hinds, P., Finlay, C. and Levine, A.J. (1989). Mutation is required to activate the p53 gene for cooperation with the *ras* oncogene and transformation. J. Virol., 63, 739–746.

Horak, E., Smith, K., Bromley, L., LeJeune, S., Greenall, M., Lane, D. and Harris, A.L. (1991). Mutant p53, EGF receptor and c-*erb*B-2 expression in human breast cancer. Oncogene, 6, 2277–2284.

Hosono, S., Chou, M.-J., Lee, C.-S. and Shih, C. (1993). Infrequent mutation of p53 in hepatitis B virus positive primary hepatocellular carcinoma. Oncogene, 8, 491–496.

Hsu, I.C., Metcalf, R.A., Sun, T., Welsh, J.A., Wang, N.J. and Harris, C.C. (1991). Mutational hotspot in the p53 gene in human hepatocellular carcinomas. Nature, 350, 427–428.

Hubbert, N.L., Sedman, S.A. and Schiller, J.T. (1992). Human papillomavirus Type 16 E6 increases the degradation rate of p53 in human keratinocytes. J. Virol., 66, 6237–6241.

Huibregtse, J.M., Scheffner, M. and Howley, P.M. (1993). Cloning and expression of the cDNA for E6-AP, a protein that mediates the interaction of the human papillomavirus E6 oncoprotein with p53. Mol. Cell. Biol., 13, 775–784.

Hulla, J.E. and Schneider, R.P. (1993). Structure of the rat p53 tumor suppressor gene. Nucleic Acids Res., 21, 713–717.

Hupp, T.R., Meek, D.W., Midgley, C.A. and Lane, D.P. (1992). Regulation of the specific DNA binding function of p53. Cell, 71, 875–886.

Iggo, R., Gatter, K., Bartek, J., Lane, D. and Harris, A.L. (1990). Increased expression of mutant forms of p53 oncogene in primary lung cancer. Lancet, 335, 675–679.

Ishioka, C., Sato, T., Gamoh, M., Suzuki, T., Shibata, H., Kanamaru, R., Wakui, A. and Yamazaki, T. (1991). Mutations of the P53 gene, including an intronic point mutation, in colorectal tumors. Biochem. Biophys. Res. Commun., 177, 901–906.

Iwabuchi, K., Li, B., Bartel, P. and Fields, S. (1993). Use of the two-hybrid system to identify the domain of p53 involved in oligomerization. Oncogene, 8, 1693–1696.

Jackson, P., Bos, E. and Braithwaite, A.W. (1993). Wild-type mouse p53 down-regulates transcription from different virus enhancer/promoters. Oncogene, 8, 589–597.

Jego, N., Thomas, G. and Hamelin, R. (1993). Short direct repeats flanking deletions, and duplicating insertions in p53 gene in human cancers. Oncogene, 8, 209–213.

Jenkins, J.R., Rudge, K., Redmond, S. and Wade-Evans, A. (1984). Cloning and expression analysis of full length mouse cDNA sequences encoding the transformation associated protein p53. Nucleic Acids Res., 12, 5609–5626.

Kastan, M.B., Onyekwere, O., Sidransky, D., Vogelstein, B. and Craig, R.W. (1991). Participation of p53 protein in the cellular response to DNA damage. Cancer Res., 51, 6304–6311.

Kastan, M.B., Zhan, Q., El-Deiry, W.S., Carrier, F., Jacks, T., Walsh, W.V., Plunkett, B.S., Vogelstein, B. and Fornace, A.J. (1992). A mammalian cell cycle checkpoint pathway utilizing p53 and *GADD45* is defective in ataxia-telangietasia. Cell, 71, 587–597.

Kern, S.E., Kinzler, K.W., Bruskin, A., Jarosz, D., Friedman, P., Prives, C. and Vogelstein, B. (1991). Identification of p53 as a sequence-specific DNA-binding protein. Science, 252, 1708–1711.

Kern, S.E., Pietenpol, J.A., Thiagalingam, S., Seymour, A., Kinzler, K.W. and Vogelstein, B. (1992). Oncogenic foms of p53 inhibit p53-regulated gene expression. Science, 256, 827–830.

Kessis, T.D., Slebos, R.J., Nelson, W.G., Kastan, M.B., Plunkett, B.S., Han, S.M., Lorincz, A.T., Hedrick, L. and Cho, K.R. (1993). Human papillomavirus 16 E6 expression disrupts the p53-mediated cellular response to DNA damage. Proc. Natl Acad. Sci. USA, 90, 3988–3922.

Khochbin, S. and Lawrence, J.-J. (1989). An antisense RNA involved in p53 mRNA maturation in murine erythroleukemia cells induced to differentiate. EMBO J., 8, 4107–4114.

Lamb, P. and Crawford, L. (1986). Characterization of the human p53 gene. Mol. Cell. Biol., 6, 1379–1385.

Lechner, M.S., Mack, D.H., Finicle, A.B., Crook, T., Vousden, K.H. and Laimins, L.A. (1992). Human papillomavirus E6 proteins bind p53 *in vivo* and abrogate p53-mediated repression of transcription. EMBO J., 11, 3045–3052.

Lees-Miller, S.P., Sakaguchi, K., Ullrich, S.J., Appella, E. and Anderson, C.W. (1992). Human DNA-activated protein kinase phosphorylates serines 15 and 37 in the amino-terminal transactivation domain of human p53. Mol. Cell. Biol., 12, 5041–5049.

Lin, D., Shields, M.T., Ullrich, S.J., Appella, E. and Mercer, W.E. (1992). Growth arrest induced by wild-type p53 protein blocks cells prior to or near the restriction point in late G_1 phase. Proc. Natl Acad. Sci. USA, 89, 9210–9214.

Liu, X., Miller, C.W., Koeffler, P.H. and Berk, A.J. (1993). The p53 activation domain binds the TATA box-binding polypeptide in holo-TFIID, and a neighboring p53 domain inhibits transcription. Mol. Cell. Biol., 13, 3291–3300.

Livingstone, L.R., White, A., Sprouse, J., Livanos, E., Jacks, T. and Tlsty, T.D. (1992). Altered cell cycle arrest and gene amplification potential accompany loss of wild-type p53. Cell, 70, 923–935.

Louis, J.M., McFarland, V.W., May, P. and Mora, P.T. (1988). The phosphoprotein p53 is down-regulated post-transcriptionally during embryogenesis in vertebrates. Biochim. Biophys. Acta, 950, 395–402.

Lowe, S.W., Schmitt, E.M., Smith, S.W., Osborne, B.A. and Jacks, T. (1993). p53 is required for radiation-induced apoptosis in mouse thymocytes. Nature, 362, 847–849.

Lozano, G. and Levine, A.J. (1991). Tissue-specific expression of p53 in transgenic mice is regulated by intron sequences. Mol. Carcinog., 4, 3–9.

Mack, D.H., Vartikar, J., Pipas, J.M. and Laimins, L.A. (1993). Specific repression of TATA-mediated but not initiator-mediated transcription by wild-type p53. Nature, 363, 281–283.

McBride, O.W., Merry, D. and Givol, D. (1986). The gene for human p53 cellular tumor antigen is located on chromosome 17 short arm (17p13). Proc. Natl Acad. Sci. U.S.A, 83, 130–134.

Maestro, R., Dolcetti, R., Gasparotto, D., Doglioni, C., Pelucchi, S., Barzan, L., Grandi, E. and Boiocchi, M. (1992). High frequency of p53 alterations associated with protein overexpression in human squamous cell carcinoma of the larynx. Oncogene, 7, 1159–1166.

Malkin, D., Li, F.P., Strong, L.C., Fraumeni, J.F., Nelson, C.E., Kim, D.H., Kassel, J., Gryka, M.A., Bischoff, F.Z., Tainsky, M.A. and Friend, S.H. (1990). Germ line p53 mutations in a familial syndrome of breast cancer, sarcomas and other neoplasms. Science, 250, 1233–1238.

Marshak, D.R., Vandenberg, M.T., Bae, Y.S. and Yu, I.J. (1991). Characterization of synthetic peptide substrates for p34^{cdc2} protein kinase. J. Cell. Biochem., 45, 391–400.

Martin, H.M., Filipe, M.I., Morris, R.W., Lane, D.P. and Silvestre, F. (1992). p53 expression and prognosis in gastric carcinoma. Int. J. Cancer, 50, 859–862.

Mashiyama, S., Murakami, Y., Yoshimoto, T., Sekiya, T. and Hayashi, K. (1991). Detection of p53 gene mutations in human brain tumors by single-strand conformation polymorphism analysis of polymerase chain reaction products. Oncogene, 6, 1313–1318.

Matlashewski, G., Lamb, P., Pim, D., Peacock, J., Crawford, L. and Benchimol, S. (1984). Isolation and characterization of a human p53 cDNA clone: expression of the human p53 gene. EMBO J., 3, 3257–3262.

Maxwell, S.A., Ames, S.K., Sawai, E.T., Decker, G.L., Cook, R.G. and Butel, J.S. (1991). Simian virus 40 large T antigen and p53 are microtubule-associated proteins in transformed cells. Cell Growth Differ., 2, 115–127.

Medcalf, E.A., Takahashi, T., Chiba, I., Minna, J. and Milner, J. (1992). Temperature-sensitive mutants of p53 associated with human carcinoma of the lung. Oncogene, 7, 71–76.

Meek, D.W., Simon, S., Kikkawa, U. and Eckhart, W. (1990). The p53 tumour suppressor protein is phosphorylated at serine 389 by casein kinase II. EMBO J., 9, 3253–3260.

Mercer, W.E., Avignolo, C. and Baserga, R. (1984). Role of the p53 protein in cell proliferation as studied by microinjection of monoclonal antibodies. Mol. Cell. Biol., 4, 276–281.

Mercer, W.E., Shields, M.T., Amin, M., Sauve, G.J., Appella, E., Romano, J.W. and Ullrich, S.J. (1990). Negative growth regulation in a glioblastoma tumor cell line that conditionally expresses human wild-type p53. Proc. Natl Acad. Sci. USA, 87, 6166–6170.

Mercer, W.E., Shields, M.T., Lin, D., Appella, E. and Ullrich, S.J. (1991). Growth suppression induced by wild-type p53 protein is accompanied by selective down-regulation of proliferating-cell nuclear antigen expression. Proc. Natl Acad. Sci. USA, 88, 1958–1962.

Michalovitz, D., Halevy, O. and Oren, M. (1990). Conditional inhibition of transformation and of cell proliferation by a temperature-sensitive mutant of p53. Cell, 62, 671–680.

Mietz, J.A., Unger, T., Huibregtse, J.M. and Howley, P.M. (1992). The transcriptional transactivation function of wild-type p53 is inhibited by SV40 large T-antigen and by HPV-16 E6 oncoprotein. EMBO J., 11, 5013–5020.

Milne, D.M., Palmer, R.H., Campbell, D.G. and Meek, D.W. (1992a). Phosphorylation of the p53 tumour-suppressor protein at three N-terminal sites by a novel casein kinase I-like enzyme. Oncogene, 7, 1361–1369.

Milne, D.M., Palmer, R.H. and Meek, D.W. (1992b). Mutation of the casein kinase II phosphorylation site abolishes the anti-proliferative activity of p53. Nucleic Acids Res., 20, 5565–5570.

Milner, J. and Cook, A. (1986). Visualisation, by immunocytochemistry, of p53 at the plasma membrane of both nontransformed and SV40-transformed cells. Virology, 150, 265–269.

Milner, J. and Medcalf, E.A. (1990). Temperature-dependent switching between "wild-type" and "mutant" forms of p53-val135. J. Mol. Biol., 216, 481–484.

Milner, J. and Medcalf, E.A. (1991). Cotranslation of activated mutant p53 with wild type drives the wild-type p43 protein into the mutant conformation. Cell, 65, 765–774.

Milner, J. and Watson, J.V. (1990). Addition of fresh medium induces cell cycle and conformation changes in p53, a tumour suppressor protein. Oncogene 5, 1683–1690.

Milner, J., Cook, A. and Mason, J. (1990). p53 is associated with p34cdc2 in transformed cells. EMBO J., 9, 2885–2889.

Milner, J., Medcalf, E.A. and Cook, A. (1991). Tumor suppressor p53: analysis of wild-type and mutant p53 complexes. Mol. Cell. Biol., 11, 12–19.

Milner, B.J., Allan, L.A., Eccles, D.M., Kitchener, H.C., Leonard, R.C.F., Kelly, K.F., Parkin, D.E. and Haites, N.E. (1993). p53 mutation is a common genetic event in ovarian carcinoma. Cancer Res., 53, 2128–2132.

Mitsudomi, T., Steinberg, S.M., Nau, M.M., Carbone, D., D'Amico, D., Bodner, S., Oie, H.K., Linnoila, R.I., Mulshine, J.L., Minna, J.D. and Gazdar, A.F. (1992). p53 gene mutations in non-small-cell lung cancer cell lines and their correlation with the presence of ras mutations and clinical features. Oncogene, 7, 171–180.

Moles, J.-P., Moyret, C., Guillot, B., Jeanteur, P., Guilhou, J.-J., Theilet, C. and Basset-Seguin, N. (1993). p53 gene mutations in human epithelial skin cancers. Oncogene, 8, 583–588.

Momand, J., Zambetti, G.P., Olson, D.C., George, D. and Levine, A.J. (1992). The mdm-2 oncogene product forms a complex with the p53 protein and inhibits p53-mediated transactivation. Cell, 69, 1237–1245.

Mulligan, L.M., Matlashewski, G.J., Scrable, H.J. and Cavenee, W.K. (1990). Mechanisms of p53 loss in human sarcomas. Proc. Natl Acad. Sci. USA, 87, 5863–5867.

Munroe, D.G., Peacock, J.W. and Benchimol, S. (1990). Inactivation of the cellular p53 gene is a common feature of Friend virus-induced erythroleukemia: relationship of inactivation to dominant transforming alleles. Mol. Cell. Biol., 10, 3307–3313.

Oliner, J.D., Kinzler, K.W., Meltzer, P.S., George, D.L. and Vogelstein, B. (1992). Amplification of a gene encoding a p53-associated protein in human sarcomas. Nature, 358, 80–83.

Oliner, J.D., Pietenpol, J.A., Thiagalingam, S., Gyuris, J., Kinzler, K.W. and Vogelstein, B. (1993). Oncoprotein MDM2 conceals the activation domain of tumour suppressor p53. Nature, 362, 857–860.

O'Rourke, R.W., Miller, C.W., Kato, G.J., Simon, K.J., Chen, D.L., Dang, C.V. and Koeffler, H.P. (1990). A potential transcriptional activation element in the p53 protein. Oncogene, 5, 1829–1832.

Pennica, D., Goeddel, D.V., Hayflick, J.S., Reich, N.C., Anderson, C.W. and Levine, A.J. (1984). The amino acid sequence of murine p53 determined from a cDNA clone. Virology 134, 477–482.

Picksley, S.M., Meek, D.W. and Lane, D.P. (1992). The conformational change of a murine temperature-sensitive p53 protein is independent of a change in phosphorylation status. Oncogene, 7, 1649–1651.

Portier, M., Moles, J.-P., Mazars, G.-R., Jeanteur, P., Bataille, R., Klein, B. and Theillet, C. (1992). p53 and *RAS* gene mutations in multiple myeloma. Oncogene, 7, 2539–2543.

Prosser, J., Porter, D., Coles, C., Condie, A., Thompson, U., Steel, C.M. and Evans, H.J. (1992). Constitutional p53 mutation in a non-Li-Fraumeni cancer family. Brit. J. Cancer, 65, 527–528.

Puisieux, A., Ponchel, F. and Ozturk, M. (1993). p53 as a growth suppressor gene in HBV-related hepatocellular carcinoma. Oncogene, 8, 487–490.

Ramqvist, T., Magnusson, K.P., Wang, Y., Szekely, L., Klein, G. and Wiman, K.G. (1993). Wild-type p53 induces apoptosis in a Burkitt lymphoma (BL) line that carries mutant p53. Oncogene, 8, 1495–1500.

Raycroft, L., Wu, H. and Lozano, G. (1990). Transcriptional activation by wild-type but not transforming mutants of the p53 anti-oncogene. Science, 249, 1049–1051.

Reisman, D. and Rotter, V. (1993). The helix-loop-helix containing transcription factor USF binds to and transactivates the promoter of the p53 tumor suppressor gene. Nucleic Acids Res., 21, 345–350.

Rideout, W.M., Coetzee, G.A., Olumi, A.F. and Jones, P.A. (1990). 5-methylcytosine as an endogenous mutagen in the human ldl receptor and p53 genes. Science, 249, 1288–1290.

Rigaudy, P. and Eckhart, W. (1989). Nucleotide sequence of a cDNA encoding the monkey cellular phosphoprotein p53. Nucleic Acids Res., 17, 8375.

Rivas, C.I., Wisniewski, D., Strife, A., Perez, A., Lambek, C., Bruno, S., Darzynkiewicz, Z. and Clarkson, B. (1992). Constitutive expression of p53 protein in enriched normal human marrow blast cell populations. Blood, 79, 1982–1986.

Rodrigues, N.R., Rowan, A., Smith, M.E.F., Kerr, I.B., Bodmer, W.F., Gannon, J.V. and Lane, D.P. (1990). p53 mutations in colorectal cancer. Proc. Natl Acad. Sci. USA, 87, 7555–7559.

Rogel, A., Popliker, M., Webb, C.G. and Oren, M. (1985). p53 cellular tumor antigen: analysis of mRNA levels in normal adult tissues, embryos and tumors. Mol. Cell. Biol., 5, 2851–2855.

Ronen, D., Rotter, V. and Reisman, D. (1991). Expression from the murine p53 promoter is mediated by factor binding to a downstream helix-loop-helix recognition motif. Proc. Natl Acad. Sci. USA, 88, 4128–4132.

Ruggeri, B., Zhang, S.-Y., Caamano, J., DiRado, M., Flynn, S.D. and Klein-Szanto, A.J.P. (1992). Human pancreatic carcinomas and cell lines reveal frequent and multiple alterations in the p53 and Rb-1 tumor-suppressor genes. Oncogene, 7, 1503–1511.

Ruppert, J.M. and Stillman, B. (1993). Analysis of a protein-binding domain of p53. Mol. Cell. Biol., 13, 3811–3820.

Ryan, J.J., Danish, R., Gottlieb, C.A. and Clarke, M.F. (1993). Cell cycle analysis of p53-induced cell death in murine erythroleukemia cells. Mol. Cell. Biol., 13, 711–719.

Samad, A. and Carroll, R.B. (1991). The tumor suppressor p53 is bound to RNA by a stable covalent linkage. Mol. Cell. Biol., 11, 1598–1606.

Samad, A., Anderson, C.W. and Carroll, R.B. (1986). Mapping of phosphomonoester and apparent phosphodiester bonds of the oncogene product p53 from Simian virus 40-transformed 3T3 cells. Proc. Natl Acad. Sci. USA, 83, 897–901.

Santhanam, U., Ray, A. and Sehgel, P.B. (1991). Repression of the interleukin 6 gene promoter by p53 and the retinoblastoma susceptibility gene product. Proc. Natl Acad. Sci. USA, 88, 7605–7609.

Scharer, E. and Iggo, R. (1992). Mammalian p53 can function as a transcription factor in yeast. Nucleic Acids Res., 20, 1539–1545.

Scheffner, M., Werness, B.A., Huibregtse, J.M., Levine, A.J. and Howley, P.M. (1990). The E6 oncoprotein encoded by human papillomavirus types 16 and 18 promotes the degradation of p53. Cell, 63, 1129–1136.

Scheidtmann, K.H., Mumby, M.C., Rundell, K. and Walter, G. (1991). Dephosphorylation of Simian virus 40 large-T antigen and p53 protein by protein phosphatase 2A: inhibition by small-t antigen. Mol. Cell. Biol., 11, 1996–2003.

Seto, E., Usheva, A., Zambetti, G.P., Momand, J., Horikoshi, N., Weinmann, R., Levine, A.J. and Shenk, T. (1992). Wild-type p53 binds to the TATA-binding protein and represses transcription. Proc. Natl Acad. Sci. USA, 89, 12028–12032.

Shaulian, E., Zauberman, A., Ginsberg, D. and Oren, M. (1992). Identification of a minimal transforming domain of p53: negative dominance through abrogation of sequence-specific DNA binding. Mol. Cell. Biol., 12, 5581–5592.

Shaulsky, G., Ben-Ze'ev, A. and Rotter, V. (1990). Subcellular distribution of the p53 protein during the cell cycle of Balb/c 3T3 cells. Oncogene, 5, 1707–1711.

Shaulsky, G., Goldfinger, N., Tosky, M.S., Levine, A.J. and Rotter, V. (1991). Nuclear localisation is essential for the activity of p53 protein. Oncogene, 6, 2055–2065.

Shaw, P., Bovey, R., Tardy, S., Sahli, R., Sordat, B. and Costa, J. (1992). Induction of apoptosis by wild-type p53 in a human colon tumor-derived cell line. Proc. Natl Acad. Sci. USA, 89, 4495–4499.

Shiio, Y., Yamamoto, T. and Yamaguchi, N. (1992). Negative regulation of Rb expression by the p53 gene product. Proc. Natl Acad. Sci. USA, 89, 5206–5210.

Shohat, O., Greenberg, M., Reisman, D., Oren, M. and Rotter, V. (1987). Inhibition of cell growth mediated by plasmids encoding p53 anti-sense. Oncogene, 1, 277–283.

Soussi, T., Caron de Fromentel, C., Mechali, M., Hay, P. and Kress, M. (1987). Cloning and characterization of a cDNA from Xenopus laevis coding for a protein homologous to human and murine p53. Oncogene, 1, 71–78.

Soussi T., Caron de Fromentel, C., Breugnot, C. and May, E. (1988a). Nucleotide sequence of a cDNA encoding the rat p53 nuclear oncoprotein. Nucleic Acids Res. 16, 11384.

Soussi, T., Begue, A., Kress, M., Stehelin, D. and May, P. (1988b). Nucleotide sequence of a cDNA encoding the chicken p53 nuclear oncoprotein. Nucleic Acids Res., 16, 11383.

Srivastava, S., Zou, Z., Pirollo, K., Blattner, W. and Chang, E.H. (1990). Germ-line transmission of a mutated *p53* gene in a cancer-prone family with Li-Fraumeni syndrome. Nature, 348, 747–749.

Sturzbecher, H.-W., Maimets, T., Chumakov, P., Brain, R., Addison, C., Simanis, V., Rudge, K., Philp, R., Grimaldi, M., Court, W. and Jenkins, J.R. (1990). p53 interacts with p34[cdc2] in mammalian cells: implications for cell cycle control and oncogenesis. Oncogene, 5, 795–801.

Sturzbecher, H.-W., Brain, R., Addison, C., Rudge, K., Remm, M., Grimaldi, M., Keenan, E. and Jenkins, J.R. (1992). A C-terminal α-helix plus basic region motif is the major structural determinant of p53 tetramerization. Oncogene, 7, 1513–1523.

Takahashi, T., Nau, M.M., Chiba, I., Birrer, M.J., Rosenberg, R.K., Vinocour, M., Levitt, M., Pas, H., Gazdar, A.F. and Minna, J.D. (1989). p53: a frequent target for genetic abnormalities in lung cancer. Science, 246, 491–494.

Takahashi, T., Takahashi, T., Suzuki, H., Hida, T., Sekido, Y., Ariyoshi, Y. and Ueda, R. (1991). The p53 gene is very frequently mutated in small-cell lung cancer with a distinct nucleotide substitution pattern. Oncogene, 6, 1775–1778.

Tuck, S.P. and Crawford, L. (1989). Characterization of the human p53 gene promoter. Mol. Cell. Biol., 9, 2163–2172.

Ullrich, S.J., Mercer, W.E. and Appella, E. (1992). Human wild-type p53 adopts a unique conformational and phosphorylation state *in vivo* during growth arrest of glioblastoma cells. Oncogene, 7, 1635–1643.

Unger, T., Nau, M.M., Segal, S. and Minna, J.D. (1992). p53: a transdominant regulator of transcription whose function is ablated by mutations occurring in human cancer. EMBO J., 11, 1383–1390.

Varley, J.M., Brammar, W.J., Lane, D.P., Swallow, J.E., Dolan, C. and Walker, R.A. (1991). Loss of chromosome 17p13 sequences and mutation of p53 in human breast carcinomas. Oncogene, 6, 413–421.

Wagner, P., Simanis, V., Maimets, T., Keenan, E., Addison, C., Brain, R., Grimaldi, M., Sturzbecher, H.W. and Jenkins, J. (1991). A human tumour-derived mutant p53 protein induces a p34[cdc2] reversible growth arrest in fission yeast. Oncogene, 6, 1539–1547.

Wang, Y. and Eckhart, W. (1992). Phosphorylation sites in the amino-terminal region of mouse p53. Proc. Natl Acad. Sci. USA, 89, 4231–4235.

Wang, N.P., To, H., Lee, W.-H. and Lee, E.Y.-H.P. (1993). Tumor suppressor activity of *RB* and *p53* genes in human breast carcinoma cells. Oncogene, 8, 279–288.

Wiman, K.G., Magnusson, K.P., Ramqvist, T. and Klein, G. (1991). Mutant p53 detected in a majority of Burkitt lymphoma cell lines by monoclonal antibody PAb240. Oncogene, 6, 1633–1639.

Yew, P.R. and Berk, A.J. (1992). Inhibition of p53 transactivation required for transformation by adenovirus early 1B protein. Nature, 357, 82–85.

Yin, Y., Tainsky, M.A., Bischoff, F.Z., Strong, L.C. and Wahl, G.M. (1992). Wild-type p53 restores cell cycle control and inhibits gene amplification in cells with mutant p53 alleles. Cell, 70, 937–948.

Yonish-Rouach, E., Resnitzky, D., Lotem, J., Sachs, L., Kimchi, A. and Oren, M. (1991). Wild-type p53 induces apoptosis of myeloid leukaemic cells that is inhibited by interleukin-6. Nature, 352, 345–347.

Zakut-Houri, R., Oren, M., Bienz-Tadmor, B., Lavie, V., Hazum , S. and Givol, D. (1985). A single gene and a pseudogene for the cellular tumor antigen p53. Nature, 306, 594–597.

Zakut-Houri, R., Bienz-Tadmor, B., Givol, D. and Oren, M. (1983). Human p53 cellular tumor antigen: cDNA sequence and expression in COS cells. EMBO J., 4, 1251–1255.

Zerrahn, J., Deppert, W., Weidemann, D., Patschinsky, T., Richards, F. and Milner, J. (1992). Correlation between the conformational phenotype of p53 and its subcellular location. Oncogene, 7, 1371–1381.

Zhang, W., Hu, G., Estey, E., Hester, J. and Deisseroth, A.B. (1992). Altered conformation of the p53 protein in myeloid leukemia cells and mitogen-stimulated normal blood cells. Oncogene, 7, 1645–1647.

Zhang, W. and Deisseroth, A.B. (1993). Stability of p53 protein in normal and leukemic blood cells. Oncogene, in press.

Neurofibromatosis Type 1 and Type 2

The most frequent forms of neurofibromatosis are peripheral neurofibromatosis (*NF1*) and central neurofibromatosis (*NF2*). *NF1* (von Recklinghausen neurofibromatosis) affects about 1 in 3500 individuals and arises in cells derived from the embryonic neural crest, causing benign growths including neurofibromas and café-au-lait spots on the skin, pheochromocytomas and malignant Schwannomas and neurofibrosarcomas. The *NF1* gene is always inherited as a mutant allele, unlike *RB1*. *NF2* (incidence 1 in 40 000) gives rise to acoustic neuromas, Schwann cell-derived tumours and meningiomas.

Related genes

NF1 shares a region of homology with *Saccharomyces cerevisiae* IRA1 and IRA2 and mammalian GAP (GTPase-activating protein; Ballester *et al.*, 1989; Tanaka *et al.*, 1990; Xu *et al.*, 1990a,b; Garrett *et al.*, 1991). NF1 contains a short region of homology with the microtubule-associated proteins MAP2 and TAU.

The candidate *NF2* gene product merlin (moesin–ezrin–radixin-like protein) shares 45–47% amino acid identity with the cytoskeleton-associated proteins from which its name is derived (Trofatter *et al.*, 1993).

Cross-species homology

NF1 is highly conserved (95% human and chicken). Similar loci occur on human chromosomes 14, 15 and 22.

	NF1 (neurofibromin)	*NF2* (merlin)
Nucleotides (kb)	300	
Chromosome		
Human	17q11.2	22q12
Exons	49/50	5
mRNA (kb)		
Human	13	
Amino acids		
Human	2818/2839	587
Mass (kDa)		
(predicted)	327	69
(expressed)	250	
Protein half-life (h)	>8	

Cellular location

Neurofibromin: Particulate cellular fraction (cf. GAP which is soluble). In NIH 3T3 fibroblasts neurofibromin associates with cytoplasmic structures distinct from actin or tubulin filaments (Golubic *et al.*, 1992).

Merlin: Cytoskeleton/plasma membrane (Rouleau *et al.*, 1993).

Tissue location

Cells of neural crest origin are most commonly affected in both forms of NF.

Neurofibromin: This is detected in most tissues and is highly expressed in brain (Hattori *et al.*, 1992). An alternatively spliced *NF1* gene product (type II) encoding an additional 21 amino acids is widely expressed in vertebrates (Andersen *et al.*, 1993) and has been reported to be differentially expressed in neuronal cells stimulated to differentiate by retinoic acid (Nishi *et al.*, 1991) and in brain tumours (Suzuki *et al.*, 1991).

Merlin: This is detected in *NF2* lymphoblast cell lines. Non-overlapping germ line deletions in the merlin gene in two independent families that remove the N-terminus or the C-terminus suggests that merlin is the *NF2* tumour suppressor (Trofatter *et al.*, 1993).

Protein function

Neurofibromin contains a GTPase-activating protein (GAP)-related domain (NF1 GRD) that stimulates the GTPase activity of normal but not oncogenic $p21^{ras}$. It binds to $p21^{ras}$ with 300-fold greater affinity than $p120^{GAP}$ (Bollag and McCormick, 1991) and the dissociation of the complex is dependent on GTP hydrolysis, in contrast to that of $p21^{ras}$–GAP complexes (Dibattiste *et al.*, 1993). In tumour cells from *NF1* patients $p21^{ras}$ is activated even though $p120^{GAP}$ is present (Basu *et al.*, 1992). The introduction of the 38 kDa catalytic C-terminus of GAP reduces the level of GTP bound to $p21^{ras}$ and causes morphological reversion of the tumour cells (DeClue *et al.*, 1992). Thus *RAS* appears to promote *NF1*-linked malignancy and *NF1* itself may function as a recessive oncogene, its normal gene product converting $p21^{ras}$ to the inactive form. Neurofibromin interacts with the effector domain of $p21^{ras}$, however, and may thus be the target of RAS rather than its regulator (see **RAS**). Neurofibromin GAP activity is inhibited by arachidonate, phosphatidate or $PtdIns(4,5)P_2$ (1 μM), to which $p120^{GAP}$ is insensitive (Golubic *et al.*, 1991) and by tubulin (Bollag *et al.*, 1993). Neurofibromin undergoes serine/threonine phosphorylation in cells stimulated by growth factors.

The 21 amino acid insertion in neurofibromin type II is conserved across species but is not present in GAP, IRA1 or IRA2 and has the effect of decreasing the GTPase activity of the protein (Andersen *et al.*, 1993).

Gene structure

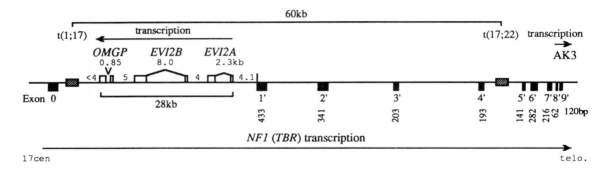

In *NF1* patients two translocations (t(1;17) and t(17;22), shaded boxes) and a number of deletions have been detected in the *NF1* (or translocation breakpoint (*TBR*)) gene. The breakpoints flank a 60 kb segment of DNA that contains the *EVI2A*, *EVI2B* and oligodendrocyte-myelin glycoprotein (*OMGP*) loci (Cawthon *et al.*, 1991; Viskochil *et al.*, 1991). *EVI2A*, *EVI2B* and *OMGP* have the same transcriptional orientation, similar genomic organization and are contained within one intron of *NF1*, which is transcribed from the opposite strand (each transcript ~2 kb: intron size shown above each gene). A pseudo-gene of the adenylate kinase 3 family (ψAK3) maps to a site distal to the breakpoints. Nine of the 49 *NF1* exons (black boxes) are represented (designated here as 0 and 1'–9'): their sizes are shown below each exon.

EVI2A (or *EVI2*), the human homologue of mouse *Evi-2A* (see Table 2.2 Supplement), is highly expressed in brain, bone marrow and peripheral blood.

EVI2B contains a 57 bp 5' non-coding exon, an 8 kb intron and a 2078 bp 3' exon that includes the entire open reading frame encoding a putative 448 amino acid, proline-rich, transmembrane protein expressed in bone marrow, peripheral blood mononuclear cells and fibroblasts.

OMPG, expressed only in oligodendrocytes, is a glycosylphosphatidylinositol-anchored protein.

Some but not all of the deletions detected in *NF1* affect the *EVI2A*, *EVI2B* or *OMPG* genes.

Sequence of human neurofibromin

```
   (1)   MAAHRPVEWVQAVVSRFDEQLPIKTGQQNTHTKVSTEHNKECLINISKYKFSLVISGLTTILKNVNNMRIFGEAAEKNL
  (80)   YLSQLIILDTLEKCLAGQPKDTMRLDETMLVKQLLPEICHFLHTCREGNQHAAELRNSASGVLFSLSCNNFNAVFSRIST
 (160)   RLQELTVCSEDNVDVHDIELLQYINVDCAKLKRLLKETAFKFKALKKVAQLAVINSLEKAFWNWVENYPDEFTKLYQIPQ
 (240)   TDMAECAEKLFDLVDGFAESTKRKAAVWPLQIILLILCPEIIQDISKDVVDENNMNKKLFLDSLRKALAGHGGSRQLTES
 (320)   AAIACVKLCKASTYINWEDNSVIFLLVQSMVVDLKNLLFNPSKPFSRGSQPADVDLMIDCLVSCFRISPHNNQHFKICLA
 (400)   QNSPSTFHYVLVNSLHRIITNSALDWWPKIDAVYCHSVELRNMFGETLHKAVQGCGAHPAIRMAPSLTFKEKVTSLKFKE
 (480)   KPTDLETRSYKYLLLSMVKLIHADPKLLLCNPRKQGPETQGSTAELITGLVQLVPQSHMPEIAQEAMEALLVLHQLDSID
 (560)   LWNPDAPVETFWEISSQMLFYICKKLTSHQMLSSTEILKWLREILICRNKFLLKNKQADRSSCHFLLFYGVGCDIPSSGN
 (640)   TSQMSMDHEELLRTPGASLRKGKGNSSMDSAAGCSGTPPICRQAQTKLEVALYMFLWNPDTEAVLVAMSCFRHLCEEADI
 (720)   RCGVDEVSVHNLLPNYNTFMEFASVSNMMSTGRAALQKRVMALLRRIEHPTAGNTEAWEDTHAKWEQATKLILNYPKAKM
 (800)   EDGQAAESLHKTIVKRRMSHVSGGGSIDLSDTDSLQEWINMTGFLCALGGVCLQQRSNSGLATYSPPMGPVSERKGSMIS
 (880)   VMSSEGNADTPVSKFMDRLLSLMVCNHEKVGLQIRTNVKDLVGLELSPALYPMLFNKLKNTISKFFDSQGQVLLTDTNTQ
 (960)   FVEQTIAIMKNLLDNHTEGSSEHLGQASIETMMLNLVRYVRVLGNMVHAIQIKTKLCQLVEVMMARRDDLSFCQEMKFRN
(1040)   KMVEYLTDWVMGTSNQAADDDVKCLTRDLDQASMEAVVSLLAGLPLQPEEGDGVELMEAKSQLFLKYFTLFMNLLNDCSE
(1120)   VEDESAQTGGRKRGMSRRLASLRHCTVLAMSNLLNANVDSGLMHSIGLGYHKDLQTRATFMEVLTKILQQGTEFDTLAET
(1200)   VLADRFERLVELVTMMGDQGELPIAMALANVVPCSQWDELARVLVTLFDSRHLLYQLLWNMFSKEVELADSMQTLFRGNS
(1280)   LASKIMTFCFKVYGATYLQKLLDPLLRIVITSSDWQHVSFEVDPTRLEPSESLEENQRNLLQMTEKFFHAIISSSSEFPP
(1360)   QLRSVCHCLYQ VVSQRFPQNSIGAVGSAMFLRFINPAIVSPYEAGILDKKPPPRIERGLKLMSKILQSIANHVLFTKEEH
                   ΔΔ
(1440)   MRPFNDFVKSNFDAARRFFLDIASDCPTSDAVNHSLSFISDGNVLALHRLLWNNQEKIGQYLSSNRDHKAVGRRPFDKMA
(1520)   TLLAYLGPPEHKPVADTHWSSLNLTSSKFEEFMTRHQVHEKEEFKALKTLSIFYQAGTSKAGNPIFYYVARRFKTGQING
(1600)   DLLIYHVLLTLKPYYAKPYEIVVDLTHTGPSNRFKTDFLSKWFVVFPGFAYDNVSAVYIYNCNSWVREYTKYHERLLTGL
(1680)   KGSKRLVFIDCPGKLAEHIEHEQQKLPAATLALEEDLKVFHNALKLAHKDTKVSVGSTAVQVTSAERTKVLGQSVFLN
(1760)   DIYYASEIEEICLVDENQFTLTIANQGTPLTFMHQECEAIVQSIIHIRTRWELSQPDSIPQHTKIRPKDVPGTLLNIALL
(1840)   NLGSSDPSLRSAAYNLLCALTCTFNLKIEGQLLETSGLCIPANNTLFVSISKTLAANEPHLTLEFLEECISGFSKSSIE
(1920)   LKHLCLEYMTPWLSNLVRFCKHNDDAKRQRVTAILDKLITMTINEKQMYPSIQAKIWGSLGQITDLLDVVLDSFIKTSAT
(2000)   GGLGSIKAEVMADTAVALASGNVKLVSSKVIGRMCKIIDKTCLSPTPTLEQHLMWDDIAILARYMLMLSFNNSLDVAAHL
(2080)   PYLFHVVTFLVATGPLSLRASTHGLVINIIHSLCTCSQLHFSEETKQVLRLSLTEFSLPKFYLLFGISKVKSAAVIAFRS
(2160)   SYRDRSFSPGSYERETFALTSLETVTEALLEIMEACMRDIPTCKWLDQWTELAQRFAFQYNPSLQPRALVVFGCISKRVS
(2240)   HGQIKQIIRILSKALESCLKGPDTYNSQVLIEATVIALTKLQPLLNKDSPLHKALFWVAVAVLQLDEVNLYSAGTALLEQ
(2320)   NLHTLDSLRIFNDKSPEEVFMAIRNPLEWHCKQMDHFVGLNFNSNFNFALVGHLLKGYRHPSPAIVARTVRILHTLLTLV
(2400)   NKHRNCDKFEVNTQSVAYLAALLTVSEEVRSRCSLKHRKSLLLTDISMENVPMDTYPIHHGDPSYRTLKETQPWSSPKGS
(2480)   EGYLAATYPTVGQTSPRARKSMSLDMGQPSQANTKKLLGTRKSFDHLISDTKAPKRQEMESGITTPPKMRRVAETDYEME
(2560)   TQRISSSQQHPHLRKVSVSESNVLLDEEVLTDPKIQALLLTVLATLVKYTTDEFDQRILYEYLAEASVVFPKVFPVVHNL
(2640)   LDSKINTLLSLCQDPNLLNPIHGIVQSVVYHEESPPQYQTSYLQSFGFNGLWRFAGPFSKQTQIPDYAELIVKFLDALID
(2720)   TYLPGIDEETSEESLLTPTSPYPPALQSQLSITANLNLSNSMTSLATSQHSP GIDKENVELSPTTGHCNSGRTRHGSASQ
                                                                 Δ
(2800)   VQKQRSAGSFKRNSIKKIV (2818)
```

Alternative processing causes either 54 bp or 63 bp insertions coding for an additional 18 (ASLPCSNSAVFMQLFPHQ (Δ)) or 21 (ATCHSLLNKATVKEKKENKKS (ΔΔ)) amino acids, respectively. Italics: regions of similarity to the GAP family. Underlined residues: 6 potential cAMP-dependent protein kinase recognition sites. Underlined italicized region: a potential tyrosine kinase recognition site.

Substitution of Lys1423, detected in colon adenocarcinoma, myelodysplastic syndrome, anaplastic astrocytoma and NF1, decreases the GAP activity of neurofibromin by 200- to 400-fold without affecting the binding affinity for RAS–GTP (Li *et al.*, 1992; Gutmann *et al.*, 1993).

Sequence of merlin

```
  (1)  MSFSSLKRKQPKTFTVRIVTMDAEMEFNCEMKWKGKDLFDLVCRTLGLRETWFFGLQYTI
 (61)  KDTVAWLKMDKKVLDHDVSKEEPVTFHFLAKFYPENAEEELVQEITQHLFFLQVKKQILD
(121)  EKIYCPPEASVLLASYAVQAKYGDYDPSVHKRGFLAQEELLPKRVINLYQMTPEMWEERI
(181)  TAWYAEHRGRARDEAEMEYLKIAQDLEMYGVNYFAIRNKKGTELLLGVDALGLHIYDPEN
(241)  RLTPKISFPWNEIRNISYSDKEFTIKPLDKKIDVFKFNSSKLRVNKLILQLCIGNHDLFM
(301)  RRRKADSLEVQQMKAQAREEKARKQMERQRLAREKQMREEAERTRDELERRLLQMKEEAT
(361)  MANEALMRSEETADLLAEKAQITEEEAKLLAQKAAEAEQEMQRIKATAIRTEEEKRLMEQ
(421)  KVLEAEVLALKMAEESERRAKEADQLKQDLQEAREAERRAKQKLLEIATKPTYPPMNPIP
(481)  APLPPDIPSFNLIGDSLSFDFKDTDMKRLSMEIEKEKVEYMEKSKHLQEQLNELKTEIEA
(541)  LKLKERETALDILHNENSDRGGSSKHNTIKKLTLQSAKSRVAFFEEL (587)
```

The common moesin–ezrin–radixin domain spans residues 1–350. In the sequence of Rouleau *et al.* (1993) eight additional residues (MAGAIASR) precede the first methionine.

Databank file names and accession numbers

	GENE	EMBL	SWISSPROT	REFERENCES
Human	NF1	Hsnf1b M60496	NF1 HUMAN P21359	Marchuk *et al.*, 1991
Human	NF2	L11353		Trofatter *et al.*, 1993
Human	EV12B	Schwannom Z22664		Rouleau *et al.*, 1993
Human	EV12B3P	Hsevi2b M60829		Cawthon *et al.*, 1991
Human	OMG	Hsevi2b3 M60830		Cawthon *et al.*, 1991
		Hsneurof L05367; L03723		Cawthon *et al.*, 1990
				Viskochil *et al.*, 1991

Papers

Andersen, L.B., Ballester, R., Marchuk, D.A., Chang, E., Gutmann, D.H., Saulino, A.M., Camonis, J., Wigler, M. and Collins, F.S. (1993). A conserved alternative splice in the von Reckinghausen neurofibromatosis (*NF1*) gene produces two neurofibromin isoforms, both of which have GTPase-activating protein activity. Mol. Cell. Biol., 13, 487–495.

Ballester, R., Michaeli, T., Ferguson, K., Xu, H.-P., McCormick, F. and Wigler, M. (1989). Genetic analysis of mammalian GAP expressed in yeast. Cell, 59, 681–686.

Basu, T.N., Gutmann, D.H., Fletcher, J.A., Glover, T.W., Collins, F.S. and Downward, J. (1992). Aberrant regulation of *ras* proteins in malignant tumour cells from type 1 neurofibromatosis patients. Nature, 356, 713–715.

Bollag, G. and McCormick, F. (1991). Differential regulation of *ras*GAP and neurofibromatosis gene product activities. Nature, 351, 576–579.

Bollag, G., McCormick, F. and Clark, R. (1993). Characterization of full-length neurofibromin: tubulin inhibits Ras GAP activity. EMBO J., 12, 1923–1927.

Cawthon, R.M., Weiss, R., Xu, G., Viskochil, D., Culver, M., Stevens, J., Robertson, M., Dunn, D., Gesteland, R., O'Connell, P. and White, R. (1990). A major segment of the neurofibromatosis type 1 gene: cDNA sequence, genomic structure, and point mutations. Cell, 62, 193–201.

Cawthon, R.M., Andersen, L.B., Buchberg, A.M., Xu, G.F., O'Connell, P., Viskochil, D., Weiss, R.B., Wallace, M.R., Marchuk, D.A., Culver, M., Stevens, J., Jenkins, N.A., Copeland, N.G., Collins, F.S. and White, R. (1991). cDNA sequence and genomic structure of EV12B, a gene lying within an intron of the neurofibromatosis type 1 gene. Genomics, 9, 446–460.

DeClue, J.E., Papageorge, A.G., Fletcher, J.A., Diehl, S.R., Ratner, N., Vass, W.C. and Lowy, D.R. (1992). Abnormal regulation of mammalian p21^{ras} contributes to malignant tumor growth in von Recklinghausen (type 1) neurofibromatosis. Cell, 69, 265–273.

Dibattiste, D., Golubic, M., Stacey, D. and Wolfman, A. (1993). Differences in the interaction of p21$^{c-Ha-ras}$-GMP-PNP with full-length neurofibromin and GTPase-activating protein. Oncogene, 8, 637–643.

Garrett, M.D., Major, G.N., Totty, N. and Hall, A. (1991). Purification and N-terminal sequence of the p21^{rho} GTPase-activating protein, *rho*GAP. Biochem. J., 276, 833–836.

Golubic, M., Tanaka, K., Dobrowolski, S., Wood, D., Tsai, M.H., Marshall, M., Tamanoi, F. and Stacey, D.W. (1991). The GTPase stimulatory activities of the neurofibromatosis type 1 and the yeast IRA2 proteins are inhibited by arachidonic acid. EMBO J., 10, 2897–2903.

Golubic, M., Roudebush, M., Dobrowolski, S., Wolfman, A. and Stacey, D.W. (1992). Catalytic properties, tissue and intracellular distribution of neurofibromin. Oncogene, 7, 2151–2159.

Gutmann, D.H., Boguski, M., Marchuk, D., Wigler, M., Collins, F.S. and Ballester, R. (1993). Analysis of the neurofibromatosis type 1 (NF1) GAP-related domain by site-directed mutagenesis. Oncogene, 8, 761–769.

Hattori, S., Maekawa, M. and Nakamura, S. (1992). Identification of neurofibromatosis type I gene product as an insoluble GTPase-activating protein toward *ras* p21. Oncogene, 7, 481–485.

Li, Y., Bollag, G., Clark, R., Stevens, J., Conroy, L., Fults, D., Ward, K., Friedman, E., Samowitz, W., Robertson, M., Bradley, P., McCormick, F., White, R. and Cawthon, R. (1992). Somatic mutations in the neurofibromatosis 1 gene in human tumors. Cell, 69, 275–281.

Marchuk, D.A., Saulino, A.M., Tavakkol, R., Swaroop, M., Wallace, M.R., Andersen, L.B., Mitchell, A.L., Gutmann, D.H., Boguski, M. and Collins, F.S. (1991). cDNA cloning of the type 1 neurofibromatosis gene: complete sequence of the *NF1* gene product. Genomics, 11, 931–940.

Nishi, T., Lee, P.S.Y., Oka, K., Levin, V.A., Tanase, S., Morino, Y. and Saya, H. (1991). Differential expression of two types of the neurofibromatosis type 1 (*NF1*) gene transcripts related to neuronal differentiation. Oncogene, 6, 1555–1559.

Rouleau, G.A., Merel, P., Lutchman, M., Sanson, M., Zucman, J., Marineau, C., Hoang-Xuan, K., Demczuk, S., Desmaze, C., Plougastel, B., Pulst, S.M., Lenoir, G., Bijlsma, E., Fashold, R., Dumanski, J., de Jong, P., Parry, D., Eldrige, R., Aurias, A., Delattre, O. and Thomas, G. (1993). Alteration in a new gene encoding a putative membrane-organizing protein causes neuro-fibromatosis type 2. Nature, 363, 515–521.

Suzuki, Y., Suzuki, H., Kayama, T. and Shibahara, S. (1991). Brain tumors predominantly express the neurofibromatosis type 1 gene transcript containing the 63 base insert in the region coding for GTPase activating protein-related domain. Biochem. Biophys. Res. Commun., 181, 95–961.

Tanaka, K., Nakafuku, M., Satoh, T., Marschall, M.S., Gibbs, J.B., Matsumoto, K., Kaziro, Y. and Toh-e, A. (1990). S. cerevisiae genes IRA1 and IRA2 encode proteins that may be functionally equivalent to mammalian *ras* GTPase activitity protein. Cell, 60, 803–807.

Trofatter, J.A., MacCollin, M.M., Rutter, J.L., Murrell, J.R., Duyao, M.P., Parry, D.M., Eldridge, R., Kley, N., Menon, A.G., Pulaski, K., Haase, V.H., Ambrose, C.M., Munroe, D., Bove, C., Haines, J.L., Martuza, R.L., MacDonald, M.E., Seizinger, B.R., Short, M.P., Buckler, A.J. and Gusella, J.F. (1993). A novel moesin-, ezrin-, radixin-like gene is a candidate for the neurofibromatosis 2 tumor suppressor. Cell, 72, 791–800.

Viskochil, D., Buchberg, A.M., Xu, G., Cawthon, R.M., Stevens, J., Wolff, R.K., Culver, M., Carey, J.C., Copeland, N.G., Jenkins, N.A., White, R. and O'Connell, P. (1990). Deletions and a translocation interrupt a cloned gene at the neurofibromatosis type 1 locus. Cell, 62, 187–192.

Viskochil, D., Cawthon, R., O'Connell, P., Xu, G.F., Stevens, J., Culver, M., Carey, J. and White, R. (1991). The gene encoding the oligodendrocyte-myelin glycoprotein is embedded within the neurofibromatosis type 1 gene. Mol. Cell. Biol., 11, 906–912.

Xu, G., O'Connell, P., Viskochil, D., Cawthon, R., Robertson, M., Culver, M., Dunn, D., Stevens, J., Gesteland, R., White, R. and Weiss, R. (1990a). The neurofibromatosis type 1 gene encodes a protein related to GAP. Cell, 62, 599–608.

Xu, G., Lin, B., Tanaka, K., Dunn, D., Wood, D., Gesteland, R., White, R., Weiss, R. and Tamanoi, F. (1990b). The catalytic domain of the neurofibromatosis type 1 gene product stimulates *ras* GTPase and complements *ira* mutants of *S.cerevisiae*. Cell, 63, 835–841.

Von Hippel–Lindau disease

Von Hippel–Lindau disease (VHL) is a dominantly inherited familial cancer syndrome that predisposes individuals most frequently to haemangioblastomas of the central nervous system and retina, renal cell carcinoma and pheochromocytoma. The incidence at birth is at least 1 in 36 000.

Related genes

VHL has no significant homology to known proteins although it includes eight copies of a tandemly repeated pentamer similar to that present in the surface membrane protein of *Trypanosoma brucei*.

Cross-species homology

VHL is highly conserved from mammals to *Drosophila* and sea urchin (Latif *et al.*, 1993).

	VHL
Nucleotides (kb)	<20
Chromosome	
Human	3p25–p26
mRNA (kb)	
Human	6.0/6.5
Amino acids	
Human	284
Mass (kDa) (predicted)	
Human	28

Cellular location

Possibly plasma membrane.

Tissue location

VHL is widely expressed. Only one of the 6.0 or 6.5 kb mRNA species are expressed in fetal brain and fetal kidney; both are expressed in adult tissues.

Protein function

Unknown. The repeated acidic domain resembling that of the *Trypanosoma brucei* surface membrane protein suggests that VHL may be involved in signal transduction or cell–cell contacts.

Sequence of VHL

```
  (1)  PRLRYNSLRCWRILLRTRTASGRLFPRARSILYRARAKTTEVDSGARTQLRPASDPRIPR
 (61)  RPARVVWIAEGMPRRAENWDEAEVGAEEAGVEEYGPEEDGGEESGAEESGPEESGPEELG
                                  *      ***
(121)  AEEEMEAGRPRPVLRSVNSREPSQVIFCNRSPRVVLPVWLNFDGEPQPYPTLPPGTGRRI
(181)  HSYRGHLWLFRDAGTHDGLLVNQTELFVPSLNVDGQPIFANITLPVYTIKERCLQVVRSL
(241)  VKPENYRRLDIVRSLYEDLEDHPNVQKDLERLTQERIAHQRMGD (284)
```

Underlined: The tandemly repeated acidic domain Gly–X–Glu–Glu–X. Major deletions or insertions in the gene occur with high frequency (>12%) in VHL patients. One intragenic 8 bp frameshift insertion and two intragenic deletions (removing amino acids 153–154 {***} or Ile146 {*}) have also been detected in VHL families. In sporadic renal cell carcinomas, four small intragenic frameshift deletions and one nonsense mutation have been detected. The effects of these mutations are the replacement of residues 246–284 with 28 new amino acids, the replacement of residues 238–284 with 32 new residues, the replacement of residues 212–284 with 62 new residues or the generation of a truncated protein caused by mutation in codon 254.

Databank file names and accession numbers

	GENE	EMBL	SWISSPROT	REFERENCES
Human	VHL	L15409		Latif *et al.*, 1993

Paper

Latif, F., Tory, K., Gnarra, J., Yao, M., Duh, F.-M., Orcutt, M.L., Stackhouse, T., Kuzmin, I., Modi, W., Geil, L., Schmidt, L., Zhou, F., Li, H., Wei, M.H., Chen, F., Glenn, G., Choyke, P., Walther, M.M., Weng, Y., Duan, D.S.R., Dean, M., Glavac, D., Richards, F.M., Crossey, P.A., Ferguson-Smith, M.A., Le Paslier, D., Chumakov, I., Cohen, D., Chinault, C.A., Maher, E.R., Linehan, W.M., Zbar, B. and Lerman, M.I. (1993). Identification of the von Hippel–Lindau disease tumor suppressor gene. Science, 260, 1317–1320.

Wilms' tumour

Wilms' tumour is an embryonal renal neoplasm that occurs in sporadic and familial forms and affects 1 in 10 000 children. Approximately 2% of Wilms' tumours occur in association with aniridia, genitourinary anomalies and mental retardation (WAGR syndrome) in which deletions of 11p13 were first detected.

Related genes

WT1 is a member of the early growth response family (*EGR1, EGR2, EGR3, EGR4*).

Cross-species homology

The human and mouse proteins are >95% identical.

Transformation

Wilms' tumour, like retinoblastoma, occurs in unilateral or bilateral early onset forms but may involve three loci rather than one. Deletions at 11p13 are associated with the bilateral form but in the sporadic forms allelic loss occurs at 11p15 (*WT2*), exclusively in the maternal allele, and a third locus may be involved in the familial forms. Insertion of a normal human chromosome 11 into Wilms' tumour cells causes their reversion to normal, non-tumorigenic cells (Stanbridge, 1988).

	WT1
Nucleotides (kb)	50
Chromosome	
Human	11p13
Exons	10
mRNA (kb)	
Human	3.2
Amino acids	
Human	449/446/432
Mass (kDa)	
(predicted) Human	45–49
(expressed) Human	52/54

Cellular location

Nuclear (Telerman et al., 1992).

Tissue location

WT1 is expressed in the developing kidney, gonads, spleen and mesothelium and brain (Huang *et al.*, 1990; Pritchard-Jones *et al.*, 1990). All these tissues are mesodermally derived and undergo a mesenchymal–epithelial transition.

Protein function

WT1 proteins are transcription factors. The minor form represses transcription by binding to the sequence 5'-CGCCCCCGC-3' (Call *et al.*, 1990; Morris *et al.*, 1991), to which EGR1 binds as a transcriptional activator (Madden *et al.*, 1991). The major form (+KTS, see below) binds to a different DNA sequence (Bickmore *et al.*, 1992). The N-terminal (leucine zipper) region of WT1 is required for repression although the protein does not form (homo)dimers. Human PDGFA transcription is strongly repressed by WT1 interaction with two binding sites that lie 5' and 3' relative to the transcription start site (Gashler *et al.*, 1992; Wang *et al.*, 1993). When WT1 binds to only one of these sites it functions as a *trans*-activator (Wang *et al.*, 1993). *IGF2*, which encodes an autocrine growth factor expressed at high levels in Wilms' tumour, may also be a target gene. *IGF2* is expressed from the paternal allele in normal human fetal tissue but expression can occur biallelically in Wilms' tumour (Ogawa *et al.*, 1993). The *H19* gene is also monoallelically expressed in normal tissue but can show biallelic expression in Wilms' tumour (Rainer *et al.*, 1993). Both *IGF2* and *H19* are located at 11p15 and the relaxation of genomic imprinting may therefore be involved in the development of Wilms' tumour.

Point mutations that occur in Denys–Drash syndrome (see below; Bruening *et al.*, 1992) appear to be dominant in their mode of action and lead to severe developmental abnormalities of the gonads and kidney as well as to Wilms' tumour (Pelletier *et al.*, 1991). Together with the developmental expression pattern, this suggests that WT1 has a crucial role in normal genitourinary development.

Gene structure

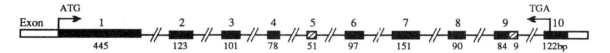

The alternatively spliced exons are cross-hatched. All four possible variants are expressed in normal developing kidney, that including both alternative sequences being most common (Haber *et al.*, 1991). The isoforms contain four Cys$_2$–His$_2$ zinc fingers: the variants having a 3 amino acid insertion at exon 9 cannot bind the *EGR* recognition element (Madden *et al.*, 1991). Mutations within intron 9 that prevent alternative splicing and in the zinc finger domains occur in Denys–Drash syndrome (Bruening *et al.*, 1992) and in Wilms' tumour DNA (Little *et al.*, 1992). A 10 bp insertion in exon 7 and a single base pair change in exon 8 that generate truncated proteins lacking part of the zinc finger domain have also been detected in unilateral Wilms' tumours (Baird *et al.*, 1992). All four *WT1* transcripts are expressed in Wilms' tumours (Brenner *et al.*, 1992).

Sequences of human and mouse WT1

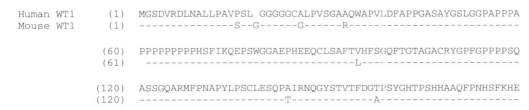

```
Human WT1   (1)    MGSDVRDLNALLPAVPSL GGGGGCALPVSGAAQWAPVLDFAPPGASAYGSLGGPAPPPA
Mouse WT1   (1)    ---------------S--G------G------R---------------------------

            (60)   PPPPPPPPPHSFIKQEPSWGGAEPHEEQCLSAFTVHFSGQFTGTAGACRYGPFGPPPPSQ
            (61)   ----------------------------------L------------------------

            (120)  ASSGQARMFPNAPYLPSCLESQPAIRNQGYSTVTFDGTPSYGHTPSHHAAQFPNHSFKHE
            (120)  ----------------------T------------A------------------------
```

```
(180)  DPMGQQGSLGEQQYSVPPPVYGCHTPTDSCTGSQALLLRTPYSSDNLYQMTSQLECMTWN
(180)  ------------------------------------------------------------

(240)  QMNLGATLKGVAAGSSSSVKWTEGQSNHSTGYESDNHTTPILCGAQYRIHTHGVFRGIQD
(240)  ---------M---------------GI--------A------------------------

(300)  VRRVPGVAPTLVRSASETSEKRPFMCAYPGCNKRYFKLSHLQMHSRKHTGEKPYQCDFKD
(300)  ----S-------------------------------------------------------

(360)  CERRFSRSDQLKRHQRRHTGVKPFQCKTCQRKFSRSDHLKTHTRTHTGKTSEKPFSCRWP
(360)  -------------------------------------------------------------H

(420)  SCQKKFARSDELVRHHNMHQRNMTKLQLAL (449)
(420)  --------------------------HV-- (449)
```

Dashes indicate identical amino acids. Human 27–83: proline-rich domain. Underlined: zinc finger regions (323–347, 353–377, 383–405, 414–438). Underlined italics: alternative splice regions (250–266 and 408–410); these introduce 17 amino acids after 249 or three amino acids between the third and fourth zinc fingers and are conserved between humans and mice. The variant containing the KTS sequence is the predominant form in all cells that express WT1 (Haber *et al.*, 1991). Residues 84–179 of the 429 amino acid form mediate *trans* repression: 180–294 *trans* activation (Wang *et al.*, 1993).

Databank file names and accession numbers

	GENE	EMBL	SWISSPROT	REFERENCES

Human	WT1	Hswt1 X51630
		Hswt33 M30393
		Hswt101–Hswt105 M80217–
		  M80221
		Hswt106 M80228
		Hswt109/110 M80231/32;
		  M74917
			WT1_HUMAN
			P19544
				Gessler *et al.*, 1990
				Call *et al.*, 1990
				Haber *et al.*, 1991
				Buckler *et al.*, 1991
				Little *et al.*, 1992
				Pelletier *et al.*, 1991
				Baird *et al.*, 1992

Mouse	Wt-1	Mmwt1 M55512	WT1_MOUSE P22561	Buckler *et al.*, 1991

Reviews

Haber, D.A. and Buckler, A.J. (1992). WT1 — a novel tumor suppressor gene inactivated in Wilms' tumor. New Biologist, 4, 97–106.
van Heyningen, V. and Hastie, N.D. (1992). Wilms' tumour: reconciling genetics and biology. Trends Genet., 8, 16–21.

Papers

Baird, P.N., Groves, N., Haber, D.A., Housman, D.E. and Cowell, J.K. (1992). Identification of mutations in the *WT1* gene in tumours from patients with the WAGR syndrome. Oncogene, 7, 2141–2149.
Bickmore, W.A., Oghene, K., Little, M.H., Seawright, A., van Heyningen, V. and Hastie, N.D. (1992). Modulation of DNA binding specificity by alternative splicing of the Wilms' tumor *wt1* gene transcript. Science, 257, 235–237.

Brenner, B., Wildhardt, G., Schneider, S. and Royer-Pokora, B (1992). RNA polymerase chain reaction detects different levels of four alternatively spliced *WT1* transcripts in Wilms' tumors. Oncogene, 7, 1431–1433.

Bruening, W., Bardeesy, N., Silverman, B.L., Cohn, R.A., Machin, G.A., Aronson, A.J., Housman, D. and Pelletier, J. (1992). Germline intronic and exonic mutations in the Wilms' tumour gene (*WT1*) affecting urogenital development. Nature Genomics, 1, 144–148.

Buckler, A.J., Pelletier, J., Haber, D.A., Glaser, T. and Housman, D.E. (1991). Isolation, characterization and expression of the murine Wilms' tumor gene (WT1) during kidney development. Mol. Cell. Biol., 11, 1707–1712.

Call, K.M., Glaser, T., Ito, C., Buckler, A.J., Pelletier, J., Haber, D.A., Rose, E.A., Kral, A., Yeger, H., Lewis, W.H., Jones, C. and Housman, D.E. (1990). Isolation and characterization of a zinc finger polypeptide gene at the human chromosome 11 Wilms' tumor locus. Cell, 60, 509–520.

Gashler, A.L., Bonthron, D.T., Madden, S.L., Rauscher, F.J., Collins, T. and Sukhatme, V.P. (1992). Human platelet-derived growth factor A chain is transcriptionally repressed by the Wilms tumor suppressor WT1. Proc. Natl Acad. Sci. USA, 89, 10984–10988.

Gessler, M., Poustka, A., Cavenee, W., Neve, R.L., Orkin, S.H. and Bruns, G.A.P. (1990). Homologous deletion in Wilms tumours of a zinc-finger gene identified by chromosome jumping. Nature, 343, 774–778.

Haber, D.A., Sohn, R.L., Buckler, A.J., Pelletier, J., Call, K.M. and Housman, D.E. (1991). Alternative splicing and genomic structure of the Wilms tumor gene *WT1*. Proc. Natl Acad. Sci. USA, 88, 9618–9622.

Huang, A., Campbell, C.E., Bonetta, L., McAndrews-Hill, M.S., Chilton-MacNeill, S., Coppes, M.J., Law, D.J., Feinberg, A.P., Yeger, H. and Williams, B.R.G. (1990). Tissue, developmental, and tumor-specific expression of divergent transcripts in Wilms tumor. Science, 250, 991–994.

Little, M.H., Prosser, J., Condie, A., Smith, P.J., van Heyningen, V. and Hastie, N.D. (1992). Zinc finger point mutations within the *WT1* gene in Wilms tumor patients. Proc. Natl Acad. Sci. USA, 89, 4791–4795.

Madden, S.L., Cook, D.M., Morris, J.F., Gashler, A., Sukhatme, V.P. and Rauscher, F.J. (1991). Transcriptional repression mediated by the WT1 Wilms tumor gene product. Science, 253, 1550–1553.

Morris, J.F., Madden, S.L., Tournay, O.E., Cook, D.M., Sukhatme, V.P. and Rauscher, F.J. (1991). Characterization of the zinc finger protein encoded by the WT1 Wilms' tumor locus. Oncogene, 6, 2339–2348.

Ogawa, O., Eccles, M.R., Szeto, J., McNoe, L.A., Yun, K., Maw, M.A., Smith, P.J. and Reeve, A.E. (1993). Relaxation of insulin-like growth factor II gene imprinting implicated in Wilms' tumour. Nature, 362, 749–751.

Pelletier, J., Bruening, W., Kashtan, C.E., Mauer, S.M., Manivel, J.C., Striegel, J.E., Houghton, D.C., Junien, C., Habib, R., Fouser, L., Fine, R.N., Silverman, B.L., Haber, D.A. and Housman, D. (1991). Germline mutations in the Wilms' tumor suppressor gene are associated with abnormal urogenital development in Denys–Drash syndrome. Cell, 67, 437–447.

Pritchard-Jones, K., Fleming, S., Davidson, D., Bickmore, W., Porteous, D., Gosden, C., Bard, J., Buckler, A., Pelletier, J., Housman, D., van Heyningen, V. and Hastie, N. (1990). The candidate Wilm's tumour gene is involved in genitourinary development. Nature, 346, 194–197.

Rainer, S., Johnson, L.A., Dobry, C.J., Ping, A.J., Grundy, P.E. and Feinberg, A.P. (1993). Relaxation of imprinted genes in human cancer. Nature, 362, 747–749.

Stanbridge, E.J. (1988). Genetic analysis of human malignancy using somatic cell hybrids and monochromosome transfer. Cancer Surv., 7, 317–324.

Shirodkar, S., Ewen, M., DeCaprio, J.A., Morgan, J., Livingston, D.M. and Chittenden, T. (1992). The transcription factor E2F interacts with the retinoblastoma product and a p107-cyclin A complex in a cell cycle-regulated manner. Cell, 68, 157–166.

Telerman, A., Dodemont, H., Degraef, C., Galand, P., Bauwens, S., Van Oostveldt, P. and Amson, R.B. (1992). Identification of the cellular protein encoded by the human Wilms' tumor (*WT1*) gene. Oncogene, 7, 2545–2548.

Wang, Z.-Y., Qiu, Q.-Q. and Deuel, T.F. (1993). The Wilms' tumor gene product WT1 activates or suppresses transcription through separate functional domains. J. Biol. Chem., 268, 9172–9175.

Familial adenomatosis polyposis

Familial adenomatosis polyposis (FAP) arises from the inheritance of one abnormal *APC* (adenomatous polyposis coli) allele. The incidence is 1 in 8000 and it causes the development of hundreds of colonic polyps in early life and leads, in untreated individuals, to colorectal cancer. *APC* is mutated in the germ line of FAP patients, virtually all mutations inactivating the gene (Miyoshi *et al.*, 1992). The locus is involved in other forms of colorectal cancers although in these cases the incidence of allelic losses from chromosome 5q is very variable (Fearon and Vogelstein, 1990). The *MCC* (*m*utated in *c*olorectal *c*ancer) gene, ~180 kb from *APC*, is not mutated in the germ line but undergoes somatic mutations in FAP and colon cancer (Bourne, 1991). Deletions in the 5q21 region also occur in ~25% of lung cancers (Ashton-Rickardt *et al.*, 1991).

Related genes

There are no closely related genes but both *APC* and *MCC* contain heptad repeats that give predicted coiled domains, similar to those in myosins and keratins and the *Ski* family.

	APC	*MCC*
Nucleotides (kb)	120	170
Chromosome	5q21	5q21
Exons	15	17
mRNA (kb)	~10	5–10
Amino acids	2843/2743	829
Mass (kDa)		
(predicted)	312	93
(expressed)	~300	

Cellular location

APC: cytoplasmic, concentrated in the basolateral portion of the crypt epithelial cells (Smith *et al.*, 1993).

Tissue location

Lymphoblastoid cell lines; both forms (see below) probably ubiquitous.

Protein function

Unknown: contains multiple serine phosphorylation, glycosylation and myristylation sites. Forms dimers via the leucine zipper region. Transgenic mice homozygous for the null *APC* allele develop normally, indicating that in mice this gene is not essential for proliferation and differentiation.

Gene and protein structure of *APC*

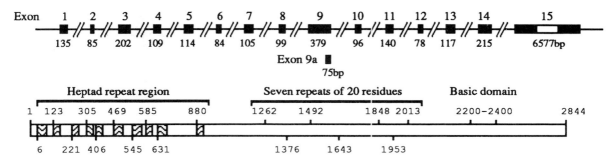

The alternatively spliced form (exon 9a) has a deletion of bases 934–1236 that removes 101 amino acids. The initial amino acids of the ten heptad repeats and the seven 20 residue repeats (consensus F–VE–TP–CFSR–SSLSSLS) are numbered. The last 14 amino acids of the fourth and the first 7 amino acids of the fifth heptad repeats are present only in the longer gene product (containing exon 9).

Sequence of human APC

```
  (1)    MAAASYDQLLKQVEALKMENSNLRQELEDNSNHLTKLETEASNMKEVLKQLQGSIEDEA
 (60)    MASSGQIDLLERLKELNLDSSNFPGVKLRSKMSLRSYGSREGVSSRSGECSPVPMGSFP
(120)    RRGFVNGSRESTGYLEELEKERSLLLADLDKEEKEKDWYYAQLQNLTKRIDSLPLTENFS
(180)    LQTDMTRRQLEYEARQIRVAMEEQLGTCQDMEKRAQRRIARIQQIEKDILRIRQLLQSQA
(240)    TEAERSSQNKHETGSHDAERQNEGQGVGEINMATSGNGQGSTTRMDHETASVLSSSSTHS
(300)    APRRLTSHLGTKVEMVYSLLSMLGTHDKDDMSRTLLAMSSSQDSCISMRQSGCLPLLIQL
(360)    LHGNDKDSVLLGNSRGSKEARARASAALHNIIHSQPDDKRGRREIRVLHHLLEQIRAYCET
(420)    CWEWQEAHEPGMDQDKNPMPAPVEHQICPAVCVLMKLSFDEEHRHAMNELGGLQAIAELL
(480)    QVDCEMYGLTNDHYSITLRRYAGMALTNLTFGDVANKATLCSMKGCMRALVAQLKSESED
(540)    LQQVIASVLRNLSWRADVNSKKTLREVGSVKALMECALEVKKESTLKSVLSALWNLSAHC
(600)    TENKADICAVDGALAFLVGTLTYRSQTNTLAIIESGGGILRNVSSLIATNEDHRQILREN
(660)    NCLQTLLQHLKSHSLTIVSNACGTLWNLSARNPKDQEALWDMGAVSMLKNLIHSKHKMIA
(720)    MGSAAALRNLMANRPAKYKDANIMSPGSSLPSLHVRKQKALEAELDAQHLSETFDNIDNL
(780)    SPKASHRSKQRHKQSLYGDYVFDTNRHDDNRSDNFNTGNMTVLSPYLNTTVLPSSSSSRG
(840)    SLDSSRSEKDRSLERERGIGLGNYHPATENPGTSSKRGLQISTTAAQIAKVMEEVSAIHT
(900)    SQEDRSSGSTTELHCVTDERNALRRSSAAHTHSNTYNFTKSENSNRTCSMPYAKLEYKRS
(960)    SNDSLNSVSSSDGYGKRGQMKPSIESYSEDDESKFCSYGQYPADLAHKIHSANHMDDNDG
(1020)   ELDTPINYSLKYSDEQLNSGRQSPSQNERWARPKHIIEDEIKQSEQRQSRNQSTTYPVYT
(1080)   ESTDDKHLKFQPHFGQQECVSPYRSRGANGSETNRVGSNHGINQNVSQSLCQEDDYEDDK
(1140)   PTNYSERYSEEEQHEEEERPTNYSIKYNEEKRHVDQPIDYSLKYATDIFSSQKQSFSFSK
(1200)   SSSGQSSKTEHMSSSSENTSTPSSNAKRQNQLHPSSAQSRSGQPQKAATCKVSSINQETI
(1260)   QTYCVEDTPICFSRCSSLSSLSSAEDEIGCNQTTQEADSANTLQIAEIKEKIGTRSAEDP
(1320)   VSEVPAVSQHPRTKSSRLQGSSLSSESARHKAVEFSSGAKSPSKSGAQTPKSPPEHYVQE
(1380)   TPLMFSRCTSVSSLDSFESRSIASSVQSEPCSGMVSGIISPSDLPDSPCQTMPPSRSKTP
(1440)   PPPPQTAQTKREVPKNKAPTAEKRESGPKQAAVNAAVQRVQVLPDDADTLHFATESTPDG
(1500)   FSCSSSLSALSLDEPFIQKDVELRIMPPVQENDNGNETESEQPKESNENQEKEAEKTIDS
(1560)   EKDLLDDSDDDDIEILEECIISAMPTKSSRKAKKPAQTASKLPPPVARKPSQLPVYKLLP
(1620)   SQNRLQPQKHVSFTPGDDMPRVYCVEGTPINFSTATSLSDLTIESPPNELAAGEGVRGGA
(1680)   QSGEFEKRDTIPTEGRSTDEAQGGKTSSVTIPELDDNKAEEGDILAECINSAMPKGKSHK
(1740)   PFRVKKIMDQVQQASASSSAPNKNQLDGKKKKPTSPVKPIPQNTEYRTFVRKNADSKNNL
(1800)   NAERVFSDNKDSKKQNLKNNSKDFNDKLPNNEDRVRGSFAFDSPHHYTPIEGTPYCFSRN
(1860)   DSLSSLDFDDDDVDLSREKAELRKAKENKESEAKVTSHTELTSNQQSANKTQAIAKQPIN
(1920)   RGQPKPILQKQSTFPQSSKDIPDRGAATDEKLQNFAIENTPVCFSHNSSLSSLSLSDIDQEN
(1980)   NNKENEPIKETEPPDSQGEPSKPQASGYAPKSFHVEDTPVCFSRNSSLSSLSLSIDSEDDLL
(2040)   QECISSAMPKKKKPSRLKGDNEKHSPRNMGGILGEDLTLDLKDIQRPDSEHGLSPDSENF
(2100)   DWKAIQEGANSIVSSLHQAAAAACLSRQASSDSDSILSLKSGISLGSPFHLTPDQEEKPF
(2160)   TSNKGPRILKPGEKSTLETKKIESESKGIKGGKKVYKSLITGKVRSNSEISGQMKQPLQA
(2220)   NMPSISRGRTMIHIPGVRNSSSSTSPVSKKGPPLKTPASKSPSEGQTATTSPRGAKPSVK
```

```
(2280)  SELSPVARQTSQIGGSSKAPSRSGSRDSTPSRPAQQPLSRPIQSPGRNSISPGRNGISPP
(2340)  NKLSQLPRTSSPSTASTKSSGSGKMSYTSPGRQMSQQNLTKQTGLSKNASSIPRSESASK
(2400)  GLNQMNNGNANKKVELSRMSSTKSSGSESDRSERPVLVRQSTFIKEAPSPTLRRKLEES
(2460)  ASFESLSPSSRPASPTRSQAQTPVLSPSLPDMSLSTHSSVQAGGWRKLPPNLSPTIEYND
(2520)  GRPAKRHDIARSHSESPSRLPINRSGTWKREHSKHSSSLPRVSTWRRTGSSSSILSASSE
(2580)  SSEKAKSEDEKHVNSISGTKQSKENQVSAKGTWRKIKENEFSPTNSTSQTVSSGATNGAE
(2640)  SKTLIYQMAPAVSKTEDVWVRIEDCPINNPRSGRSPTGNTPPVIDSVSEKANPNIKDSKD
(2700)  NQAKQNVGNGSVPMRTVGLENRLNSFIQVDAPDQKGTEIKPGQNNPVPVSETNESSIVER
(2760)  TPFSSSSSSKHSSPSGTVAARVTPFNYNPSPRKSSADSTSARPSQIPTPVNNNTKKRDSK
(2820)  TDSTESSGTQSPKRHSGSYLVTSV(2843)
```

The 101 amino acids missing in the alternatively spliced form (312–412) are italicized. The 10 heptad repeat regions are underlined. The heptad repeats may mediate oligomer formation between full-length and truncated APC (Smith *et al.*, 1993).

Sequence of human MCC

```
(1)    MNSGVAMKYGNDSSAELSELHSAALASLKGDIVELNKRLQQTERERDLLEKKLAKAQCE
(60)   QSHLMREHEDVQERTTLRYEERITELHSVIAELNKKIDRLQGTTIREEDEYSELRSELSQ
(120)  SQHEVNEDSRSMDQDQTSVSIPENQSTMVTADMDNCSDLNSELQRVLTGLENVVCGRKKS
(180)  SCSLSVAEVDRHIEQLTTASEHCDLAIKTVEEIEGVLGRDLYPNLAEEERSRWEKELAGLR
(240)  EENESLTAMLCSKEEELNRTKATMNAIREERDRLRRRVRELQTRLQSVQATGPSSPGRLT
(300)  STNRPINPSTGELSTSSSSNDIPIAKIAERVKLSKTRSESSSSDRPVLGSEISSIGVSSS
(360)  VAEHLAHSLQDCSNIQEIFQTLYSHGSAISESKIREFEVETERLNSRIEHLKSQNDLLTI
(420)  TLEECKSNAERMSMLVGKYESNATALRLALQYSEQCIEAYELLLALAESEQSLILGQFRA
(480)  AGVGSSPGDQSGDENITQMLKRAHDCRKTAENAAKALLMKLDGSCGGAFAVAGCSVQPWE
(540)  SLSSNSHTSTTSSTASSCDTEFTKEDEQRLKDYIQQLKNDRAAVKLTMLELESIHIDPLS
(600)  YDVKPRGDSQRLDLENAVLMQELMAMKEEMAELKAQLYLLEKEKKALELKLSTREAQEQA
(660)  YLVHIEHLKSEVEEQKEQRMRSLSSTSSGSKDKPGKECADAASPALSLAELRTTCSENEL
(720)  AAEFTNAIRREKKLKARVQELVSALERLTKSSEIRHQQSAEFVNDLKRANSNLVAAYEKA
(780)  KKKHQNKLKKLESQMMAMVERHETQVRMLKQRIALLEEENSRPHTNETSL(829)
```

The underlined region is similar to amino acids 249–272 of the G protein-coupled m3 muscarinic acetylcholine receptor. Variants in colorectal cancer: 486 (P → L), 506 (R → Q), 698 (A → V).

Databank file names and accession numbers

	GENE	EMBL	SWISSPROT	REFERENCES
Human	APC	Hsfapapc M74088	APC_HUMAN P25054	Joslyn *et al.*, 1991
Human	MCC	Hscrcmut M62397	CRCM_HUMAN P23508	Kinzler *et al*, 1991

Papers

Ashton-Rickardt, P.G., Wyllie, A.H., Bird, C.C., Dunlop, M.G., Steel, C.M., Morris, R.G., Piris, J., Romanowski, P., Wood, R., White, R. and Nakamura, Y. (1991). *MCC*, a candidate familial polyposis gene in 5q21, shows frequent allele loss in colorectal and lung cancer. Oncogene, 6, 1881–1886.

Bourne, H.R. (1991). Suppression with a difference. Nature, 353, 696–698.

Fearon, E.R. and Vogelstein, B. (1990). A genetic model for colorectal tumorigenesis. Cell, 61, 759–767.

Kinzler, K.W., Nilbert, M.C., Vogelstein, B., Bryan, T.M., Levy, D.B., Smith, K.J., Preisinger, A.C., Hamilton, S.R., Hedge, P., Markham, A., Carlson, M., Joslyn, G., Groden, J., White, R., Miki, Y., Miyoshi, Y., Nishisho, I. and Nakamura, Y. (1991). Science, 251, 1366–1370.

Joslyn, G., Carlson, M., Thliveris, A., Albertsen, H., Gelbert, L., Samowitz, W., Groden, J., Stevens, J.,

Spiro, L., Robertson, M., Sargeant, L., Krapcho, K., Wolff, E., Burt, R., Hughes, J.P., Warrington, J., McPherson, J., Wasmuth, J., LePaslier, D., Abderrahim, H., Cohen, D., Leppert, M. and White, R. (1991). Identification of deletion mutations and three new genes at the familial polyposis locus. Cell, 66, 601–613.

Miyoshi, Y., Ando, H., Nagase, H., Nishisho, I., Horii, A., Miki, Y., Mori, T., Utsunomiya, J., Baba, S., Petersen, G., Hamilton, S.R., Kinzler, K.W., Vogelstein, B. and Nakamura, Y. (1992). Germ-line mutations of the *APC* gene in 53 familial adenomatous polyposis patients. Proc. Natl Acad. Sci. USA, 89, 4452–4456.

Smith, K.J., Johnson, K.A., Bryan, T.M., Hill, D.E., Markowitz, S., Willson, J.K.V., Paraskeva, C., Petersen, G.M., Hamilton, S.R., Vogelstein, B. and Kinzler, K.W. (1993). The *APC* gene product in normal and tumor cells. Proc. Natl Acad. Sci. USA, 90, 2846–2850.

DCC

Allelic loss of chromosomes 17p or 18q occurs in 70% of colorectal carcinomas and with high frequency in ovarian adenicarcinomas (Chenevix-Trench *et al.*, 1992). The 17p region contains *P53*; the 18q region contains a putative tumour suppressor gene, *DCC* (deleted in colorectal carcinomas, 18q21–qter; Fearon *et al.*, 1990) and also includes *BCL2* and *YES1*. The predicted sequence of the DCC protein is homologous to neural cell adhesion molecules (NCAMs). Its loss in many colorectal carcinomas may reflect alterations in cellular attachment; antisense RNA to *DCC* inhibits cell adhesion *in vitro* (Narayanan *et al.*, 1992). In addition to mutations in *P53*, *DCC*, *APC* and *MCC*, colorectal carcinomas also accumulate mutations in *RAS*. Mutations in *DCC* also occur in breast carcinomas (Devilee *et al.*, 1991). At least four scrambled transcripts are present at low concentrations in normal and neoplastic cells in which *DCC* exons are joined accurately at consensus splice sites but in a different order to that in the primary transcript (Nigro *et al.*, 1991). *DCC* expression is reduced in HPV-18 immortalized human keratinocytes transformed to tumorigenicity by NMU (Klingelhutz *et al.*, 1993).

Papers

Chenevix-Trench, G., Leary, J., Kerr, J., Michel, J., Kefford, R., Hurst, T., Parsons, P.G., Friedlander, M. and Khoo, S.K. (1992). Frequent loss of heterozygosity on chromosome 18 in ovarian adenocarcinoma which does not always include the DCC locus. Oncogene, 7, 1059–1065.

Devilee, P., van-Vliet, M., Kuipers-Dijkshoorn, N., Pearson, P.L. and Cornelisse, C.J. (1991). Somatic genetic changes on chromosome 18 in breast carcinomas: is the DCC gene involved? Oncogene, 6, 311–315.

Fearon, E.R., Cho, K.R., Nigro, J.M., Kern, S.E., Simons, J.W., Ruppert, J.M., Hamilton, S.R., Preisinger, A.C., Thomas, G., Kinzler, K.W. and Vogelstein, B. (1990). Identification of a chromosome 18q gene that is altered in colorectal cancers. Science, 247, 49–56.

Klingelhutz, A.J., Smith, P.P., Garrett, L.R. and McDougall, J.K. (1993). Alteration of the DCC tumor-suppressor gene in tumorigenic HPV-18 immortalized human keratinocytes transformed by nitroso-methylurea. Oncogene, 8, 95–99.

Narayanan, R., Lawlor, K.G., Schaapveld, R.Q.J., Cho, K.R., Vogelstein, B., Tran, P.B.-V., Osborne, M.P. and Telang, N.T. (1992). Antisense RNA to the putative tumor-suppressor gene DCC transforms rat-1 fibroblasts. Oncogene, 7, 553–561.

Nigro, J.M., Cho, K.R., Fearon, E.R., Kern, S.E., Ruppert, J.M., Oliner, J.D., Kinzler, K.W. and Vogelstein, B. (1991). Scrambled exons. Cell, 64, 607–613.

Cell Adhesion Regulator (*CMAR/CAR*)

The *CMAR/CAR* gene (chromosome 16q) encodes an 82 amino acid protein containing an N-terminal myristylation signal and a C-terminal tyrosine kinase phosphorylation consensus sequence that enhances cell attachment to collagen types I and IV and laminin (Pullman and

Bodmer, 1992). CAR is unrelated to any known integrins nor does it modulate the expression of integrin heterodimers. The high levels of allelic loss on 16q that occur in breast and prostate cancers indicate that *CAR* may be a tumour suppressor gene, its normal function being to repress tissue invasiveness.

Sequence of CMAR/CAR

```
(1)   MLRGSDMKGPCEPIVLSPAALSSSSLINGASQAQALGSGGLTTAPCCHVDWCKLRTSCWS
(60)  SHACSVGDALVFTALRIVEILY (82)
```

Underlined: myristylation site. Bold type: tyrosine phosphorylation site.

Paper

Pullman, W.E. and Bodmer, W.F. (1992). Cloning and characterization of a gene that regulates cell adhesion. Nature, 356, 529–532; correction ibid., 361, 564.

α-Inhibin (*INHA*)

Inhibin A and inhibin B are growth factors that suppress the secretion of follicle stimulating hormone (FSH). Both forms of inhibin contain an α subunit linked via one or more disulfide bridges to one of two types of β subunit (βA or βB).

Transgenic mice homozygous for the null allele of α-inhibin develop normally but all animals, both male and female, eventually develop mixed or incompletely differentiated gonadal stromal tumours (Matzuk *et al.*, 1992). Thus inhibin is not essential for normal sexual differentiation and development in the mouse but is a negative regulator of gonadal stromal cell proliferation.

Paper

Matzuk, M.M., Finegold, M.J., Su, J.-G.J., Hsueh, A.J.W. and Bradley, A. (1992). α-Inhibin is a tumour-suppressor gene with gonadal specificity in mice. Nature, 360, 313–319.

RNA-activated protein kinase (*PKR*)

PKR (also called PK_{ds}, p68, dsI, P1 kinase or dsRNA-activated inhibitor (DAI)) is a cytoplasmic, ribosome-associated enzyme that is activated by double-stranded RNA. PKR is activated by dsRNA produced during viral replication and it phosphorylates the initiation factor eIF-2, thereby inhibiting protein synthesis. A number of viral genomes encode RNAs or proteins that inhibit the activation of PKR (Imani and Jacobs, 1988; Gunnery *et al.*, 1990; Mathews and Shenk, 1991; Davies *et al.*, 1992). The overexpression of mutant, inactive PKR renders NIH 3T3 fibroblasts highly tumorigenic in nude mice (Koromilas *et al.*, 1992; Meurs *et al.*, 1992). This indicates that inactive *PKR* may function as a dominant negative tumour suppressor gene.

Review

Mathews, M.B. and Shenk, T. (1991). Adenovirus virus-associated RNA and translational control. J. Virol., 65, 5657–5662.

Papers

Imani, F. and Jacobs, B.L. (1988). Inhibitory activity for the interferon-induced protein kinase is associated with the reovirus serotype 1 σ3 protein. Proc. Natl Acad. Sci. USA, 85, 7887–7891.

Gunnery, S., Rice, A.P., Robertson, H.D. and Mathews, M.B. (1990). Tat-responsive region RNA of human immunodeficiency virus 1 can prevent activation of the double-stranded-RNA-activated protein kinase. Proc. Natl Acad. Sci. USA, 87, 8687–8691.

Davies, M.V., Elroy-Stein, O., Jagus, R., Moss, B. and Kaufman, R.J. (1992). The vaccinia virus K3L gene product potentiates translation by inhibiting double-stranded-RNA-activated protein kinase and phosphorylation of the alpha subunit of eukaryotic initiation factor 2. J. Virol., 66, 1943–1950.

Koromilas, A.E., Roy, S., Barber, G.N., Katze, M.G. and Sonenberg, N. (1992). Malignant transformation by a mutant of the IFN-inducible dsRNA-dependent protein kinase. Science, 257, 1685–1689.

Meurs, E.F., Galabru, J., Barber, G.N., Katze, M.G. and Hovanessian, A.G. (1992). Tumor suppressor function of the interferon-induced double-stranded RNA-activated protein kinase. Proc. Natl Acad. Sci. USA, 90, 232–236.

Metastasis Suppressor Genes (Cadherins, *TIMP, NME*)

A crucial step in the metastasis of tumour cells is the invasion of the basement membrane, which requires both adhesion by specific tumour cell surface proteins and enzymatic degradation of the underlying membrane.

Cadherins

Cadherins are a multigene family of transmembrane glycoproteins (125–140 kDa) that mediate Ca^{2+}-dependent intercellular adhesion and are thought to be essential for the control of morphogenetic processes, including myogenesis (Takeichi, 1991). The family includes B-cadherin, E-cadherin (also known as uvomorulin (*UVO*, chromosome 16q22.1), *Arc-1* or cell-CAM 120/80), EP-cadherin, M-cadherin, N-cadherin (A-CAM), P-cadherin, R-cadherin, T-cadherin, U-cadherin, cadherins 4–11 and L-CAM (Suzuki *et al.*, 1991). Cadherin function is regulated by cytoplasmic proteins including a vinculin-like protein, α-catenin (or CAP102), and β-catenin, a homologue of plakoglobulin (Knudsen and Wheelock, 1992).

The loss of cell–cell adhesion caused by the selective downregulation of E-cadherin expression can cause de-differentiation and invasiveness of human carcinoma cells. Impaired E-cadherin expression has been detected in 53% of a sample of primary breast cancers (Oka *et al.*, 1993) and human cell lines derived from bladder, breast (Sommers *et al.*, 1991), lung and pancreatic carcinomas that have an epithelioid phenotype, are non-invasive and express E-cadherin but those with a fibroblastoid phenotype are invasive and have lost E-cadherin expression. Invasiveness is blocked by transfection with E-cadherin cDNA and re-induced by treatment of the transfected cells with anti-E-cadherin monoclonal antibodies (Frixen *et al.*, 1991). E-Cadherin protein expression is also lost in primary hepatocellular carcinomas (Shimoyama and Hirohashi, 1991a), metastatic squamous cell carcinomas (Schipper *et al.*, 1991) and prostate cancers (Umbas *et al.*, 1992; Bussemakers *et al.*, 1992) and mRNA levels are lower in squamous cell carcinoma lines than in normal keratinocytes, whereas P-cadherin levels are similar (Nicholson *et al.*, 1991). In gastric carcinomas, however, P-cadherin expression is either downregulated or unstable whereas that of E-cadherin is normal (Shimoyama and Hirohashi, 1991b).

In vitro assays indicate that induction of high E-cadherin expression by transfection of cDNA into highly invasive epithelial tumour cell lines causes loss of invasiveness, and the expression of E-cadherin-specific antisense RNA in non-invasive *RAS*-transformed cells with high endogenous E-cadherin expression renders the cells invasive (Vleminckx *et al.*, 1991). Expression of E-cadherin inhibits the migration of cells into three-dimensional collagen gels (Chen and Obrink, 1991). v-*src* causes tyrosine phosphorylation of cadherin-associated proteins (catenins) that correlates with the metastatic potential of the transformed cells and may reflect the modulation of cell–cell adhesion by tyrosine phosphorylation of the cadherin–catenin system (Matsuyoshi *et al.*, 1992; Hamaguchi *et al.*, 1993). E-Cadherin thus appears to act as an invasion suppressor.

Tissue inhibitors of metalloproteinases (*TIMP*)

Cell lines with high metastatic capacity synthesize abnormally large amounts of matrix metalloproteinases (MMPs). The MMP family includes interstitial collagenase, type IV collagenases (progelatinases (72 and 92 kDa)) and stromelysin. These enzymes are secreted as zymogens and their active forms are subject to regulation by tissue inhibitors of metalloproteinases (TIMPs, 21/28 kDa) present in normal bone and cartilage cells and secreted by a variety of cells in culture. The transfection of Swiss 3T3 fibroblasts with a vector conferring constitutive expression of TIMP antisense deoxyoligonucleotide renders these cells tumorigenic and metastatic in mice (Khokha *et al.*, 1989) and transfection of tumour cells with a vector expressing TIMP-2 (Curry *et al.*, 1992) decreases the activity of secreted MMPs and the growth rate of the cells *in vivo* as well as suppressing the invasive capacity of the cells for surrounding tissue (DeClerck *et al.*, 1992; Khokha *et al.*, 1992). However, the expression of TIMP also increases transcription of several proteinases, of osteopontin and *Spp* and of the Ca^{2+} binding protein calcyclin (Khokha *et al.*, 1991), although the significance of these effects is unclear. TIMP-3 promotes the detachment of cells from the extracellular matrix and may promote the development of the transformed phenotype (Yang and Hawkes, 1992).

NM23–1/NME2 and *NM23–2/NME1*

The putative metastasis-suppressor genes *NME1* (non-metastatic cells 1, expressed) and *NME2* (formerly *NM23* (non-metastatic 23), chromosome 17q21.3) encode nucleoside diphosphate (NDP) kinases (17 kDa) expressed on the cell surface (Urano *et al.*, 1993). The concentration of NDP kinase A (encoded by human *NME1* and 88% identical to NDP kinase B (*NME2*)) increases in proliferating normal cells (Keim *et al.*, 1992) and reduced *NM23* expression correlates with high metastatic potential in some tumours and cell lines. The transfection of murine *Nm23-1* cDNA reduces primary tumour formation and metastasis *in vivo*. However, *NM23* expression is increased in some neoplastic tissues, although in ductal breast carcinomas this increase does not appear to correlate with tumour size, estrogen or progesterone receptor expression, lymph node metastases or other prognostic factors (Sastre-Garau *et al.*, 1992). Amplification and overexpression of *NM23* has been detected in childhood neuroblastomas, but this is accompanied by a point mutation in the gene (Leone *et al.*, 1993) and mutations have also been detected in colorectal adenocarcinoma (Wang *et al.*, 1993). The 17q21 region carries the locus for early onset familial breast and ovarian cancer (Hall *et al.*, 1990; Narod *et al.*, 1991) and several other genes involved in tumorigenesis, namely *HER2*, *HOX2*, *RARA*, *MYL* and *PHB* (Backer *et al.*, 1993).

Reviews

Nicolson, G.L. (1991). Gene expression, cellular diversification and tumor progression to the metastatic phenotype. BioEssays, 13, 337–342.

Takeichi, M. (1991). Cadherin cell adhesion receptors as a morphogenetic regulator. Science, 251, 1451–1455.

Papers

Backer, J.M., Mendola, C.E., Kovesdi, I., Fairhurst, J.L., O'Hara, B., Eddy, R.L., Shows, T.B., Mathew, S., Murty, V.V.V.S. and Chaganti, R.S.K. (1993). Chromosomal localization and nucleoside diphosphate kinase activity of human metastasis-suppressor genes *NM23–1* and *NM23–2*. Oncogene, 8, 497–502.

Bussemakers, M.J.G., van Moorselaar, R.J.A., Giroldi, L.A., Ichikawa, T., Isaacs, J.T., Takeichi, M., Debruyne, F.M.J. and Schacker, J.A. (1992). Decreased expression of E-cadherin in the progression of rat prostatic cancer. Cancer Res., 52, 2916–2922.

Chen, W.C. and Obrink, B. (1991). Cell–cell contacts mediated by E-cadherin (uvomorulin) restrict invasive behavior of L-cells. J. Cell. Biol., 114, 319–327.

Curry, V.A., Clark, I.M., Bigg, H. and Cawston, T.E. (1992). Large inhibitor of metalloproteinases (LIMP) contains tissue inhibitor of metalloproteinases (TIMP)-2 bound to 72000-*Mr* progelatinase. Biochem. J., 285, 143–147.

DeClerck, Y.A., Perez, N., Shimada, H., Boone, T.C., Langley, K.E. and Taylor, S.M. (1992). Inhibition of invasion and metastasis in cells transfected with an inhibitor of metalloproteinases. Cancer Res., 52, 701–708.

Frixen, U.H., Behrens, J., Sachs, M., Eberle, G., Voss, B., Warda, A., Lochner, D. and Birchmeier, W. (1991). E-Cadherin-mediated cell–cell adhesion prevents invasiveness of human carcinoma cells. J. Cell Biol., 113, 173–185.

Hall, J.M., Lee, M.K., Newman, B., Morrow, J.E., Anderson, L.A., Huey, B. and King, M.-C. (1990). Linkage of early-onset familial breast cancer to chromosome 17q21. Science, 250, 1684–1689.

Hamaguchi, M., Matsuyoshi, N., Ohnishi, Y., Gotoh, B., Takeichi, M. and Nagai, Y. (1993). p60[v-src] causes tyrosine phosphorylation and inactivation of the N-cadherin-catenin cell adhesion system. EMBO J., 12, 307–314.

Keim, D., Hailat, N., Melhem, R., Zhu, X.X., Lascu, I., Veron, M. and Strahler, J. (1992). Proliferation-related expression of p19/nm23 nucleoside diphosphate kinase. J. Clin. Invest., 89, 919–924.

Khokha, R., Waterhouse, P., Yagel, S., Lala, P.K., Overall, C.M., Norton, G. and Denhardt, D.T. (1989). Antisense RNA-induced reduction in murine TIMP levels confers oncogenicity on Swiss 3T3 cells. Science, 243, 947–950.

Khokha, R., Waterhouse, P., Lala, P.K., Zimmer, M.J. and Denhardt, D.T. (1991). Increased proteinase expression during during tumor progression of tissue inhibitor of metalloproteinases cell lines down-modulated for levels: a new transformation paradigm? J. Cancer Res. Clin. Oncol., 117, 333–338.

Khokha, R., Zimmer, M.J., Graham, C.H., Lala, P.K. and Waterhouse, P. (1992). Suppression of invasion by inducible expression of tissue inhibitor of metalloproteinase-1 (TIMP-1) in B16-F10 melanoma cells. J. Natl Cancer Inst., 84, 1017–1022.

Knudsen, K.A. and Wheelock, M.J. (1992). Plakoglobulin, or an 83-kD homologue distinct from β-catenin, interacts with E-cadherin and N-cadherin. J. Cell Biol., 118, 671–679.

Leone, A., Seeger, R.C., Hong, C.M., Hu, Y.Y., Arboleda, M.J., Brodeur, G.M., Stram, D., Slamon, D.J. and Steeg, P.S. (1993). Evidence for *nm23* RNA overexpression, DNA amplification and mutation in aggressive childhood neuroblastomas. Oncogene, 8, 855–865.

Matsuyoshi, N., Hamaguchi, M., Taniguchi, S., Nagafuchi, A., Tsukita, S. and Takeichi, M. (1992). Cadherin-mediated cell-cell adhesion is perturbed by v-*src* tyrosine phosphorylation in metastatic fibroblasts. J. Cell Biol., 118, 703–714.

Narod, S.A., Feunteun, J., Lynch, H.T., Watson, P., Conway, T., Lynch, J. and Lenoir, G.M. (1991). Familial breast–ovarian cancer locus on chromosome 17q12-q23. Lancet, 338, 82–83.

Nicholson, L.J., Pei, X.F. and Watt, F.M. (1991). Expression of E-cadherin, P-cadherin and involucrin by normal and neoplastic keratinocytes in culture. Carcinogenesis, 12, 1345–1349.

Oka, H., Shiozaki, H., Kobayashi, K., Inoue, M., Tahara, H., Kobayashi, T., Takatsuka, Y., Matsuyoshi, N., Hirano, S., Takeichi, M. and Mori, T. (1993). Expression of E-cadherin cell adhesion molecules in human breast cancer tissues and its relationship to metastasis. Cancer Res., 53, 1696–1701.

Sastre-Garau, X., Lacombe, M.-L., Jouve, M., Veron, M. and Magdelenat, H. (1992). Nucleoside diphosphate kinase/NM23 expression in breast cancer: lack of correlation with lymph-node metastasis. Int. J. Cancer, 50, 533–538.

Schipper, J.H., Frixen, U.H., Behrens, J., Unger, A., Jahnke, K. and Birchmeier, W. (1991). E-cadherin expression in squamous cell carcinomas of head and neck: inverse correlation with tumor dedifferentiation and lymph node metastasis. Cancer Res., 51, 6328–6337.

Shimoyama, Y. and Hirohashi, S. (1991a). Cadherin intercellular adhesion molecule in hepatocellular carcinomas: loss of E-cadherin expression in an undifferentiated carcinoma. Cancer Lett., 57, 131–135.

Shimoyama, Y. and Hirohashi, S. (1991b). Expression of E- and P-cadherin in gastric carcinomas. Cancer Res., 51, 2185–2192.

Sommers, C.L., Thompson, E.W., Torri, J.A., Kemler, R., Gelmann, E.P. and Byers, S.W. (1991). Cell adhesion molecule uvomorulin expression in human breast cancer cell lines: relationship to morphology and invasive capacities. Cell Growth Differ., 2, 365–372.

Suzuki, S., Sano, K. and Tanihara, H. (1991). Diversity of the cadherin family: evidence for eight new cadherins in nervous tissue. Cell. Regul., 2, 261–270.

Umbas, R., Schalken, J.A., Aalders, T.W., Carter, B.S., Karthaus, H.F.M., Schaafsma, H.E., Debruyne, F.M.J. and Isaacs, W.B. (1992). Expression of the cellular adhesion molecule E-cadherin is reduced or absent in high-grade prostate cancer. Cancer Res., 52, 5104–5109.

Urano, T., Furukawa, K. and Shiku, H. (1993). Expression of nm23/NDP proteins on the cell surface. Oncogene, 8, 1371–1376.

Vleminckx, K., Vakaet, L., Mareel, M., Fiers, W. and van Roy, F. (1991). Genetic manipulation of E-cadherin expression by epithelial tumor cells reveals an invasion suppressor role. Cell, 66, 107–119.

Wang, L., Patel, U., Ghosh, C., Chen, H.-C. and Banerjee, S. (1993). Mutation in the nm23 gene is associated with metastasis in colorectal cancer. Cancer Res., 53, 717–720.

Yang, T.-T. and Hawkes, S.P. (1992). Role of the 21-kDa protein TIMP-3 in oncogenic transformation of cultured chicken embryo fibroblasts. Proc. Natl Acad. Sci. USA, 89, 10676–10680.

Integrins

The integrins are a family of cell-surface proteins that mediate cell–substratum and cell–cell adhesion. Integrins are heterodimers of non-covalently linked α and β subunits, each of which is a transmembrane protein. Eleven α and six β subunits have been identified that give rise to at least 16 distinct integrins and, in addition, a single α or β subunit can associate with more than one β or α chain, respectively. Although no integrin has yet been shown to be a tumour suppressor gene, they mediate some of the processes involved in metastasis and changes in integrin expression accompany malignant transformation (Plantefaber and Hynes, 1989). However, thus far it has been difficult to discern correlations between altered patterns of integrin expression and tumorigenicity.

In some cells in vivo tumorigenicity is reduced by the expression of the $\alpha_5\beta_1$ integrin (fibronectin) receptor (Giancotti and Ruoslahti, 1990). However, the capacity of human lung adenocarcinoma cells to adhere to endothelial cells is increased when the latter are treated with interleukin-1. This increases the expression of both the fibronectin receptor and the vitronectin receptor ($\alpha_v\beta_3$ integrin) and the latter appears to be responsible for the increased adhesiveness of the cells (Lafrenie et al., 1992).

Human melanoma cells are stimulated to proliferate by fibronectin acting via the $\alpha_5\beta_1$ receptor (Mortarini et al., 1992). The tumorigenicity of these cells correlates with the expression of $\alpha_v\beta_3$ integrin (Marshall et al., 1991). The invasiveness in vitro of human melanoma cells is inhibited by antibody directed against $\alpha_v\beta_3$ integrin that also inhibits the adhesive activity of the receptor (Seftor et al., 1992). However, an anti-α_v antibody that does not affect adhesive capacity also promotes invasion, as does the ligand vitronectin. This suggests that ligation of the vitronectin receptor activates a cellular response that promotes invasion by melanoma cells through the basement membrane matrices, a conclusion consistent with the finding that these cells increase secretion of type IV collagenase in response to $\alpha_v\beta_3$ antibody.

In primary breast carcinomas the expression of $\alpha_6\beta_4$ integrin is either reduced or modulated such that the polarized pattern of distribution at the basolateral aspect of the epithelium occurring in normal tissue is lost (Natali et al., 1992). The expression of a functional $\alpha_2\beta_1$ integrin receptor in rhabdomyosarcoma cells correlates with increased formation of metastatic tumours in nude mice (Chan et al., 1991) and there is evidence that the expression of integrin β_3 correlates with melanoma metastasis (Albeda et al., 1990). In human E1A-transformed tumour cells the overexpression of active $TGF\beta_1$ enhances the tumorigenicity of the cells in nude mice and causes increased adhesiveness in vitro that correlates with the increased expression of $\alpha_1\beta_1$, $\alpha_2\beta_1$ and $\alpha_3\beta_1$ integrins, all of which recognize laminin (Arrick et al., 1992).

The aggregation of platelets mediated by the binding of fibrinogen to $\alpha_{IIb}\beta_3$ integrin stimulates the tyrosine phosphorylation and kinase activity of p125^{FAK} (Lipfert et al., 1992) and p125^{FAK} phosphorylation has been observed in a variety of other types of cells undergoing attachment to extracellular matrix proteins (Burridge et al., 1992; Guan and Shalloway, 1992; Hanks et al., 1992; Kornberg et al., 1992). p125^{FAK} is also activated by v-src transformation and by a number of normal growth factors, including bombesin, vasopressin or endothelin (Zachary et al., 1992) but not by oncogenic Ras (Guan and Shalloway, 1992). Thus pp125^{FAK} and truncated forms of FAK termed FRNK (FAK-related non-kinase), both of which are localized in focal adhesions (Schaller et al., 1993), may mediate signals initiated by integrin-dependent cell adhesion and by growth factors as well as providing a cytoplasmic target for tyrosine kinase oncoproteins.

Review

Hynes, R.O. (1992). Integrins: versatility, modulation, and signaling in cell adhesion. Cell, 69, 11–25.
Pigott, R. and Power, C. (1993). The Adhesion Molecule FactsBook. Academic Press, London.

Papers

Albeda, S.M., Mette, S.A., Elder, D.E., Stewart, R., Damjanovich, L., Herlyn, M. and Buck, C.A. (1990). Integrin distribution in malignant melanoma: association of the β_3 subunit with tumor progression. Cancer Res., 50, 6757–6764.

Arrick, B.A., Lopez, A.R., Elfman, F., Ebner, R., Damsky, C.H. and Derynck, R. (1992). Altered metabolic and adhesive properties and increased tumorigenesis associated with increased expression of transforming growth factor β1. J. Cell Biol., 118, 715–726.

Burridge, K., Turner, C.E. and Romer, L.H. (1992). Tyrosine phosphorylation of paxillin and pp125FAK accompanies cell adhesion to extracellular matrix: a role in cytoskeletal assembly. J. Cell. Biol., 119, 893–903.

Chan, B.M.C., Matsuura, N., Takada, Y., Zetter, B.R. and Hemler, M.E. (1991). In vitro and in vivo consequences of VLA-2 expression on rhabdomyosarcoma cells. Science, 251, 1600–1602.

Giancotti, F.G. and Ruoslahti, E. (1990). Elevated levels of the $\alpha_5\beta_1$ fibronectin receptor suppress the transformed phenotype of Chinese hamster ovary cells. Cell, 60, 849–859.

Guan, J.-L. and Shalloway, D. (1992). Regulation of focal adhesion-associated protein tyrosine kinase by both cellular adhesion and oncogenic transformation. Nature, 358, 690–692.

Hanks, S.K., Calalb, M.B., Harper, M.C. and Patel, S.K. (1992). Focal adhesion protein-tyrosine kinase phosphorylated in response to cell attachment to fibronectin. Proc. Natl Acad. Sci. USA, 89, 8487–8491.

Kornberg, L., Earp, H.S., Parsons, J.T., Schaller, M. and Juliano, R.L. (1992). Cell adhesion or integrin clustering increases phosphorylation of a focal-adhesion associated tyrosine kinase. J. Biol. Chem., 267, 23439–23442.

Lafrenie, R.M., Podor, T.J., Buchanan, M.R. and Orr, F.W. (1992). Up-regulated biosynthesis and expression of endothelial cell vitronectin receptor enhances cancer cell adhesion. Cancer Res., 52, 2202–2208.

Lipfert, L., Haimovich, B., Schaller, M.D., Cobb, B.S., Parsons, J.T. and Brugge, J.S. (1992). Integrin-dependent phosphorylation and activation of the protein tyrosine kinase pp125^{FAK} in platelets. J. Cell. Biol., 119, 905–912.

Marshall, J.F., Nesbitt, S.A., Helfrich, M.H., Horton, M.A., Polakova, K. and Hart, I.R. (1991). Integrin expression in human melanoma cell lines: heterogeneity of vitronectin receptor composition and function. Int. J. Cancer, 49, 924–931.

Mortarini, R., Gismondi, A., Santoni, A., Parmiani, G. and Anichini, A. (1992). Role of the $\alpha_5\beta_1$ integrin receptor in the proliferative response of quiescent human melanoma cells to fibronectin. Cancer Res., 52, 4499–4506.

Natali, P.G., Nicotra, M.R., Botti, C., Mottolese, M., Bigotti, A. and Segatto, O. (1992). Changes in expression of α_6/β_4 integrin heterodimer in primary and metastatic breast cancer. Brit. J. Cancer, 66, 318–322.

Plantefaber, L.C. and Hynes, R.O. (1989). Changes in integrin receptors on oncogenically transformed cells. Cell, 56, 281–290.

Schaller, M.D., Borgman, C.A. and Parsons, J.T. (1993). Autonomous expression of a noncatalytic domain of the focal adhesion-associated protein tyrosine kinase pp125[FAK]. Mol. Cell. Biol., 13, 785–791.

Seftor, R.E.B., Seftor, E.A., Gehlsen, K.R., Stetler-Stevenson, W.G., Brown, P.D., Ruoslahti, E. and Hendrix, M.J.C. (1992). Role of the $\alpha_v\beta_3$ integrin in human melanoma cell invasion. Proc. Natl Acad. Sci. USA, 89, 1557–1561.

Zachary, I., Sinnett-Smith, J. and Rozengurt, E. (1992). Bombesin, vasopressin, and endothelin stimulation of tyrosine phosphorylation in Swiss 3T3 cells. J. Biol. Chem., 267, 19031–19034.

Prohibitin

The prohibitin gene (*PHB*) encodes a mammalian anti-proliferative protein (Nuell *et al.*, 1991) and maps to human chromosome 17q21. The gene is mutated in some sporadic breast cancers that show loss of heterozygosity on 17q and may be a tumour suppressor gene (Sato *et al.*, 1992).

Papers

Nuell, M.J., Stewart, D.A., Walker, L., Friedman, V., Wood, C.M., Owens, G.A., Smith, J.R., Schneider, E.L., Dell'Orco, R., Lumpkin, C.K., Danner, D.B. and McClung, J.K. (1991). Prohibitin, an evolutionarily conserved intracellular protein that blocks DNA synthesis in normal fibroblasts and HeLa cells. Mol. Cell. Biol., 11, 1372–1381.

Sato, T., Saito, H., Swensen, J., Olifant, A., Wood, C., Danner, D., Sakamoto, T., Takita, K., Kasumi, F., Miki, Y., Skolnick, M. and Nakamura, Y. (1992). The human prohibitin gene located on chromosome 17q21 is mutated in sporadic breast cancer. Cancer Res., 52, 1643–1646.

WNT1/WNT3

Wnt-1/Int-1 was originally identified as a frequent target for MMTV insertion in mammary carcinomas (Nusse and Varmus, 1982). *Int-2* (Peters *et al.*, 1983) and *Int-3* are additional, unrelated mouse genes activated by MMTV proviral insertion (see Table 2.2). *Wnt-3* is related to *Wnt-1* and also activated by proviral insertion (Roelink *et al.*, 1990). The known related human genes are *WNT1*, *WNT2* and *WNT3*.

Related genes

There are at least 10 genes in the mouse *Wnt-1/Int-1* family (Nusse and Varmus, 1992). On the basis of their similarity to the *Drosophila melanogaster vingless* gene product (Rijsewijk *et al.*, 1987a), *Int-1* and related genes have been re-classified as *Wnt* (*wingless*-type MMTV integration site; Nusse *et al.*, 1991). In addition to *Wnt-1*, *Wnt-2* (Int-1 related protein, *Irp*) and *Wnt-3* (see below), this family includes *Wnt-3A* (chromosome 11), *Wnt-4* (chromosome 4), *Wnt-5A* (chromosome 14), *Wnt-5B* (chromosome 6), *Wnt-6* (chromosome 1), *Wnt-7A* (chromosome 6) and *Wnt-7B* c (chromosome 15).

The murine WNT proteins share many structural features and are between 50% and 85% identical in sequence with the exception of the most divergent, WNT1, that is 38% identical to WNT2.

At least 12 *Xenopus laevis Xwnt* genes have been detected (Noordermeer *et al.*, 1989; Christian *et al.*, 1991; Wolda and Moon, 1992) and a homologue of *Wnt-5B* has been detected in *Caenorhabditis elegans* (Waterston *et al.*, 1992).

Cross-species homology

WNT1: 99% identity (human and mouse). WNT2: 97% identity (human and mouse). All known members of the WNT family contain 22 absolutely conserved cysteine residues (see **Protein structure**, below).

Transformation

MAN

WNT1 is amplified in some primary retinoblastoma tumours (Arheden *et al.*, 1988). Amplification or rearrangement of *WNT1* has not been detected in human breast carcinomas, even in samples in which amplification of *INT2*, *MYC* or *HER2* occurs (Meyers *et al.*, 1990).

ANIMALS

Wnt-1/Int-1 and *Int-2* are the most frequent targets in MMTV-induced tumours (see Table 2.2). Either *Wnt-1* or *Int-2* or both may be activated (Gray *et al.*, 1986) and insertion at each site has been detected in both pre-malignant lesions and in malignant tumours (Morris *et al.*, 1990). The frequency with which the *Wnt-1* and *Int-2* loci are rearranged by MMTV insertional mutagenesis is a function of the host genetic background (Escot *et al.*, 1986; Etkind, 1989; Marchetti *et al.*, 1991). Thus in the C3H mouse strain *Int-1* and *Int-2* rearrangements occur in 80% and 10% of tumours, respectively, whereas in GR strain tumours the corresponding figures are 25% and 44%. This indicates that strains inbred for a high incidence of mammary tumours have acquired host mutations that complement the activity of specific *Wnt/Int* genes. It has been found that 5% of mammary tumours induced in GR strain mice contain a provirus at *Wnt-3* (Roelink *et al.*, 1990). In transplants of mammary tumours from GR mice, *Wnt-3* can become activated in clones that no longer express *Wnt-1* or *Int-2* (Roelink *et al.*, 1992). Hormone-independent tumours derived in a similar manner may contain an amplified and overexpressed *Wnt-2* gene.

IN VITRO

Wnt-1 transforms fibroblasts with very low efficiency but expression of the gene by fibroblasts causes morphological transformation of co-cultured mammary epithelial cells (Jue *et al.*, 1992). Thus WNT1 protein may participate in a paracrine mechanism.

Wnt-1 partially transforms the C57 mammary epithelial cell line (Blasband *et al.*, 1992) and renders the RAC mammary cell line tumorigenic (Rijsewijk *et al.*, 1987b).

TRANSGENIC ANIMALS

Wnt-1 causes hyperplasia in the mammary glands of male and female mice which can progress to mammary and salivary adenocarcinomas (Tsukamoto *et al.*, 1988; Edwards *et al.*, 1992). Bi-transgenic mice carrying both *Wnt-1* and *Int-2* transgenes regulated by the MMTV LTR develop mammary carcinomas more rapidly and with higher frequency than when either gene is expressed alone (Kwan *et al.*, 1992). This indicates that *Wnt-1* and *Int-2* cooperate in mammary tumorigenesis.

	WNT1/Wnt-1 (INT1/Int-1)	WNT2/Wnt-2 (IRP/Irp)	WNT3/Wnt-3 (INT4/Int-4
Nucleotides (kb)	30		>50
Chromosome			
Human	12q13	7q31	17q21–q22
Mouse	15		11
Exons	4		5
mRNA (kb)	2.6		3.8
Amino acids			
Human	370	360	
Mouse	370	360	355
Mass (kDa)			
(predicted)	40	41	40
(expressed)	gp44	gp35	

Cellular location

Wnt-1 encodes a secreted glycoprotein (Papkoff and Schryver, 1990). The *Drosophila wingless* gene product has been detected in the intercellular space in *Drosophila* embryos (Van den Heuvel *et al.*, 1989).

Tissue location

All murine *Wnt* genes are expressed in a variety of embryonic and adult tissues, particularly in brain and lung. *Wnt-1* is also expressed in the adult testis (Jakobovits *et al.*, 1986). *Wnt-3* is expressed in mouse embryos and in the adult mouse brain (Roelink *et al.*, 1990).

Protein function

Secreted WNT1 glycoprotein binds to the extracellular matrix (van Ooyen and Nusse, 1984; Papkoff and Schryver, 1990). Secretion of WNT1 is inefficient and substantial amounts are present in the endoplasmic reticulum associated with Bip (Kitajewski *et al.*, 1992). It is probably a growth factor but its receptor is unknown. Normal function is in embryogenesis: in the mouse it is required for development of the mid-brain and anterior hindbrain.

In PC12 cells *Wnt-1* expression enhances cell–cell adhesion and correlates with increased expression of E-cadherin and plakoglobulin and decreased expression of N-CAM.

Expression of *Wnt-1* in embryos can reproduce the effects of lithium treatment, suggesting that WNT-1 may modulate the way cells respond to inducing agents by suppressing the concentration of phosphoinositides available to generate second messenger signals (Sokol *et al.*, 1991; Olson *et al.*, 1991).

These observations are generally consistent with the evidence that *Drosophila* and *Xenopus* wnt genes are involved in the generation of the central nervous system (Christian *et al.*, 1991).

Wnt-1 gene structure

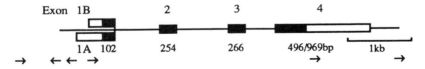

The sequence and organization of the *Wnt-1* gene is highly conserved in organisms ranging from man to *Drosophila*. The conservation between human *WNT1* and mouse *Wnt-1* includes extensive intronic regions as well as 5′ and 3′ non-translated regions (van Ooyen *et al.*, 1985).

The 5′ exon has two forms (1A and 1B) with identical 3′ ends but different 5′ ends, the start site of exon 1A being 160 nucleotides 5′ of that for 1B (Nusse *et al.*, 1990). There are two TATA boxes upstream of the 1B start site at –35 and –25. The region upstream of 1A contains no TATA boxes but is very GC-rich and includes at least two Sp-1 binding sites.

Arrows indicate integrations sites and orientations of MMTV proviruses in a variety of tumours, the majority being orientated away from *Wnt-1*. For *Wnt-1*, *Int-2*, *Hst-1* and *Int-4* proviral integration of MMTV does not perturb the DNA encoding these genes (Roelink *et al.*, 1990; Peters *et al.*, 1989). For *Wnt-1*, when the insertion site of MMTV is outside the immediate vicinity of the *Wnt-1* promoter, the two start sites of transcription are quantitatively unaffected.

When insertion replaces the *Wnt-1* promoters with proviral DNA, read-through over the right MMTV LTR into the *Wnt-1* gene generates transcripts of 10.0 and 6.0 kb. However, the normal *Wnt-1* 2.6 kb transcript is still produced as a consequence of start in the right LTR and gives rise to the normal WNT1 protein.

The structure of *Wnt-3* is similar to that of *Wnt-1*. All introns are at homologous positions compared with *Wnt-1* except for a unique intron before a fifth exon that is completely non-coding (Roelink *et al.*, 1990).

Protein structure

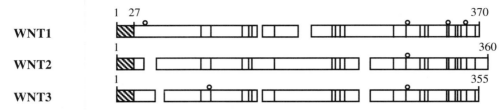

The vertical bars represent the 22 cysteine residues conserved throughout the WNT family. Circles indicate potential *N*-glycosylation sites. The cross-hatched box indicates the signal sequence.

Sequence of human WNT1 (INT1)

```
  (1)  MGLWALLPGWVSATLLLALAALPAALAANSSGRWWGIVNVASSTNLLTDSKSLQLVLE
 (60)  SLQLLSRKQRRLIRQNPGILHSVSGGLQSAVRECKWQFRNRRWNCPTAPGPHLFGKIVNR
(120)  GCRETAFIFAITSAGVTHSVARSCSEGSIESCTCDYRRRGPGGPDWHWGGCSDNIDFGRL
(180)  FGREFVDSGEKGRDLRFLMNLHNNEAGRTTVFSEMRQECKCHGMSGSCTVRTCWMRLPTL
(240)  RAVGDVLRDRFDGASRVLYGNRGSNRASRAELLRLEPEDPAHKPPSPHDLVYFEKSPNFC
(300)  TYSGRLGTAGTAGRACNSSSPALDGCELLCCGRGHRTRTQRVTERCNCTFHWCCHVSCRN
(360)  CTHTRVLHECL (370)
```

Sequence is identical to that of mouse WNT1 (INT1) except that the substitutions of S for G, T for A, T for A and I for V occur in the mouse protein at amino acids 9, 13, 20 and 40, respectively. The signal sequence is underlined.

Sequences of human and mouse WNT2

```
Human WNT2    (1)  MNAPLGGIWLWLPLLLTWLTPEVNSSWWYMRATGGSSRVMCDNVPGLVSSQRQLCHRHP
Mouse WNT2         --V-------------------S-----------------------------------

            (60)  DVMRAISQGVAEWTAECQHQFRQHRWNCNTLDRDHSLFGRVLLRSSRESAFVYAISSAGV
                  ------GL--------------------------------------------------

           (120)  VFAITRACSQGEVKSCSCDPKKMGSAKDSKGIFDWGGCSDNIDYGIKFARAFVDAKERKG
                  -----------L---------K-------T----------------------------

           (180)  KDARALMNLHNNRAGRKAVKRFLKQECKCHGVSGSCTLRTCWLAMADFRKTGDYLWRKYN
                  ---------------------------------------------------E-------

           (240)  GAIQVVMNQDGTGFTVANERFKKPTKNDLVYFENSPDYCIRDREAGSLGTAGRVCNLTSR
                  ----------------K-----------------------------------------

           (300)  GMDSCEVMCCGRGYDTSHVTRMTKCGCKFHWCCAVRCQDCLEALDVHTCKAPKNADWTTAT (360)
                  -----------------------E---------------------------S---A-P- (360)
```

Dashes indicate identical amino acids.

Sequence of mouse WNT3

```
  (1)  MEPHLLGLLLGLLLSGTRVLAGYPIWWSLALGQQYTSLASQPLLCGSIPGLVPKQLRFC
 (60)  RNYIEIMPSVAEGVKLGIQECQHQFRGRRWNCTTIDDSLAIFGPVLDKATRESAFVHAIA
(120)  SAGVAFAVTRSCAEGTSTICGCDSHHKGPPGEGWKWGGCSEDADFGVLVSREFADARENR
(180)  PDARSAMNKHNNEAGRTTILDHMHLKCKCHGLSGSCEVKTCWWAQPDFRAIGDFLKDKYD
(240)  SASEMVVEKHRESRGWVETLRAKYALFKPPTERDLVYYENSPNFCEPNPETGSFGTRDRT
(300)  CNVTSHGIDGCDLLCCGRGHNTRTEKRKEKCHCVFHWCCYVSCQECIRIYDVHTCK(355)
```

The potential signal sequence is underlined.

Databank file names and accession numbers

	GENE	EMBL	SWISSPROT	REFERENCES
Human	WNT1 (INT1)	Hsint1g X03072	WNT1_HUMAN P04628	Van Ooyen et al., 1985 Nusse et al., 1990
Human	WNT2	Hsirp X07876	WNT2_HUMAN P09544	Wainwright et al., 1988
	(IRP: INT1 related protein)			
Mouse	Wnt-1 (Int-1)	Mmint1m M11943	WNT1_MOUSE P04426	Van Ooyen and Nusse, 1984
		Mmint1 M34750, K02593		Fung et al., 1985
Mouse	Wnt-2		WNT2_MOUSE P21552	McMahon and McMahon, 1989
				Gavin et al., 1990
Mouse	Wnt-3	Int4 M32502	WNT3_MOUSE P17553	Roelink et al., 1990
Xenopus	Xwnt-3	Xlxwnt3a M55054		Noordermeer et al., 1989
	Xwnt-4	Xlxwnt4a M55055		Christian et al., 1991
	Xwnt-5A	Xlxwnt5aa M55056		Wolda and Moon, 1992
	Xwnt-8	Xlxwnt8 X57234		
	Xwnt-8A	Xlxwnt8a M55058		
Caenorhabditis elegans	Wnt-5B	ce9h7 Z14953		Waterston et al., 1992

Review

Nusse, R. and Varmus, H.E. (1992). *wnt* genes. Cell, 69, 1073–1087.

Peters, G. (1991). Inappropriate expression of growth factor genes in tumors induced by mouse mammary tumor virus. Seminars Virol., 2, 319–328.

Papers

Arheden, K., Tommerup, N., Mandahl, N., Heim, S., Winther, J., Jensen, O.A., Prause, J.U. and Mitelman, F. (1988). Amplification of the human putative oncogene INT1 in primary retinoblastoma tumors. Cytogen. Cell Genet., 48, 174–177.

Blasband, A., Schryver, B. and Papkoff, J. (1992). The biochemical properties and transforming potential of human *wnt-2* are similar to *wnt-1*. Oncogene, 7, 153–161.

Christian, J.L., Gavin, B.J., McMahon, A.P. and Moon, R.T. (1991). Isolation of cDNAs partially encoding four *Xenopus wnt-1/int-1*-related proteins and characterization of their transient expression during embryonic development. Devel. Biol., 143, 230–234.

Edwards, P.A.W., Hiby, S.E., Papkoff, J. and Bradbury, J.M. (1992). Hyperplasia of mouse mammary epithelium induced by expression of the *wnt-1* (*int-1*) oncogene in reconstituted mammary gland. Oncogene, 7, 2041–2051.

Escot, C., Hogg, E. and Callahan, R. (1986). Mammary tumorigenesis in feral *Mus cervicolor popaeus*. J. Virol., 58, 619–625.

Etkind, P., (1989). Expression of the *int-1* and *int-2* loci in endogenous mouse mammary tumor virus-induced mammary tumorigenesis in the C3Hf mouse. J. Virol., 63, 4972–4975.

Fung, Y.K.T., Shackleford, G.M., Brown, A.M.C., Sanders, G.S. and Varmus, H.E. (1985). Nucleotide sequence and expression in vitro of cDNA derived from mRNA of *int-1*, a provirally activated mouse mammary oncogene. Mol. Cell. Biol., 5, 3337–3344.

Gavin, B.J., McMahon, J.A. and McMahon, A.P. (1990). Expression of multiple novel *wnt-1/int-1*-related genes during fetal and adult mouse development. Genes Devel., 4, 2319–2332.

Gray, D.A., Jackson, D.P., Percy, D.H. and Morris, V.L. (1986). Activation of *int-1* and *int-2* loci in GRf mammary tumors. Virology, 154, 271–278.

Jakobovits, A., Shackelford, G.M., Varmus, H.E. and Martin, G.R. (1986). Two protooncogenes implicated in mammary carcinogenesis, int-1 and int-2, are independently regulated during mouse development. Proc. Natl Acad. Sci. USA, 83, 7806–7810.

Jue, S.F., Bradley, R.S., Rudnicki, J.A., Varmus, H.E. and Brown, A.M.C. (1992). The mouse *wnt-1* gene can act via a paracrine mechanism in transformation of mammary epithelial cells. Mol. Cell. Biol., 12, 321–328.

Kitajewski, J., Mason, J.O. and Varmus, H.E. (1992). Interaction of *wnt-1* proteins with the binding protein BiP. Mol. Cell. Biol., 12, 784–790.

Kwan, H., Pecenka, V., Tsukamoto, A., Parslow, T.G., Guzman, R., Lin, T.-P., Muller, W.J., Lee, F.S., Leder, P. and Varmus, H.E. (1992). Transgenes expressing the *wnt-1* and *int-2* proto-oncogene cooperate during mammary carcinogenesis in doubly transgenic mice. Mol. Cell. Biol., 12, 147–154.

McMahon, J.A. and McMahon, A.P. (1989). Nucleotide sequence, chromosomal localization and developmental expression of the mouse *int-1*-related gene. Development, 107, 643–650.

Marchetti., A., Robbins, J., Campbell, G., Buttitta, F., Squartini, F., Bistocchi, M. and Callanhan, R. (1991). Host genetic background effect on the frequency of mouse mammary tumor virus-induced rearrangements of the *int-1* and *int-2* loci in mouse mammary tumors. J. Virol., 65, 4550–4554.

Meyers, S.L., O'Brien, M.T., Smith, T. and Dudley, J.P. (1990). Analysis of the *int-1*, *int-2*, c-*myc*, and *neu* oncogenes in human breast carcinomas. Cancer Res., 50, 5911–5918.

Molven, A., Njolstad, P.R. and Fjose, A. (1991). Genomic structure and restricted neural expression of the zebrafish *wnt-1* (*int-1*) gene. EMBO J., 10, 799–807.

Morris, D.W., Barry, P.A., Bradshaw, H.D.J. and Cardiff, R.D. (1990). Insertion mutation of the *int-1* and *int-2* loci by mouse mammary tumor virus in premalignant and malignant neoplasms from the GR mouse strain. J. Virol., 64, 1794–1802.

Noordermeer, J., Meijlink, F., Verrijzer, P., Rijsewijk, F. and Destree, O. (1989). Isolation of the *Xenopus* homolog of *int-1/wingless* and expression during neurula stages of early development. Nucleic Acids Res., 17, 11–18.

Nusse, R. and Varmus, H.E. (1982). Many tumors induced by the mouse mammary tumor virus contain a provirus integrated in the same region of the host genome. Cell, 31, 99–109.

Nusse, R., van Ooyen, A., Cox, D., Fung, Y.K.T. and Varmus, H.E. (1984). Mode of proviral activation of a putative mammary oncogene (*int-1*) on mouse chromosome 15. Nature, 307, 131–136.

Nusse R., Theunissen, H., Wagenaar, E., Rijsewijk, F., Gennissen, A., Otte, A., Schuuring, E. and van Ooyen, A. (1990). The *wnt-1* (*int-1*) oncogene promoter and its mechanism of activation by insertion of proviral DNA of the mouse mammary tumor virus. Mol. Cell. Biol., 10, 4170–4179.

Nusse, R. Brown, A., Papkoff, J., Scambler, P., Shackleford, G., McMahon, A., Moon, R. and Varmus, H.E. (1991). A new nomenclature for *int-1* and related genes: the *Wnt* gene family. Cell, 64, 231.

Olson, D.J., Christian, J.L. and Moon, R.T. (1991). Effect of Wnt-1 and related proteins on gap junction communication in *Xenopus* embryos. Science, 252, 1173–1176.

Papkoff, J. and Schryver, B. (1990). Secreted *int-1* protein is associated with the cell surface. Mol. Cell. Biol., 10, 2723–2730.

Pathak, V.K., Strange, R., Young, L.J.T., Morris, D.W. and Cardiff, R.D. (1987). Survey of *int* region DNA rearrangements in C3H and BALB/cfc3H mouse mammry tumor system. J. Natl Cancer Inst., 78, 327–331.

Peters, G., Brookes, S., Smith, R. and Dickson, C. (1983). Tumorigenesis by mouse mammary tumor virus: evidence for a common region for provirus integration in mammary tumors. Cell, 33, 369–377.

Peters, G., Kozak, C. and Dickson, C. (1984). Mouse mammary tumor virus integration regions *int-1* and *int-2* map on different mouse chromosomes. Mol. Cell. Biol., 4, 375–378.

Peters, G., Lee, A.E. and Dickson, C. (1986). Concerted activation of two potential proto-oncogenes in carcinomas induced by mouse mammary tumor virus. Nature, 320, 628–631.

Peters, G., Brookes, S., Smith, R., Placzek, M. and Dickson, C. (1989). The mouse homolog of the *hst/k-FGF* gene is adjacent to *int-2* and is activated by proviral insertion in some virally induced mammary tumors. Proc. Natl Acad. Sci. USA, 86, 5678–5682.

Rijsewijk, F., Schuermann, M., Wagenaar, E., Parren, P., Weigel, D. and Nusse, R. (1987a). The Drosophila homolog of the mouse mammary oncogene *int-1* is identical to the segment polarity gene *wingless*. Cell, 50, 649–657.

Rijsewijk, F., van Deemter, L., Wagenaar, E., Sonnenberg, A. and Nusse, R. (1987b). Transfection of the *int-1* mammary oncogene in cuboidal RAC mammary cell line results in morphological transformation and tumorigenicity. EMBO J., 6, 127–131.

Roelink, H., Wagenaar, E., Lopes da Silva, S. and Nusse, R. (1990). *Wnt-3*, a gene activated by proviral insertion in mouse mammary tumors, is homologous to *int-1/Wnt-1* and is normally expressed in mouse embryos and adult brain. Proc. Natl Acad. Sci. USA, 87, 4519–4523.

Roelink, H., Wagenaar, E., and Nusse, R. (1992). Amplification and proviral activation of several *wnt* genes during progression and clonal variation of mouse mammary tumors. Oncogene, 7, 487–492.

Sokol, S., Christian, J.L., Moon, R. and Melton, D.A. (1991). Injected WntRNA induces a complete body axis in *Xenopus* embryos. Cell, 67, 741–752.

Tsukamoto, A.S., Grosschedl, R., Guzman, R.C., Parslow, T. and Varmus, H.E. (1988). Expression of the *int-1* gene in transgenic mice is associated with mammary gland hyperplasia and adenocarcinomas in male and female mice. Cell, 55, 619–625.

Van den Heuvel, M., Nusse, R., Johnston, P. and Lawrence, P.A. (1989). Distribution of the *wingless* gene product in *Drosophila* embryos: a protein involved in cell-cell communication. Cell, 59, 739–749.

van Ooyen, A. and Nusse, R. (1984). Structure and nucleotide sequence of the putative mammary oncogene *int-1*; proviral insertions leave the protein-encoding domain intact. Cell, 39, 233–240.

van Ooyen, A., Kwee, V. and Nusse, R. (1985). The nucleotide sequence of the human *int-1* mammary oncogene; evolutionary conservation of coding and non-coding sequences. EMBO J., 4, 2905–2909.

Wainwright, B.J., Scambler, P.J., Stanier, P., Watson, E.K., Bell, G., Wicking, C., Estivill, X., Courtney, M., Boue, A., Pedersen, P.S., Williamson, R. and Farrall, M. (1988). Isolation of a human gene with protein sequence similarity to human and mouse int-1 and the *Drosophila* segment polarity mutant *wingless*. EMBO J., 7, 1743–1748.

Waterston, R., Martin, C., Craxton, M., Huynh, C., Coulson, A., Hillier, L., Durbin, R., Green, P., Shown-keen, R., Halloran, N., Metzstein, M., Hawkins, T., Wilson, R., Berks, M., Du, Z., Thomas, K., Thierry-Mieg, J. and Sulston, J. (1992). A survey of expressed genes in *Caenorhabditis elegans*. Nature Genetics, 1, 114–123.

Wolda, S.L. and Moon, R.T. (1992). Cloning and developmental expression in *Xenopus laevis* of seven additional members of the *wnt* family. Oncogene, 7, 1941–1947.

YES1

v-*yes* is the oncogene of two avian sarcoma viruses, Esh sarcoma virus (ESV) and Y73. Esh was isolated from a tumour arising in a White leghorn owned by Mr Esh of Pennsylvania (Wallbank *et al.*, 1966). Y73 was isolated from a transplantable tumour arising in a chicken of the same strain on a farm in Yamaguchi Prefecture (Iothara *et al.*, 1978).

YES genes encode membrane-associated protein tyrosine kinases.

Related genes

Yes is a member of the *Src* tyrosine kinase family (*Blk, Fgr, Fyn, Hck, Lck/Tkl, Lyn, Src, Yes*). Chicken *Yrk* (Yes-related kinase) encodes a protein 72.4% identical to chicken YES (Sudol *et al.*, 1993). *YESP/YES2* is a human pseudogene that maps to chromosome 22q11–q12.

Cross-species homology

Yes genes are highly conserved: three domains (exon 2, exons 3–6 and exons 7–12) evolved at different rates. YES: 73%, 85% and 93%, similarity respectively in these domains (human and *Xiphophorus*). Overall sequence identities with the mouse protein: 96% (human), 91% (chicken) and 87% (*Xenopus*).

Transformation

MAN

Moderate to strong expression of *YES1* has been detected at relatively low frequency in a variety of cancers including fibrosarcoma, malignant lymphoma, glioblastoma, breast cancer, colorectal cancer, head and neck cancer, renal cancers, lung cancers and stomach cancer (Sugawara *et al.*, 1991). Amplified *YES1* has been detected in one gastric carcinoma (Seki *et al.*, 1985). In some types of follicular lymphomas there is a high correlation with t(14;18)(q32.3;q21.3) translocations in which a breakpoint occurs nears the *YES1* locus. However, the *BCL2* locus also lies in this region and may be the gene involved.

ANIMALS

Y73 and ESV induce sarcomas in chickens (Kawai *et al.*, 1980).

IN VITRO

Y73 and ESV transform fibroblasts (Ghysdael *et al.*, 1981).

	YES1/Yes-1	v-*yes*
Nucleotides		
	>30 kb	1755 (cell-derived)
		3718 (Y73)
Chromosome		
Human	18q21.3	
Exons	12	
mRNA (kb)		
Human	2.3, 4.8	4.8
	(Reed *et al.*, 1986; Semba *et al.*, 1985)	
Chicken	3.7, 3.9	
Amino acids		
Human	543	528 (v-*yes*)
Chicken	541	812 (Y73 *gag–yes*)
Murine	541	
Xenopus	537	
Mass (kDa)		
Predicted	61	
Expressed	pp62	pp90[gag-yes] (Y73)
		pp80[gag-yes] (ESV)

Cellular location

YES1: Plasma membrane and attached to the cytoskeleton.
v-YES: More diffusely distributed but concentrated in cell junction and adhesion plaques, similarly to SRC.

Tissue location

YES mRNA is widely distributed. In humans expression is high in the brain and kidney and low in spleen, muscle and thymus (Semba *et al.*, 1985; Reed *et al.*, 1986; Sukegawa *et al.*, 1990). p62[YES] kinase activity is high in platelets, peripheral blood T cells and natural killer cells but low in monocytes and B lymphocytes (Eiseman and Bolen, 1990; Zhao *et al.*, 1990). In chickens there is substantial expression in brain, liver and kidney (Semba *et al.*, 1985, 1988; Zhao *et al.*, 1991). In rats *Yes* is expressed in the lungs, kidney, liver, skin and testes and in specific types of neural tissues (Zhao *et al.*, 1990, 1991; Azuma *et al.*, 1991). Expression is stimulated during lymphocyte mitogenesis (Reed *et al.*, 1986).

Protein function

The YES proteins are tyrosine kinases, functionally related to SRC. As for SRC there is evidence implicating YES in the tyrosine phosphorylation of multiple substrates and in the modulation of phosphatidylinositol metabolism that occurs during the activation of many normal cell types and in transformed cells.

In normal quiescent fibroblasts stimulated by PDGF a small proportion of YES associates with the PDGF receptor and phosphatidylinositol kinase (Kypta *et al.*, 1990). This complex formation is correlated with a transient increase in the activity of the pp62 kinase. For transforming mutants of polyomavirus middle T antigen the extent of association of middle T antigen with YES and phosphatidylinositol kinase correlates with transforming capacity (Kornbluth *et al.*, 1990).

In the mouse mast cell line PT-18 the kinase activity of YES is increased after cellular stimulation via the high-affinity IgE receptor (Eiseman and Bolen, 1992). YES immunoprecipitates with the receptor and may therefore be responsible for the tyrosine phosphorylation of proteins that occurs when these cells are activated. In these cells YES is the only SRC family kinase that is activated but in another mast cell line the equivalent response may be mediated by p56^{lyn} and pp60^{src}. Association of pp62^{yes} (together with pp60^{fyn}, p54^{lyn} and p58^{lyn}) with a major signalling receptor also occurs in human platelets and in the cell lines C32 (human melanoma) and HEL (human erythroleukaemia). The receptor is the membrane glycoprotein IV (CD36) and, as in mast cells, the SRC family kinases appear to be involved in generating the pattern of protein tyrosine phosphorylation that occurs after cell stimulation (Huang *et al.*, 1991).

In epidermal keratinocytes the YES protein content and kinase activity is decreased during differentiation (Zhao *et al.*, 1992) and in neoplastic keratinocytes in basal cell carcinomas (Krueger *et al.*, 1991).

In Y73-transformed cells vinculin (Sefton *et al.*, 1981, 1982) and integrin (Hirst *et al.*, 1986) are phosphorylated on tyrosine residues and the concentrations of PtdIns(3)P, PtdIns(3,4)P_2 and PtdIns(3,4,5)P_3 are increased (Fukui *et al.*, 1991).

Structure of the Y73 proviral genome

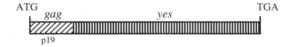

The 5' recombination site with *Yes* occurs between p19^{gag} and p27^{gag} such that Y73 includes the intact p19^{gag} sequence. An out of frame termination codon is used within gp37^{env} on the 3' side, 21 nucleotides 3' of the recombination site. The chicken YES and v-YES sequences differ by six substitutions and the replacement of 8 amino acids at the extreme of the C-terminus of YES by three *env*-encoded residues. This modification may be the major feature responsible for the transforming properties of v-*yes* (see **SRC**).

The *Yes* promoter contains six GC box-like sequences but no TATA box (Matsuzawa *et al.*, 1991). Four of the GC boxes immediately 5' of the gene bind Sp-1 and affect *Yes* transcription.

Sequences of human and chicken YES and v-YES

```
Human YES    (1)   MGCIKSKENKSPAIKYRPENTPEPVSTSVSHYGAEPTTVSPCPSSSAKGTAVNFSSLSM
Chicken YES  (1)   --------D-G--M---TD-----I-SH-----SD SSQATQ -PAI--S----NSH--
v-YES        (1)   VGCIKSKENKGPAMKYRTNNTPE***** ****** ****************
```

```
Human YES    (60)  TPFGGSSGVTPFGGASSSFSVVPSSYPAGLTGGVTIFVALYDYEARTTEDLSFKKGERFQ
Chicken YES  (58)  -----P--M-----------A---P--ST------V-----------D-----------
v-YES        (51)  **************************************G*****************G*****
```

```
Human YES    (120) IINNTEGDWWEARSIATGKNGYIPSNYVAPADSIQAEEWYFGKMGRKDAERLLLNPGNQR
Chicken YES  (118) ------------------T-----------------------------------------
v-YES        (111) ********************************E************************
```

```
Human YES    (180) GIFLVRESETTKGAYSLSIRDWDEIRGDNVKHYKIRKLDNGGYYITTRAQFDTLQKLVKH
Chicken YES  (178) ----------------------V-----------------------ES-------
v-YES        (171) *********************************************************
```

```
Human YES    (240) YTEHADGLCHKLTTVCPTVKPQTQGLAKDAWEIPRESLRLEVKLGQGCFGEVWMGTWNGT
Chicken YES  (238) -R----------------------------------------------------------
v-YES        (231) S***********************************************************
```

```
Human YES    (300) TKVAIKTLKPGTMMPEAFLQEAQIMKKLRHDKLVPLYAVVSEEPIYIVTEFMSKGSLLDF
Chicken YES  (298) -------------------------------------------------T------
v-YES        (291) ********L**************************************************
```

```
Human YES    (360) LKEGDGKYLKLPQLVDMAAQIADGMAYIERMNYIHRDLRAANILVGENLVCKIADFGLAR
Chicken YES  (358) ----E--F--------------------------------------D------------
v-YES        (351) **********************************************************
```

```
Human YES    (420) LIEDNEYTARQGAKFPIKWTAPEAALYGRFTIKSDVWSFGILQTELVTKGRVPYPGMVNR
Chicken YES  (418) --------------------------------------------L---------------
v-YES        (411) **********************************************************
```

```
Human YES    (480) EVLEQVERGYRMPCPQGCPESLHELMNLCWKKDPDERPTFEYIQSFLEDYFTATEPQYQPGENL (543)
Chicken YES  (478) ------------------------K-----------------------------D-- (541)
v-YES        (471) ***********************************************A**SGY (529)
```

Dashes indicate identity with human YES. * Indicates identity with chicken YES. The human SH3 domain and the ATP binding site (GXGXXG: 284–289 and 305 (YES); 559–564 and 580 (v-*yes*)) are underlined.

DOMAINS OF p62*yes*

Residues 1–7: necessary and sufficient for myristylation (glycine 2).
Residues 8–93: unique domain variable between non-membrane receptor tyrosine kinases.
Residues 94–144: SH3 domain.
Residues 145–256: SH2 domain.
Residues 256–524: catalytic domain, which shares sequence homology with other tyrosine kinases and contains an ATP binding site surrounding Lys302.
Residues 525–543: regulatory domain.

Databank file names and accession numbers

	GENE	EMBL	SWISSPROT	REFERENCES
Human	*YES1*	Hscyes1 M15990	KYES_HUMAN P07947	Sukegawa *et al.*, 1987
Chicken	*Yes*	Ggyes X12461	KYES_CHICK P0934	Zheng *et al.*, 1989
		Ggcyes X13207		Sudol *et al.*, 1988
Chicken	*Yrk*	Ggyrka X67786; X68973		Sudol *et al.*, 1993
Murine	*Yes*	X67677		Klages *et al.*, 1993
Xenopus laevis	*Yes*	Xlyes X14377	KYES_XENLA P10936	Steele *et al.*, 1989
Xiphophorus helleri	*Yes*	Xhcyes X54970		Hannig *et al.*, 1991
ASV (strain Y73)	*v-yes*	Reasvy V01170	KYES_AVISY P00527	Kitamura *et al.*, 1982

Review

Eiseman, E. and Bolen, J.B. (1990). *src*-related tyrosine protein kinases as signaling components in hematopoietic cells. Cancer Cells 2, 303–310.

Papers

Azuma, K., Ariki, M., Miyauchi, T., Usui, H., Takeda, M., Semba, K., Matsuzawa, Y., Yamamoto, T. and Toyoshima, K. (1991). Purification and characterization of a rat liver membrane tyrosine-protein kinase, the possible protooncogene c-*yes* product, p60$^{c\text{-}yes}$. J. Biol. Chem., 266, 4831–4839.

Eiseman, E. and Bolen, J.B. (1992). Engagement of the high-affinity IgE receptor activates *src* protein-related tyrosine kinases. Nature, 355, 78–80.

Fukui, Y., Saltiel, A.R. and Hanafusa, H. (1991). Phosphatidylinositol-3 kinase is activated in v-*src*, v-*yes* and v-*fps* transformed chicken embryo fibroblasts. Oncogene, 6, 407–411.

Ghysdael, J., Neil, J.C., Wallbank, A.M. and Vogt, P.K. (1981). Esh avian sarcoma virus codes for a *gag*-linked transformation-specific protein with an associated protein kinase activity. Virology, 111, 386–400.

Hannig, G., Ottilie, S. and Schartl. M. (1991). Conservation of structure and expression of the c-*yes* and *fyn* genes in lower vertebrates. Oncogene, 6, 361–369.

Hirst, R., Horwitz, A., Buck, C. and Rohrschneider, L. (1986). Phosphorylation of the fibronectin receptor complex in cells transformed by oncogenes that encode tyrosine kinases. Proc. Natl Acad. Sci. USA, 83, 6470–6474.

Huang, M.-M., Bolen, J.B., Barnwell, J.W., Shattil, S.J. and Brugge, J.S. (1991). Membrane glycoprotein IV (CD36) is physically associated with fyn, lyn, and yes protein-tyrosine kinases in human platelets. Proc. Natl Acad. Sci. USA, 88, 7844–7848.

Iothara, S., Hirata, K., Inone, M., Hatsuoka, M. and Sato, A., (1978). Isolation of a sarcoma virus from a spontaneous chicken tumor. Jpn J. Cancer Res. (Gann), 69, 825–830.

Kawai, S., Yoshida, M., Segawa, K., Sugiyama, H., Ishizaki, R. and Toyoshima, K. (1980). Characterization of Y73, an avian sarcoma virus: a unique transforming gene and its product, a phosphopolyprotien with protein kinase activity. Proc. Natl Acad. Sci. USA, 77, 6199–6203.

Kitamura, N., Kitamura, A., Toyoshima, K., Hirayama, I. and Yoshida, M. (1982). Avian sarcoma virus

Y73 genome sequence and structural similarity of its transforming gene product to that of Rous sarcoma virus. Nature, 297, 205–208.

Klages, S., Adam, D., Eiseman, E., Fargnoli, J., Dymecki, S.M., Desiderio, S.V. and Bolen, J.B. (1993). Molecular cloning and analysis of cDNA encoding the murine c-*yes* tyrosine protein kinase. Oncogene, 8, 713–719.

Kornbluth, S., Cheng, S.H., Markland, W., Fukui, Y. and Hanafusa, H. (1990). Association of p62^{c-yes} with polyomavirus middle T-antigen mutants correlates with transforming ability. J. Virol., 64, 1584–1589.

Krueger, J., Zhao, Y.-H., Murphy, D. and Sudol, M. (1991). Differential expression of p62^{c-yes} in normal, hyperplastic and neoplastic human epidermis. Oncogene, 6, 933–940.

Kypta, R.M., Goldberg, Y., Ulug, E.T. and Courtneidge, S.A. (1990). Association between the PDGF receptor and members of the *src* family of tyrosine kinases. Cell, 62, 481–492.

Matsuzawa, Y., Semba, K., Kawamura-Tsuzuku, J., Sudo, T., Ishii, S., Toyoshima, K. and Yamamoto, T. (1991). Characterisation of the promoter region of the c-*yes* proto-oncogene: the importance of the GC boxes on its promoter activity. Oncogene, 6, 1561–1567.

Reed, J.C., Alpers, J.D., Nowell, P.C. and Hoover, R.G. (1986). Sequential expression of protooncogenes during lectin-stimulated mitogenesis of normal human lymphocytes. Proc. Natl Acad. Sci. USA, 83, 3982–3986.

Sefton, B.M., Hunter, T., Ball, E.H. and Singer, S.J. (1981). Vinculin: a cytoskeletal target of the transforming protein of Rous sarcoma virus. Cell, 24, 165–174.

Sefton, B.M., Hunter, T., Nigg, E.A., Singer, S.J. and Walker, G. (1982). Cytoskeletal targets for viral transforming proteins with tyrosine protein kinase activity. Cold Spring Harbor Symp. Quant. Biol., 46, 939–951.

Seki, T., Fujii, G., Mori, S., Tomaoki, N. and Shibuya, M. (1985). Amplification of c-*yes* proto-oncogene in a primary human gastric cancer. Jpn J. Cancer Res. (Gann), 76, 907–910.

Semba, K., Yamanashi, Y., Nishizawa, M., Sukegawa, J., Yoshida, M., Sasaki. M., Yamamoto, T. and Toyoshima, K. (1985). Location of the c-*yes* gene on the human chromosome and its expression in various tissues. Science, 227, 1038–1040.

Semba, K., Nishizawa, M., Satoh, H., Fukushige, S., Yoshida, M.C., Sasaki. M., Matsubara, K., Yamamoto, T. and Toyoshima, K. (1988). Nucleotide sequence and chromosome mapping of the human c-*yes*-2 gene. Jpn J. Cancer Res. (Gann), 79, 710–717.

Steele, R.E., Irwin, M.Y., Knudsen, C.L., Collett, J.W. and Fero, J.B. (1989). The *yes* proto-oncogene is present in amphibians and contributes to the maternal RNA pool in the oocyte. Oncogene Res., 4, 223–233.

Sudol, M., Kieswetter, C., Zhao, Y.-H., Dorai, T., Wang, L.-H. and Hanafusa, H. (1988). Nucleotide sequence of a cDNA for the chick *yes* proto-oncogene: comparison with the viral *yes* gene. Nucleic Acids Res., 16, 9876.

Sudol, M., Greulich, H., Newman, L., Sarkar, A., Sukegawa, J. and Yamamoto, T. (1993). A novel Yes-related kinase, Yrk, is expressed at elevated levels in neural and hematopoietic tissues. Oncogene, 8, 823–831.

Sugawara, K., Sugawara, I., Sukegawa, J., Akatsuka, T., Yamamoto, T., Morita, M., Mori, S. and Toyoshima, K. (1991). Distribution of c-*yes*-1 gene product in various cells and tissues. Brit. J. Cancer, 63, 508–513.

Sukegawa, J., Semba, K., Yamanashi, Y., Nishizawa, M., Miyajima, N., Yamamoto, T. and Toyoshima, K. (1987). Characterization of cDNA clones for the human c-*yes* gene. Mol. Cell. Biol., 7, 41–47.

Sukegawa, J., Akatsuka, T., Sugawara, I., Mori, S., Yamamoto, T. and Toyoshima, K. (1990). Monoclonal antibodies to the amino-terminal sequence of the c-*yes* gene product as specific probes of its expression. Oncogene, 5, 611–614.

Wallbank, A.M., Sperling, F.G., Hubben, K. and Stubbs, E.L. (1966). Isolation of a tumor virus from a chicken submitted to a Poultry Diagnostic Laboratory – Esh sarcoma virus. Nature, 209, 1265.

Zhao, Y.-H., Krueger, J.G. and Sudol, M. (1990). Expression of cellular-*yes* protein in mammalian tissues. Oncogene, 5, 1629–1635.

Zhao, H.-Y., Baker, H., Walaas, S.I. and Sudol, M. (1991). Localization of p62^{c-yes} protein in mammalian neural tissues. Oncogene, 6, 1725–1733.

Zhao, Y., Sudol, M., Hanafusa, H. and Krueger, J. (1992). Increased tyrosine kinase activity of c-src during calcium-induced keratinocyte differentiation. Proc. Natl Acad. Sci. USA, 89, 8298–8302.

Zheng, X., Podell, S., Sefton, B.M. and Kaplan, P.L. (1989). The sequence of chicken c-*yes* and p61^{c-yes}. Oncogene, 4, 99–104.

Appendix

The Life Cycle of Retroviruses; HIV and HTLV

The Life Cycle of Retroviruses

Retroviral infection only occurs in cells that are actively replicating, the block to infection in quiescent cells probably occurring after virus entry (Miller *et al.*, 1990). Viruses bind to cells through interactions between the surface proteins of the virion and structures on the target cell surface that act as viral receptors. Retroviral glycoproteins are polymorphous and viruses of each viral envelope class use a different host cell receptor. The specificity of interaction with host cell proteins gives rise to three classes of retrovirus: ecotrophic (replicate only in cells from the host animal and closely related species), xenotrophic (replicate only in heterologous cells) and amphotrophic (replicate in cells of natural host and in heterologous cells). The high specificity of host cells in which retroviruses may replicate derives from three basic causes (1) absence of host cell surface receptors for the viral glycoprotein (no infection), (2) non-survival of the viral genome after penetration and reverse transcription and (3) inability to assemble complete, infectious virions (non-permissive infection). In mouse cells a post-penetration block to integration occurs via the host *Fv-1* gene (2 allelles *Fv-1^{nn}* and *Fv-1^{bb}*): a murine leukaemia virus (MuLV) is said to be N-trophic if *Fv-1^{nn}* cells are permissive and *Fv-1^{bb}* cells restrictive; B-trophic if the reverse and NB-trophic if both types of cells are permissive. Following binding, most retroviruses enter cells by membrane fusion, as do some DNA viruses (e.g., herpesviruses). Some retroviruses appear to undergo receptor-mediated endocytosis. These include murine leukaemia viruses and human immunodeficiency viruses, and adenoviruses and polyomaviruses are also internalized by endocytosis, subsequently appearing in coated pits and endosomes.

Retroviruses contain two large (~30 000 nucleotides), identical, single-stranded RNA molecules, together with the enzyme reverse transcriptase, an RNA-directed DNA polymerase. Following uptake by the host cell, reverse transcriptase catalyses the formation of double-stranded DNA from the RNA of the virion (Temin and Baltimore, 1972). The enzyme possesses three enzymatic activities in its two polypeptide chains: it copies RNA to give double-stranded DNA–

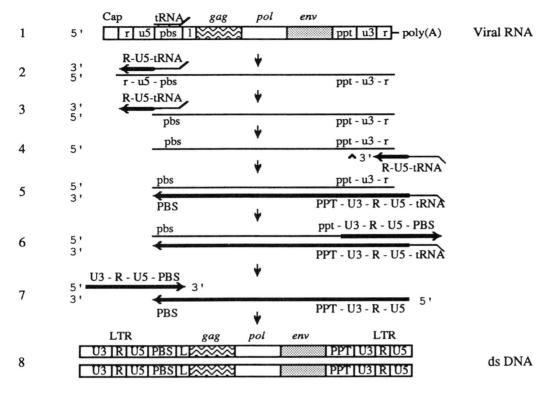

Fig. A1. The mechanism of reverse transcriptase.
1. Structure of one of the two identical strands of retroviral RNA. In diagrams 2–6 this is represented by thin lines. tRNA annealed to the primer binding site (pbs) is used as a primer for DNA synthesis.
2. Reverse transcriptase extends one of the tRNA molecules from its 3'-OH end to form a minus strand strong stop DNA copy of r–u5.
3. The RNAase H activity in reverse transcriptase degrades the r–u5 sequence of the template RNA exposing minus strand DNA.
4. This DNA transfers to the 3' end of the RNA genome (presumably using the complementarity between the R regions).
5. Minus strand DNA synthesis continues. RNAase H makes a specific nick (∧) just 5' of the u3 sequence at the polypurine tract (ppt) and u3–r is digested.
6. The nicked viral RNA acts as a primer to initiate plus strand DNA synthesis. The minus strand U3–R–U5 DNA, as well as the portion of the primer tRNA that is complementary to pbs, is copied, forming plus strand DNA.
7. This DNA transfers to the almost completed minus strand DNA, presumably by the complementarity to the pbs region. All RNA is digested by RNAase H.
8. Reverse transcriptase adds nucleotides to both the plus and minus strand 3' termini to form a complete copy of the retroviral RNA terminated at each end by an LTR.
Lower case and capital letters: RNA and DNA, respectively. Bold lines with solid arrows indicate the direction of DNA synthesis.
(From Hu and Temin, 1990.)

RNA, it copies primed single-stranded DNA to form double-stranded DNA and it degrades RNA in DNA–RNA hybrids (Fig. A1). The resulting dsDNA sequence is not an exact copy of the viral RNA: sequences from the 5' and 3' ends of the RNA are combined and duplicated to form a long terminal repeat (LTR) at both ends of the double-stranded DNA molecule. The general structure of LTRs is U3–R–U5, representing copies of untranslated sequences originally at the 3' and 5' ends of the viral RNA genome and a sequence repeated at both ends (R). This double-stranded DNA then circularizes before being inserted into the host chromosome to form a DNA provirus. In the growth cycle of a retrovirus, integration of viral DNA in the host chromosome is obligatory, in contrast to that of DNA viruses.

In the second stage of the life cycle the machinery of the host cell is employed to generate multiple copies of single transcripts to provide both viral RNA and, after cleavage, mRNA from which the viral proteins are translated. The viral genes are *gag, pol* and *env*, the latter encoding the viral envelope proteins (Fig. A1). A polyprotein translated from the *gag* (group-specific *anti-*gens: viral capsid proteins) and *pol* (*polymerase*) regions is cleaved to yield four core proteins from the *gag* region whilst the *pol* protein, which constitutes the β subunit of reverse transcriptase, may also be hydrolysed to release the smaller, α subunit of reverse transcriptase (which aggregates with the β chain) and the integrase protein.

MMTVs are unlike other murine retroviruses in that, in addition to the multiple polypeptides encoded by the *gag, pol* and *env* genes, they have an open reading frame (ORF) in the 3' LTR (Choi *et al.*, 1991). The ORF genes are highly conserved among MMTVs and mediate the minor lymphocyte-stimulating (Mls) response by which Vβ-bearing autoreactive T cells are eliminated in the thymus during the establishment of tolerance (Acha-Orbea *et al.*, 1991). Endogenous MMTV proviruses are present in the germ line of all inbred mice and the action of the ORF protein confers resistance to exogenous MMTV infection (Golovkina *et al.*, 1992).

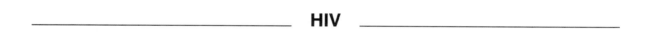

HIV

The structural complexity that may evolve in retroviruses is best illustrated by the human immunodeficiency viruses (HIV) and the human T-lymphotropic viruses (HTLV-1 and HTLV-2). It should be noted, however, that although infection with these viruses frequently correlates with neoplasia, there is no evidence that any of their gene products are themselves oncogenic. HIV is associated with acquired immunodeficiency syndrome (AIDS) and with a variety of neoplasms including Kaposi sarcoma, malignant B cell lymphomas, small-cell cancers and oropharyngeal and perirectal carcinomas. The many different isolates of HIV have been broadly classified as HIV-1 and HIV-2. The HIV-1 genome (Fig. A2) utilizes a variety of alternative splicing patterns to encode four virion core proteins, a protease, reverse transcriptase, integrase, two envelope proteins, two *trans*-activators and at least four other proteins. It is the specific binding of the viral envelope glycoprotein gp120 to the CD4 receptor that mediates the selective destruction of CD4+ subsets of T lymphocytes characteristic of AIDS.

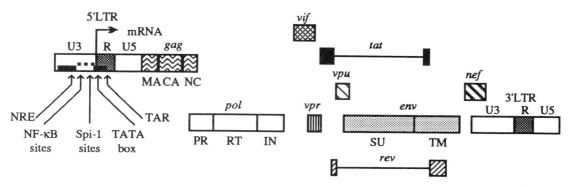

Fig. A2. The HIV-1 genome (9.5 kb). Boxes represent the LTRs (each 634 bp) and coding sequences and the displaced horizontal alignments permit the representation of alternative, overlapping splicing patterns.

The primer binding site at the 5' end of R is an 18 bp sequence complementary to the 3' terminus of tRNA-lysine: $tRNA_{lys}$ is also used by mouse mammary tumour virus but all other retroviruses have a $tRNA_{pro}$ primer.

Each LTR contains: a negative regulatory element (NRE) through which the *nef* gene product acts as a *trans*-repressor; an NF-κB binding site (tandem repeat) to which HIVEN 86A also binds; Spi-1 binding sites (triple repeat); a TATA box 27 bp 5' of the cap site (the U3–R boundary); a CCAAT sequence 178 bp 5' of R, *trans-acting* response element (TAR) within the R region of the LTRs to which the *tat* gene product binds to enhance transcription of viral genes. Additional factors known to interact with this region are CTF/NFI (binds to CCAAT) EBP-1, LBP-1 and/or UBP-1. The HTLV *tax* protein (see HTLV-1 below) stimulates transcription of HIV genes by increasing NF-κB binding to the LTR.

The abbreviations for gene products indicate the following protein functions: (other designations that have been used are shown in brackets): p55*gag* is the precursor for the MA, CA and NC proteins: MA: matrix protein (p16, myristylated); CA: capsid protein (p24); NC: nucleocapsid proteins (p15, cleaved to yield p7/p9); p160*pol* is the precursor for the PR, RT and IN proteins: PR: protease (p10); RT: reverse transcriptase (p61) and RNAase H (p52); IN: integrase (p31); SU: surface glycoprotein (gp120); TM: transmembrane glycoprotein (gp41); *rev*: regulator of virion production (art, trs, p16); *tat*: trans-activating transcriptional regulation factor essential for HIV-1 replication (tat-III, p14); *nef*: negative regulatory factor with GTPase activity (3'-orf, orf-B, p27); *vif*: viral infectivity factor (sor (short open reading frame), orf-A, p23); *vpr*: viral protein R, transcription activator (orf-R, p15); *vpu*: viral protein U, particle release factor (orf-U, p16), encoded only by HIV-1, not HIV-2; *vpx*: viral protein X, function unknown (orf-X, p14), encoded only by HIV-2, not HIV-1. The *pol* ORF overlaps that of *gag* by 80 amino acids, rather more than the overlap in most other retroviruses (Cann and Karn, 1989; Vaishnav and Wong-Staal, 1991).

HTLV-1

HTLV-1 and HTLV-2 are C-type retroviruses that have ~45% sequence homology, the major region of difference between them being the *env* gene sequence. HTLV-1 is associated with adult T cell leukaemia (ATL) and tropical spastic paraparesis (TSP). HTLV-2 has been isolated from individuals with hairy cell leukaemia. *In vitro* HTLV-1 immortalizes human T cells but does not induce the chromosomal abnormalities (14q11, 3 and 6) that characterize ATL cells. HTLV infection may therefore merely facilitate neoplastic transformation, rather than act as the principal transforming agent.

The LTR sequences occurring in HTLV-1 are typical of those found in retroviruses (Fig. A3). Each LTR consists of 754 bp including inverted repeats of 2 bp at the ends, an example of the minimal inverted repeat presumed to be necessary for proviral DNA integration. The seven bases of the adjacent host sequence are in direct repeat. This pattern of LTR structure is ubiquitous and includes invariant proviral termini of 5'-TG and CA-3', although the extent of the host repeat sequence may vary between viruses, as does the size of the sequence of the viral genes, which is approximately 7.3 kbp in HTLV-1. The R sequence in HTLV-1 (229 bp) is longer than in most retroviruses (97 bp in HIV-1, 173 bp in HIV-2, 67 bp in FBR-MuSV).

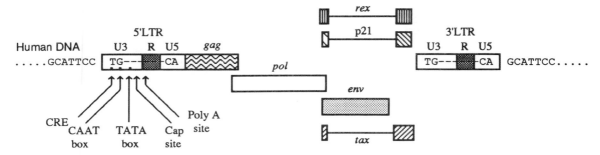

Fig. A3. The HTLV-1 genome (8.7 kb). Boxes represent the LTRs and coding sequences and show regions of overlap. Each LTR contains three imperfect repeats that include a cAMP response element (CRE, TGACG). *gag* encodes p19, p24 and p15; the partially overlapping second reading frame encodes the proteinase and reverse transcriptase (p99); the *env* precursor (p62) is cleaved to yield p46 and p21. Translation of *tax* is from the *env* initiation codon in a doubly spliced mRNA to yield p40 (p40^{tax} activates transcription from the HTLV-1 LTR indirectly via the CRE); *rex* (pp27) initiates 56 nucleotides upstream of the *env* initiation codon and a protein of unknown function (p21) is also translated from the same reading frame as *rex* but commencing 78 codons downstream. pp27^{rex} prevents splicing of the primary transcript into subgenomic mRNAs, i.e. it suppresses the production of itself, p40^{tax} and p21 in a manner analogous to the action of the HIV *rev* protein.

The organizations of the closely related bovine leukaemia virus (BLV) and simian T-lymphotropic virus 1 (STLV-1) are similar.

Reviews

Hu, W.-S. and Temin, H.M. (1990). Retroviral recombination and reverse transcription. Science, 250, 1227–1233.

Temin, H.M. and Baltimore, D. (1972). RNA-directed DNA synthesis and RNA tumor viruses. Adv. Virus Res., 17, 129–186.

Vaishnav, Y.N. and Wong-Staal, F. (1991). The biochemistry of AIDS. Annu. Rev. Biochem., 60, 577–630.

Papers

Acha-Orbea, H., Shakhov, A.N., Scarpellino, L., Kolb, E., Muller, V., Vessaz-Shaw, A., Fuchs, R., Blochlinger, K., Rollini, P., Billotte, J., Sarafidou, M., MacDonald, H.R. and Diggelmann, H. (1991). Clonal deletion of Vβ14-bearing T cells in mice transgenic for mammary tumor virus. Nature, 350, 207–211.

Cann, A.J. and Karn, J. (1989). Molecular biology of HIV: new insights into the virus life-cycle. AIDS, 3, S19–S34.

Choi, Y., Kappler, J.W. and Marrack, P. (1991). A superantigen encoded in the open reading frame of the 3' long terminal repeat of mouse mammary tumour virus. Nature, 350, 203–207.

Golovkina, T.V., Chervonsky, A., Dudley, J.P. and Ross, S.R. (1992). Transgenic mouse mammary tumor virus superantigen expression prevents viral infection. Cell, 69, 637–645.

Miller, D.G., Adam, M.A. and Miller, D. (1990). Gene transfer by retrovirus vectors occurs only in cells that are actively replicating at the time of infection. Mol. Cell. Biol., 10, 4239–4242.

Glossary and Abbreviations

Acoustic neuroma	See Schwannoma.
Acute erythroleukaemia	See Leukaemias.
Adenoma	Benign tumour derived from (secretory) epithelial cells.
AEV	Avian erythroblastosis virus: family *Retroviridae*, subfamily *Oncovirinae*, genus Type C oncovirus. Acute leukaemia retrovirus carrying the v-*erbB* oncogene (strain AEV-H) or v-*erbB* and v-*erbA* (strain AEV-ES4).
AIDS	Acquired immune deficiency syndrome. Clinical syndrome caused by infection with human immunodeficiency virus. Diagnostic criteria include opportunistic infections, abnormal T helper/T suppressor ratio and malignancies including Kaposi's sarcoma and lymphoma.
ALL	See Leukaemias.
ALV	Avian leukaemia virus. C-type retroviruses (*Oncovirinae*) that cause leukaemias and other tumours in birds, including avian erythroblastosis virus (AEV), avian myeloblastosis virus (AMV) and myelocytomatosis viruses.
AML	See Leukaemias.
Amphotrophic virus	Virus that can replicate in cells of either its normal host or of other species.
Amplification	Increase in gene copy number. Enhanced expression of the gene is a general consequence but the increase in mRNA concentration is not always proportional to the number of gene copies.
AMV	Avian myeloblastosis virus: family *Retroviridae*, subfamily *Oncovirinae*, genus Type C oncovirus. Causes myeloblastosis, osteopetrosis, lymphoid leukosis and nephroblastosis in chickens.
ANLL	See Leukaemias.

Antisense oligodeoxynucleotide (ODN)	Synthetic nucleotide sequence (usually 15 or 18 bases) complementary to RNA or DNA sequences used to inhibit specifically the translation or transcription of a gene. In addition to unmodified oligonucleotides, classes of ODN include methylphosphonates, phosphorothioates and α-oligonucleotides. Antisense RNA with sequences complementary to some mRNAs has been detected in prokaryotes and eukaryotes (see *P53*) and transcription of regions of the negative strand has also been detected in eukaryotes (see *EGFR/HER2* and *MYC*).
APL	See Leukaemias.
Astrocytoma	Tumour arising from astrocytes, the major structural brain cell type. Range from benign to highly malignant. They are the most common form of primary brain tumour. Rarely metastasized beyond the central nervous system.
ASV	Avian sarcoma virus: *Retroviridae* causing tumours in chickens (e.g. Rous sarcoma virus, RSV).
Ataxia telangiectasia	Autosomal recessive disorder involving defective DNA repair. Characterized by serious degenerative changes in the central nervous system, skin lesions, immune deficiency and an increased incidence of malignancy, particularly leukaemia or lymphoma. Up to 40% of patients with the syndrome develop a malignancy.
ATL	Adult T cell lymphoma leukaemia. An aggressive form of T cell lymphoma leukaemia characterized by the proliferation of mature $CD4^+$ cells. Associated with HTLV-1 infection and occurring particularly in individuals born in the Caribbean, West Africa and southern Japan.
Autosomal	Arising from the expression of a gene carried on any chromosome that is not a sex chromosome.
B-trophic	The integration of viral DNA into the genome of mouse cells is controlled by the host *Fv-1* gene (2 alleles *Fv-1^{nn}* and *Fv-1^{bb}*). A murine leukaemia virus (MuLV) is B-trophic if *Fv-1^{nn}* cells are restrictive and *Fv-1^{bb}* cells permissive, N-trophic if *Fv-1^{nn}* cells are permissive and *Fv-1^{bb}* cells restrictive and NB-trophic if both types of cells are permissive.
Benign tumour	Such tumours may arise in any tissue and cause local damage by pressure or obstruction but does not spread to other sites or invade adjoining tissues.
Bloom's syndrome	One of three autosomal recessive diseases commonly associated with unrepaired chromosomal breaks (the others are Fanconi's anaemia and ataxia telangiectasia). It is associated with telangiectatic redness of the skin in photo-exposed areas and stunted growth with a propensity to develop acute myeloblastic leukaemia or lymphoma.
Burkitt's lymphoma	Human B cell malignancy having 20- to 50-fold higher incidence in tropical Africa than elsewhere. Characterized by chromosomal translocations involving the *MYC* locus (see *MYC*). Almost all African forms of Burkitt's lymphoma carry Epstein–Barr virus (EBV) DNA and express at least one viral antigen (see **DNA Tumour Viruses: EBV**).

cMGF	Chicken myelomonocytic growth factor. Stimulates the growth of normal, bone-marrow-derived myeloid cells and is required for the proliferation *in vitro* of *myb*-transformed myeloblasts and *myc*-transformed macrophages.
Carcinoma	Malignant tumour of epithelial cells. Characterized by ability to invade adjacent tissues and to undergo metastasis. The term includes malignant tumours of glandular epithelial tissue that are termed adenocarcinomas.
Carcinosarcoma	A rare form of malignant tumour containing both epithelial and sarcomatous elements.
Casein kinase I	Mg^{2+}-dependent cytoplasmic (30–37 kDa) and nuclear (25–55 kDa) monomeric enzymes for which glycogen synthase and SV40 T antigen are substrates.
Casein kinase II	Ca^{2+} and cAMP-independent serine/threonine kinase (α_2/β_2, α 37–44 kDa, β 24–28 kDa) that is widely distributed in eukaryotic cells. Activity is stimulated by growth factors (insulin, TPA, serum) and may be involved in the regulation of cell proliferation. Amino acid substrates must lie within acidic domains. Consensus phosphorylation sequences occur in FOS, JUN, MYC, MYCN, MYCL, MYB, p53, ERBA, v-ETS, adenovirus E1A, SV40 T antigen and HPV E7 proteins. (For a review see Tuazon, P.T. and Traugh, J.A. (1991). Casein kinase I and II – multipotential serine protein kinases: structure, function, and regulation. Adv. Second Mess. Phosphoprot. Res., 23, 123–164.)
CLL	See Leukaemias.
CML	See Leukaemias.
cis activation	Stimulation of gene transcription by a DNA sequence located on the same chromosome, i.e. not by a diffusible agent.
CRE	Cyclic AMP responsive element. An upstream DNA sequence (TGACGTCA) regulating the transcription of some eukaryotic genes.
CREB	A family of genes encoding proteins (transcription factors) with leucine repeats that bind as dimers to the CRE.
De-differentiation (or retro-differentiation)	Reversion of cells possessing characteristics of a mature phenotype to a form of immature, precursor cell.
Denys–Drash syndrome	Rare human developmental disorder affecting the urogenital system and leading to renal failure, intersex disorders and Wilms' tumour.
Direct repeat sequence	Identical or virtually identical DNA sequence present as two or more copies in the same orientation in the same molecule. Direct repeats may be adjacent or widely separated.
Dominant (allele)	An allelic form of a gene expressed in a given cell phenotype as distinct from the other allele carried on the homologous chromosome. Dominant alleles are thus expressed in the homozygous or heterozygous condition: recessive alleles are expressed only when both members of a pair of alleles (or sets of alleles at corresponding loci) are identical.

E74	The ecdysone-inducible *Drosophila* transcription factor required for metamorphosis.
Ecotropic virus	Virus that can only replicate in cells of its normal host.
Enhancer	Eukaryotic promoter element that increases the transcriptional efficiency of a gene. Often present as short tandem repeats of 50–100 bp (e.g. the 72 bp repeat of SV40 virus). Enhancers may be located upstream or downstream of the gene they control at distances of up to several thousand nucleotides from the gene and in some genes (e.g. chicken β-globin) the enhancer is located within the gene. Enhancers are equally effective in either orientation.
Enhanson	Multiple functional elements that together comprise an enhancer and act synergistically to stimulate transcription from an associated promoter. Three classes of enhanson have been defined on the basis of the *trans*-activating capacity of repeated sequences of the enhanson, independent of other enhancer elements (proto-enhancer activity). Class A: proto-enhancer activity as a tandem repeat or when associated with a class B enhanson (e.g. Sph-I, Sph-II, GT-IIC). Class B: no proto-enhancer activity alone but cooperate with class A enhansons (e.g. GT-I). Class C: independent proto-enhancer activity (e.g. TC-II, octamer). Class D enhansons act independently as monomers, e.g. the response elements activated by steroid hormone–receptor complexes. Each enhanson binds at least one *trans*-activating factor. For example, Sph-I, Sph-II and GT-IIC bind TEF-1, GT-I binds TEF-2, TC-II binds TC-IIA/NF-κB-like and TC-IIB/KBF1/H2TF1-like proteins (that also bind to the κ light chain κB proto-enhancer and the H-2K^b proto-enhancer in the MHC H-2K^b promoter) and the octameric proto-enhancer binds a variety of lymphoid cell-specific factors. Enhanson sequences: Sph-I: AAGCATGCA; Sph-II: AAG-TATGCA; GT-IIC: GTGGAATGT; GT-I: GGGTGTGG; TC-II: GGAAAGTCCCC; H-2K^b: TGGGGATTCCCCA; SV40-P (AP-1 binding): TTAGTCA; human metallothionein IIA (AP-1 binding): TGACTCA.
Epstein–Barr virus	Burkitt's lymphoma virus: virus of the family *Herpesviridae*, subfamily *Gammaherpesvirinae*. Isolated from the endemic (African) form of Burkitt's lymphoma that primarily afflicts children.
Erythroleukaemia	See Leukaemias.
Ewing's sarcoma	The second most common primary bone tumour in children and young adults. Cell of origin is unknown. Highly malignant. t(11;22)(q24;q12) translocation identified, resulting in the fusion of *ETS* and *EWS* genes (see Table 2.3 Supplement).
Expression vector	A plasmid-like construct the DNA sequence(s) of which can be transcribed and translated when the vector is taken up by an appropriate host cell. Vectors may include a constitutively active or an inducible promoter.
gag	See Retroviral genome.
pol	See Retroviral genome.

env	See Retroviral genome.
Fibrosarcoma	Malignant tumour of mesenchymal fibrous tissue.
Glioma	Tumour of the glial tissues (non-neuronal cells present within the CNS) that accounts for ~60% of all primary CNS tumours. Gliomas comprise five distinct types: astrocytomas, oligodendrogliomas, medulloblastomas, ependymomas and spongioblastomas.
Glycosaminoglycans	Polysaccharide sidechains of proteoglycans made up of >100 repeating disaccharide units of amino sugars, at least one having a negatively charged side-group (carboxylate or sulfate; e.g. heparin). Formerly called mucopolysaccharides.
Granulocyte-macrophage colony stimulating factor (GM-CSF)	A cytokine stimulating the formation of granulocyte or macrophage colonies from myeloid stem cells isolated from bone marrow.
Hairy cell leukaemia	See Leukaemias.
Helix–loop–helix	A domain occurring in some proteins (e.g. OCT1, OCT2, MYC, MYCN and MYCL) that regulate transcription. It is composed of two α-helical regions separated by a β-turn. Helix–loop–helix proteins bind to DNA as dimers and use both subunits to recognize target sequences and stabilize DNA–protein interactions.

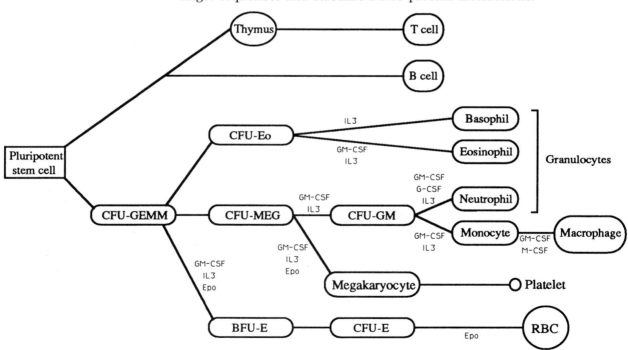

Haematopoietic differentiation pathways	(Adapted from Clark, S.C. and Kame, R. (1987). The human hematopoietic colony-stimulating factors. Science, 236, 1229–1237.)
Heterozygosity	Possession of one or more dissimilar pairs of alleles of particular genes.

HIV	Human immunodeficiency virus (HTLV-3, human lymphotropic virus type 3, lymphadenopathy-associated virus (LAV)). Family *Retroviridae*, subfamily *Lentivirinae*.
Hodgkin's lymphoma	See Lymphoma.
Homologous recombination	Recombination at regions of homology between chromosomes by breakage and reunion of DNA allowing direct replacement of the original DNA sequence with an exogenous segment.
HTLV-1, HTLV-2	Human T cell leukaemia/lymphotropic viruses types 1 and 2. Family *Retroviridae*, subfamily *Lentivirinae*. Replication-competent retroviruses. HTLV-1 is the apparent causal agent of ATL and is also associated with a variety of non-neoplastic immunological diseases including TSP.
Inhibin	Inhibins (31 kDa) are α/β heterodimeric glycoproteins secreted by the Graafian follicle and Sertoli cells that selectively suppress the secretion of pituitary follicle-stimulating hormone (FSH). There are two homologous forms of the β subunit (βA and βB) that give rise to two heterodimeric forms (inhibinA and inhibinB). The β subunits have a high degree of homology with TGFβ (see **Tumour Suppressor Genes: α-inhibin**).
Insertional mutagenesis	Alteration of a gene as a consequence of inserting nucleotide sequences from viruses or transposons or by transfection or microinjection of DNA.
Kaposi's sarcoma	Malignant tumour, probably arising from blood vessels. Rare, endemic form is a slowly progressing disease of the elderly. Epidemic Kaposi's sarcoma occurs in patients with HIV infection and pursues a more aggressive course.
LCR	Long control region: regulatory region in viral genomes. In human papillomaviruses the LCR encompasses 5–12% of the viral genome and contains an intricate network of *cis* responsive elements.
Leucine zipper	A protein sequence of five leucine amino acids each separated by six residues. It mediates dimer formation via a coiled-coil arrangement of parallel α helices and is normally adjacent to a basic, DNA binding domain. The leucine zipper family includes C/EPB, FOS, JUN, CREB and GCN4. In CREB and GCN4 the fifth leucine is substituted by arginine and lysine respectively.
Leucocyte	Any colourless, amoeboid cell mass, including lymphocytes, monocytes and granulocytes (neutrophils, basophils and eosinophils).
Leukaemias	Malignant proliferation of bone marrow cells which are the precursors of normal elements of the blood, e.g. lymphocytes, erythrocytes, etc. Classified according to lineage of origin (see Haematopoietic differentiation pathways) and degree of differentiation of the tumour cells, which often predicts clinical behaviour. The major consequences of leukaemia arise from overgrowth of malignant cells in the bone marrow leading to reduction in production of normal bone marrow and blood components. The infiltration of other organs (e.g. spleen, skin) can also occur. Acute leukaemias have features of cells early in the differentiation pathway, and often have an explosive clinical course.

Chronic leukaemia cells appear more closely related to fully differentiated blood cells, and pursue a more indolent course, sometimes spanning many years.

The major subdivisions of leukaemias are those with lymphoid features (ALL, acute lymphoblastic leukaemia; CLL, chronic lymphocytic leukaemia) and those with myeloid features (AML, acute myeloblastic leukaemia; AMML, acute myelomonocytic leukaemia; APL, acute promyelocytic leukaemia; CML, chronic myeloid leukaemia). The acute myeloid leukaemias are also termed acute non-lymphoblastic leukaemias (ANLL).

Acute lymphoblastic leukaemia is the most common leukaemia in childhood, while the myeloid leukaemias predominate in adulthood. Analysis of cell surface markers allows ALL to be subdivided according to precursor lineage (B cell, T cell) though some forms of the disease lack such markers, suggesting an earlier cell of origin. The clinical features of each type of ALL are subtly different.

Acute myeloid leukaemias are subdivided according to morphology. The major subtypes are:

M1: Myeloblastic leukaemia (AML) without maturation in which myeloblasts predominate.

M2: Acute myeloblastic leukaemia with maturation in which more than 50% of cells are myeloblasts or promyelocytes. About 15% of cases show a t(8;21) (t8q– 21q+).

M3: Hypergranular promyelocytic leukaemia in which the majority of cells are generally abnormally granulated and in which translocation between 15q and 17q may occur.

M4: (similar to M2): Myelomonocytic leukaemia in which more than 20% of cells are monocytes and pro-monocytes.

M5: Monocytic leukaemia (AMOL) in which monocytoid cells predominate.

M6: Erythroleukaemia: an acute leukaemia characterized by proliferation of red blood cell precursors (erythroblasts). Megakaryoblastic leukaemia is an acute leukaemia in which platelet precursors (megakaryoblasts) predominate. Both are rare. Clinical features of acute myeloid leukaemias differ according to cell type.

CLL (chronic lymphocytic leukaemia) is the commonest leukaemia in the elderly. It is characterized by proliferation of mature lymphocytes in the bone marrow, with increased white cell count in the blood and infiltration and enlargement of lymph nodes, spleen and liver. In the majority of cases clonal proliferation is of B cell lineage. Hairy cell leukaemia is also a proliferation of cells with B cell characteristics which results in massive spleen enlargement and bone marrow suppression.

CML (chronic myelogenous leukaemia, also known as chronic granulocytic leukaemia) is a proliferation of mature granulocytes resulting in bone marrow infiltration and suppression, spleen and liver infiltration. In the majority of cases tumour cells have a consistent chromosomal abnormality (the Philadelphia (Ph[1]) chromosome: see **ABL**). Transformation from chronic leukaemia to an aggressive acute leukaemia occurs in the majority of cases after a period of years. In approximately 20% of cases acute leukaemic cells appear to have lymphoid rather than myeloid features.

Leukosis
Proliferation of leukocyte-forming tissue: includes myelosis and lymphadenosis and forms the basis of leukaemia. In chickens, fowl leukosis refers to the proliferation of immature myeloid or lymphoid cells, including erythroblastosis, granuloblastosis, lymphomatosis and myelocytomatosis.

LFA-1
Lymphocyte function-associated antigen-1: involved in adhesion of B cells to cytotoxic T cells, natural killer cells and vascular endothelium.

LOH
Loss of heterozygosity. Complete absence of one allele at a given locus. Any somatic alteration arising in a tumour in the relative abundance of two alleles should be identifiable from a Southern blot comparing normal and tumour DNA samples.

LTR
Long terminal repeat. Identical (may include some inverted repeats) DNA sequences of several hundred base pairs (~270–1300) of the structure U3–R–U5 (5' to 3') at both ends of the unintegrated linear DNA product of reverse transcription, at both ends of integrated proviral DNA and in closed circular retroviral DNA.

Inverted repeats (I.R.) occur at the ends of LTRs and are perfect (or slightly imperfect) inverted repeats of ~3–25 bp that form a palindrome when two complete LTRs are joined in circular DNA. Integration of proviral DNA results in the loss of 2 bp from the I.R.s (see **Introduction**, page 3).

Lung cancer
Major subdivisions are small-cell lung cancer and the non-small-cell cancers, namely squamous (epidermoid) carcinoma, adenocarcinoma and large-cell undifferentiated carcinoma. Tumours with mixed histology may occur. Uncommon lung neoplasms include carcinoid tumours and bronchioalveolar carcinoma.

Lymphoid cells
One of the major classes of cells derived from bone marrow stem cells (see Haematopoietic differentiation pathways).

Lymphoid tissues
Lymphatic system tissue predominantly arranged in lymph glands but also found in bowel wall and other sites.

Lymphoma
Malignant proliferation of lymphoid cells. Major divisions of the disease are Hodgkin's disease (Hodgkin's lymphoma) and non-Hodgkin's lymphomas.

Hodgkin's disease is characterized by the presence of binucleate or multinucleate Sternberg–Reed cells, though the cell of origin of Hodgkin's disease is unknown. The disease predominantly presents as lymph node swellings, which may be isolated or, in more extensive disease, involve multiple lymph node sites, liver, spleen, bone marrow and other organs. Hodgkin's disease is subdivided according to histological appearance into groups which have differing clinical behaviour and prognosis. In the majority of cases Hodgkin's disease is curable with chemotherapy and/or radiotherapy.

The non-Hodgkin's lymphomas present a varied spectrum of histological features and clinical behaviour, ranging from Burkitt's lymphoma which has a doubling time shorter th human tumour to well-differentiated lymphocytic which has a natural history which may span decades. non-Hodgkin's lymphoma into high-grade, intermediate grade disease, based on morphological and surface expression, identifies groups with differing prognosis and th Some types of non-Hodgkin's lymphoma are curable with chemotherapy and/or radiotherapy.

Malignant tumour Uncontrolled cell growth characterized by invasion through the basement membrane into surrounding tissue and a propensity to spread (metastasize) by blood or lymphatic routes to other sites.

MAP kinases Mitogen-activated kinases, also known as extracellular signal-related kinases (ERKs): highly conserved cellular enzymes that are activated by a variety of extracellular signals that cause their phosphorylation on serine and tyrosine residues. MEK1 (*M*AP kinase or *E*RK *k*inase) stimulates the activity of MAP kinase (Crews, C.M. *et al.*, 1992, Science, 258, 478–480).

Melanoma Malignant tumour of melanocytes (pigmented skin cells). A benign proliferation of such cells is termed a naevus.

MEN 1 Multiple endocrine neoplasia type 1 (Wermer's syndrome). Inherited autosomal dominant trait distinguished by the occurrence of multiple tumours of the anterior pituitary and pancreatic islet cells and parathyroid hyperplasia.

MEN 2A/MEN 2B Multiple endocrine neoplasia type 2A is a cancer inherited as an autosomal dominant trait involving malignant tumours of the "C" cells of the thyroid (medullary carcinoma of the thyroid, MTC) and usually benign tumours of the adrenal medulla (phaeochromocytoma). MEN 2B is similar to MEN 2A but is characterized by earlier tumour onset, ganglioneuromatosis of the intestine and Marfanoid habitus.

Metastasis Spread of malignant cells from the site of origin to other sites. Cells usually migrate via the bloodstream or lymphatics but spread can also occur directly (within the abdominal cavity) or via the cerebrospinal fluid from one site in the central nervous system to another.

Minimal inverted repeat Inverted repeat, or palindromic, sequences of nucleic acids in which the code reads the same from each end on complementary strands.

Mink cell focus-forming viruses (MCF) A class of murine leukaemia viruses (MuLVs) that induces cytopathic changes in mink lung fibroblasts. MCF viruses are dual-trophic: they grow in mouse cells (like ecotrophic MuLVs) and induce thymomas in mice and in cells of non-murine species (like xenotrophic MuLVs) but differ from amphotrophic MuLVs in their properties, notably their effects on mink lung fibroblasts. MCF viruses probably arose by recombination between ecotrophic and xenotrophic MuLVs within the envelope (*env*) gene.

MMTV Murine mammary tumour virus. Family *Retroviridae*, subfamily *Oncovirinae*, genus Type B oncovirus. Tumorigenic virus transmitted in milk.

MNNG	*N*-Methyl-*N'*-nitrosoguanidine: chemical mutagen.
Monocytes	Mononuclear blood phagocytes that migrate into tissues and differentiate into macrophages.
MuLV	Murine leukaemia virus.
MuSV	Mouse sarcoma virus. Family *Retroviridae*, sub-family *Oncovirinae*, genus Type C oncovirus. All strains rapidly induce sarcomas in mice.
Multiple myeloma (myelomatosis)	Malignant proliferation of plasma cells.
Myeloblasts	Bone marrow cells which are the precursors of myelocytes (see Haematopoietic differentiation pathways).
Myeloblastoma	Myeloblast tumour: e.g. myelogenous leukaemia and chloroma.
Myelocytes	Bone marrow cells that develop into granular leucocytes (polymorphonuclear leucocytes) in the blood and are present in certain forms of leukaemia (see Haematopoietic differentiation pathways).
Myelocytomatosis	Leukosis involving myelocytes; in fowl: tumours composed of myeloid cells.
Myeloid cells	One of the two classes of cells derived from bone marrow stem cells (the other being lymphoid cells) and comprising megakaryocytes, erythroid precursors, monocytes and polymorphonuclear leucocytes (granulocytes).
Myeloid tissue	Erythrocyte- and leucocyte-producing tissue in fetal liver and spleen and in the bone marrow.
Myoblast	Muscle cell (myocyte) precursor.
N-trophic/NB-trophic	See B-trophic.
N-CAM	Neural cell adhesion molecule. Cell surface glycoprotein: anti-N-CAM antibody inhibits cell–cell adhesion.
Neoplasm	New or abnormal cell growth, e.g. a tumour.
Neuroblastoma	Malignant tumour derived from primitive ganglion cells. Together with nephroblastoma (Wilms' tumour), one of the most common solid tumours of childhood.
Neural crest	Transient embryonic structure of the neural epithelium that is converted to a mesenchymal state: these cells subsequently migrate throughout the embryo to give rise to many derivatives including most of the peripheral nervous system and melanocytes.
Neurofibromatosis Type 1 (Von Recklinghausen's disease or multiple neuroma)	Familial condition caused by germ line mutations at the *NF1* locus that give rise to developmental changes in the nervous system, muscle, bones and skin. Tumours of nerve sheaths (neurofibromas) may occur in multiple sites. Occurs in 1 in 30 000 births.
NGF	Nerve growth factor: 118 amino acid polypeptide (13 kDa) with chemotropic properties for sympathetic and sensory neurons. In peripheral tissues it attracts neurites to form synapses.
ORD	Oncogene responsive domain. Promoter sequence of polyoma virus gene.

ORF

Open reading frame: a sequence of nucleotides in DNA that can be read as codons, does not contain a termination codon and potentially encodes a polypeptide. ORF also denotes a highly conserved gene present in the 3′ LTR of mouse mammary tumour viruses (MMTVs; see **Appendix**, page 590).

ori

Replication origin: distinct chromosomal site at which DNA replication is thought to be initiated by the binding of cellular factors.

Osteosarcoma

Malignant tumour of bone, particularly occurring in childhood and early adulthood.

Papilloma

Benign tumour of epithelial cells of skin, alimentary tract or bladder. The corresponding malignant forms are carcinomas.

PDGF

Platelet derived growth factor. Dimer of A and/or B polypeptide chains. PDGFB chain is almost identical to the v-SIS oncoprotein. The PDGFA gene is 60% similar to the B chain gene. AA, AB and BB dimers occur in normal and transformed cells. There are two distinct types of receptor: PDGF-α and PDGF-β. PDGF-β receptors bind only PDGF-BB. PDGF-α receptors bind PDGF-AA, PDGF-AB or PDGF-BB with high affinity. PDGF-$\alpha\beta$ receptors bind PDGF-AB or PDGF-BB.

Phaeochromocytoma

See MEN 2.

Plasmacytoma

Localized malignant tumour of plasma cells (i.e. B lymphocytes). Multiple myeloma is a disseminated form of plasmacytoma. Plasmacytoma in rodents is caused by injection of complete Freund's adjuvant. The hybridoma cells from which monoclonal antibodies are obtained are produced by fusion of plasmacytoma cells and primed lymphocytes.

Plasmid

Small, circular, double-stranded DNA (up to 200 kb) that can replicate independently and be transferred from one organism to another. Widely used as carriers of cloned genes.

Polymorphonuclear leucocytes (granulocytes)

Mammalian blood leucocytes of the myeloid lineage. The subclasses of PMNLs are neutrophils (short-lived phagocytic cells), eosinophils (poorly phagocytic) and basophils (non-phagocytic histamine containing).

Proviral integration

The acquisition of virally encoded DNA by a host cell genome. Genes activated or mutated by proviral integration may be identified by cloning somatic proviral DNA–host cellular DNA junction fragments from retrovirally induced tumours. DNA probes for the regions flanking the provirus are then used to screen DNA from other tumours.

Proviral tagging

Use of proviral DNA as a probe to isolate flanking DNA from tumour cell libraries. Activated cellular proto-oncogenes and previously unknown genes have been detected by this means. Analogous to transposon tagging.

Provirus

Viral DNA that has become integrated into a host cell's chromosomal DNA. The RNA genome of *Retroviridae* must first be transcribed to DNA by the action of reverse transcriptase. Proviral genes may be expressed or latent. Proviral integration of oncogenic viruses may cause cell transformation.

Pseudogene	Non-functional DNA sequences closely similar to those of expressed genes (e.g. see **RAS**). May be the result of gene duplications in which loss of promoters or other mutations prevent expression.
Reticuloendotheliosis virus (REV)	Oncogenic virus that induces reticuloendotheliosis in chickens, quail, ducklings, goslings and guinea keets. The REV group includes REV-T (carries the v-*rel* oncogene), spleen necrosis virus (SNV), duck infectious anaemia virus (DIAV) and chicken syncytial virus (CSV).
Retinoblastoma	Malignant tumour of the retina composed of primitive retinal cells and usually occurring in children less than five years old. Occurs as sporadic or familial forms. In the familial form a germ line mutation of the *RB* gene is found and retinoblastoma occurs bilaterally in approximately one-third of cases. There is a high incidence of second malignancy in these patients, particularly osteosarcoma.
Retinoic acid	Vitamin A precursor. Dietetic deficiency causes visual impairment. Influences cell differentiation. Used therapeutically in some forms of leukaemia and epithelial pre-malignancy.
Retroviruses	Family of spherical enveloped viruses divided into three subfamilies: *Oncovirinae* (includes all oncogenic and closely related non-oncogenic viruses), *Lentivirinae* (the "slow" viruses, e.g. visna virus) and *Spumavirinae* ("foamy" viruses that cause persistent infections without any clinical disease). The genome consists of an inverted dimer of linear (+)-sense RNA. All viruses contain an RNA-dependent DNA polymerase activity (reverse transcriptase). Viruses are 80–100 nm in diameter with surface glycoprotein projections of 8 nm. The helical ribonucleoprotein is contained in an icosahedral capsid. Transmission is both vertical and horizontal.

A-, B-, C- and D-type virus particles: Morphologically defined groups of retrovirus particles. The three types of murine retroviruses are classified as: A-type: double-shelled spherical particles of diameter 65–75 nm (outer shell) and 50 nm (inner shell) often found as intracellular particles in tumour cells; B-type: dense core of 40–60 nm diameter within a 90–120 nm diameter envelope seen outside mouse mammary carcinoma cells after budding through the cell membrane (e.g. MMTV); C-type: 90–110 nm diameter particles seen in association with leukaemic tissue and with sarcomas (e.g. ALV). D-type: observed both intracellularly (60–90 nm diameter) and extracellularly (100–120 nm diameter). The electron-dense nucleoid of the extracellular form is located eccentrically but the glycoprotein spikes are shorter than those of B-type particles. The nucleoid region is located acentrically in B-type particles and concentrically in C-type particles.

Retroviral genome (elements)	
R	A short sequence (20–80 nucleotides) directly repeated at both ends of each retroviral RNA subunit that excludes the cap nucleotide at

	the 5′ terminus and the poly(A) tract at the 3′ terminus. Present in each LTR in viral DNA.
U5	Sequence (80–100 nucleotides) between R and PBS. Present once in viral RNA and in each LTR of viral DNA.
PBS	Primer binding site for the initiation of negative strand synthesis.
L	Untranslated sequence (~250 nucleotides) preceding the coding region of *gag* that may determine the packaging of virion RNA.
gag	*G*roup-specific *a*nti*g*en: the first of the three coding domains of a replication competent retroviral genome. *gag* (~2 kb) encodes a polyprotein whose products form the major structural proteins of the virus.
pol	RNA-directed DNA *pol*ymerase (reverse transcriptase): the second coding domain of a replication competent retroviral genome (~3 kb). *pol* encodes a polyprotein that generates *gag* peptides as well as reverse transcriptase and RNAase H.
env	*Env*elope: the third coding domain (~2 kb) of a replication competent retroviral genome the product of which is a polyprotein from which the major structural proteins of the viral envelope are generated.
onc	Generic region found in many oncogenic retroviruses that encodes an oncoprotein. May be 3′ to *env* or replace some or all of the normal retroviral genes resulting in a replication defective virus.
PB+	Undefined site for primer binding for the positive strand.
U3	Untranslated region at the 3′ end of the viral genome (~170–1200 nucleotides) that contains the viral promoter. Present once in viral RNA and in each LTR of viral DNA.
Retrovirus vector	Retroviruses from which all viral genes have been removed or altered and which contain the foreign gene to be expressed, usually with a selectable marker (typically neomycin phosphotransferase).

Retroviral vector: the lines represent viral sequences; the arrows indicate transcription initiation sites:

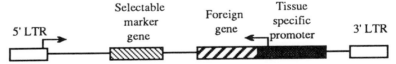

To prepare virus stocks cloned proviral DNA is transfected into a packaging cell that contains an integrated provirus with intact genes but lacking the sequence recognized by the packaging apparatus. Thus packaging cells cannot produce infectious virus but can package RNA transcribed from the transfected vector into virions that are released from the cell and can infect target cells. This virus stock should be helper-free, i.e. lack wild-type replication-competent virions.

Reverse transcriptase	RNA-dependent DNA polymerase: an enzyme of retroviruses that synthesizes a single strand of DNA using an RNA template.
Rhabdomyosarcoma	Malignant tumour of striated muscle, particularly occurring in childhood.

Sarcoma	Tumours of tissue derived from the mesenchymal layer (connective tissue, bone, cartilage, muscle, fat, blood vessels) as distinct from carcinomas which are derived from epithelial cells. Often highly malignant.
Schwannoma	Tumour of the nerve sheath. Termed acoustic neuroma when the tumour occurs on the auditory nerve, the most common site.
Splice donor site (SD)	Site at which a 5' portion of the integrated proviral genome is joined to a 3' region to form spliced, subgenomic mRNA. The major SD occurs near the 5' terminus, either within *gag* or in the untranslated region upstream of the first *gag* initiation codon.
Splice acceptor site (SA)	3' site at which viral RNA is joined to a SD to form subgenomic mRNA.
Squamous carcinoma	Malignant tumour of squamous epithelial cells.
Teratocarcinoma	See Teratoma.
Teratoma	Tumours comprised of tissues that are derived from three germinal layers, the endoderm, mesoderm and ectoderm. These may be solid or cystic and are classified histologically as mature, immature and malignant. The term teratocarcinoma is used to describe tumours in which malignant teratoma tissue coexists with material which histologically resembles epithelial malignancy.
Terminal differentiation	Regulated progression of eukaryotic cells through successive steps of differentiation and growth inhibition resulting in growth arrest.
Thyroid hormones	Thyroxine and triiodothyronine: iodinated aromatic amino acid compounds produced and secreted by the thyroid gland.
THR	Thyroid hormone receptor.
trans activation	Modulation of gene transcription by the product of a locus on another chromosome, usually by a regulatory protein.
Transduction	Acquisition of cellular genes by recombination with a viral genome: as a result the cellular genes may become oncogenic.
Transfection	Introduction of DNA into a eukaryotic cell and its subsequent integration into that cell's chromosome. Techniques for transfection include precipitation of DNA onto the cell surface by Ca^{2+} ions and electroporation.
Transformation	Conversion of a cell to a state of unregulated growth resembling that of a cancer cell. This meaning is distinct from the permanent change in one or more genetic parameters of a cell following the acquisition of novel DNA, e.g. by transfection of DNA.
Transforming growth factors (TGFα, TGFβ)	TGFα (50 amino acids) binds competitively to the EGFR, causing tyrosine autophosphorylation and receptor-mediated endocytosis, although there is evidence that the latter process is not identical for the two ligands. In general, TGFα activates similar cell responses to EGF, although it is more potent than EGF in stimulating bone resorption. Induces features of the transformed cell phenotype (growth in semi-solid agar): together with oncogenic *ras* causes full transformation. Five distinct TGFβs have been detected in vertebrates: $TGF\beta_1$, $TGF\beta_2$ and $TGF\beta_3$ occur in man and several other species; $TGF\beta_4$

and TGFβ$_5$ have been detected in the chicken and frog, respectively. TGFβs are secreted by many types of cell and are potent inhibitors of proliferation of most cell types *in vitro*. TGFβ$_1$ is a homodimer (two 112 amino acid chains: 25 kDa), the monomers of which are derived by proteolytic cleavage of a 390 amino acid precursor. TGFβ$_1$ stimulates connective tissue formation and is expressed during cellular injury and repair and TGFβ$_2$ and TGFβ$_3$ during differentiation. Elevated levels of TGFβ$_1$ and TGFβ$_3$ mRNA have been detected in some human tumours.

Transgenic organism	Organism transformed by the introduction of novel DNA into its genome, e.g. by the injection of cloned DNA sequences into fertilized eggs. Transgenic mice are usually created by establishing a permanent embryonic stem cell line with cells taken from a blastocyst. These cells are transfected with a vector carrying the gene (or modified gene) to be introduced and cloned cells expressing that gene are injected into a blastocyst for incubation in a foster mother to obtain a chimeric founder. Heterozygous and homozygous recombinants are then generated by breeding with wild-type animals.
TSP	Tropical spastic paraparesis. HTLV-1-linked disease of the CNS, also called HTLV-1-associated myelopathy (HAM). Similar to the chronic progressive form of multiple sclerosis.
Tyrosine kinases	There are five classes of receptor-type tyrosine kinases based on organization and sequence similarities. Prototypes are the EGF receptor (class I), the insulin receptor (class II), the PDGF-AA, PDGF-BB, CSF-1, c-KIT and FLT1 receptors (class III), the FGF receptors (class IV), neurotropin receptors (class VI) and the *EPH/ECK*-encoded receptors (class VII). (For references see Ullrich, A., and Schlessinger, J. (1990). Cell, 61, 203–212; Cadena, D.L. and Gill, G.N. (1992). Receptor tyrosine kinases. FASEB J., 6, 2332–2337.)

Additional receptor forms are represented by:
Ark (Rescigno, J., Mansukhani, A. and Basilico, C. (1991). A putative receptor tyrosine kinase with unique structural topology. Oncogene, 6, 1909–1913;

KDR (Terman, B.I., Carrion, M.E., Kovacs, E., Rasmussen, B.A., Eddy, R.L. and Shows, T.B. (1991). Identification of a new endothelial cell growth factor receptor tyrosine kinase. Oncogene, 6, 1677–1683);

TIE (Partanen, J., Armstrong, E., Makela, T.P., Korhonen, J., Sandberg, M., Renkonen, R., Knuutila, S., Huebner, K. and Alitalo, K. (1992). A novel endothelial cell surface receptor tyrosine kinase with extracellular epidermal growth factor homology domains. Mol. Cell. Biol., 12, 1698–1707);

Tyk2 (Bernards, A. (1991). Predicted *tyk*2 protein contains two tandem protein kinase domains. Oncogene, 6, 1185–1187; Firmbach, K.I., Byers, M., Shows, T., Dalla, F.R. and Krolewski, J.J. (1990). *tyk*2, prototype of a novel class of non-receptor tyrosine kinase genes. Oncogene, 5, 1329–1336);

Jak1/Jak2 (Harpur, A.G., Andres, A.-C., Ziemiecki, A., Aston,

R.R. and Wilks, A.F. (1992). JAK2, a third member of the JAK family of protein tyrosine kinases. Oncogene, 7, 1347–1353; Howard, O.M.Z., Dean, M., Young, H., Ramsburg, M., Turpin, J.A., Michiel, D.F., Kelvin, D.J., Lee, L. and Farrar, W.L. (1992). Characterization of a class 3 tyrosine kinase. Oncogene, 7, 895–900);

Tek/HPK-6 (Dumont, D.J., Yamaguchi, T.P., Conlon, R.A., Rossant, J. and Breitman, M.L. (1992). *Tek*, a novel tyrosine kinase gene located on mouse chromsome 4, is expressed in endothelial cells and their presumptive precursors. Oncogene, 7, 1471–1480; Ziegler, S.F., Bird, T.A., Schneringer, J.A., Schooley, K.A. and Baum, P.R. (1993). Molecular cloning and characterization of a novel receptor protein tyrosine kinase from human placenta. Oncogene, 8, 663–670).

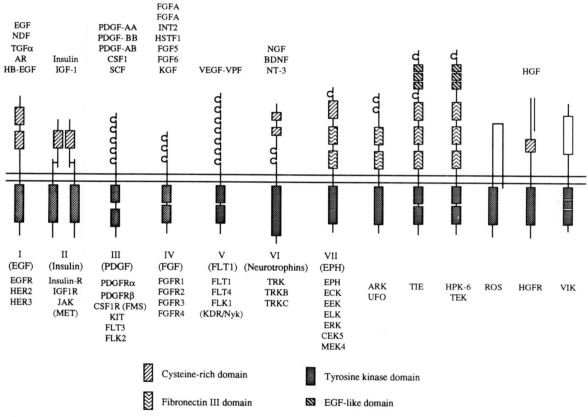

Wilms' tumour (nephroblastoma)

Childhood solid tumour arising from renal tissue. Most Wilms' tumours are sporadic and unilateral but some are bilateral and approximately 1% are familial.

Xenotrophic

Virus that can only replicate in cells of species other than its normal host.

Index

(All oncogenes, tumour suppressor genes, viral integration sites and breakpoint region genes are included in the appropriate tables of Chapter 2, in addition to any other locations shown in this index. Bold entries indicate individual section for that subject)

3-methoxybenzamide 189
3'-orf (HIV gene) 590–591
3BP-1 (SH3 binding protein) 459
225 (T cell early response gene) 10

A-CAM (N-cadherin) 569
A-MYB 293, 295, 302
α-Spectrin 448
A23187 191, 192, 296, 338
Abelson murine leukaemia virus (AbMuLV) 76–85
Abelson virus-induced myeloid lymphosarcoma (ABML) 38, 76–92, 294, 295, 299
ABL 11, 12, 17–19, 38, **76–92**, 203, 253, 315, 361, 367, 373, 383, 393, 500
ABL2 (ARG) 76, 82
ABP1p 107, 449
Achaete scute (*Drosophila*) 245
Acidic fibroblast growth factor (*FGFA* or HBGF-1) 222–224, 226–228, 368
Actin 123, 173
Acute lymphocytic leukaemia (ALL) *see under* Cancers
Acute myelogenous leukaemia (AML) *see under* Cancers
Acute non-lymphocytic leukaemia (ANLL) *see under* Cancers
Acute promyelocytic leukaemia (APL) *see under* Cancers
Adenocarcinoma *see under* Cancers
Adenoma *see under* Cancers
Adenovirus 135–140
see also E1A *and* E1B
Adenylate kinase 3 family (ψAK3) 554
ADP-ribosyltransferase (ADPRT) 189
ADP-ribosyltransferase (ADPRT) inhibitor 189, 305, 340
Adrenal tumours *see under* Cancers
Adult T cell leukaemia (ATL) *see under* Cancers

AF4 (also known as *MLLT2*) 47–48
AF9 (also known as *MLLT3*) 47–48
Ahi-1 5, 25
Akt-1 51–52
AML1 48
Amphiregulin 495
Amphotropic virus 588, 593
Anaplastic astrocytoma 556
Angiotensin 192, 244
Angiotensin receptor 272
Anion transport protein (Band III) 439, 488
Ankyrin 93, 97
Annexin II (p36, calpactin I or lipocortin II) 468, 495
Antisense (negative strand) transcription 322, 323, 335, 491
AP-1 137, 142, 148, 164, 181, 184, 185, 188, 238–245, 369, 386, 399
AP-2 128, 164, 220, 387
APC 17, **563–567**
Apoptosis 96, 97, 136, 149, 181, 238, 319, 541
Ara 378
Arachidonic acid 192, 386
Arc-1 (E-cadherin) **569–572**, 577
ARG 76, 82
Ark 607
art (HIV gene) 590
AS42 virus 59
Asbestos 245
ASH (abundant SRC homology protein) 449
Astrocytoma *see under* Cancers
Ataxia telangiectasia 159, 541
ATF-2 240
ATF-like transcription factor 530
Atk 449
Avian erythroblastosis virus (AEV) 5, 11, 15, 485, 489, 490, 496, 497, 593